D1266084

MEDICAL DEPARTMENT
UNITED STATES ARMY
IN WORLD WAR II

MEDICAL DEPARTMENT, UNITED STATES ARMY

SURGERY IN WORLD WAR II

ACTIVITIES OF SURGICAL CONSULTANTS

Volume II

Prepared and published under the direction of

Lieutenant General LEONARD D. HEATON
The Surgeon General, United States Army

Editor in Chief
Colonel JOHN BOYD COATES, Jr., MC, USA

Editor for Activities of Surgical Consultants
B. NOLAND CARTER, M.D.

Associate Editor
ELIZABETH M. McFETRIDGE, M.A.

OFFICE OF THE SURGEON GENERAL

DEPARTMENT OF THE ARMY

WASHINGTON, D.C., 1964

SURGERY IN WORLD WAR II

Advisory Editorial Board

MICHAEL E. DeBAKEY, M.D., *Chairman*

FRANK B. BERRY, M.D.	JOHN B. FLICK, M.D.
BRIAN BLADES, M.D.	FRANK GLENN, M.D.
J. BARRETT BROWN, M.D.	M. ELLIOTT RANDOLPH, M.D.
STERLING BUNNELL, M.D. (dec.)	ISIDOR S. RAVDIN, M.D.
NORTON CANFIELD, M.D.	JOSEPH R. SHAEFFER, M.D.
B. NOLAND CARTER, M.D.	ALFRED R. SHANDS, Jr., M.D.
EDWARD D. CHURCHILL, M.D.	HOWARD E. SNYDER, M.D.
MATHER CLEVELAND, M.D.	R. GLEN SPURLING, M.D.
DANIEL C. ELKIN, M.D. (dec.)	BARNES WOODHALL, M.D.

ROBERT M. ZOLLINGER, M.D.

Brigadier General JAMES E. GRAHAM, USA (ex officio)
Brigadier General DOUGLAS B. KENDRICK, Jr., USA (ex officio)
Colonel JOHN BOYD COATES, Jr., MC, USA (ex officio)

The Historical Unit, United States Army Medical Service

Colonel JOHN BOYD COATES, Jr., MC, USA, *Director*
CHARLES J. SIMPSON, *Executive Officer*
Lieutenant Colonel DOUGLAS HESFORD, MSC, USA, *Chief, Special Projects Branch*
CHARLES M. WILTSE, Ph. D., Litt. D., *Chief, Historians Branch*
ERNEST ELLIOTT, Jr., *Chief, Editorial Branch*
Lieutenant Colonel JEROME RUDBERG, MSC, USA, *Chief, Information Activities Branch*
RODERICK M. ENGERT, *Chief, General Reference and Research Branch*
HAZEL G. HINE, *Chief, Administrative Branch*

Library of Congress Catalog Card Number: 62–60004

For sale by the Superintendent of Documents, U.S. Government Printing Office
Washington, D.C., 20402 · Price $8.50

ACTIVITIES OF
SURGICAL CONSULTANTS

Volume II

MEDICAL DEPARTMENT, UNITED STATES ARMY

The volumes comprising the official history of the Medical Department of the United States Army in World War II are prepared by The Historical Unit, United States Army Medical Service, and published under the direction of The Surgeon General, U.S. Army. These volumes are divided into two series: (1) The administrative or operational series; and (2) the professional, or clinical and technical, series. This is one of the volumes published in the latter series.

VOLUMES PUBLISHED

ADMINISTRATIVE SERIES

Hospitalization and Evacuation, Zone of Interior
Organization and Administration in World War II
Personnel in World War II

CLINICAL SERIES

Internal Medicine in World War II:

Vol. I. Activities of Medical Consultants
Vol. II. Infectious Diseases

Preventive Medicine in World War II:

Vol. II. Environmental Hygiene
Vol. III. Personal Health Measures and Immunization
Vol. IV. Communicable Diseases Transmitted Chiefly Through Respiratory and Alimentary Tracts
Vol. V. Communicable Diseases Transmitted Through Contact or By Unknown Means
Vol. VI. Communicable Diseases: Malaria

Surgery in World War II:

Activities of Surgical Consultants, vol. 1
General Surgery, vol. II
Hand Surgery
Neurosurgery, vol. I
Neurosurgery, vol. II
Ophthalmology and Otolaryngology
Orthopedic Surgery in the European Theater of Operations
Orthopedic Surgery in the Mediterranean Theater of Operations
The Physiologic Effects of Wounds
Thoracic Surgery, vol. I
Vascular Surgery

Miscellaneous:

Cold Injury, Ground Type
Dental Service in World War II
Veterinary Service in World War II
Wound Ballistics

Authors

EUGENE M. BRICKER, M.D.

Associate Professor of Clinical Surgery, Washington University School of Medicine, St. Louis, Mo. Chief Consultant in Plastic Surgery to the Chief Surgeon, European Theater of Operations, U.S. Army, 1943–45. Formerly Colonel, MC, AUS.

NORTON CANFIELD, M.D.

Associate Clinical Professor in Otolaryngology, Yale University School of Medicine, New Haven, Conn.; Consultant in Otolaryngology, U.S. Veterans' Administration Center, San Patricio Hospital, San Juan, P.R., and Rodriguez U.S. Army Hospital, Antilles Command, U.S. Army Caribbean; Consultant in Audiology to The Surgeon General, U.S. Army, Washington, D.C., since 1946. Senior Consultant in Otolaryngology, Office of the Chief Surgeon, European Theater of Operations, U.S. Army, 1943–45; Chief, Otolaryngology Branch, Surgical Consultants Division, Office of The Surgeon General, 1945–46; Chief Consultant in Audiology, Veterans' Administration, Washington, D.C., 1946–55. Formerly Colonel, MC, AUS.

MATHER CLEVELAND, M.D., Sc.D.

Consulting Orthopaedic Surgeon, St. Luke's Hospital and Presbyterian Hospital, New York, N.Y.; Civilian Consultant in Orthopedic Surgery to The Surgeon General, U.S. Army. Orthopedic Consultant, Fourth Service Command, 1943–44; Senior Consultant in Orthopedic Surgery, European Theater of Operations, U.S. Army, 1944–45. Formerly Colonel, MC, AUS.

ELLIOTT C. CUTLER, M.D. (Deceased)

Moseley Professor of Surgery, Harvard Medical School, Boston, Mass., 1932–47; Surgeon-in-Chief, Peter Bent Brigham Hospital, 1932–47; Civilian Consultant to the Secretary of War, 1946–47; Chief Consultant in Surgery, Office of the Chief Surgeon, European Theater of Operations, U.S. Army, 1942–45; Chief, Professional Services Division, Office of the Chief Surgeon, European Theater of Operations, 1945. Formerly Brigadier General, AUS.

LOYAL DAVIS, M.D.

Professor and Chairman, Department of Surgery, Northwestern University Medical School, Chicago, Ill. Senior Consultant in Neurological Surgery to the Chief Surgeon, European Theater of Operations, U.S. Army, 1942–43. Formerly Colonel, MC, AUS.

REX L. DIVELEY, M.D.

Associate Professor of Orthopaedic Surgery, Kansas University School of Medicine, Kansas City, Kans.; Area Orthopedic Consultant, Veterans' Administration, St. Louis, Mo. Senior Consultant in Orthopedic Surgery, Office of the Chief Surgeon, and, later, Chief, Rehabilitation Division, Office of the Chief Surgeon, European Theater of Operations, U.S. Army, 1942–45. Formerly Colonel, MC, AUS.

GEORGE O. EATON, M.D., C.M.

Associate Professor of Orthopedic Surgery, The Johns Hopkins University School of Medicine, Baltimore, Md. Orthopedic Consultant for the Southwest Pacific Area, 1943–45; Civilian Consultant in Orthopedic Surgery to The Surgeon General, 1953–58. Formerly Lieutenant Colonel, MC, AUS.

JOHN B. FLICK, M.D., C.M.

Consulting Surgeon, Pennsylvania Hospital, Philadelphia, Pa., and Bryn Mawr Hospital, Bryn Mawr, Pa.; Consultant in Surgery, Valley Forge Army Hospital, Phoenixville, Pa.; Secretary-Treasurer, The American Board of Surgery, since 1952. Consultant in Surgery, Ninth Service Command, 1942–45; Consultant in Surgery, Pacific Ocean Areas, 1945. Formerly Colonel, MC, AUS.

A. STEPHENS GRAHAM, M.D., M.S. (In Surgery)

Associate Clinical Professor of Surgery, Medical College of Virginia; Chief, Surgical Service, Stuart Circle Hospital; Surgical Consultant, Veterans' Administration Hospital, Richmond, Va. Chief, Surgical Service, 45th General Hospital, Camp Lee, Va., and Rabat, French Morocco, 1942–43; Surgical Consultant, First Service Command, 1943–44; Surgical Consultant, India-Burma and China Theaters, 1945. Formerly Colonel, MC, AUS.

JAMES N. GREEAR, Jr., M.D.

Area Consultant in Ophthalmology, Veterans' Administration, for States of Oregon, Washington, Idaho, Utah, Nevada, and northern California; President, Nevada State Medical Association. Chief, Eye Center, Valley Forge General Hospital, Phoenixville, Pa., 1943–45; Senior Consultant in Ophthalmology, European Theater of Operations, 1945. Colonel, MC, USAR (Ret.).

PAUL R. HAWLEY, M.D., LL.D., Sc. D.

Chief Surgeon, Special Observer Group, London, England, 1941–42; Chief Surgeon, U.S. Army Forces in the British Isles and European Theater of Operations, U.S. Army, and later Chief, Medical Services, Services of Supply, European Theater of Operations, U.S. Army, 1942; Chief Surgeon, European Theater of Operations, U.S. Army, 1943–45; concurrently Chief Surgeon, Services of Supply (later Communications Zone), European Theater of Operations, U.S. Army, 1944–45. Chief Medical Director, Department of Medicine and Surgery, U.S. Veterans' Administration, 1945–47; Chief Executive Officer, Blue Cross and Blue Shield Commissions, 1948–50; Director, American College of Surgeons, 1957–61. Major General, USA (Ret.).

JAMES C. KIMBROUGH, Colonel, MC, USA (Ret.) (Deceased)

Chief, Professional Services Division, Office of the Chief Surgeon, European Theater of Operations, U.S. Army, 1942–45; Commanding Officer, Percy Jones Convalescent Hospital, 1945–46; Chief, Genito-Urinary Service, Walter Reed Army Hospital, Washington, D.C., 1946–53; Consultant in Urology, Walter Reed Army Medical Center, 1953–56.

ASHLEY W. OUGHTERSON, M.D. (Deceased)

Clinical Professor of Surgery, School of Medicine, Yale University, New Haven, Conn., 1943–56. Formerly Colonel, MC, USAR.

WM. BARCLAY PARSONS, M.D.

Professor Emeritus of Clinical Surgery, College of Physicians and Surgeons, Columbia University, New York, N.Y. Surgical Consultant, Services of Supply, Southwest Pacific Area, 1942–44; Surgical Consultant, Sixth Service Command, 1944–45. Formerly Colonel, MC, AUS.

BERNARD J. PISANI, M.D.

Director, Obstetrics and Gynecology, St. Vincent's Hospital, New York, N.Y., since 1953; Assistant Visiting Obstetrician and Gynecologist, Bellevue Hospital Center, New York, N.Y., since 1946; Chairman Advisory Committee, and Consultant in Gynecology, Veterans' Administration Hospital, East Orange, N.J., since 1954; Special Consultant in Gynecology, Department of Medicine and Surgery, Veterans' Administration, Washington, D.C., since 1954; Consultant in Obstetrics and Gynecology, Community Hospital, Glen Cove, N.Y., and St. Francis Hospital, Poughkeepsie, N.Y., since 1955; Associate Clinical Professor of Obstetrics and Gynecology, New York University, since 1951. Chief, Surgical Service, 1219th Corps Area Service Command, 1942; Commanding Officer, 16th Station Hospital, 1942; Post Surgeon, and later Chief of Mess School, Headquarters, American School Center, Services of Supply, European Theater of Operations, U.S. Army, 1942–43; Director, Medical Field Service School, Shrivenham, 1944; Executive Officer, Professional Services Division, Office of the Chief Surgeon, European Theater of Operations, U.S. Army, 1944–45. Formerly Lieutenant Colonel, MC, AUS.

FORRESTER RAINE, M.D. (Deceased)

Consultant in Surgery, Central Pacific Area, 1942–45. Formerly Colonel, MC, AUS.

ROBERT CRAWFORD ROBERTSON, M.D., M.S.

Orthopaedic Surgeon, Chattanooga, Tenn. Chief Orthopedic Consultant to the Surgeon, Hawaiian Department, Central Pacific Area, Pacific Ocean Area, and Mid-Pacific, 1942–45; Orthopedic Consultant to The Surgeon General (Mobilization Designation), 1951–55. Colonel, MC, USAR (Ret.).

JOHN N. ROBINSON, M.D.

In private practice of urology. Formerly Associate Professor of Clinical Urology, College of Physicians and Surgeons, Columbia University, New York, N.Y. Chief of Urology, 2d General Hospital, 1942; Chief Consultant in Urology, Office of the Chief Surgeon, European Theater of Operations, U.S. Army, 1942–45. Formerly Lieutenant Colonel, MC, AUS.

RALPH M. TOVELL, M.D., M. Sc., F.F.A.R.C.S. (London)

Director, Department of Anesthesiology, Hartford Hospital, Hartford, Conn.; Special Consultant in Anesthesiology to Central Office, Veterans' Administration, Washington, D.C. Senior Consultant in Anesthesia, European Theater of Operations, U.S. Army, 1942–45. Formerly Colonel, MC, AUS.

I. RIDGEWAY TRIMBLE, M.D.

Associate Professor of Surgery, The Johns Hopkins School of Medicine, Baltimore, Md.; Civilian Consultant in Surgery to The Surgeon General. Chief of Surgical Service, 118th General Hospital, 1942–44; Chief Consultant in Surgery, Army Forces Western Pacific and Army Forces Pacific, 1944–46. Formerly Colonel, MC, AUS.

ROBERT M. ZOLLINGER, M.D.

Professor and Chairman, Department of Surgery, The Ohio State University, Columbus, Ohio. Senior Consultant in Surgery, European Theater of Operations, 1943–44; Commanding Officer, 5th General Hospital, 1944–45. Formerly Colonel, MC, AUS.

Foreword

This volume, the twenty-sixth to be published in the total series relating the history of the U.S. Army Medical Department in World War II, is the second of the two volumes dealing with the activities of surgical consultants. Volume I, published in 1962, describes the work of these consultants in the Office of The Surgeon General, the extension of the system to the service commands in the Zone of Interior, and its operation in U.S. field armies overseas. This second volume deals with the activities of the surgical consultants on the theater level overseas.

As is indicated in the first of these volumes, no formal provision for the consultant system existed in the Office of The Surgeon General before the outbreak of World War II, and this situation delayed its development and created many kinds of difficulties. A major problem was that consultants overseas were hampered in their activities, at least initially, by the inconvenience and actual inefficiency caused by the lack of direct channels of communication between themselves and the consultants in the Office of The Surgeon General. The situation led one consultant in the European theater to complain that the theater had had little from the Zone of Interior in the way of directives or other information on the treatment of casualties.

Just as in the Zone of Interior, so overseas the surgical consultants occupied themselves, with the full approval of those in authority, not only with clinical matters but with a variety of related administrative matters. They evaluated the qualifications of personnel and advised their assignment. They planned specialized treatment centers and helped to implement the planning. They supervised such professional training programs as were practical in an active theater of operations. They organized meetings and conferences on local and general levels and planned the agenda for them. They prepared circular letters and ETMD's (essential technical medical data). They planned such clinical studies and analyses as were practical in wartime. Finally, they held themselves on constant call to aid in the solution of problems on any level within their competence.

In short, consultants overseas followed the same pattern of endeavor as the consultants in the Zone of Interior, expanding their functions, and adapting them as necessary, in relation to the special conditions which they encountered. As I noted in the foreword to the first of these two volumes, it is a tribute to the tact of the consultants as well as to their competent performance that the original opposition to them gradually died away. It is an even greater tribute to them that, in the areas in which the consultant system did not operate, the desire for it was frequently expressed and that, when consultants were not formally appointed, acting consultants served in various specialties for longer or shorter periods of time.

There is a certain amount of overlapping of other volumes by this volume, but it is almost inevitable and warrants no apologies. To have avoided it would have meant the setting up of rigid and artificial distinctions. It would also have meant the loss of something of real value, the presentation of material on the same subject from different, but equally competent, points of view.

I am impressed in this volume, as I have been in all previous volumes, by the amount of factual material it contains and by the frankness with which the story is told. The consultant system did not always operate smoothly. There were many difficulties, some of them created by personalities, others by circumstances, and no purpose would be served by ignoring them. In fact, because these problems have been brought out into the open, it should be possible to cope better with similar situations in the future.

I am also impressed in this volume, as I have been in previously published volumes, by the wisdom of the basic editorial policy of utilizing the personal experiences of present and former medical officers who recorded, and often created, the data upon which this whole history is based. It is desirable, of course, to make a record of events as they occur, with an eye to the future use of these documents, but in wartime the ideal frequently gives way to the practical, and records, if they exist, are often no more than sketchy notes. If a formal record exists, that is good. If it does not, then we must rely upon the recollections of the medical officers who were there. There is scarcely a volume in this series in which there are not recorded one or more major events for which there is no formal documentation. In some instances there is no documentation at all for decisions that altered the whole course of therapy. I cannot share the pedantic view of the so-called historiographers who regard nothing as reliable unless it is corroborated by a bit of paper. To my mind, there are no more valid sources of data than the medical officers who served in World War II, who saw events happen, and who often played a part in their creation.

For that reason I applaud the unorthodox method used in this volume of telling the story of the surgical consultant service in the European Theater of Operations and in the Pacific by publishing the (edited) diaries of Brig. Gen. Elliott C. Cutler and Col. Ashley W. Oughterson, MC, who served as surgical consultants in those locations. Both officers died after the war ended, General Cutler before he had done any work at all on the history and Colonel Oughterson when his work on it was barely started.

The information which both of these officers possessed was essential for the history of the consultant system in both the European theater and the Pacific. It would have been unthinkable not to write this history. The solution was to use their official diaries, which, like most official diaries, often served as personal diaries as well. The material has been edited to eliminate irrelevant and extraneous material, perhaps not as drastically as it should have been, but the editorial work was done from the standpoint of deleting nothing that would alter the meaning or intent of the writers.

Unfortunately, certain passages in these diaries require elucidation that cannot now be secured. In other passages, one wonders whether the diarists, had they had the opportunity, might have wished to modify certain of their statements, or perhaps to comment on them. For these and other reasons, the diaries were submitted to the theater (area) surgeons under whom the writers served. Maj. Gen. Paul R. Hawley, MC, USA (Ret.), Chief Surgeon, European theater, has read and commented on the Cutler diary, while Brig. Gen. Earl Maxwell, USAF (MC) (Ret.), Maj. Gen. John M. Willis, MC, USA (Ret.), now deceased, and Maj. Gen. Guy B. Denit, MC, USA (Ret.), under all of whom Colonel Oughterson served, have done the same for his diary.

After World War I ended, a board of medical officers, appointed to investigate and report upon the conduct of the Medical Department, Allied Expeditionary Forces, and to recommend improvements in it, stated that the chief consultant in surgery in an oversea theater should be a medical officer of the highest surgical attainments. Wittingly or unwittingly, that recommendation must have been borne in mind over the years. The consultant system in the European theater in World War II began with the appointment in June 1942 of Col. James C. Kimbrough, MC, as Chief of the Professional Services Division, Office of the Chief Surgeon, and the appointment the following month of Col. (later Brig. Gen.) Elliott C. Cutler, MC, as Senior Consultant in Surgery. It is hard to imagine more fortunate selections.

In February 1945, just before Colonel Kimbrough left the theater and General Cutler succeeded him as Chief of Professional Services, General Cutler paid tribute to him as a man possessed of "a canny imagination." He gave no better proof of his canniness than in the imaginative use he made of his Senior Consultant in Surgery. General Cutler also paid tribute to the Theater Chief Surgeon who, while demanding the standardization of methods required in wartime, was always willing to allow changes, once a better way had been demonstrated.

In his comments on General Cutler's diary, General Hawley noted that, while some of the observations in it are based upon incomplete or erroneous information, they had been allowed to stand, with appropriate footnotes, because everything in the diary "* * * portrays faithfully his dedication to his task, his resentment of everything which impeded its accomplishment, and what he regarded as unjustifiable requirements of military administration. * * * he was a devoted and loyal soldier, who contributed more than his share to the success of the medical service of the European Theater of Operations."

Of all General Cutler's functions, perhaps the most important was his evaluation and assignment of professional personnel. It was an extremely difficult task, for needs far outran qualified personnel. It was doubly difficult for him, for, as General Hawley also pointed out, "an innate honesty often compelled his professional judgments to be severe," and he was "intolerant of mediocrity."

Immediately upon his appointment Colonel Cutler noted that while soldiers in base hospitals were well provided for, the care of the soldier "up the line" was entirely inadequate. For this lack he had a number of solutions including, first of all, mobility, which "must be forced on all medical services." As early as August 1942 he declared that the chief need was for auxiliary surgical groups. From the experience at Dieppe he concluded that if undue delay in treatment were to be avoided, hospitals must be set up near points at which casualties would be returned and that the successful operation of these hospitals would require the addition of surgical and shock teams to the normal hospital complement. The later establishment of transit hospitals can perhaps be traced to this concept. Colonel Cutler also stressed the importance of triage of casualties, and he thought that surgeons at the front must be general surgeons, not specialists in any particular field. He never lost sight of the fact that it was in forward areas that the end results of injuries were determined in terms of survival, morbidity, and permanent deformity versus complete restoration to normal.

In the courses of instruction that he planned and the circular letters that he prepared, in the lectures and talks that he gave, in fact, at every opportunity, General Cutler lost no chance of emphasizing the correct initial management of wounds in general and of regional wounds, with special reference to initial wound surgery. He found the almost universal ignorance of such surgery extremely depressing. Every young physician, he said, should be taught how to handle trauma, for it would constitute 20 to 30 percent of his peacetime practice. It would be better, in fact, if medical students were taught the principles of debridement in their undergraduate days. Certainly they should learn them as soon as they entered the Army. Traumatic surgery, he emphasized again and again, is not a separate specialty, and he could not see the logic— apparently he clearly saw the possible harm—of a special society devoted to it.

He suffered many frustrations in his attempts to solve the early problems associated with medical supplies and equipment. There were critical shortages of both. Planning impressed him as totally unrealistic. Battle provisions for 10,000 men a month included three litters, several thousand rolls of toilet paper, and one bedpan, but no oxygen tanks and no tetanus toxoid or antitoxin. An infantry division of 17,000 men was authorized two sphygmomanometers. Closure of sucking wounds would save lives (and make casualties transportable), but the proper needles and silkworm gut required to close the wounds were not provided. General Cutler was perfectly aware that in wartime it is frequently necessary to accept what is available rather than what is desirable, but compromise with him went only so far, and his initial supply activities marked the beginning of the later superbly operated supply service in the European theater.

The provision of blood for forward casualties was one of General Cutler's major preoccupations, as it was of General Hawley, and it is interesting to note how his thoughts on this subject evolved. In 1942, after hearing a discussion on blood and plasma at a meeting of the Royal Canadian Medical Corps Pathological Club, he wrote in his diary that it seemed to him that "the rise of plasma, etc., had let all forget the benefit of transfusion." "Our soldiers," he continued, "are all grouped. They should be the best vehicle for getting blood forward. No bottles to carry." He was soon to learn that it was not so simple, and it was only two years later that he was among the first to insist that local provision of whole blood was entirely inadequate and that the only satisfactory solution was an airlift of blood from the Zone of Interior.

His conversion to the perils of trenchfoot was similar. When he first observed it in Italy, in the fall of 1943, it seemed to him that the victims were "using their pain very hard to get out of fighting." Later, when the troops in the European theater were hard hit by cold injury, there was no more vigorous proponent of preventive measures than he was.

General Cutler approved of making casualties ambulatory as rapidly as possible after surgery, but he viewed early ambulation, which became popular in civilian circles in the course of the war, with considerable suspicion, terming it "a questionable acceleration of professional care."

He made plans for special studies on abdominal wounds, thoracic wounds, and other regional wounds, and for studies on gas gangrene, which fortunately proved unnecessary. He also planned special studies on penicillin therapy, again emphasizing that penicillin must be administered against a background of good surgery if it was to fulfill its usefulness. He concerned himself with securing texts and journals for hospital and other libraries. He directed the preparation of the "Manual of Therapy, European Theater of Operations," so successfully that during the war, and at the end, very few changes were required to bring it into conformity with current practices.

General Cutler was instrumental in forming the American Medical Society, ETOUSA, to which all U.S. medical officers in the theater automatically belonged. He also played a large part in founding the Inter-Allied Conferences on War Medicine, convened by the Royal Society of Medicine, and he lost no opportunity to stress the importance of liaison with our Allies, particularly the British. After his death, Sir Gordon Gordon-Taylor wrote: "The death of Elliott Cutler * * * will occasion deep sorrow in the hearts of his many friends in the United Kingdom. Perhaps no surgeon of the United States ever yearned or strove more earnestly to forge lasting bonds of friendship, not only between the surgeons, but between the peoples of the great English-speaking countries on either side of the North Atlantic, and to this end he directed both written and spoken word."

The special reports by consultants in the various specialties in the European theater all deserve careful reading. It is perhaps invidious to mention special chapters because space does not permit me to comment on them all, but attention must be called to:

1. The investigations by Col. Loyal Davis, MC, of high altitude frostbite; his development of protective helmets for Air Force crews; and his stabilization of policies concerning herniated nucleus pulposus.

2. The advances in rehabilitation, which permitted the return to duty, often to full duty, of greatly increased numbers of men.

3. The development of policies of rehabilitation for deafened and blinded casualties.

4. The miracles wrought by plastic surgery.

5. The enormous advances in surgical therapy made possible by the enormous advances in anesthesia under Col. Ralph M. Tovell, MC.

General Cutler and Colonel Oughterson were totally different persons and yet, oddly, much that has been said about General Cutler could well be said about Colonel Oughterson. Both were brilliant surgeons, whose technical dexterity was based on sound judgment. Both were born teachers. Both were men of ideas who were not satisfied until their ideas were translated into actions.

The comments of the surgeons under whom Colonel Oughterson served—and who did not always agree with his ideas—indicate the kind of medical officer he was. General Maxwell wrote that his diary represented the thoughts of a great organizer, "the thinking of a mature mind on a very difficult subject." It was written, he said, by a man who, if he had had the opportunity to edit it, would still think and write the same way.

General Denit was even more explicit. "I am not inclined," he wrote, "* * * to take exception to anything he has to say. After all he gives the picture as he sees it * * *. No one who hasn't experienced it [war in the jungle] can believe the difficulties encountered * * *. I had a great admiration for Colonel Oughterson and gave him the job of 'thinking' and advising me on how surgery and care of the wounded could be improved. I didn't want him to have any administrative authority. I wanted him to (1) see, (2) think and (3) advise. Often when one tries to correct he loses his value as an adviser."

The wars in which General Cutler and Colonel Oughterson served were utterly different in many respects. In the European theater, for instance, evacuation of casualties was often a matter of hours. In the Pacific areas, it was usually a matter of days and sometimes a matter of weeks. The Pacific War was a war of incredible distances, which had to be taken into account in every aspect of medical care. In the European theater, coincidental disease seldom complicated the management of wounds. In the Pacific, malaria was a possible concomitant of every wound until the war was more than half over, and other tropical diseases were a possibility all through the war. Gas gangrene, which proved no problem in the European theater, was sometimes a serious problem in the Pacific. And so it went.

Nevertheless, in spite of the differences in the wars that were fought in Europe and the Pacific, it is surprising how squarely the views of these two eminent surgeons corresponded with each other in basic principles if not always in details.

Colonel Oughterson's constant plea was for the placing of qualified surgeons well forward in combat areas, where their talents were required because of the inevitable delays in evacuation. The shortage of qualified surgeons, however, in a theater in which each island was a unit in itself was always extreme and was enhanced by the concentration of talent in affiliated units, from which it was often detached with great difficulty. Shortages of anesthesiologists with proper training and qualifications further complicated shortages of surgeons. At one time, when Colonel Oughterson surveyed six portable hospitals, he found three of them competently staffed and three others completely unusable because of lack of qualified personnel. The portable hospital, he noted, was excellent in jungle warfare but ill adapted and wasteful when communications were good. When it was not properly staffed, he said, "It gives the dangerous illusion that a surgical hospital is available."

His comments were always to the point. The incidence of gas gangrene, he noted, was an index of the kind of surgery being performed at the front, but the omission of plaster because gas gangrene might occur was simply the correction of one surgical mistake by making another. His comments on "moderate debridement" were caustic. He had never seen a surgeon who did good surgery at home do bad surgery in the Army. Almost as soon as he arrived in the Pacific, in November 1942, he began to comment that the principal cause of war neurosis was weak leadership, that men who were not happy were men who were not kept busy, and that the way to correct poor morale and poor surgery in a hospital was to provide it (1) with a strong commanding officer and (2) with a good surgeon. Whether Colonel Oughterson was evaluating surgical qualifications, correcting surgical errors, or trying to provide washing machines for hospital linens, screens for operating rooms, or hobnailed shoes for litter carriers, he was both practical and perceptive, and many of his comments might well become aphorisms.

The brilliant study of casualties in the Bougainville Campaign, which he initiated and directed, is a lasting addition to the science of wound ballistics. The conclusions he derived, and the lessons he drew, from medical care in each campaign in the Pacific deserve the most careful reading and reflection. Like the Cutler diary, the Oughterson diary is a real contribution to military medicine.

The consultant system was introduced late in the China-Burma-India theater, but the chapter describing it, the final chapter in this volume, is another experience well worth recording of medical care in inhospitable terrain, with constant shortages of personnel and supplies, in which not the least of the problems was the attempt to improve the efficiency of the Chinese Army Medical Service.

Again and again General Cutler mentions in his diary how desirable it would have been to have worked in peacetime on the problems he encountered during the war. He reminded himself frequently that one of his responsibilities as surgical consultant in the European theater would be to write the story of the consultant service. The chief problems of this service, as he saw it, were the relations of the consultants with each other and the relations be-

tween Regular Army medical officers and the officers who had just come into
service from what he called "the well-oiled machinery of civilian practice."
He found more patient those who, like himself, had served in World War I—
though it might come as a surprise to some of his associates to hear the word
patience attached to any activity of General Cutler's. At any rate, it was
his urgent wish that a permanent consultant system be established as an integral part of the Army Medical Department. He would have been happy,
had he lived, to know that this ardent desire of his has been translated into
reality.

As in all volumes in this series for which it is my privilege to write the
foreword, it is a pleasure to express my gratitude to the editors and authors
who wrote and directed this volume, particularly the special editor for the
two volumes dealing with the activities of surgical consultants, the former
Col. B. Noland Carter, MC; to the Advisory Editorial Board for Surgery;
and to the personnel in my office who are helping me to carry out what I regard
as one of my truly important missions, the preparation and publication of the
history of the U.S. Army Medical Department in World War II.

LEONARD D. HEATON,
Lieutenant General,
The Surgeon General.

Preface

This volume is an account of the activities of surgical consultants in oversea theaters of operations excluding field armies. The experiences of surgical consultants attached to field armies and of those in the Zone of Interior were recorded earlier in volume I. The experiences recounted in this volume are both interesting and instructive and will undoubtedly be invaluable to those individuals who may be called upon at some future time to serve as oversea consultants. Two of the chapters consist of diaries of consultants who have died since the war. These diaries have been edited in an effort to preserve the more interesting portions and to delete personal and nonessential details. It is most unfortunate that an account of the experiences of the Chief Surgical Consultant to the North African (later Mediterranean) theater could not be obtained, since so many of the surgical concepts of the care of the wounded were developed in that theater. The chapters in volume I by Col. Frank B. Berry, MC, Consultant in Surgery to the Seventh U.S. Army, and by Col. Howard E. Snyder, MC, Consultant in Surgery to the Fifth U.S. Army, however, give an excellent account of the surgical problems encountered and of how they were met in portions of that theater.

It has been rightfully stated on many occasions that surgical consultants in theaters of operations were potent factors in reducing the mortality rate. Their services were invaluable and became increasingly appreciated as the war progressed. Consultants to the oversea theaters came from civilian life and, for the most part, had been connected with important teaching centers in the United States. They were untiring in their efforts, dedicated to their duties, and magnificent in their accomplishments. One is impressed, as one reads of their experiences, that all of them felt that they could have performed their duties more efficiently if they had had better indoctrination, if there had been a definite place for them in the organizations to which they were assigned, and if they had been given rank commensurate with the rank of their counterparts in the Allied Armies and with the responsibilities which they had assumed. The manner in which these men performed their duties has demonstrated to the Armed Forces the necessity for surgical consultants and, it is believed, has done much to establish them as important and permanent additions to the military effort.

In addition to acknowledgments appearing elsewhere to the various authors, deep appreciation is expressed to the following individuals who have contributed materially toward the compilation of this volume.

Mrs. Elliott C. Cutler, widow of the late Brig. Gen. Elliott C. Cutler, MC, AUS, made available her husband's personal diaries, without which the chapter covering the activities of General Cutler could never have contained the personal insight it now has.

Dr. Bernard J. Pisani and Mrs. Pisani, to whom General Cutler's personal diary was entrusted, together accomplished the laborious task of extracting matters pertinent to this history from that handwritten diary. Dr. Pisani also reviewed in detail the entire chapter pertaining to General Cutler's activities and contributed one of the epilogues.

Maj. Gen. Paul R. Hawley, MC, USA (Retired), carefully reviewed the chapter concerning General Cutler; initiated inquiries on questionable matters to Dr. Loyal Davis, Sir Gordon Gordon-Taylor, and others; contributed the prologue; added annotations (now included as footnotes) which greatly amplify the text; and graciously and firmly insisted that General Cutler's remarks remain in the text, whether or not complimentary to the Chief Surgeon, ETOUSA (General Hawley).

Dr. Robert M. Zollinger, in addition to contributing his own chapter, reviewed the chapter pertaining to General Cutler's activities and wrote one of the epilogues.

The late Dr. Marion E. Howard (Mrs. Ashley W. Oughterson) gathered together the personal papers of Dr. Oughterson upon his untimely death in an airplane crash and presented them to The Historical Unit, U.S. Army Medical Service. She also loaned The Historical Unit the personal war journal of Dr. Oughterson. Without these contributions on Dr. Howard's part, the chapter pertaining to the wartime activities of Col. Ashley W. Oughterson, MC, could not have been compiled.

Maj. Gen. Guy B. Denit, MC, USA (Retired) ; Maj. Gen. John M. Willis, MC, USA (Retired) ; Brig. Gen. Earl Maxwell, USAF (MC, Retired) ; and Dr. Maurice C. Pincoffs reviewed the chapter pertaining to Colonel Oughterson's activities and made comments included as introductory matter and footnotes thereto.

Dr. Julian A. Sterling very generously reviewed the manuscript of chapter VI, which records the experiences of the consultants in orthopedic surgery and rehabilitation in the European theater.

Miss Elizabeth M. McFetridge provided invaluable advice and help in preparing portions of the chapter pertaining to surgical consultant activities in the Southwest Pacific Area.

Maj. James K. Arima, MSC, in addition to functioning in other capacities, searched out the photographs from which the illustrations for this book were selected. Sp4c. Jacques Kornberg also helped.

Mr. Melvin J. Hadden prepared the excellent layouts for the illustrations in this volume and handled the artwork and the preparation of the illustrations for printing.

Miss Elizabeth P. Mason, Chief, Cartographic Section, and Miss Jean A. Saffran, Cartographic Section, of the Special Projects Branch, The Historical Unit, prepared the maps.

Mrs. Claire M. Sorrell, Historian, of the General Reference and Research Branch, The Historical Unit, rendered research assistance.

Miss C. Louise Brady, Editor (Printed Media), Editorial Branch, The Historical Unit, U.S. Army Medical Service, edited and prepared the manuscript for printing and prepared the index for this volume.

B. Noland Carter, M.D.

Contents

Part II

THE PACIFIC AND ASIA

Illustrations

Charts

Maps

Tables

Part I

EUROPE

CHAPTER I

Surgical Consultants in the European Theater of Operations

Col. James C. Kimbrough, MC, USA (Ret.)

It may be said that the foundation for the consultant system in the European theater of World War II was laid during World War I. Many of the campaigns in Europe in the Second World War were fought over the same battlegrounds of the only major theater in which American Forces were involved in the First World War. The AEF (American Expeditionary Forces) in World War I eventually developed a full-fledged system of consultation in both medicine and surgery. Lessons learned in the metamorphosis of the consultant system during the first great conflict were recorded and available for reference in the medical history of that war. Thus, a review of consultation in surgery in the European theater during World War II must begin with World War I.

CONSULTANT SYSTEM IN WORLD WAR I

At first glance, it would appear that the AEF in World War I was amply supplied with consultants.[1] At various times, consultants were assigned to every echelon of command from combat divisions to the Chief Surgeon's Office and in headquarters and hospital centers of the base sections. The system under which the consultants were appointed, organized, and operated took two quite distinct forms during the war. The earlier of the two may be simply characterized as a more-or-less unsystematic form in which consultants worked independently and entirely on their own. The second, and later, form may be said to have been an attempt at systematization and unification of the professional services.

Under the first system, there were eight "directors" in the Office of the Chief Surgeon, AEF. A director was appointed for each of the following: General medicine; general surgery; orthopedic surgery; surgery of the head; urology, and skin and genitourinary diseases; laboratories; psychiatry; and roentgenology. This "director" system was implemented throughout the army corps, administrative sections of the lines of communications, larger hospitals, and other commands. Many assistant consultants were appointed in various eche-

---

[1] Most of the material in this section is based on the discussion of the professional services, AEF, contained in "The Medical Department of the United States Army in the World War, Volume II, Administration, American Expeditionary Forces" (Washington: U.S. Government Printing Office, 1927).

lons of the medical service. At the start, each infantry division also had a surgical consultant. The assistants and consultants at the division level were commonly known as junior consultants.

Under this system, each consultant was directly under either the surgeon of a command or the commander of a hospital center. The Chief Surgeon's circular establishing the system emphasized that professional authority did not include administrative control. This was indeed an open-end statement since nothing was said as to what, specifically, "professional authority" entailed. At General Headquarters, AEF, the directors were supposedly under the control of the Hospitalization Division of the Chief Surgeon's Office at Chaumont, some 45 kilometers from where the directors were stationed at Neufchateau. Their activities were uncoordinated. Each director sought to solve in his own way the very different and difficult problems which confronted him. No specific instructions had been issued governing their status.

The confusion which often resulted is readily understandable under the circumstances. First, the new professional directors did not have the military background and experience which would have made their tasks easier of accomplishment. Moreover, there was really nobody to help them. Each director was an enthusiast in his own specialty, and his zeal—as well as the misnomer of his title, "director"—not infrequently led him to misdirected activities. Some of the best clinicians were assigned to divisions and other commands which had little need or use for their talents during most of this period. Even the seemingly simplest matters became problems of no small proportions. For example, someone in authority had most generously ruled that each director at General Headquarters, AEF, was authorized the use of an automobile for unlimited periods of time! Considerable embarrassment was caused by a shortage of automobiles for this purpose and by the absence of an arbiter to coordinate the use of the few vehicles that were available from time to time.

In spite of the difficulties encountered, the initial work accomplished by the specialists was of very great importance, and there were many basic similarities in their modes of operation. As their functions became more clearly defined, it was evident that consultants were expected to direct and supervise the professional services in all echelons of the medical service, to provide for continuity of treatment from front to rear, to modify, as need be, accepted methods of treatment, and to inaugurate new treatment methods.

On 18 April 1918, the Chief Surgeon appointed Lt. Col. (later Col.) William L. Keller, MC, Director of Professional Services for the purpose of coordinating professional medical activities. Among the missions given Colonel Keller, the following were most significant:

> By virtue of this appointment, you are empowered to represent the chief surgeon, A.E.F., in all matters pertaining to the administration, direction, and coordination of the professional services. You are responsible for such professional matters relating to hospitalization, evacuation, laboratories, sanitation, and other activities as may pertain to the proper sorting, distribution, and evacuation of sick and wounded through the channels that will best insure efficient treatment from the front to the rear.

All requests for the movement of personnel and supplies originating in the professional services will be forwarded by or through you to the chief surgeon, A.E.F., or to some one designated by him.

      *   *   *   *   *   *   *

You will direct the compilation of a classified roster by each chief consultant, of all professional personnel, such as specialists, consultants, or surgical teams among the various army units of our own and allied formations, so as to facilitate their proper distribution and utilization in emergencies as well as in routine. When the organization of the professional service is completed, you will direct its workings, either from general headquarters or such other places as best serves the interests of the service.

With the three original divisions, medicine, surgery, and laboratories as a basis, you will so coordinate the activities of the subdivision thereof that scientific research and clinical proficiency may be effectually promoted.[2]

With the appointment of the Director of Professional Services, a reorganization—actually an organization—of the rest of the professional services was directed on a trial basis. The organization was fully adopted and officially announced by General Orders No. 88, General Headquarters, AEF, on 6 June 1918. This was the beginning of the second system previously referred to, that of a coordinated professional service for the AEF. The titles of directors were at this time changed to consultants. The publication of these general orders gave them a status which they had not previously enjoyed and promoted broader appreciation of their responsibilities.

Under the Director of Professional Services, who, incidentally, was still under the Hospitalization Division, were a Chief Consultant in Surgery and a Chief Consultant in Medicine. The Chief Consultant in Surgery was Brig. Gen. John M. T. Finney, MC. He was given the overall responsibility for supervising the professional activities of the surgical subdivisions in the AEF. He was instructed to organize and coordinate these subdivisions in a manner whch would permit him to anticipate and request, as far in advance as possible, necessary changes in personnel. He was charged with the formation and functioning of surgical teams and collecting timely reports from them. He was to make recommendations for inspections as to technical procedure and instruction in the specialty of surgery.

Under the Chief Consultant in Surgery were nine senior consultants in various specialties representing the subdivisions of surgery which were to be recognized in the AEF. These were surgical research; roentgenology; neurosurgery; orthopedic surgery; ear, nose, and throat surgery; general surgery; venereal and skin diseases and genitourinary surgery; maxillofacial surgery; and ophthalmology. The mission of these senior consultants was to coordinate professional activities relating to their specialties in subordinate commands. They were specifically instructed to make recommendations to the Chief Consultant so that instructions relative to professional subjects could be directed to subordinate commands with dispatch and executed promptly.

---

[2] Letter, Chief Surgeon, AEF, to Lt. Col. W. L. Keller, MC, 18 Apr. 1918, subject: Detail as Director of Professional Division, A.E.F.

A consultant who reported directly to the Chief Consultant in Surgery on professional matters was appointed in each army corps. His title was senior divisional surgical consultant. He was responsible for the supervision and direction of all surgical activities in the infantry divisions, a responsibility, formerly, of the division surgical consultant. It was the duty of the senior divisional surgical consultant to relieve division surgeons of the necessity for supervising strictly technical work, since it was considered that division surgeons would have their hands full with other operational and administrative matters. Aiding the senior divisional surgical consultant—who, it is to be remembered, was assigned to an army corps—were divisional surgical consultants. These were assigned to the corps, usually on the basis of one per division, to supervise the immediate surgical activities of operating teams within the divisions. Toward the end of hostilities, these divisional surgical consultants were withdrawn as superfluous when the First and Second U.S. Armies were organized with their full complement of consultants.

To round out the surgical services of the AEF, there were consultants at hospital centers, specialists in base hospitals and tactical divisions, and surgical teams. Consultants at the hospital centers were named in the various specialties, as required, and were available for consultation to nearby units as well as within the hospitals of the center. While the need for them was evident early, it was not until near the end of hostilities that they could be supplied in any number. At the end of 1918, 16 hospital centers had surgical consultants. Specialists were also designated at hospitals in eight of the nine surgical specialties previously mentioned. (There were no consultants or specialists locally designated in surgical research.) Each infantry division had a specialist in orthopedic surgery and one in urology. In 1918, surgical teams were first organized from personnel of base hospitals. These teams, numbering some three hundred by the end of October 1918, were used wherever necessary, including the division areas, and were composed of one operator, an anesthesiologist, two nurses, and two orderlies.

The Chief Surgeon, AEF, subsequent to the signing of the armistice, convened a board of officers to investigate and report upon the conduct of the Medical Department, AEF, and to make recommendations with a view to the improvement of that department. This board approved fully the system of professional services which had been developed during the war. Specifically, it stated that the Director of Professional Services should be a colonel selected from that scarce category of Regular Army medical officers who knew the routine of Army administration well and, at the same time, were well informed as to the professional qualifications of large numbers of civilian practitioners so that they could be assigned to duties wherein the greatest efficiency in performance would result. The board went on to say that the Chief Consultant in Surgery should be a medical officer of the highest surgical attainments and that his surgical subdivision of professional services should be further subdivided into the nine surgical specialties heretofore mentioned. The board also recommended assignment of consultants to field armies, corps, and divisions only during active campaigns. Assuming that the theater surgeon would also function as Surgeon, SOS (Services of Supply), for the administration of base sections, the board emphasized the need for consultants in general surgery and orthopedic surgery to supervise and direct all surgical activities throughout base sections of the Services of Supply.

CONSULTANT SYSTEM IN WORLD WAR II

Organization

The activities of the surgical consultants of ETOUSA (European Theater of Operations, U.S. Army) were coordinated by the Chief Consultant in Surgery, Col. (later Brig. Gen.) Elliott C. Cutler, MC. These surgical consultants functioned under the Division of Professional Services, Office of the Chief Surgeon, ETOUSA (chart 1).

CHART 1.—*Organization of the Division of Professional Services, Office of the Chief Surgeon, ETOUSA, in 1942*

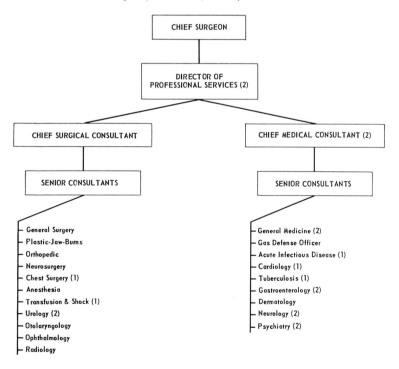

(1) Part-time positions held by medical officers assigned permanent duties elsewhere than in the Office of the Chief Surgeon.

(2) Dual positions. Director of Professional Services was also consultant in urology; likewise, neurology and psychiatry were handled by one officer, and general medicine and gastroenterology by the chief medical consultant.

The Division of Professional Services was activated on 19 June 1942 with Col. James C. Kimbrough, MC, as chief (fig. 1). The consultant organization was set up according to the Regular Army surgical service in the large Army hospitals. In such an organization, the general surgeon was chief of the surgical service and the specialist surgeons—such as those in orthopedics, ophthalmology, and neurosurgery—were chiefs of the various surgical sections. (Later, about 1945, specialties in army hospitals were given the status of a service, or department, similar to the organization in large civilian hospitals.) Since all the consultants in the European theater held high positions in university hospitals and medical schools in the United States, this subordination to a general surgeon caused some dissatisfaction. The specialist surgeons objected to the designation "senior consultant," as contrasted to the title "chief consultant." They were, however, all such patriots and of such high caliber as surgeons that this regimentation at no time interfered with their efficiency or their devotion to duty.

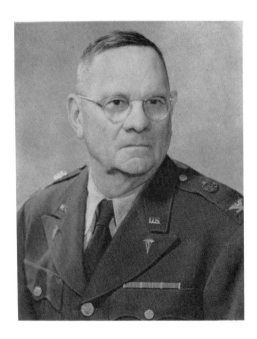

Figure 1.—Col. James C. Kimbrough, MC.

Anesthesia was represented by a senior consultant functioning under general surgery. In like manner, radiology became a part of the surgical service.

After the Professional Services Division had been established and medical officers to fill the consultant positions began to arrive in the theater, it was necessary to promulgate an official statement relating to the organization for consultation in medicine and surgery. This was done by an unaddressed document, signed by the Chief Surgeon, Col. (later Maj. Gen.) Paul R. Hawley, MC (fig. 2), and dated 18 August 1942. Titled "Organization of Professional Services E.T.O.U.S.A., Services of Supply," the pronouncement read:

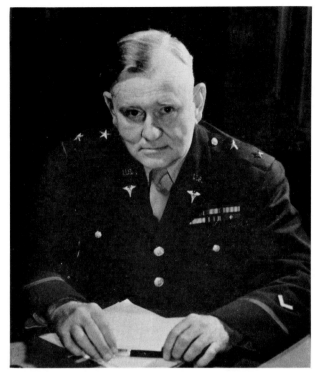

FIGURE 2.—Maj. Gen. Paul R. Hawley.

In order to utilize the professional services of the consultants and the specialists of the Medical Department, E.T.O.U.S.A., in a manner that will best facilitate the coordination between the forces, from front to rear, the following instructions are issued:

1. *Director of Professional Services*—The Director of Professional Services, under the Chief Surgeon, E.T.O.U.S.A. will supervise the professional activities of the Medical Department, E.T.O.U.S.A., and coordinate the work of the consultants and specialists of this department.

2. *Chief Consultants*—The Chief Consultant, surgical service, will supervise the professional work of the surgical sub-divisions. He will organize and coordinate these sub-divisions in such manner that will permit them to function at the greatest efficiency in carrying out surgical treatment.

Chief Consultant, medical service, will supervise the medical sub-divisions. He will organize and coordinate these sub-divisions in such manner as to ensure the highest possible standard of professional endeavour.

3. *Senior Consultants*—Under the supervision of the Director of Professional Services and the Chief Consultants in medicine and surgery, consultants for the special sub-division of the Chief Surgeon's office will coordinate the activities relating to their respective specialties.

They will make such recommendations to the Chief Consultants as are considered necessary for the instructions of consultants and specialists in hospitals, divisions and other army formations.

4. *Consultants*—Under the supervision of the Senior Consultants, the Consultants for the army, corps, divisions, hospitals, base sections and other formations will supervise and coordinate the work of the specialists under their respective sub-divisions.

5. *Specialists*—Under the supervision of the Consultants, the specialists on duty with hospitals, divisions and other formations will organize and carry out the work of their respective specialties in the most efficient manner possible.

The surgical consultants in the European theater were eventually arranged in five groups (chart 2) :

1. Consultants assigned to the Chief Surgeon's Office. This group consisted of Col. Elliott C. Cutler, MC, as chief and the surgical specialists functioning under the overall supervision of the Chief Surgeon.

2. Base section surgical consultants. These changed frequently and functioned under the direction of the base surgeons.

3. Regional consultants and coordinators in the hospital centers. These were usually the senior outstanding surgeons of one of the general hospitals of the center who performed the duties of consultant in addition to their duties as chiefs of the surgical services or sections of the hospitals to which they were assigned.

CHART 2.—*Organization of the consultant system in ETOUSA, 1944*

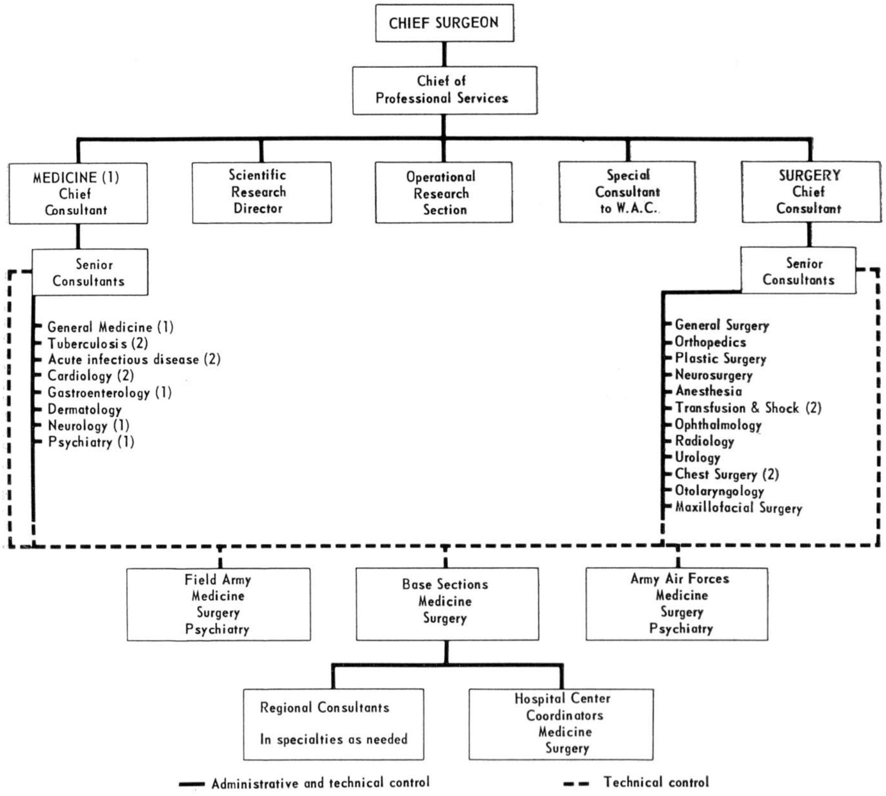

(1) Dual positions. Chief medical consultant was also consultant in general medicine and gastroenterology; neurology and psychiatry were handled by one officer.

(2) Part-time positions held by medical officers assigned permanent duties elsewhere than in the Office of the Chief Surgeon.

4. Army surgical consultants. Each field army had an assigned surgical consultant who functioned under the direction of the army surgeon.

5. The Army Air Forces developed a limited system of consultation as necessary within their own commands.

As the continental activities increased, appropriate continental base sections and advance sections were set up after the Chief Surgeon's headquarters was moved to continental Europe. All activities in the United Kingdom were consolidated under Headquarters, United Kingdom Base Section.

Personnel

The following individuals were consultants to the Chief Surgeon:

1. Col. Elliott C. Cutler, MC, Moseley Professor of Surgery, Harvard Medical School, was chosen Chief Consultant in Surgery and reported to Headquarters, ETOUSA, on 9 August 1942.

2. Lt. Col. (later Col.) James B. Brown, MC, professor of clinical and oral surgery, Washington University, St. Louis, Mo., reported for duty as Consultant in Plastic Surgery on 8 June 1942.

3. Colonel Brown was accompanied by Maj. (later Lt. Col.) Eugene M. Bricker, MC, from Washington University, who eventually succeeded Colonel Brown on 12 January 1943 and rendered superior service in that department.

4. Lt. Col. (later Col.) Loyal Davis, MC, professor of surgery, Northwestern University, Evanston, Ill., reported as Consultant in Neurosurgery in September 1942.

5. Lt. Col. (later Col.) Ralph M. Tovell, MC, Hartford Hospital, Hartford, Conn., arrived on 28 September 1942 and was placed in charge of anesthesia.

6. Lt. Col. (later Col.) Derrick T. Vail, MC, professor of ophthalmology, University of Cincinnati, came in on 5 October 1942 to become Consultant in Ophthalmology.

7. During the fall of 1942, Lt. Col. (later Col.) Rex L. Diveley, MC, of Kansas City reported to take over the role of orthopedic consultant.

8. Lt. Col. (later Col.) Norton Canfield, MC, professor of otolaryngology, Yale University School of Medicine, came in to take charge of otolaryngology in January 1943.

9. Lt. Col. (later Col.) Kenneth D. A. Allen, MC, radiologist, Presbyterian Hospital and other hospitals of Denver, reported on 9 February 1943 in charge of radiology.

10. Maj. (later Lt. Col.) William J. Stewart, MC, reported on 17 January 1943 and acted as the consultant in orthopedic surgery when Colonel Diveley was absent in North Africa and continued to assist in orthopedics until the arrival of Lt. Col. Mather Cleveland, MC.

11. Maj. (later Lt. Col.) Ambrose H. Storck, MC, Charity Hospital, New Orleans, reported on 2 March 1943 as Consultant in General Surgery.

12. Lt. Col. (later Col.) Robert M. Zollinger, MC, professor of surgery, Harvard Medical School, took over from Colonel Storck on 1 July 1944.

13. Maj. (later Lt. Col.) John E. Scarff, MC, assistant professor of neurosurgery, Columbia University, succeeded Colonel Davis on 10 September 1943.

14. Col. Roy A. Stout, DC, was placed in charge of maxillofacial surgery on 8 November 1943.

15. Capt. (later Maj.) Charles D. Rancourt, MC, was designated Assistant Consultant in Radiology, on 14 June 1943.

16. Lt. Col. (later Col.) Mather Cleveland, MC, assistant professor of anatomy and instructor of orthopedic surgery, College of Physicians and Surgeons, Columbia University, was placed in charge of orthopedic surgery after Colonel Diveley became chief of the separate Rehabilitation Division on 3 January 1944.

17. Lt. Col. (later Col.) R. Glen Spurling, MC, clinical professor of surgery (neurosurgery), University of Louisville School of Medicine, became Consultant in Neurosurgery on 15 March 1944.

18. Maj. (later Lt. Col.) John N. Robinson, MC, Columbia University, was designated Consultant in Urology in the spring of 1943.

19. Lt. Col. (later Col.) Paul C. Morton, MC, was designated surgical consultant for the United Kingdom Base Section on 10 September 1944.

20. Lt. Col. James N. Greear, Jr., MC, came in as Consultant in Ophthalmology, succeeding Colonel Vail in March 1945.

In considering the great achievements of this group of eminent surgeons, it is believed that never before has an army at any time had available such expert advice in caring for and treating every type of casualty (fig. 3).

Base section and regional consultants.—The base section and regional consultants changed so many times that it is impracticable to attempt to list them by name. They all rendered superior service.

Surgical consultants to the field armies.—Each field army had a surgical consultant whose duty it was to supervise the treatment and transportation of patients from aid stations through the evacuation hospitals. They had technical control of the auxiliary surgical groups assigned to the army and in general were advisers to the army surgeons concerning the treatment and transportation of surgical casualties.

Col. J. Augustus Crisler, Jr., MC, was consultant surgeon for the First U.S. Army; Lt. Col. Thomas B. Jones, MC, and later Col. Charles B. Odom, MC, for the Third U.S. Army; Col. Frank B. Berry, MC, for the Seventh U.S. Army; Col. Gordon K. Smith, MC, for the Ninth U.S. Army; and Col. William F. MacFee, MC, for the Fifteenth U.S. Army.

The great responsibility of the surgical consultants can best be appreciated when it is realized that approximately 80 percent of the battle casualties in the European theater required surgical management. The excellent results obtained are everlasting testimony to the outstanding ability of these surgeons who supervised and directed the transportation and treatment of the wounded. The great personal and professional sacrifices made by this group in voluntarily leaving their families and professional activities is outstanding evidence of their great patriotism and their intense desire to serve their country.

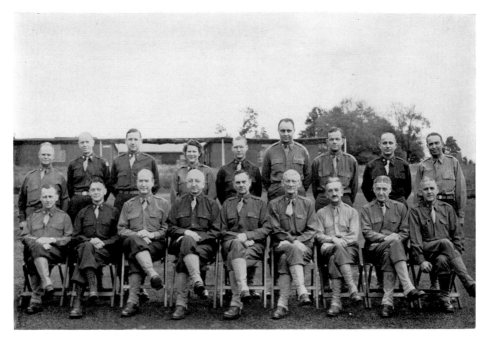

FIGURE 3.—Consultant group at Cheltenham, England, mid-1944, before the move of the Office of the Chief Surgeon, ETOUSA, to the Continent. First row, left to right, Lt. Col. Ralph M. Tovell, MC, Col. Donald M. Pillsbury, MC, Col. Derrick T. Vail, MC, Col. Roy A. Stout, DC, Col. James C. Kimbrough, MC, Col. Elliott C. Cutler, MC, Col. Lloyd J. Thompson, MC, Col. Thomas H. Lanman, MC, and Lt. Col. Mather Cleveland, MC. Second row, left to right, Lt. Col. Gordon E. Hein, MC, Lt. Col. Kenneth D. A. Allen, MC, Lt. Col. Norton Canfield, MC, Capt. Marion C. Loizeaux, MC, Capt. Wayne H. Jonson, MAC, Lt. Col. Eugene M. Bricker, MC, Maj. John N. Robinson, MC, Lt. Col. Robert M. Zollinger, MC, and Lt. Col. R. Glen Spurling, MC.

Policies

Policies for the operation of the Professional Services Division were established early and set the pattern for the many activities in which the various surgical consultants later became engaged (fig. 4).[3] These policies were stated as follows:

1. *Supervision of Professional Services:*

a. It is the policy of this division to implement plans whereby the personnel of the American forces shall receive promptly the highest standard of medical and surgical care.

b. The Consultants' Section will ascertain as often as necessary the condition of all patients reported seriously ill in U.S. Army hospitals.

c. The condition of all patients admitted to British hospitals will be verified as often as necessary.

d. In order to maintain adequate bed capacity for the sick and wounded, only the complicated venereal diseases and those intolerant to the usual therapy will be hospitalized

---

[3] Letter, Director, Professional Services (Col. James C. Kimbrough, MC) to Chief Surgeon, SOS, ETOUSA, 9 Dec. 1942, subject: Policies for the Operation of the Division of Professional Services.

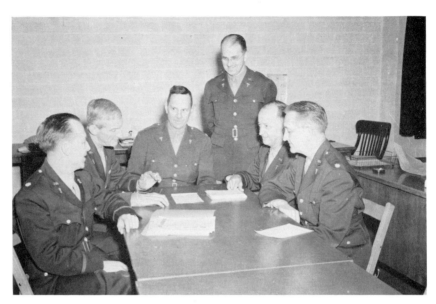

FIGURE 4.—Weekly meetings of the consultant group were initiated early in the European theater to discuss and solve problems and to establish policy.   Left to right, Lieutenant Colonel Tovell, Colonel Cutler, Colonel Kimbrough, Lt. Col. James B. Brown, MC, Lt. Col. William S. Middleton, MC, and Lieutenant Colonel Thompson, Cheltenham, England, 6 January 1943.

in station and general hospitals.   Uncomplicated venereal disease will be treated at the local infirmaries.

e. In order to maintain and stimulate professional morale and disseminate recent medical information, it is considered advisable that medical meetings be held regularly at general hospitals and station hospitals.   The type and frequency of these meetings will depend on local conditions at each hospital and the general condition of the activities of the armed forces.

f. It is desired that Commanding Officers of general and station hospitals prepare plans for the management of casualties in large numbers, possibly in train load lots.

g. It is hoped that the Commanding Officers and Chiefs of Professional Services in all medical installations in the European Theater of Operations will stimulate and encourage among the officers in their commands the compilation of medical data for publication whenever such data would seem to be of interest to members of professional medicine either here or at home.

h. Each general hospital will maintain a blood bank.

i. United States Army Medical Officers will be encouraged to register with the British Medical Council and to become members of the Royal Society of Medicine.

2. *Co-ordination of Consultants.*

a. The Consultants in Medicine and Surgery will make written reports daily of their activities to Director of Professional Services through the Chief Consultants in Medicine and Surgery.   These reports will be consolidated by the Chief Consultants and Director of Professional Services for transmission to the Chief Surgeon.

b. Request for consultation service for medical units in the SOS, ETO, will be made to the Division of Professional Services, Chief Surgeon's Office.   The manner and time of transmitting these requests will be determined by the merits in each individual case. At night the request for such service may be made to the Consultant concerned at his billet.

It is the policy of this division to have consultation service immediately available at all times.

c. Arrangements have been made with the British authorities whereby the consultants are made available to American personnel in the hospitals of the British Naval, Army and Air Forces and the Emergency Medical Service hospitals, and the Canadian Military hospitals.

3. *Liaison with British Research and Development in Professional Services.*

a. The appropriate personnel of the Division of Professional Services will be authorized to attend the meetings of the British Medical Research Council and other medical conferences pertaining to their respective specialty.

b. The attendance of meetings and conferences and professional contact with British personnel and institutions with a view to promoting general good will and obtaining professional knowledge is encouraged.

4. *Physical Standards.*

a. In reviewing the physical examination of applicants for commission, promotion, re-classification, etc., the standards provided in Army Regulations governing each type of case will be maintained.

5. *Professional Training.*

a. Arrangements will be encouraged whereby United States Medical Officers may be assigned to British hospitals for the observation of their activities for periods of one to two weeks. Allotment of United States Medical Officers to British service and civilian medical courses has been arranged.

b. Courses of instruction for the medical department personnel of base section, divisions, station and general hospitals will be carried out.

Duties and Functions

To implement the policies mentioned, the Director of Professional Services circulated the following statement of the duties of consultants for the information and guidance of all concerned and as a directive to the consultants themselves:

1. The consulting staff of the Chief Surgeon's Office will function under the direction of the Division of Professional Services and are the responsible advisers to the Chief Surgeon on all professional and technical matters pertaining to their particular branch of medicine.

2. They will submit their reports and recommendations, thru the Director of Professional Services to the Chief Surgeon.

3. They will be available to visit Medical Department Units for the purpose of giving their opinion and assistance with regard to technical and professional matters.

4. They will advise on the selections and assignment of junior consultants and specialists and will report from time to time on the standard of professional efficiency maintained by such officers.

5. They will be instrumental, in collaboration with the Operations Division, Chief Surgeon's Office, in arranging Courses of Instruction, Medical Meetings, and Training Schools, and will keep the officers of the Medical Department in touch with the latest developments in medical science.

6. They will initiate and carry out research and investigations with a view to conserving manpower in the field and restoring to health the sick and wounded.

7. They will maintain liaison with consultants and specialists in all branches of medicine of the British armed forces and civilian practice.

8. They will advise as to the suitability of drugs, instruments, equipment, and accommodations and on other matters pertaining to the health of the Armed Forces.

Specifically for the Chief Consultant in Surgery, the Director of Professional Services dictated the following duties:

1. He will advise the Chief Surgeon thru the Director of Professional Services on questions of surgical policy.

2. He will advise on the selection and allocation of surgical equipment.

3. He will advise, in collaboration with the Chief Consultant in Medicine, on the selection of drugs for use in the ETOUSA.

4. He will advise the Chief Surgeon regarding the selection and duties of surgical consultants and specialists.

5. He will visit Medical Department Units and correlate the military surgical procedure as a whole.

6. He will establish liaison with the surgical service of the Medical Department of other U.S. Forces and with the medical service of the British Forces both civilian and military.

Significant Activities

It was the chief concern of the surgical consultants to initiate and implement the policies of surgical treatment for the theater. This duty involved the methods of transportation of the wounded and the selection and allocation of surgical equipment.

Contact was maintained with the hospitals in England, and the surgical procedures and end results of treatment were supervised. After landing on the Continent, they followed the armies in the field and supervised the treatment and methods of evacuation. On several occasions, they made visits to the Zone of Interior in order to ascertain the condition in which the wounded reached the Zone of Interior hospitals.

Upon arrival in the theater, each medical unit was visited, the qualifications of the personnel were verified by the appropriate consultant, and recommendations were made to effect the most efficient assignments.

Special treatment facilities were set up in hospitals under the supervision of the appropriate consultant for patients requiring highly specialized treatment such as those with cold injury and burns and those requiring neurosurgical, urological, and plastic procedures. These special hospitals were usually located in the hospital centers.

During the summer of the Normandy invasion, it was realized that the supply of blood for transfusion which was obtainable in the European theater would be inadequate and that supplies from the Zone of Interior would be necessary. Colonel Cutler, Colonel MacFee, and Maj. (later Lt. Col.) Robert C. Hardin, MC, returned to Washington to inform The Surgeon General of the urgent need for whole blood from the United States. The plan for procurement, preservation and transportation of this blood from the Zone of Interior to the European theater was implemented by the Office of The Surgeon General under the supervision of Lt. Col. (later Col.) Douglas B. Kendrick, Jr., MC. The actual transportation of blood early became a function of the supply service. At no time was there an overall shortage in the supply of whole blood for the American wounded.

Rehabilitation

In June 1942, at the time of arrival of the U.S. Army in the United Kingdom, the rehabilitation facility had become a well-established institution of the British Army Medical Service. These rehabilitation hospitals were visited and the organization was reviewed by Colonel Cutler and Colonel Diveley. Under the supervision of Colonel Diveley, a rehabilitation "camp" was set up at Bromsgrove, England, on 1 April 1943. In the beginning, an 8 weeks' course of training was carried out, designed to prepare the recently recovered wounded for the hardships of field duty. The activities increased so rapidly that it was necessary to move the "camp" to more extensive quarters at Stoneleigh, which had a capacity of 300 (fig. 5). Rehabilitation activities were released from the Professional Services Division and established in a separate division—the Rehabilitation Division—on 3 January 1944 under the direction of Colonel Diveley, who was replaced by Colonel Cleveland as Consultant in Orthopedic Surgery.

Colonel Diveley visited the Zone of Interior to advise The Surgeon General on the establishment of rehabilitation facilities in the Zone of Interior. These facilities were the forerunners of the convalescent hospitals in the United States.

Miscellaneous Activities

In order to insure a uniformity in the management of the wounded, the European Theater Manual of Therapy was prepared by the consultants of the Chief Surgeon's Office. The manual was published before D-day (6 June 1944) and made available to all medical officers of the theater. The value of this booklet justified the great amount of labor expended in its preparation and publication.

The Medical Department supply tables of surgical instruments and drugs were reviewed with a view to eliminating unnecessary items. The equipment obtained from the British was cataloged to correspond to the item numbers of the U.S. Army supply tables. This work was carried out by the consultants in cooperation with the medical supply service.

It was noted early that the Zone of Interior clinical record for patients was too extensive for use in the European theater. A special clinical record was prepared. This record was of such size that it could be carried in the field medical record envelope so that, on return to the Zone of Interior, the entire history and record of treatment were in a single cover.

The European Theater School of Medicine and Surgery and the Medical Field Service School at Shrivenham were contributed to in great measure by the surgical consultants who served as supervisors and instructors in these schools.

The auxiliary surgical groups were under the control of the Operations Service of the Chief Surgeon's Office and were allotted to field armies where their activities were administered by the army surgical consultants. Teams

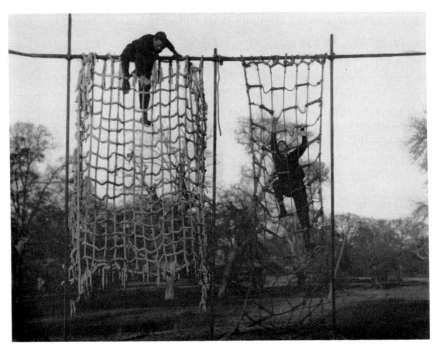

FIGURE 5.—Convalescent patients at 307th Station Hospital, Stoneleigh Park, Warwickshire, England, negotiate a Jacob's ladder on the obstacle course.

from the auxiliary surgical groups functioned at the evacuation hospitals or field hospitals of a field army.

A mobile field surgical unit was implemented by Colonel Zollinger at the 5th General Hospital. This unit was completed in November 1943 and delivered to the 3d Auxiliary Surgical Group. The plan eventually evolved into the mobile army surgical hospital later adopted by the Army. The unit was complete with equipment, tentage, beds, and the like, to care for emergency surgical cases at the frontline level.

Colonel Allen, Senior Consultant in Radiology, assembled a mobile field X-ray unit which was delivered to the 3d Auxiliary Surgical Group of the First U.S. Army in November 1943.

A simple field blood transfusion unit was created by Maj. (later Lt. Col.) Charles P. Emerson, Jr., MC, and Maj. (later Lt. Col.) Richard V. Ebert, MC, of the 5th General Hospital.

Liaison with the British medical service.—In 1942, the surgical consultants had arranged with the medical services of the British Army and Royal Air Force for the attendance of U.S. Army medical officers at the following schools and courses: Antigas school at Aldershot; London School of Hygiene and Tropical Medicine; Army School of Hygiene; gas school, Leeds University; blood transfusion school, Southmead Hospital, Bristol; and neurosurgical training at Oxford. These courses were arranged by the surgical consultants in their individual fields.

Liaison with the Russian medical service.—In order to obtain information regarding the medical service of the Soviet Army and to promote amicable diplomatic relations with the U.S.S.R., a commission of prominent surgeons from the Allied armies was selected to visit Russia. The United States was represented by Colonel Cutler and Colonel Davis.

Major Robinson, Consultant in Urology, visited the Zone of Interior in November and December 1944 for the purpose of presenting information to the Office of The Surgeon General regarding the management of wounds of the urogenital tract.

Medical Society, ETOUSA.—Early in the medical activities of the European theater, the Medical Society, ETOUSA, was organized. Meetings were held at general hospitals until the dispersion of the facilities made such meetings impractical, at which time the meetings were conducted under the direction of the base surgeons. The surgical consultants contributed materially to the programs of this society.

Operational research.—In May 1944, the Operational Research Section of the Professional Services Division was established at Cambridge Military Cemetery. With the cooperation of quartermaster graves registration personnel, facilities were established for studying the killed-in-action with a view to determining the types of wounds causing deaths, the missiles producing fatal wounds, and the circumstances under which death occurred. This operation was supervised by the surgical consultants who assembled a great deal of valuable information.

D-day activities on 6 June 1944.—During the early part of the continental liberation the members of the consultant group were present at the reception points on the beaches in England and at the transit hospitals supervising the care of the wounded transported back from Normandy. As a result of this observation, Circular Letter 101, Office of the Chief Surgeon, ETOUSA, concerning care of battle casualties was published on 30 July 1944.

Liaison with the French.—On arrival of the Office of the Chief Surgeon in Paris, the surgical consultants were welcomed to the French National Academy of Surgery and the Val de Grâce Military Hospital (French).

SUMMARY

It is not practicable to mention even a few of the numerous outstanding contributions rendered by individual consultants. All surgical consultants were on duty constantly, giving the American soldier the best surgical care that has ever been recorded in the history of warfare (fig. 6).

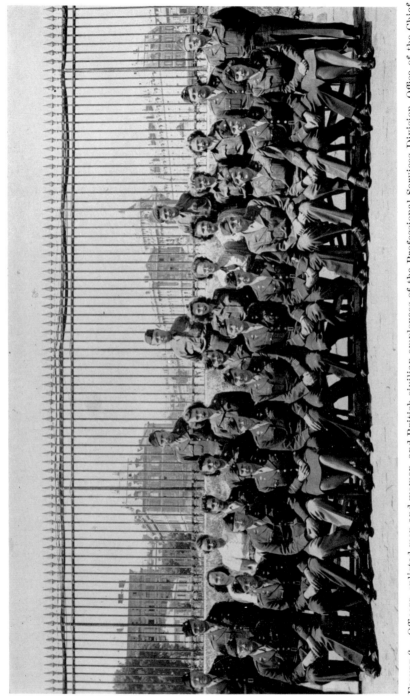

FIGURE 6.—Officers, enlisted men and women, and British civilian employees of the Professional Services Division, Office of the Chief Surgeon, ETOUSA, after V–E Day, Versailles, 1945.

CHAPTER II

The Chief Consultant in Surgery

Elliott C. Cutler, M.D.[1]

PROLOGUE

The war diary maintained by Brigadier General Elliott C. Cutler, MC (fig. 7) is an invaluable contribution to the overall history of the medical service in the European Theater of Operations. As Chief Consultant in Surgery, General Cutler occupied a position in which he could observe the many activities of the medical service in the theater, and this position, combined with an inquisitive mind, and limitless energy, enabled him to pursue the paths which his observations—including those not confined to his immediate field of responsibility—opened up.

Some of his observations were based upon incomplete or erroneous information. To have edited or deleted such entries would have marred the reflection of his strong personality in his writing. Where an inaccuracy may present a distorted picture of an important event, an appropriate footnote has been supplied.

Cutler's diary portrays faithfully his dedication to his task, his resentment of everything which impeded its accomplishment, and his intolerance of what he regarded as unjustifiable requirements of military administration. Notwithstanding his occasional caustic criticisms, he was a devoted and loyal soldier who contributed more than his share to the success of the medical service of the European Theater of Operations.

PAUL R. HAWLEY
Major General, MC, USA (Ret.)
October 1958

1942: GETTING STARTED

The Beginning

Dr. Elliott Carr Cutler, Moseley Professor of Surgery at the Harvard University School of Medicine and Surgeon-in-Chief, Peter Bent Brigham Hospital, Boston, was at Martha's Vineyard, Mass., when, quite by coincidence,

---

[1] Except where other sources are specifically cited, this account has been compiled and edited from the official diaries maintained by Elliott C. Cutler, M.D., deceased, as well as from other records, by Maj. James K. Arima, MSC, The Historical Unit, U.S. Army Medical Service.

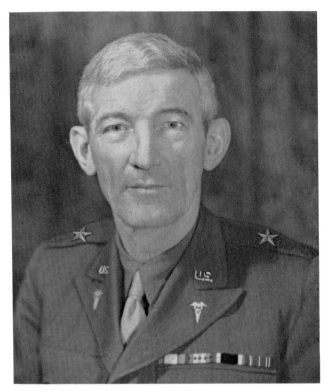

FIGURE 7.—Brig. Gen. Elliott Carr Cutler.

he received on the Fourth of July 1942, orders to report for active duty on 15 July 1942.

It was understood that he was to become Chief Consultant in Surgery in the European Theater of Operations, a position similar to that held by Brig. Gen. John M. T. Finney, MC, with the AEF (American Expeditionary Forces) in World War I. The reasons why Dr. Cutler was chosen for this position were inextricably rooted in that first great conflict.[2] In 1915, he was in Paris working with the French. He returned to the United States and received a commission in the Medical Corps Reserve as first lieutenant on 2 June 1916. He sailed for France on 11 May 1917 with Base Hospital No. 5, a unit affiliated with the Harvard Medical School. He served in various capacities, one of which was as adjutant of an evacuation hospital. Dr. Cutler was associated closely with Dr. Harvey Cushing throughout World War I, but his most significant experiences probably were those gained while working directly with Dr. Cushing on surgical teams, particularly in neurosurgery.[3]

Dr. Cutler was discharged as a major on 29 April 1919. He returned to the Medical Corps Reserve in 1921 and, from then on, kept in constant close touch with Army Medical Department affairs. One of The Surgeons General,

[2] Annual Report, Chief Consultant in Surgery, European Theater of Operations, U.S. Army, 1942.
[3] Cushing, Harvey: From a Surgeon's Journal, 1915–1918. Boston: Little, Brown & Co., 1936.

Maj. Gen. Robert U. Patterson, was Dr. Cutler's commanding officer while he was with Base Hospital No. 5. Subsequent Surgeons General were well known to Dr. Cutler, and The Surgeon General at this time (1942), Maj. Gen. James C. Magee, was also a close acquaintance from World War I days.

The immediate relation of Dr. Cutler to the present conflict came in the fall of 1941 when he was asked by the dean of the Harvard University Medical School to reactivate Base Hospital No. 5 as the 5th General Hospital. This was readily accomplished, but by the time the unit was pressed into active service in February 1942, The Surgeon General had requested that Dr. Cutler be relieved of his post as commanding officer and await further assignment. Shortly thereafter, Dr. Cutler was offered the position of Chief Consultant in Surgery, ETOUSA (European Theater of Operations, U.S. Army), a post which he eagerly accepted in spite of the objections by the president of Harvard University and the trustees of Peter Bent Brigham Hospital.

Washington Orientation, 18 July to 5 August 1942

The first 10 days in Washington were crammed full of instruction, news, and renewing, and making new, acquaintances. Dr. Cutler's rank was the problem of immediate concern. While he had been a lieutenant colonel since 1924 and had been offered a colonelcy for lesser assignments on three prior occasions, there had been no choice but to come on active duty as a lieutenant colonel. The situation was soon rectified, however, and Dr. Cutler's promotion to colonel reached him on 22 July 1942.

While he was getting ready mentally and equipping himself with all the information he could gather, plans gradually emerged. At this time, 29 July 1942, Colonel Cutler learned that the consultant group for the European theater would probably consist of the following compartments and subdivisions:

Medicine	*Surgery*	*Neuropsychiatry*
William S. Middleton	Elliott C. Cutler	Lloyd J. Thompson
	Orthopedic Surgery	
	Rex L. Diveley	
	Neurosurgery	
	Loyal Davis	
	Otolaryngology	
	Lyman G. Richards	
	Ophthalmology	
	Derrick T. Vail	
	Anesthesia	
	Ralph M. Tovell	
Blood and Plasma	*Venereal Disease*	*Laboratories*
Cornelius P. Rhoads	James C. Kimbrough	Ralph S. Muckenfuss

Colonel Kimbrough, he thought, might be changed and placed over the whole group, and perhaps Dr. A. Winternitz could be called for later to augment the laboratory group.

He felt that the group should be a cabinet of advisers to the Chief Surgeon and that its members should report as a group, and, therefore, have frequent common gatherings and meetings. He thought that the Chief Surgeon should send them into the field for specific information and should ask them to give him specific advice. Success, he calculated, would depend on relationships with the Chief Surgeon and on the men in the field equally. He reasoned that contacts with professional colleagues in England would also be highly desirable.

The problem which bothered him most was that almost no provision had been made for the professional care of the American soldier "up the line" or at "the front." He wrote in his diary:

It seems to me that the base area has had lots of thought. Base or general hospitals are well set up and well equipped. I have studied in detail lists of equipment until my eyes are sore—lists of drugs never to be used.

But what of the front where it seems to me men are saved or marred for life? I cannot find any happy solution here. There is loose talk of station hospitals broken up, and of new but never assembled mobile evacuation hospitals, but the latter depend on 10-ton trailer trucks which will probably never be delivered. And there is talk of a light field hospital of 400 beds.

Moreover, in a study of teams (surgical affiliated units) I find a tendency to make them rigid and to set them up here equipped in diverse ways with a basic general equipment and then separate equipment for chests—neurosurgery, maxillofacial surgery, orthopedic teams, etc.

1. It is certain the old fixed American hospitals (evacuation, mobile, or surgical hospitals, U.S. Army; casualty clearing stations, British) have been of little use and dangerous in the present mobile, fluid conflict.

2. I believe the above is true and that early surgical therapy, if properly set up, may save many lives—perhaps the lives of my children.

3. If the above two are true, we must organize something new for the U.S. Army Medical Department.

4. I believe the answer lies in putting surgical teams in the clearing station area.

    a. Perhaps female nurses should not go.

    b. Perhaps the new field hospital can go there.

    c. The team personnel should be general surgery, not specialists.

    d. The team should be completely equipped; i.e., surgeon should have instruments for head, chest, abdominal, and peripheral surgery. The team should also carry dry goods, supplies, anesthesia outfits, splints, etc.[4]

As a result of voicing his thoughts on this question, Colonel Cutler was instructed to draw up an equipment list for teams serving the frontlines. But where were the teams to come from? Affiliated groups being organized? Excess in general hospitals? There appeared to be no immediate answer. At any rate, Colonel Cutler received his baptism into the complexities of supply procedures

---

[4] "This diary entry was made in Washington before General Cutler came to the E.T.O. He never had any such concern after arrival in the E.T.O. You may be sure that I had no thought of going into combat without the very type of mobile medical units which we did have. The only new unit added after I left the U.S. was the field hospital—and I never thought very much of it as a front-line unit." (Letter, Paul R. Hawley, M.D., to Col. John Boyd Coates, Jr., MC, 25 Aug. 1958.)

while working on the equipment for these teams, and the difficulties of medical supply continued to challenge him on many occasions thereafter.

As the long summer days of July turned into August and Colonel Cutler found himself still in Washington, he became increasingly restless and anxious to leave. He recorded:

As a matter of fact, Washington is slow, let down, or, if not worse, full of inefficient people. No one quite at it hammer and tongs, unless it is * * *. I cannot write more but it is awful slow when our country is in danger—grave danger. How few seem to realize the seriousness of this! We are all too old, and yet the old men seem to have the right spirit. That's what the country needs, a spiritual uplift! * * * If I had time, I should sit down and cast into Shakespearean English what stirs my "innards" and stimulates my days. As it is, I'm off for action. Perhaps that's my cue. Now to serve my country.

London

While the last few days in Washington were long, the last was barely long enough. In something less than 12 hours from the time he received notification that travel priorities had been established for him, Colonel Cutler had to obtain his Government transportation requests and tickets, clear administratively for departure, finish packing, bid farewell to friends and family, run the last half mile to the Washington station, and be at La Guardia Airport in New York for a flight at 0100 hours on 6 August 1942. The Pan-American "Clipper" discharged its passengers at Limerick Airport, Foynes, Ireland, the next day. After two unsuccessful attempts to fly from Limerick to Bristol, owing to the fog, the third attempt resulted in the aircraft's being grounded suddenly at an intermediate airport because "Jerry" was reported overhead. Colonel Cutler finally reached his destination, London, at 2350 hours, 8 August 1942, and was billeted at the Claridge Hotel.

Early the next morning, he was off to 20 Grosvenor Square (fig. 8), headquarters of ETOUSA, where he registered, turned in his passport, and filled out the numerous blank forms required upon arriving at a new command.

The next stop was 9 North Audley Street (fig. 9), the London office of the Chief Surgeon, Col. (later Maj. Gen.) Paul R. Hawley, MC. There he met another acquaintance, Col. Charles B. Spruit, MC, (fig. 10) who was now Deputy Surgeon and represented the Chief Surgeon at Headquarters, ETOUSA. Colonel Hawley had moved to Cheltenham, headquarters of SOS (Services of Supply), ETOUSA, when he was also designated Surgeon, SOS. All the medical officers Colonel Cutler met here, just as in Washington, were bitterly critical of this new organization which ostensibly subordinated the Medical Department to an overall supply service. It seemed to leave no provision for integrating services, such as medical, for the Services of Supply and the army in the field. The reorganization appeared to mean that there was no job to correspond to that of Maj. Gen. Merritte W. Ireland with the AEF in World War I. If anything, the squabble over this reorganization was worse in England than in Washington. The immediate question confronting Colonel Cutler as a result of this situation was whether he was to stay in London or go to Cheltenham.

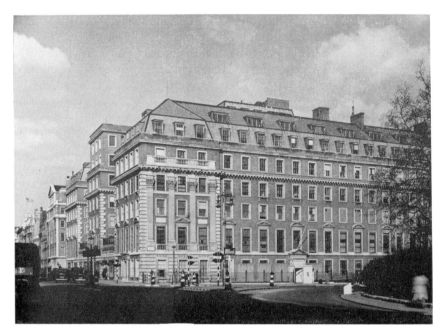

FIGURE 8.—Headquarters, ETOUSA, at 20 Grosvenor Square, London.

He soon learned the answer. The next day, Colonel Hawley arrived in London, and Colonel Cutler was able to meet with him. Colonel Cutler was to be located with the Chief Surgeon at Cheltenham. He was given his mission in simple terms. As the chief consultant in surgery, he was to see that the American soldier received the best medical care that the tactical situation and local circumstances would permit. Colonel Hawley also expressed his policy of fostering the best of relations between the Americans and the British and working closely with them. Colonel Hawley also thought that the consultants should have and bring up their own ideas as well as carry out orders from him.

"I think we will get on," Colonel Cutler wrote after the meeting, "Indeed, we must."

The next few days were exceedingly busy as Colonel Cutler set out to make his contacts with other American agencies and the British offices in London.

Among the Americans he met again was Maj. (later Col.) Herbert B. Wright, MC, who was chief of the Professional Services for the Eighth Air Force surgeon and the latter's liaison officer with the Office of the Chief Surgeon, ETOUSA. Colonel Cutler learned a great deal from Major Wright about medical organization, procedures, and functions in the Eighth U.S. Air Force.

Colonel Cutler also met Dr. Kenneth Turner, liaison officer of the American National Research Council with the British National Research Council. Dr. Turner was attached to and lived with the American Embassy staff in London.

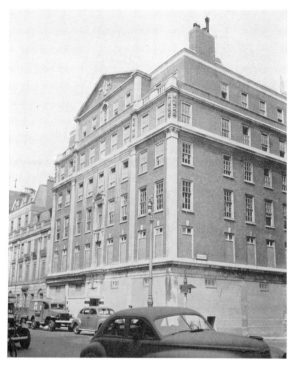

FIGURE 9.—Office of the Chief Surgeon, ETOUSA, at
9 North Audley Street, London.

Among other things, Colonel Cutler discovered that Dr. Turner had a very complete file of National Research Council reports and publications and received new items frequently and promptly. These papers were obviously of critical importance to the maintenance of highest standards of medical practice among the American forces in the United Kingdom. Dr. Turner, however, informed Colonel Cutler that he was not permitted to release them to the U.S. Army. They were strictly for his information to facilitate his dealings with the British counterpart of the American National Research Council. This situation was disappointing, to say the least, and entirely at odds for the best conduct of the war effort. Colonel Cutler later made a strong appeal to have the unfortunate situation rectified. As a result, Dr. Turner was able to obtain State Department approval for receiving extra copies of the American National Research Council publications to be turned over to the Chief Surgeon, ETOUSA. In exchange therefor, Dr. Turner was later invited to attend all strictly professional meetings and conferences held under auspices of the Chief Surgeon.

In the next few days, Colonel Cutler went about the most pleasant task of establishing himself with the staff of the AMD (British Army Medical Directorate) and the Canadian medical staff in England. Lunch on two occasions at the RAMC (Royal Army Medical Corps) School in one fell swoop placed Colonel Cutler in the midst of their activities. It was the custom of the DGMS (Director General, Medical Service) to hold a monthly meeting of his consul-

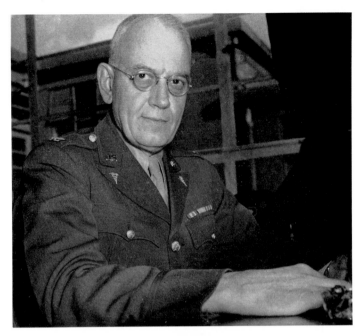

FIGURE 10.—Col. Charles B. Spruit, MC.

tants, advisers, and directors of medical services in area commands. Consultants from the RCAMC (Royal Canadian Army Medical Corps) were already participating in these meetings. The chief surgical consultant, Brigadier J. M. Wedell, RAMC, and the chief medical consultant, Maj. Gen. Sir Alexander Biggam, RAMC, held meetings of consultants in their respective branches the day preceding the Director General's meeting. Colonel Cutler was asked to, and later became a regular participant in, the meetings of the surgical group and those of the DGMS, Lt. Gen. Sir Alexander Hood, RAMC.

The subject of particular concern, on the occasion of Colonel Cutler's first visit, was that of rehabilitating men in convalescent camps rather than occupying beds in hospitals. The proposal was to provide plenty of exercise and physical training, perhaps under the direction of line officers, and encourage men to fight their way back to health. The British hoped to make extensive use of physiotherapists in this organization. The civilian-directed hospitals of the EMS (Emergency Medical Service), in which British soldiers were hospitalized for long-term definitive treatment, had been much too lenient in the past.

On his last day in London, 13 August 1942, Colonel Cutler, with an old-time acquaintance, Brigadier (later Maj. Gen.) William Anderson, dined as guests of Surgeon Rear Admiral Gordon Gordon-Taylor (later knighted) (fig. 11), another good friend from pre-World War II days. Brigadier Anderson was surgeon of the Scottish Command and Admiral Gordon-Taylor was Chief Consultant in Surgery to the Royal Navy. Brigadier Anderson later became Chief Surgical Consultant of the British Army.

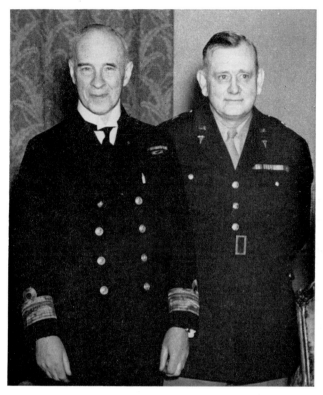

FIGURE 11.—Surgeon Rear Admiral Gordon Gordon-Taylor, Royal Navy, with General Hawley.

In addition to these representatives of the British Army and the Royal Navy, Colonel Cutler also met and spoke at length with Tudor Gardiner of the Royal Air Force and Prof. J. Patterson Ross, neurosurgical consultant to the Emergency Medical Service.

Colonel Cutler felt that he had accomplished much in a mere few days as he left London by train in the early afternoon of 14 August 1942 and arrived at Cheltenham some 5 hours later. In a memorandum, a copy of which went to the Chief Surgeon, Colonel Cutler presented these impressions of his first few days in England:

Observations on military surgery at this time—

a. The Combat Divisional Medical setup is O.K., though we need to get directives to the medical units as to proper professional handling (i.e., very simple, but to include use of sulfonamides, splints and evacuation).

b. The Base Area Hospitals (Station and General) are admirable and when brought up to the T.O. with American equipment cannot be bettered.

c. The area between the tail of the Division and the Base Area is a so far uncharted area. It appears at first glance that the British may be getting themselves too *set* on following up their Libyan experiences which practically leaves a plan that throws out the C.C.S.'s [Casualty Clearing Stations] and other forward hospital units and relies almost entirely on the utilization of surgical teams in independent, self-contained, motor-transported small units.

I believe we must be prepared both for the above mobile, surgical team set-up, utilizing this close to a Clearing Company and possibly with part of our new field hospital, as well as for putting in our evacuation hospitals, though they must be stripped and cut down in weight for mobility. No one now can predict when and where, therefore, we must have alternate plans.

And when we come to contemplate a beach-head and medical care, the matter is further complicated * * *.

A final thought brings up the major problems of evacuation from the forward area. Try as one will there is no escaping the conviction which becomes even firmer that the *optimum solution is in the air.*[5]

Cheltenham, Headquarters, SOS

Cheltenham, Colonel Cutler found, was quite pleasant. He was given a tiny, but adequate, top-floor room at the Hotel Ellenborough. The officers were awakened at 0630, breakfast was at 0700, a bus transported them to the office at 0745, and working hours were from 0800 to 1700 daily. Saturdays, however, began an hour later, and on Sundays the officers were required to work only in the forenoon. The office facilities, unfortunately, were not the best, and later, when the full complement of consultants was on duty, the noise was said to be akin to a boiler factory (p. 362).

Col. James C. Kimbrough, MC, had been made Director of Professional Services, Office of the Chief Surgeon, Services of Supply, ETOUSA, as Colonel Cutler had anticipated, and was thus placed over all the consultants. He was also acting as consultant in urology, his specialty, and was responsible for the quality of treatment being given patients with venereal disease.

Lt. Col. (later Col.) William S. Middleton, MC, was Chief Consultant in Medicine. The only other consultant present at the headquarters at this time was Lt. Col. (later Col.) James B. Brown, MC, Consultant in Plastic Surgery and Burns. Colonel Middleton, as he had explained to Colonel Cutler at their first meeting in London, did not expect to have a large full-time staff. He was operating under the principle that men of special abilities and qualifications in the general hospitals could be designated theater and area consultants in addition to their regular duties in most of the specialties of medicine. He planned to have full-time consultants only in dermatology and neuropsychiatry. The consultants who were to make up the initial group of surgical consultants in the European theater were expected (and did arrive) in the next few weeks. They were Lt. Col. (later Col.) Rex L. Diveley, MC, Senior Consultant in Orthopedic Surgery; Lt. Col. (later Col.) Loyal Davis, MC, Senior Consultant in Neurological Surgery; Lt. Col. (later Col.) Ralph M. Tovell, MC, Senior Consultant in Anesthesia; and Lt. Col. (later Col.) Derrick T. Vail, MC, Senior Consultant in Ophthalmology.

---

[5] Memorandum, Col. E. C. Cutler, MC, to Col. J. C. Kimbrough, MC, 16 Aug. 1942, subject: Report of Activities, Aug. 9–14, 1942.

Colonel Cutler had just arrived in Cheltenham late Friday, 14 August; but Sunday, 16 August, found him off again to London. Innumerable trips to London were to follow.

On Monday, he called on Air Marshal Sir Harold Whittingham, DGMS of the RAF (Royal Air Force), and Sir Francis Fraser, director of the Emergency Medical Service. He also dined and had conferences with Col. (later Maj. Gen.) Malcolm C. Grow, MC, Surgeon, Eighth Air Force, and the aforementioned Major Wright. The conferences with Colonel Grow and other members of the Eighth Air Force concerned the curriculum of a proposed course of instruction for medical officers with no previous training in aviation medicine. The Eighth Air Force hoped to open a provisional medical school at High Wycombe by the end of August.

The following day, Tuesday, 18 August, was a preview of things to come and the first trip in the field for the recently arrived Chief Consultant in Surgery. With Sir Harold Whittingham, Colonel Hawley, Colonel Grow, Colonel Spruit, Major Wright, and an engineer officer of the Eighth Air Force, he visited Hendon Airport, London, to inspect the litter arrangements for transport aircraft. The demonstration showed only one thing of significance. It was very apparent that more work would have to be done to make the conversion of transport aircraft into evacuation aircraft an efficient and simple operation. The aircrew required 10 minutes to position each of 18 litter racks. It took some 20 minutes for a British ambulance crew to load 10 litter cases. Much time was wasted because the litter racks were made to take small-pole litters and not the American or British Army wooden litters. With properly modified litter racks and a trained crew, Colonel Cutler thought that the whole operation of setting up the litter racks and loading patients could be accomplished in 30 minutes.[6]

After the demonstration, Colonel Cutler inspected a dispensary located at Hendon Airport and then journeyed back to Cheltenham. There, he proceeded to write up reports of the trip to London and to put down on paper the type of education and training that would be necessary for medical officers in the immediate future. He envisaged three areas upon which emphasis in this training program could be placed: (1) Early treatment at the front, (2) treatment during the evacuation phase, and (3) the type of treatment to be given in base hospitals. He stressed particularly the following point:

Chief emphasis must be placed upon choice of soldier upon whom surgery is to be carried out in the forward areas. A directive regarding this can be written but will have to be modified by the necessity. Precedence should be given to haemorrhage, shock, sucking chest wounds, major compound fractures. The military surgeon must learn that the quickest way to win the war (and this in the end saves the most suffering) is to get back to duty as many men as possible. Abdominal cases and time consuming major surgical procedures that offer little or no hope of return to duty can never have first call on the efforts of the good military surgeon.[7]

---

[6] Memorandum, Col. E. C. Cutler, MC, to Col. J. C. Kimbrough, MC, 19 Aug. 1942, subject: Report re Visit to London August 17 and 18, 1942.
[7] See footnote 6.

This bit of advice was something which many medical officers, including some of the specialist senior consultants in surgery, were going to find most difficult to accept.

In this same paper on medical courses to be conducted in the theater, Colonel Cutler also stated: "I consider an Auxiliary Surgical Group our chief necessity at this time!" He went on to report that the component teams were being carefully picked in the office of Brig. Gen. Charles C. Hillman, Chief, Professional Service Division, Office of The Surgeon General.

Having finished his London report and the suggestion for courses in military medicine, Colonel Cutler found solace and cheer in the accomplishments of his first few days in the European theater. His diary entry read:

> For the first time I feel orderly and as if something had been done. Of course, I have only been here 10 days. Since I've cemented myself with the RAMC, the RAF, and our own Air medical people, I must have gotten something done. Also in touch with the Royal Navy through Gordon-Taylor and the EMS through Francis Fraser.

Solitary reflection on the general outlook, however, caused Colonel Cutler to philosophize:

> The doctor at war is worth thought. He cools his heels in this preparatory phase with those whose entire thoughts are directed toward implementing conditions he is already trying to oppose. True, the common fear binds them together. All must visualize the necessity of the undertaking lest a greater evil befall our people. But unmistakably, he is set aside—sometimes just as chaff, sometimes in undue respect as the necessity for his ministrations seems more imminent, or as the limited imagination of his colleagues looks to the future.

There was yet another reason for cheer on this day, Colonel Cutler's 10th day of duty in the Office of the Chief Surgeon, ETOUSA. The British and Canadians, with a few attached Americans, had staged a major raid at Dieppe.

Dieppe and Its Aftermath

The raid at Dieppe sounded good to Colonel Cutler. It showed that a landing could be achieved. It proved that tanks could be landed. Was it worthwhile? Yes, for any offensive, no matter how small, would upset the Germans.

A Canadian from Saskatchewan who had just returned from the raid told Colonel Cutler that it was a cinch. He had gone in 2 miles. It was easy. No one was frightened. This young man went on to say that the Allies might as well tell Hitler when an attack was coming because nothing could stop it. He asserted that the Germans knew 5 days beforehand of the Dieppe attack.

But there were casualties, American casualties. The Chief of Staff, ETOUSA, upon learning of the seriousness of their wounds, became extremely concerned over the care the Americans were receiving in the Canadian Army hospitals to which they had been taken. Colonel Cutler, together with Colonel Middleton, visited each of the three Canadian general hospitals in which the American casualties were hospitalized and carefully reviewed each case. The treatment and care being provided them was excellent. To a man, each patient refused to be transferred to an American hospital when the choice of remaining in the Canadian hospital or being transferred was proffered. They were happy where they were and had utmost confidence in the Canadian medical officers into whose care they had been entrusted.

There was one seriously ill case, a Colonel "H." Colonel "H." had been on the bridge of a destroyer when a direct hit blew off the bridge and amputated most of his left foot. He tied on a necktie as a tourniquet and hobbled to the gunwales of the sinking ship. As he was preparing to go overboard, a gunboat hove alongside and Colonel "H." was handed over to it. "Go aft," he was ordered, but, seeing that the forward gunner was leading enemy aircraft badly, he crawled forward and continued to direct the gunner's fire. Some 30 hours elapsed before he was put ashore at Portsmouth, England. Another 24 hours passed before he reached the Canadian General Hospital where he received his first surgical treatment.

At the hospital, Colonel "H." 's lower left leg had been amputated 5 inches below the knee. Sulfonamide had been placed in the wound, which was left open. The wound was clean. He had been given doses of sulfanilamide for 24 hours, but this was stopped because of nausea, mental confusion, and his general poor condition. In the 3 postoperative days, he had been given 2,800 cc. of whole blood and 3,000 cc. of plasma. Repeated, continued transfusions were urged by both Colonel Cutler and Colonel Middleton, and the professional staff at the Canadian hospital concurred.

Ten days after injury, the patient's condition continued extremely grave. Colonel Cutler was directed to review the case personally. In a midnight visit to the hospital on 30 August, he found Colonel "H." somewhat improved but still apparently dying of a peculiar syndrome. His kidneys and heart were failing, and the etiology indicated multiple transfusions with reaction which had compounded the effects of original blood loss. Colonel Cutler followed the case daily, thereafter, until the patient was out of danger. This courageous officer made an excellent recovery, was returned to duty, and continued to serve in the European theater after having been fitted with an artificial limb. His case became an object lesson for much of the planning that followed.

As the initial sensational aspects of the Dieppe raid wore off, there were doubts in some circles as to its effectiveness or worthwhileness. The force had sustained 55 percent casualties. The lessons for the Medical Department were clear. An analysis of the situation in England revealed the following facts:

If things could have been done better our Canadian colleagues were the first to recognize it. They pointed out to us * * * that it would have been better if all of the wounded had been kept near the landing areas [in England], even if additional teams had been focussed there, or the local hospitals enlarged to care for such an influx * * * . It was thought that there would be a larger number of wounded than could be handled locally, and therefore the first to arrive were sent by train to the Midlands, which was perhaps a mistake for they went without surgery, even after arriving in England, for a considerable period of time. The Canadians themselves were the first to be self-critical about this, but since * * * they handled individual cases so well, we can have nothing but gratitude for their care.[8]

This analysis indicated that, with a Continental invasion, hospitals would have to be set up near the points where casualties would be returned to England in order to preclude undue delay in treatment as was experienced by Colonel "H." If general hospitals were to function in this capacity of receiving evacuees from an over-water operation, they could only do so after provision had been made for some 10 or more surgical teams to work at one time. The surgical teams, too, would have to be added to the normal surgical complement of a general hospital.

On the far shore, it was clear that small medical units with attached surgical teams would have to be deployed near all possible landing sites. The Dieppe raid proved once again that confusion reigns supreme in war. Owing to many factors, significant among which was the destruction of small landing craft, landing serials found themselves at points completely foreign to their original intent, upsetting the most carefully prepared plans.

Finally, the important part which sorting or triage would play could not be minimized. Sorting at the invasion beaches and the receiving areas in England had to be done expertly and quickly so that the seriously wounded would receive immediate attention, as would also the lightly wounded in order that they might be returned to duty as early as possible.[9]

British Army Blood Supply Depot at Bristol

One of the first items of official correspondence directed to Colonel Cutler for action was a report on the British Army Blood Supply Depot submitted by Capt. (later Lt. Col.) Robert C. Hardin, MC, who was the American liaison officer at the depot. Colonel Hawley, in turning over the report to Colonel Cutler, signified that the Chief Consultant in Surgery would be responsible for the technical aspects of providing blood, blood substitutes, crystalloids, and related substances to the U.S. Army medical units in the theater.[10]

Colonel Cutler, at the first opportunity, on 26 August 1942, made a trip to Southmead Hospital, Bristol, where the depot was located. Colonel Kimbrough and Colonel Middleton accompanied him. Brigadier L. E. H. Whitby, RAMC, the officer in charge of the depot and Director, Army Blood Transfusion Service, was absent in London, but the visiting officers were received by Major Maycock, RAMC, and Captain Hardin. They learned that the center prepared all plasma and arranged for the supply of blood transfusion kits for the British Army (fig. 12). The general setup was obviously geared for production. In the previous one year, the depot had supplied over 110,000 pints of plasma.

---

[8] See footnote 2, p. 20.

[9] (1) See footnote 2, p. 20. (2) Memorandum, Col. E. C. Cutler, MC, and Lt. Col. W. S. Middleton, MC, to Col. J. C. Kimbrough, MC, 26 Aug. 1942, subject: Report of Survey of American and Canadian Casualties From Dieppe Operations, August 25, 1942, by Members of Professional Services Division.

[10] Medical Department, United States Army. Blood Program in World War II. Washington: U.S. Government Printing Office, 1964.

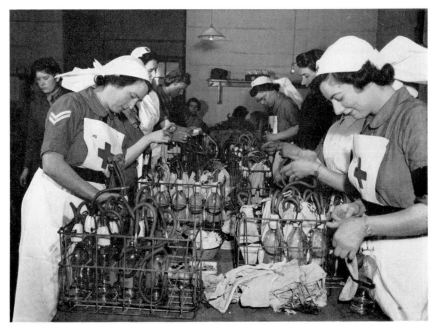

FIGURE 12.—Blood transfusion kits being packed at the British Army Blood Supply Depot.

Citrated whole blood was supplied only for limited use. A cream separator was used in the preparation of a wet plasma, the red cells being thrown away. The plasma was bottled and stored at room temperature and not subsequently checked for sterility unless the solution became turbid (fig. 13). It was obvious to the officers from Cheltenham that the onus of applying proper precautions in the use of British wet plasma rested with the user. The visit to this center did not allay their fears of the propriety of telling American medical installations to use British plasma liberally. Colonel Cutler and Colonel Middleton recommended that, as soon as possible, all American medical installations be supplied with the American standard dried plasma units.[11]

A short time later, on 7 October 1942, Colonel Cutler met with Maj. Gen. L. T. Poole, RAMC, director of pathology, AMD, and Brigadier Whitby to work out for the interim an understanding between the American and British Forces in England with respect to the supply of blood and blood substitutes. At this conference, it was agreed that:

1. The American Forces would be glad to use British supplies of dry or wet plasma, but the amounts required would be no greater than for a British hospital in the same circumstances.

2. Should the American Forces leave for operations outside of England, they would take American plasma which was already stocked in quantity and would not require crated British stocks.

---

[11] Memorandum, Col. E. C. Cutler, MC, to Col. J. C. Kimbrough, MC, 27 Aug. 1942, subject: Visit to Central British Blood Procurement Center, Bristol, August 26, 1942.

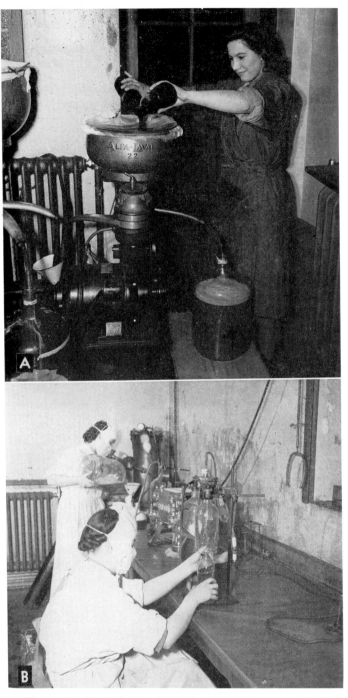

Figure 13.—Bottled wet plasma being prepared at the British Army Blood Supply Depot. A. A cream separator being used to separate blood cells and plasma. B. The filtering of plasma.

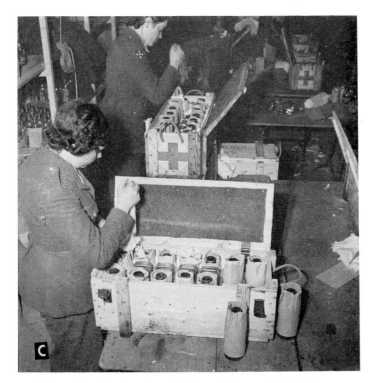

Figure 13.—Continued.   C. Plasma being packed for issue.

3. Individual American units would be prohibited from requesting blood or plasma directly from British centers but would submit requisitions to American medical supply sources which would stock these items received in bulk from the British.

4. Far greater use would be made of Captain Hardin in the future as an assistant to the theater consultants and to help with the organization and training of shock teams. Brigadier Whitby stated that Captain Hardin was essential both in running the plant and in the large teaching load which was carried there, and had requested that he continue in his present duties and assignment.

5. American hospitals would cooperate with the British blood bank program. That is, U.S. Army hospitals would bleed a few donors each week from a prepared panel of donors representing the community in which the hospital was located and turn the blood over to the appropriate bank.

6. It would be inadvisable to use American troops as donors for this blood bank program because of the political implications. It was believed that Americans at home might resent giving blood for the American soldier when he, in turn, was being bled for the citizens of another country. Moreover, there was the possibility that the combination of blood from Negro and white troops might complicate the situation.

7. Finally, Colonel Cutler promised to try to obtain additional American personnel to help staff the British Army Blood Supply Depot.[12]

This was indeed a humble beginning to a project which was to become, literally, the lifeblood of the theater's medical efforts, and Colonel Cutler's perspicacity with regard to the greater use to be made of Captain Hardin was to be most amply vindicated.

First Supply Problem

On 24 August, just before he was called upon to inspect the Canadian hospitals harboring American casualties from the Dieppe raid, Colonel Hawley had summoned the Chief Consultant in Surgery. Colonel Cutler was directed to draw up a list of medical supplies necessary for the routine maintenance of a field force of 770,000 with 140,000 SOS troops. This was no small task. Colonel Cutler started Colonel Brown, Consultant in Plastic Surgery and Burns, on the list before embarking on the all-night trip to the Canadian hospitals.

A few days later, Colonel Cutler met with Lt. Col. (later Col.) George W. Perkins, Jr., CWS, in London. Colonel Perkins worked with the central procurement office of the ETOUSA staff and was concerned with the procurement of medical supplies and equipment from British sources. This officer politely informed Colonel Cutler that the Medical Department was "all wet" on its figures. "I've no doubt," Colonel Cutler noted in his diary, "and this puts me in a difficult spot * * * [with respect to Colonel Hawley's request]."

Another aspect of the problem was what was needed now—at this time— as compared to what, ideally, might be required in a hypothetical operation. Phrased in another way, the problem became a matter of what was available as compared to what was desired. Consultants visiting and inspecting hospitals had found critical shortages of necessary equipment and the prevailing use of many unsatisfactory items. On the other hand, the U.S. Army medical supply depot at Thatcham was, from all reports, quite well stocked. The fact remained that necessary equipment for hospitals was, for reasons unknown to Colonel Cutler, not getting out. Colonel Cutler wanted particularly to have the three general hospitals in the theater brought up to their full authorized equipment, preferably their original American equipment. These general hospitals had professional talent of the highest caliber, but they could not be expected to provide services of a similar high caliber without the proper equipment. Should U.S. Army sources in the theater not be able to provide this equipment, it was evident that British sources would have to be tapped. And thus, Colonel Cutler had arranged the foregoing meeting with Colonel Perkins.

On 3 September, Colonel Cutler and Colonel Brown visited Ludgershall, the largest British Army medical supply depot, to pick out instruments suitable

---

[12] Memorandum, Col. E. C. Cutler, MC, to Col. J. C. Kimbrough, MC, 9 Oct. 1942, subject: Report on Meeting With British Officers Concerned With the Supply of Blood and Plasma for the Armed Forces.

for interchange with American instruments. Colonel Diveley and Colonel Perkins had journeyed to the depot from London. In addition to the RAMC officers concerned with the depot, representatives from three British instrument manufacturers were present. The entire day was spent in going over item by item the instruments listed in American supply tables so that determination could be made as to whether a satisfactory substitute British item existed. On the whole, the British instruments were excellent, and, although somewhat heavier than American instruments, each item accepted was a satisfactory substitute. There was some question, however, as to whether some items could be produced in sufficient quantity. There was a particular lack of production in England of all electrical apparatus, and only a negligible supply of heavy X-ray apparatus. Generally, instruments not being produced in England were not essential, and a good surgeon could do a satisfactory job without them. Colonel Cutler was particularly impressed with the cleanliness and orderliness of this depot and the wonderful selection of materiel offered.[13]

Upon returning to Cheltenham, Captain Martin, in charge of the American depot at Thatcham, was contacted. Arrangements were made for Colonel Brown to visit the depot the next day to have a firsthand look at what was actually available and could be counted upon.

Before the Chief Surgeon's first problem could be answered, another was posed. This time, it was not hypothetical, and it was urgent.

Second Supply Problem

A persistent rumor had been that any attack on the Continent from England had been called off for the time being, and the basis of this rumor soon became clear. BOLERO, the buildup for invading the Continent was being subordinated to Operation TORCH, an attack in Africa which was to come off in the very near future. With this as a background, the following came about on 5 and 6 September, as chronicled by Colonel Cutler.

We work daily and seem to make no progress, largely because, as will be clear below, we are caught in a mess! Our army is still being trained broadly and absolutely lacks specialists. Take supply as an example. Here is our chief, Major General Lee [Maj. Gen. (later Lt. Gen.) John C. H. Lee, USA, Commanding General, SOS, ETOUSA], a very bright man and well equipped with native intelligence. Moreover, he is an engineer, but here his problem is supply. It is a professional job. His training in supply and logistics is more than mine, but not complete. His transport office has the job of the New York Central RR. Of course he isn't equipped. We must change this, and our army must have specialists!

In the Medical Corps, it is just puerile.

Take the last 24 hours. At 9:00 last night, Colonel Hawley's sergeant came here with a note from the Chief that the heads of his offices come to him at 9:00 AM. It was a supply problem. JCK, WSM, and ECC [Cols. Kimbrough, Middleton, and Cutler] were given a list of medical maintenance units for 10,000 men per month. We were informed on Africa. We were warned about secrecy, of course. Then we took the list and put 10 hours on it.

---

[13] Memorandum, Col. E. C. Cutler, MC, Lt. Col. J. B. Brown, MC, and Lt. Col. R. L. Diveley, MC, to Col. J. C. Kimbrough, MC, 4 Sept. 1942, subject: Report of Visit by Col. Cutler, Lt. Col. Brown and Lt. Col. Diveley to British Medical Supply Depot, Ludgershall.

We could make additions and increase the number of items, but there could be no deletions. It was a tough job. The list was a riot. It was supposed to be under battle conditions for 1 month. There were 3 litters, no tetanus toxoid or antitoxin, no instruments (were they supposed to last forever?), no oxygen tanks, but several thousand rolls of toilet paper! One bedpan!

The next day, 7 September, Colonel Hawley asked Colonel Cutler to drive to Oxford (2d General Hospital) with him. The Chief Surgeon seemed to have much on his mind. He explained what hospitals would be going to Africa, a relatively small force from England. He said that they would be sent well and fully equipped, but otherwise didn't seem overly interested in them. The 2d and 5th General Hospitals, two of the best units, were to stay. Colonel Hawley implied that when the Operation TORCH forces had gone he would settle down and clean up in England, and he realized there was much to do. As to Colonel Cutler, the Chief Surgeon said that he would like to see him make weekly visits to all hospitals, develop the instructional program (schools), and stimulate high professional work.

It is elsewhere recorded that, as plans progressed further for Operation TORCH, the European theater had to request that replenishment supplies to support the operation be sent directly from the Zone of Interior. The basis for this request was the realization that it would be more feasible to furnish these supplies from the distant Zone of Interior than to attempt to find them in the depots in England.[14]

Introduction to 1st Infantry Division

On 15 September 1942, a Captain Miller, MC, from the 1st Infantry Division visited Cheltenham to further activities for the professional education of the division's medical personnel. He represented Lt. Col. (later Col.) James C. Van Valin, MC, division surgeon, who had previously written Col. Oramel H. Stanley, MC, the Chief Surgeon's executive officer, on this matter.

Captain Miller was referred to Colonel Cutler. When Captain Miller revealed the fact that the medical officers of the division would not be permitted to attend the surgical courses being established in London, Colonel Stanley proposed that the consultants give a brief series of lectures at the division. This suggestion was quickly accepted by Colonel Van Valin and the II Corps surgeon, Col. Richard T. Arnest, MC.

The lectures were conducted at Tidworth Barracks during 16, 17, and 18 September. On the first day, Colonel Cutler gave two exercises which covered first aid surgical measures in the first and second echelons of medical service within the division. There was no attempt to discuss definitive surgery as carried out in the evacuation, surgical, or general hospitals. He stressed the fact that the primary requisites for adequate initial surgical care of the wounded soldier were the control of hemorrhage, relief of pain, adequate dressing of the wound and use of sulfonamides to prevent further contamination, booster dose

---

[14] Medical Department, U.S. Army. Medical Supply in World War II. [In preparation.]

of tetanus toxoid, proper splinting, closure of sucking chest wounds, and an adequate appreciation of shock, crush, and blast so that proper therapy could be started as far forward as possible.

On the following days, Colonel Brown presented talks on injuries to the face and jaw, care of burns, and care of injuries in Air Force personnel; Colonel Diveley spoke on care of fractures and their transport and evacuation; Colonel Davis discussed neurosurgery in war; and Lt. Col. (later Col.) Lloyd J. Thompson, MC, Senior Consultant in Neuropsychiatry, gave a talk on neuropsychiatric problems in the field.

The talks were well received, but this course of instruction, which had begun as a one-way flow of information, provided a wealth of instruction to the consultants themselves. When Colonel Cutler had completed his portion of the program and a discussion of the basic first aid surgical measures had ensued, it became remarkably clear that the 1st Infantry Division was not equipped with instruments or drugs of the type to best facilitate and carry out these necessary measures. This alarmed Colonel Cutler. There were no morphine Syrettes for forward work, no sulfonamide powder for dusting wounds, and no local or intravenous anesthetics. There were only two blood pressure apparatuses within this division of 17,000 men. The instrument kits were inadequate, and the equipment on hand was, in many cases, nearly useless. A simple procedure which could be carried out by almost anyone and would save life was that of closing sucking chest wounds, but there was no supply of the necessary needles and silkworm gut sutures.

As a further check on the statements made by the medical officers, Colonel Cutler inspected the equipment and supplies on hand in the division's medical supply section. He also went over, item by item, the No. 2 medical chests which were being used in the division's dispensaries and which were also meant to be used under battle conditions for the care of casualties. Colonel Cutler was again struck by the lack of equipment and supplies which he now knew from personal experience were available and could be supplied from sources in England.

Upon returning to Cheltenham, he dictated a memorandum in which he detailed simple, but specific measures which could be accomplished to correct these deficiencies. He closed the memorandum with the following:

I consider these recommendations of vital importance. The material essential is all here. We have been instructed to see that the care of the American soldier is as adequate as it can be made under the conditions imposed by battle. The requests above are simple, but may be life saving, and if they are neglected we should be and will be severely criticised.[15]

Once back in his room, he wrote:

Well, I have been told my job is to see that the Americans get the best professional care under circumstances presented by terrain, enemy resistance, etc. So I handed

---

[15] Memorandum, Col. E. C. Cutler, MC, to Col. J. C. Kimbrough, MC, 18 Sept. 1942, subject: Teaching Exercises With the First Division at Tidworth Barracks, Sept. 16, 1942. (Copies to Colonel Hawley, Colonel Stanley, and Colonel Middleton.)

in a memo today practically stating that, if an American newspaper knew 17,000 picked men were going into battle with simple things lacking which every American hospital had, then we all would be fixed.

This was the beginning of extensive medical supply operations in the European theater in which many individuals participated following the realization that elements of the U.S. Army were not adequately provided with modern medical equipment and supplies.

Inter-Allied Conferences on War Medicine

While Colonel Cutler and the consultants were planning the teaching exercises for the 1st Infantry Division, a secretary in another office of the headquarters was transcribing a telephone message from N. B. Parkinson, Director, Home Division of the British Council. Mr. Parkinson's message stated that the British Medical Association had recently been in touch with the British Council and had expressed their earnest desire that the Association do all it could to assist members of the medical professions of the allied nations now resident in England and to insure that British members of the profession benefit from the presence of so many medical persons from all over the world. To further this end, the British Medical Association was willing to provide certain facilities and privileges under its control. It had been suggested that an association or society be formed which would serve to bring together medical men of the allied nations and promote a sense of professional unity among them. Before any further steps were taken, Mr. Parkinson was suggesting that leading members of the various national groups meet to express their views at the offices of the British Council.

Colonel Cutler had been aware of the fact that the Belgians had initially attempted to form such an inter-Allied medical organization. It was brought to his attention in Colonel Spruit's office when he had first arrived in London, but Colonel Cutler had since given it little thought. This time, he and Colonel Kimbrough were selected to attend the proposed meeting to represent the American point of view. The meeting was held as scheduled at the offices of the British Council on 23 September 1942. In attendance were representatives from Canada, Belgium, the Free French, Czechoslovakia, Norway, and The Netherlands in addition to the British and American delegates. The Poles could not come but telephoned expressing their interest.

Most of the participants at the meeting expressed a desire to have joint meetings, but there was little enthusiasm for a separate dues-paying association with a name, officers, journal, and permanent fixtures The Belgians reported that an organization had already been formed, under the honorary presidency of Mr. Biddle and the active presidency of General Hood, which was to hold its first open meeting in December. These deliberations were duly reported back to the British Medical Association by the British Council, but the matter again fell through. Apparently, the British thought a club and home were desired—the Belgians and Czechoslovaks had said so—and, in their usually astute way, questioned whether such an affair could be properly financed.

Curiously enough, it was at a meeting of the editorial board of the *British Journal of Surgery*, on 12 October 1942, that the matter was again brought up. (Colonel Cutler had accepted the invitation to become a member of this board, a signal honor, since previously the journal was concerned only with publishing efforts from British surgeons.) The chairman of the board, Prof. George Gask, took keen interest in the proposed inter-Allied medical meetings. He arranged for Colonel Cutler to meet with Maj. Gen. H. L. (later Sir Henry) Tidy, President, Royal Society of Medicine, on Wednesday, 21 October. The Honorary Secretary, Mr. Broster, and Sir Geoffrey Edwards, Secretary, also attended the meeting. The officers of the Royal Society of Medicine were most willing and pleased to be able to sponsor such military medical meetings of the Allies.

Colonel Cutler was greatly encouraged by the outcome of this conference. Formerly, attempts to hold medical meetings of the Allies had been thwarted. These meetings now had a sponsor with the facilities and organization to see the desires through to fruition. "I think I kicked it on its way," he noted, "and I believe these meetings will serve not only to educate us now for the war, but will be a bridging force for all the Allies, helping us to organize the world and civilization which is to follow."

On Tuesday of the following week, 27 October 1942, a meeting was held at the Royal Society of Medicine attended by representatives of all His Majesty's services and representatives from each of the Allied countries. It was passed unanimously that monthly meetings should be held at the Royal Society of Medicine, under the sponsorship of this organization, to which members from all the Allied forces would go. The Directors General of His Majesty's medical services promised every assistance in the way of speakers and advice.

To carry the story a little further, the first meeting was held auspiciously enough on 7 December 1942, the first anniversary of the entry of the United States into the war. There was a large attendance, and comments were very favorable. Colonel Cutler thought the meeting was only fair and would have to be better in the future. Towards this end, he had already persuaded General Tidy to set up an executive committee to lend closer direction to program and coordinating activities. The meetings continued to improve and were held in series throughout the years of the war. Medical officers of the U.S. Army contributed in no small measure to the success of the meetings. Selected lectures from the entire series were published after the war under the honorary editorship of General Tidy.[16]

Operation TORCH: Hopes for an Early End

The attack on North Africa, to those in England, came off quietly and with some surprise insofar as the actual timing was concerned (fig. 14). True, the consultants had been called upon for advice on specific, limited aspects, but

---

[16] Tidy, Sir Henry (Ed.). Inter-Allied Conferences on War Medicine, 1942–1945, Convened by the Royal Society of Medicine. New York, Toronto, London: Staples Press, Ltd., 1947.

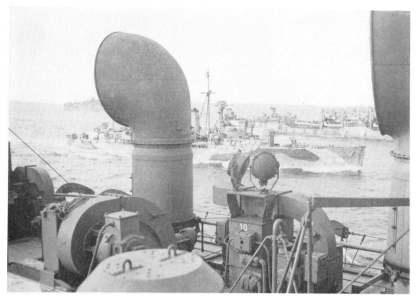

FIGURE 14.—The Royal Navy cruiser *Aurora*, escorting a convoy to North Africa from the United Kingdom.

they had neither been taken into complete confidence on the plans nor asked to participate to the extent that they might have been able. Colonel Cutler, himself, asked on at least three separate occasions for permission to go with the force from England but was turned down. Unless he acquired experience in an actual combat area soon, he reasoned, then his words would eventually become empty and devoid of any worth, at least so far as this war was concerned.

As it was, Colonel Cutler realized that the attack was on only after some of the combat elements in England had pulled out of their stations for the staging areas. When news of the assault on 8 November 1942 arrived (fig. 15), it was through the public press, and it was good news. The news led to considerable optimism, which, as it eventually turned out, was rather premature. But, at the moment, Colonel Cutler was quite elated. Writing on 9 November, he said:

All the time the good news was waiting and tonight it is still better. It looks as if all Africa would shortly fall. This is the big thing we've been so secret about. Now it has really come off well. What next, Italy? Or an attack here by spring? It's the turn of the war. Victory and release all in the air. Home seems near us and smiles should grace our faces. I once said 5 years and thought of 3. But now, who can deny us hope that the ETO will be over within a year?

The Surgeon General Visits the European Theater

The first visit to the European theater from anybody in the Office of The Surgeon General which concerned the chief consultant in surgery was that of The Surgeon General, Maj. Gen. James C. Magee (fig. 16). General Magee

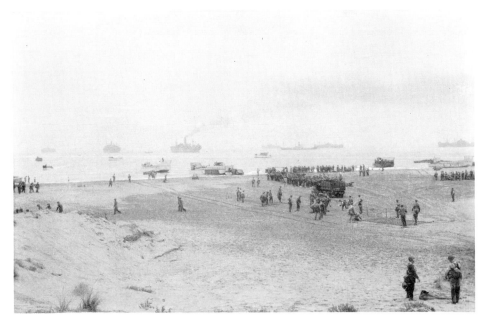

FIGURE 15.—The beach at Saint-Leu, Algeria, North Africa, on D-day, 8 November 1942.

arrived at 9 North Audley Street on 20 November 1942, accompanied by General Hawley. Appointments were made by Colonel Spruit for General Magee to meet with the medical heads of the British services, and preliminary discussions were held with General Hawley and Colonel Spruit.

At 1500 hours, 21 November, a business meeting and dinner were held for The Surgeon General at Thurlestaine Hall, Hotel Cheltenham. Guests were the four base section surgeons, the V Corps surgeon, and from the Army Air Forces, Colonel Grow, Col. Harry G. Armstrong, MC, Col. Edward J. Tracy, MC, and Colonel Wright. As expected, The Surgeon General's chief interest in this trip was to iron out difficulties and to arbitrate differences in opinion for providing medical support to Air Force units. With no warning, Colonel Cutler was the first to be asked for an opinion. "I was pretty noncommittal," he later wrote, "except for saying Air Force was sustaining first casualties and, therefore, the men needed the first help." The problems were brought well into the open, however, and Colonel Cutler thought the meeting was very good. The aspects of the discussions which concerned Colonel Cutler were the desires by the Army Air Forces for recognition and support of the Air Force medical school, better equipment at Air Force stations, hospitals to care for casualties at the operational airfields, and consultants, or their equivalent, within the Air Force medical organization in England.

The following day, Sunday, 22 November, Colonel Cutler motored to "Pinetree," Eighth Air Force headquarters at High Wycombe, with Colonel

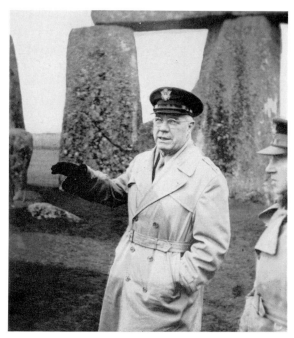

FIGURE 16.—Maj. Gen. James C. Magee, The Surgeon
General, visiting Stonehenge on the Salisbury Plain,
Wiltshire, England, November 1942.

Grow, Colonel Armstrong, and Colonel Wright. "To my consternation,"
Colonel Cutler found, "Grow was very bitter. Said the Medical Corps wouldn't
help him. He hereafter wouldn't help them. It may have been 'a show' for
Daddy. I played it safe." Upon reaching "Pinetree," the party lunched with
Maj. Gen. Ira C. Eaker, Commanding General, Eighth Air Force. After the
luncheon, Colonel Cutler discussed possible means of satisfying Air Force desires but found Colonel Grow not easily convinced that a happy and cordial
relation with the Ground Forces could be established.[17]

Colonel Cutler proposed that, if the Air Forces desired consultants, they
would be most welcome to serve within the framework of the theater consultant plan and that the provisional school which was now being carried
on could be integrated into a school for medical officers in general, as distinct
from a school just for the Army Air Forces. The Eighth Air Force also desired that a separate treatment facility be established for the care of aircrews
with flying fatigue or threatened with actual neurosis. Colonel Cutler suggested that Colonel Middleton and Colonel Thompson, in whose hands this
responsibility lay, would be most willing to cooperate in this project.

"The answer to all this," Colonel Cutler reported, "depends upon whether
the Air Force will accept the intimate relation to the Professional Services

---

[17] Letter, Col. E. C. Cutler, MC, to Col. J. C. Kimbrough, MC, 27 Nov. 1942, subject: Relations of
Your Office to Air Force.

as outlined above, but until such time as we are instructed not to serve the Air Force it appears to me that we should lend every effort to keep together the entire medical service."

During the next 2 weeks of General Magee's visit, it was Colonel Cutler's privilege to accompany The Surgeon General on some of his visits to nearly all the major American medical installations in the United Kingdom and many of the British installations as well. In talks with General Magee, Colonel Cutler had the opportunity to approach him about the field dressing in the individual soldier's first aid packet. This was a matter to which Colonel Cutler had given considerable thought. Colonel Cutler had been able to obtain much information on the efficacy and requirements of field dressings as a result of an invitation to participate in the British First Field and Shell Dressing Committee. The British committee had decided that their dressing had to be larger and had recommended that it be put in a cellophane packet. Colonel Cutler believed that the U.S. Army field dressing, which was still packed in a metal container, could also profit by similar modifications and advised The Surgeon General so. He recommended that further studies be made under The Surgeon General's direction in the Zone of Interior to see whether a cellophane packaging could not replace the metal container and the bandage itself be made larger. The Surgeon General was given a sample of the new British packet to take back with him.[18]

Colonel Cutler was also able to ask General Magee for an assistant. He informed General Magee that such increasing needs for consultants as going into EMS and RAF hospitals at night as well as during the day made it impossible for Colonel Cutler to fulfill completely his obligations in such matters because of other and more weighty engagements which could not be broken. He asked that Maj. (later Lt. Col.) Ambrose H. Storck, MC, in Brig. Gen. Charles C. Hillman's office be selected for this position as assistant to the Chief Consultant in Surgery in the European theater. General Magee, in return, suggested that it would be nice if the European theater would invite Col. (later Brig. Gen.) Fred W. Rankin, MC, Chief Consultant in Surgery in the Office of The Surgeon General, to visit the theater.[19]

In a more formal vein, Colonel Middleton was given the project of collecting answers from the Professional Services Division to a list of questions which The Surgeon General had brought with him from members of his office. Questions which concerned the Chief Consultant in Surgery and his answers to Colonel Middleton on this occasion in effect provided a résumé of consultant activities to date. They were:

1. Education and training.
Many courses in medico-military subjects are being given to U.S. Medical Department officers, to both those in the combat [units] and * * * those in the station, evacuation, and general hospitals, as well as to the Air Force.

---

[18] Memorandum, Col. E. C. Cutler, MC, to Col. J. C. Kimbrough, MC, 27 Nov. 1942, subject: First Aid Packet for the American Soldier.
[19] Letter, Col. E. C. Cutler, MC, to Director of Professional Services, 30 Nov. 1942, subject: Additional Consultant in General Surgical Field.

As a part of the above general courses, special attention has been paid to the proper treatment of the wounds in general, largely by Colonel Cutler, and wounds in special surgical fields by the senior consultants in orthopedic surgery, neurological surgery, maxillo-facial and plastic surgery and burns, ophthalmology, anesthesia, thoracic surgery, and transfusion and shock. These surgical courses have been given in turn at the Air Force school, to the medical officers of two American divisions, to groups of doctors in our base section areas, and to individual hospital assemblages.

2. Activities of surgical consultants.

All of the surgical consultants have the closest relationships with their opposite members in the British military set-up, including Army, Navy and Air Force. The Chief Consultant in Surgery attends the meeting of the British Surgical Consultant Group each month, and the meeting of the Director General of Medical Services, RAMC. He has a similar relationship with the EMS, RAF, and Royal Navy. Through this liaison we have been permitted to enter and study all of the organizations of the British Services, and have thereby profited greatly.

Another activity of the consultants has been to aid in establishing the high level of professional work in all of the American hospitals—station, evacuation or general, in ETOUSA. This has meant constant visits to institutions, the stimulation of ward rounds, clinical meetings, and assistance in acquiring the necessary material for proper professional endeavour. This activity goes on constantly, and I am sure that much benefit has accrued from this intimate contact of the Consultant Group with the hospital setup.

A special field might be said to be our relation with the American Air Force. We understand that we serve them as well as the Ground Forces, and we have been happy to teach in their schools and to look after their wounded as they enter our hospitals.

An unexpected labor to the Consultant Group has been the constant demands made upon them to assist in straightening out the medical supply situation in ETOUSA. A tremendous amount of labor and time have had to go into supplying proper lists for the medical requirements of both divisions and static hospitals, and a constant liaison has had to be established with those who purchased British medical material for the use of the American Forces.

3. Unit assemblages.

The answer to this is complicated, for the Consultant Group is not entirely familiar with unit assemblages. It should be said, however, that we have been instructed by General Hawley to go over the arrangements and material in medical chests Nos. 1 and 2 and delete certain items and add others that are necessary * * *. We believe that there should be another complete revision, by a group familiar with this matter, of material required in [an] active theater of war * * *. It appears that some of the material being sent, which was of value twenty years ago, is now out-moded.

4. Dried serum plasma.

The situation * * * is as follows. On hand Nov. 15—4,224 units. Issued in September—10,238 units. Issued in October—2,735 units. We need more plasma immediately, in view of the fact that combat forces are instructed to take such material with them.

5. Intravenous fluids.

The answer * * * is simple. If hospitals were supplied with adequate stills it would be unwise to send over bottled intravenous fluids. Stills, however, cannot be acquired in Great Britain, at this time, in sufficient number and of the type desired. They should therefore be sent with a high priority rating.

6. Physical standards for induction.

From visits to all of our hospitals, it is apparent to the Surgical Group that a considerable number of physically unfit enlisted men are arriving in ETOUSA. I have personally seen two individuals in a single hospital with large defects in their skulls produced by terrific accidents in youth, and I have seen large scrotal hernias in individuals taken into the Army; also two severe cases of Dupuytren's contracture of the hand. Another matter commented upon by Colonel Diveley is the failure, apparently, to examine the feet properly before induction.

7. Weekly medical newsletter from the Office of The Surgeon General.

It is my impression that a weekly medical newsletter would be highly acceptable. Note that the Canadians do this, and do it very well. Undoubtedly a copy of their Newsletter is available from General Hillman.[20]

There were a few sidelights which appeared during General Magee's visit which Colonel Cutler found inviting to reflect upon but which were quite serious matters at the time of their occurrence, particularly to those involved. For example, he recorded:

But now this curious story: Yesterday was Thanksgiving. I had worked hard and hadn't paid any attention to an invitation by Lady Harding at St. James's Palace. Colonel Stanley saw me and asked why I was here [Cheltenham] when the King had sent for me. He said I couldn't refuse and had to go. So I worked all day, forewent lunch to get more done, and left by car at 2:00 PM for London. By then I had found out that Harding was the King's secretary. So I reported to C. Spruit and found General Hawley there just in from Buckingham Palace. He looked sick and promised to let Bill [Colonel Middleton] examine him tomorrow (i.e., today, which has been done, and he goes in hospital, 2d GH, tomorrow). Then C. S. [Charles Spruit] and I went to St. James's. Great crush of people, all tired, and I was hungry.

Unfortunately, the Royalty were unable to appear, and the two colonels later found it necessary to search elsewhere for food, but it was a unique honor to have been invited to the Palace and a privilege to have met the important personages of the era who were there. Concerning General Hawley, Colonel Cutler noted on a visit to the 2d General Hospital, 30 November 1942:

Came here [London] yesterday, stopping at the 2d General to see General Hawley and to get my X-rays. The former is better, but his laryngitis is bad and his temper is bad; the latter, beautiful and I have hardly coughed recently. Had long discussion re sitting of party for General Magee. There will be 13 with ECC, so I was out.

Avonmouth, Disembarkation of Hospital Ship No. 38, the *Newfoundland*

With the attack on North Africa, it was inevitable that casualties would sooner or later arrive in England. Colonel Kimbrough and Colonel Cutler journeyed to Avonmouth on the English south coast on 17 December 1942, to see one of the first shiploads disembark. Colonel Cutler's account follows:

Arrived in time to see her dock. It was the *Newfoundland* of Liverpool; all white with red crosses and a black "38" on her side (fig. 17). Could see American soldiers at the rail as she came in. Then we boarded. We were shown about by the RAMC major in charge. The men were in swivel beds that were set like tables in yachts so that when the boat rolled, the bed did not. They, about 400, were packed pretty close (fig. 18). Saw the sickest eight; just had morphine, so were comfortable. About one-half were Americans and one-half British. There were a few British marines and a handful of prisoners. Just through a stormy trip back. The unloading went on smoothly. There were plenty of ambulances; separate ones from the Royal Navy for the Marines! All other wounded went to the 298th GH (Michigan). The British were later sent to their own hospitals. We went to the 298th and had a nice chat with Colonel Kirksey and Walter Maddock. Am going to get them three teams from the 3d Auxiliary Surgical Group tomorrow. (Unit just in at Oxford.) Will set up a questionnaire to study effects of sulfonamides.

---

[20] Letter, Col. E. C. Cutler, MC, to Lt. Col. W. S. Middleton, MC, 20 Nov. 1942, subject: Memo for General Magee.

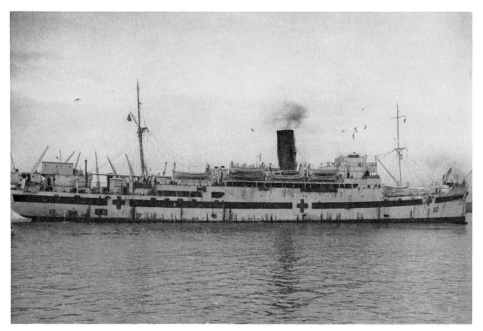

FIGURE 17.—Hospital Ship No. 38, the *Newfoundland* of Liverpool.

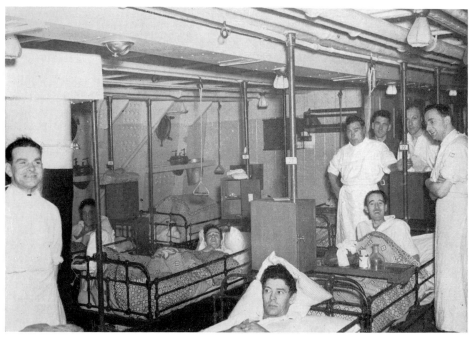

FIGURE 18.—The interior of the *Newfoundland*.

Upon returning to Cheltenham, Colonel Cutler reported to the Director of Professional Services, as follows:

The most interesting phase was the visit to the ward containing seriously wounded or sick people. I talked to six seriously wounded Americans. My questions, other than their general condition to cheer them up, were objected solely as to whether they had taken the sulfonamides which each American soldier presumably carries on his person. Not one individual had either taken tablets by mouth or dusted the powder into his wounds. They seemed to know what these medicines were for but had not bothered to use them, partly because in each case the individual was apparently unconscious following the accident, or spitting up blood if injured in the chest, or was so near the first aid man or first aid post [aid station] that he preferred to have the latter give him the medicine. The individuals I talked to came from the 16th and 18th Infantry [Regiments] and 39th Engineers.

This lack of our men taking sulfonamides brings up the problem repeatedly put to the British, that it is not wise or intelligent to tie up such a vast amount of a precious drug in packets for soldiers when the drug can be better and more securely given by the first aid posts. The only criticism of this British attitude is that there may be a long interval between being wounded and reaching a first aid post.

The arrival of these American casualties in the United Kingdom gives us an opportunity to put out a questionnaire and study the matter of (a) whether sulfonamides were used [and] (b) the interval after being wounded and the use of sulfonamides [in order] to check on their value by study of the conditions of the wounds now, since many of the wounds were sealed up in plaster almost from the beginning. Thus, the danger of secondary infection dismissed, we may be able to arrive at some fairly satisfactory scientific data.[21]

3d Auxiliary Surgical Group

On 18 December, the day following the visit to Avonmouth, Colonel Cutler, in the company of Colonel Kimbrough, hastened to visit the 3d Auxiliary Surgical Group, newly arrived at Cowley Barracks, Oxford, from a temporary station in Scotland. A pleasant meeting was held with the group's commanding officer, Lt. Col. (later Col.) John F. Blatt, MC. The problem was how to use the officers of the group in gainful pursuits in order to maintain their morale and spirits at as high a level as possible. The visitors explained how these officers could be used in hospitals, both British and American, and sent to American and British schools. Arrangements were made for the immediate dispatch of four teams to the 298th General Hospital and for Capt. (later Maj.) Benjamin R. Reiter, MC, to initiate the sulfonamide study. Colonel Cutler was particularly impressed by the high professional caliber of the group as a whole. He noted: "Some were among the best surgeons in the United States, and it is a great credit to those who assembled such a group that so many A–1 surgeons could be gotten together." [22]

It was just about Christmas Eve when General Hawley and Colonel Cutler conferred further on utilization of teams from the 3d Auxiliary Surgical Group. General Hawley decided to offer to the British up to 20 general surgical teams from the group for use with British Forces in North Africa. Both Gen-

[21] Letter, Col. E. C. Cutler, MC, to Col. J. C. Kimbrough, MC, 18 Dec. 1942, subject: Visit to Hospital Ship Disembarkation, Avonmouth, Dec. 17, 1942.

[22] Memorandum, Col. E. C. Cutler, MC, 19 Dec. 1942, subject: Visit to No. 3 Auxiliary Surgical Group, Cowley Barracks, Oxford, 18 Dec. 1942.

eral Hawley and Colonel Cutler were aware of the acute shortage of doctors in the British Army and knew that, in characteristic fashion, the British had tightened their belts and had not asked the United States for additional medical personnel, even though this possibility had been suggested. They realized, too, that the experience which these teams might gain would be most valuable. It was Christmas Eve when Colonel Cutler approached Brigadier Anderson, chief surgical consultant, RAMC, on the loan of these 20 surgical teams to the British Army.

On 28 December, Brigadier Anderson telephoned Colonel Cutler and relayed General Hood's message accepting this offer. The Director General was very grateful and most complimentary. Colonel Blatt also happened to visit General Hawley's office on this day, and he was fully oriented on the forthcoming dispatch of these teams to Africa.

The following day, Colonel Cutler returned to Cowley Barracks and gave the group an hour's talk on professional matters—their job at the front, the importance of debridement, their equipment, history of medical activities in the theater to date, and so forth. At lunch with the group, Colonel Cutler was dismayed to find a strong anti-British sentiment among members of the group. "Made me mad," he later wrote, "* * * laid it down a bit, as gently as possible. Told them it's no way to begin a war by criticizing a generous ally."

The administrative difficulties in providing these teams for the British proved most formidable, and final arrangements had to be worked out personally by General Hawley and Colonel Spruit with higher echelons of command.

Summary of Miscellaneous Activities During 1942

In his annual report of activities for 1942, Colonel Cutler stated:

The multitudinous duties which confront a consultant group are hard to categorize, for, with our broad instructions to see that each individual soldier has the best medical or surgical therapy possible under the conditions imposed in this theater, we naturally cut across all the usual boundaries of Army organization.

Thus, while the highlights of Colonel Cutler's first year in the European theater, 1942, have been briefly described in the foregoing pages, a still briefer word in passing must be devoted to some of his other multifarious activities in order to provide a faithful account.

American women doctors in England.—For various administrative and political reasons resulting from the war, General Hawley asked Colonel Cutler to investigate the status of women doctors in England of American citizenship and to look into the possibility of their employment as contract surgeons in the U.S. Army. In conferences with Sir Francis Fraser, director, EMS, and Dr. Murchie, the EMS personnel officer, Colonel Cutler was able to determine that most of these women doctors were advantageously employed by the British in their EMS installations. One was a major in the RAMC, Maj. Barbara

Stimson, cousin of the U.S. Secretary of War. The women were happy where they were and did not want to become contract surgeons, especially since, as they later learned, the pay was less than that being received from the British. What was required was a mechanism for their commissioning in the U.S. Army Medical Corps. Eventually, after many conferences and considerable give-and-take by all concerned, most of the women were made contract surgeons and loaned to the British EMS to continue in their jobs. Major Stimson remained in the RAMC and was sent to an active British theater, the Middle East. Colonel Cutler's final comment on this problem was:

> Barbara Stimson back from talk with her cousin HLS [Henry L. Stimson, Secretary of War] and Somervell [Lt. Gen. Brehon B. Somervell, Commanding General, SOS]. Guess women will get in Medical Corps soon. I have long advised they be taken in gracefully before they are put in against wishes of the Medical Corps. They will get in for sure.

Acting senior consultants.—Senior consultants for the theater in radiology and otolaryngology were expected momentarily, but, in the interim, individuals qualified and physically on duty in England had to be designated to act in such capacities as the needs arose. In accordance with the policy of grouping all professional medical specialties under the Chief Consultant in Medicine or the Chief Consultant in Surgery, radiology had been designated to come under the purview of Colonel Cutler. Accordingly, Lt. Col. Robert P. Ball, MC, and Capt. (later Maj.) Edmond P. Fowler, Jr., MC, both of the 2d General Hospital, were appointed to act as senior consultants in radiology and otolaryngology, respectively, in addition to their regular duties.

British Medical Research Council.—Attendance at and membership on the various committees of the British Medical Research Council "* * * have been extraordinarily enlightening * * *. Here one sees science applied to this devastating matter of war in an extraordinarily intelligent manner. * * * The writer is satisfied that great progress has been made by the intelligent few who sit with the British Medical Research Council." [23]

In particular, Colonel Cutler found attendance at meetings of the War Wounds Committee and its subcommittees most profitable. It was through this committee that he effected the promulgation of instructions to the British Army Medical Service and the EMS to use tetanus toxoid prophylactic doses rather than antitoxin in the prevention of tetanus in wounded or injured American soldiers. The British habitually used antitoxin for their wounded or injured soldiers in danger of tetanus infection. When antitoxin had been used on American soldiers, some serious reactions had occurred. Conversely, Colonel Cutler was able to have a circular letter published by the Chief Surgeon, ETOUSA, which instructed American medical units treating British soldiers on the proper prophylactic dose of antitoxin to be given.

Return postcard (surgical).—From his World War I days, and from what he had seen so far in World War II, Colonel Cutler realized that there

---

[23] See footnote 2, p. 20.

was very little interchange of information between the first echelons of medical service and those conducting definitive treatment in the rear. Yet, it was important that there be a constant flow of information between those first treating a patient and those who saw him later. Colonel Cutler had mentioned this need to the Chief Surgeon at one of their first conferences and had received his approval to design and have printed a postcard form for this purpose.

When the card was printed, the only casualties occurring in England were among operational aircrews. Medical officers in the Eighth Air Force, when asked, showed a keen desire to give the return postcard system a trial use. Accordingly, Circular Letter No. 79 was issued on 17 December 1942 by the Chief Surgeon. A portion of it follows:

Follow-up cards (ETOUSAMD Form 303) are being distributed to unit surgeons of the 8th Air Force. These are pre-addressed cards designed for the purpose of transmitting back to the medical officer who first treats an injury or battle casualty information concerning the subsequent progress of the case.

The medical officer giving immediate treatment at the station dispensary will print his name, grade, and A.P.O. number on the address side of the card. * * * and the card * * * will accompany injured and wounded patients to hospital.

The medical officer treating such cases at the receiving hospital will complete the reverse side of the card as soon as immediate therapy has been instituted, sign, and mail [it] * * *. A card will not be held at hospitals until completion of the case.

When ground hostilities were later engaged in on the Continent, this directive was modified to permit use of the card by all units initially treating casualties. This simple system worked with considerable success.

Special studies.—In addition to the sulfonamide study initiated with the first receipt of casualties from North Africa, limited studies in other areas were also begun.

The problem of fatigue in long training marches was being investigated by the 29th Infantry Division. Blood pressure, pulse rate, and blood sugar levels before, during, and after the training efforts were being recorded in order to obtain reliable data upon which could be based proper decisions as to the optimum amount of physical effort which could be expended without an inordinate increase in fatigue and morbidity.

Maj. (later Lt. Col.) Rudolph N. Schullinger, MC, 2d General Hospital, at his own request, was permitted to procure penicillin in small amounts from Prof. Howard E. Florey at Oxford and to experiment on its clinical application.

The consultants were asked to evaluate the efficacy of gas gangrene antitoxin and to make recommendations for its use in the theater. In this case, no actual experimentation could be initiated at the time, but expert opinion in the available literature and that obtained from interviews with members of the Allied forces and the British Medical Research Council indicated no conclusive results as to its efficacy. Since, however, there were implications in laboratory experiments that the antitoxin might assist in preventing the development of infection, Colonel Cutler recommended that a small stock be kept in the medical supply depots where it would be available to surgeons who wished to make use of it or who would like to make special studies on its efficacy and use. He recommended that gas gangrene antiserum not be included as a regular supply item for all medical installations at this time.[24]

Journals, books, and headquarters' library.—While the need for books, journals, and libraries was universally accepted, there was no professional library at the Cheltenham headquarters, and the sets of basic texts and journals for hospitals were lost in the depots. Colonel Cutler continually pressed the issue until the hospital sets were found and could be distributed, and one of the last things he did in 1942 was to appoint himself as librarian in order to establish a professional medical library at the headquarters in Cheltenham. A system was initiated whereby hospitals would get copies of journals routinely and reserve sets would be maintained for the hospitals which were later to arrive in the theater.

On visiting the British libraries, particularly those of the Royal Society of Medicine and the Royal College of Surgeons, it was most disconcerting to Colonel Cutler to find that American medical journals were arriving in England badly mutilated by the American censors. He took it upon himself to invite the attention of the War Department to this deplorable situation. He stated:

* * * Copies of these journals come to the Chief Surgeon's Office uncensored, and the Division of Professional Services * * * has never been able to find any article in these journals in which censorship could in any way affect the war * * * The extent to which such censorship is carried out is out of reason as well as robbing American doctors in this country of the ability to keep abreast of modern medicine.

It is recommended that the War Department take steps to see that American medical journals now going to the United Kingdom for use in public libraries * * * be uncensored. Thousands of these journals are freely distributed in America where their contents can easily be studied. It seems unnecessary to censor these journals because they travel across the Atlantic to an allied nation with whom we should have the most cordial and friendly relations.[25]

Medical field service school.—As indicated in the preceding narrative, there were many educational opportunities afforded the medical officer in the United Kingdom. Most of the contacts with the teaching institutions had been established before Colonel Cutler's arrival in England. After his arrival, he had continued to supervise the input of surgical officers to the various courses and had himself, or in cooperation with his senior consultants, created other training opportunities in British schools and hospitals and in certain of the U.S. Army hospitals. The instruction being received by officers attending these courses was of great value in keeping up and developing skills in certain aspects of medicine and surgery. There was needed, however, a centralized and coordinated instruction of the civilian doctor in military uniform as to the many duties expected of him in which he had little or no prior experience. It was also necessary to indoctrinate him on the accepted, basic tenets of medical

---

[24] Memorandum, Col. E. C. Cutler, MC, to Col. J. C. Kimbrough, MC, 1 Sept. 1942, subject: Gas Gangrene Anti-Toxin.
[25] Letter, Col. E. C. Cutler, MC, to the War Department, 26 Dec. 1942, subject: The Censoring of Medical Journals Now Being Forwarded to Libraries of Medical Installations in Great Britain.

and surgical practice in the theater in order to standardize the treatment of the more common conditions found as a result of military service or injuries incurred in combat. This obvious need was being met by plans to establish a medical field service school in conjunction with the SOS American School Center at Shrivenham, Berkshire.

Colonel Cutler had started work on the curriculum and courses of study for this school as soon as he had oriented himself in the theater. By early September, he had completed the courses of study in the surgical topics to be covered. He then discussed them and arranged for their incorporation into the overall curriculum with Lt. Col. George D. Newton, MC, who was initially in charge of establishing the school at Shrivenham.

Observations at Year's End

By the end of 1942, most of the positions for which senior consultants were contemplated had been filled. The many duties and responsibilities of a consultant had gradualy evolved through his day-to-day commerce with fellow officers in the headquarters and in the field and through his concern in the medical matters of the theater. It was possible, at this time, to reflect on the activities of the year and to make recommendations which only the knowledge gained through experience could make possible.

Colonel Cutler had the following thoughts for The Surgeon General:

The memorandum has been on my desk three months; it has been fully considered by most of the present Consultant Group who give it their warm approval. It is presented without bias or criticism as a piece of constructive thinking which has arisen during the day's work. To my way of thinking, it is the most important contribution I can make in my present office.

*   *   *   *   *   *   *

In this thinking, observation of and discussion with our British and Canadian colleagues have been helpful for medical and surgical problems are universal and do not belong to nationalities. Always in these discussions the remark arises in those who are not members of a Regular Army Medical Corps but who have left their civilian positions to help as best they can at this time, "I wish we could have worked on these problems in peace time!"

And this desire to have played a role in peace time has many beginnings. It arises in part from the findings that the Regular Corps are not on a whole, though there be brilliant exceptions, as much abreast of modern medical and surgical practice as the civilian profession is. It arises because what to the military doctor is an essential apparatus or medication long since was dropped from use in medical practice. And it arises because the civilian doctor finds he thinks and talks even a little different medical philosophy from his regular colleague and wishes they had had more in common in the past.

I believe that were an arrangement set up with a permanent Advisor or Consultant Group established as a part of the Army Medical Department there would result a steady flow of benefit to our Army Medical Corps. Such a Board would bring an immediate close relationship between civilian doctors and the Medical Corps. Each would be led to the other's domain. Each would attend the medical meetings of the other group. The interest of the public as a whole would be aroused and once again the Army medical man would be the real and actual colleague of his civilian prototype.

This would be especially true if a method of appointment to this Board was utilized which [would] put the responsibility for appointment on the leading medical and surgical societies in the USA * * *. This would put these leading societies squarely behind the Medical Department of the U.S. Army, for having assumed responsibility for an appointment the associations would inevitably follow through with an abiding interest. This alone would be a great step forward. * * *

Such a Board with the great clinical societies squarely behind it would result in a new attitude of civilian doctors to military doctors. The two would closely approach each other, the civilian group would feed personnel into the Army group. The advantage from common meeting grounds in each other's associations and societies would have incalculable benefits. And all the time the Consultant Group could be kept working on medical supplies and methods for military movements. It is not proper to wait until we go to war to prepare to bring proper medical and surgical relief to our soldiers. We must be prepared always with material and methods. We must practice lest we fail in our responsibility. What amount of labor by a doctor can equal the offering to his country of an infantry man, an aviator, or any member of the fighting forces? There can be no demands upon his time and skill in peace time along these lines that our profession would not gladly give.

The fact that the British Navy and the British Army have had for years civilian consultants in times of peace and the role they now play and all benefits to their service which have flowed from this arrangement strengthens my temerity in offering this memorandum.

In closing, Colonel Cutler made the following specific recommendations:

1. That an Advisory or Consultant Board in the fields of Medicine and Surgery be set up as a Permanent Part of the U.S. Army Medical Department. This is to function in times of Peace as well as War.

2. That the Senior Consultants in Medicine and Surgery be nominated respectively by the American Association of Physicians and the American Surgical Association. That the Senior Consultants in the Medical and Surgical Specialties be nominated by their respective Associations or Societies in the USA.

3. That confirmation of these nominations rest in the hands of the Surgeon General.

4. That this Board be a continuously active part of the medical department and be consulted freely and continuously on all matters pertaining to the fields covered by its membership.[26]

1943 TO EARLY 1944: PLANNING, BUILDING UP, AND WAITING

The First Half, 1943

The new year began with quite an experience for the Chief Consultant in Surgery. He left by auto from Cheltenham for London on 3 January in order to attend the second session of the Inter-Allied Conferences on War Medicine. "The high point of 3 January," he later reported to Colonel Kimbrough, "was the unfortunate fact that my car rolled over on me while driving from Cheltenham to Swindon. Fortunately, no one was hurt, but I reported the accident immediately by telephone and dispatch rider to Headquarters and to the Inter-Allied Medical Meeting." The meeting, however, was very successful, and many favorable comments were made on General Hawley's presentation and upon that by Colonel Diveley, Senior Consultant in Orthopedic Surgery.

---

[26] Letter, Col. E. C. Cutler, MC, to the Chief Surgeon, ETOUSA, and The Surgeon General, 13 Jan. 1943, subject: A Plan for an Advisory or Consultant Board in Medicine and Surgery as a Part of the US Army MD in Peace as Well as in War.

Problems of interpersonal relationships

Perhaps the one thing which characterized the life and pursuits of the consultants during the greater part of 1943 was their attempt to acclimatize themselves to the military, professional, and social milieu which prevailed in the Chief Surgeon's Office and among its members. This constant effort to adjust was still an undertone to the bustle of activity which marked later, more active periods in the life of the theater and remained a matter of deep concern to the consultants even after the fight was won. It was, however, during this period of relative calm—a long, frustrating period of waiting for the big things to happen—that these interpersonal relationships arose as manifest problems to the welfare of the individuals involved and to the overall effort of the medical headquarters in the European theater.

Had Colonel Cutler been able to take the time to write this consultant story, as he called it, he undoubtedly would have placed great emphasis on this aspect of the total picture. His diary contained frequent reminders to himself that he would have to write the consultant story some day, reminders inevitably tied in with these problems of interpersonal relations. Unfortunately—or for that matter, fortunately—Colonel Cutler was, rather, a man who preferred to do something about these things, and, thus, they were never written.

Briefly put, there were two problem areas. One problem was the relationship between the officers who had only recently come on active duty and the officers of the Regular Establishment. The other problem concerned the relationships of the consultants with one another. The officers in the Chief Surgeon's Office had come from many walks of life with greatly varying backgrounds and experiences. The consultants were men of outstanding ability and prominence who, to a great extent, owed their success to their unique individuality. It was to be expected that a great amount of give and take had to occur and that true communication was to be most difficult. In his annual report for 1942, Colonel Cutler gave the following indication of the rising problem:

> It is fair to state that on the whole the consultants have been patient and forgiving. We who are used to the fast well-oiled machines of civilian life have often been irked at the slowness of action or certain hidebound regulations which do not seem to allow us to put the best man in the right place, or the right material where it is necessary. Curiously, those who went through the last war in this group seem more patient than those who did not. Perhaps we learnt something about the Army in the last war. I am sure that all the consultants see eye to eye in their main desire to render expert surgical and medical care to every American soldier. Our own Chief of the Professional Services, and, in particular, the Chief Surgeon, have been immensely patient with us, and we are happy to have this opportunity to give them our gratitude in return.

The weather, among other things, had been "rotten," rainy, cold and miserable, and Colonel Cutler, himself, had felt no better. He noticed that the morale of his consultants was particularly low. On Sunday, 25 October, he recorded: "In the afternoon, the boys * * * gave me hell; said we weren't getting anywhere and suggested it was partly my fault!" The following day, he wrote: "Staff meeting, 4:00 to 5:00, and this time the boys took it out on JCK [Colonel Kimbrough]. I think they are wrong, petulant, and a bit childish. Anything they can do will help our soldiers, but they seem to feel that, unless it is a great big job, they might demean themselves by doing it." A few days later, he commented: "I appreciate they have little to do that looks important, but why cannot they see that everyday they serve their country, it is a privilege. Why must all think: What are we doing? What do we get out of it? Perhaps I'm just a stupid little boy, but anyway, I'm happy to serve."

After these really uncalled for, but understandable, outbursts of temperament, Colonel Cutler tried, he believed successfully, to mend damaged feelings and arrive at a better understanding among the consultants. On occasions, however, things seemed to go from bad to worse.

The new year held no promise for improving the situation. On New Year's Day, Colonel Cutler entered this rather despondent statement: "I seem to feel that we are all stagnating and going to seed, though we work steadily at organization." And on 4 February he recorded: "All day I've felt bad, and now I feel just rotten. Discouraged with a system which isn't calculated to help a country at war, though that obviously is the reason for its existence.[27]

That this matter of interpersonal relationships was no trivial matter can well be attested by the attrition rate among the surgical consultants. During 1943, four of the senior consultants in surgery returned to the Zone of Interior for permanent change of assignment. Among reasons for their reassignment was that of failing health brought on by the environment and circumstances under which they worked. One of the consultants was seriously ill. Another had to be removed from the Professional Services Division and given a division of his own in order for the Service to obtain the maximum contribution that was expected and needed of him and that he was fully qualified to give. Apparently, from the written record, Colonel Cutler was able to contain himself remarkably well, considering the circumstances.

Another phase of this struggle, particularly as it might be applicable to the professional personnel who made up the group of surgical consultants, was the personality of Colonel Cutler, himself. These statements made by General Hawley, however, could have applied to each of the other consultants as well. Speaking in retrospect of Colonel Cutler, he wrote the following:

* * * An innate honesty often compelled his professional judgments to be severe; but, whenever possible, they were softened with praise of other qualities. His high ideals and his devotion to duty made him, in his younger and formative years, somewhat intolerant of mediocrity; and this occasionally brought him into conflict with others. But the years brought him the wisdom that recognizes the impossibility of universal perfection, and

---

[27] "Much of this was written in late 1942 and early 1943. At that time there was no firm war plan for the E.T.O., and none of us knew what the eventual plan would be. Plans were changed every week. The Air Force was still promising to 'bomb Germany to her knees'; and certainly no ground forces of the magnitude which were assembled in late 1943 and in 1944 were then planned." (Letter, Paul R. Hawley, M.D., to Col. John Boyd Coates, Jr., MC, 25 Aug. 1958.)

a tolerance for human weakness that fell short only of abridging his high principles. He required a lot of knowing, did Elliott Cutler; and casual contact rarely revealed the true fineness of his character.[28]

It may be said with considerable certainty that Colonel Cutler's attitude on the position of general surgery vis-à-vis the specialized branches of surgery in war was an important factor in the conflict of ideas and aspirations among the surgical consultants (pp. 167–168). In a broader sense, this attitude could be related to Colonel Cutler's convictions on the surgery of trauma and the position of those in the fields of the more limited surgical specialties.

During the doldrums which gripped the consultants in late October 1942, Colonel Cutler found it necessary to comment on the place of surgical specialists in an oversea theater. His memorandum, presented to Colonel Kimbrough, read, in part, as follows:

1. This is a careful and thorough study deserving the most thorough consideration. It reveals careful consideration of the problem not only of this surgical specialty but of all surgical specialties.

2. The basic consideration that specialists are undesirable in the forward areas has my entire approval as does the corollary that the Surgeon General's Office, Washington, does not appreciate this since it is committed to a heavy training program, expensive and probably of no value.

3. * * * I have myself always been of the opinion that this is a small island and that if transportation is available (and safe) all who can no longer serve here should be evacuated to the Zone of Interior immediately.

4. The final suggestion that narrow specialists be sent home is not for my decision but this may be said:

    a. Any good citizen now here can be of immense service to his country and replacement is difficult.

    b. Lt. Col. — has been a major element in whatever value the Chief Surgeon may put upon his Surgical Consultants because he is loyal, faithful, a hard worker and a man of sound judgment.

    c. Patience is a noble virtue and far transcends surgical specialization.[29]

The problem of traumatic surgery was not limited to the American forces in England. If anything, it was apparently a greater problem among the British medical profession. The 2 February meeting of EMS consultant advisers with the director, Sir Francis Fraser, brought out a heated argument on traumatic surgery and the orthopedists' claim to it. Colonel Cutler was asked to speak, and he did. As a result, he was asked to speak on the same subject at a forthcoming meeting of the British Surgical Association, particularly with reference to the educational system and the organization of a university teaching clinic. In his memorandum of 5 February 1943, reporting the meeting to Colonel Kimbrough, Colonel Cutler stated:

In furtherance of the discussions that took place, it seemed to me obvious that a psychological barrier has arisen between my general surgical colleagues and my orthopedic

[28] Hawley, Paul R.: Obituary—Brigadier General Elliott Carr Cutler, Med. Res. U.S. Army, Mil. Surgeon, 101 : 351–352, October 1947.
[29] Memorandum, Col. E. C. Cutler, MC, to Col. J. C. Kimbrough, MC, 30 Oct. 1942, subject: Comment on Contribution of Lt. Col. —.

colleagues in Great Britain, in that the orthopedist has come to think he is the only one who can look after trauma. Of course, this is ridiculous. He cannot care for trauma of the head, nor care for the ruptured kidney or ruptured spleen, nor would he have any idea of what to do with nonperforating thoracic injury.

With the aforementioned memorandum of February 5, Colonel Cutler submitted also a memorandum which he had written, he stated, for his own thinking after the last meeting of "this Committee." The substance of this memorandum was as follows:

A disturbing finding in England is the professional thinking, which seems general, that only orthopedic surgeons can treat fractures and other forms of trauma. This seems to me to create a grave danger in the broad outlook of medical practice, both for the people we treat and for the profession.

It creates immediately a fundamental new speciality in that it carries the indication that every fracture incurred on the street must go to an orthopedic specialist. Such a fundamental breakdown of medical practice is just the sort of treatment for the people that is sure to give rise to new cults. * * * It is always our mistakes which give rise to new cults. Yet we keep blaming the people for accepting them when we, the profession which should have the responsibility of the people always at heart, have been responsible for the change.

A study of what happened in Britain reveals the following. With the great blitz, it was found that fractures were badly treated by the ordinary doctor. Therefore, those responsible ruled that only experts should treat fractures, and they thought that only orthopedic surgeons were experts in fractures. As a result, Britain now finds herself with only a few people able to treat fractures, and the young man going out into the field with the Army has no training in trauma because at home such work has been not a part of his general surgical education but a specialty. What Britain should have done when the blow came was to have impressed upon the schools, the leaders, and the teachers that all doctors must learn adequately the care of trauma. Trauma constitutes between 20 and 30 percent of every young doctor's work, and the schools should drill the students completely in its handling and care. Had this been done in England, she would now have thousands of people trained in trauma, and not just a pitiful handful ready. It is the long run view which saves both people and the profession.

We can take a lession from this—a lesson not taken in any schools from a critical point of view—because we can benefit from the experience of our colleagues and our sister nation. We must now see that every young surgeon is taught trauma. If we do not do this, the foolish separation already occurring in our country of a specialty for traumatic surgeons, giving rise to even a society with this name, will jeopardize the care of the people, which is our complete responsibility.

Colonel Kimbrough forwarded both of the aforementioned memorandums to General Hawley who, in turn, had them copied and forwarded to General Hillman in the Office of The Surgeon General.

On 12 April, Colonel Cutler presented a talk to the British Consultants Club on organization for surgical teaching clinics in the future. "Really an attempt to hold specialization in place," he wrote. In a letter to Colonel Kimbrough, dated 16 April 1943, he mentioned the following points made in his talk:

> The real problem relates to the role to be played by specialists and the question is becoming more urgent whether there should be separate clinics or institutes for the specialties in medicine and surgery, or whether they should form part of a general clinic. The reasons for a general clinic seem to be many, but in particular are included in the statement that a general clinic, especially where the patients are mixed in vast wards and not segregated in special wards, is best:
>
> For the patient, since this permits simple cases which are recoverable to be next to more serious people whose outlook is hopeless.
>
> For the students, and the Oath of Hippocrates states that every doctor must assist in educating students—since if the patients of all specialties, etc. mix in wards, the students' mental exercise in entering the ward is not simplified as it is when he knows that all cases in that ward are restricted to diseases in a certain domain.
>
> For the doctor, for under these circumstances the specialists and the general surgeons find themselves willy-nilly next to each other in an open ward discussing their problems. If they run separate institutes then they are shut away from each other, and open discussion and common problems [are] lost.

As for the Chief Surgeon, General Hawley announced on numerous occasions his policies on the use of specialists. Notes from a conference of 19 April 1943 show that General Hawley emphasized the following points:

> That it was not his policy to train specialists in the E.T.O.: that he considered a world war and a theatre of operations were neither the time nor the place for medical education. He had found from experience in the last war that General Practitioners, nervous of conditions when they returned home from the Army, had been anxious to specialize. They had attended short courses in varied medical fields and had then considered themselves specialists. The outcome was that the men were useless in the theatre during the time of their so-called training; that the soldier suffered and eventually the civilian population from "half-baked" specialists. General Hawley agreed * * * that some differentiation should be made concerning those men who were either in the midst of training or about to embark upon training as specialists when they entered the Army.

Significant activities

The first half of 1943 found Colonel Cutler engaged in three primary projects. These were: (1) Preparations for participation in a British-American surgical mission to the U.S.S.R. (Union of Soviet Socialist Republics), (2) providing a means for assuring the supply of whole blood in combat, and (3) creating mobile surgical units. These subjects will be discussed separately, but it should be noted here that they were interrelated in one respect. As plans materialized for the trip to the U.S.S.R., it became evident that the mission would leave some time near midyear. There was a risk involved in making such an extended trip, particularly when plans called for visits to the combat zone. The risk, small as it may have been, could not be ignored. At the same time, it became increasingly evident to Colonel Cutler that there would have to be a bountiful supply of whole blood in the combat zone and surgical units as far forward as feasible in order to provide the optimum care for battle casualties. The combination of these factors meant one thing to the Chief

Consultant in Surgery: He had to complete plans for the provision of whole blood and surgical units before he departed for the U.S.S.R. This objective became an inescapable, moral obligation to which he rigidly adhered. Otherwise, the Chief Consultant in Surgery, in addition to carrying on with the routines and programs already in effect, was directly involved in the following noteworthy developments.

Change and expansion of consultant system.—Colonel Diveley, Senior Consultant in Orthopedic Surgery, visited NATOUSA (the North African Theater of Operations, U.S. Army), during the period 16 February to 19 March 1943. Maj. (later Lt. Col.) William J. Stewart, MC, was appointed Acting Consultant in Orthopedic Surgery on 1 March 1943. Major Stewart remained on duty with the theater consultant staff after Colonel Diveley's return. His services were most valuable because Colonel Diveley was required to give a great amount of time to rehabilitation activities and the making of training films. Lt. Col. (later Col.) Kenneth D. A. Allen, MC, upon arrival from the Zone of Interior, was appointed Senior Consultant in Radiology on 9 February 1943. Colonel Brown was returned to the Zone of Interior on 29 March, and Maj. (later Lt. Col.) Eugene M. Bricker, MC, of the 298th General Hospital, was appointed Senior Consultant in Plastic and Maxillofacial Surgery and Burns in his stead. Lt. Col. Norton Canfield, MC, arrived from the Zone of Interior in January and was appointed Senior Consultant in Otolaryngology on 1 July 1943.

During this period were initiated the beginnings of a system of consultation at the local level. Colonel Cutler explained the basis of the system at a meeting of the Chief Surgeon's Consultants' Committee on 30 April 1943 as follows:

With the desire to be prepared for a maximum load in the near future, the surgical consultants are submitting * * * a list of consultants in general surgery and the surgical specialties which consist of officers now on the roster of our general hospitals but who are of such professional standing that they might well be used in a consultative capacity. Note that in some specialties they are spaced at the rate of one to each base section; in some, less frequently; and in major fields for work for a consultant from each general hospital and evacuation hospital.

* * * The surgical Sub-Committee feels that by making this matter a permanent one now they may be protecting the patients subsequently to come to this theater, ensuring them adequate surgical care.

General Hawley approved of the idea wholeheartedly and urged that more than the number presently necessary be appointed to plan for the future and to assure the availability of an alternate consultant in the event the regularly designated consultant could not answer a call.

Another change which occurred late in this period was a reorganization of the theater command structure which involved the establishment of base commands and a change in the internal organization and arrangement of the Chief Surgeon's Office. The principal change in the latter was the reestablishment of General Hawley in London and the subsequent shifting of the

deputy surgeon, Colonel Spruit, to Cheltenham. The former change complicated matters greatly, but was an obvious necessity, just as it had been in the
First World War. It brought to the fore the question of who had the operational responsibility for consultations at the local level, since the base commander was to be supreme in his area, as Colonel Spruit informed the
consultants.

The change involving General Hawley and Colonel Spruit, it soon became
obvious, was the reorganization which had been required to improve the management of the Chief Surgeon's Office. General Hawley was one of the first
to admit this, for he observed at a conference held by him on 28 June 1943:

> The only other thing that I want to say is that it is very obvious to me that this
> office is working much better and that Colonel Spruit is doing [more] * * * to get [mat-
> ters] working smoothly than I was ever able to do.
>
> We are going to expand and decentralize, and more and more responsibility is going
> to division chiefs. Obviously the time is coming very, very soon when many things come up
> that cannot all be decided centrally. We are going to make mistakes. I have made several
> mistakes and you are going to make mistakes. I think we can all forgive mistakes that
> are honestly made but I cannot forgive a mistake that is camouflaged. Many of the mis-
> takes in this office, many of the failures in this office, I feel personally, result from poor
> leadership on my part. There are certain things that are not the result of that, and that is
> absolute and flagrant disobedience of a direct order. I can forgive almost anything else,
> but when I tell someone that I want something done I expect that to be done and done
> promptly.

Expert surgical observation from battlefront to base hospital.—A
letter on this subject, dated 6 January 1943, was submitted by Colonel Cutler to
Colonel Kimbrough. The letter read as follows:

> 1. I have long been of the opinion that the next step forward in military surgery will
> only come when experts can be placed in the forward elements of the Division, and can
> observe the wounded soldier from the time he is hit until he is convalescing. You will
> recall that it was the observations of a British R.A.M.C. Captain behind Ypres in the sum-
> mer of 1917 that gave us the complete evidence of a poisonous substance manufactured in
> a traumatized extremity on the way from front to rear.
>
> 2. I believe we should at this time have the privilege of sending into Division teams:
>
>> a. In general surgery,
>> b. In orthopedic surgery,
>> c. In thoracic surgery,
>> d. In neurological surgery,
>> e. In maxillo-facial surgery,
>
> who should observe cases on the battlefield, certainly at the battalion aid station, and then
> travel down the line at least through to the hospital where the first definitive surgical treat-
> ment is given. These men should have the privilege of operating upon individuals if in
> their judgment that seems wise.
>
> 3. I am sure that observations made by real experts even on 50 cases in each category
> would open up a new release for the wounded soldier.
>
> 4. I have been in long consultation with Colonel Holtz, Chief Surgical Officer of the Nor-
> wegian Forces, who went through the Finnish campaigns as well as the present struggle.
> He is an expert chest surgeon, and should such a group of American officers be allowed
> to go it would be a great benefit to us as well as to him if he could accompany this group.
> His government would be willing to give him two or three months leave for this purpose.

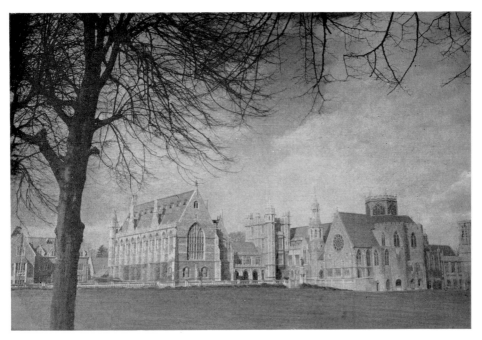

FIGURE 19.—Headquarters, V Corps, U.S. Army, at Clifton College, Bristol, England, 16 March 1943.

Colonel Kimbrough forwarded the letter to General Hawley who commented: "Noted with interest and will be applied when we start fighting." General Hawley also had his executive officer, Colonel Stanley, provide the Surgeon, V Corps (fig. 19), with a copy of the letter.

American Board of Surgery examinations.—Colonel Cutler was most happy when the American Board of Surgery, in answer to his request, replied favorably in regard to examinations in the European theater. He wrote to the deputy surgeon on 20 February:

The officers of the American Board of Surgery have just corresponded with me and given permission for the examinations * * *, providing members of the Founders Group can give the examination. There are sufficient members of the Founders Group in the theater * * *.

Will you please study the requirements submitted with this, and then send in the names of any men who would like to be candidates and are suited to the requirements. At a later date we will settle the examination time and place.

I am pleased at the action taken by the Board at home, because at least it does not militate against the young surgeon, when he becomes a good patriot, and we should have a lift in surgical morale through this action.

Record forms were secured, and the matter was publicized in the theater through notices in the *Medical Bulletin, ETOUSA*. Later, however, the Board in the United States felt that it was impossible to have these examinations conducted away from the United States. "This is a regrettable decision," Colonel Cutler stated in his annual report for 1943, "for it might appear that the young citizen who is willing to offer his services to his country should not thus be additionally penalized for patriotism. Our advice was to give the examinations either here or neither here nor in the U.S.A. for the period of the war."

Elective surgery.—As the troop and medical strength of the theater increased and more station hospitals came to England, the unqualified personnel performing surgery in these hospitals became a problem. The theater policy, established by General Hawley personally, was that no major elective surgery would be permitted except at the 10th Station Hospital and in general hospitals. Furthermore, there was a policy that patients who required more than 30 days of hospitalization would not be held in station hospitals. There was, however, the large realm of cases which, conceivably, could have surgery and be out of the hospital within this period. There were also station hospitals assigned to bases of the Army Air Forces to which skilled personnel had been assigned in order to provide definitive treatment for air casualties and the treatment of essential personnel which the Air Forces did not want to lose through ordinary replacement channels. In addition, there was the string of station hospitals which had been strategically placed in southern England with the idea that they not only serve troops in that area but also take care of evacuation from beaches upon the commencement of hostilities on the Continent. Colonel Vail, Senior Consultant in Ophthalmology, was of the opinion that ophthalmologists presently in the station hospitals were perfectly capable of performing the usual surgical procedures involving the eye. The real difficulty lay in trying to define elective surgery accurately and so that the definition would be uniformly understood, particularly in such operations as the repair of hernias. General Hawley's opinion was that, when something could not be defined accurately, it was impossible to enforce and control it rigidly. In the matter of station hospitals being permitted to perform special types of surgery, such as major ophthalmic procedures, the General stated that the surgeons in the theater at this time (March 1943) might be competent but this would not hold always.[30]

A policy was then agreed upon that no major elective surgery would be allowed in station hospitals except when application was submitted by the hospital for special permission to perform them, and the application was approved by the consultants concerned in the Professional Services Division.

The problem was not one of great magnitude, but it continued to occupy the time of the consultants because so many specific incidents continued to arise in which differences of opinion resulted in an apparent breach in theater policy and because the status of station hospitals had to be constantly reviewed to ascertain whether they could be permitted to perform or continue to perform operations of election.

The Chief Surgeon, during this period, did not choose to accept Colonel Cutler's definition of elective surgery based on the criterion of time; that is, that surgery covering those conditions where delay in transport does not endanger

---

[30] Minutes, Chief Surgeon's Consultants' Committee meeting, 5 Mar. 1943.

the patient's welfare.[31]   Neither did he permit the publication of a directive on certain types of elective operations which could be performed in station hospitals.

American Medical Society, ETOUSA.—At the suggestion of the Chief Surgeon, Colonel Cutler was given the responsibility for creating a medical society in which all American medical officers in the European theater would have automatic membership.   General Hawley specifically prescribed that the management of the society should rest in the hands of officers outside the Office of the Chief Surgeon.   Accordingly, Colonel Cutler further delegated to Lt. Col. (later Col.) Robert M. Zollonger, MC, the responsibility for forming the organization.   An organizational meeting was held on 14 May 1943 in conjunction with the meeting in Cheltenham of the chiefs of medical and surgical services of all general hospitals.   Lt. Col. Gordon E. Hein, MC, and Lt. Col. (later Col.) Wale Kneeland, Jr., MC, chiefs of the medical services of the 30th and 2d General Hospitals, respectively, and Colonel Zollinger were elected as a temporary executive committee.   The 298th General Hospital offered to sponsor the first meeting of the proposed society.

This initial meeting was held on 23 June 1943.   A business meeting was held preceding the meeting proper.   A simple constitution and bylaws were drawn up which stated the purpose of the society to be as follows:

> Upon authority of the Chief Surgeon, European Theater of Operations, this Society is formed for the purpose of disseminating current professional ideas and methods of military significance among officers of the Medical Corps of the United States Army in this theater.
>
> This Society shall be known as The American Medical Society, European Theater of Operations, United States Army.

The following officers were elected: President, Colonel Zollinger, 5th General Hospital; Vice President, Lt. Col. (later Col.) William F. MacFee, MC, 2d Evacuation Hospital; Secretary-Treasurer, Maj. Clifford L. Graves, MC, 3d Auxiliary Surgical Group; and Executive Committee at Large, Col. Edward J. Tracy, MC, Surgeon, Bomber Command, Eighth Air Force, and Lt. Col. Ralph S. Muckenfuss, MC, 1st Medical General Laboratory.   Monthly meetings on a rotational basis at general hospitals were planned.   Mornings were to be devoted to clinical ward rounds in the various sections followed by short presentation of topics related to the sections, and afternoon sessions were to be given over to topics of general interest.   Provision was made for the submission of papers from individual medical officers for presentation and the invitation of well-known guest speakers.   The chiefs of the medical and surgical services of the sponsoring hospital were designated the program committee for the meeting to be held at any particular installation.

Honorary Fellowship in Royal College of Surgeons.—While dining with Surgeon Rear Admiral Gordon Gordon-Taylor on the evening of 16 March 1943, Colonel Cutler was informed by Admiral Gordon-Taylor that he was to be made an Honorary Fellow of the Royal College of Surgeons in

---

[31] Draft, by Col. E. C. Cutler, MC, of proposed circular letter, 5 Mar. 1943, subject: Policy Regarding Surgical Therapy in Station Hospitals.

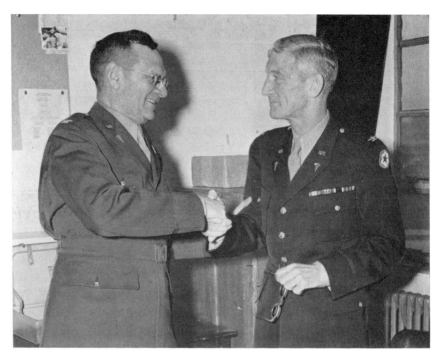

FIGURE 20.—Col. James C. Kimbrough, MC, congratulating Colonel Cutler upon his being made an Honorary Fellow of the Royal College of Surgeons.

July at London.   Colonel Cutler was very pleased, but he could not help but think: "It seems less important during a war, however."   On 9 April, Admiral Gordon-Taylor informed Colonel Cutler that he had been elected an Honorary Fellow of the Royal College of Surgeons.   On this occasion, Colonel Cutler wrote: "I am and should be immensely proud—greatest honor yet."   The appointment was conferred on 26 May 1943, rather than in July, because of the impending trip to the U.S.S.R. (fig. 20).

Sulfonamide studies.—The sulfanomide study (pp. 49, 52) initiated by Colonel Cutler and carried out by Capt. Benjamin R. Reiter, MC, at the 298th General Hospital on returning wounded from North Africa proved quite disappointing at first.   After going over the results with Captain Reiter on 7 January, Colonel Cutler had to conclude: "The information on sulfonamides from Africa is a fizzle.   There are too few figures and [they] proved nothing."

The study was continued, however, and expanded to other hospitals treating battle casualties from North Africa.   Eventually, 259 cases were studied in addition to Captain Reiter's original 73 cases, making a total of 332 cases—essentially all American wounded from North Africa evacuated to hospitals in the United Kingdom.   With this number of cases, it was possible for Colonel Cutler to say with some confidence in his letter of 24 May 1943 to Colonel Kimbrough:

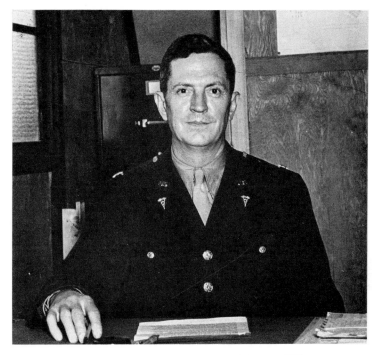

FIGURE 21.—Lt. Col. William F. MacFee, MC.

The statistics show that the sulfonamides, even taken and given under the optimum conditions, do not keep infection away from wounds.

The presence of infection, however, does not mean that the wounds would not have been more highly infected had sulfonamide not been used, and in fact we have every reason to believe that people who might have died of infection are now saved by the use of sulfonamide. * * *

Even transcending the above deductions of importance are the psychological effects upon the troops themselves. Almost to a man the soldiers have said, when questioned, that their lives were saved by the use of sulfa drugs. Experienced clinicians will recognize the value of this mental attitude * * *, and whether recognized or not by the physical scientists of this generation, [it] is something no good physician would be willing to set aside as a highly beneficial agent in the recovery from any physical ill.

Quite by coincidence, on the day Colonel Cutler submitted the foregoing conclusions, he was called upon to answer a question which had been presented in the British Parliament. A member of Parliament had asked from the floor: "Can it be said that sulfonamides as used by the U.S. Armed Forces have saved life?"

Colonel Cutler's reply was: "The answer is difficult but, put that way, must be 'No'."

Other studies were encouraged and carried on by individual medical officers. Notable among these was that by Lt. Col (later Col.) William F. MacFee, MC (fig. 21), at the 2d Evacuation Hospital on fresh Air Force casualties at an American airbase in England. Of some 250 whose wounds had been

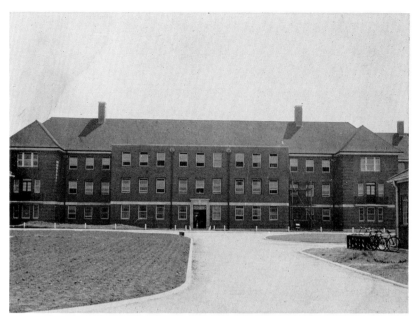

FIGURE 22.—Medical Field Service School, ETOUSA, at Shrivenham Barracks, England.

closed per primam after debridement and who had been administered sulfonamides, there were only four cases of infection, none serious. "This,"
Colonel Cutler wrote in his annual report for the year 1943 to the Chief Surgeon, "is an accomplishment that a good surgeon with a fresh casualty might
have without any chemotherapy * * *."

Penicillin.—Penicillin from the United States first arrived in England
only a short while before Colonel Cutler's departure for the U.S.S.R. First,
there was a radio message from General Rankin in the Office of The Surgeon
General that a shipment was on its way. Then, on 5 May, upon notification,
Colonel Cutler hurried to Widewing, Air Force headquarters in the theater.
There he discovered a crate marked for his attention from Merck & Co., Rah-
way, N.J. The crate inclosed 180 boxes, each containing 10 ampules with
10,000 Florey units of penicillin per ampule—a grand total of 18,000,000 Florey
units.

Colonel Cutler took, what was at this time, "a great load of penicillin" to
the 2d General Hospital. He immediately arranged with Professor Florey
of Oxford to standardize the efficiency of this shipment. Three days later,
with Professor Florey's guidance, Colonel Cutler made arrangements for
one laboratory officer in turn from each general hospital to come to the 2d
General Hospital and learn the laboratory procedures necessary to use and
store penicillin and to recover it from the urine of patients treated with it.
Other arrangements were made with the supply division for special tubing
and refrigeration equipment.

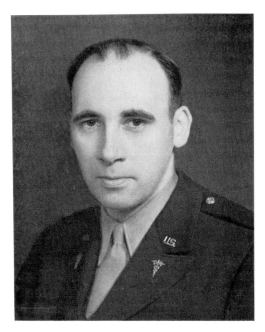

FIGURE 23.—Maj. Bernard J. Pisani, MC.

When, after correspondence with General Rankin, it was apparent that considerable amounts of penicillin would continue to arrive in England, Colonel Cutler met with General Hawley on the morning of 19 May to determine how the new drug would be used. General Hawley approved it for situations where its use might be lifesaving. He did not approve its use, at this time, for sulfonamide-resistant gonorrhea, as recommended. Some of the more specific uses of penicillin agreed upon by General Hawley and Colonel Cutler were for:

1. All cases with gas gangrene.

2. Serious general infections, usually with osteomyelitis and preferably infected with *Staphylococcus aureus*.

3. Eye infections (in a special ointment to be prepared by Colonel Vail).

4. Septic hands.[32]

Serious investigation into the efficacy of penicillin in surgical conditions had to await Colonel Cutler's return from the U.S.S.R. and larger more frequent shipments from the Zone of Interior. As precious as it was at this time, a generous amount of the drug was taken by the mission to Russia as a gift to the Soviet peoples.

Schools and professional training.—A milestone in the theater's medical educational activities was the opening of the European theater Medical Field Service School at the American School Center, Shrivenham Barracks (fig. 22), under the direction of Capt. (later Lt. Col.) Bernard J. Pisani, MC (fig. 23).

---

[32] Letter, Col. E. C. Cutler, MC, to Col. J. C. Kimbrough, MC, 22 May 1943, subject: Talk With General Hawley re Penicillin, Wednesday, 19 May.

The first course convened on 8 March 1943 and continued for 3 weeks.[33] The purpose of the school, as announced, was to train medical officers, particularly those serving with field units, in aspects of military medical practice not ordinarily familiar to civilian physicians. Included in the curriculum were 22 hours of lectures and conferences on problems of combat as they affected surgery, acute medical conditions, and neuropsychiatry.

Before the opening of the school, Colonel Cutler had worked many hours on the surgical courses of study, but an item of immediate concern to him shortly before the opening was the appointment of instructors on professional subjects. Some, apparently, had been appointed without knowledge of the Professional Services Division, and Colonel Cutler informed the Chief Surgeon of his concern over this situation.

In reply, the Chief Surgeon stated at the February meeting of his Consultants' Committee the policy that all instruction in clinical medicine at the school, except chemical warfare, would be controlled by the Professional Services Division and that no instructors on professional subjects would be sent to Shrivenham without that division's approval. General Hawley further explained that he wanted the course at Shrivenham for the man in the field, but also wanted it to include essential teaching on frontline treatment to avoid the necessity of sending officers to two separate courses.

Partially as a result of this policy, professional training at the school retained a high level, and instruction could be varied as circumstances indicated. Most of the teaching on strictly professional subjects was given by the various theater consultants concerned.

Another course, initiated during this period, became known as the London tours course. This program was created at Colonel Cutler's request by Surgeon Rear Admiral Gordon Gordon-Taylor, consulting surgeon to the Royal Navy. A limited number of officers was accepted for a 1-week schedule of visits to a different British hospital in the environs of London each day—to London, Guy's, Middlesex, St. Mary's, and St. Bartholomew's Hospitals. Luncheon was provided at each hospital, and, on certain afternoons, the American Red Cross in London provided transportation and guides for tours to interesting points in the city. The professional interests of candidates selected were relayed to the hospital directors in advance.

Finally, an administratively difficult, but most worthwhile, program was begun of exchanging for short periods of time medical officers in line units with those in hospitals. This program fulfilled the dual purpose of providing a more varied experience in clinical practice for medical officers of line units and served to acquaint medical officers in hospitals with the problems of providing medical service in line units. The plan was a good precursor for the system later adopted of rotating combat- and service-element medical officers when active hostilities ensued on the Continent.

---

[33] Circular No. 22, Headquarters, ETOUSA, 23 Feb. 1943.

Blood

Back in 1942, upon hearing a discussion on blood and plasma at a meeting of the Royal Canadian Medical Corps Pathological Club, Colonel Cutler had recorded: "Very interesting. It seemed to me that the rise of plasma, etc., had let all forget the benefit of transfusion. Our soldiers are all grouped. They should be the best vehicle for getting blood forward. No bottles to carry!" But, comments he heard later and reflection on the transfusion problems of World War I convinced him that the matter was not as simple as this. The problem lay in the area of a practical unit usable under the conditions of combat to effect transfusions.

In a letter to the Chief Surgeon on 27 March 1943, concerning standardization of the portable transfusion unit for combat areas, Colonel Cutler wrote the following:

The information we have from the present battle fronts of all nations including our own in Africa and elsewhere, is that transfusion as a method of resuscitation is steadily on the increase. Colonel Diveley brings us this information from our own troops in North Africa and Brigadier Whitby tells me that the use of wet plasma has practically been given up, and transfusion used in its stead in the British Army.

He then proposed a simple transfusion kit to be used by American units in the European theater (fig. 24). The kit was composed of items of standard equipment available in the theater, and, when packed in a chest, made it possible for a shock team to provide a large number of transfusions. This kit, developed by Capt. (later Lt. Col.) Richard V. Ebert, MC, and Capt. (later Lt. Col.) Charles P. Emerson, MC, 5th General Hospital, included equipment for grouping donors rapidly and satisfactorily, for these officers had discovered that a 10-percent error existed on the blood types stamped on identification tags of individuals.

Colonel Cutler recommended that a number of units of this type be assembled, packed, and held for distribution in the medical depots. There was no immediate need for the item, since the British taking and giving sets currently in use were satisfactory for the type of medical service being provided.

Colonel Cutler, on 31 March 1943, was given a firsthand explanation of a system used by the British in Africa. At the Post-Graduate Medical School, RAMC, in London, Col. A. E. Porritt, RAMC (later Brigadier and consulting surgeon, 21 Army Group), gave a splendid discussion on how the British Forces in the Middle East drew blood in Cairo, flew it to a distributing point behind the lines, and then transported it in refrigerated vehicles to forward units, such as field ambulances and advanced surgical centers.

In a letter, dated 2 April 1943, concerning his 30 March–1 April tour of duty, Colonel Cutler reported to Colonel Kimbrough: "With us, we had expected to send expert teams up the line who would then draw sufficient blood at each medical installation from lightly wounded or hospital personnel." He continued: "Both systems are open to the criticism that adequate studies of the blood for syphilis, malaria and other diseases are not made, and this needs critical thinking."

IMPROVISED BLOOD TAKING AND GIVING SETS

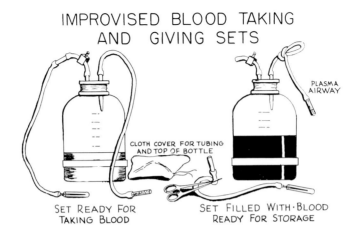

IMPROVISED BLOOD TAKING AND GIVING SETS

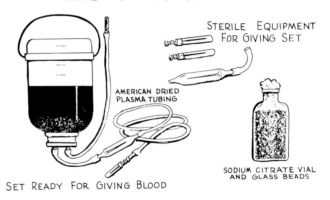

FIGURE 24.—A transfusion set improvised by Capt. Richard V. Ebert, MC, and Capt. Charles P. Emerson, MC, of the 5th General Hospital.

On 7 May, Colonel Cutler had a long session with Brigadier Whitby and others at the British Army Blood Supply Depot, Bristol. This meeting served to review and consolidate all previous thinking which had been given to the problem of supplying U.S. Army units with blood and protein fluids when the invasion began. The core of the problem was expressed in the following three questions and answers:

1. Are a common apparatus and a common source of blood and plasma essential for proper liaison between the British and American Armies?

Answer: Should we invade the Continent, the answer to this is that a common kit is not essential, for units using the materials would never be so closely mixed. Also, the British would have great difficulty in supplying us with material in this field.

2. What is the optimum time for resuscitation?

Answer: The answer is early, rapidly and adequately. British figures show 10 percent of wounded require transfusion. The Russian figure is 11 percent. Transfusion means blood or plasma, or both. These figures may rise to greater heights. For example, in a private letter from the Tunisian front to Brigadier Whitby 42 out of 180 serious casualties in an M.D.S. required transfusion, roughly 23 percent.

3. What is the problem in forward areas?

Answer: Everyone has agreed it is difficult to procure blood for transfusion in the most forward elements and the value of plasma is not fully appreciated by most medical officers. For example, word has come back both from the American and British sources in North Africa that plasma was no good and blood should be used. There can be no question but what replacement with plasma is highly efficacious and the opinions from frontline surgeons do not represent scientific evidence to the contrary but seem to be mostly hunches. It is as if these forward surgeons thought that certain serious casualties to whom plasma was given might have been saved if blood had been given. True, when massive hemorrhage has occurred blood is essential, but we should have a directive concerning the use of blood and plasma and the conservation of these.[34]

The British system contemplated for a continental invasion, as described by Brigadier Whitby, was to follow closely the North African experience. Freshly drawn refrigerated whole blood was to be delivered to the Continent by air. Thence, refrigerated trucks carrying 400 bottles each were to supply forward transfusion teams which, in turn, were to be equipped with 3-ton refrigerated trucks holding 80 bottles of blood and 200 units of plasma. The British graciously offered to fly U.S. Army blood to the Continent, but from there on the responsibility would have to rest with U.S. Army elements. Moreover, it was impressed on the conferees that the British planned to draw only 200 pints a day, which could be boosted with difficulty to 400. This absolutely prohibited the U.S. Army from counting on the British for a supply of fresh blood.

Considering the foregoing factors, the logical conclusions were fourfold, and these Colonel Cutler expressed as his recommendations to Colonel Kimbrough and the Chief Surgeon on 10 May 1943. First, there was the need to publish a directive concerning the proper use of blood and plasma in combat. Secondly, he stated that plasma was now being supplied to divisional medical elements, mobile hospitals, and fixed hospitals and required no further elaboration except that ample stocks had to be made ready. The third and fourth recommendations concerned the supply of whole blood and were divided into means of providing whole blood (1) from donors in the field and (2) from sources in the United Kingdom or the United States proper. They were as follows:

We recommend that a satisfactory bleeding and giving set with the equipment for gross agglutination to determine compatibility of blood be assembled and set up in the United Kingdom, this unit to go forward with our transfusion teams and be available for other medical use also. The equipment is contained in the T/BA of the mobile surgical unit already submitted. We feel that the transfusion team "up the line" can bleed the lightly

---

[34] Letter, Col. E. C. Cutler, MC, to Brig. Gen. P. R. Hawley (through Col. J. C. Kimbrough, MC), 10 May 1943, subject: The Use and Procurement of Blood and Plasma for the E.T.O.

wounded in sufficient supply for most of the needs for blood, provided plasma and blood are intelligently used.

It would seem desirable to have an additional supply of refrigerated fresh whole blood originating either in the U.S.A. or in the SOS or the U.S. Army in the United Kingdom. This would require the setting up in the U.S.A. or in the United Kingdom of 1) Bleeding centers, 2) the transport of such blood in a refrigerated aeroplane to the Continent, 3) the use of refrigerated automobiles to take the blood up the line to medical installations who would have refrigeration in which to keep it. Blood, when refrigerated, has been used up to 2, 4 and even 6 weeks after withdrawal, but it is perhaps not wisely used after 2 weeks. (Calculating 72 hours from bleeding in U.S.A. to the Continent we would have plenty of time to follow the English and Russian system and have blood drawn in America reach this forward area before any deleterious changes had taken place. If the air transportation of freshly drawn blood is too unreliable, blood could be secured from the U.S. Army SOS installations in the United Kingdom.)

The same day that the preceding recommendations were prepared, 10 May 1943, Colonel Cutler briefly apprised the Chief Surgeon and his staff on the problems of providing blood to combat forces. He emphasized particularly, at this informal conference, the difficulties attendant on the air transportation of blood from the United States and the fact that there was no machine suitable for the use of U.S. Forces in the European theater for properly giving and taking blood. The American equipment, Colonel Cutler told the conferees, was excellent, but when the slightest repairs became necessary, the equipment had to be returned to the Zone of Interior.

On 5 June 1943, Col. Walter L. Perry, MC, Major Storck, and Captain Hardin met with Colonel Cutler in Cheltenham. Colonel Perry (fig. 25) was the theater medical supply officer, and Major Storck, the recently appointed Senior Consultant in General Surgery. The meeting was arranged to expand further the proposals submitted by Colonel Cutler on 10 May 1943 and to recommend more specific steps necessary for the implementation of Colonel Cutler's suggestions.

The matter of obtaining blood from the Zone of Interior was left in abeyance since it was obviously a separate problem from that of obtaining, processing, storing, and distributing blood within the theater. Moreover, once blood from the United States had arrived in the theater, it presented a problem no different from that for blood collected and processed in the theater. Therefore, the conferees concentrated on facilities and programs to be developed within the capabilities of the theater itself—the only basis on which *absolutely reliable* plans could be made. They made the following decisions:

1. A depot-type unit would be necessary in the United Kingdom to centralize and direct the many activities involved.

2. Bleeding of American troops and/or British civilians would be necessary.

3. American bleeding teams and facilities would have to be used.

4. Provision had to be made for a unit to receive and further distribute blood on the Continent, once a firm beachhead had been established.

5. Proper refrigeration equipment would be necessary throughout all phases of the program.

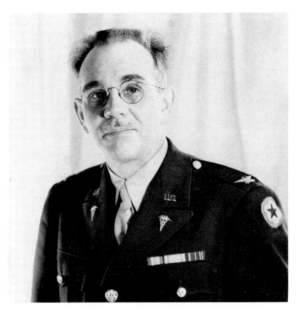

FIGURE 25.—Col. Walter L. Perry, MC.

Also discussed was the progress which had been made in establishing blood banks and donor panels at each active general hospital and the work yet remaining to accomplish this objective.[35]

On 10 June, Colonel Cutler had a conference with General Hawley in London. The general, after first expressing his surprise at finding Colonel Cutler still in London, directed him to finish by all means the plans for providing blood and plasma before leaving for the Soviet Union.

June 11, Colonel Cutler's diary reveals, was spent "all day at work on memo re blood, plasma, and crystalloids; all done."

"The purpose of this memo," he wrote General Hawley, "is to bring together all data concerning intravenous therapy for shock and allied conditions, and to conserve the use of these precious materials (blood, plasma and crystalloid solutions) which are often misused and wasted at the present time." [36]

Colonel Cutler listed for General Hawley all the directives which had been published to date on blood, plasma, and crystalloid solutions; presented an inventory of all plasma and crystalloids on hand, both American and British; and reviewed procurement demands still outstanding on the British for these items. He provided General Hawley proposed directives on the making of crystalloids by general hospitals for their own use and on the economic use of

[35] (1) Letter, Capt. R. C. Hardin, MC, to Col. E. C. Cutler, MC, 5 June 1943, subject: A Plan for the Procurement and Delivery of Whole Blood for a Continental Task Force From the U.S.A. or U.K. (2) Letter, Capt. R. C. Hardin, MC, to Col. E. C. Cutler, MC, 5 June 1943, subject: Provision for Procurement of Whole Blood for Transfusion in General Hospitals in the E.T.O.

[36] Letter, Col. E. C. Cutler, MC, to Brig. Gen. P. R. Hawley (through channels), 11 June 1943, subject: The Procurement and Use of Blood, Plasma and Crystalloid Solutions (Saline and Sugar) for Intravenous Use in the E.T.O.

blood and plasma by units in the field. He stated that the general medical laboratory, when established, should also have as one of its duties the manufacture of crystalloid solutions.

On the matter of supplying whole blood, Colonel Cutler again referred General Hawley to the basic tenets made in his letter of 10 May 1943; namely, that a simple field-transportable transfusion set was necessary for bleeding "on the hoof," and supplemental sources of blood were required within the theater or the Zone of Interior. He submitted copies of the 10 May 1943 letter, a revised and final version of plans for the field transfusion set, and letters prepared by Captain Hardin on the 5 June 1943 meeting.

In submitting plans for the transfusion set, Colonel Cutler noted:

1. The following TB/A for a Whole Blood Transfusion unit is the final product of months of experimentation with Major Emerson and Major Ebert of the 5th General Hospital.

2. In discussion with Colonel Perry we propose that if Field Medical Chests are scarce the wooden boxes in which our U.S. Army plasma arrives would act as suitable containers.

3. Two types of units may be dispensed.

a. The complete unit as listed for teams going into combat area.

b. A unit for hospital use consisting only of those items not available in static hospitals (chiefly bleeding and giving sets with citrate and large needles).

4. We believe the officers responsible for this standardization, Majors Emerson and Ebert, would be happy to assist in the original packaging.

Captain Hardin's letter reviewed the following necessities for any plan by which whole blood could be supplied to a continental force:

Blood from the Zone of Interior

Blood collected in the Zone of Interior can be delivered to the E.T.O. only by air transport. The collection, processing, and initial delivery to a depot in the United Kingdom would be a function of an agency in the Zone of Interior. Its reception, internal storage, and distribution to the base unit and/or * * * transfusion teams would be the responsibility of the depot located in the United Kingdom * * *. The depot would necessarily be located near an airport and would provide adequate refrigeration for the blood throughout its entire handling from the time of unloading the plane.

Collection of Blood in the U.K.

Blood can be obtained from two sources in the U.K.:

1. Base and SOS Troops.

2. Civilians (British).

The first * * * is somewhat problematical since the troops * * * are scattered over a wide area and because the bleeding would take place during periods of activity when those troops will be least available. The second source is probably the better. To put it into operation would entail taking over an area in the U.K. where the civilians could be bled. This area must be outside of the British Army Area (roughly Southern Command) and * * * the London area where the EMS bleed heavily to secure plasma for drying.

Organization of such an area would include enrolling of donors and procurement of bleeding centers. * * *

Bleeding Teams

These teams must be mobile and carry with them all of the equipment necessary to do one day's bleeding. Such a team when bleeding military personnel can bleed 150 per day provided that a constant stream of donors is made available. British teams bleeding civilians average 75 per day.

Depot

This unit serves as a base from which the mobile [bleeding] teams work. It supplies the teams with all the apparatus needed and maintains * * * vehicles. Records are kept of the bleeding, apparatus [is] reconditioned and assembled, and blood [is] processed. This includes serologic tests, typing, addition of glucose, and bacteriologic control. Here also internal storage of blood must be undertaken, which requires the provision of adequate refrigeration.

Distribution to the Field

Behind any force there must be a base unit which draws blood from the depot and distributes it to the shock teams. This unit may be small and simply concerned with supply of blood or like the British unit be capable of producing crystalloid solutions as well as distributing blood and plasma. It must be equipped adequately to be able to recondition apparatus and carry out sterilization. It must also have mobile refrigeration.

Refrigeration

Blood is ideally kept at $+3°$ to $+6°C$. It must not be frozen and undergoes considerable deterioration if the temperature of storage fluctuates greatly. Two types of refrigeration may be used:

1. Ordinary refrigerator capable of maintaining the required temperature. This type of refrigeration calls for fitting of airplanes and trucks with refrigerators. It is the type of refrigeration used by the British Army Transfusion Service and has worked well in practice.

2. Refrigeration by melting ice: Ice melts at $+4°C$ which is the ideal temperature for blood storage. By the utilization of compartment boxes into which ice and bottled blood can be placed in separate chambers an adequate but simple type of refrigeration is obtained. To utilize this to the fullest extent, lightweight well insulated containers could be built to hold 10 to 20 bottles of blood. Such containers under ordinary temperature conditions will hold ice for 72 hours.

Advantages: Simple, accurate refrigeration, with no machinery to break down. Dispersal of stores possible. Containers can be carried in any plane or vehicle without special installation.

Disadvantages: Procurability of ice. Ice making machines would be necessary in the base unit and perhaps in the depot.[37]

In summary, Colonel Cutler had shown how transfusions could be accomplished by "bleeding on the hoof," by obtaining whole blood from the Zone of Interior, by bleeding British civilians, and by bleeding U.S. Army service troops. Each of these proposals posed an enormous logistical undertaking to implement. It was certainly beyond the prerogatives of the Chief Consultant in Surgery to decide which steps would be taken. Hence, his closing words to the Chief Surgeon asked for "instruction to Professional Services concerning the method selected for supplying a Continental Task Force with whole blood that we may assist in implementing such decision * * *."

During Colonel Cutler's absence in the Soviet Union, General Hawley approved the construction and assembly of the field transfusion units. At his regular monthly conference with the consultants on 23 July 1943, General Hawley told them that blood should not be transported from the United

---

[37] See footnote 35(1), p. 75.

States.[38] He directed that the consultant group go ahead with plans for collection and distribution of blood and that the British be consulted with reference to preservation and storage.

In reply to a question by General Hawley as to the development, procurement, and distribution of blood transfusion kits for mobile medical units, his executive officer provided him with the following answers:

1. A blood transfusion chest had been designed and had been approved for clearing companies, evacuation hospitals, field hospitals, and auxiliary surgical groups. One hundred of these chests were being packed at Medical Depot G–35. Clearing companies and evacuation hospitals were to receive 2 chests each, while field hospitals were to receive 3 chests, and auxiliary surgical groups, 10.

2. A smaller unit had also been designed which was built around a new quartermaster item known as the "man pack carrier." Two hundred of these man-pack-carrier, blood-transfusion sets were to be assembled as soon as the pilot model was approved and the quartermaster carriers became available. Two of these kits were to be distributed to each collecting company and regimental medical detachment.

3. The standard, approved transfusion bottles for both the chests and the man-pack-carrier units were being assembled at the 5th General Hospital.[39]

Mobile surgical units

From his first days in Washington, Colonel Cutler had realized that the key to providing optimum care for battle casualties lay in taking the surgeon to the wounded man instead of bringing him back to the surgeon. This could only be accomplished, he believed, by a truly mobile, self-contained surgical team. At every opportunity, he had discussed this possibility with the Chief Surgeon and his colleagues, both British and American. One of the first things he had asked of General Hawley was that the latter request Washington for the assignment of an auxiliary surgical group to the European theater. By early 1943, he had gained considerable experience in current Army ways and felt quite capable of coping with the problems involved in coming forward with specific recommendations for the organization and equipment of a surgical team such as he had in mind.

In early February 1943, two things happened which encouraged Colonel Cutler to embark immediately upon the formation of a mobile surgical team. On 16 February, he attended a session at the RAMC College during which Maj. Gen. David C. Monro, RAMC, newly appointed consulting surgeon to the British Army, gave a brilliant discourse on his experiences of 2 years in

---

[38] "There is strong implication in the early part [of the manuscript] that the Chief Surgeon's disapprovals of some of the recommendations of the consultants were purely arbitrary and capricious. The truth is that, throughout the war, the Chief Surgeon had top secret information which he could not share even with his deputy; and many of these adverse decisions were based upon such information.

"One example of this is the account of the reluctance of the Chief Surgeon early in the war to attempt to obtain whole blood from the Zone of Interior. The reasons for this were (1) that the transatlantic airlift at that time was so limited, and so restricted to other priorities, that it could not take on such a load; and (2) The Surgeon General had told the Chief Surgeon flatly that he would not approve." (Letter, Paul R. Hawley, M.D., to Col. John Boyd Coates, Jr., MC, 17 Sept. 1958.)

[39] (1) Operational Directive No. 28, Office of the Chief Surgeon, ETOUSA, 10 July 1943. (2) Letter, Col. J. H. McNinch, MC, to Chief Surgeon, ETOUSA, 26 July 1943, subject: Status of Development, Procurement and Distribution of Blood Transfusion Kit for Mobile Medical Units.—Operational Dir. #28.

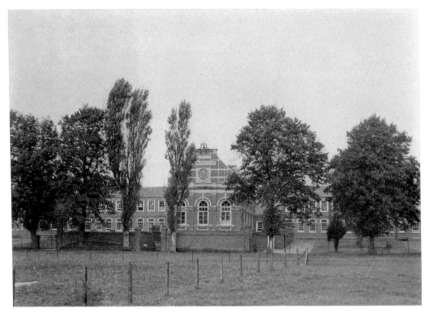

FIGURE 26.—The 36th Station Hospital, Exeter, England.

the Middle East. He traced the development of the field surgical unit and its successor, the mobile surgical unit, as constituted in that British theater of operations. General Monro emphasized the requirements for mobility, stated that team members had to be surgeons of outstanding ability and mature judgment, and warned that teams with equipment fitted (built-in) to vehicles were undesirable. The latter, he suggested, could be disabled with a single gunshot in the radiator.

Upon returning from this session at the RAMC College, Colonel Cutler recommended that (1) mobility must be forced on all of the medical services, (2) this could probably be best achieved by mobile surgical units based on parent units which would continue to supply and administer them, and (3) a certain amount of segregation of casualties by anatomical groups would be necessary in the rear areas for better surgical therapy. He concluded: "I believe that there are many lessons in this talk from which we should benefit, and benefit now. * * * Perhaps this first-hand experience will bring the Medical Corps of our Army face to face with what I believe to be a major issue, which must be solved before we get into a real battle." [40]

At about that time, Lt. Col. Herbert Wright of the Eighth Air Force had submitted a special report to the Chief Surgeon in which he brought General Hawley's attention to the situation which confronted the Air Forces in Cornwall. Many crippled aircraft returning from combat missions were landing at RAF fields in this area with frequent serious casualties among their crews. The nearest American hospital at Exeter (fig. 26) was some distance away from

---

[40] Letter, Col. E. C. Cutler, MC, to Col. J. C. Kimbrough, MC, 16 Feb. 1943, subject: Summary of Talk by Maj. Gen. D. C. Monro, 11 Feb. 1943, at the RAMC College.

this area, thus precluding the transfer of American casualties to it. More-over, this was the only specialized hospital in the theater, a neuropsychiatric facility with but a small surgical staff. Colonel Wright recommended the procurement of certain buildings just outside of Truro and requested the assignment of surgical specialists to staff a medical facility to be activated there.

Colonel Cutler found many objections to the plans submitted by Colonel Wright. He proposed, instead, that the U.S. Army obtain from 10 to 20 beds at the EMS Royal Cornwall Infirmary at Truro, send a surgical team there, and, in recompense, offer the services of the team to the infirmary when it was not fully engaged in treating U.S. Army Air Forces casualties.

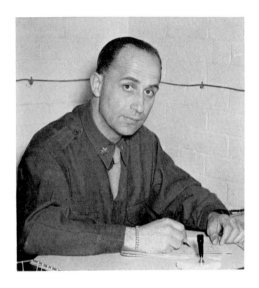

FIGURE 27.—Maj. Robert M. Zollinger, MC.

When this suggestion received General Hawley's approval, Colonel Cutler asked Maj. (later Col.) Robert M. Zollinger, MC (fig. 27), of the 5th General Hospital to work on a mobile surgical unit with the following guidance in mind: (1) The equipment should not be built in a truck, (2) the equipment and tentage should be for a mobile surgical team, such as a team from an auxiliary surgical group, and (3) the team should take all the materials necessary for lighting and for surgery to cover 50 to 100 major surgical casualties or 200 minor casualties.[41]

As things turned out, it was the obtaining of beds at the Royal Cornwall Infirmary at Truro which proved to be the greatest obstacle to this program. It was only through the intercession of Colonel Cutler's close friends, Prof. George Gask and Mr. Rock Carling, that an allocation of 12 beds was obtained at the Royal Cornwall Infirmary for the hospitalization of U.S. Army Air Forces casualties. The trustees of the infirmary approved Colonel Cutler's plan on 25 February, but the space was not immediately available because repair

---

[41] Annual Report, Chief Consultant in Surgery, ETOUSA, 1943.

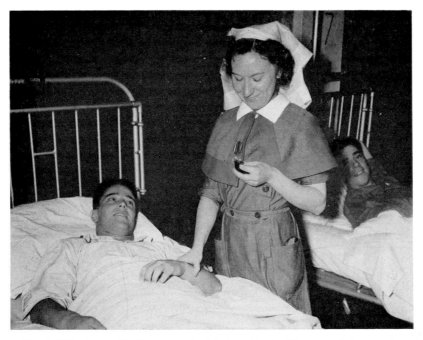

FIGURE 28.—A U.S. Army Air Forces patient being attended by one of the nursing sisters
at Royal Cornwall Infirmary, Truro, Cornwall, England.

of the buildings was underway following a bombing of the infirmary. When
reporting the approval received from the trustees, Colonel Cutler added that a
surgical unit consisting of two surgeons, one operating room nurse, four ward
nurses, and their necessary equipment was ready to go at the 5th General Hospital. General Hawley and Colonel Cutler visited the 5th General Hospital
on 6 March and looked over the equipment for the team. On 14 March, the
director of the Royal Cornwall Infirmary telephoned Colonel Cutler that the
institution was ready to receive the American contingent. The next day, Col.
Maxwell G. Keeler, MC, commanding officer of the 5th General Hospital, and
Major Zollinger went to Truro to make final arrangements. Ten days later,
the surgical unit was well established and working. Their work and attitude
created a most favorable impression at the infirmary (fig. 28). Within a month,
as planned, this unit from the 5th General Hospital was relieved and returned to
its parent unit, and a team of similar composition from the 3d Auxiliary Surgical Group took over its functions.

In the meanwhile, suggestions to provide surgical teams to other areas
in which the Air Forces were operating did not materialize since Colonel
Grow, after considerable thought on the matter, felt that the use of these
teams might erroneously suggest to the British that their services were inferior.

In London on 31 March, Colonel Cutler was privileged to attend another
brilliant discussion on mobile surgical units, given, this time, by Col. Arthur E.
Porritt, RAMC, at the RAMC Post-Graduate Medical School (p. 71). On

6 April 1943, Colonel Cutler received a communication from the British War Office, issued by the consulting surgeon, General Monro, which quoted items of information from the Middle East theater on the outstanding success the field surgical units had encountered. General Monro, in commenting on the reports, agreed that lighting was one of the main problems since, as one unit reported, 80 percent of the work had been during hours of darkness. A most important point, General Monro noted, was as follow: "If F.S.U.'s are to give of their best, they *must train together not only in field exercises but in the operating theatre.* Commands should be instructed to see to it, that the F.S.U.'s now mobilized in this country, relieve, as a team, one of the existing surgical teams in a static unit, for a period of 3 to 4 weeks." [42]

Finally, on 12 April, Colonel Cutler heard General Hood, DGMS, British Army, explain to a group of medical officers in the British Southern Command the new organization of the RAMC field medical service which currently featured an advanced surgical center. This advanced surgical center, comprised of a field dressing station, a field surgical unit, and a field transfusion unit, had 20 cots and many litters and was to perform only urgent surgery— abdominals, sucking chest wounds, wounds of the buttocks, and compound fractures, especially in the joints. They were assignable on the basis of two per combat division.

Armed with this wealth of recent information on the efficacy of mobile surgical units in combat plus detailed and complete reports on the workings of the team at Truro, submitted by Colonel Keeler and Major Zollinger, Colonel Cutler dictated a memorandum, dated 18 April 1943, to the Chief Surgeon (through Colonel Kimbrough) which brought up to date his complete thinking on the matter of mobile surgical teams for the U.S. Army in the European theater. The body of the memorandum follows:

1. *Introductory.*

This memorandum on surgical teams is added to those which have preceded it because the need for mobility in our forces is increasing, and because of recent attempts to reorganize the teams as they now appear in the Auxiliary Surgical Group.

2. The regrouping of teams in the Auxiliary Surgical Group was submitted to the Chief Surgeon by Colonel Mason. In this regrouping it was made clear that practical experience in this war had but corroborated the experience obtained in the last war, that the surgeon in the forward area must be a general surgeon. In the last war we had: *a.* General surgical teams, *b.* Shock teams, *c.* Splint teams. This resulted because experience showed that the general surgeon must be the one to do the work in the forward area. Also it was found he needed as a colleague somebody to help put on the splints when compound fractures existed, just as he will today need such an expert colleague to put on the plaster for immobilization rather than the Thomas' splint used in the last war. Also, if the general surgeon is to be kept busy all the time at what he is bound to do, i.e. surgical operations, he should have as a further colleague a man trained in resuscitation and shock who can treat the cases before an operation and then care for them afterwards, thus freeing the surgeon's time for constant application to his handicraft in the operating theater. This combination of experts needs highly trained personnel working at top speed in their selected fields, and accomplishes the maximum overturn of labor in the shortest period of time. It would appear to me that the Auxiliary Surgical Group

---

[42] Dispatch, The War Office, London, 2 April 1943, subject: Field Units (F.S.U.'s. M.E.F.W.E.).

teams should be re-organized on a basis similar to the thinking above. In my mind, the best team would be one in which the surgeon was a general surgeon, the assistant surgeon, however, an orthopedic individual or at least a surgeon properly trained in plaster technique. In addition, each surgical team would need a man trained in shock * * * though I believe that where two surgical teams were out together to a single installation, one shock team might care for the work of two surgical teams. The defect in the Auxiliary Group is that they only carry with them their instruments and would have to be given all of the rest of the impedimenta of operating theaters by the hospital to which they were attached.

3. *Mobile surgical teams.*

The use of the term "mobile surgical team" is coined to describe a setup somewhat different to that above, for in this setup the team is to have its own transport and take with it everything it needs in the way of professional supplies to cover the completion of 100 major surgical operations. This is to include lights, bandages, a shock team setup, plasma, saline, basins to scrub up their hands in, soap, drugs, anesthetics, etc. Such a team could be sent at a moment's notice because it has its own transportation to any point desired by the corps or army surgeon. To my way of thinking it might best be placed at the clearing company of a division, and the only matter which is not settled in our minds is whether this mobile surgical group, with its team and shock men and supplies should take its own tentage or not * * *.

As stated in previous memoranda, I am opposed to building in of the apparatus into the truck, feeling that something might happen to the truck and thus immobilize the team. If the material can be easily put into a truck and then taken out, then any truck will suffice, and complete freedom and mobility is assured. The TB/A of such a mobile surgical team as opposed to the teams now organized in our Surgical Group is appended. It is largely the system set up by the group from the 5th General Hospital, with changes, both deletions and additions, as suggested in our Consultant Group and by our British colleagues.

On 21 April 1943, Colonel Cutler conferred with General Monro and Maj. Gen. Max Page, RAMC, at the British AMD, 39 Hyde Park Gate, London (fig. 29). He discussed with them the matter of tents for a mobile surgical unit, a part of the plans which had not been firmed. He was also shown a lantern which burned kerosene under pressure with a brilliance of some 400 cp. It seemed to be the ideal unit for providing emergency lighting for the mobile surgical team in the event of power failure, and Colonel Cutler on his return immediately ordered a sample unit for trial and study. Later that week, he was able, with the cooperation of Col. Charles E. Brenn, MC, the U.S. V Corps surgeon, to select and set up tenting for the proposed mobile surgical team. The feasibility of the tents for operating pavilions was tested, particularly under blackout conditions.

In a letter, dated 6 May 1943, to General Hawley through Colonel Kimbrough, Colonel Cutler submitted complete proposed tables of organization and equipment for a mobile surgical unit composed of a surgical team and a transfusion-laboratory team. The proposed organization included:

For the surgical team:

   1 general surgeon, chief
   1 assistant surgeon, preferably trained in plaster technique
   1 anesthetist, officer or enlisted
   3 operating room technicians, enlisted

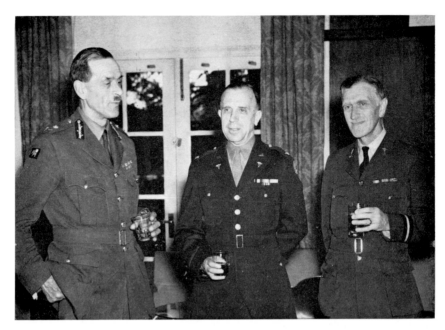

FIGURE 29.—Maj. Gen. Max Page, RAMC (left), and Air Commodore Geoffrey Keynes, consulting surgeon to RAF (right), with Col. Oramel H. Stanley, MC, at the reception and dinner given in their honor by General Hawley and his consultant group.

For the shock team:
    1 officer, preferably a physician
    2 technicians, enlisted
The organization also called for two drivers to drive and maintain the unit's vehicles, one 2½-ton truck, and one ¾-ton weapons carrier (fig. 30). Assistant drivers, he stated, could be trained from among the enlisted men of the surgical and shock teams.

With reference to the shock team (fig. 31), Colonel Cutler explained:

We have called the second group a transfusion-laboratory group because as we visualize the work of a surgical team in the forward area it will require a transfusion team to attend to the resuscitation of its patients before the operation and to care for them afterwards. Moreover, this group will do work such as blood counts, examination of the urine, determination of hemoglobin for better treatment of shock, occasional microscopic examination of smear preparations from joints, spinal canal, etc., and occasional microscopic examination of the bacterial flora in the wound, where the finding of gas bacillus forms might strengthen one's hands before amputation.

All the medical supplies and equipment were packed into 18 trunks with a total weight of approximately one ton, except for a few bulky items such as splints and litters. Of these 18 trunks, 16 used the container for medical chest number 1 with a total packed weight of approximately 1,800 pounds, and 2 used the container for medical chest number 2 with a total packed weight of approximately 250 pounds. The basic instrument set, stock number 93212, 1942 model,

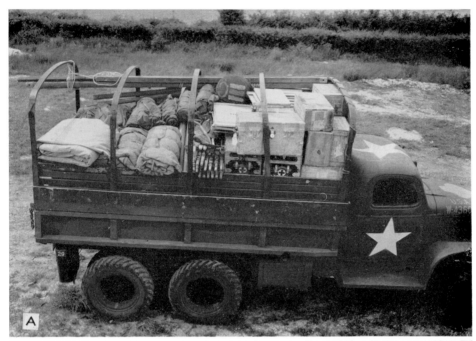

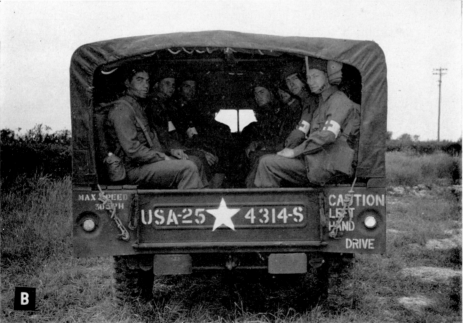

FIGURE 30.—Transport for a mobile surgical unit. A. A truck loaded with the complete equipment and supplies for a unit. B. A weapons carrier used for the transport of personnel.

was used with a few extra instruments from special sets for neurosurgery, orthopedic surgery (fig. 32), abdominal surgery, et cetera. Included also was a complete anesthesia set, stock number 93512, endotracheal, inhalation, intravenous, regional, and spinal, 1942 model (fig. 33), and a suction machine, complete, stock number 37750 (fig. 34). Expendables, such as dressings, bandages, adhesive tape, gauze, cotton, plaster, towels, sponges, suture material, anesthetics, medicinals, crystalloids, and the like, were packed in quantities sufficient for 200 surgical operations (fig. 35).

The tent decided upon for the operating theater was that known as a tent, storage, camouflaged, with fly (fig. 36). All possible equipment and supplies for emergency sources of lighting—battery-operated lanterns and surgical lights and a 2.5 kw. gasoline-operated generator—were included (fig. 37). The common oil-burning pot-bellied stoves were added for heating purposes. The final list of supplies and equipment, Colonel Cutler advised the Chief Surgeon, was made in conjunction with the members of the 5th General Hospital who assisted in the preparation of the list and had some further suggestions after returning from their temporary duty at Truro. He suggested that the responsibility for replenishing supplies of any particular team would rest with the parent unit from which the team personnel were derived (for example, an auxiliary surgical group), and the parent unit would be based for supply support on a field army.

On Tuesday, 18 May, General Hawley and Colonel Cutler journeyed to the 5th General Hospital and held a showdown inspection of the mobile surgical unit as constituted in the 6 May letter to the Chief Surgeon. After their return from the hospital, General Hawley and Colonel Cutler had a long talk on the proposed unit. General Hawley's opinions follow:

1. The 5th General Hospital should assemble in Salisbury (where the hospital was located) all the equipment finally selected for a mobile surgical unit.

2. The 5th General Hospital should secure still and moving pictures of this unit in all phases, including putting up tents and operating upon a patient.

3. Officers in the 5th General Hospital should write up separately how the unit functions as a whole and how the transfusion-laboratory team is to function.

4. The equipment for a single mobile surgical unit should then be transferred to the 3d Auxiliary Surgical Group after they have been taught how it functions, including the putting up and taking down of the tents.

5. It will be the responsibility of the 3d Auxiliary Surgical Group to teach the rest of their teams this same matter and to teach in the Medical Field Service School at Shrivenham, if that was desired.

6. The headquarters of the auxiliary surgical group should acquire facilities for sterilizing dry goods so that, as the parent organization, it could keep the dispersed units supplied with materials.[43]

---

[43] Letter, Col. E. C. Cutler, MC, to Col. J. C. Kimbrough, MC, 22 May 1943, subject: Further Regarding Mobile Surgical Unit.

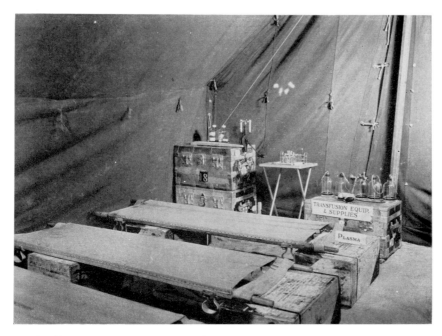

FIGURE 31.—The equipment and supplies for a shock team, mobile surgical unit, set up for use. The boxes on which the cots rest are plasma cartons.

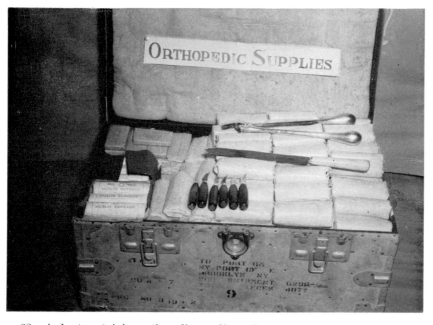

FIGURE 32.—A chest containing orthopedic supplies and equipment for a mobile surgical unit.

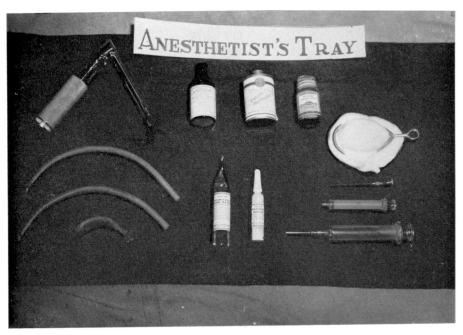

FIGURE 33.—A tray used by the anesthetist of a mobile surgical unit.

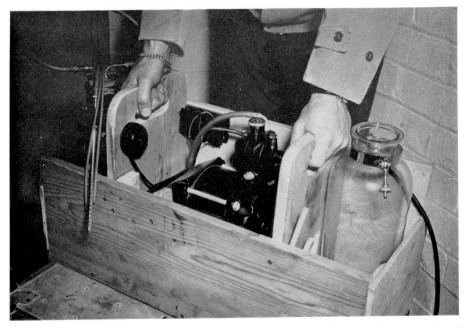

FIGURE 34.—A suction apparatus with an improvised holder, used by a mobile surgical unit.

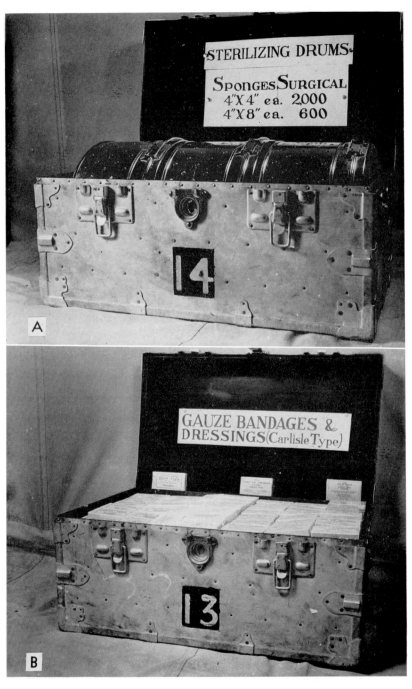

FIGURE 35.—Expendables and a sterilizing drum of a mobile surgical unit. A. A steriliz-ing drum, packed in a Medical Department chest and containing surgical sponges. B. Gauze bandages and dressings sufficient for 200 surgical operations.

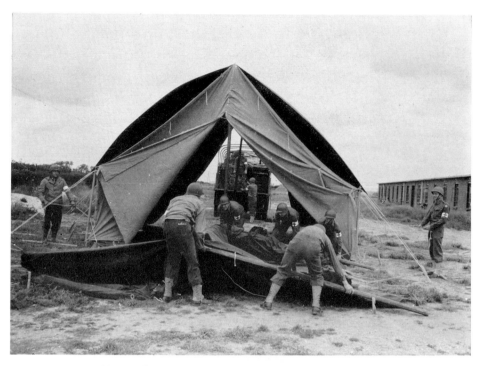

FIGURE 36.—Pitching an operating room tent of a mobile surgical unit.

Finally, in a hectic rush to complete all aspects of the mobile surgical unit plan prior to his trip to the U.S.S.R., Colonel Cutler was able to report to the Chief Surgeon by letter, on 15 June 1943, the following:

Certain changes have been made in the TBA submitted [6 May 1943], and we now submit TBA in final form after repeated experimentation in packing and unpacking and experimentation with tents.

Many photographs have been taken of the unit * * * during processes of assembly and with patients being operated upon in the tent (fig. 38). These should arrive shortly. A film including the setting up operation and taking down of the unit, has been made and is now being put in order by the Signal Corps, and should also be in your hands shortly.

Lt. Col. Robert Zollinger who has been experimenting with this problem under our guidance since February 1943, is writing up the complete functioning of the unit in the hope that you will send this back to The Surgeon General for his information and publication.

We have arranged with Major Pisani, E.T.O. Medical Field Service School, that this unit be demonstrated as a part of the exercises in the next classes.

While the principles of assembling the necessary equipment for the supply of a surgical team in the performance of at least a hundred major operations was followed by auxiliary surgical groups, it was rarely, if ever, necessary for a surgical team to function as an isolated unit during the combat period of operations on the Continent during 1944–45. Instead of utilizing their own tentage, lighting, and other heavy equipment, surgical teams invariably utilized the facilities of the unit to which they were attached; that is, field and evacuation

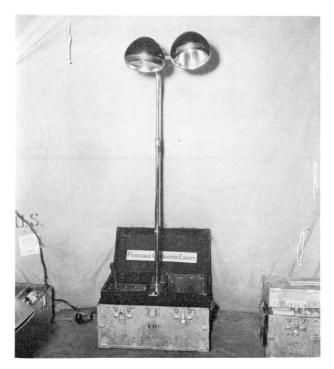

FIGURE 37.—Portable operating light, equipment of a mobile surgical unit.

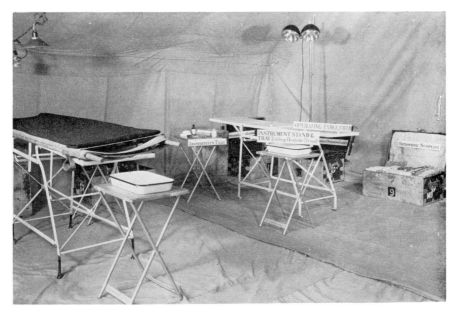

FIGURE 38.—The arrangement of the operating tables of a mobile surgical unit.

hospitals. The teams carried with them and frequently utilized certain surgical instruments and other small medical supply items organic to the auxiliary surgical group.

Surgical mission to Union of Soviet Socialist Republics

Background.—Colonel Cutler, in a memorandum, dated 15 January 1943, advised General Hawley as follows:

Some months ago when you were ill, I attended a dinner given by Mr. Broster, following his first Inter-Allied Medical Meeting. In responding for you I thanked President Tidy and the group in the Royal Society of Medicine of our colleagues for all that they have done for us. I then pointed out what I thought might be the value of all the Allied people getting to know something of each other. At that time I said I was greatly concerned that I had been unable to meet a Russian, and I thought this was a pity, and wondered if there are any Russians in London. Sir Wilson Jameson and Sir Alfred Webb-Johnson and other people who knew all about the Russian difficulty, and that a British hospital ship had even reached Murmansk and had been turned back again, were much upset. They have talked to me repeatedly about this, and apparently had been to the Foreign Office again. I learned yesterday that a request might shortly be made for three British medical officers, and three American medical officers, to visit Russia. I thought you should be apprised of this possibility early. It appears to me that a country who must have had millions of casualties should be able to teach us a good deal about military surgery and military medicine.

Colonel Cutler's diary states, for 29 January: "I'm getting worse at this [keeping up the diary], just when it is getting interesting. For example, Russia. I have long been worried I couldn't find a Russian. I've spoken of it as a reason for the Inter-Allied Conferences. I spoke of it at a dinner with Fraser, Sir Wilson Jameson, Sir Alfred Webb-Johnson, Dean * * * of the Graduate Schools, and Broster (his dinner). As a result, I now have a commission of 3 British and 3 American medical officers to be asked to go to Russia."

Colonel Cutler had just returned to Cheltenham from a trip to London, Basingstoke, and Chatham on the morning of Saturday, 10 April, when General Hawley called him to his office in the afternoon and instructed him to see the U.S. Ambassador in London about the trip to the Soviet Union. Dutifully, Colonel Cutler turned around, went back to London the next day, and saw John G. Winant, U.S. Ambassador to the Court of St. James's (fig. 39), in the late afternoon. On 16 April, he reported on this meeting by letter to General Hawley (through Colonel Kimbrough). A portion of this letter follows:

We discussed at great length the rumored joint medical mission of British and American service personnel to Russia. He reported previous discussions re Russia and happenings in Russia that bore small relation to this problem. He reported the Typhus Commission was turned down. * * * The urgency of the matter was again brought to his attention when I told him that on April 16 Surgeon Rear Admiral Gordon-Taylor was lunching with M. Maisky, the Russian Ambassador, * * *, and that members of the British Commission were now instructed to get their passports. (British Commission headed by Surgeon Rear Admiral Gordon-Taylor, other members, Maj. Gen. Monro, Mr. Rock Carling.) Finally he promised * * * to see M. Maisky, Mr. Eden, and Sir Edward Mellanby [on 15 April], and give you a final report.

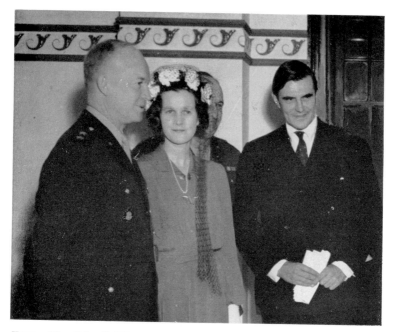

FIGURE 39.—John G. Winant, U.S. Ambassador to the Court of St. James's, and Mrs. Winant with Gen. Dwight D. Eisenhower.

Mission established.—On 19 April, Colonel Cutler was given a message to call Admiral Gordon-Taylor. Mrs. Gordon-Taylor answered and informed Colonel Cutler that he and Lt. Col. Loyal Davis, MC, were to go to the Soviet Union with the English mission (fig. 40). Colonel Cutler was elated. He recorded: "This is something I have been working on for 4 weeks and indeed feel partly responsible for. Now I am getting somewhere! We're to go in about 3 weeks; in May. Know nothing more. Of course it is a risk, but that is small compared to what others are doing. I'm happy for a moment."

Preparations for departure.—The next few weeks were kaleidoscopic for the Chief Consultant in Surgery. There was so much to be done before leaving, and yet details concerning the mission to the U.S.S.R. took time in themselves.

On Wednesday, 21 April, he had tea with Admiral Gordon-Taylor who informed Colonel Cutler that the mission would depart on or about 15 May; that the English members would be Admiral Gordon-Taylor, General Monro, Mr. R. (later Sir Reginald) Watson-Jones, Civilian Consultant in Orthopedic Surgery to the Royal Air Force, and Mr. Ernest Rock Carling; and that the U.S. representatives would be Colonel Cutler and Colonel Davis. Admiral Gordon-Taylor also confided to Colonel Cutler that he was learning Russian. Later that day, Colonel Cutler had a talk with General Hawley, after which he recorded: "[General Hawley] informed me that the Ambassador thought: (1) There should be separate missions, and (2) three U.S. members. General Hawley and I agreed the joint mission was best. As to the third member, the

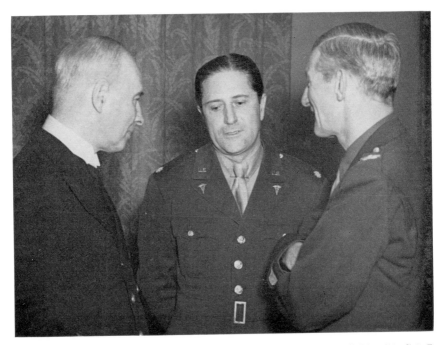

Figure 40.—American members of the surgical mission to the U.S.S.R., Lt. Col. Loyal Davis, MC (center), and Colonel Cutler, with Surgeon Rear Admiral Gordon Gordon-Taylor, RN, head of the mission.

Russians would like men of high academic standing in surgery [professors of surgery]. The General thought Loyal Davis and I were the only ones here who filled the bill."

The next day, because there was some uncertainty as to who was to head the American representation, Colonel Cutler spoke again with General Hawley who confirmed the fact that Colonel Cutler would head the American representation. He then saw Admiral Gordon-Taylor again. The admiral approved the giving of fellowships to two famous Soviet surgeons, N. Burdenko and Serge Yudin,[44] by the American College of Surgeons, and Colonel Cutler went back to General Hawley with this information.

By the middle of May, Colonel Cutler and Colonel Davis had written to the American College of Surgeons for permission to bestow the honorary fellowships. The ceremonial hoods had been borrowed from two Englishmen, Admiral Gordon-Taylor and Mr. Harry Platt, with the promise that these would later be replaced. The speech of investiture was then approved by General Hawley. There was also some confusion as to the diplomatic channels through which the names of the American representatives would be submitted to the Soviet Government, but the matter was eventually taken care of and

---

[44] The variation in the spelling of the names of Russian individuals in this volume is due to the fact that there are two systems of transliteration in use.

passports were obtained on 11 May. On 13 May, Professor Sarkisov, an assistant to Academician Burdenko, arrived in England from Vladivostok and was introduced at a luncheon held at the Royal College of Surgeons. He gave the most comforting assurance that the mission would, in all probability, be warmly welcomed in the Soviet Union. And, finally, word was received that Prof. Wilder G. Penfield of McGill University, Montreal, Canada, would be added to the mission.

There was no further clarification, as of 15 May, as to when the mission would leave. But, with the arrival of Professor Penfield, the membership of the mission was complete, and amenities preparatory to departure continued at a high pace. As an example, on 24 May there was a luncheon given by the British Council for the mission at Claridge's in London. There was also a serious talk with the U.S. Ambassador on what to do and not to do while in the Soviet Union. Finally, there was tea at the Soviet Embassy, 13 Kensington Palace Gardens, given by Ambassador Maisky. With respect to the Soviet ambassador's tea, Colonel Cutler's comment was: "Tremendous." As to the meeting with Ambassador Winant, Colonel Cutler reported as follows in a letter to Colonel Kimbrough, dated 30 May 1943:

* * * He gave Colonel Davis and myself explicit verbal instructions, but said he did not wish to give us anything in writing, emphasizing that we should use our own discretion, and hoping that we would get on well with our Russian colleagues. The latter was emphasized as highly important, since if this mission is happily received others of great importance may be allowed to follow. Ambassador Winant made it very clear that the instructions to which we should adhere closely were to discuss nothing except professional medical matters. He emphasized this point by stories of diplomacy wrecked on the rocks of missions going beyond their protocol. He urged us to take anything with us that could enlighten the Russians on American surgical methods, and hoped we might bring back matters of importance to our people.

The Ambassador also promised Colonel Cutler a list of American diplomatic officials in the countries through which the mission would travel en route to and from the Soviet Union.

Soviet motion picture.—On 31 May 1943, Colonel Cutler was privileged to see, at the Soviet Embassy, a motion picture depicting the care given the wounded Soviet Army soldier during his evacuation from the front to the rear and through his rehabilitation. His account of the film showing in a letter to Colonel Kimbrough, dated 5 June 1943, follows:

This was a battle picture and most interesting. Soldiers were picked up on the battlefield and given preliminary First Aid by a trained first aider. They then passed through battalion and divisional aid posts and to hospitals similar to our surgical hospitals, where definitive surgery was carried out. Certainly a great attempt was made to give as adequate care as possible, and every effort was made to restore the soldier to active duty as soon as possible.

The most important observations of interest to me were:

The use of women in the forward area. Women were even in the divisional aid posts of casualty clearing companies, and from the expressions on soldiers' faces, even without the spoken word, one felt sure that their presence was of great moral value. * * *

Cleaning and bathing facilities. Here, the Russians, whom we have not thought of as a clean people, can give all of us a very good lesson. They had excellent bathing facilities in their most forward hospitals, and spoke of such facilities as equally important to good surgery. * * *

Air transport. This was greatly emphasized in the film, and is used in the care of wounded amongst the guerillas, which is a part of the obligation of the Russian Medical Corps.

"Like politics at home."—The motion picture served to increase the desires of the mission members to see the Soviet medical service first hand, but the actual departure was not to be for quite some time. Partially, perhaps, as a result of this interminable waiting, the solidarity among the members became strained. By the time 13 June arrived and the mission was still awaiting travel instructions, Colonel Cutler was quite concerned. So, apparently, was General Hawley, for he called Colonel Cutler by telephone and asked him about the situation. There were varying claims as to how the mission had originated and who was responsible for its establishment. There was a question as to who was going to head the mission. Instead of the senior military members from the United States and the United Kingdom, there were strong indications that Colonel Davis was being selected to represent the National Research Council of the United States and that Mr. Ernest Rock Carling would represent the British Medical Research Council.

"Real trouble is my worry over the Russian mission," the diary entry for 13 June reads, "Have warned General Hawley and C. Spruit—the whole thing is loaded with dynamite."

The following inkling of this warning is mentioned in the diary on 17 June:

Conference with Ambassador, 2:30 PM, and then with General Hawley. General Hawley is to see the Ambassador at 4:30. No definite news, but PRH wrote our orders: "To help Gordon Gordon-Taylor, head of mission, and to carry out mission's protocol * * *." Also, I saw PRH's wire to The Surgeon General (written after phone call with me 2 or 3 days ago). Stated:
   1. Mission arranged by British
   2. American members invited by British
   3. Professional protocol (not military)
   4. Advises against further powers mixing into this.

The next day, Friday, 18 June, Colonel Cutler reviewed General Hawley's meeting with Ambassador Winant, as follows:

Saw General Hawley after he saw Ambassador Winant. As I thought, the Ambassador wants Loyal [Davis] to represent National Research Council in mufti. General Hawley told the Ambassador that was a mistake. The Ambassador asked if he could go to Devers! Of course, General Hawley said yes. General Hawley also saw a letter from Eden saying we leave in about a week via Cairo. Good.

So strong was this rumor about members of the mission going to the Soviet Union in mufti that Admiral Gordon-Taylor had gone to Surgeon Vice Admiral S. (Sir Sheldon) Dudley, DGMS, Royal Navy, and had asked him about it. Sir Sheldon had simply stated that Admiral Gordon-Taylor would go in uniform or else he would not go at all.[45]

---

[45] Letter, Sir Gordon Gordon-Taylor to Paul R. Hawley, M.D., 9 October 1958.

Finally, on Sunday, 20 June, after receiving a message from Mr. Carling, Colonel Cutler felt constrained to admit that it was all "too bad—like politics at home."

Departure.—The mission finally departed on 28 June 1943 with the military members in uniform. Admiral Gordon-Taylor, as one of the two ranking military members of the mission and representing the senior British service, the Royal Navy, had been officially recognized as the head of the mission. Colonel Davis had been confirmed as the representative of the Committee for Medical Research of the National Research Council, U.S.A.; Mr. Carling, as the representative for the Medical Research Council of Great Britain; and Professor Penfield, for the Medical Research Council of Canada. Mr. Watson-Jones was going as a civilian consultant to the Royal Air Force. General Hawley had approved the taking of 2,000,000 units of penicillin from the stockpile at the 2d General Hospital as a gift for the Soviet peoples. And, finally, all official papers which were to be taken by the mission had been censored and sealed.[46]

Desires of mission expressed.—The mission, upon arriving in Moscow, was delayed in getting about its business for reasons unknown. The members of the mission took the opportunity to compose a memorandum to the Soviet authorities on its intents and desires, as follows:

The Delegation of American, British and Canadian surgeons wishes to thank the Soviet authorities for having so kindly made possible their visit to the Soviet Union, and hopes during its stay to study the methods used by Soviet surgeons in the treatment of battle casualties, reports on the success of which have made so deep an impression on the medical authorities in Canada, Great Britain and the United States.

The study of the methods used by Soviet surgeons for the treatment of fractures caused by weapons of war is the primary object of the Delegation.

The second object of the Delegation is to confer on Professors Burdenko and Yudin, who are known abroad as two of the most distinguished surgeons of the Soviet Union, Honorary Fellowships of the Royal College of Surgeons of England and Honorary Fellowships of the American College of Surgeons.

As regards the second of these objects, the Delegation is anxious to come to an agreement with the People's Commissariat regarding the date and place of the ceremony at which the Fellowships will be conferred. The Delegation trusts that the ceremony will be conducted with due dignity and publicity and that the People's Commissariat will agree that the diplomatic representatives of Great Britain and the United States should be invited to attend. For purposes of record in Great Britain and the United States it would be appreciated if the ceremony could be photographed and prints made available to the Delegation before its departure.

As regards the first object of the mission, the study of Soviet methods of treating fractures caused by weapons of war, the Delegation trusts that it will be given opportunities of seeing the work of Soviet surgeons at all stages in the treatment of battle casualties, and that each member of the Delegation will be able to discuss with Soviet

---

[46] An account of the observations of Lt. Col. Loyal Davis, while he was en route to the Soviet Union, his commentary on activities engaged in while he was in that country, and his remarks concerning the return trip comprise pages 420–439 of this volume. Any personal papers which Colonel Cutler may have maintained during the trip to the U.S.S.R. were not available to the compilers of this chapter. The full official report prepared jointly by Colonel Cutler and Colonel Davis is added to this volume as appendix A. It should be referred to as an integral part of Colonel Davis' chapter as well as of this chapter.—J. B. C., Jr.

surgeons specializing in his field the problems in which he is particularly interested. The Delegation believes that this could best be accomplished if facilities were granted for visiting forward medical units, inspecting methods for the evacuation of the wounded, and visiting hospital units, medical institutions and rehabilitation centres in the base area.

The Delegation, in addition to fulfilling the two basic objects described above, would be glad to learn of any other surgical procedures which the Soviet authorities may consider of interest in the treatment of battle casualties, and the members of the Delegation, if requested to do so, will gladly furnish any information which they may themselves possess.

The British members of the Delegation have been requested by various medical organizations in the United Kingdom to present to the Soviet authorities a list of medical questions which it has not been possible to raise hitherto owing to the absence of any convenient channel of communication. The Delegation would be most grateful if facilities could be offered to its members to study these questions during their visit.

The Delegation has brought a number of publications and photographs which may be of interest not merely to individual surgeons, but to the Soviet medical authorities in general, who may already have been made acquainted with them by their representatives abroad, such as Professor Sarkisov in Great Britain and Professor Lebedenko in the United States. The Delegation would be glad to learn whether books and journals of this nature are of assistance to the Soviet authorities and if so whether the Soviet authorities would like to be regularly supplied with similar publications.

The Delegation has brought 2,000,000 units of Penicillin which the United States Medical Corps wish to present to the Soviet medical authorities.

Certain members of the Delegation have also brought a number of new surgical instruments for presentation to the appropriate medical authorities at the discretion of the People's Commissariat.

Several members of the Delegation carry with them letters of introduction and greeting addressed to prominent Soviet surgeons. They would be grateful for advice as to the correct procedure for transmitting these letters to the addressees.

A number of members of the Delegation have also brought in their individual capacities certain publications on surgery which they would like to present to individual Soviet surgeons interested in the various fields of surgery which the publications cover. In some instances the members of the Delegation have in mind the individual Soviet surgeons to whom they wish to present these publications. In others they would welcome the advice of the People's Commissariat regarding the most suitable candidate for presentation. In both cases the advice of the People's Commissariat is sought regarding the procedure to be followed.

The Ministry of Supply have requested the Soviet Trade Delegation in London to clear up certain questions connected with medical supplies ordered by the Soviet authorities. While not wishing to duplicate their request for elucidation of certain items which they have not properly understood, the Ministry have informed Mr. Rock Carling of the points on which they require further information, and Mr. Rock Carling would be glad to discuss these points with the competent Soviet authorities if the latter should consider it desirable. There are in addition one or two other questions of detail regarding medical supplies to the Soviet Union which the Delegation is anxious to raise.

General Monro has brought with him certain memoranda regarding the work of the Directorate of Army Psychiatry. If the Soviet military authorities are interested in this branch of medicine he would be glad to make available to them the material which he has brought with him.

Lastly, if the Soviet authorities should wish to discuss questions of medical research or explore the possibility of establishing closer medical liaison between the Union of Soviet Socialist Republics and the countries represented by the Delegation, the Delegation would be glad to discuss these questions with them. The surgeons who represent the

Surgical Committee of (1) The Medical Research Council of Great Britain (Mr. Rock Carling) ; (2) The Committee for Medical Research and the National Research Council, U.S.A. (Lt. Col. Loyal Davis) ; (3) The National Research Council of Canada (Prof. Wilder Penfield) will also gladly discuss the work of these Committees and the methods by which surgical information is now being exchanged between these three countries for the use of the various combatant services.

Investiture of Burdenko and Yudin into Royal College of Surgeons and American College of Surgeons.—One of the highpoints of the delegation's visit to the Soviet Union was the conferring of honorary fellowships to Academician Lt. Gen. Nicolai Nilovich Burdenko and Prof. Serge S. Yudin in the Royal College of Surgeons and the American College of Surgeons. Academician Burdenko occupied a position in the Soviet Army Medical Service equivalent to that of chief consultant in surgery. Professor Yudin had been outstanding for his surgical accomplishments at the Sklifossowsky Institute. The investiture of these two eminent Soviet surgeons into the American College of Surgeons was accomplished by Colonel Cutler and Colonel Davis. The formalities were preceded by the following address presented by Colonel Cutler:

This gathering is momentous. We doctors now signify to the solidarity and common purpose of a majority of living peoples. The occasion justifies the hope that this junction of our races is but the beginning of a friendly and cooperative liaison for all time. As a token of this spiritual union Colonel Davis and I are empowered to grant Honorary Fellowships in the American College of Surgeons to two distinguished Russian surgeons, a function which heretofore has never occurred beyond the confines of our own country.

     *   *   *   *   *   *   *

We congratulate ourselves that in this tumultuous world men of such eminence have found in service to the State a way of life that brings satisfaction to all.

Academician General Burdenko's acknowledgment (fig. 41) of this unprecedented and unique honor of being made a member of both these great organizations simultaneously and on soil foreign to the sponsoring organizations follows:

I am deeply moved by the honor of electing me member of the American College of Surgeons.

I understand this honor as a generous approval of my papers and my work in the past and present. It makes me think about my work in the future, particularly now when the fight against Fascists has reached a decisive stage.

I recognize this election to be of deep and wide meaning.

The last decade has shown that the United States is now the center of medical science, and scientific problems are to be solved from the point of view of American science.

During this year I have received very many proofs of attention from the United States.

My contributions to world science and field surgery are but modest. It pleases me to share this great honor with all surgeons of my country.

The acknowledgment by Professor Yudin (fig. 42) of the honor bestowed upon him follows:

You will easily understand my animation when immediately after one high honor the surgeons of a second great Allied country—the U.S.A.—bestow on me another.

Illustrious Colleague,

I am deeply moved by the honour of electing me member of the American Surgeon Society.

I understand this honour as a generous approval of my papers and my work in the past and present. It makes me think about my work in the future, particularly now when the fight against fascists has reached a decisive stage.

I recognise this election to be of deep and wide meaning.

Last decade has shown that the United States is now the center of medical science and scientific problems are to be solved from the point of view of American Science.

During this year I have received very many proves of attention from the United States.

My tributions to world science and field surgery are but modest. It tends me to share this great honour with all surgeons of my country.

Yours very respectfully,

Academician, General

N. Burdenko

15. VII. 43

FIGURE 41.—A copy of Academician Lt. Gen. Nicolai N. Burdenko's speech upon his being made an Honorary Fellow of the American College of Surgeons.

I know little of your beautiful country. I am proud of my personal acquaintance-ship—and even friendship—with George Crile, Howard Kelly, the late Mayo brothers, and some other American surgeons of world fame.

But could I dream 15 years ago that the time would come when I should not only become an honorary fellow of the American College of Surgeons, but should also receive my degree and this diploma from the hands of the great Harvey Cushing's successor.

By the way, it is an astonishing fact that the day of my decoration by the Allies completely coincides with the day I was severely wounded by a German shell on the eve of July 15, 1915.

For the second time in the same quarter of a century our nations are united in their hard efforts to save their countries and the world's civilization. Now, just as it was the first time, we are fighting with the same eternal dangerous enemy—Germany. But as it was on the first occasion, our British Allies are fighting again on our side.

Victory will be ours. Nobody has any doubts about it, even our enemies. Let our scientific relations which have begun in a time of such strained military needs get stronger and flourish more and more after this victory and the won peace.

In the time of struggle, surgery is as necessary for victory as arms, transport, and all kinds of supplies. But when the last gun of the enemy ceases and released humanity turns with hope to the restoration of great destruction caused by the war, we surgeons will have to heal the wounds and injuries of hundreds of thousands of people, who have won for us this victory.

Your high election of me as honorary fellow of the American College of Surgeons will serve as a new additional stimulus for further development of my scientific work in sur-gery, which has already received from you such high estimation.

I once more deeply and sincerely thank you.

The official acknowledgment of this auspicious event on behalf of the So-viet Government was made by Vice Commissar Kolesnikov, who said:

The admission today of two outstanding Russian surgeons, Academician Burdenko and Professor Yudin to the honorary fellowship of the Royal College of Surgeons of Eng-land presents itself to us, witnesses of this act, as an occasion of great cultural and po-litical meaning.

The Royal College of Surgeons of England since long ago has been famed as an orga-nization, responsible in no small way for the development of surgery both in England and outside her boundaries. Amongst the fellows of this College have been, and are now some of the outstanding representatives of English surgical thought. The greatest ex-ponents of surgery of other countries have earned the honor of being honorary fellows of this College since its creation, in accordance with its established and glorious traditions. On every occasion the selection of honorary fellows amongst foreign scientists has been an unbiased and just appreciation of their really great technical contributions. Therefore, selection to an honorary fellowship of the Royal College of Surgeons of England has always been a distinction in the eyes of the world's scholars. Similarly, the glory of the American College of Surgeons is well known.

We are glad in the knowledge that, today, the choice of the Royal College of Surgeons and the American College of Surgeons should have fallen on the two best representatives of our native surgery. Both the new honorary fellows of the Colleges, Academician Bur-denko and Professor Yudin, are deservedly famed in our country, and outside her boundaries, as leading experts in the realm of their specialties. Not for nothing are they both worthy of the highest scientific decoration of our country—the Stalin Prize; whilst Academician Burdenko with honor holds the title of Hero of Socialist Work.

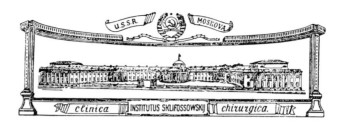

Colonel Cutler, Gentlemen,

You will easily understand my animation when immediately
after one high honor the surgeons of a second Great Allied Country
- U.S.A. - bestow on me another one.

I know a little your beautiful country. I am proud of
my personal acquantance - and even friendship - with Geoge CRILE,
Howard KELLY,the late MAYO brothers and some other American surgeons
with the world fame.

But could I dream 15 years ago that time would come when
I should not only become an Honorary Fellow of the American College
of Surgeons,but also should recieve my degree and this diploma from
the hands of the great Harvey CUSHING'S successor.

By the way, it is an astonishing fact that the day of my decoration by the Allies completely coinsid's wmith the day I was severely wounded by a german shell on the eve of July 15-th 1915.

For the second time in the same quarter of a century our
nations are united in their hard efforts to save their countries and
the world's civilisation.Now, just as it was f or the first time,we are
fighting with the same eternal dangerous enemy - Germany. But as it
was on the first occassion,our British Allies are fighting again on
our side.

FIGURE 42.—A copy of Prof. Serge Yudin's speech upon his being made an Honorary Fellow
   of the American College of Surgeons.   The letterhead is of the Sklifossowsky Institute.

Victory will be ours.Nobody has any doubts about it, even our enemies...And l et our scientific relations which have begun in time of such strained military needs,get stronger and flourish more & more after this victory and the won peace.

In time of struggl e surgery is as necessary for victory as arms,transports and all kinds of supplies.But when the last gun of enemy will cease and the released humanity will turn with hope to the restoration of great destroyments caused by the war, we,surgeons will have to heal the wounds and injuries of hundreds of thousands of people,who have won for us this victory.

Your high election of me as Honourary Fellow of the American College of Surgeons will serve as a new additional stimulus for further development of my scientific work in surgery,which has already received from you such high estimation.

I once more deeply and sincerely thank you.

Serge Yudin

FIGURE 42.—Continued.

The outstanding contributions of Academician Burdenko in the development of neuro-surgery, his brilliant experimental work, and his elaboration of the basic principles of a new type of field surgery, which have proved so brilliantly successful in the present war, make us certain that he will be a worthy member of the glorious family of the finest repre-sentatives of contemporary surgery that is combined in the Royal College of Surgeons and the American College of Surgeons. Professor Yudin will bear the title of Fellow of the Colleges with equal honor and worthiness. His name is tied with great successes in abdominal surgery, in plastic operations on the alimentary tract, in blood transfusion, and in the prophylaxis and treatment of infected wounds, etc.

We, the representatives of the family of Soviet medical workers, are today justifiably proud of the great honor bestowed on Academician Burdenko and Professor Yudin. At the same time we express our sincerest appreciation to the Royal College of Surgeons of England and to the American College for this mark of distinction. In the name of the People's Commissar and in our name I ask you, Mr. Vice-President and Colonel Cutler, to convey our thanks to your organizations. In the name of the People's Commissar and in our name I congratulate Academician Burdenko and Professor Yudin on their selection for the honorary fellowship of the Colleges.

Today's occasion takes place in days of bitter warfare against the cruel enemy of progressiveness—Hitler's Fascism! In this war, our medical teaching has extensively become the teaching of war medicine, and it helps our armies in their struggle against this cruel foe. The admission of the most famous Soviet scientists to the honorary fellowship of the Colleges marks in itself a strengthening of the scientific ties between the allied nations. I am certain that those ties will strengthen further in the continuation of this struggle to complete victory over our common enemy.

Summary of observations on military medicine and surgery in U.S.S.R.—On their return to the United Kingdom, Colonel Cutler and Colonel Davis prepared jointly a concise summary of their full report (appendix A, p. 953) for General Hawley. They asked that special consideration be given the following topics because they appeared to be of chief value to the Medical Department of the U.S. Army.

Care of the lightly wounded.

These are early segregated into special hospitals and are preferably kept in these hospitals in the forward area, not sent to the base. Secondary suture of all wounds is practiced early. Rehabilitation and reconditioning exercises begin at once and the men are restored often within a month to active duty.

Cleansing facilities, i.e., bath and barbers in all hospitals.

This is a great contribution to military surgery * * * every soldier, unless he be urgently required in the operating room, goes first to the barber and a room where he can be washed. This is sincerely appreciated by the troops and is something we should emulate in our opinion.

Facilities for Blood Transfusion.

The [full] report emphasizes the great amount of blood used in the Russian Army and its easy availability. Though this doubtless wasted some blood it made it certain that every wounded man could get blood if that was desirable. We should establish a system making blood as well as plasma available to our forward hospitals.

Laundry facilities.

In the Russian Army the medical department controls laundries serving the hospitals. In the Russian Army laundries are set up and serve a group of adjacent hospitals. We suggest that a similar set up be provided for the medical department U.S. Army. This might be in the ratio of one laundry to a Corps surgeon.

Surgical specialization.

The Russians begin major specialization at the forward hospital level. This provides that in the more important fields of surgery soldiers are given what the specialist thinks is wisest from the very beginning of his treatment.

Sorting and triaging.

This is carried out beautifully at the forward hospitals and emphasizes the organization of forward hospitals found necessary in the last Great War. If large numbers of wounded people are to be competently cared for, some systematic sorting must occur. In the Russian Army this permitted the segregation of slightly wounded in hospitals in the forward area and their rapid restoration to duty; it facilitated the care by specialists of those needing special care and it greatly facilitated the major problem of evacuation.[47]

Soviet Union and its people.—Colonel Cutler could not help but be impressed with the Soviet scene in general, and, patriot that he was, he felt it his duty to make these impressions known to those who might be able to take advantage of them in their official duties. He realized that his opportunities for ob-

---

[47] Letter, Col. E. C. Cutler, MC, and Col. L. Davis, MC, to Chief Surgeon, ETOUSA, 7 Aug 1943, subject: Surgical Mission to Russia.

serving the Soviet people and their ways were quite unique at this time—a time when the Soviet Union was allied with the free world against a common enemy, when its people had undergone an untold amount of suffering, yet had remained steadfast in their determination to resist the Nazi aggressor and had actually begun to turn the tables on the Wehrmacht on the Eastern front. Under the dateline of 7 August 1943, Colonel Cutler wrote the following to Ambassador Winant:

The opportunity to enter Russia and contact people there inevitably led to certain impressions' being created in the mind of the visitor and since these thoughts may be of value to the State Department I have tried to put them into writing.

We were shown every courtesy officially and we gathered the impression that those with whom we came into contact were delighted that we had come. Intimate contacts and dinners up the line with the army officers of our own rank and responsibilities made us feel quite at home and at ease. Every opportunity was given us to see the things we asked to see, both in Moscow and when forward with Army hospitals, but all the time one felt that there lay over the officials taking us about an iron hand, which made them cautious in their remarks and which often led to a change of conversation in an abrupt fashion. Thus, on several occasions when we asked questions and the conversation started to give us the answer, the Vice Commissar who accompanied us would make a remark and the conversation on the question ceased and began on some totally unrelated matter. It was as if only special people could speak on special problems and that no one was ever allowed to express an opinion beyond his own special field where the problem had been set to him by someone "on top."

This impression of a strong "fist" on top was strengthened by observation of the mission in Moscow itself. The people were not cheerful. They kept their eyes fixed on the ground as a rule. Of course no independent Russian could talk to us, because were a Russian seen talking to a foreigner he would immediately be taken aside and, if not punished, certainly have a difficult time. Up in the army there was a different feeling. It was as if they were away from that threatening something overhead. The people were cheerful; they laughed; they had simple dances, and seemed entirely happy.

The power of this something overhead turned up in many ways. In intimate discussions with General Martel, the British military attache or observer in Moscow, who Seemed to get on very well with the Russian Army officers, it was quite clear that his dealings with the army were very satisfactory, but that when something had to come out of the army and go to the Government in Moscow, then everything was different.

A further sense of the overhead power came to the mission directly. We flew into Russia in a British plane, which was I believe the second plane on this southern route, and which we were told had all been arranged for through the Ministries. Our plane was to return for us in 2½ weeks. It reached Teheran but was never allowed to enter Russia and a great deal of diplomatic tangling went forward. Apparently the British had signed the agreement for this southern route but had not signed the agreement for the northern route. The Russians wanted certain things added to the northern route agreement and when the British refused to sign this, then they refused to sign the southern route agreement.

*   *   *   *   *   *   *

My own personal observations of the Russian character were that he was really [a] pretty frank, open, very direct and entirely rational person. He had not forgotten the official attitudes of the U.S.A. and Britain toward his country a few years back. He was not going to be fooled again, and he was going to stand on his own feet. Moreover, he had suffered horribly during this war, certainly more than 6 million casualties and perhaps 8 million. He confidently expected to win the war, and to win the war alone if necessary, but would like our help. Everyone spoke of our starting a second front. They don't think the Mediterranean fights were much, and were glad to quote to us the battle casualty figures as measurements of that effort. They refused to speak of the Japanese war, though they knew of its existence. However, it should be said in defense of the opinion of the ordinary Russian that their newspapers and their radio announcements don't give very much information concerning what was going on in the war except in Russia. The propaganda about Russia was tremendous and the personal propaganda for Stalin and Molotov was equally conspicuous. Each room in every hospital up the line, let alone the places in Moscow, contained a picture of very large size of both Stalin and Molotov.

I took the occasion to remind the Commissar, when he spoke as though we were doing nothing, of the efforts of ourselves and our allies, the British. I must say he took this smilingly, said he knew of all our efforts and thanked us. At the same time I am sure none of this would ever get to the people.

My impression of Russian medicine was that it was good, not excellent, but surprisingly good in view of what we had been led to think of them. Their effort in medical education is enormous, and though 90 percent of medical graduates are women, 40,000 were graduated from Government medical schools last year, and these students go through a six year course.

Finally, I came back with a very strong impression that Russia is a really good country with fine people in it, who are bound to take their rightful place as one of the great peoples in the coming civilization. Anyone who fails to take this into consideration and who deals with them with old fashioned diplomacy and not honesty and directly will fail miserably and to the discomfort of his country. We are fortunate in having in Moscow such a directly spoken man as Ambassador [William H.] Standley. He serves his purpose well and is regarded with affection and esteem by the Russians. They like his honesty and frankness and even when he speaks to them contrary to their desires they take it well because of that honesty and frankness. Because of this he stands out among the diplomats at Moscow. He has of course a tremendous advantage in having in Moscow General Faymonville, who apparently is admitted by the British as well as the American people there [to be] the one person persona grata with the Russian people, both the ordinary people and the government. One cannot speak too highly of the eminent qualities of these two citizens who serve our country so well in Russia.

Late 1943—Early 1944

Thus wrote Colonel Cutler in his diary on 15 May 1944, a few weeks before D-day in Europe: "Time flies with increasing agility. The deluge will be upon us soon and will we be ready? No, never fully satisfied, but to begin is something."

These few words truly characterize this period for the Chief Consultant in Surgery. The pace was quickening upon his return from the Soviet Union. At the turn of the year, it had definitely accelerated. By May 1944, the surge of activity was a headlong gallop to the day of destiny—D-day, Europe, 6 June 1944.

During this period, American Forces in the United Kingdom were built up from a few divisions to those making up the First U.S. Army with supporting troops and the nucleus of the Third U.S. Army. In August 1943, upon his return from the U.S.S.R., there were 6 general hospitals, 17 station hospitals, and 2 evacuation hospitals in operation. A few months later, at the beginning of 1944, these had been increased to 17 general hospitals and 34 station hospitals actually in operation. The final SOS plan for mounting the assault on fortress Europe called for 79 fixed hospitals in the United Kingdom alone. This figure did not include those medical units staging to be moved to the Continent at the first opportunity or the evacuation, field, and convalescent hospitals assigned to the armies.[48]

This expansion of the theater troop basis required reorganization and decentralization. Hospital centers were created to operate groups of hospitals. Base section surgeons were given almost complete control over medical facilities in their areas, except for the control of beds in general hospitals. Colonel Cutler had to expand the consultant system to provide for consultants in these centers and base sections. The growth in numerical strength of troops and units and the delegation of many functions to lower echelons shifted the emphasis of activities in the Office of the Chief Surgeon, including those of the Chief Consultant in Surgery, from direct supervision to that of liaison, coordination, and the development and enunciation of policies.

Conferences.—This change in emphasis meant that Colonel Cutler had to attend more routine staff conferences. Weekly meetings of all the consultants in the Professional Services Division were held, preceded by preliminary meetings of the surgical and medical consultants held separately. On each fourth Monday of the month the consultants and the Chief of Professional Services met with the Chief Surgeon. There were also fortnightly meetings of base section surgeons, and the weekly staff meetings instigated by Colonel Spruit after he became Deputy Chief Surgeon at Cheltenham. Starting in January 1944, General Hawley held weekly meetings with his division chiefs, which Colonel Cutler usually attended with Colonel Kimbrough.

In addition, there were the regular RAMC meetings which Colonel Cutler attempted to attend with regularity, especially as the day for the invasion drew ever nearer. There was no consultant in surgery appointed by the Americans at the Allied Supreme Headquarters level, and Colonel Cutler, by mutual understanding of all concerned, acted in that capacity: (1) Through his superior officers and staff at the theater level, (2) through Maj. Gen. Albert W. Kenner, MC, USA, Chief Medical Officer, SHAEF (Supreme Headquarters, Allied Expeditionary Force) (fig. 43) and (3) in meetings of the various committees of the British AMD and EMS.

Changes in senior consultants.—Colonel Zollinger served as Acting Chief Consultant in Surgery in the European theater during Colonel Cutler's visits to the U.S.S.R. and, later, to NATOUSA (the North African Theater of Operations, U.S. Army). After Major Storck's return to the United States, Colonel Zollinger was appointed Senior Consultant in General Surgery. Maj. (later Lt. Col.) John N. Robinson, MC, 2d General Hospital, was appointed Senior Consultant in Urology, in addition to his other duties, since the supervision of urological activities in the theater had grown to be too great an activity

---

[48] (1) Annual Report, Chief Consultant in Surgery, ETOUSA, 1943. (2) Annual Report, Professional Services Division, Office of the Chief Surgeon, ETOUSA, 1944. (3) SOS, ETOUSA Mounting Plan, Medical Corps, Annex No. 8: Medical Plan—Mounting the Operation.

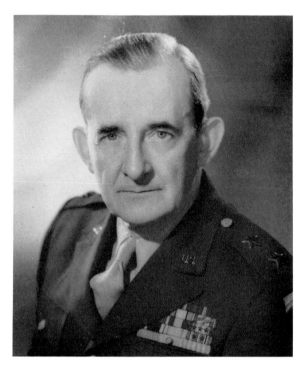

FIGURE 43.—Maj. Gen. Albert W. Kenner.

for Colonel Kimbrough to perform in addition to being Chief of Professional
Services. Col. Roy A. Stout, DC, was appointed Senior Consultant in Maxillo-
facial Surgery on 8 November 1943, relieving Colonel Bricker of these duties;
Colonel Bricker remained Senior Consultant in Plastic Surgery and Burns.
Maj. (later Lt. Col.) John E. Scarff, MC, 2d General Hospital, served for
a considerable time as Acting Senior Consultant in Neurosurgery during
Colonel Davis' trip to the U.S.S.R. and after his return to the United States.
Finally, on 15 March 1944, Lt. Col. (later Col.) R. Glen Spurling, MC, arrived
in the theater and was appointed Senior Consultant in Neurosurgery. Lt. Col.
(later Col.) Mather Cleveland, MC, arrived from a previous assignment as a
service command consultant in the Zone of Interior and in May 1944 was
appointed Senior Consultant in Orthopedic Surgery replacing Colonel Diveley,
who, in turn, became chief of the Rehabilitation Division.

    Significant activities.—Items of significance during this period, insofar
as they involved Colonel Cutler, included various measures to get ready for the
invasion of the Continent—Operation OVERLORD, further developments in
the effort to provide whole blood for combat operations, extensive study of
the efficiency of penicillin, a trip to the North African theater, discussions
with The Surgeon General on the closure of wounds and amputations, and the
expansion of the consultant system. These are discussed separately, but the

following items of no less importance, though perhaps more limited in scope in some instances, were also his concern.

American Medical Society, ETOUSA.—Following the August general meeting of the American Medical Society, ETOUSA, General Hawley informed Colonel Cutler that the general monthly meeting of the society could no longer be held after the one for the current month. He suggested means of having smaller, decentralized meetings. As a result, the responsibility for forming local societies and holding meetings was eventually decentralized to the base sections. With decentralization, however, there was a lack of coordination with the result that areas for local societies were overlapping, and so forth. Originally, Colonel Cutler had been told, the intent was to have a society completely independent of any control from the Chief Surgeon's Office, but a coordinating center had to be established. Actually, this coordination, Colonel Cutler thought, benefited the local groups since it provided services such as helping to formulate programs, obtaining guest speakers, and collecting papers from local meetings for forwarding to appropriate individuals and offices within the theater and, in some cases, to the Office of The Surgeon General. The last general meeting during this period was held in January 1944 at Widewing, Eighth Air Force headquarters. At a business session of this general meeting, Colonel Wright, Chief of Professional Services for the theater Army Air Forces, was elected president of the society.

Throughout this period, there were many stimulating meetings held locally in the various base sections (fig. 44). Colonel Cutler and his consultants were able to attend many of these local meetings and were gratified to find participation at the grass-roots level extremely healthy.

Education and training.—The European theater Medical Field Service School at Shrivenham continued with its full curriculum, as did the Air Force school at "Pinetree." The London tours course was discontinued before the Americans "wore out their welcome" at the busy London hospitals. In spite of some initial reticence on the part of the Chief Surgeon and his Education and Training Branch, a very extensive program in the training of anesthetists was begun under the direction of Colonel Tovell, Senior Consultant in Anesthesia. Colonel Diveley, as Senior Consultant in Orthopedic Surgery, initiated a badly needed course of instruction in plaster work (fig. 45). This instruction was carried out in 3-day periods, mostly for medical officers of the First U.S. Army.

Selected U.S. Army medical officers were sent to the various courses at the British Post-Graduate Medical School in continuation of a program which had been established in the very earliest days of the theater. The courses which were being offered during this time in successive weekly intervals were: Recent advances in war injuries, treatment of fractures, war surgery of the nervous system, war medicine, war surgery of the extremities, surgical care of the soldier in training, war surgery of the abdomen, and war surgery of the

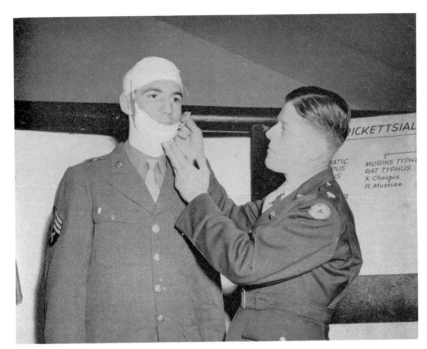

FIGURE 44.—A demonstration of an improvised splint for a fractured jaw at the meeting of the American Medical Society, ETOUSA, at the 315th Station Hospital, Axminster, Devon, England, on 22 March 1944.

chest. Mr. Tudor Edwards' 2-week course in thoracic surgery for American medical officers was likewise continued at several British thoracic surgery centers in and around London. The British Army Blood Supply Depot continued to accept a limited number of U.S. Army medical officers for training in the principles and techniques of bleeding, processing, storing, refrigerating, and shipping whole blood—together with the clinical aspects of shock, whole blood transfusion, and resuscitation.

The previously stated policy of General Hawley that specialists would not be trained in the theater had to be modified, upon the insistence of Colonel Cutler and the other consultants, to allow for the further training of those who had had some preliminary training in a surgical specialty. The instruction was conducted at selected station and general hospitals for individuals or small groups. The length of instruction was flexible, as was the scope of instruction, and was dependent upon the advice of the senior consultant concerned.[49]

Monthly report of surgical service.—In order to maintain a closer touch on the pulse of surgical activities in the theater—something which was exceed-

---

[49] Circular Letter No. 174, Office of the Chief Surgeon, Headquarters, European Theater of Operations, U.S. Army, 28 Nov. 1943.

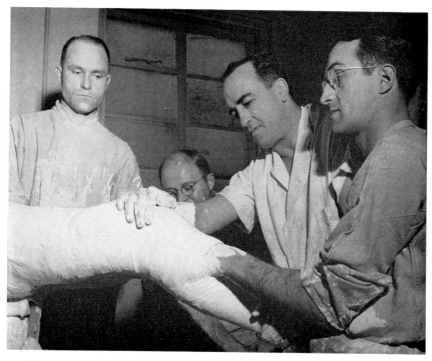

FIGURE 45.—Training in the application of plaster at the 298th General Hospital, Bristol, England.

ingly necessary because of the decentralization of activities and the impossibility of the theater-level consultants personally supervising all surgical activities—Colonel Cutler had Colonel Zollinger, Senior Consultant in General Surgery, devise a monthly report of surgical services to be submitted by all fixed hospitals in the theater. A daily operating room log was also devised to be used as a standardized record in these hospitals, a log which would permit easy compilation of the monthly surgical report. The reporting requirement was approved by the Chief Surgeon and promulgated on 12 March 1944.[50]

From the outset, the report proved very satisfactory, and Colonel Cutler was most pleased by the control it offered. He reported in the monthly Essential Technical Medical Data report for April 1944, as follows:

The report may from time to time be inaccurate, but it should prove informative and should provide us with information concerning the relative incidence of wound infections, battle injuries and nonbattle injuries in the various specialties.

In a recent report * * * the number of whole blood transfusions amounted to 172. Of these, 168 came from stored blood in a blood bank in a hospital. At the same time 637

---

[50] Administrative Memorandum No. 29, Office of the Chief Surgeon, Headquarters, European Theater of Operations, U.S. Army, 12 Mar. 1944 (Amended by Administrative Memorandum No. 134 and Administrative Memorandum No. 144, Office of the Chief Surgeon, Headquarters, European Theater of Operations, U.S. Army, 1944).

units of dried plasma were given. In this first monthly surgical report we computed the incidence of wound infections in six of the seven hospitals in East Anglia where airmen injured in missions over enemy territory are treated:

*Battle injuries*_____	214
Number infected_____	15
Incidence _____	7 percent
*Nonbattle injuries*_____	388
Number infected_____	8
Incidence _____	2 percent
*Clean operations*_____	730
Number infected_____	3
Incidence _____	0. 4 percent

The above is a sample of the control such a simple report has on professional work.

This report was received from all hospitals in the communications zone for the entire period of the war—hospitals in which most of the reparative surgery provided in the theater was conducted. The last report submitted by these hospitals was for the month of May 1945.

Activities in conjunction with Army Air Forces.—One of the first things Colonel Cutler did upon his return from the U.S.S.R. was to tour each of the hospitals which had been established primarily to serve the Air Force (fig. 46). These were at this time either in full operation or just about ready to start operations, and the Air Force medical staff in the theater was very pleased with the results. For one thing, the surgical service at these hospitals had to be first rate because they were treating air combat casualties, and Colonel Cutler had done everything in his power to make them so. However, the growth of the air arm, which paralleled the buildup in the theater of the other arms and services, soon outstripped the services these hospitals could provide. As more heretofore standby airfields were activated, their distance to hospitals became a serious problem in the eyes of the Air Forces, and, in spite of other priorities, General Hawley gave first consideration to building and activating additional hospitals to serve them. The duty of seeing that the surgical service in these hospitals included the required high-grade professional personnel befell to Colonel Cutler and his consultants. The providing of this personnel became a most difficult undertaking when well-qualified individuals were required to augment the staffs of newly arriving hospitals with very little specialized talent and when surgical teams which had been attached to the hospitals serving the Air Forces had to be withdrawn in preparation for the land campaign on the Continent.

In addition, as the Air Forces in the theater grew, it became necessary for the theater Air Force medical staff to supervise activities on a broader, less personal scale. Consequently, the theater consultant staff was called upon from time to time to help formulate policy and write professional directives which were issued by the theater Air Force commander, or by the Surgeon, General Grow. One of these, personally worked out by Colonel Cutler, was a basic directive on the reception and initial treatment of casualties at airbases.

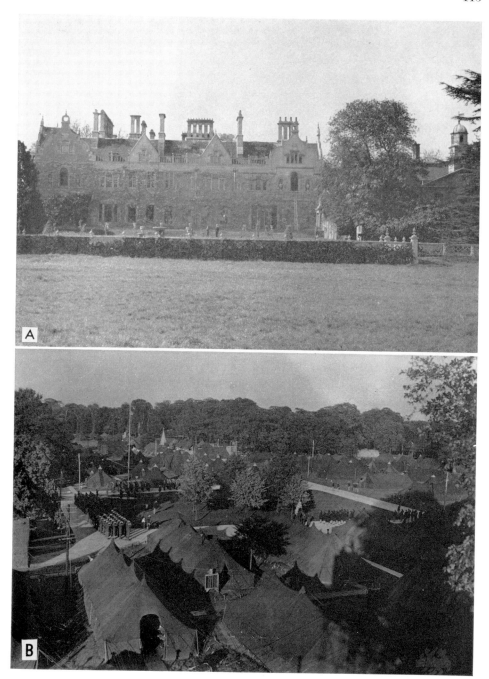

FIGURE 46.—Hospitals established primarily to serve Army Air Forces in England.
A. The 160th Station Hospital in Lilford Hall, Northamptonshire, England. B. The 348th
Station Hospital, Grantham, Lincolnshire, England, a model tented hospital. All concrete
pathways and flooring were planned and laid before the tenting was erected.

Maj. Gen. David N. W. Grant, the Air Surgeon, visited the theater in September 1943 and in March 1944. General Grant was an avowed advocate of a separate medical service for the Air Forces, but he was forced to admit—upon advice of the Eighth Air Force medical personnel—that arrangements in the theater were as satisfactory as they could be under existing circumstances and did not require any immediate major change. Colonel Cutler was pleased at this outcome and felt pride in having done much to cement this cooperative close relationship—largely through his associations with Colonel Wright and, also, through his intense interest in the combat casualties of the Eighth Air Force (fig. 47).[51]

Study of casualties with respect to causes of death and causative agent.—Colonel Cutler had urged since his early days in the theater that provision be made for the study of wounds and wounding, the distribution of wounds, and the relationship of wounds to the causative agents. In his reports to the Chief Surgeon and The Surgeon General, he had always tried to indicate at least the distribution of wounds (regional frequency) whenever the data were amenable to such a tabulation. In his trip to the U.S.S.R., he had made it a point to obtain some data on the Soviet experience in the frequency by which various regions of the body were hit. Shortly after his return from the Soviet Union, he formally suggested that a group be established for the purpose of studying the wounds of war. The minutes of the Chief Surgeon's 23 August 1943 meeting with his consultants show the following discussion on this proposal:

> The Surgical Subcommittee's proposal to establish a pathological group for the study of fatality statistics in the army was discussed. Colonel Cutler pointed out that the group might serve a double purpose; i.e., to find out what kind of wound causes death, and what kind of missile causes the wound. He felt that some valuable findings might result, and that the group might work with the graves registration people. Colonel Spruit said that the responsibilities of the medical department were directed in one line—to get men back to duty. He felt that there were two aspects of the proposal, (a) That this pathological group would have to be put in the front line, and that the Division would have the burden of carrying them along, and (b) That if the scheme was practicable it might prove valuable, but that at present it was only possible to formulate ideas.

Finally, Maj. Gen. Norman T. Kirk, The Surgeon General, officially announced the need for obtaining such information in an article prepared for the *Bulletin of the U.S. Army Medical Department*.[52] In January 1944, however, before publication, copies of the article were sent to all theaters of operations requesting that programs for the collection of data on missile wounds be set up.

Colonel Cutler again recommended that teams consisting of pathologists and enlisted men be set up to collect and make studies along these lines. But it was not until The Surgeon General visited the theater in March 1944 that

---

[51] Minutes, Conference of the Deputy Chief Surgeon, 12 Sept. 1943.
[52] Office of The Surgeon General: Need for Data on the Distribution of Missile Wounds. Bull. U.S. Army M. Dept., No. 74, March 1944, pp. 19–22.

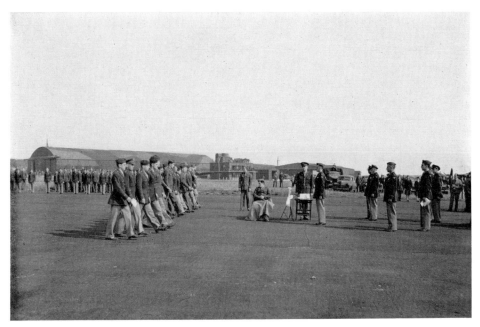

FIGURE 47.—Maj. Gen. Carl Spaatz, Commanding General, Army Air Forces, ETOUSA, awarding the order of the Purple Heart to men of the 97th Bombardment Group, Polebrook, England, September 1942.

sufficient impetus was given to the program to bring forth General Hawley's approval for the establishment of a casualty survey team in the theater. On 2 April, Colonel Cutler stated in a memorandum to Colonel Kimbrough:

> For about a year the Professional Services group have, at the approval of General Hawley, continued studies of how to implement a group of people acquiring information as to what killed men in battle, and where they were hit when injured. During the recent visit of The Surgeon General and General Grant, a discussion of deaths in airplanes while on missions over enemy territories led to the finding that personnel arriving dead were not autopsied. I was then instructed by General Hawley to set up a group for such studies.

It so happened that Maj. Allan Palmer, MC, chief of the pathology service, 30th General Hospital, had accompanied Prof. S. (later Sir Solly) Zuckerman of Oxford University on a special casualty survey mission to Italy and was well initiated in the procedures involved in conducting with rigid scientific precision the necessary studies to provide useful and meaningful data on war wounds. Major Palmer was assigned to Colonel Cutler to undertake the organization and establishment of a team to study casualties and the killed in action. Since, at this time, the only fresh casualties being received in the theater were the result of air combat, Major Palmer's unit—called the Medical Operational Research Section, Professional Services Division, Office of the Chief Surgeon—was established at the Cambridge American Military Cemetery with full facilities for conducting autopsies of the Air Forces' dead, making photographic studies, and preserving specimens.

One stumbling block in the building of the laboratory, it is interesting to note, was the fact that there was a stately and ancient tree growing exactly in the middle of the plot of ground which had been designated for the laboratory building. Apparently, Dr. Rosamond E. M. Harding, the owner of Madingley Hall, Cambridgeshire—the estate within which the cemetery was located, had specified that the U.S. Army could use the grounds but that no trees would be cut down. The U.S. Army Engineers, accordingly, steadfastly refused to cut down this particular tree so that Major Palmer's laboratory could be built. Finally, it was necessary for Colonel Cutler to call on Dr. Harding personally. This he did on 30 April 1944. The visit, which was most pleasant, ended with talk over the possibility of Dr. Harding's coming to America to see Colonel Cutler after the war in order to continue certain studies she was interested in. The tree was cut, but such were the duties of a Chief Consultant in Surgery that they often carried him far afield from the hospital operating rooms.[53]

Free-French surgical teams.—Late in this period, a group of eminently qualified French surgeons, refugees in England, volunteered their services for the impending attack on the European mainland. They were welcomed by the Chief Consultant in Surgery who initiated the necessary steps to organize, activate, and equip them as mobile surgical teams. It was contemplated that they could most gainfully be employed in support of the Free-French Forces which were scheduled for participation as a part of the Allied effort.[54]

"Vetting" newly arrived units.—Especially characteristic of this period was the necessity on the part of all the theater-level consultants to meet and evaluate the professional capabilities of the numerous medical units newly arriving in the theater. This became known as "vetting." Of particular importance was the need to assess carefully the merits of the professional personnel, since the supply of well-qualified physicians and surgeons was beginning to run low and many units were being sent overseas with the assumption that key professional personnel could be supplied from units already in the theaters.

There were many problems associated with the vetting and subsequent need for exchanging personnel. First of all, Colonel Cutler reiterated, it was imperative that unqualified officers arriving with these new units be in the lower grades because the theater could not assimilate well those who were in higher grades. This was true because, in many cases, a professionally well-qualified individual being sent into these new units as the chief of a service or section was himself a relatively young, junior officer. Furthermore, most of the well-qualified talent was in the affiliated units, and they believed they were being "robbed" of their better personnel, and, of course, resented it. Before long,

---

[53] Results of the studies conducted by the Medical Operational Research Section at the Cambridge American Military Cemetery as well as Major Palmer's casualty survey report on his Italian experiences are published in full in: Medical Department, United States Army. Wound Ballistics. Washington : U.S. Government Printing Office, 1962, pp. 547–611.

[54] Memorandum, Col. E. C. Cutler, MC, to Chief, Professional Services Division, 3 June 1944, subject : French Surgeons.

these units recognized the overall needs of the theater and responded well. Colonel Cutler was deeply gratified by this response and never ceased to commend these units which were called upon again and again to give up personnel and yet continued to maintain their high standards. In a way, it was to the benefit of these units because such transfers permitted their junior officers to be promoted, whereas promotion possibilities were extremely limited if the junior officers continued to stay with the original units. Finally, there was the matter of command authority to effect transfers between units to spread the talent more equally. On more than one occasion, a consultant had to be reprimanded for giving instructions which—in many cases unwittingly—were taken at the local level to be commands. The desired changes in personnel had to be offered as suggestions to the base section surgeons, who were usually very cooperative in accepting and implementing them. It was more difficult, Colonel Cutler noted, when two or more base sections were involved in a series of transfers, as was often the case.

General Hawley took a very firm position on this matter of exchanging personnel, realizing full well the necessity for it, while also recognizing the need to respect the authority of commanders at the lower levels. He made the following statement at his 25 October 1943 conference with base section surgeons:

I do not need to tell you all, that we are never building up one Base Section at the expense of another and if these changes that we have are advisable, while you may get a little shortchange on one change you are going to make it up on the next. We are trying to get a balanced setup. The thing which concerns us very largely is to get thoroughly competent Chiefs of Services in these hospitals.

Col. David E. Liston, MC, Chief, Personnel Division (later Deputy Chief Surgeon) (fig. 48), was most helpful in undertaking the necessary details to coordinate and effect the transfers which were desired by the professional consultants. At a conference with base section surgeons on 2 August 1943, he made the following statement:

Sometimes we are told to move three men who have a spark of genius and it means we have to move three men who do not have this spark of genius. * * * Nobody wants these people [without the spark of genius] but we have to do something with them. If we are going to make a captain a major, that is an easy decision. The difficult decision is where to put that man we kicked out where he can get proper training.

Eventually, the need to provide not only chiefs of service but nearly all the specialists as well for the newly arriving units became a very serious problem. Colonel Cutler and Colonel Zollinger could meet this problem only by preparing lists in advance of those officers in the theater who were qualified to become chiefs of surgical services in hospitals and those in the various specialties who could be used to bolster the incoming units. This foresight on the part of the Chief Consultant in Surgery and the Senior Consultant in General Surgery proved particularly effective when, as D-day neared, many of the better, more experienced medical units of the theater were earmarked for movement to the Continent and their personnel were frozen. Officers in these units

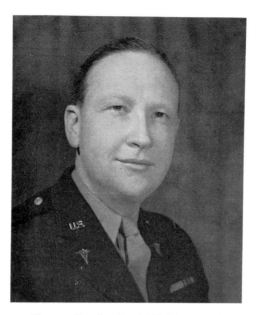

FIGURE 48.—Col. David E. Liston, MC.

who had been selected to become chiefs of surgical service or specialists in other units were relieved from assignment to their units before the personnel freeze was effected and remained with their units after they were alerted on an attached unassigned basis until the need for a particular individual arose.

As time went on, assaying and recommending the shifting of personnel became one of the primary functions of consultants at the theater headquarters, in the base sections, and in the field armies.

Expansion of the consultant system

An attempt to establish a system of consultation at the local level was mentioned as having been initiated immediately before Colonel Cutler's trip to the Soviet Union. This embryonic system of regional consultants and the "mother hospital" scheme was further expanded during this period, which also saw the appointment of coordinators in medicine and surgery at hospital centers and surgical and medical consultants at the base section level. The changes and innovations which were made during this immediate preinvasion period formed the framework for the duration of the war in the European theater, and it was not until well after V–E Day that that this consultant system required a complete overhaul, and then only to gear it to the needs of an army of occupation.

Regional consultants.—At General Hawley's insistence, more than enough regional consultants in the various specialties had been appointed. They were first announced by the Chief Surgeon's Circular Letter No. 89, dated 21 May 1943. At that time, the directive listed eight regional consultants in general surgery, one in plastic surgery and burns, five in neurosurgery, two in orthopedic surgery, seven in otolaryngology, nine in urology, and four in anesthesiology. This directive required immediate amendment later in May and in early June to provide for additional consultants in ophthalmology, roentgenology, orthopedic surgery, and plastic surgery. From the outset, this method of appointing and controlling regional consultants centrally from the Office of the Chief Surgeon was doomed to be unwieldy. When, in June, the operation of medical facilities in the United Kingdom was delegated to base sections, the system became all the more cumbersome—a point which was consistently belabored by the newly appointed base section surgeons. From time to time, Colonel Kimbrough reported that the surgical consultants were attempting to bring the original directive up to date, but changes were occurring so fast that revisions never passed the draft stage. Eventually, General Hawley directed that consultation at the local level be made a responsibility of the base section surgeon and that the Office of the Chief Surgeon be informed of the actions taken.

Accordingly, Circular Letter No. 21, Office of the Chief Surgeon, 7 February 1944, was published and set the policy for consultative services for the American Forces which remained in effect for the duration of the war in Europe. It stated:

5. *Regional Consultants.* The personnel of general hospitals and specially designated stations hospitals will be available for consultation in the vicinity of their stations and will conduct their activities under the direction of the base section surgeons. Base Section surgeons will inform each hospital where it will apply for consultant service in each of the several specialties.

In actual practice, the system of regional consultants did not work out quite as simply as may be implied in the foregoing excerpt. First of all, as Colonel Cutler explained on one occasion, there were not enough good men to place in all the general hospitals so that every general hospital could be a mother hospital to station hospitals in its vicinity for every specialty. Consequently, specific hospitals had to be designated for certain specialties as the mother hospital. In cases, this crossed boundaries of base sections so that, in some fields, surgeons of two or more base sections had to agree on the area to be covered by a particular regional consultant. Finally, the hospitals which had designated regional consultants were hard pressed for transportation and could not afford to maintain a standby vehicle for the consultants—a problem which had existed in World War I. On this occasion, however, an extra jeep was eventually authorized for each general and station hospital having regional consultants for the specific use of these consultants. The reader is also asked to note that this system of administering regional consultants could not have been established without creating base section consultants in general surgery and medicine, a program which was carried out concurrently with the development of the regional consultant system.

Base section consultants.—By far the most important step taken during this period in expanding the consultant system was the appointment of base section consultants. At first, base section surgeons objected to their appointment, for no positions had been established in their tables of organization for consultants. There was also considerable question in the minds of the base section surgeons as to what such a consultant would do, or as to whether he would even have anything to do. On 20 December 1943, General Hawley, said, at his regular meeting of base section surgeons; "There is scarcely a base section whose job is not going to be bigger in a month than the whole theater was in the beginning of this month. I think your consultants for the time being should be limited to medicine and surgery, but I do feel that you need consultants for medicine and surgery. It may be that, in Southern Base, you will need more than one."

The need for having base section consultants, when considered in this light, was apparent. For the time being, there was no other course but to appoint them in addition to their other duties in hospitals to which they were assigned. The policy concerning base section consultants was announced in aforementioned Circular Letter No. 21, emanating from the Office of the Chief Surgeon. It stated:

4. Base Section Consultants

a. Upon recommendation of the Office of the Chief Surgeon, base section surgeons will appoint consultants in general medicine and general surgery for their respective base sections. These consultants will be available to all organizations of the American Forces in their base sections. They may render service, on request of the commanding officers, to Canadian and British Hospitals in which patients of the U.S. Forces are under treatment. They may be obtained by request made to the office of the base section surgeons. In urgent cases this request should be made by telephone.

b. *Reports.* The base section consultants will render reports as required by the base section surgeons and will send a copy to the Office of the Chief Surgeon.

At a somewhat later date, Colonel Cutler found it necessary to state his policy with regard to the duties of base section consultants. In a memorandum dated 2 April 1944, which was apparently issued to each base section consultant personally, he wrote:

1. Keep familiar with level of professional work carried out at all hospitals in your base section. This means constant personal visits. Written directions and circulars can never take the part of the influence of a real surgeon at the bedside of the patient.

2. As a part of the above you must see all new units which enter your base section shortly after arrival, and evaluate the personnel. Your opinions should be turned into the Office of the Chief Surgeon, attention of Chief Consultant in Surgery, as soon as investigation has been completed. In addition to your evaluation of new units representatives of the consultant group in the Division of Professional Services will also make their own appraisal. Copies of these opinions will be forwarded to you.

3. Attend all meetings of the Professional Services Division. This includes automatically: a. General Hawley's monthly meeting with the Professional Services Division, b. Meeting of the Professional Services Division each Saturday morning at 10 a.m., Headquarters, SOS. If you wish to bring up special subjects for discussion at either meeting send notice for agenda one week in advance. At the weekly Division meeting you will be expected to make a brief report.

4. In your visits you should see that the professional directives are lived up to, that station hospitals in particular do not do major elective surgery or undertake professional matters beyond their professional capacity. You should also keep an eye on evacuation and see that hospitals are prompt in evacuating people either to the Zone of Interior, if they are of the type that should be returned to the Zone of Interior, or to the rehabilitation

hospitals, that their hardening process may begin as promptly as possible. In particular you must keep an eye on inter-hospital consultations. Encourage this, and see that reports made by your regional consultants come to you promptly.

5. All of your hospital reports should be rendered to the Base Section surgeon, but copies should come to the Chief Consultant in Surgery.

Coordinators in hospital centers.—In the overall decentralization program, it was necessary to establish hospital centers to administer and operate groups of hospitals and to bring together under one administration the facilities and personnel required to treat any type of injury. Hospital centers established in the United Kingdom during this period were at Malvern Wells, Worcestershire (12th Hospital Center); Cirencester Park, Gloucestershire (15th Hospital Center); and Whitchurch, Flintshire (6810th Hospital Center, Provisional). There were, in each of these centers, hospitals provided with equipment and personnel for highly specialized treatment in neurosurgery, thoracic surgery, plastic and maxillofacial surgery, urological surgery, and the surgical treatment of extensive burns.[55] It is readily apparent that, with such extensive facilities in men and equipment, the center commander required an officer to manage the surgical care carried out in the center. To differentiate this officer from the regional and base section consultants, he was called a coordinator in surgery, and such coordinators were appointed at each hospital center at this time and in those established later during the operations that followed.

Visit to North African Theater of Operations and Fifth U.S. Army

Perhaps one of the wisest moves made by the Chief Surgeon in preparation for the eventual assault on continental Europe was to send key medical personnel to the North African theater to observe firsthand the combat and support activities in progress. Colonel Cutler's turn came in November 1943. He departed by air from Prestwick, Scotland, on 27 November and returned to London on 24 December 1943.

During his visit, Colonel Cutler was able to observe a hospital train movement; general, station, and convalescent hospitals in the base sections; and clearing stations (fig. 49), surgical teams, and field, evacuation, and convalescent hospitals in the Fifth U.S. Army area. He noted the great differences between the North African theater and the European theater, and, on his return, reported, as follows:[56]

In NATOUSA the distances are great, the transport problem a nightmare (fig. 50), the hospitalization with the difficulties of evacuation (fig. 51) seemed inadequate and the supply problem is magnified by the above considerations. In spite of all this the medical department of NATOUSA must have our warm congratulations. Hospitals assume tremendous loads; for example General Hospital No. 21 (fig. 52) once had as many as 2,600 patients and many 500 bed station hospitals went over 1,000 patients! * * * In the Army area, even greater loads were necessary. Moreover, a large share of this load were battle casualties demanding on admission immediate attention and many requiring careful daily care.

---

[55] See footnote 48 (2), p. 107.
[56] Letter, Col. E. C. Cutler, MC, to Chief Surgeon, ETOUSA, 27 Dec. 1943, subject: Report on Visit to NATOUSA and Fifth U.S. Army.

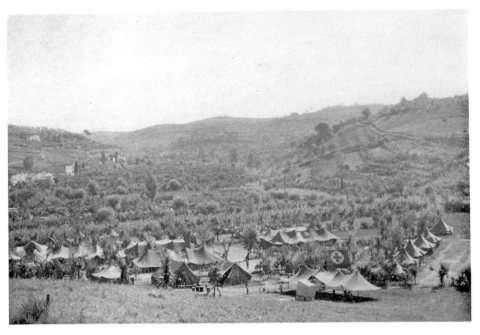

FIGURE 49.—A clearing station of the 85th Infantry Division in Italy.

Colonel Cutler observed that, in the Fifth U.S. Army, a platoon from a field hospital was usually established adjoining a division clearing station. Casualties who might be endangered by further transportation were carried by litter from the clearing stations to these field hospital platoons, which were set up with from 40 to 100 beds (fig. 53). Four or five surgical teams from the 2d Auxiliary Surgical Group were attached to the field hospital platoons. Colonel Cutler was most favorably impressed by this system. He stated in his report:

I heartily approve the system for the care of the heavily damaged nontransportables in Field Hospital platoons. I even would urge an extension of this forward surgery, believing that "surgery should be brought to the soldier," not the soldier to the surgeon. In addition to chests and abdomens, perhaps all the femurs, all the lower leg wounds with vascular damage and some of the heads should be done here.

On the use of evacuation hospitals in Fifth U.S. Army (fig. 54), Colonel Cutler commented:

In Fifth Army, 400 to 750 bed Evacs were used interchangeably (* * * 750 Evac excellent and no one in this theater understands why Washington (S.G.O.) thinks they are bad). As a matter of fact 400 and 750 Evacs soon overflowed even with low percentage casualties coming in. * * * Evac Hospitals taking seriously wounded were unable to hold patients for sufficient time to ensure safe evacuation. It seemed to me that the forward hospitals did not keep a sufficient number of empty beds but this is not offered as a serious criticism since only those on top can gauge the necessity for free beds. In relation to my experience in forward hospitals in the last war where Evacs frequently took 1,000 cases a day and were only able to dress and pass on the bulk of the wounded,

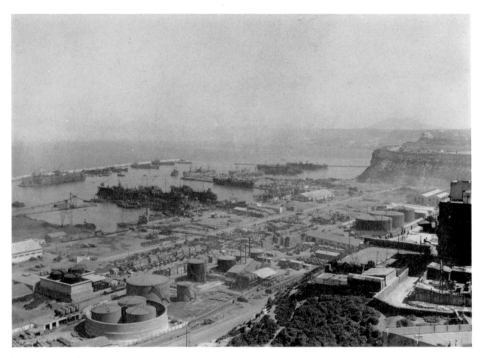

FIGURE 50.—Part of the tremendous transport network in the North African theater, Oran Harbor, Algeria, North Africa.

I was favourably impressed with the far greater percentage of surgery now done in the forward area. This is of course where it should be done.

In conjunction with the evacuation hospitals, he also noted that they had too much paper work in the way of required reports. There were 8 daily, 7 weekly, 9 periodic, and 12 monthly reports required of them. There was also a bottleneck in the radiology service. The equipment was adequate, but the personnel soon tired when overworked, indicating a need for at least double the X-ray personnel in an evacuation hospital. Colonel Cutler's views reflected in the following observation in his report were to become the cause for vigorous action on his part upon his return to the European theater:

I believe separate Evacs should be used for the care of *lightly wounded*. These are the men we should restore to duty, these deserve our best surgeons, these can be evacuated direct to a convalescent hospital. This means good sorting at the clearing station, but that is a function of clearing stations and if sorting is well done the multiple hospital transfers now going on will be minimized.

Other aspects of the professional service in the North African theater were reported by Colonel Cutler as follows:

The professional care of neurological cases is excellent. These can as a rule reach an Evac Hospital for definitive surgery. There are criticisms in the forward areas of the tripod incision as practiced by Harvey Cushing in the last war but I saw no adequate tripod wounds and am writing to remind the Surgeons of this war that the flap method

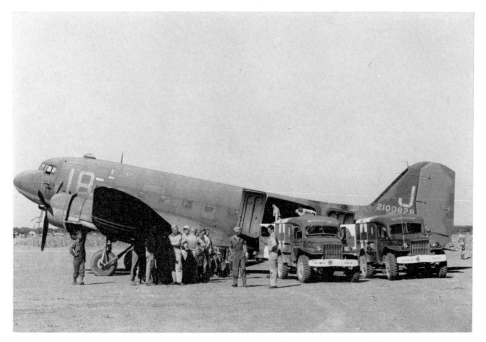

FIGURE 51.—Air evacuation from the Fifth U.S. Army area by C–47 aircraft.

now in use was given an adequate try in the last war and found unsatisfactory. The secret of success in this field lies in careful, thorough and gentle debridement of the inter-cranial wound and especially in the removal of indriven bone fragments, followed by closure of the wound. I am not convinced the Bovie instrument is necessary and its use adds to the injury and reaction. Also, I believe strong suction is a danger rather than an advantage.

The care of thoracic and the combined thoraco-abdominal injury is admirable and a chief advance. Emphasis on the chest wall rather than the lung as a chief source of hemorrhage has been proven and leads to competent debridement of chest wall with hemostasis and minimal pulmonary surgery. Early repeated evacuation of blood before clotting and infection will avoid many empyemata. Emphasis on frequency of the combined abdomino-thoracic injury is excellent and radiologic control needs continual emphasis.

Early abdominal surgery is the only road to success in this field. Resections of small bowel have been rarely necessary and exteriorization of large bowel injuries or closure rectosigmoid and colostomy above have given good results. I am not convinced that bowel surgery through the thorax via an injured diaphragm is wise, but the number of splenec-tomies via this route speaks for itself.

Extremity surgery—Here adequate debridement, preservation of bone, holding cases with vascular damage for fear of clostridium infections and transportation in plaster seems well done. The low-waisted spica sometimes including sound thigh seems better than the Tobruk plaster though Brigadier Weddell still votes for the latter except in upper femur cases.

Surgical Teams—These are essential and now that the Evacuation Hospitals have learned under pressure that with their intrinsic personnel only they cannot do the job, they will be in greater demand. In fact I am willing to *recommend* that an active army of 3 active corps or more needs two auxiliary surgical groups or an increase in the number of the teams as at present authorized.

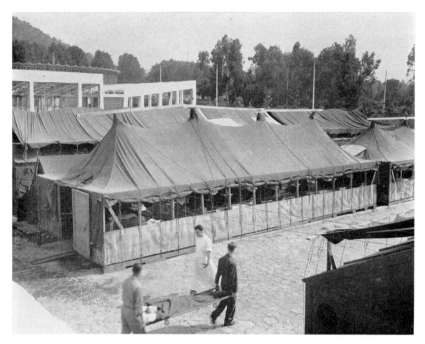

FIGURE 52.—A tented expansion area of the 21st General Hospital, Italy.

Colonel Cutler also saw the advantages of having specialized hospitals in each base area and recommended that a similar organization be established in the European theater, including a convalescent hospital in each base section. Professional work in the base sections, he advised, had been greatly clarified and improved by the setting up of special centers. Not only were the individual cases better handled this way, he believed, but concentrating material at special centers was certain to develop new methods and policies.

Colonel Cutler closed his report to the Chief Surgeon, ETOUSA, with the following note of warning on the handling of fractures:

Fractures—This field needs further study. The tendency with femurs is to use skeletal traction at the base. This throws out the work of the Spanish and Russian schools and greatly increases professional labor. We had traction in the last war, we had some hope that early reduction and plaster might reduce work as well as give better results. I am not myself convinced that we are yet masters of the plaster technique. When we are, I have a suspicion less skeletal traction will be practiced.

Sometime after his return from North Africa and Italy, Colonel Cutler was reminded of certain observations he had made there and had, possibly, neglected to emphasize sufficiently. But, on 9 April 1944, he wrote the following memorandum, which was directed to the Chief Quartermaster, ETOUSA, through the Executive Officer, Office of the Chief Surgeon:

1. During December '43 I had the opportunity of visiting the U.S. Fifth Army and made a particular point while there of studying with my colleague, Colonel Churchill,

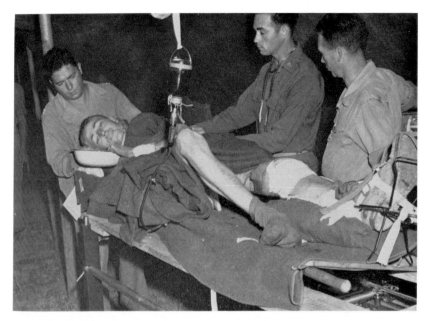

FIGURE 53.—A seriously wounded soldier receiving transfusion of whole blood while his gastric contents are aspirated, at the 33d Field Hospital, Italy.

Consultant in Surgery, NATOUSA, the many men coming out of [the] line complaining of painful and swollen feet. The condition is not exactly similar to the "trench feet" of the last war, nor to the many cases of "immersion feet" so carefully studied by Navy medical personnel. It is however a great and growing concern to the U.S. Army, for the loss of manpower from this source alone is disturbing.

2. Studies by medical personnel of the feet of such casualties up to this time have not brought forward any method of therapy likely to restore the individual to combat duty in a short period of time. The general medical opinion is that prevention is the best method of treatment.

3. Colonel Holst, formerly Professor of Surgery at Oslo, Norway (now Chief Consultant in Surgery to the Norwegian Forces in the United Kingdom), has just returned from a two months' visit with the Fifth U.S. Army and the British VIIIth [Eighth] Army. He too made an exhaustive study of these "cold wet feet" and passed some remarks to me which should be in your possession. Note that Colonel Holst is a Norwegian, who participated in the Finnish-Russian War, and has had as great an experience with cold wet feet as any competent medical officer living.

It is Colonel Holst's opinion that :—

a. The sock furnished the U.S. Army does not have a sufficient content of wool.

b. That a rigid discipline must be enforced within combat companies insisting on the changing of socks daily, even if it only means wringing out the wet sock and putting it on again.

c. That our soldiers are invariably fitted with shoes too small for them.

Later in the month, Colonel Cutler was asked to furnish suggestions for line officers whose responsibility it was to insure that proper disciplinary measures were carried out in order to prevent cold injury. Accordingly, in a memorandum, dated 25 April 1944, he provided the following suggestions:

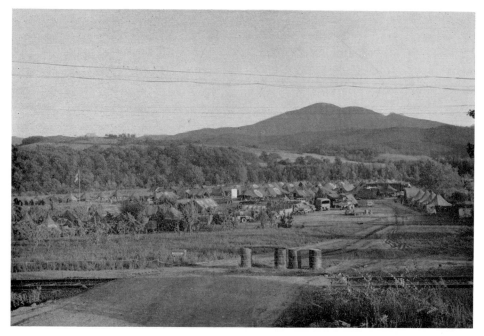

FIGURE 54.—The 94th Evacuation Hospital, Fifth U.S. Army, Italy.

Care of the feet is the responsibility of the company commander, but we are glad to furnish this draft for their use as they see fit.

1. The condition of trench or immersion foot incapacitates the soldier for one or more months and we have no specific therapy for this condition.

2. Prevention of the conditions giving rise to trench foot is largely possible if the following instructions are carefully adhered to.

a. Every attempt should be made to keep the feet warm and dry, using overshoes where possible and encouraging mobility.

b. Shoes should not be tight, and when fitted are preferably fitted over 2 pairs of heavy *all-wool* socks.

c. Canvas leggings, when worn, should not be tightly laced.

d. *All-wool* socks should be provided troops in areas where immersion or wetting is common.

e. Socks and shoes should be changed daily, even if at the change the soldier does nothing more than wring out the wet pair of socks, rub his feet and put on the wet pair of socks again. This routine, if the socks are all-wool, will be a major factor in the prevention.

f. When wet shoes and socks are changed it is advisable to rub in lanolin or Vaseline lightly after drying the skin.

It is not within the scope of this chapter to discuss further what actions were taken at this time on these recommendations by the Chief Consultant in Surgery. This is done elsewhere, but it is significant to note that the matter had been brought up and that simple remedial measures had been suggested.[57]

---

[57] Medical Department, United States Army. Cold Injury, Ground Type. Washington: U.S. Government Printing Office, 1958, pp. 127–210.

Closure of wounds

In a global war, such as World War II, it was indeed difficult for those at the hub in Washington to establish policies which would be applicable under most circumstances anywhere. Even if it was possible to do so, there remained the major problem of communicating the ideas in such a manner that all would receive them and interpret them identically. The incident next to be reported, in which Colonel Cutler was involved, brought out these problems well.

Colonel Cutler had attended a meeting of the surgical consultants subcommittee of the British Army consultants committee on 12 January 1944. He was impressed by remarks made by Sir Harold Gillies. He reported the following to Colonel Kimbrough by letter on 16 January 1944:

> Sir Harold Gillies, Hon. Consultant, RAMC, was present at a Consultants' Meeting for the first time in four years. He came to emphasize the value of early covering of surface wounds. He emphasized that there was great delay in the use of either plastic procedures or skin grafting, and urged that the Consultant Group promulgate through all theaters the desirability of utilizing modern ideas of plastic surgery. I felt he made a good point and will some day try and write a note for the Bulletin of the Chief Surgeon concerning covering of wounds, whether by delayed primary suture, secondary sutures, skin grafting or flaps.

These observations by Sir Harold Gillies were most apropos at this time since the early closure of wounds had only recently been a matter of concern to the Chief Consultant in Surgery. The causes for his concern resulted from two directives which had been issued by The Surgeon General. The earlier of the two, Circular Letter No. 91, dated 26 April 1943, concerning amputations, stated: "Primary suture of all wounds of the extremities under war conditions is never to be done; it is permitted after debridement in certain abdominal, chest, and maxillofacial injuries only." The directive further stated that the guillotine or open circular method of amputation was the procedure of choice in traumatic surgery under war conditions and permitted the flap-type open operation to "be done only in cases in which early evacuation is not contemplated and subsequent closure at the same station is deemed possible."

The later directive, Circular Letter No. 189, concerning surgery of the extremities, was a followup of the earlier. Issued on 17 November 1943, it noted that cases of gas gangrene infection were still occurring as a result of treatment of compound fractures and wounds of the extremities with closure of the wound and without thorough debridement. The directive made the following clear statements: "It is *STRICTLY FORBIDDEN* that any compound fracture or extensive wound of the extremities be treated with closure of the wound. * * * It is *STRICTLY FORBIDDEN* that * * * amputation be done higher than necessary or that the stump be closed." The directive, in closing, warned: "Commanding officers of all general and station hospitals will be held responsible for the abandonment of the improper procedures described above and for the necessary instruction and compliance with these directives."

On 30 December 1943, Colonel Cutler, in a memorandum to Colonel Kimbrough, called his attention to the fact that these circulars had not been reproduced in the theater as theater directives. Colonel Cutler informed Colonel Kimbrough that they had reached commanding officers of hospitals, however, and that, if they were blindly followed, certain cases would be forced to have two operations where one would suffice. He asked whether it would not be proper to request The Surgeon General to reconsider these directives as they might apply to casualties occurring in the Army Air Forces and to nonbattle injuries. He suggested that perhaps The Surgeon General had not given full consideration to the casualty of the Army Air Forces. In explanation of his stand, Colonel Cutler wrote:

In both of these categories previously healthy and often clean, vigorous young men reach a hospital within two hours of injury thus simulating civilian hospital practice. Several have had to have immediate amputation and in selected cases short flap amputation has permitted early secondary closure and even primary closure with highly satisfactory results. It appears to us that there should be a difference in therapy according to terrain and environment. Thus, a sailor knocked into the sea water by a shell fragment and immediately picked up and taken to a hospital ship and an aviator wounded in clean clothes, in a clean airplane and reaching a hospital within three hours and a wounded infantry soldier who has lived in a foxhole, covered with mud and clothes in filthy garments for one or two weeks and who reaches a hospital in 6–12 hours need entirely different treatment at the hand of the surgeon.

Colonel Kimbrough passed Colonel Cutler's memorandum to General Hawley. The general's decision was to leave matters where they stood with respect to the directives and to take care of the exceptions to The Surgeon General's policies by personal instruction within the theater.

Colonel Cutler, however, did not believe that the Chief Surgeon's decision went far enough. In a memorandum to the Chief Surgeon, dated 24 January 1944, concerning the amputation circular, he made the following suggestion:

I believe it would be unwise to issue confidential instructions which are in any way contrary to those recommended by The Surgeon General. It was the intent of my memo of 30 December that you might send a professional opinion to The Surgeon General outlining the situation concerning amputations. I have tried to outline this for you in the attached letter. Would not this be the wisest policy?

General Hawley accepted Colonel Cutler's recommendations and sent the letter to The Surgeon General asking the question of whether casualties of the Army Air Forces, for example, did not justify a different type of therapy according to the environment in which they were wounded and the prompt availability of surgical care. The letter also inclosed a "short note" prepared by Colonel Cutler for publication in the *Medical Bulletin, ETOUSA*. Titled "The Importance of Wound Closure," this article read as follows:

"Do not suture" is accepted as a major principle in the surgery of battle casualties. It, however, must be applied intelligently. For example, it does not mean, never, at any time hereafter, suture these wounds, nor does it mean keep this wound open forever. Yet the dictum has had the above unfortunate connotation. In fact, many surgeons, once a wound has been debrided, seem to relax their interest in the wound unless it becomes septic. This leads to long hospitalization and late return to duty. Moreover, to let a wound heal by cicatrization often leads to unnecessary stiffness in the part and even limitation of function.

We must all consider another principle when we leave a wound open, which is, the best way to sterilize a wound is to close it. No antiseptic is equal to overlying complete epithelization, whether it be achieved by delayed primary suture, early secondary suture, skin graft or flap procedures. Indeed, we owe much to our plastic surgical colleagues who constantly reiterate the importance of a closed wound.

With these two principles in mind let us return to a consideration of the battle casualty and the relation of his injury to terrain and environment. The man wounded in the battlefield where he has been wearing the same suit of clothes for three weeks and who is covered with mud and dirt experiences the same wounds as an airman in his clean clothes, fresh from a bath, or the sailor blown off the deck of his ship by a bomb splinter. True, when surgery is first applied it is wiser to follow the dictum "do not suture the wound". But there analogy ceases; the foot soldier's wound is inevitably seriously contaminated, that of the airman or the sailor swimming in salt water has a minimum of infection. In the case of the foot soldier, delayed primary suture or secondary suture can only be practiced infrequently; in the case of the airman and the sailor it should be practiced almost as the rule.

A recent study in E.T.O. with early closure yields light upon this point. A study was made of the wounds of casualties who had been given penicillin therapy, or sulfonamide therapy, or no chemotherapy. An outstanding observation was that those wounds closed early, irrespective of chemotherapy or none, healed well. When there was delay in closure, infection resulted. And no great choice was made which wounds to close early and which to leave open.

This matter is again brought forward because it appears that the inestimable advantages of an epithelial covering are not generally recognized. If early closure cannot be accomplished, then early grafting or even flap procedures should be carried out. The difficulties of these latter procedures are increased by cicatrization.

Not to suture a wound initially is good practice. To fail to close it at the first safe moment is neglecting an opportunity to protect the soldier against further infection and loss of function.

The reaction in Washington, upon receipt of General Hawley's letter and Colonel Cutler's inclosure, was quick and sensational. First, there was a reply from General Rankin, Chief Consultant in Surgery, Office of The Surgeon General. The letter, dated 3 February 1944, stated:

General Kirk showed me your letter of January 24th relative to amputations and, since there was an enclosure from Cutler on *The Importance of Wound Closure*, he asked me to drop you a line relative to this. I believe he intends to answer your letter, insofar as amputations are concerned, himself.

In a word, we neither of us agree with the modification of the amputation program. I am sure that the wide experience of General Kirk and other men from the last war who dealt with amputations has resulted in giving us a program which is pretty nearly as satisfactory as one can have, and when it comes to fashioning flaps, et cetera, I think that we will have to disagree with our colleagues. I just can't go along with the hypothetical case of the young airman, either in the question of flaps for his amputation or in the proposed wound closure such as Elliott Cutler outlines. If there is one thing that I thought we had learned from the past war and from our experiences in this war, it is *do not close wounds primarily*. I don't believe there is any evidence at all that this should be deviated from. I cannot agree with Cutler that infection results when there is delayed closure because of the delayed closure only. Infection results because infection is there. I am perfectly sure that any deviation from this principle will be followed by profound repercussions. There may be 1 percent, or even 5 percent, of wounds which, when operated upon early, may be closed with relative safety, but the 95 percent (and probably 99 percent) of war wounds, regardless of what service they are in, are better left open, in my judgment. One cannot visualize experienced surgeons always present when people are wounded under seemingly satisfactory conditions for closure and the great difficulty, as I see it, is that the example will be followed by inexperienced men in unfavorable conditions. We had the same thing to deal with here in the States in the treatment of compound fractures occurring near camps produced by accidents in motor vehicles. These fractures resembled in all details those of civil life and were frequently gotten into hospital within one to three hours. It was with the greatest difficulty and only after numerous directives that the Surgeon General's Office was able to compel the surgeons to leave these wounds open, more as an example and a lesson than anything else because many of them could be closed safely, but not in war wounds. I have no hesitation in placing myself on record that we still adhere to the principle of no closure. I think that I can buttress this with the experience of the surgeons in the Tunisian and Sicilian campaigns and I am sure that their records show that a great many people developed serious complications both in the closure of wounds and in the packing of wounds, which is equally undesirable.

On 4 February 1944, Maj. Gen. Norman T. Kirk wrote a letter to General Hawley containing the following:

Much bone length has been sacrificed by these methods. I am sure that the chances of infection are less in Air personnel and in the Navy with men aboard ships. However, I have seen many infections occur in operating rooms under what were supposed to be ideal aseptic conditions and when elective rather than emergency surgery was being performed. I don't believe that a wound has to be full of mud, manure or cinders to have streptococcus, staphylococcus or even gas bacillus present in it. Peterson, in a recent tour of our hospitals, found three amputations here at home where debridement and primary suture were carried out within the critical period and gas gangrene occurred requiring amputation to save life. I have seen other cases so treated and the wound closed. The doctor said he took a chance and got away with it. The patient took the chance, not the doctor. Also, the patient didn't have a vote and wouldn't have known how to vote.

The Consultant in North Africa finds that many of these wounds, at the end of eight or ten days, with the assistance of penicillin, sulfa drugs or none of these agents, may be safely excised and secondary suture performed. I am in accord with this, particularly in superficial wounds, to get men back to duty earlier. It may be applicable to compound fractures with destruction of large muscle masses. I am not too sure about this, however.

It is accepted that the flap type guillotine may initially be performed if that patient is not to be transported and can be held under observation in a given hospital but the following must be weighed and when this is considered: traction is applied with difficulty and traction made by the use of sutures through flaps causes necrosis of tissue followed by infection. Bone length almost always has to be sacrificed when this method is employed. We are getting back too many below-knee stumps from overseas that are too short to be fitted with prosthesis. We are also getting many back with skin grafts. This is not at all necessary. The circular type guillotine of the thigh with proper traction will be healed in six weeks and will stay healed. If it is closed primarily, too many cases of osteomyelitis will develop, too much shortening will be occasioned and the resulting stumps will frequently not be satisfactory from the prosthetic standpoint.

As you can see from the above, I am not at all in accord with your policy of handling your Air casualties. I know everything is going to speed these days and speed is a great thing but no matter how fast a plane can fly if the motor is cut out in flight it soon flops and it doesn't arrive at its destination. A lot more speed can be obtained if sound principles of surgery are at the same time observed. In the last war lives were lost, as well as extremities, from primary closure as well as too early secondary closures. No surgeon, no matter how expert, can always do a complete debridement of a wound. If that were true we would not be having the increase in the incidence of gas gangrene in Italy. And I am very afraid of what that incidence is going to be when we get into the Continent. I am also afraid that a lot of it is going to develop under plaster, with disastrous results.

Under these circumstances, General Hawley's instructions to the Chief, Professional Services Division, on 16 February 1944, were simply: "This policy will be followed in ETO. Implement."

The implementation was done by publishing The Surgeon General's Circular Letter No. 91 as Circular Letter No. 28, Office of the Chief Surgeon, ETOUSA, 1 March 1944, Section I of which was titled "Surgery of the Extremities." On 21 February 1944, Colonel Cutler informed General Rankin by letter that this was being done. He explained as follows:

I fear you did not quite understand my little note on "The importance of wound closure". It begins with the sentence: "'Do not suture' is accepted as the major principle in the surgery of battle casualties". What I was interested in was to have our surgeons remember that there also was something to be desired in closing the wound eventually so that the man could be returned to duty. Everyone has emphasized "do not suture a wound" so much that the young surgeon takes no interest in his wound after it is once made, and wounds which could be closed on the second to fifth day by delayed secondary suture or by skin grafts during the same period are left to slowly granulate, thus keeping a man in hospital sometimes a month or more after he should have been discharged. I hope you and the Surgeon General do not for a moment think that we are practicing the primary closure of wounds.

The Surgeon General in his letter says: "I am not at all in accordance with your policy of handling your air casualties". I cannot find we have done anything he would not approve of. There have been few amputations with the Air Force and only one in which very short flaps were made. In this case the wound was closed by delayed secondary suture the next day, and healed forthwith. It was an arm which had been blown off by rocket shell in the Schweinfurt raid, at about the junction of the middle and upper third. Every attempt is made here to leave as much bone as possible and I feel certain that if you and the Surgeon General could visualize our work in those hospitals serving the Air Force you would be most happy, as are General Grow and those responsible for the medical care of the Air Force itself.

Fortunately, only a few weeks later, General Kirk and General Grant (fig. 55), the chief medical officers of the Army and the Army Air Forces, respectively, were sent to the European theater for the specific purpose of reviewing hospitalization facilities for the Army Air Forces in the United Kingdom. It was Colonel Cutler's privilege to accompany and guide them through the many installations devoted to the care of air casualties. In their tour of the hospitals, which began on 9 March 1944 and continued almost without a break through 17 March, there was complete satisfaction in the surgical care which was being provided.[58]

---

[58] Memorandum, Col. E. C. Cutler, MC, for Maj. Gen. N. T. Kirk, 20 Mar. 1944, subject: Tour of Medical Units, E.T.O., March 8, 1944–March 17, 1944.

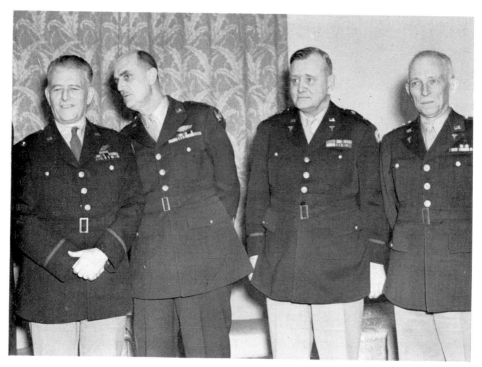

FIGURE 55.—Left to right, Maj. Gen. Malcolm C. Grow, Maj. Gen. David N. W. Grant, Maj. Gen. Paul R. Hawley, and Maj. Gen. Norman T. Kirk.

Penicillin

Spurred on by the war effort, knowledge concerning penicillin increased by leaps and bounds. There grew an ever-hopeful attitude that here was a new medical implement which would have profound effects in improving the care which could be given the wounded. There were indications that it might prove to be the greatest bacteriological agent yet produced, although Colonel Cutler thought it needed further assay in the human body before final opinion could be hardened. There were indications, also, that great strides were being made in devising methods for producing penicillin, methods which, early in this period, were still laborious and time-consuming processes. Thus, for the Chief Consultant in Surgery, ETOUSA, it was imperative that he gain all the data he could in order to be able with some confidence to advocate a stand-ardized regimen of treatment using penicillin and to insure that adequate sup-plies of the antibiotic would be available to carry out the treatment recom-mended. Moreover, the opportunity to study the efficacy of penicillin in the European theater was unparalleled, for here in the United Kingdom were some of the persons who were at the forefront in its development.

As reported previously (p. 52), a beginning in this direction had been made by the studies which Lt. Col. Rudolph N. Schullinger, MC, was conducting at the 2d General Hospital with the advice and help of Prof. Howard E. Florey and Dr. Mildred Florey, his wife. By the opportune arrival of more penicillin in September 1943, Colonel Schullinger was able to continue his work and bring it to a conclusion in March 1944. Colonel Schullinger gave the following account of these early experiences: [59]

Shortly after the Second General Hospital arrived at Heddington, Oxford, in July 1942, the University faculty as well as some of the hospital staff members held a reception for the "invaders" at Christ College. It was a most interesting and enjoyable occasion. Here it was my good fortune and privilege to meet Professor Howard Florey, Director of the Sir William Dunn Research Laboratory, and his wife, Doctor Mildred Florey. In the course of our conversation, they spoke of their exciting studies with penicillin and invited me to visit their laboratory. The invitation was eagerly accepted. The attractive and well built laboratory was situated on a quiet street not far from Rhodes House. Once inside, the visitor could sense an atmosphere of considerable activity. As one passed the various research units, it was apparent that doctors and technicians were busy and intent on their work. Professor Florey's study was a spacious oval room on the second floor flanked with bookshelves and files. In the center was a large table covered with papers and periodicals in "orderly disorder" and, at the end, nearest the window, was Professor Florey's chair. No matter how busy he was with his studies, correspondence, and writings, the visitor was always received with a welcome smile and an invitation to join his company.

It soon became apparent that here a great project was in full play. Professor Florey was at the helm, directing the technical aspects in the production and refinement of penicillin, and consulting with his wife, who carried out the clinical application of this new antibiotic. The process of preparing penicillin was so laborious in the early phases of this work that only carefully selected cases could be chosen for this therapy. In fact, the amount of penicillin was so limited that the urine of patients undergoing treatment was saved and returned to the laboratory for extraction and repurification of the penicillin for subsequent use. Sometimes the supply of penicillin gave out completely, thus necessitating temporary discontinuance in critically ill patients. These were trying and discouraging moments.

Thus, during the autumn and winter months of 1942–1943, the writer enjoyed the unusual privilege of witnessing the clinical application of penicillin to patients in some of the British military, civilian, and E.M.S. hospitals. Several trips were also made to the RAF Hospital at Holton. Wherever she went, Doctor Florey took careful notes and measured out the dosages with precision (perhaps two to five thousand units per dose) for the next two or three days. The results were usually dramatic. Here was a boy with a fulminating hematogenous osteomyelitis who responded promptly to "large doses" (10,000 units every four hours) of penicillin and required no operative interference. In the Radcliffe Infirmary a young army officer with cavernous sinus thrombosis and sepsis recovered after a fortnight of penicillin therapy. Infected wounds seemed to improve rapidly with local applications of penicillin. A penicillin cream was used for certain types of burns.

Observing the clinical aspects with Doctor Florey, and discussing the overall problem at various times with Professor Florey, it was obvious that here was an agent that would be of enormous benefit both for military and civilian purposes. Colonel Elliott Cutler was consulted and it was decided to requisition a supply of penicillin "through channels" via the Chief Surgeon, E.T.O. Unfortunately, the supply in U.S.A. was quite limited and

---

[59] This account was obtained from Dr. Schullinger by William S. Middleton, M.D., Chief Medical Director, Veterans' Administration. Dr. Middleton, who was formerly a colonel in the Medical Corps and Chief Consultant in Medicine in the European theater forwarded the paper to Col. J. B. Coates, Jr., MC, by letter, 26 August 1957.

there was none available through British sources. After a considerable interval another attempt was made to obtain the precious material by enlisting the British Research Council to make a direct appeal to the O.S.R.D. Meanwhile, Professor Florey had flown to the Eighth Army in North Africa to study the effect of penicillin in its local application to septic war wounds.

Finally, on 8 May 1943 a consignment of one million units, valued at one thousand dollars, arrived at the Second General Hospital. It was prepared in powder form, sealed in 10,000 unit vials. The consignment was locked in the ice-box next to the main kitchen. A consultation was then held with Professor Florey, Colonels Cutler, Kimbrough, and Storck, as well as Major Sloan and the writer, in order to formulate certain policies on usage and dosage.

Although the penicillin was to be administered only to members of the U.S. Forces, it was difficult indeed to deny urgent requests from neighboring British military and civilian hospitals. The first case to be treated was a young Air Force lieutenant with staphylococcus osteomyelitis of the left femur secondary to flak and shrapnel wounds of the thigh and pelvis. Other cases soon followed, chiefly infections secondary to injuries and wounds. This continued through the late spring and summer of 1943. At the same time, instruction courses on the use and preservation of penicillin were given at the Second General Hospital to officers on detached service, and this was continued well into the spring of 1944.

During the winter of 1943–1944 the writer presented results of penicillin therapy administered to patients in General Hospital Number Two at various U.S. Army Installations in England (Tavistock, Winchester, Leamington, etc.). Of considerable interest was the reported recovery in January 1944 of a British soldier, at the military hospital in Shaftsbury, stricken with *Staphylococcus aureus* pyemia and endocarditis. He received a total dosage of five million units. Finally, on 11 February 1944, through the kind offices of the late Sir Arthur Hurst, it was the writer's privilege and honor to address the faculty and students at Guy's Hospital on penicillin therapy, based on clinical studies at the Second General Hospital.

During March 1944, sufficient penicillin had been received as to permit formulation of directives for its use at various U.S. military hospitals in the United Kingdom. Already plans were being drawn up for penicillin therapy in advance combat areas.

On 29 March, the documented report on penicillin therapy at the Second General Hospital was submitted to Colonel Elliott Cutler.

Thus, in brief, the reader may appreciate the role played by one of the U.S. Army hospitals in Britain in the clinical application of penicillin therapy during the earlier years of its development (1943–1944). It would be impossible to give adequate expression of appreciation and gratitude to Sir Howard and Lady Mildred Florey for their many kindnesses, gracious hospitality, and warm friendship, not to mention their unselfish expenditure of time and interest in counseling and encouraging the writer during this stirring period of study at the Second General Hospital in Oxford.

An abbreviated version of Colonel Schullinger's final report was forwarded by Colonel Cutler to The Surgeon General.[60] The summary portion of the report read, in part, as follows:

A somewhat varied group of forty cases, treated with penicillin in this theater between May 1943 and March 1944, has been collected and presented. Twenty-six were improved or cured, seven had doubtful or equivocal results and seven were failures. Five deaths occurred, in which three may have succumbed to other causes or, at best, to distantly related circumstances. * * * The forty cases comprised two main categories, namely

---

[60] Essential Technical Medical Data, European Theater of Operations, U.S. Army, for May 1944, dated 14 June 1944.

infections and prophylactically treated wounds. This report does not include sulfa-resistant gonococcal urethritis, lues, fresh battle wounds or medical infections, such as meningitis or pneumonia. * * *

An effort has been made to point out the necessity for strict adherence to the criteria governing proper penicillin therapy. The indications for therapy should be carefully considered and evaluated, before resorting to active treatment. Actual dosage should not be according to fixed or dogmatic rules, but should be governed by careful bacteriostatic control, because of the variability in excretion rate. Inadequate dosage predisposes to the development of penicillin-fast strains. However, complete bacteriostasis, throughout the *whole* interval between doses, may not be essential. On the other hand, some strains have a natural resistance even though the family is ordinarily sensitive. Contrariwise, we have encountered two sensitive strains of *Streptococcus viridans*. The duration of treatment should be ample, particularly in the staphylococcal infections. * * * Many of the patients, with successfully treated infections, followed a fairly typical pattern: the improvement was gradual, the temperature fell by lysis, they looked and felt better, the appetite increased, sometimes quite markedly; there was less need for opiates, and the hemogram became normal. In those cases with infected wounds there was a marked diminution in pain, swelling and discharge, with rapidly appearing healthy granulations and accelerated healing. The route of penicillin administration was intramuscular, intravenous or local, sometimes in two, or even all three combinations. * * * The locally treated infections illustrate the remarkable efficacy of relatively small amounts of penicillin. * * * The number of equivocal results and failures in the present series suggests a lack of proper selection or inadequate therapy or poor management.

　　*　　　　　*　　　　　*　　　　　*　　　　　*　　　　　*　　　　　*

The prophylactic treatment of the group of compound fractures was most encouraging. This was due, in large part, to the short duration between injury and operation, the relative cleanliness of the wounds in the successfully treated patients, the skillful management by the experienced surgeons, and the local and parenteral administration of penicillin. The advantages of converting a compound fracture into a simple one is obvious. * * * The treatment of these compound fractures unfolds new possibilities in war, as well as civil surgery. Nevertheless, with few exceptions, primary closure of compound fractures must *never* be practiced in the forward areas.

Elsewhere in the report, Colonel Schullinger warned: "* * * the writer cannot too strongly emphasize the importance of adhering to sound surgical principles in the treatment of patients with penicillin. To neglect such practice, with the expectation that penicillin can perform miracles, is pernicious, and may even jeopardize a patient's life. It demands too much of penicillin and nothing could place it more readily into disrepute."

The study by Colonel Schullinger was, actually, a clinical trial of penicillin and not an experiment in the classic sense. The question of the efficacy of penicillin when used prophylactically was a paramount one because of its great implications for surgery in the field. True, Colonel Schullinger's studies had included eight compound fractures in which penicillin had been administered prophylactically. Six of the eight had improved or been cured, one was a failure, and the other resulted in death in which the result of the prophylactic use of penicillin was equivocal. Furthermore, except for a clinical appraisal, there was no way to be absolutely certain that the improvement or cure of the six cases was due as much to other extenuating circumstances and the expert surgery available as it was to the prophylactic use of penicillin. Therefore, on 10 September 1943, Colonel Cutler conferred with General Hawley and later the same day reported to Colonel Kimbrough by memorandum, as follows:

> The experience thus far in the use of this bactericidal agent has been largely in the treatment of chronically infected wounds. Our own experience as well as that of Mrs. Florey does not reveal that this agent is as universally satisfactory as has been written. Recently, Professor Florey and Brigadier Hugh Cairns have returned from North Africa and Sicily, where penicillin is now being placed in fresh battle casualty wounds with a sulfonamide. Thus there is no proper control of the efficacy of the agent.
>
> We have an opportunity with fresh battle casualties in our Eighth Air Force of testing out the value of implanting penicillin shortly after wounding. I have proposed to General Hawley, and it has his approval, that we conduct proper controlled experiments with casualties from the above source, treating every other battle casualty in each of our 6 station hospitals with the 8th Air Force with penicillin.

The proposal was also approved by General Grow, Surgeon, Eighth Air Force. Initially, Lt. Col. (later Col.) William F. MacFee, 2d Evacuation Hospital, was placed on one month's temporary duty as a special consultant with the Eastern Base Section to supervise and control the study. Later, as the project continued with the advent of more penicillin, Lt. Col. (later Col.) Paul C. Morton, MC, and Capt. (later Maj.) William R. Sandusky, MC, were assigned to the project. Colonel Morton eventually assumed primary responsibility for the study after the relief of Colonel MacFee.

The first problem in getting the study started was penicillin itself. Where was the supply to come from? Of the original supply which had arrived in May 1943, there was little left. In the London depot, however, there were 7,200,-000 units remaining of a supply which had been sent to be used for sulfonamide-resistant gonorrhea. The only other purpose for which this could be used was in cases of overwhelming infection where the saving of life was involved. Colonel Cutler calculated that 5,100,000 units of the original penicillin had been used for lifesaving purposes or for the treatment of gonorrhea and was able to recoup this amount, in exchange, from the stock in the depot.[61] This supply enabled the study to get underway. Shortly thereafter, General Hawley ruled that any amount of the penicillin being received for the treatment of sulfonamide-resistant gonorrhea could be used for the surgical penicillin work.[62] This decision permitted the distribution of 5,000,000 additional units to the study made on air force personnel and the 5,000,000 units previously mentioned to the 2d General Hospital for Colonel Schullinger's project.

Meanwhile, to insure a continuing supply of penicillin for the limited purposes for which it was then being used, over and beyond that which had been requested for sulfonamide-resistant gonorrhea, Colonel Cutler had advised the Chief Surgeon to make a request for an increase in the proposed

---

[61] Memorandum, Col. E. C. Cutler, MC, to Col. J. C. Kimbrough, MC, 14 Sept. 1943, subject: Re Withdrawal of 5,100,000 Units of Penicillin Now in London Medical Depot.

[62] Memorandum, Col. E. C. Cutler, MC, to Col. J. C. Kimbrough, MC, 18 Sept. 1943, subject: Penicillin Supply.

monthly allotment of penicillin for the theater. When the Chief Surgeon accepted this advice, the following letter was prepared by Colonel Cutler for General Hawley to send to General Kirk:

This communication relates to additional supplies of penicillin desired in the ETO. Our instructions from your office are that you will send us a supply of penicillin for treatment of sulfa-resistant gonorrhea only. We have already submitted data on the number of units of penicillin necessary to treat the expected incidence of this disorder according to the troop basis. You have already shipped to the ETO for this purpose 20 million units. Preliminary reports suggest highly beneficial results.

In addition to the above supply for "sulfa-resistant gonorrhea only" there was donated to this theater, on 3 May 1943, 18 million units. This has been used in close cooperation with Professor Florey and at present writing less than 2 million units remain on hand. Our Professional Services Division are extremely anxious that additional supplies of penicillin be avaliable for use in the ETO for the following purposes:

   a. Treatment of cases with gas gangrene
   b. Pyococcal septicemia and serious osteomyelitis cases
   c. Treatment of certain of the meningitides
   d. For a study of the value of penicillin when instilled into freshly acquired battle wounds.

We feel that we have an ideal set-up for properly controlled studies in the last category. Amongst casualties returning daily in our "bombers" the flow of patients is steady but not so pressing as to detract from the careful care and consideration. No other group of patients will present a better opportunity. We would like to treat every other patient without choice by placing penicillin in the wound and using a certain amount parenterally. We will have the opportunity to conduct proper bacteriological and other laboratory tests.

Heretofore in this theater the use of penicillin has largely been carried out in chronically infected wounds where the multiplicity of organisms and the extent of infection mitigate against great success by any single remedy.

The British penicillin group, of which Professor Florey and Brigadier Hugh Cairns are the leaders, have just returned from the active theater below us. There, penicillin is being instilled into fresh battle casualties, but always in conjunction with a sulfonamide, which will give us no absolutely positive evidence.

Supply

For the above categories of penicillin therapy we would like a monthly supply amounting to 50 million units a month for the present, in addition to that sent for the treatment of sulfa-resistant gonorrhea. We could easily use more and we are disturbed that our Canadian colleagues have been promised large amounts when it appears to us that we have a great opportunity for a competent study. If this request is granted, could a preliminary fraction be flown over shortly?

Because penicillin loses potency rapidly after being removed from the refrigerator and when in any other form than when dried and hermetically sealed, we would greatly prefer our units to come in the 10 thousand unit ampoules, as in our first lot, than in the 100 thousand unit ampoules, as in the second lot.[63]

The supply of penicillin seemingly assured, the controlled study on the efficacy of penicillin used prophylactically in combat-incurred wounds of aircrews was continued until March 1944, as was the study being conducted by Colonel Schullinger. The March termination of these studies was decided upon in order that final reports could be prepared for inclusion in a penicillin

---

[63] Letter, Brig. Gen. P. R. Hawley to Maj. Gen. N. T. Kirk, 17 Sept. 1943.

fasciculus to the April issue of the *British Journal of Surgery*. (The fasciculus was later postponed to the July issue.)

In the study made on air force personnel, there were eventually 250 wounds occurring in 146 patients which were available for comparison. In the penicillin treated group, there were 68 patients with 123 wounds; in the control group, 78 patients with 127 wounds (table 1).

The final report of the studies mentioned some of the following observations:

It should be clearly understood that the object of this study is not to determine whether penicillin is effective in established wound infections, but rather to learn whether penicillin, used prophylactically, will prevent or lower the incidence of infection in the wounds of aerial combat in a theater of war where early definitive surgery and continued observation can be carried out.

The wounded patients were divided into two groups. Those in one group were given parenteral and local penicillin prophylactically * * *. Those in the other group received no chemotherapeutic agent and serve as controls.

TABLE 1.—*Comparison of infection rates, with respect to wounds, in patients receiving penicillin prophylactically and in controls (patients receiving no chemotherapeutic agent)*

Wound category and patient group	Wounds	Infections	Infection rate
	Number	*Number*	*Percent*
Compound fractures:[1]			
Penicillin-treated patients	38	6	15. 8
Controls	28	5	17. 9
All patients	66	11	16. 7
Soft-part wounds:			
Penicillin-treated patients	85	5	5. 9
Controls	99	6	6. 1
All patients	184	11	6. 0
Total wounds:[1]			
Penicillin-treated patients	123	11	8. 9
Controls	127	11	8. 7
All patients	250	22	8. 8

[1] Excluding skull fractures.

Penetrating wounds of the abdomen or thorax or burns are not included in this study. The policy has been to administer sulfonamides or penicillin or both to all such patients, therefore no group of control cases is available for comparison.

The local dosage for wounds involving only soft tissue varied from 5,000 to 20,000 units in accordance with the size of the wound. Wounds associated with compound fracture and soft part wounds in the region of the anus or buttocks received from 10,000 to 40,000 units. In a limited number of instances, doses as great as 100,000 units were administered.

The usual method of preparation for local application has been to dissolve the sodium salt of penicillin in sterile physiological saline solution in amounts of 1,000 units of penicillin per cubic centimeter. This solution was sprayed on the wound by means of an atomizer. Another method only recently developed has been the insufflation of a mixture of penicillin powder and dehydrated human plasma on the wound surface. Ten thousand to 20,000 units of the sodium salt of penicillin to 0.1 to 0.2 gm of plasma has been found to be a satisfactory combination.

The local use of penicillin was combined with parenteral administration. The practice was to give intramuscularly 10,000 units of the sodium salt dissolved in 1 cc of physiological saline solution. This dosage was given immediately following operation and was repeated at three-hour intervals. Early in the study parenteral administration was continued for three days, but subsequently this was reduced to 48 hours.

At the time of operation the debrided tissue from the majority of the wounds was placed in sterile wide mouthed bottles and saved for culture. Following debridement and irrigation the wound was again sampled for bacteriologic examination. This was done by gently and thoroughly passing, over all parts of the wound, a sterile cotton swab, which was later cultured. In the beginning of the study only aerobic cultures were done. Later, four of the hospitals had facilities for anaerobic, as well as aerobic cultural methods.

The results have been judged solely from the standpoint of wound infection. The criteria for infection required the presence of one or more clinical signs such as tenderness, swelling, redness, lymphangitis, lymphadenitis, the presence of purulent discharge or infected hematoma. In wounds which were left open a distinction has been made between those having simple surface contamination and those showing clinical infection. The presense of organisms on the surface of an otherwise healthy wound is not considered infection of that wound.

The findings are presented in the tables [table 1]. The differences in percentage between the infection rates in the penicillin group and control group in each instance are not of statistical significance.

The results indicate that penicillin, used in conjunction with early definitive surgery did not lower the incidence of infection in such wounds. We cannot too strongly emphasize that our findings are not to be compared nor confused with other studies in which penicillin has been used to treat established surgical infections.

It is obvious that penicillin used prophylactically in the manner herein described did not prevent the development of gas gangrene in two patients. The role of this agent in modifying the infection, altering the toxicity, or in combatting secondary invaders cannot be evaluated at the present time.

* * * there are several points of interest from the bacteriologic standpoint. One has been the finding of a high percentage of contaminated wounds in aerial casualties [85 percent.] * * * The predominant organism has been the staphylococcus. Another contaminant worthy of note is the clostridium. The incidence of this organism in cultures of the debrided tissue increased as improvements were made in the anaerobic methods in the different laboratories. In one of the laboratories, when anaerobic as well as aerobic cultures were done routinely the incidence of clostridia (anaerobic gram positive bacilli) in the debrided tissue was 24 percent. Equally noteworthy has been the infrequent recovery of streptococci and enterobacilli. Another interesting finding has been the persistence of contaminating organisms in almost three-fourths [71 percent] of the wounds after debridement and irrigation.[64]

Early in the course of these studies, three cases of gas gangrene developed, and ultimately, there were seven cases of gas gangrene occurring in patients who had received therapeutic penicillin. Six of the seven were in wounds in-

---

[64] Essential Technical Medical Data, European Theater of Operations, U.S. Army, for May 1944, dated 14 June 1944. Inclosure 9, subject: Observations on the Prophylactic Use of Penicillin in the Wounds of Aerial Warfare.

curred as a result of air combat or air crashes, and five of the seven had also received penicillin prophylactically at the time of initial definitive treatment.

The occurrence of these cases, Colonel Cutler knew, was very significant since, at this time, many had high hopes that penicillin could forestall or prevent the serious complications of gas gangrene in war wounds. Penicillin in vitro had exhibited a bacteriostatic effect upon the organisms frequently associated with gas gangrene. Certain clostridial infections, experimentally induced in laboratory animals, had also been treated as well as prevented by the inoculation of penicillin. On the other hand, there were very little data on its effects on clinical gas gangrene.

At the first opportunity, Colonel Cutler presented a report on the findings in the three early cases. This was at a meeting of the Section of Experimental Medicine, Royal Society of Medicine, on 9 November 1943. A final report of all seven cases was prepared by Colonel Cutler and Captain Sandusky to accompany the reports of the other two studies—those of Colonel Schullinger and Colonel Morton. The early report and the final report emphatically brought out that the use of penicillin in these cases had not prevented the development of gas gangrene.

The final report observed:

While it is unwise to draw conclusions from so small a group of cases, we are so impressed with the fact that out of seven cases of gas gangrene, only one proved fatal and two recovered without loss of limb. [The fatality occurred after amputation as a result of uremia. Microscopically the kidneys showed hemoglobinuric nephrosis. At time of death, the local clostridial infection appeared to have been controlled.]

Equally impressive is the fact that of the recovered cases in no instance was a fatality apprehended. Each of the seven patients had the benefit of early diagnosis, prompt surgical extirpation of the infected tissue, therapeutic penicillin, large amounts of gas gangrene antitoxin and frequent blood transfusions. With so many factors tending to influence the outcome, it is difficult to estimate the value of any single one. * * *

For the group as a whole one conclusion is obvious and outstanding: Penicillin used prophylactically in the manner herein described did not prevent the development of gas gangrene. * * *

There can be little doubt but that penicillin is effective against many of the organisms which are found amongst the multiple contaminants in the wounds of battle casualties. Also a reduction in the devitalizing and even destructive effects of such other organisms tends to prevent a suitable medium for growth of the clostridia. At the same time this small experience does not fall in line with published and confidential reports to us that "penicillin is extremely effective in gas gangrene." [65]

In addition to these experiments, Colonel Cutler had information from many other sources, chiefly from the British. Of particular importance, in this respect, were meetings of the Penicillin Clinical Trials Committee and the War Wounds Committee of the Medical Research Council. As early as the 12 October 1943 meeting of the Penicillin Trials Committee, there was already information available to Colonel Cutler on the results of penicillin used prophy-

---

[65] Essential Technical Medical Data, European Theater of Operations, U.S. Army, for May 1944, dated 14 June 1944. Inclosure 10, subject: Treatment of Clostridial Infections With Penicillin.

lactically and therapeutically in actual combat, for much of this meeting was spent in discussion of the Florey-Cairns report.[66] In a memorandum, dated 16 October 1943, Colonel Cutler wrote to Colonel Kimbrough:

Professor Florey gave us a summary of the report of the Penicillin Commission which recently visited North Africa and Sicily. He made it clear that experience in that area had shown that placing some 50,000 units of penicillin even in a septic wound as late as 3 days allowed a great percentage of the wounds to close immediately and prevented the occurrence of osteomyelitis in compound fractures. This report will be of the utmost importance to us, for the matter of dosage now assumes a major problem. Professor Florey reported that calcium salt was as a rule used in conjunction with a sulfonamide in soft part injuries, but that where fractures were present larger amounts were used up to 750,000 units, and here sodium salt is used.

While these efforts were being made to gain as much information as possible on penicillin, Colonel Cutler also had to define the purposes for which it could be used, who could use it, and how it was to be used as greater amounts became available.

The first "penicillin circular," prepared in draft by Colonel Cutler, was Circular Letter No. 176, Office of the Chief Surgeon, ETOUSA, issued on 7 December 1943. The circular letter stated that penicillin was being issued to all general hospitals and the 49th and 121st Station Hospitals. It limited therapy to: (1) Patients suffering from overwhelming infections whose lives might be saved by the use of penicillin, (2) patients suffering from sulfon-amide-resistant gonorrhea, and (3) patients suffering from infections which, although not immediately endangering life, manifested symptoms which did not respond to the usual treatment. The selection of patients at hospitals supplied with penicillin was made a responsibility of the commanding officer. In hospitals not supplied with penicillin, commanding officers were instructed to request base section surgeons for permission to use penicillin in any particular case. If the request was approved, penicillin could be obtained from the nearest hospital supplied with it. The circular letter further stated that instructions regarding local and systemic administration of penicillin would be issued, as necessary.

The instruction to using hospitals was, of course, given to individuals concerned at the 2d General Hospital, as previously mentioned. Obviously, too, this extended use of penicillin provided an opportunity to expand the clinical studies being conducted at the 2d General Hospital, and, accordingly, elaborate laboratory checks and records were required.

The minutes of the 17 January 1944 conference of base section surgeons state that Colonel Kimbrough made the following announcement at the conference:

The supply of penicillin has increased so that it has become available for more general treatment. The plan now, and the Circular No. 6 has just been issued, is that a supply

---

[66] Preliminary Report to the War Office and the Medical Research Council, H. W. Florey and Hugh Cairns, October 1943, subject: Investigations Concerning the Use of Penicillin in War Wounds.

will be kept in all hospitals—field, evacuation, convalescent, station and general. The only check this office keeps on it is that all requisitions will be referred to the Chief Surgeon's Office for approval.[67]

The still wider use of penicillin within the theater made it necessary for Colonel Cutler to have the original penicillin circular changed. This was accomplished by Circular Letter No. 22, Office of the Chief Surgeon, ETOUSA, 8 February 1944, concerning penicillin therapy. The new circular rescinded the former and designated the following conditions for which penicillin therapy could be given:

1. Patients with serious infection, which will include injury and battle casualty cases as well as pneumonias, septicaemias, meningitides, etc., proven to be sulfa-resistant.

2. Patients with gonorrhea proven to be sulfa-resistant, and patients with gonorrhea untreated by sulfonamides, the importance of whose duties make it desirable that they should be absent from duty for the shortest period of time.

3. Patients suffering from chronic infections, usually osteomyelitis or prolonged wound sepsis, where the condition though not endangering life greatly prolongs convalescence.

It was now necessary to train nearly all of the medical officers in hospitals in the use of penicillin. Procedures to be used in carrying this out were announced by Colonel Kimbrough at a conference of base section surgeons on 31 January 1944, as follows:

Previously our plan was to have * * * a new hospital that was authorized to use penicillin send personnel to the nearest general hospital to be indoctrinated. It has gone so far now that all the personnel of the station hospitals need some training and it seems advisable to have an officer from the Medical Service, Surgical Service, and Laboratory Service visit their nearest general hospital for maybe a day or two's indoctrination in the methods of penicillin therapy. As a rule, all the general hospitals have officers that are trained. Rather than have one officer responsible for all penicillin, it was thought better to have medical, surgical, and laboratory officers. I was trying to avoid having penicillin put out to hospitals whose personnel were not familiar with its use and laboratory check.

Commenting on this statement, General Hawley warned:

The conditions for which penicillin can be used in this theater are very definitely laid down. I am going to take very severe and very summary action against any medical officer and any hospital commander and the Chief of Service that wastes stocks of penicillin in personal experimentation: I do not want any mistake about that. We need all the penicillin we can get for the use for which we have authorized it.

Assured by Colonel Kimbrough that the selection of cases had been definitely stipulated, the Chief Surgeon continued:

Professional policies are laid down by this office and will be carried out. We have got the best professional advice in the world and that is the way we are going to practice medicine in this theater.

With so many medical officers who would now be using penicillin receiving instruction from various sources, it was evident, this time, that a statement of official policy on methods of therapy was necessary. In consideration of this

---

[67] Circular No. 6 pertained to the extension of penicillin treatment for sulfonamide-resistant gonorrhea.

need, the Chief Consultant in Surgery submitted the following instructions on the local and parenteral treatment of wounds which were included in the afore-mentioned new directive Circular Letter No. 22.

Methods of therapy
*   *   *   *   *   *   *

(2) *Local and general therapy* * * *

(a) Make aerobic and anaerobic cultures of the wound before and after debridement.

1. All debrided tissue will be placed in a sterile jar and sent to the laboratory for study * * *.

2. After debridement and irrigation, wound to be swabbed with cotton swab which should be sent to laboratory for making cultures * * *.

(b) The debridement should be conservative with respect to living tissues particularly skin and bone fragments.

(c) Irrigate the wound thoroughly with physiological salt solution at body temperature during and at the end of debridement; penicillin works best in a slightly alkaline medium.

(d) Penicillin will be provided as a powder in ampules of 10,000 units or 100,000 units each.

(e) *Local* use of penicillin: For local use in wounds 10,000 units are dissolved in 10 cc. of sterile physiological salt solution, (strength 1,000 units per cc.).

1. For small wounds of the soft parts 5,000 units are sprayed into the wound.

2. For wounds of medium size 10,000 units should be used in the same manner.

3. For wounds of large size 20,000 units are similarly employed.

4. For compound fractures of the large bones the dose should be from 30,000 to 60,000 units * * *.

(f) After debridement and treatment with penicillin, the wound may be closed by primary suture, by secondary suture, or left open as circumstances warrant.

(g) *Parenteral* use of penicillin: For parenteral use, 10,000 units of penicillin are dissolved in one (1) cc. of physiological salt solution immediately before injection * * *.

1. For small wounds of the soft parts and medium sized wounds with little contamination, no parenteral use of penicillin is necessary.

2. In large wounds, in compound fractures, and in badly contaminated wounds of any size, the patient should receive 20,000 units intramuscularly every three (3) hours for two (2) days.

(h) If the wound has been left open following debridement, as in a compound fracture, the initial treatment of the wound with penicillin is followed by further penicillin sprayed into the wound as well as by intramuscular injection * * *. The wound dosage in such cases is 5,000 units sprayed twice a day.

(i) For wounds in the vicinity of the anus, buttocks, perineum, upper inner side of thigh and lower back, the standard dosage should be doubled.

(j) The initial dressing of the wound should be ample in size and well secured. Frequent changes of dressing are undesirable because of the risk of secondary contamination.

(k) In solution, penicillin deteriorates rapidly. It should be freshly prepared before each use. It is unfavorably affected by heat in both powder and liquid form and should be kept in the refrigerator or in the coolest place available. The solution will remain potent however, for 5 or 6 days, if prepared under aseptic conditions and kept in the refrigerator.

(1) Penicillin is a bacteriostatic agent and not a bactericide. It is excreted rapidly in the urine; fluids, therefore, should be moderately restricted unless other considerations preclude this measure.

(m) Penicillin affects particularly staphylococci, streptococci, gonococci, meningococci, pneumonococci and the clostridii. It is most effective in unmixed infections. It does not affect the colon group of gram negative organisms, the diphtheroids nor pyocyanus.

(n) Sensitivity and bacteriostatic tests must be carried out in every case.

(o) *Records.* All observations of wounds treated with penicillin will be recorded on the forms provided, in order to determine applicability of this drug in the treatment of war wounds. * * * All three forms will become part of the Clinical Record of the patient.

(p) All clostridii isolated in bacteriological laboratories at station or general hospitals * * * will be sent to the 1st General Medical Laboratory for final identification.

(q) *Laboratory instructions, wound treatment.* These instructions may be obtained from the Office of the Chief Surgeon * * *.

As the second long English winter ended for the Chief Consultant in Surgery, there was no doubt that the new spring would finally see an invasion of the Continent by the Allies. The production of penicillin at home had been stepped up tremendously. The shipment to the European theater for the month of March was 500,000,000 units. There were indications that this would be increased soon to 3,000,000,000 units. Other sources had said that the supply was now unlimited. Col. Silas B. Hays, MC, the new theater medical supply officer, said at the conference of base section surgeons on 13 March 1944: "In fact I would not be at all surprised if by the summer time we don't get too much penicillin."

In spite of the great amount of data on penicillin now available, much of it was tentative and some of it, contradictory. Current instructions on the use of penicillin were obviously neither intended for, nor applicable to, a combat situation. But what were the instructions to be? This question was of constant concern to Colonel Cutler, and there was not much time left. In a memorandum, dated 3 April 1944, he wrote the following to Colonel Kimbrough:

On 29 March 1944, I held a meeting in the Office of the Chief Surgeon of a group consisting of Colonel Schullinger, Colonel Morton and myself in order to discuss the present situation of penicillin in this theater.

In particular we met to discuss the material being assembled for publication in the British Journal of Surgery.

     *   *   *   *   *   *

The Committee took up further the matter of revising our penicillin circular. This is much too bulky and demands too much for actual battle conditions, and by the time we have the next meeting we must have a simple circular telling the surgeon just how much penicillin to put in the wound, and we must rid ourselves of elaborate laboratory tests. Such a circular is now being drawn up.

And, on 10 April 1944, he wrote to Colonel Morton:

I have sent you a copy of the Florey & Cairns report. There is no one here much to help you with gas gangrene, though if we can arrange some kind of a meeting with MacLennan, who is back from the Mediterranean now, I will see you are implicated.

     *   *   *   *   *   *

We will call another meeting about the end of the month, but before then harden your mind as to exactly what you wish to put in a circular covering the use of penicillin in Army hospitals. My own ideas are crystallized as follows:

a. It will not be used in small wounds.

b. In large wounds of soft parts 20,000 units will be given in some suitable vehicle, and I presume this will have to be sulphanilamide.

    c. In all fractures we will lift the dose to 40,000 units.

    d. I am dubious about additional dosage by intramuscular injection, but perhaps we should attempt it, and you must specify over how many doses this is to be used.

The meeting alluded to was convened on 18 April. In his diary, Colonel Cutler noted that he worked with Colonel Schullinger on the penicillin directive and with Colonel Morton on the gas gangrene directive. But he informed Colonel Kimbrough by memorandum on 22 April 1944:

    18 and 19 April was put in mostly working on penicillin, the greater part of the time with Lieutenant Colonels Schullinger and Morton.

    *   *   *   *   *   *   *

    Attached to this is a fairly final draft of the use of penicillin for battle casualties as it will be incorporated in the professional directive now being drawn up for our combat forces. In general I would like to state that we have presented in this document the optimum method; that is, we begin the parenteral use of penicillin as far forward as it seems possible to get the drug and we continue it for as long a period as we think ideally necessary. In addition, we place penicillin in the wound. I have heard that the U.S. Army in Italy is not using penicillin in the wound and I believe we have reached that point in our knowledge of this agent where we can say it is best used as are the sulfonamides; that is, by maintaining an adequate blood level which can be done without placing penicillin in the wound. However, if we do not limit our thinking to terms of the supply of the agent, then the method cited in our draft is optimum. Note that if we utilize penicillin as outlined the amount of drug required runs in to astronomical figures.

    a. Each soft part injury requires 420,000 units.

    b. Each compound fracture, 580,000 units, and both of these amounts are doubled when the wound is about the perineum or buttocks.

    c. If we take 6,000 injuries per day, which one might say is 1,000 casualties a day from each of 6 divisions, one corps of a 3 corps army in fighting, then the requirements would be, for 4,000 soft part injuries 1,680,000,000 units, and for 2,000 fractures 1,160,000,000 units, or a total of 2,840,000,000 units, and if 10 percent of the cases were wounds of the buttock, upper thigh or perineum, i.e. 600 cases, in which the dose would be double, then these 600 cases would need roughly 300,000,000 units or a total daily demand of 3,140,000,000 units. This for one month would mean 94,200,000,000 units which would mean 940,000 vials. Recommend that you transmit a demand for at least 75,000,000,000 units per month, once operations commence.

    We believe there is no contradiction to, and indeed desire that sulfonamide therapy continue at the same time as penicillin therapy.

    In addition to the recommendations made on the attached draft concerning penicillin in the Army, we are now revamping the circular for the use of penicillin in S.O.S. installations.

On the same day, recommendations for the treatment of gas gangrene were also submitted in final form. Both the penicillin and gas gangrene statements were included in Circular Letter No. 71, Office of the Chief Surgeon, ETOUSA, dealing with the treatment of battle casualties in the combat zone (appendix B, paragraphs 7 and 10). These instructions were published on 15 May 1944, not any too soon, and only 3 weeks before D-day. The important fact, however, is that the necessary decisions had been made and the command had been informed. Moreover, the decision had been independently made. The British, at this time, had not yet hardened their minds as to what their policies would be for the use of penicillin in the continental invasion.

Status of the blood bank

A question asked on more than one occasion by the Chief Surgeon during this period was: "What is the status of the blood bank?"

And therein lies the clue to activities at this time in the field of transfusion and resuscitation for the Chief Consultant in Surgery, ETOUSA. Unlike penicillin, facts in the case had been assembled, and he had made his recommendations. He had determined that probably 1 out of every 10 casualties would require parenteral fluids for resuscitation and that the proportion of plasma to whole blood used would be about two to one. Instructions had been issued to begin making some 350 field transfusion kits of the Ebert-Emerson type, and their assembly had begun. The Chief Surgeon had decided that whole blood would not be procured from the Zone of Interior, which left only one alternative—to provide for supplemental sources of whole blood within the theater itself.

The problem at this stage was to present the overall objectives to the theater commander for his approval, since the plan involved all elements of the command. Following approval of the plan, if granted, there would be an enormous amount of staff work to set up and establish the desired organization for the whole blood service, obtain the personnel and equipment, and gain further approval for specific operations involving elements other than the medical. In other words, the problem was no longer primarily professional. It was now a matter of operations and supply. Accordingly, the guiding force in establishing a whole blood service devolved upon Lt. Col. (later Col.) James B. Mason, MC, of the Operations and Training Division, Office of the Chief Surgeon (fig. 56). Later, Lt. Col. (later Col.) Angvald Vickoren, MC (fig. 57), replaced Colonel Mason in this responsibility. Initially, the supply aspects of the problem fell upon Col. Walter L. Perry, MC, then the theater medical supply officer.

Actually, much of the work on this project was done in committee fashion with Colonel Cutler representing the professional services; Colonel Perry, medical supply; Colonel Mason, operations; Lt. Col. Ralph S. Muckenfuss, MC, the 1st Medical General Laboratory; and Captain Hardin, transfusion and resuscitation. Obviously, efforts of the operations and supply officers would have been limited without the "ammunition" and advice provided by the professional members of this committee.

The first meeting of this group was on 19 August 1943. In addition to those mentioned above, Lt. Col. Ambrose H. Storck, MC, then Senior Consultant in General Surgery, also attended. The purpose of the meeting was to consider the matter of implementing the supply of whole blood and the entire problem of blood transfusion for the European theater. Colonel Cutler's report of the meeting mentioned certain points, substantially as follows:

1. After full discussion of the present transfusion field kit set originally laid down by Majors Ebert and Emerson, of the 5th General Hospital, it was

decided to place with each kit issued a printed list of instructions of its use. In this instruction sheet it will appear that 50 cc. of 2.5 percent sodium citrate should be added to 400 cc. of whole blood, giving a final concentration of sodium citrate of 0.27 percent.   Colonel Perry believes he can now implement the securing of a sufficient number of these sets for our requirements.

2. The securing of whole blood in the SOS and its transport to combat forces on the Continent.

a. Source of blood.   The source is to be SOS troops and lightly wounded and the ground personnel of the Air Force (about 40 percent of American

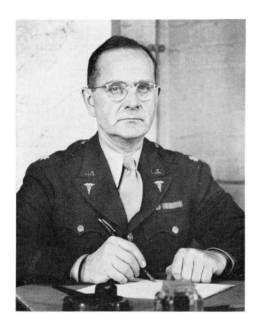

FIGURE 56.—Col. James B. Mason, MC.

troops are in Group O and are therefore satisfactory donors).   The source above should be ample for our requirements.

b. The giving of blood by the above troops should be *compulsory* (General Lee).

c. Collection of blood.   This requires mobile units with a refrigeration plant for 120 pints.   It is suggested we use 1½-ton trucks.   Personnel and T/BA of these mobile bleeding units already laid down and in the hands of Colonel Mason, and copies to be given to Colonel Muckenfuss.

d. Storage.   This should be at 1st Medical General Laboratory.   The refrigerator plant should be the large Navy refrigerators already acquired by Medical Supply.   We should need 2,000 pints in storage and should be prepared to supply 200 pints per day to the Army.   The General Medical Laboratory will need: (1) Storage space, (2) cleaning space, and (3) personnel for cleaning.   They will require 2,000 bleeding sets, 5,000 bottles, and 5,000 giving sets.

e. Delivery to the Army. Delivery from the laboratory to the Army should be by air in iced or Thermos containers. Colonel Perry is to look into the supply of these and Colonel Mason should make contact with the Air Force for the privilege of using such planes.

f. During delivery from the Army Medical Depot to the Army hospitals the blood will be kept in iced or Thermos containers. The responsibility for the returning of giving sets, bottles, and containers will be that of the Army surgeon.

g. None of this program should be implemented unless first priorities can be secured for the handling of such a precious and vital material as whole blood.

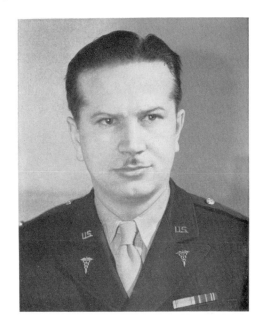

FIGURE 57.—Col. Angvald Vickoren, MC.

This includes items of collection, storage, transportation, and return of vitally important apparatus to the laboratory for cleaning and reuse.

On 24 August, Colonel Cutler and Colonel Mason visited Widewing, Eighth Air Force headquarters, for exploratory talks on the flying of blood to the Continent. At a conference on 20 September, Colonel Mason was requested by the Chief Surgeon to prepare with the least delay for submission to the Chief of Operations, SOS, details of plans for the whole blood service. After informing the medical supply officer of this requirement, Colonel Perry informed Colonel Mason that all necessary supplies were available in the theater except vehicles to be converted into refrigerated trucks. These, after Captain Hardin had checked over all types of vehicles for adaptability, were 2½-ton, 6 x 6, short-wheel-based cargo trucks. Colonel Perry initiated requests through the theater Chief of Ordnance to the Zone of Interior for 30 of these trucks. (Later, four additional trucks of this type were requested.) Provision of these trucks became known, in supply parlance, as Project GS 22 and GS 22 Supplemental.

In addition, Colonel Muckenfuss and Captain Hardin were asked to prepare a paper which would show the entire project in detail. This they did with their paper broken down into the following sections: Operating procedures, volunteer blood panel, estimate of requirements, operating agencies, the blood collection section of the base blood depot, the laboratory section of the base blood depot, distribution during the assault phase, personnel requirements, and necessary organic equipment.

Their report showed that 200 pints of blood per day would be required during the period from D-day to D+90 and that the whole blood service could collect 600 pints per day as a maximum. Beginning at about D−7, they estimated that 3,000 pints of blood could be collected by D-day. Following that, they contemplated maintaining a level of 1,000 pints at the base blood depot and 200 pints in advanced blood depots.

It was proposed that each SOS unit would maintain current lists of volunteer donors. Each SOS unit would report monthly the number of donors available to their base section commanders who, in turn, would consolidate these reports and notify the Chief Surgeon of the total number of donors available in their areas. The sum total of these volunteers would be known as the ETO Volunteer Blood Panel.

The operating agencies of the whole blood service were to consist of a headquarters section located at the 1st Medical General Laboratory, a base blood depot, and advanced blood depots. The headquarters would include the director of the whole blood service; a Medical Administrative Corps or Sanitary Corps officer in charge of administration, records, and supply; and clerks, orderlies, drivers, and automotive and refrigeration mechanics.

Under the headquarters, there would be a base blood depot with four bleeding teams and a laboratory section. The base blood depot was to be located at the 1st Medical General Laboratory with additional refrigerators at the 5th General Hospital for emergency storage and dispersion. The blood collecting section was to be composed of four bleeding teams, each having one Medical Corps officer and seven enlisted men with a refrigerated truck and other equipment necessary to operate mobile bleeding stations. The laboratory section was to recondition, clean, assemble, and sterilize equipment; process and store the blood; and prepare blood for shipment. One officer, an expert in transfusion and resuscitation, was to head the laboratory service and the base blood depot. He was to have 33 enlisted men to operate the washing room; the assembly room; the supply, still, and sterilizer facilities; the glassblowing and needle-sharpening facilities; the blood-processing facilities; and the refrigerators.

Contemplated for the other side of the channel were advanced blood depots to be attached to armies and those to be attached to communications zones. The functions of advance blood depots were solely to store and distribute blood under the supervision of the army or communications zone medical supply depot to which they would be attached. The primary difference between an army type of unit and a communications zone type of unit was that, in the former, there were to be eight refrigerated trucks and, in the latter, only four. In addition to the refrigerated trucks, each unit was to have an unmounted storage refrigerator.

The operation of each of these agencies was described in minute detail, as well as proposals for operating the service during the initial phase of the attack on the Continent.

Needless to say, preparation of a document of this sort, accompanied by charts and figures, required time. An equally lengthy period was required by the Operations Division, Office of the Chief Surgeon, to review, revise, and dress it up for formal presentation in sufficient copies.

In order to submit the proposed plan, Colonel Mason required a succinct statement as to why it was so essential, and he asked Colonel Cutler for this "ammunition." On 15 November 1943 Colonel Cutler provided Colonel Mason the following statement concerning the whole blood service in the European theater:

2. The evidence that whole blood is valuable in caring for battle casualties seems completely established.

a. We have the analysis of 30,000 givings of blood from the British North African campaigns. In these campaigns blood was drawn in Cairo, flown to forward areas and delivered by refrigerated trucks to forward medical units.

b. We have evidence that certain cases suffering from severe blood loss can only be saved by restoration of the volume through whole blood. Plasma alone may prove insufficient, and has been proven so by physiological experimentation as well as by clinical trial.

c. The Russian and British armies have a setup similar to that proposed.

d. Correspondence with our own medical units in the North African campaign shows that the forward medical units greatly desire blood in addition to plasma and some observers felt lives could have been saved had blood been supplied in sufficient quantity.

e. Direct communications from British officers follow:

From General Ogilvie, Consulting Surgeon, British M.E.F.: "Blood is being used more frequently, earlier and further forward. Blood transfusions save more useful lives than ever before."

From Colonel Porritt: "The best thing in the British medical services in North Africa was the Blood Transfusion Service."

On the same day that he submitted the foregoing information, Colonel Cutler also wrote to the chief of the Operations Division, Office of the Chief Surgeon, substantially as follows:

1. I am worried what might happen in this theater if a big attack started and great quantities of wounded people were brought to this island and our blood bank was not working.

2. Should we set up blood banks in station hospitals as well as in general hospitals now, or can we count upon our blood bank's supplying station hospitals with blood, should the necessity arise?

Colonel Mason assured Colonel Cutler that the distribution plan for whole blood provided for the emergency supply to station and general hospitals in the United Kingdom.

He also indicated that it was probable that each hospital could provide enough blood for transfusion from donors available in and about the hospital. Authorization of the Blood Panel, ETOUSA, and command arrangements for shipping, Colonel Mason stated, were being handled in the London office. As of that date, Col. Thomas J. Hartford, MC, had not sent out the letters to the Commanding General, SOS, although he had indicated this would be done in the very near future. Colonel Mason added that he would like to discuss with Colonel Cutler the matter of the supply of blood to SOS units in the United Kingdom at Colonel Cutler's earliest convenience.

The matter of supplying blood to SOS units in the United Kingdom was settled most opportunely at a later date. Meanwhile, General Hawley had submitted his recommendations (based on information submitted by the whole blood committee) for a whole blood service for the theater, as follows:

1. *The problem* To furnish fresh, whole blood for transfusion of battle casualties as far forward as division clearing stations.

2. *Facts bearing upon the problem* *a* The experience of the British and Russian Armies, as well as the experience of U.S. forces on all fighting fronts, is that dried plasma meets the requirements of only about two-thirds of all cases requiring replacement of blood volume.

b One-third of all battle casualties requiring replacement of blood volume must have whole blood as well as plasma.

c Early transfusion with whole blood in many cases greatly reduces the time spent in hospital and hastens the restoration of the casualty to full duty.

d A small amount of whole blood is available "on the hoof" in all medical installations; but this cannot meet the requirements for the following reasons:

(1) It must be typed under field conditions which favor inaccuracy, and death may result from giving unmatched blood.

(2) No tests can be made for syphilis and other communicable diseases; and the battle casualty may be given a disease by such transfusions.

(3) The efficiency of duty personnel is greatly reduced when they must donate blood.

e Fresh blood can be collected in the SOS, processed, stored and delivered to front-line divisions in small trucks carrying refrigerators.

f A total of 1 officer and 22 enlisted men, and 8 2½-ton trucks, 2 motorcycles and one ¼-ton car will be required for each field army. *All necessary personnel and equipment is already on hand in the Theater and the troop basis will not be increased.*

3. *Recommendations* *a* That the policy of furnishing refrigerated whole blood to medical units as far forward as division clearing stations, inclusive, be established in this Theater.

b That each army commander be informed that the necessary personnel and equipment * * * will be attached to the medical depot assigned to his army * * *.

c That all agencies transporting supplies be directed that refrigerated whole blood will be shipped on the highest priority.[68]

Following approval of the plan by the Commanding General, SOS, and the theater commander, the basis for the whole blood service was firmly established with instructions to the Commanding General, First U.S. Army Group, and

---

[68] Memorandum, Brig. Gen. P. R. Hawley to Commanding General, SOS, ETOUSA, 26 Nov. 1943, subject: Provision of Whole Blood for Battle Casualties.

instructions from the Commanding General, SOS, to set up the ETOUSA blood panel.

The command letter, dated 2 January 1944, from Lt. Gen. (later Gen.) Jacob L. Devers, Commanding General, ETOUSA, to the Commanding General, First U.S. Army Group, contained the following statement:

1. The provision of whole blood for the treatment of casualties in this theater, throughout all echelons down to and including division clearing stations, is approved.

2. Whole blood will be an item of medical supply and will be distributed through medical supply channels. It will be given the highest priority in transportation.

3. * * * personnel and special equipment will be furnished to each Army *without requisition* from sources available to the Commanding General, SOS, ETOUSA, * * *.

The ETOUSA blood panel was established by a command letter from Maj. Gen. John C. H. Lee's SOS headquarters, on 6 January 1944. The substance of the letter was as follows:

1. The establishment of a blood panel for the theater, to furnish whole blood in the treatment of casualties, has been approved by the theater commander.

2. It is desired that:

a. In each unit of the SOS, a nominal list of volunteer donors of TYPE O be prepared and retained in the unit headquarters.

b. A record of the *number* of TYPE O volunteers, *by unit*, in your command be maintained in your headquarters.

c. The records required by subparagraphs a and b be corrected as of the 15th of each month; and, immediately following each such correction, a report of the number of TYPE O donors in each unit of the SOS in your command be sent to the Commanding Officer, Blood Bank, ETOUSA, 1st General Medical Laboratory.

d. Upon call of the Commanding Officer, Blood Bank, ETOUSA, the volunteer TYPE O donors of the unit specified be assembled at a designated bleeding station (ordinarily the unit dispensary) at an hour, to be determined by you, which will not seriously interfere with the normal duties of the unit and which will be reasonably convenient for the bleeding team.

e. Only light duty be required of donors from the time of bleeding until reveille the following morning.

3. The general rule will be that four-fifths of a pint of blood will be taken at each bleeding, and that donors will not be bled oftener than once in each 3 months. This amount of bleeding will have no ill effect upon any donor and will neither reduce his physical capacity for work nor predispose him to illness.

4. Your active interest in obtaining as many volunteers as possible is enjoined.

As slow and ponderous as progress on the project might have seemed, there was no doubt that it was being carefully and thoroughly established. Colonel Cutler was pleased with the work being done and must have felt considerable pride in seeing what had been but a year before an idea of his maturing into a full-fledged theaterwide operation. After one apparently most satisfactory conference with General Hawley on the whole blood service, he wrote in his diary: "Blood project OK. Hope I got Jim Mason promoted."

The groundwork having been laid, there was still much to be accomplished before the whole blood service could be a reality. There was the question of how to provide the manpower for the service, and opinion varied between merely augmenting the 1st Medical General Laboratory or using a separate unit. The decision was made on the latter and a special table of distribution was made up for the 152d Station Hospital, which became the Blood Bank, ETOUSA. In December, both Colonel Mason and Colonel Cutler urged that it was high time to appoint an officer to be in charge of the whole blood service and command the 152d Station Hospital. Some names were suggested, but none proved acceptable for various reasons. The only position on which there was complete agreement was that Captain Hardin should be in charge of the base blood depot and the laboratory and bleeding sections under it. Eventually, Colonel Muckenfuss was placed in charge of the whole blood service and in command of the 152d Station Hospital. This was in addition to his duties as the commanding officer of the 1st Medical General Laboratory and as the theater consultant on laboratories. Since the headquarters and base blood depot of the whole blood service were to be located physically within the premises of the 1st Medical General Laboratory, and, since there would be no need to move either the whole blood service headquarters or the 1st Medical General Laboratory soon after the invasion, the choice was reasonable. Moreover, Colonel Muckenfuss had been acting, for all intents and purposes, as the head of the whole blood service up until this time. These arrangements solved the personnel aspects of establishing the blood project.

In late December 1943, not long after initiating the request for trucks, Colonel Perry had been notified by a message from PEMBARK, the New York oversea supply depot, that the trucks, as requested, had been approved and that 12 trucks were at the port awaiting shipment and the others soon would follow.

On 31 January 1944, General Hawley asked at the meeting of base section surgeons: "What is the status of the blood bank?"

Colonel Kimbrough, replying to the questions, said: "The last report they were 10 days from having the construction done—that was a week ago. The equipment is almost in. Refrigerators are frozen, allocated but not delivered. The people are there under the direction of Colonel Muckenfuss on the administration side, and Captain Hardin is carrying out the professional side. They have not called on us for any more personnel."

Two weeks later, at the 14 February 1944 conference of base section surgeons, General Hawley again asked: "What is the status of the blood bank?" This time, he added: "When are they going to be ready to start some bleeding?"

Colonel Kimbrough said that the physical plant was practically complete and that they should be able to begin bleeding at an early date (fig. 58). Lt. Col. (later Col.) Raymond E. Duke, MC, Operations Division, Office of the Chief Surgeon, said that, according to Colonel Muckenfuss, they should be ready to go within 2 weeks.

The bottleneck was in trucks and refrigerators. An incoming message from PEMBARK, 16 March 1944, said that the 30 trucks requested on project GS 22 were in port and were expected to go forward soon and that the four trucks requested in project GS 22 Supplemental were also in port and were

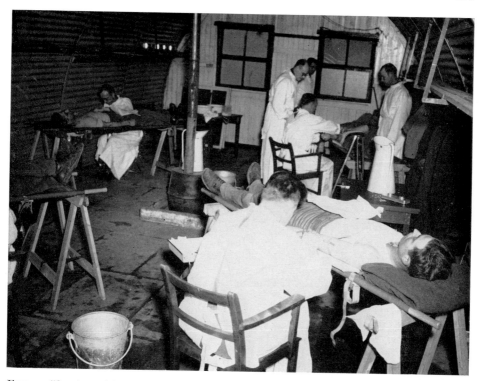

FIGURE 58.—A mobile bleeding team, beginning the first collection of blood for the European theater blood bank, Shootend Camp, Wiltshire, England, 11 March 1944.

expected to be shipped soon. It was disheartening to learn at this late date that the vehicles were still awaiting shipping. But Colonel Vickoren, with keen foresight, had anticipated such an outcome. PEMBARK had said in December 1943 that 12 trucks were ready to be shipped. As these had not arrived by the end of February 1944, Colonel Vickoren arranged to "borrow" 12 similar trucks from Ordnance maintenance stocks in the theater which were to be repaid by the 12 at New York when they arrived. These 12 were received from the theater Ordnance stocks late in March. When surveillance of the manifests revealed that none of the trucks from New York were on board any ships due to arrive soon, Colonel Vickoren requested that the remaining 22 trucks be supplied from Ordnance maintenance stocks. In the request, he stated: "These trucks are urgently needed, as approximately three (3) weeks' time is required to install refrigerators in these trucks after delivery is effected. The European theater blood bank cannot function without this vehicular equipment, yet each unit must be completely equipped prior to start of operations." [69]

---

[69] Memorandum, Chief Surgeon, European Theater of Operations, U.S. Army (by Lt. Col. A. Vickoren, MC), to G–4, G–3, Chief of Ordnance, Services of Supply, European Theater of Operations, U.S. Army, 18 Apr. 1944, subject: Vehicles for E.T.O. Blood Bank.

The story was the same with the refrigerators. They were approved and available on paper but could not be gotten physically. It was not until mid-February that the first refrigerators were received, but a relatively steady trickle continued to be received thereafter. Even at three per week, however, this represented four-fifths of the output of the British supplier. The remainder was being used by the British for maintenance of existing equipment. The delay in obtaining the original shipment was due to demands from active theaters.

At this time, when it appeared that the barest needs for establishing a whole blood service to support one army in the field seemed assured, Col. Thomas J. Hartford, MC, Executive Officer in the Office of the Chief Surgeon, London, returned from North Africa and Italy with some startling details. Certain of these bothered General Hawley and, in a memorandum to his Professional Services Division, on 28 March 1944, he wrote the following:

1. * * *
   b. *This not to be discussed outside the Division.* Less and less reliance is being placed upon plasma. Plasma seems to be quite effective if nothing is done to the patient afterwards, including transportation. But, if the patient is operated [on,] or if he is placed in an ambulance and moved, if he has had only plasma he relapses rapidly into shock.
   In the early days of the campaign, one pint of *whole blood* was used for each eight casualties. Now, one pint of whole blood is used for each 2.2 casualties (fig. 59).

*   *   *   *   *   *   *

2. The increasing use of whole blood makes me concerned about the capacity of our own blood bank.
   We cannot count upon an average useful life of more than 10 days for whole blood. I am informed that, under the best conditions, we cannot deliver whole blood to the front in less than 4 days after procurement. This means that an average life of *usable* whole blood is not more than 6 days; and, to be safe, we should not count on more than 5 days.
   This, in turn, means that the blood bank must be able to replace the total demands for blood at the front every 5 days.
   Can it do it?

Colonel Kimbrough optimistically replied that plans were being made to furnish whole blood in the ratio mentioned and that the blood bank would be able to replace whole blood in the time and amount required. Colonel Liston, acting for General Hawley while the latter was in the United States, insisted, however, that a firm figure for planning purposes be provided of the ratio of whole blood required to the number of casualties.

The problem was put to Colonel Cutler, who advised as follows:

British plans (from talk with Colonel Benstead in office of Major General Poole, British War Office, 6 April 1944)
   1. *Original British planning* after North African campaign was that *1 in every 10 casualties* would require fluid replacement including *blood.* When this is necessary, give 1 pint blood and 2 pints plasma—repeat S.O.S.
   2. *Recent planning* calls for *greater use of blood.* Colonel Boyd who was in charge of British Medical Blood Banks, favors 1.5 pints for every 10 casualties.
   U.S. Army plans
   1. Originally we planned as in paragraph 1 [Under British plans], 1 pint for every 10 casualties, supplemented with plasma.

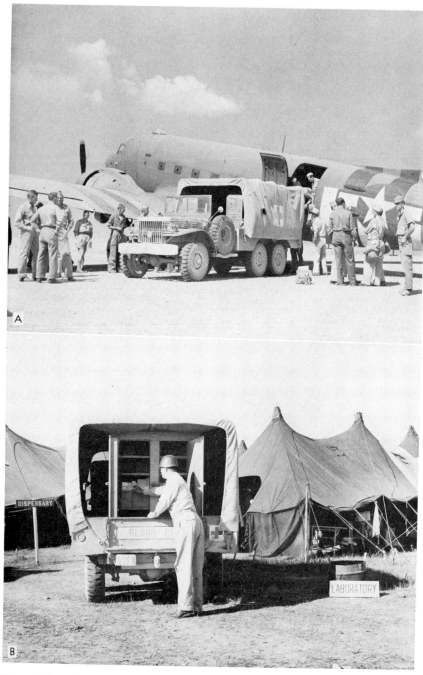

FIGURE 59.—Whole-blood service in the Mediterranean theater. A. Blood Transfusion Unit refrigerated truck, delivering blood to planeside for transportation to the Fifth U.S. Army area. B. A refrigerated truck delivering blood to a Fifth U.S. Army evacuation hospital.

2. Colonel Hartford, recently returned from Italy and North Africa, brings back use of blood after establishment of blood bank at Naples in Army Med. Lab.

Recent 5th Army beachhead statistics show: U.S. Forces used 1 pint blood to each 1.85 casualties, British used 1 pint blood to each 2.79 casualties. Total 5th Army statistics equal 15,000 casualties, show use of 1 pint of blood to each 2.2 casualties (this is field hospital and evacuation hospitals).

Comment: (1) Note Colonel Hartford's figures are for pints used, not blood per casualty. Thus, if 2 pints per casualty, it would be at following rate: blood would be required by each 4.4 casualty.

(2) In Italy donors are paid $10 per bleeding.

Recommend: U.S. Army E.T.O. Blood Bank be equipped to supply combat force with whole blood at rate 1 pint for every 5th casualty.[70]

While this recommendation and the logic by which it was attained might appear to be not entirely satisfactory, the fact of the matter was that the demand for a new planning ratio was merely an academic question at this time. It was obvious enough that the original objective of one pint of blood for every 10 casualties was going to be difficult to realize. Moreover, it had been necessary for the Commanding General, SOS, ETOUSA, to issue another command letter, on 6 April 1944, notifying SOS subordinate commanders that the number of donors had fallen far short of expectations and requirements and that action would be taken to increase the number of whole blood donors.

On the brighter side of the picture, however, were these factors. When Colonel Cutler had visited the blood bank on 31 March 1944 to discuss the possible extension of blood production, he had learned that six of the large walk-in type of storage refrigerators had been installed at the 1st Medical General Laboratory and were ready for use. Eleven trucks had been fitted with refrigerators and were also ready for use. And, with these facilities available, the blood bank was ready to engage in trial distributions of blood to the East Anglia area as an experiment—to ascertain how the service was actually going to function. Colonel Cutler noted, too, with pleasure, that Captain Hardin had finally been promoted to major.

Arrangements for the air delivery of blood to the Continent had long since been completed by Colonel Mason. In conference with Col. Edward J. Kendricks, MC, Surgeon, Ninth U.S. Air Force, Colonel Mason had obtained complete agreement on the following procedures: (1) Troop carrier aircraft from the Ninth Air Force would deliver blood from the vicinity of the base blood depot to the vicinity of the army medical supply depot on the Continent, (2) an enlisted man from the base blood depot could accompany a shipment of blood to insure proper handling and delivery, and (3) aircraft would return empty containers and equipment from the far shore and bring back the

---

70 (1) Memorandum, Col. E. C. Cutler, MC, to Col. J. C. Kimbrough, MC, 7 Apr. 1944, subject: Demands for Whole Blood. (2) "If the full truth be told, it was not until fighting was well under way that the consultants discovered that their estimates on the amount of blood needed were far too low. Until that time, they had thought that the capacity of the ETO blood bank would be sufficient." (Letter, Paul R. Hawley, M.D., to Col. John Boyd Coates, Jr., MC, 17 Sept. 1958.)

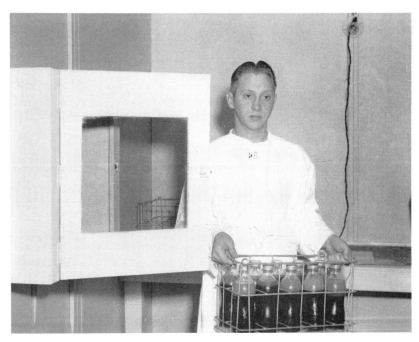

FIGURE 60.—Bottled whole blood from the Blood Bank, ETOUSA, ready for delivery or storage.

enlisted men who had accompanied the blood shipments. Colonel Kendricks also revealed the encouraging note that the Troop Carrier Command of the Ninth Air Force was quite familiar with the transportation of blood, since they had transported blood for the British Eighth Army during the North African campaign.

As D-day approached, there was no longer any doubt that the whole blood service was ready and able to conduct its initial mission of supplying whole blood in support of the invasion of the Continent (fig. 60).

While the whole blood service was being developed in this manner, there were also significant development in the matter of transfusion sets for "bleeding on the hoof."

Individuals in the Office of The Surgeon General saw certain difficulties and undesirable characteristics in the Emerson-Ebert transfusion unit, when they received details of the set. They realized that it had been devised with consideration for material available in the theater and for use, possibly, in areas forward of hospitals where autoclaving facilities would not be available. But they did not believe that directions given for cleansing and sterilizing the set would eliminate pyrogens and contaminants. The special representative to The Surgeon General on transfusions and intravenous solutions, Lt. Col. (later Col.) Douglas B. Kendrick, Jr., MC, suggested that it might be better to follow the system using empty plasma containers as described in Circular Letter No. 108, Office of The Surgeon General, 1943. The ideal solution to the problem, he suggested, was the expendable vacuum bottles and expendable recipient sets with filters, which were being proposed as regular medical supply items. Unfortunately, however, these recommendations could not be applied until the necessary equipment could be obtained.[71]

There were disadvantages, too, to the method recommended by The Surgeon General in Circular Letter No. 108, 27 May 1943, utilizing the dried plasma apparatus. Major Emerson brought these to Colonel Cutler's attention. The objections were pointed out in a memorandum, dated 27 Sept. 1943, to Maj. (later Lt. Col.) Michael E. DeBakey, MC, in the Surgeon General's Office, and included the following: (1) Cross-matching, as recommended, was not feasible with equipment available in the field, (2) the open technique was liable, in the field, to introduce appreciable amounts of foreign matter into the blood, (3) the type of airway in the apparatus would cause air pressure in the bottle to be below atmospheric pressure, and this, plus a layer of glass beads, two needles, and filter, would materially limit the rate at which blood could be administered, and (4) the material and equipment required for the cleaning and sterilization procedures recommended would not always be available in the field. The primary objection, however, was to the fact that only 300-cc. flasks of dried plasma were available in the European theater and when these were used for collecting sets with the requisite introduction of 50 cc. of citrate solution, the amount of blood collected would scarcely make the effort worthwhile.

In view of this situation, Major Emerson was detached to the medical supply depot at Thatcham, England, with enlisted men to help him, and continued to assemble the transfusion units devised by him and Major Ebert. Some 800 sets of instruction were printed to go into the unit packing, which eventually was done in used .50 caliber ammunition cases repainted to medical standards with the Geneva Cross. A 25-minute training film in color was also made to show how the transfusion kit was to be used. With only minor problems of obtaining the necessary items at the right time, the production of these transfusion units proceeded well.

In the meanwhile, Major Ebert was sent to the Office of The Surgeon General to present the European theater plans for providing whole blood in the field. Upon his return, he prepared a report of his visit for Colonel Cutler. The report was substantially as follows:

A brief interview with The Surgeon General and a long discussion with Colonel Kendrick, Special Representative in Transfusions and Intravenous Solutions in the Surgeon General's Office, were held on 6 December 1943 and subsequent days.

The Surgeon General was of the opinion that whole blood was not necessary in the most forward areas and that plasma should be used for the treatment of

---

[71] Memorandum, Lt. Col. B. N. Carter, MC, for General Hillman, 28 Oct. 1943, subject: Essential Technical Data, ETOUSA, and inclosure thereto.

shock under these conditions. In general, he did not believe whole blood should be used forward of the evacuation or field hospital.

A complete discussion was held with Colonel Kendrick concerning the nature and relative advantages of the equipment used at present in the European theater and the equipment recommended by the Surgeon General's Office. Colonel Kendrick described the equipment for blood transfusions now in production but not available at the present time. This consists of 750-cc. vacuum bottles containing 200 cc. of sterile McGill solution (an anticoagulant containing sodium citrate and glucose which is suitable for storage and blood). These bottles are manufactured by the Baxter Co., are expendable, and are used once and then discarded. In addition, donor sets and expendable recipient sets are provided. The recipient sets are made of viscose (cellophane) tubing, are packaged under sterile conditions, and are ready for immediate use. A simple wire mesh filter is included in each recipient set. This transfusion equipment is suitable for fresh blood transfusion or for the storage of whole blood.

In the discussion with Colonel Kendrick, the advantage of having all the equipment necessary for performing a blood transfusion included in a single container was pointed out. As a consequence it was decided to package the equipment in a fiber box which will contain 11 vacuum transfusion bottles, 11 recipient sets (sterile expendable), 1 donor set, and a box each of anti-A and anti-B typing serum. This equipment will not be ready for distribution until approximately February 1944. The equipment should, however, be requisitioned immediately. The equipment has not yet been given an order number. It can be requisitioned as follows:

Complete transfusion set containing the following: 11 vacuum transfusion bottles with McGill solution, 11 recipient sets (sterile expendable), 1 donor set, 1 box of typing serum anti-A, 1 box of typing serum anti-B.

In view of the fact that the exact date of delivery could not be guaranteed, it was recommended that the present plans for transfusion equipment in the European theater should be continued until such a time as the new equipment should be substituted.

A 4-cubic-foot electric refrigerator designed for storage of whole blood is available. This has sufficient capacity to hold approximately 50 bottles of blood. The refrigerator can be operated from the usual powerline supply as well as by a small 500-watt generator which is supplied with it. It is recommended that these refrigerators be placed in all general, evacuation, and field hospitals. The refrigerators can be requisitioned as follows:

Refrigerator for storage of whole blood.

Generator for above.

It was strongly felt by all concerned in the discussion that transfusion services should be established in all hospitals under the supervision of a transfusion officer. This service would be responsible for the formation of a donor panel, typing of blood, withdrawal and administration of blood and storage of blood. It was felt that provision should be made for training men in modern transfusion technique.

Through the courtesy of Capt. John Elliott, SnC, Army Medical School, and Dr. Louis K. Diamond, of Harvard Medical School, 20 cc. of anti-Rh serum (in dried form) was obtained for use in this theater.

In accordance with Major Ebert's suggestions, Colonel Zollinger, acting for Colonel Cutler, took the necessary steps through the Operations Division and the Supply Division, Office of the Chief Surgeon, to procure 4,000 complete transfusion sets of the expendable type and some 200 refrigerators and generators for storing whole blood. Sufficient refrigerators, over and beyond those already available in the theater's hospitals, were requisitioned so that not only the general, evacuation, and field hospitals—as recommended by Major Ebert—but station and convalescent hospitals and general dispensaries as well could be equipped with blood-storage facilities.

By mid-March, the Emerson-Ebert transfusion units were ready for distribution and were issued to units of the First U.S. Army on the following basis:

First U.S. Army Unit	Transfusion sets
Evacuation Hospital (750-bed)	2
Evacuation Hospital (400-bed)	2
Field Hospital (2 each platoon)	6
Convalescent Hospital	1
Auxiliary Surgical Group	20
Clearing Company, Medical Battalion	2

Colonel Zollinger explained that these units varied from the original in that sufficient serum for typing only 25 donors was included instead of enough for the original 50. In addition, the number of transfusions possible from each kit was 10 or 11 instead of 18, as originally planned. These changes were necessitated because it was necessary to use British sodium citrate solution, which was more bulky in its packing than American supplies of the solution.[72]

On the basis of issue determined by the Operations Division, the First U.S. Army required some 175 of the transfusion units. When the decision was made that the Third U.S. Army would be equipped with the new expendable type of unit being developed by the Surgeon General's Office, the excess transfusion units developed in the European theater were provided Army Air Forces medical units at operational airbases in the United Kingdom for emergency use. It was further contemplated that replacement of the Emerson-Ebert transfusion sets would be accomplished by using the new expendable type.

The equipment and facilities for transfusion and restoration of blood having been completed, the entire program was finally tied together with intensive courses conducted throughout the medical units in the theater on the reconstitution of blood plasma for administration, attendance of First U.S. Army medical officers at the course on transfusion and resuscitation at the British Army Blood Supply Depot, and instruction on the use of the European theater transfusion unit utilizing the motion picture which had been prepared.

---

[72] Memorandum, Lt. Col. R. M. Zollinger, MC, to Lt. Col. A. Vickoren, MC, 13 Mar. 1944, subject: Concerning Field Transfusion Units.

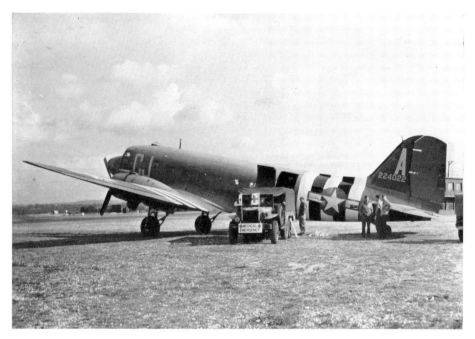

FIGURE 61.—A European theater blood bank truck at an airfield in England. Note the "Medical Emergency" sign on the truck.

Finally, permission was obtained to classify the refrigerator trucks, which would be distributing blood, as surgical trucks so that they could be painted with the Geneva cross and receive protected status—and also, so that they would be given priority on the roads in carrying out their lifesaving mission of mercy (fig. 61).

Incidental preparations for invasion—Operation OVERLORD

General Hawley continually insisted that all planning should be done with combat operations in mind. For instance, at the 30 August 1943 meeting of base section surgeons, he stressed the point that no procedures should be established which could not be followed when combat started. Thus, all planning was, or should have been, directly related to contemplated combat operations. But some things were done specifically for the first phase of combat in the European theater, the assault upon the Continent—Operation OVERLORD. Other activities, while the intent was for their continuance during and after Operation OVERLORD, nevertheless had to be completed for OVERLORD or were conducted with OVERLORD specifically in mind. Among the latter, incidental preparations which concerned the Chief Consultant in Surgery were such programs as: (1) Rehabilitation, (2) care of the lightly wounded, (3) realinement of teams within auxiliary surgical groups, and (4) preparation of documents which would be readily available and would contain all basic policies on surgical care and management of casualties.

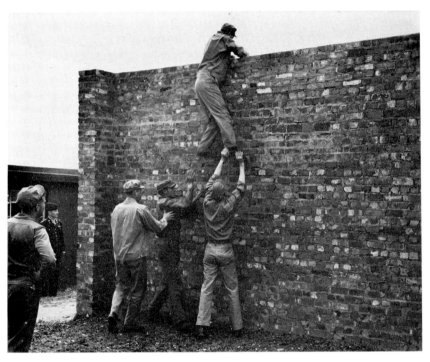

Figure 62.—Convalescent patients at the 203d Station Hospital, Stoneleigh Park, surmounting a wall in the obstacle course.

Rehabilitation.—The preliminary meeting of the surgical subcommittee preceding the meeting of the Chief Surgeon with his consultants on Monday, 22 November 1943, was lengthy and concerned chiefly the matters of rehabilitation and care of the lightly wounded. While Colonel Diveley, under General Hawley's direction, had initiated a huge, comprehensive rehabilitation program, there was yet a notable lack of agreement on many points (fig. 62). The program set up by Colonel Diveley, and at times looked upon with considerable alarm by Colonel Cutler, was based on large rehabilitation centers which were to bear the brunt of the rehabilitation program. There was also a requirement that hospital commanders, using their initiative, establish rehabilitation programs for their in-patients. Questions in this area now involved such items as (1) how much and what rehabilitation was to be conducted in hospitals, (2) who were to go to these rehabilitation centers and during what phase of their convalescence they were to go, (3) what the distinction was between hardening (reconditioning) and rehabilitation, (4) what the functions were of a replacement center as compared to those of the rehabilitation center, and (5) when a soldier was to be considered as rehabilitated? While the rehabilitation problem was of considerable concern to all the consultants during this period and had been a responsibility of the Chief Consultant in Surgery at one time, a separate portion of this chapter deals with the subject and this report on the activities of the Chief Consultant in Surgery will not belabor the subject. Let it be said, however, that Colonel Cutler and the other consultants all saw eye to eye in the needs for a sound rehabilitation program regardless of their individual differences as to how the program should be carried out. And Colonel Cutler, with characteristic energy, strove to develop the rehabilitation program while keeping it in bounds. Although the object of the rehabilitation program was to return as many patients as possible as early as possible to some useful form of duty in the theater, it is mentioned here because there was also the contingent need to make the most efficient use of hospital beds by transferring elsewhere those who were ambulant and could convalesce with little professional medical care.

Care of lightly wounded.—The care of the lightly wounded was a topic near to the heart of the Chief Consultant in Surgery, for it was in the optimum management of these cases that surgery could make its major contribution for returning the greatest number of wounded to the battlefronts. This matter had been frequently discussed within the Professional Services Division, but at the aforementioned meeting of 22 November 1943, there was enough agreement of opinion to permit Colonel Cutler to recommend that some 10 miles behind the 400-bed evacuation hospitals supporting divisions on the line, there should be a 750-bed evacuation hospital. "This," Colonel Cutler stated, "should be a hospital for the care of the lightly wounded and the nonseriously ill medical [patients]. At a moderate distance from this evacuation hospital should be the convalescent hospital, centered for the army, and the lightly wounded and nonseriously ill medical [patients] should be able to stream through this 750-bed evacuation hospital for initial treatment, and then recover in the convalescent hospital, from which they could be restored to active duty without traveling further down the line. Indeed, some personnel could go directly from this 750-bed evacuation hospital to active duty."

The overall system using platoons of field hospitals close to division clearing stations, 400-bed evacuation hospitals farther to the rear, a 750-bed evacuation hospital well in the corps rear area, and a convalescent hospital in the army service area would allow for the care of the nontransportable seriously injured individuals either in the field hospitals or small evacuation hospitals close to the line, and the care of the lightly wounded and others restorable to active duty in a 750-bed hospital and a convalescent hospital.[73]

At the 22 November afternoon meeting of all the consultants with the Chief Surgeon, the subject was again presented. Col. (later Brig. Gen.) John A. Rogers, MC, First U.S. Army surgeon, wanted to know what size army Colonel Cutler was referring to for his suggested use of 750-bed evacuation hospitals, and Colonel Spruit offered the thought that perhaps an evacuation hospital was not the correct type of unit to provide care of this sort. Colonel Cutler replied that he was thinking of one 750-bed evacuation hospital for an

---

[73] Letter, Col. E. C. Cutler, MC, to Col. J. C. Kimbrough, MC, 22 Nov. 1943, subject: Minutes of Surgical Sub-Committee Meeting, 22 Nov. 1943.

army corps.   To Colonel Spruit's assertion that the equipment of an evacuation hospital was too extensive to be used in this situation, Colonel Cutler submitted the opinion that, if these wounded were to fight again, they needed good care.

Colonel Rogers directed the attention of the conferees to the fact that there were not enough 750-bed evacuation hospitals in the theater to be used at the rate of one per corps and that the First U.S. Army was going to have only one. Colonel Cutler insisted that two would be necessary, but added that perhaps two field hospitals could replace one of them.   Colonel Cutler mentioned that there were many of the larger evacuation hospitals in North Africa.   Colonel Tovell confirmed this statement by reporting that there were 14 in the North African theater.   Colonel Cutler closed the discussion by explaining that he was not so interested in the type of unit as in the care of the lightly wounded in hospitals.

"We could save a lot of personnel for the Army," he maintained, "and it would make a big step forward."

The implementation of such a program rested squarely with the army surgeon, within the limits of facilities available to him.   And Colonel Cutler was very gratified to learn that Colonel Rogers saw the problem and its solution in much the same light as he.

Auxiliary surgical groups.—On 30 September 1943, Colonel Cutler visited the newly arrived 1st Auxiliary Surgical Group which had recently arrived in England and was quartered at the 68th Station Hospital.   He had an excellent talk with the group's commander, Col. Clinton S. Lyter, MC, who, he discovered, had some excellent ideas about the employment of mobile surgical teams. Colonel Cutler also learned, in his lengthy visit with the unit, that some of the medical officers were "pure" specialists in the sense that they were specialized in such a narrow field that they could not be employed on more general types of surgery.   For instance, there were two neurological surgeons who could not be counted on to carry out surgical procedures elsewhere than on the brain. They, obviously, would have to be removed from the group since they would be of no great use under combat conditions.   Colonel Lyter also informed Colonel Cutler that there was a new table of organization which greatly reduced the strength of the group and more or less limited teams to general surgery, a change which Colonel Cutler approved heartily and had been recommending since his first days in the Army in this war.

Later, Colonel Cutler and Colonel Lyter met with Major Graves of the 3d Auxiliary Surgical Group and planned to replace teams from the 3d Auxiliary Surgical Group on temporary duty at various installations in and about the United Kingdom by teams from the 1st Auxiliary Surgical Group.   However, on 2 October, word was received that the members of the 3d Auxiliary Surgical Group who had been loaned to the North African theater were returning.   This news necessitated cancellation of plans to exchange teams in the United Kingdom until more definite information was available as to the return of the 3d Auxiliary Surgical Group's long-absent members.

One specific measure was initiated as a result of these meetings. Under instructions from Colonel Mason, Colonel Cutler asked Major Graves to turn over the property in the hands of the 3d Auxiliary Surgical Group relating to mobile surgical teams to the 1st Auxiliary Surgical Group.[74]

At the conference of the Deputy Chief Surgeon on 3 October 1943, Colonel Cutler mentioned the arrival of the 1st Auxiliary Surgical Group and the expected return of that part of the 3d Auxiliary Surgical Group that had been in Africa and Italy. The immediate problem, he explained, was what to do with 300 doctors with nothing to do and nowhere to go.

Colonel Cutler met with General Hawley on 5 October 1943 and, among other things, there was a long discussion about auxiliary surgical groups. General Hawley asked Colonel Cutler to have the consultants draw up a comprehensive plan for the use of these groups, differentiating functions and personnel, as seemed wise, for a group with an army and for a group when employed within the SOS. Colonel Cutler advised General Hawley that he should ask the North African theater to return immediately an officer from the 3d Auxiliary Surgical Group for the purpose of training members of the newly arrived 1st Auxiliary Surgical Group. In a letter, dated 7 October 1943, written after his return to Cheltenham, Colonel Cutler informed Colonel Kimbrough of the conference with General Hawley and reported that he had drawn up a plan for the employment of auxiliary surgical groups under the dichotomous situations stipulated by the Chief Surgeon.

Colonel Cutler's recommendations entailed the following:

Regarding the use of auxiliary surgical groups with a field army, he thought that their function should be to carry out definitive surgical procedures in the forward areas by being attached to evacuation hospitals, field hospitals, and, possibly, even division clearing stations. The professional requirements for team members working in an army area and the need for specialists, he stated, were as follows:

The professional requirements of chiefs of surgical teams should be those of well trained general surgeons. The chiefs of teams should be competent to deal with injuries of any part. Strict specialists in the sense that they are competent to deal only with injuries to the brain, to the chest, to the extremities, the abdomen, the face and jaw are ideally undesirable. However, surgeons specializing in certain fields and at the same time competent to work in other fields would be desirable. And finally, the prosthetic teams, providing they were scattered and never concentrated in one place, should prove of great value to those surgeons dealing with injury to the jaws. Similarly, the orthopedic teams, as sent over with the 1st Auxiliary Surgical Group, could be of continuous value to all teams dealing with compound fractures. This was the arrangement in the last war when such teams were called splint teams.

As for the distribution of teams in any army area, he calculated that general surgical teams should be used in the ratio of two or three to one orthopedic team and that a prosthetic team was only needed for from four to six general teams. Further, he thought that the prosthetic teams would be needed only

---

[74] Letter, Col. E. C. Cutler, MC, to Col. J. C. Kimbrough, MC, 3 Oct. 1943, subject: Visit to 1st Auxiliary Surgical Group.

at very hard-pressed and active units. Neurological, chest, and maxillofacial teams would be required, according to his plans, only as the needs for them arose. This distribution of teams, Colonel Cutler stipulated, was based on the assumption that teams would be needed for 24-hour duty in the hospitals to which they would be attached, thus necessitating the assignment of two teams to every one team which would be working at any specific time and place.

Turning to the use of auxiliary surgical groups in communications zone facilities, Colonel Cutler stated that their mission would be to strengthen the professional capacity of hospitals and should be employed only in station and general hospitals. Special teams, he pointed out, could always be used to greater advantage in communications zone facilities than in those of a field army. This would be especially true if parts of several general hospitals were set aside as centers for thoracic, neurosurgical, or maxillofacial work.

After the usual Sunday meeting of the Professional Services Division on 10 October 1943, the surgical consultants, with Colonel Cutler, decided upon the temporary assignment of the various teams of the 1st Auxiliary Surgical Group to hospitals then active in the theater and turned over the plan to the Operations Division for implementation.

Later, certain specialists were gradually removed from the two groups, and, as revised tables of organization were received from the War Department, the component teams were reconstituted. The latter procedures were, primarily, a function of the Operations and Personnel Divisions and the commanders of the groups. They concerned Colonel Cutler little as the professional qualifications of those being realined within the groups was of the necessary high standard. Those qualified specialists who were dropped from the groups were reassigned most advantageously to hospital centers where their special talents were in great need. By the time D-day drew near, in addition to an auxiliary surgical group assigned to the communications zone, there was an auxiliary surgical group to be assigned to each of the two U.S. field armies—one of them to be used in the United Kingdom to augment medical facilities during the initial receipt of casualties from the far shore, as the Third U.S. Army was not scheduled for immediate participation in Operation OVERLORD, and the other to accompany the First U.S. Army during the assault on Normandy (fig. 63).

Publications and directives.—Shortly after returning from the Soviet Union, Colonel Cutler reported that the project of revising War Department TM (Technical Manual) 8–210, Guides to Therapy for Medical Officers, to make it more applicable to the European theater had been continuing for almost a year. He stated that, actually, it had been necessary to rewrite rather than revise and that there was still confusion in the revision concerning frontline care and the type of care to be given in fixed hospitals. The final revision, Colonel Cutler considered, entailed cutting down the manual still more and deleting some of the philosophical dissertations.[75]

---

[75] Minutes, 10th Meeting of the Chief Surgeon's Consultants' Committee, 23 Aug. 1943.

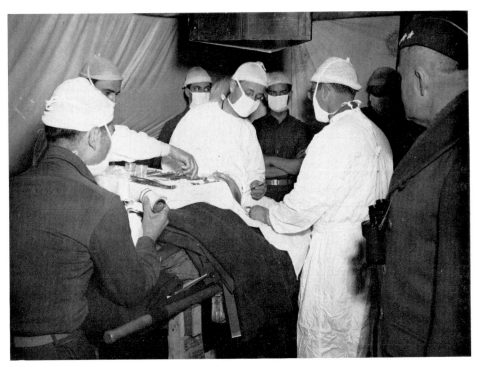

FIGURE 63.—Lt. Gen. John C. H. Lee, SOS, ETOUSA, observes a surgical team from the 3d Auxiliary Surgical Group as they train for the invasion of continental Europe with the First U.S. Army, Pentewan Beach, Cornwall, England, 12 April 1944.

At the 14th meeting of the Chief Surgeon's Consultants' Committee on 28 December 1943, Colonel Cutler reported that much additional work had been done on the manual after discussions with medical officers who had had experience in the Sicilian and Italian campaigns. The original revision had been recast in simple form with short, directive, staccato statements. He suggested that it was just about ready for the printer. In addition to this manual of therapy, which was to be printed in pocket-size editions, Colonel Cutler asked the Chief Surgeon whether it would be possible to issue a circular covering the care of battle casualties in general and applicable to the whole European theater. He said that the circular might be similar to Circular Letter No. 178, published by The Surgeon General, and NATOUSA Circular Letter No. 13 on forward surgery.[76] General Hawley approved the publication of such a circular and said that it was high time special policies were set up for the European theater.

A month later, Colonel Cutler reported that the manual was ready for the printer. He submitted, for General Hawley's consideration, remarks, from

---

[76] (1) Circular Letter No. 178, Office of The Surgeon General, 23 Oct. 1943. (2) Circular Letter No. 13, Office of the Chief Surgeon, Headquarters, NATOUSA, 15 May 1943.

which he asked the Chief Surgeon to prepare an introductory note. Colonel Cutler stated that the manual contained the principles underlying professional care of medical and surgical emergencies which may be encountered in the European theater—well-established principles which had been correlated with recent experience gained by the Americans and the Allies in the present war. Colonel Cutler further explained that the material was divided into three parts: (1) Primary surgical treatment of the soldier intended primarily for medical officers in division areas, (2) definitive surgical treatment as may be applied to hospitals regardless of type, and (3) treatment of medical emergencies. (The last part had been composed by the theater medical consultants under Colonel Middleton, the Chief Consultant in Medicine.) Lastly, it was explained, medical officers would be expected to adhere to the policies contained in the manual insofar as possible.[77]

By early May, the booklet had been received from the printer. Distribution had started. An appointment was made with General Lee for General Hawley and Colonel Cutler to present and explain the handbook to the SOS commander in the European theater. What happened at the meeting with General Lee is well explained in Chapter III of this volume (p. 366).

The same dual purpose of War Department TM 8–210 prompted the compilation of the circular for establishing policies with regard to surgical treatment and management. That is, one portion of the circular was written primarily for emergency surgical treatment and another portion was aimed at fixed facilities which would be providing definitive reparative care.

Colonel Cutler took upon himself the onus of compiling the first part on emergency surgical care. He was given help by all the surgical consultants, but particularly by Colonel Zollinger, Captain Hardin, and, as previously shown, by Colonel Morton and Colonel Schullinger on the gas gangrene and penicillin portions. Colonel Bricker, the Senior Consultant in Plastic Surgery and Burns, was given the responsibility of compiling the second portion of the proposed circular dealing with definitive care in fixed hospitals. Colonel Bricker experienced more difficulty than Colonel Cutler since his portion was of a more detailed and specific nature involving each of the specialist consultants. As a result, that portion dealing with the emergency management of battle casualties was finished first, and it became very apparent that the two parts were quite separate and distinct from each other. So, as time grew short, Colonel Cutler advised the chief of the Professional Services Division in a memorandum, dated 6 May 1944, as follows:

After a great amount of work we have decided that it is necessary to have two circular letters concerning surgical professional care. One is the major circular largely covering SOS fixed units, upon which Colonel Bricker has put so much work, and which he has

[77] Letter, Col. E. C. Cutler, MC, to Chief, Professional Services Division, subject: Minutes of Surgical Sub-Committee, 24 Jan. 1944.

about finished. The other is a circular dealing largely with battle casualties; that is, Army surgical therapy. It is attached, and I believe will be implemented immediately, as the Army needs this now.

Circular Letter No. 71, Office of the Chief Surgeon, ETOUSA, was published on 15 May 1944 and was titled "Principles of Surgical Management in the Care of Battle Casualties." It was as succinct a statement as could be made at the time on the emergency care and initial treatment of battle casualties in the combat zone. It included: (1) A definition of the functions and responsibilities of the various echelons of surgical service in the combat zone, (2) administration of morphine with particular emphasis on contraindications, as well as the causes of morphine poisoning, (3) blood transfusion, (4) definition of certain nontransportable cases, (5) dressings, debridement, and amputation, (6) sulfonamide therapy, (7) penicillin therapy, (8) closure of wounds, particularly early secondary closure, (9) general principles to be followed in the use of plaster casts, (10) treatment of anaerobic infections, (11) radiology in forward areas, and (12) identification of gases in cylinders, with particular reference to the difficulty caused by different British and American markings. The complete circular letter appears in this volume as appendix B (p. 963), and, in subsequent discussions, it may be referred to merely as Circular Letter 71.

The other circular letter entered the publication mill during the very height of activities for D-day, 6 June 1944, and did not appear until 10 June 1944. It was published as Circular Letter No. 80, Office of the Chief Surgeon, ETOUSA. It concerned policies and procedures governing care of patients in the European theater.

The new circular letter rescinded 33 prior directives which had been issued by the Office of the Chief Surgeon over a period of nearly 2 years. To place all pertinent items in these many directives into one was an accomplishment in itself which certainly helped to ensure compliance with these policies and procedures which had been built up over such a length of time—policies and procedures which many had forgotten or, as in the case of those newly arrived, had not known of their existence.

Circular Letter No. 80, calling attention to the Manual of Therapy, ETOUSA, stated:

> The Manual of Therapy, ETOUSA, sets forth principles of treatment which have been tested in active operations by both our own forces and those of our Allies. In it are incorporated many of the professional policies of the medical service of ETO. These policies will be followed habitually. Any one of them may, and should, be disregarded in an individual case where there is sound reason for departing from policy. Personal preference for other methods of treatment as a routine is not "sound reason." Departures from policies will be made *only* because of special circumstances associated with individual cases.

There was a lengthy and detailed explanation of all practices to be followed with respect to the procurement of blood and transfusions in general and station hospitals. It required all hospitals: (1) To develop a "casualty organization" to facilitate the reception, resuscitation, triage, and treatment of multiple casualties, (2) to utilize officers from the surgical, medical, and laboratory services, and (3) to make specific preparations in advance to meet great numbers of such conditions as burns, hemorrhage, profound shock, exhaustion, and chemical warfare casualties.

One of the items which had held up this directive was that of hospitals for special treatment. From the outset, General Hawley had insisted that there would be no specialized hospitals, except for treatment of the psychoneurotic and psychotic. At the 6 December 1943 meeting of base section surgeons, the only concession General Hawley would make was that in the following statement:

> Unless it can be thoroughly justified, we are not going to specialize hospitals. There may be a time, after we get trains running and battle casualties, we may specify certain hospitals for certain cases, but at the moment it is just complicating our evacuation system.

The Chief Surgeon never permitted any hospital to become "specialized," but, when the need became apparent, he eventually permitted the location of personnel and equipment at certain hospitals or hospital centers to provide special treatment. Circular Letter No. 80, compiled by Colonel Bricker, described these hospitals with facilities for special treatment as follows:

> Certain hospitals where special types of treatment are available will be designated from time to time in separate directives from this office. The policies enumerated below will govern the treatment of patients requiring therapy in which a high degree of specialization is necessary.
>
> a. Surgery: Selected patients requiring special surgical treatment will be transferred at the earliest practical time to those designated hospitals where additional facilities for their care have been provided. Such hospitals will include those for—*Neurosurgery, Thoracic Surgery, Urological Surgery, Plastic and Maxillofacial Surgery, Treatment of Burn Cases,* and other surgical specialties as may be found necessary.
>
> (1) In those hospitals designated for the treatment of cases requiring * * * [special surgical facilities], it is recommended that separate sections of the Surgical Service be formed for each specialty. Administratively, these sections would function as all other sections of the surgical service.
>
> (2) The surgical specialists in charge of these sections may be used by the Base Section Surgeons as Regional Consultants in their respective fields.

Another circular letter issued under the same date, 10 June 1944, designated the three hospital centers with special treatment facilities for neurosurgery, thoracic surgery, plastic and maxillofacial surgery, surgical treatment of extensive burns, and urological surgery. This additional directive, Circular Letter No. 81, Office of the Chief Surgeon, ETOUSA, designated other hospitals in which special facilities had been established for neurosurgery (with special urological facilities to care for the paraplegic) and for plastic and maxillofacial surgery (with special facilities for the surgical treatment of extensive burns).

Circular Letter No. 80 also specified *administrative* policies and procedures for X-ray therapy, hospitalization and disposition of neuropsychiatric patients, rehabilitation of the blind at St. Dunstan's Institute, the holding of regular medical meetings in hospitals as a part of the educational program, and care of members of the WAC (Women's Army Corps). There were also specific *professional* policies pertaining to certain conditions which were listed under the headings of general surgery, neurosurgery, orthopedic surgery, plastic surgery, and X-ray diagnosis in fixed hospitals.

In closing this section on publications and directives, a case must be noted wherein the Chief Consultant in Surgery thought he had nothing to do with a directive which to him was nearly all professional. As will be seen soon, the subjects discussed in this directive were the very items on which he and Colonel Zollinger were devoting their utmost energies at the time. And he was startled to see the directive for the first time a month after it had been written and promulgated. It was published not as a circular letter but as Administrative Memorandum No. 62, Office of the Chief Surgeon, ETOUSA, to Base Section Surgeons and Transit Hospitals. Dated 3 May 1944, it stated:

1. *General.*

a. Patients will be evacuated from the Continent to the United Kingdom in vessels manned by the Navy and in aircraft of the Troop Carrier Command. Patients returned by water will be disembarked at hards or ports having been classified into evacuable and nonevacuable patients prior to disembarkation. Evacuable patients are those who can withstand further evacuation by ambulance to "transit" hospitals (15 to 30 miles). Patients who are nonevacuable will be given emergency treatment in "holding units" in order to prepare them for further evacuation to "transit" hospitals. Patients arriving at "transit" hospitals will again be classified into evacuable and nonevacuable patients; evacuable patients being those who can travel 12 hours by train with reasonable safety. Nonevacuable patients will be prepared for further evacuation as soon as possible.

b. Patients evacuated by air will be removed to a "holding unit" at the airfield or a nearby fixed hospital, from whence evacuable patients will be evacuated to a general hospital for definitive treatment.

c. Designated general and station hospitals functioning as "transit" hospitals, will streamline their administrative procedures, and will function similarly to evacuation hospitals. "Transit" hospitals will be called upon to admit large numbers of patients expeditiously, and to evacuate them in trainload groups.

* * * * * * *

3. *Professional Care in "Transit" Hospitals.*

a. *The scope of professional care in transit hospitals will be the same as that in evacuation hospitals, bearing in mind that those wounded who may travel safely for another 12 hours will be immediately evacuated without definitive surgery.* [Italics are the editor's.] As a rule, all casualties will have their wounds debrided; no wounds will be closed; immobilization apparatus, splinting, or plaster of paris will be applied for all fractures; and patients will be given the necessary supportive treatment. Post-operative abdominal cases are usually not transportable for 7 days. Ambulatory and lightly wounded

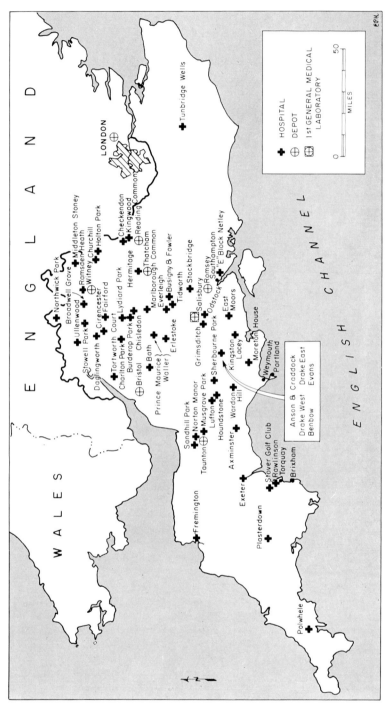

MAP 1.—Medical support in the United Kingdom for the Normandy invasion, 1 July 1944.

casualties will be evacuated through transit hospitals as rapidly as possible. This type of casualty represents a primary responsibility of the Medical Department because these patients, with good treatment, can be restored to active duty in the combat forces at an early date.

When Colonel Cutler first saw the directive on 2 June 1944, invasion fever was running high, and it was very obviously too late to do anything about it. At the same time, he was having a most difficult time trying to obtain approval for stationing his consultants in key areas during the invasion phase. It was, in a way, the last straw. He wrote most bitterly in his diary: "SOP's get written, and I never see them. God, how they have opened themselves to criticism. It is a colossal blunder. Only today I [saw] Administrative Memorandum No. 62, 3 May 1944. None of it is our responsibility [doing] and yet it is all the professional system." On second thought, he added: "Well, maybe it will be OK." And well might he add that thought, for the words in the directive were very much those of Colonel Cutler as he, from time to time, reported on the progress being made for the care of patients in transit through the evacuation chain on the southern shores of England.

However, he had advised: "* * * *Bearing in mind that if the pressure for evacuation is great, those wounded who may travel safely for another 24 hours will then be immediately evacuated without definitive surgery at the 'transit' hospitals.*" He had further qualified this statement with his definition: "An *evacuable patient* varies with the pressure of work and the demands for beds." Colonel Cutler was greatly exercised and chagrined to learn that base section surgeons and transit hospital commanders had been directed to evacuate all patients who could travel for 12 hours without definitive surgery. The clear intent of Colonel Cutler's recommended policy was that all patients in need of definitive surgery would receive such in transit hospitals except when (1) the pressure for evacuation was great at these hospitals and (2) the patient could travel safely for an additional 24 hours.

But now, more about these preparations to which the discussion of this directive has brought us.

Specific preparations for Operation OVERLORD

General Hawley explains.—Colonel Cutler attended a conference held by the Chief Surgeon at 9 North Audley Street, London, on 10 January 1944. The Deputy Chief Surgeon and executive officer, chiefs of divisions in the Chief Surgeon's Office, Col. Alvin L. Gorby, MC, from the Office of The Surgeon General, and Maj. Gen. Robert H. Mills, DC, director of the Dental Division, Office of The Surgeon General, were there. The minutes of the meeting show that General Hawley outlined plans formulated by his office for the reception, hospitalization, and evacuation of casualties in connection with the projected operations (map 1).

The plans for the medical support for the Normandy invasion included the following hospitals and depots:

General Hospitals	Location
22d & 522d (composite unit) __	Anson & Craddock Barracks, Pimperne, Dorset
22d (detachment) _____	Benbow Barracks, Pimperne, Dorset
28th _____	Kingston Lacey, Wimborne Minster, Dorset
40th _____	Daglingworth, Gloucester
48th _____	Stockbridge, West Hampshire
62d _____	Ullenwood, Cheltenham, Gloucester
62d (detachment) _____	Prince Maurice Barracks, Devizes, Wiltshire
67th _____	Musgrove Park, near Taunton, Somerset
91st _____	Churchill, Headington, Oxford
91st (detachment), augmented with a detachment of the 127th.	Norton Manor Barracks, near Taunton, Somerset
94th _____	Tortworth Court, near Falfield, Gloucester
97th _____	Holton Park, near Wheatley, Oxford
97th (detachment), augmented with a detachment of the 25th.	Waller Barracks, Devizes, Wiltshire
98th _____	Hermitage, near Newbury, Berkshire
98th (detachment) _____	Busigny & Fowler Barracks, Perham Downs, Wiltshire
106th _____	Kingston Lacey, Wimborne Minster, Dorset
141st _____	Erlestoke Park, near Erlestoke, Wiltshire
154th _____	Chiseldon Camp, Chiseldon, Wiltshire
158th _____	Odstock, near Salisbury, Wiltshire
159th _____	Houndstone Barracks, near Yeovil, South Somerset
159th (detachment) _____	Lufton Barracks, near Yeovil, South Somerset
160th _____	Stowell Park, near Stowell, Gloucester
185th and 685th (composite unit).	Sandhill Park, Bishop's Lydeard, Somerset
186th and 686th (composite unit).	Fairford Park, near Fairford, Gloucester
187th and 687th (composite unit).	Everleigh Manor, near Everleigh, Wiltshire
187th (detachment), augmented with a detachment of the 32d.	Rawlinson Barracks, near Newton Abbot, Devon
188th _____	Cirencester No. 1, Gloucester
192d _____	Cirencester No. 2, Gloucester
203d _____	Broadwell Grove, Burford, West Oxford
216th _____	Longleat Park, near Warminster, Wiltshire
216th (detachment), augmented with a detachment of the 127th.	Drake Barracks, East, Pimperne, Dorset
217th _____	Burderop Park, near Wroughton, Wiltshire
217th (detachment), augmented with a detachment of the 32d.	Drake Barracks, West, Pimperne, Dorset

Station Hospitals	Location
3d	Tidworth, Wiltshire
36th	Exeter, Devon
38th	St. Swithins School, Winchester, Hampshire
68th	Ramsden Heath, Ramsden, Oxford
77th	Erlestoke Park, Erlestoke, Wiltshire
110th	Royal Victoria, "E" Block, Netley, Hampshire
115th	Plasterdown, Tavistock, Devon
120th	Charlton Park, Charlton, Wiltshire
127th	Odstock, Salisbury, Wiltshire
130th	Chisledon, Wiltshire
152d	Odstock, Salisbury, Wiltshire
160th	Bath, Somerset
228th	Sherborne Park, Haydon, Dorset
250th	Grimsditch, Coombe Bissett, Dorset
302d	Lydiard Park, Swindon, Wiltshire
304th	Kingwood Common, Rotherfield Peppard, Oxford
306th	Checkendon, Oxford
313th	Fremington, Devon
314th	Polwhele, Truro, Cornwall
315th	Axminster, Devon
316th	Stover Golf Club, Teigngrace, Devon
318th	Middleton Stoney, near Middleton, Oxford
327th	Northwick Park, Blockley, Gloucester
347th	Marlborough Common, Marlborough, Wiltshire
365th	Ramsden Heath, Ramsden, Oxford

Field Hospitals	Location
6th	Tunbridge Wells, Kent

DEPOTS: Taunton, Bristol, Witney, Thatcham, Reading, Romsey, London

The minutes of the 10 January conference state:

He [General Hawley] gave first a broad picture of the overall plan for the reception of casualties. * * * All the hospitals, including the general hospital at Stockbridge, but excluding other general hospitals in a designated area along the south coast of England had been made available to the Southern Base Section for the purpose of receiving casualties. Casualties would be unloaded and given immediate attention on beaches and hards and then evacuated to the hospitals in this area [later called "transit" hospitals]. Evacuation of patients from these hospitals by hospital train to hospitals elsewhere in the United Kingdom would ensure that beds were constantly available in the designated area. Certain beaches and hards were to be designated as medical and the Navy would deliver casualties here as much as possible. A fixed holding unit of at least 50 beds would be placed at a maximum distance of 500 yds. from each medical beach and hard; situated preferably in whatever buildings were available. Here casualties which could not be transported by ambulance without immediate treatment would be transported by hand. These units, being so close to the beach or hard, would be exposed to bombing, but in order to deal with patients who could not be transported by ambulance without treatment, this was unavoidable. Ambulances and buses, for walking wounded, would be used to transport all other types of casualties to the nearby hospitals.

Owing to the many difficulties attendant upon bringing the casualties back—the diversion of LST's due to sudden emergencies, the possibilities of damage to the craft, the fact that trips were made at night and the crews were young and inexperienced— there would be frequent occasions on which casualties were brought to beaches and hards other than those designated as medical.   There were large numbers of such beaches and hards which would all have to be "covered."   For this purpose, with close liaison established between the Navy and [the] Southern Base Section, a large reserve of ambulances and personnel for unloading LST's would have to be kept available to move to any point on call.   It was essential that any congestion should be avoided and a considerable number, possibly as many as twenty-five, ambulances would have to be available to unload each LST, in order that all the casualties on board should be evacuated immediately.   In addition there would have to be under a central control (not that of the SBS [Southern Base Section]) two big reserve pools of ambulance and bus transportation to reinforce that for both medical and nonmedical beaches and hards and meet any sudden emergencies that might arise.

Colonel Cutler asked the general about provision for triage at the beaches and holding units.   General Hawley replied that no sorting would be done at the beaches and hards or in the "holding" units and that all those casualties that could possibly be transported would be moved immediately to hospitals.

The minutes state:

General Hawley then went on to explain, in slightly more detail, the methods for dealing with the casualties received.   All hospitals in the area would be reinforced with surgical teams and resuscitation and shock teams would be present on the beaches or hards.   To meet requirements in the initial stages of the operation, and until "the route of evacuation was canalized," teams and ambulance companies would have to be borrowed from areas north of the Southern Base Section.

    *   *   *   *   *   *   *

General Hawley explained how it was the responsibility of the Evacuation Division to keep the beds in the reception area "fluid."   It was *essential* that patients should not be immobilized in these hospitals and beds thus "frozen."   Therefore only essential surgical treatment, such as that given in Evacuation Hospitals, must be given therein. The bulk of the patients should be evacuated within 24 hours.

The Chief Surgeon then explained what measures would have to be implemented to care for the great influx of troops into the staging areas.

In the discussions that followed, Colonel Cutler again brought up the desire for sorting at the beaches and suggested that hospital trains evacuate less seriously wounded and neuropsychiatric patients from the receiving areas. General Hawley said that evacuation by hospital train of such patients could not be considered since there were no facilities for parking the trains in the vicinity of the beaches and hards.   He insisted that sorting of patients could not be done at the beaches.   He stressed that it was essential for all to be moved away immediately, and he added the conjecture that the run of neuropsychiatric cases would not be high.   He also said that very little treatment would be given by the Navy on LST's, although the Naval medical officer in charge of LST operations was most cooperative.   Colonel Spruit said that naval medical personnel might need reinforcing by Army personnel.   General Hawley agreed and directed that this question be looked into.

To a question on air evacuation by Colonel Gorby, General Hawley replied:

* * * the possibilities of Air Evacuation of casualties had been considered, but it was not estimated that it would start until D+10 or D+15. In the early stages, aircraft would have to return to specified troop carrier command airfields. Since there were no fixed hospital facilities in the vicinity of these airfields, tented hospitals would have to be used. Later it might be possible for aircraft to "touch down" near fixed hospitals. General Hawley pointed out that the demands on the air forces would be so great that it was extremely unlikely that aircraft would be available for evacuation of patients from hospitals in the reception area in the event of a dislocation of rail traffic, at any rate initially.

General Hawley concluded his explanation with comments on the supply situation and the need for decentralization. He said that supplies which would have to be furnished would be largely maintenance, but that a reserve must be kept to replace equipment lost by sinking or from other causes. For an example, he mentioned the fact that a whole evacuation hospital might be needed, and that arrangements must be made in advance to provide replacement for immediate and speedy loading on LST's. Provision must be made, he added, for the transport of blood and its storage at ports.

So this was it, pondered Colonel Cutler. The big effort was finally going to be made soon—but when? He recalled with some apprehension that, just before Christmas, General Hawley had warned the base section surgeons that in a month there would be scarcely a base section whose job would not be bigger than the theater was at the beginning of the month (December 1943). He could not help but conjure up memories of those southern shores of Devon, the European theater Assault Training Center, which he had visited not long ago.

Visit to Assault Training Center, ETOUSA.—On 5 November 1943, Colonel Cutler departed Cheltenham to visit the Assault Training Center, ETOUSA, near Braunton, Devon. On the way, he had stopped by at First U.S. Army headquarters and learned the happy news from Colonel Rogers that General Hawley had suggested Maj. William J. Stewart, MC, as orthopedic consultant for the First U.S. Army. He knew that Major Stewart would be an excellent consulting surgeon for the First U.S. Army and of great assistance to Colonel Rogers and to Maj. (later Col.) J. Augustus Crisler, Jr., MC, its surgical consultant, but this suggested appointment did not materialize.[78]

At the European theater Assault Training Center, Colonel Cutler was pleasantly surprised at the realism and practicality of the demonstration he observed on the employment of the medical services upon assaulting a hostile beach (fig. 64). However, he stated in a memorandum to Colonel Kimbrough, dated 7 November 1943, that, while the role of the Naval beach control officer had not been made entirely clear, the Chief Consultant in Surgery had been somewhat taken aback by the impression he had received that the Navy controlled entirely evacuation from the beach. Colonel Cutler also had a ride in a "duck" [DUKW (amphibious truck, 2½ ton cargo)] and found it quite a task for a healthy man unencumbered by the paraphernalia of war to mount

---

[78] Memorandum, Col. E. C. Cutler, MC, to Col. J. C. Kimbrough, MC, 6 Nov. 1943, subject: Orthopedic Consultant for the First Army.

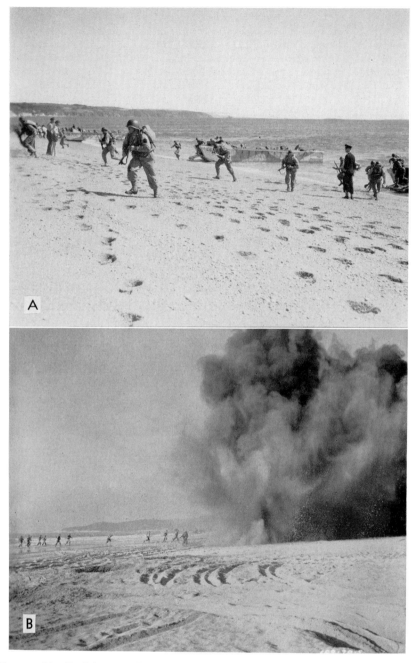

FIGURE 64.—Training at Assault Training Center, ETOUSA. A. Troops landing on the beach. B. Troops advancing inland amid clouds of bursting shells simulated by explosive charges detonated in sand.

into one. From this experience, he could not help but conclude that the means for getting walking wounded and even litter cases into a "duck" are inadequate. As a substitute, he suggested that everything should be done to land jeeps for use as light ambulances at the earliest possible time. Jeep ambulances, he said, would save much time for the wounded and perhaps make it unnecessary to set up what was called, in the demonstration, a reinforced regimental aid post.

British EMS plans.—And recently, just a few days before General Hawley's talk, Colonel Cutler had participated in a similar discussion on the British side. Mr. Willinck, the new Minister of Health, was present at the meeting of consultant advisers to the EMS held at the ministry offices, Whitehall, London, on Tuesday, 4 January 1944. The Director General, EMS, newly knighted, was chairman as usual. Sir Francis Fraser led the discussion on the care of battle casualties by the EMS when the Continent was invaded. The British were going to use three selected ports for the receipt of their wounded. The wounded, upon their return to England, would be taken to "transit" hospitals in the general locality of these ports. After surgical therapy, or immediately in medical cases, the wounded were to be sent to base hospitals in the north and west of England. They did not plan to use the great London hospitals as base hospitals, since heavy retaliation on London by the Germans was expected. Following treatment at the base hospitals, selected cases were to be sent as necessary to special hospitals for maxillofacial surgery, neurosurgery, and so forth. The need for basic surgical directives and mobile teams was cited, although it was stressed that their professional men would be sent to transit hospitals as well as the many base and special hospitals to which they were already assigned. Colonel Cutler offered to send the EMS copies of the NATOUSA circular letters on surgical therapy which he had recently brought back with him from Italy, and the EMS consultants implied that they would like to model theirs after the NATOUSA directives—just as Colonel Cutler, himself, was to do later.

After returning to Cheltenham, Colonel Cutler submitted to Colonel Kimbrough on 8 January a brief memorandum summarizing the highlights of this meeting with the EMS. He concluded his memorandum with: "I believe this meeting makes it clear that we should keep in close liaison with the British setup for the care of casualties returning from possible continental invasion."

Elsewhere, he wrote this enigmatic afterthought of the meeting: "The EMS is to look after all returned battle casualties, and, after 4 years, are still surprised over it!"

The buildup begins.—As General Hawley had foretold, the remainder of January 1944 set the pace for the busy months that were to follow. Taking a quick respite on Sunday, 23 January, Colonel Cutler noted in his diary: "Catching up; things moving. Hospitals arriving daily. Hard to keep up with work. Robert Zollinger is a great help."

Problems in Allied coordination.—Colonel Cutler had said that the American should keep close liaison with the British in the working out of procedures for the reception of casualties. It soon became apparent that the British thinking was very similar. Sir Francis Fraser asked Colonel Cutler to meet with British representatives for the joint working out of certain problems which had appeared. On 28 January, Colonel Cutler journeyed to Oxford and met with Prof. Geoffrey Jefferson, adviser in neurosurgery to the EMS, and Brigadier Hugh Cairns, Consultant in Neurosurgery to the British Army.

Professor Jefferson stated that the EMS had a very meager supply of specialists to meet the tremendous demands which were expected. While the British Army could help to a limited extent, it was particularly in neurosurgery where they feared the greatest shortage of qualified professional help. Professor Jefferson asked if the American Army would be willing to have British neurosurgical casualties sent to their hospitals for care. It was apparent to Colonel Cutler that similar decisions were desired for other types of cases as well. Significant, and most obvious, was the fact that the EMS had not been informed on these matters, and Colonel Cutler did not have the answers either. He could but say that there was an overall planning group which had probably settled these problems and that, certainly, representatives of the Canadian, British, and U.S. Army medical services had to meet, settle, and integrate plans for the care of all casualties arriving in the reception areas.

In a memorandum, written on 29 January, after his return to Cheltenham, Colonel Cutler advised the Deputy Chief Surgeon, through the chief of the Professional Services Division, that the following specific questions should be put to the Allied planning group:

1. Will U.S. Army hospitals, Canadian Army hospitals, and EMS hospitals in the reception areas take in and care for Allied casualties just like their own?

2. Can the EMS count upon U.S. Army hospitals taking in and caring for specialty injuries over and above the general run of casualties?

3. Should the answer to question 2, above, be favorable, can a list of U.S. Army hospitals in the reception areas with information as to where what specialists are assigned be submitted to the EMS so that the EMS may route patients to such hospitals?

And here, the reader should note, was the first instance where Colonel Cutler was acting as the American surgical representative for Allied planning of the invasion—a function which was to grow and become more involved as time passed and which devolved upon him naturally in the course of events without any specific orders.

At the monthly meeting of advisers and consultants to the EMS held on 8 February, it was still obvious to Colonel Cutler that the EMS was in ignorance about overall plans, and the professional board of the EMS felt that its planning could not be reasonable until they had further information. Colonel Cutler noted, too, that the specialists desired early triage so that casualties requiring special treatment could receive that care within a reasonable period of time. As it was, if the general plan were followed, 3 to 5 days would be consumed before this special care would be available to casualties needing it, and mortality and morbidity would be increased by such delay. The Director General, EMS, spoke of the need for gradually vacating beds in the better hospitals, the possibility of triage at transit hospitals, the necessity for rapid passing of cases through transit hospitals where long holdovers would be undesirable, and securing additional special instruments for work in special fields for use in transit hospitals.[79] These problems, with which the EMS was contending, were to Colonel Cutler the very problems that the U.S. Army had yet to face, and matters of serious concern.

Following this last meeting, Colonel Cutler visited the Chief Surgeon's London office and spoke with Colonel Liston, the Deputy Chief Surgeon, on the various matters which had been brought up by the EMS. Colonel Cutler told Colonel Liston that planning was not his problem and that he had asked the EMS to put in writing to him any specific desires they had so that he, Colonel Cutler, could pass them on to the Chief Surgeon, ETOUSA.

Critical shortage of qualified officers in ETOUSA.—On Thursday, 10 February, a teleprinter conference was in progress between the Chief Surgeon and the Office of The Surgeon General in Washington. Perhaps Colonel Cutler was unaware of the conference, itself, but, as has been shown, he was certainly aware of the problem which was its subject (pp. 37–38). The conference concerned personnel, particularly supply personnel. The tenor of the conference also indicated how critical activities were in this immediate preparatory period prior to launching Operation OVERLORD. An excerpt from the teleprinter conference of 10 February 1944 follows:

This is Hawley speaking: Colonel Voorhees and his group have done a splendid job in diagnosing the troubles and pointing out the cure. I am implementing their suggestions at once, but I must have help to implement them properly. Until recently this theater was of minor importance in the large picture. Realizing this, I have refrained from asking for the ablest officers available, with the result that, with a few notable exceptions, the officer personnel furnished me was not of high quality. We have tried to carry on during this period of relative inactivity and we have barely succeeded. This situation has now changed. This is the most important of all theaters and we have fully demonstrated that the quality of personnel furnished us in the past is totally inadequate for the task that lies ahead of us. We must not fail. Yet we cannot succeed unless we are given the tools to work with. The best officers to be had are none too good for the jobs to be done here.

The most critical time of all is now. After plans are made and operations are proceeding smoothly, some key personnel can be released and their places taken by subordinates who they have trained. I realize fully the many positions that have to be filled and the few really qualified people there are to fill them; and I shall be unselfish when the time comes that the need for able people is greater elsewhere than it is here. But now, for the first time in more than two years, I am really begging for assistance.

"Rotten ships for care of wounded American boys."—Colonel Cutler's impression of LST's, after his first two encounters with them, was that they

---

[79] Memorandum, Col. E. C. Cutler, MC, to Chief, Professional Services Division, 11 Feb. 1944, subject: E.M.S. Preparations.

were "rotten ships for care of wounded American boys." These initial impressions, however, were but a challenge to Colonel Cutler to make them the best possible vehicles for evacuation by sea under the circumstances. To this end, Colonel Zollinger, his consultant in general surgery, was of inestimable help.[80]

Already, on 4 February 1944, Colonel Zollinger had met with Colonel Liston, the Deputy Chief Surgeon, and Capt. George B. Dowling, MC, U.S. Navy, who was the Naval medical officer in charge of LST operations for the evacuation of casualties. On 8 February, he had met again with Captain Dowling and a Lt. William A. DuCharme, HC, U.S. Navy, to go over and evaluate medical supplies and equipment which the Navy planned to load on LST's for the care of 200 casualties. And, on 14 February, he had gone to the Southern Base Section and discussed with the base section surgeon the placing of surgical teams on LST's and the scope of treatment to be given. They had also discussed the advisability of placing general surgical and shock teams at the field hospitals to be located right at the hards for the care of nontransportable casualties. They also believed that it would be necessary to break up one or two general surgical teams to obtain experienced medical officers to supervise triage at the hards. There was talk, too, of the placement of general surgical and orthopedic teams at the transit hospitals and the use of the specialty teams in hospitals for the definitive treatment of casualties.

With this as a background, Colonel Cutler, Colonel Kimbrough, and Colonel Liston joined Colonel Zollinger on Tuesday, 15 February 1944, at Plymouth, Devonshire, to look over an LST. Colonel Muckenfuss and Captain Hardin from the Blood Bank, ETOUSA, also joined the party. The inspection of the LST, which had been arranged through Captain Dowling, was conducted by Comdr. Luther G. Bell, USN (MC). Colonel Zollinger informed the group that the ship had been used at the Salerno landings but that it was not of the type which had been converted to carrying casualties.

"We were able to inspect the entire LST," Colonel Cutler wrote of the expedition in a 15 February memorandum to the chief of the Operations Division, through Colonel Kimbrough, "including the main deck, on which was the upper battle dressing station in ward room, the middle deck, where a second battle dressing station was contemplated in the crew's messing compartment, and the lower or tank deck."

Colonel Cutler noted that the usual difficulties of movement on a ship were present. There were narrow doorways, sharp right-angled turns, and steep ladders or stairways between decks—difficulties which could not be changed but had to be recognized in the proper planning and loading of casualties on such a ship. A primary consideration underlying all planning for the care of casualties and returning sick personnel on such ships, Colonel Cutler mentioned, was the fact that "loading of casualties and patients must proceed simultaneously with the unloading of the ship." With this in mind, he believed the following sequence of care should prevail:

---

[80] See also Colonel Zollinger's personal narrative of his activities in Chapter III.

4. * * *:

a. Casualties will come up over the side in special stretcher slings developed by the Navy * * *. These deliver patients to upper deck (fig. 65).

b. From the deck the casualty may go either to: (1) The battle dressing station in the ward room, or (2) the battle dressing station in the crew's messing compartment on the middle deck. There, adequate dressing facilities for all types of wounds must be present with additional splints. There, proper notation should be made on the EMT as to some sort of categorization concerning the ability of the individual to withstand transport on reaching the near shore. If surgical procedures are necessary to save life or limb, such as ligation of a vessel or the amputation of an extremity hanging on by a few parts, then the FMR must be begun and proper notation made on it.

c. After primary first aid care has been given, as above, the casualties will then go either to the area known as the crew's quarters, which is adjacent to their messing compartment, or to the tank deck, if they are on stretchers. As there is space for some 78 stretchers in the crew's quarters it would be advisable for all stretcher cases to be held in this area if possible. Those who are ambulatory, both sick and wounded, can go down to the middle deck and be held in the space allotted as "troop quarters," which can provide for 175 men. The number of stretchers or other casualties which can be placed on the tank deck will depend upon whether we are utilizing a converted ship with wall brackets for stretchers or not (fig. 66).

5. *Comment on battle dressing stations or first aid posts:* Of the two areas provided for this service, i.e., the wardroom on the upper deck and the crew's messing compartment upon the middle deck, the latter would seem more reasonable, for if there be only one surgeon he would have near him in the adjacent crew's room (sleeping quarters) practically all of his stretcher or seriously injured people. Both stations, however, are suitably lighted and supplies could be assembled there. Moreover, both stations have tables which could serve as operating tables. The crew's quarters stations are near the kitchen, so that sterilization by boiling would be more simple, unless an electrical hotplate is added to the wardroom, where there is a plug for such a receptacle on a table.

The visitors, particularly the two from the blood bank, observed that there were two types of cold rooms on the ship. One was for meats where the temperature was kept at 20° F. This room was obviously unsuitable for storing blood. But there was another space for storing vegetables and fruits where the temperature was held at 48° F. Fortunately, they discovered, the temperature could be adjusted to 40° F. which would be appropriate for storing blood and still not hurt the fruits or vegetables.

On his return from Plymouth, Colonel Cutler reported: "No intelligent regulation can be drawn up concerning the care of casualties on such ships until knowledge is available as to time limitations." Time, he showed, would affect considerations in professional care on LST's in the following manner:

If casualties will be on such ships up to and beyond 20 hours after being wounded, then one would have to advise and provide for abdominal surgery, since the percentage of recovery in the cases of abdominal injury becomes almost nil after 24 hours. A similar attitude on definitive surgery of all types must be dictated according to the time interval. If instructions are to be given to medical officer personnel on LST's as to what they are to do, that would depend entirely upon this time interval, and if indoctrination courses are to be given to the medical officer personnel who are to be on LST's, some rough estimate of this time interval should be known to the instructor before speaking, else his advice will be inappropriate and possibly damaging to the American soldier.

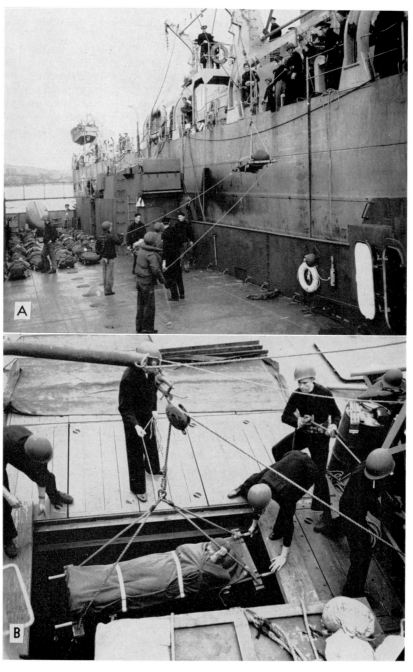

FIGURE 65.—Special slings on LST's for handling litter patients. A. A sling being used to hoist a litter from the deck of an LST. B. A sling being used to lower a litter.

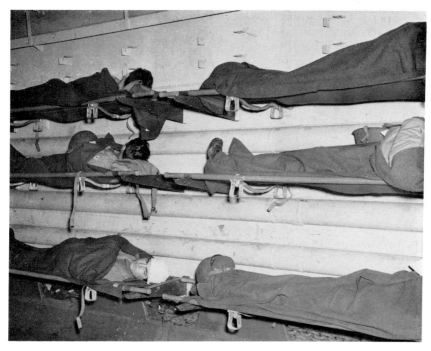

FIGURE 66.—Litter patients in an LST that had been converted with wall brackets to hold litters.

It is my hope that the interval will be so short that the professional work on an LST will be largely first aid, i.e.:

1. Control of hemorrhage.
2. Treatment of shock (for which blood and plasma will be provided).
3. Proper dressing of wounds.
4. Proper splinting of fractures.
5. The elimination of pain through medication.
6. The giving of tetanus toxoid.

If, however, the time is to be over 24 hours, or even if there is danger that it is to be over 24 hours, then an entirely different set of circumstances will prevail and different instructions must be given the medical officers in charge. We would be committing a wrong against the American soldier in this event if we did not provide for definitive surgery in the care of cases on the LST's.

On the Monday following, 21 February, Colonel Cutler joined a most illustrious group in the inspection of an LST at the chief British naval base, Portsmouth. The American representation, in addition to Colonel Cutler, included Maj. Gen. Albert W. Kenner, Chief Medical Officer, SHAEF, and Col. Alvin L. Gorby, MC, who was now assigned to the First U.S. Army Group, the overall planning organization on the American side for Operation OVERLORD. The directors general of the Royal Navy and the British Army medical services headed the British delegation, with their respective surgical consultants, Admiral Gordon-Taylor and Maj. Gen. David C. Monro. There were also Surgeon Rear Admiral Cecil P. G. Wakeley, a consulting surgeon to the Royal Navy; Brigadier Arthur E. Porritt, RAMC, then consulting surgeon with the British 21 Army Group, the British counterpart of the First U.S. Army Group; and other officers from the British 21 Army Group.

Colonel Cutler was quite disconcerted with the British attitude toward the handling and care of casualties on LST's, since, if their opinions were to prevail, much of the planning and work so far accomplished by Colonel Zollinger would have been for nought. Yet, there was on evading the fact that this particular inspection of LST's was conducted primarily from the viewpoint of the British Army and the Royal Navy medical services. Colonel Cutler's 28 February report of the trip to the Chief of the Operations Division in General Hawley's office contained the following statement:

1. The British seemed to have hardened their opinion even before visiting the ship that:

a. The ship must load casualties via the ramp through the bows.

b. They prefer not to use the ship's company's quarters, as these people will be working very hard and should not be disturbed.

c. They wish to keep all casualties on the tank deck and have plans to construct a small first-aid post, screened off, at the rear end of the tank deck.

d. The medical personnel for an LST will consist of two general duty medical officers, one qualified surgeon, one anesthetist and 32 men of noncommissioned ranks, about 20 of whom would be trained Navy medical personnel. Others would be largely used to clean the tank deck after tanks have left and before the casualties are brought in.

2. The British group felt certain that it would be impossible to take casualties up over the side in units or by any other method. They believe it will be necessary to beach the vessel, leave her on the beach throughout the fall and flow of one tide and take her off afterwards. This opinion is contrary to that of American Naval officers when inspecting.

3. On travelling back with Lt. Gen. Hood [DGMS, British Army], he expressed the opinion that the LST was an unsuitable vessel for carrying back wounded people, that it was outrageous that better provision could not be made, and that he might take this to the Prime Minister and General Eisenhower. He expressed the opinion that an LST was a "cold, dirty trap."

4. Out of the above objections, many of the professional people present, notably General Monro and Brigadier Porritt, as well as myself, felt it might be better to try and hold certainly all litter cases on the far shore, rather than accept the risks of transport back on these vessels. Certainly the "Collecto-clearing company" or the platoon of the field hospital could be landed with the second wave and give the necessary surgical care.

Much of the meeting of the Chief Surgeon's Consultants' Committee on 25 February 1944 was taken up with the subject of care of casualties on LST's. Colonel Zollinger gave a summary of the existing problems and plans which, so far, had been worked out with the Navy. One of the remaining problems was the treatment of abdominal wounds, he reported. The Navy was estimating a 16-hour journey on LST's, once they were loaded, but risk of mortality in abdominal cases rose precipitously after 6 hours. There was a general desire to do abdomens, if necessary, on the LST's, but there were no provisions for the equipment or personnel. Furthermore, planning to operate on abdomens on the far shore had its disadvantages in the initial stages because there would not be facilities to perform such operations and, because it was the general policy not to move for about a week either abdominal or chest cases which had been operated upon. Of the situation at the time, Colonel Zollinger said: "If a man happens to be qualified to operate on [board] LST's, good; if not, he will have to depend upon morphine."

General Hawley was quite taken aback by the prospect, and said: "These are young chaps—recent graduates. They will not have done any kind of residency. To operate on a belly on an LST!! The question is whether it is better to operate on the far shore and put him immediately on an LST; is that worse than operating on an LST?"

In answer to his own question, General Hawley said that it would be better to operate anyway rather than go so long as 16 hours and that it would probably be better to operate on the far shore and then have the patient taken aboard, with special care available on the ship. The reason, he said, was that there would be a better concentration of talent on the far shore and "we have to think of the most good for the largest number and establish a ruling for it."

Colonel Kimbrough, however, insisted: "I would like to stick to the recommendation that there be facilities to operate on any case that might arise on an LST."

"I agree," General Hawley replied.

The discussion on LST's was closed with strong exhortation from the Chief Surgeon that the consultants crystallize their opinions on what had to be done and how and to "get it down into an operating procedure that the Navy thoroughly understands." [81]

The reader may recall that shortly after this, in March 1944, The Surgeon General and the Air Surgeon arrived in the theater for an extended tour of medical facilities serving the Army Air Forces and that Colonel Cutler was required to accompany the visiting officers. The inspection tour and its aftermath required the services of the Chief Consultant in Surgery for the best part of a month at this critical time. The bulk of the work to develop the necessary operative procedures with the Navy fell on Colonel Zollinger.

Physical standards and disposition boards.—At the aforementioned meeting of the Chief Surgeon's Consultants' Committee on 25 February, General Hawley said, "Now I have a problem. What can we do to get these disposition boards to realize more fully their responsibilities in the conservation of manpower. I think it is getting better, but I think we are still evacuating too many people. What can we do about that?"

The disposition boards had been established at most general hospitals and certain station hospitals in August 1943.[82] Each board consisted of the

---

[81] "The emergency operating rooms on the LST's were built in the center of the tank deck along the after bulkhead. Each such room took up the space of one vehicle, but the combat troops were not advised by general headquarters of this alteration. The loading tables had been prepared for each unit; so, when the troops embarked, each unit had one truck, or other vehicle, which could not be loaded and had to be left behind. There was a lot of hell raised about this, but nobody ever criticized the Chief Surgeon. These changes had been made through command channels." (Letter, Paul R. Hawley, M.D., to Col. John Boyd Coates, Jr., MC, 17 Sept. 1958, and personal conferences, Dr. Hawley and Colonel Coates, during October 1958.)

[82] Circular Letter No. 122, Office of the Chief Surgeon, Headquarters, European Theater of Operations, U.S. Army, 17 Aug. 1943.

chief of medical service, the chief of surgical service, and the ward officer of the particular patient. If a chief of service was unavailable, the appropriate assistant chief was directed to act for his chief. The directive further required a review by a disposition board of all cases in which it was believed a patient should be returned to the United States for further observation, treatment, and disposition. The recommendations of the boards required final approval by the hospital commander.

The action of these boards had been notably inconsistent and, in many cases, unduly delayed. To General Hawley's question, Colonel Kimbrough replied that the appropriate consultants had been reviewing reports and spot checking final recommendations. He said that a great many cases which the consultants felt could be retained for duty in the theater were still being sent to the Zone of Interior. In such cases, Colonel Kimbrough continued, telephone calls were being made to hospitals involved to check on the validity of the decisions.

General Hawley then instructed the professional services to continue just that action and to submit recommendations for improving the procedures.

The emphasis at this time was on the conservation of manpower, and General Hawley's feelings were well expressed at this meeting as follows:

* * * The point is this. We all want to protect ourselves. We have to conserve manpower. We have to stop getting people out of the Army who can do any kind of a job at all. Can we be in a position to say there is nothing wrong with this man? He might walk right out and drop dead. That is just too bad. We have done everything we can, but it is going to save hundreds of other people for duty if we establish a policy and stick to it. I want you to think it over. We have, all of us, to get out of the family doctor's psychology here and we have to know that we are going to make some mistakes. Can we keep those mistakes down within reason and can we assure our preventing a lot of mistakes being made on the other side? If we can almost break 50/50 on it I think it will be worth trying because we have to preserve manpower.

Colonel Cutler, in his visits to hospitals, had found that one source of the problem lay in the lack of guidance to disposition boards. For example, he had found that many officers would have liked a list of conditions which would be appropriate for returning a soldier to the Zone of Interior. With his senior consultants, the Chief of Consultant in Surgery worked out such a list, as did the medical consultants. The list was submitted, but General Hawley was reluctant about publishing a list of this type because he thought that each individual case had to be judged on its own merits, especially with regard to the duty which the patient would be expected to perform should he be retained in the theater. Yielding to the advice of his consultants, however, the Chief Surgeon permitted the list to be published on 24 March 1944, as Circular Letter No. 45, with the following qualification: "It is to be remembered that this list is to be used only as a guide, each case to be decided on its individual merits."

Aftermath of Operation CRACKSHOT.—When the general plan for medical operations in England to support the invasion had been more or less firmly established, General Hawley had called for trial evacuations from transit hospitals to the southern belt of general hospitals which were being designated for the primary definitive treatment of patients. These were actual movements of real patients using ambulance and hospital train units which had been earmarked for the evacuation mission in England (fig. 67). One of these trials was Operation CRACKSHOT. The Chief Surgeon was quite pleased with CRACKSHOT because it showed where weaknesses in the plan were and because the observers of the trials had made such a thorough and careful analysis of these weaknesses. The Chief Surgeon called a meeting of his key staff officers on 24 March 1944 at which he opened proceedings by saying:

We have to button up some things here before operations.

There will be a stenographic report made of this but * * * anything decided here ought to be put out as a directive and by the time I get back [from the Zone of Interior] I would like to see most of it either accomplished or well on the way. We have not much longer now. All our mistakes have to be behind us.

The first thing is this report in detail on the Operation CRACKSHOT. I understand that we have had, in a few days, something which has pointed out the weakness of things in general.

From this beginning, the conference proceeded in rapid-fire fashion, most of the decisions being made by the Chief Surgeon followed by his specific directions as to the actions to be taken. The following topics concerned the Chief Consultant in Surgery.

"Here is a very important thing," said General Hawley reading from the Operation CRACKSHOT report, "Recommend that the scope of treatment given at these transit hospitals be definitely outlined and that Professional Services be consulted as to the necessity for augmenting personnel with surgical teams." The Chief Surgeon continued: "Now, these are evacuation hospitals and they have definitely to limit the amount of work that is done. You cannot immobilize patients there any more than in any other evacuation hospital."

"That has been considered," Colonel Kimbrough answered, "and that is a general policy."

General Hawley then directed, "Will you give us something that can be published that we can hold them to?"

And then a little while later, "Question of procedure," said General Hawley, "slightly wounded ambulatory patients to be separated from serious cases."

Colonel Kimbrough explained, "That triaging is planned to start on LST's."

General Hawley's comment: "It will work on LST's, but it won't be complete and final. Every hospital has to triage its own patients. Hospitals cannot depend upon triaging on LST's; every unit has to do its own."

Colonel Kimbrough then made a recommendation which had continually been made by his division. He stated: "It is recommended that a responsible medical officer, not just a junior officer, be at the hard to do triaging."

Thinking aloud, General Hawley said:

When these patients get to a general hospital they have to be triaged again. We have to keep those beds for seriously wounded. If a patient does not get definitive treatment in transit hospital he has to get completely definitive treatment in some station hospital some place else to clear that bed for a seriously wounded man who cannot be moved.

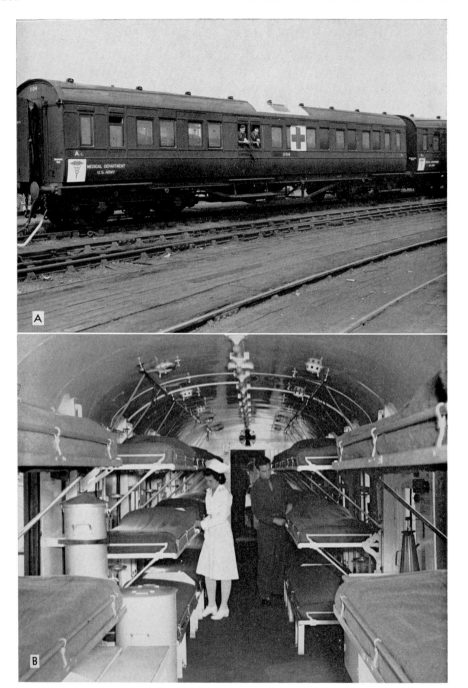

FIGURE 67.—U.S. Army hospital train ward cars in the United Kingdom.   A. The exterior
of a ward car. B. The interior of a ward car.

Our first run of patients will be from transit hospitals to the southern belt of general hospitals. We cannot let that southern belt of general hospitals get full of minor casualties. We have to keep those beds for people who cannot be moved any farther than that.

We have a lot of beds in East Anglia not going to be full, perfectly competent for taking care of arms and things after first definitive treatment. The point is, you have to keep those southern belt general hospitals for serious cases that cannot be moved after definitive surgery.

And then, after a very brief discussion, General Hawley made a decision and issued to the Operations Division the following instructions: "Incorporate in the plan the further evacuation to station hospitals of slightly wounded whose initial definitive treatment has been completed, in order to keep the

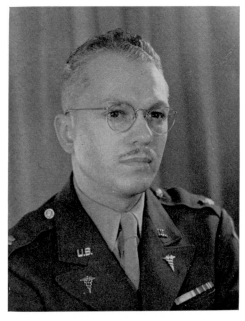

FIGURE 68.—Lt. Col. Fred H. Mowrey, MC.

beds in the first row of general hospitals fluid for serious cases that cannot be moved."

This discussion brought to General Hawley a thought on the spur of the moment. "A second thing on that," he added, "it is to keep these general hospitals indoctrinated that as soon as the patient can safely be moved to the Zone of Interior he is out and on his way home. I cannot impress that too much."

"I would like to emphasize that they do that now," explained Lt. Col. (later Col.) Fred H. Mowrey, MC, the hospitalization and evacuation officer (fig. 68). "However, some of them have been keeping patients more than 180 days. I would like to have all of those boarded so that we get rid of them within the next 6 weeks."

"I approve of that," agreed the Chief Surgeon, "In every case right now, let's start unloading beds—every case that will not be fit for duty in 180 days to be boarded and reported for evacuation." Then, addressing Colonel Kimbrough, he stated: "Responsibility of Professional Services. The hospitals are keeping up their bed strength unnecessarily. Professional Services, you have to stop that."

"We have been working on that both with hospital commanders and at base section meetings," Colonel Kimbrough assured the general, "We checked up to see about it. When we find they are not doing it we tell them to get this man or that man out."

General Hawley warned with portent, "We have to get tough with somebody here—or else."

Colonel Kimbrough took these and other discussions at this meeting to mean that his division would have to work out an SOP for the care of patients in near-shore installations and transit hospitals. He also emphasized the necessity for checking on and instructing hospital disposition boards, not only in their responsibilities for conserving manpower, but for acting quickly and early on all cases to keep their hospital beds free.

General Hawley went one step further. He issued a directive applicable to each consultant in the Chief Surgeon's Office which made it his personal responsibility to check on disposition board procedures at each hospital visited, regardless of the original purpose of the visit, and to see that hospitals were not keeping patients who should have been transferred elsewhere.

SOP (standing operating procedure) for professional care of casualties.—Three days after the Operation CRACKSHOT meeting, Colonel Zollinger had prepared and submitted to Colonel Kimbrough, with Colonel Cutler's approval, a statement of the professional care to be provided casualties in the various echelons in England during the attack on the Continent. Colonel Zollinger also prepared the necessary correspondence for obtaining the personnel required to provide the care stipulated.

With respect to surgical treatment on board LST's, the substance of the SOP was as follows:

Surgical treatment on board LST's will be similar to that of a divisional clearing station. Definitive surgery is not contemplated except in those instances in which it is necessary to receive patients with abdominal wounds, or similar casualties, occurring on board ship as a result of direct enemy action. The decision to perform major definitive surgery on board LST's will be governed by the type of wound, the estimated time interval from wounding until near shore definitive treatment is available, the professional qualifications of medical personnel, and, finally, the volume of casualties.

The casualties will be triaged on board ship into two major classes, ambulatory and stretcher cases. The stretcher cases will be further triaged into "transportable" and "nontransportable" * * *. The nontransportable casualty will be defined as a casualty requiring immediate resuscitation or surgical intervention after unloading from the LST.

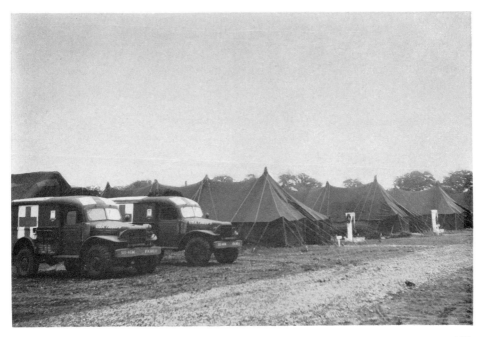

FIGURE 69.—The 46th Field Hospital at Chandler's Ford, Hampshire, England, June 1944.

At the hard, the plan called for two or three experienced surgeons for triage. These officers with mature surgical judgment were to reevaluate casualties into transportable and nontransportable cases. The plan also noted that ambulance evacuation was now going to be necessary from ships to the nearest medical facility, of which there were to be two types—field hospital platoons augmented by surgical teams and full field hospitals also augmented by surgical teams. The scope of treatment at these facilities was to be substantially as follows:

Field hospital platoons of 100-bed capacity will be located near three of the major hards. These units will receive the nontransportable casualties and other casualties which might occur about the hard. Such cases should be of the type requiring resuscitation as well as definitive surgery. It has been suggested that two general surgical teams and two shock teams be assigned to each of these units.

A tented field hospital with a capacity of 400 beds, will be located 5 or 7 miles from each of the three major hards (fig. 69). Because of the urgency of unloading LST's rapidly, it is anticipated that it will be necessary for the ambulance companies to unload the majority of the casualties at these stations. Major definitive surgery of all types, chiefly on those casualties labeled nontransportable, except neurosurgery, maxillofacial surgery, and the less urgent chest surgery, will be performed in these units. It will be necessary, therefore, that these units be heavily reinforced with surgical teams. It has been suggested that three surgical teams and one splint team be assigned.

For the general and station hospitals designated to act as transit hospitals, the plan called for procedures substantially as follows:

If time permits and the condition of the patient warrants, the ambulance companies will deliver casualties directly to these hospitals. Furthermore, they will evacuate the casualties from the field hospitals to these units as soon as possible. Casualties will be subsequently transported inland from the transit hospitals by hospital train.

It is essential that the professional qualifications of the medical personnel of these designated transit hospitals be evaluated by the Professional Services Division. Furthermore, it has been suggested that three surgical teams be assigned to each of the nine transit hospitals to insure adequate personnel to cover the 24-hour period. The surgical chief of one of the three teams assigned to each unit should be an orthopedic surgeon.

The plan was forwarded by Colonel Kimbrough to the Operations Division, Office of the Chief Surgeon, on 3 April 1944 for guidance and information in the formulation of operational plans and directives.

On 27 March 1944, when the SOP was prepared, Colonel Zollinger addressed a memorandum to Colonel Kimbrough through Colonel Cutler requesting the augmentation of transit hospital staffs so that the care called for in the plan could be carried out. In this communication, Colonel Zollinger mentioned that personnel of the 1st Auxiliary Surgical Group could not be considered for these augmentations, since most of the teams would be assigned to the field hospitals and field hospital platoons working independently. A surgical team for transit hospitals, Colonel Zollinger recommended, should consist of two surgeons, one anesthetist, one nurse, and two surgical technicians. He reiterated the portion of the SOP which called for three teams to be assigned to each transit hospital, the chief of one of the teams to be an orthopedic surgeon. He asked also for two or three experienced surgeons for triage of casualties at each of the hards. Finally, the recommendation was made that these teams be organized sufficiently in advance of their actual employment to permit individual members to learn to function as a unit.

The request was forwarded to the Personnel Division, Office of the Chief Surgeon, which assessed quotas to each of the four base sections for 18 surgical teams and 9 orthopedic teams. The requirement for providing triage officers at the hards was placed on the Southern Base Section.

When Colonel Cutler finally had more time to devote to these plans, he submitted additional items for the SOP on the care of casualties in the forthcoming operations.

With respect to transit hospitals, he offered the following in a memorandum to Colonel Kimbrough, dated 10 April 1944:

In the event that the transit hospitals are crowded with casualties needing definitive surgery then the ambulatory and lightly wounded personnel should immediately be evacuated to the General Hospitals in the base area in order that there should be no great delay in their surgical treatment. This category of casualty represents a primary responsibility of the Medical Department, for these men with good surgery at an early date can be restored to active duty in the combat forces.

In the same memorandum, he submitted the following item, with respect to general hospitals in the base area:

The general hospitals in the base area will carry out primary definitive surgical treatment on all casualties reaching them in whom such care has not already been given. This may largely consist of the lightly wounded ambulatory cases who are expected to stream through the transit hospitals without opportunity for definitive surgery at that level. These are extremely valuable personnel and deserve optimum surgical care since they represent returnable manpower to the combat forces.

Cases also will reach the general hospitals after definitive surgery has been carried out at the transit hospitals. Many of these with the assistance of chemotherapy, either the sulfonamides or penicillin, or both, will be found suitable for secondary suture of the wound and thus have the period of disability limited.

Another function at the general hospital level will be the transfer of Allied forces casualties, chiefly British, to their own hospitals. This function will be implemented through the Office of the Base Section Surgeon. Transfer of the British casualties to British hospitals must not occur until the base area has been reached.

Personnel requirements confirmed.—At about the same time that Colonel Cutler was dictating these additions to the standing operating procedure for professional care during the invasion, Colonel Zollinger notified the Chief Consultant in Surgery, in a memorandum, dated 8 April 1944, that there was some question as to the number of surgical teams required or desirable in the transit hospitals. Colonel Zollinger said that there might be changes, also, in the final number of transit hospitals. Colonel Cutler informed the chief of the Professional Services Division that there was no reason to change the original professional opinion for two general surgical teams and one orthopedic team to augment each of the transit hospitals.

Exercise SPLINT.—A few days later, Colonel Cutler was able to catch up with the most recent planning on the contemplated LST operations. With Colonel Liston, he journeyed to the southern port of Newquay on 12 April 1944. There, the entire morning was spent in observing an exercise involving beach operations and the loading of casualties into LST's (fig. 70). In the afternoon, General Kenner, Chief Medical Officer, SHAEF, presided over a critique of the exercise, following which General Lee flew Colonel Liston and Colonel Cutler back to London in his private aircraft.

Among other matters, there was a good discussion on the time required to load an LST with casualties. The Navy pointed out that it took 3 hours to unload an LST, and perhaps more. With the proposed single-sling loading of casualties over the sides of LST's from small boats, one casualty could be loaded each minute, thus making a good load of 180 casualties in 3 hours. Furthermore, the Navy pointed out, there was no reason to load the LST any faster because there was no room for casualties until the material on the ship was moved out.

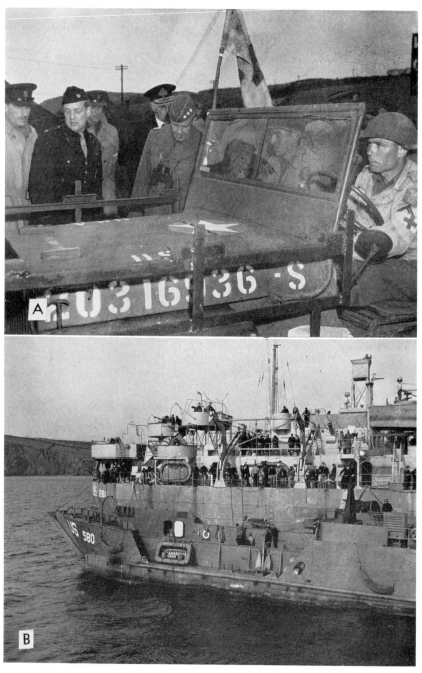

FIGURE 70.—Exercise SPLINT in and about Newquay, Cornwall, England, April 1944.
A. Gen. John C. H. Lee and Allied officials inspecting a jeep, modified in the European
theater with brackets to hold litters. B. An LCT (landing craft, tank) tying up to an
LST to transfer casualties for further evacuation.

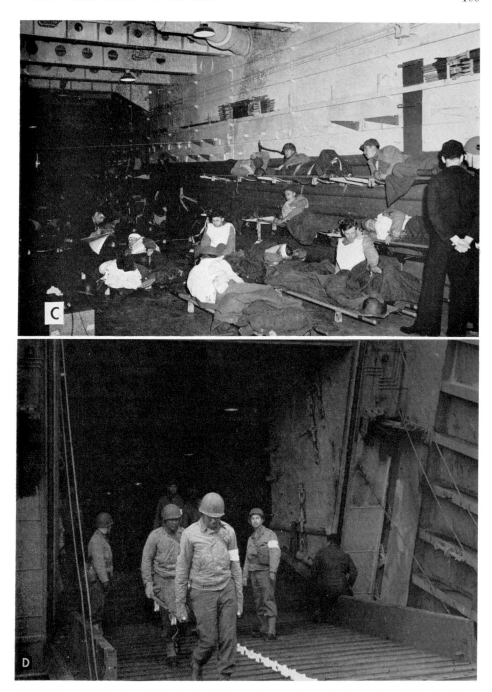

FIGURE 70.—Continued.   C. Simulated litter patients in the tank deck of an LST.   D. Litter
patients being taken off a beached LST through the open bow and ramp.

With respect to the weather hampering operations, the Navy stated that, if LST's could be unloaded, they could be loaded. That is, if the operation was on, casualties could be returned. But, perturbing, at this critique, was the estimate now entertained by some that casualties would be on LST's for 48 and even 72 hours!

"The above expectation of the time a man awaits surgery," warned Colonel Cutler, "*demands the presence of a good surgeon on each LST*." "Moreover," he added, "we must remember that the first casualties, irrespective of the condition, will be shovelled into the nearest boat and, also, serious casualties may occur on any ship."

Colonel Cutler was pleased to learn, however, that the Navy would provide 2 general medical officers for each LST and would accept a complement of 100 Army surgeons, with assistants, for assignment to these ships. Col. (later Brig. Gen.) Thomas D. Hurley, MC, Surgeon, Third U.S. Army, said that he was providing 45 good surgeons for this purpose. The others were to come from Air Force and Service units in the United Kingdom. Captain Dowling of the Navy stated that a course of instruction would be given these surgeons, who would be doing the major work on the LST's, some 4 or 5 days before the operation.[83]

However, on 24 April, at the conference of base section surgeons, it was necessary for Colonel Cutler to make this rather dismal announcement:

With reference to furnishing the Navy fully qualified surgeons for LST's, a directive was sent out asking for nominations, and we have been checking on those we have received. We promised the Navy well-qualified surgeons. I think the Base Section Surgeons may not have fully appreciated this as we have received nominations of very young and inexperienced men.

"I think everybody understood thoroughly," commented General Hawley pointedly. And then to Colonel Cutler, he said: "I think you are going to have to get those people by looking over their * * * cards in this office, deciding whether they can be spared from that unit or not and ordering them."

Early ambulatory management.—General Hawley—ever concerned with having a sufficient number of available beds before and during the continental invasion—directed the Professional Services Division to look into the matter of accelerating professional care by early ambulatory management of postoperative patients. He referred to precedents' having been established in the United States in this direction and suggested that it might even be better for the patient, himself. The matter was brought to the attention of Colonel Cutler, who stated in a memorandum to the chief of the Professional Services Division, dated 24 April 1944, that the Professional Services Division exerted constant pressure to assure that personnel hospitalized for surgical reasons were out of bed at the earliest possible moment. He continued:

The tendency in the U.S.A. to get people up on the first or second day is now widespread. * * * In the Peter Bent Brigham Hospital, Boston, Mass., I have heard recently

---

[83] Memorandum, Chief Consultant in Surgery to Chief, Professional Services Division, 16 Apr. 1944, subject: Comment on Exercise SPLINT.

with joyous comments from my junior associates that the average patient is out of bed the day after his surgical ordeal. This I consider to be unfortunate and an undesirable practice for the advance of surgery. We must remember that the art of medicine and surgery has attached to it just as many fads and fancies as other walks in life, and we must recall that it take time for wounds to heal. We know many ways by which wound healing is prevented, but we have as yet discovered no agent and no method for hastening Nature's process. Certainly to keep people in bed unnecessarily long merely weakens their general condition and probably therefore somewhat delays healing, but to force Nature beyond her powers is even more foolish.

The U.S. Navy has stated that they get people out of bed earlier than we do in the Army. Maybe they do. That does not make the wound heal faster, and moreover we must recollect the people in the Navy and in the Air Force do not have to walk with 50 odd pounds on their back over great distances. Rehabilitation for the soldier is rehabilitation for the maximum effort, and that is not true with other branches.

Colonel Cutler then called attention in the memorandum to the fact that a manual for bed exercises was being prepared and that the period of bed rest could probably be considerably shortened with specific setting-up exercises. He also made the following recommendations:

That the Division of Professional Services continue their influence to reduce the period of bed rest to the shortest period of time compatible with solid healing of the wound, and this of course varies with the position of the wound, for all those except those with wounds of the abdomen and lower extremity may be out of bed within a few days of their surgical ordeal.

While these recommendations were no doubt acceptable, there was apparently a decision that a directive was also necessary to make a program of accelerated care mandatory upon hospitals in the theater. Accordingly, under dateline of 14 May 1944, Colonel Cutler submitted in draft a directive entitled "Early Ambulatory Management Following Surgical Procedure." In submitting the proposed directive, Colonel Cutler advised Colonel Kimbrough: "When the document is presented to General Hawley I believe it should contain a statement that 'Professional Services Division believes that a greater contribution to the saving of time in hospitals will result from acceleration of the administrative program than from this questionable acceleration of professional care.'"

With minor modifications, Colonel Cutler's document was published as Administrative Memorandum No. 74, Office of the Chief Surgeon, ETOUSA, 22 May 1944, and directed that all patients be made ambulatory as soon as possible following surgical procedures. Certain obvious exceptions to the policy were specified, and the directive warned that abdominal incisions, except for the McBurney type, now had to be supported by "through and through" or retention sutures. Colonel Cutler was able, however, to have inserted in the directive instructions requiring the number of days of total bed rest to be noted on each patient's record. General and station hospitals were also required to make an evaluation of the results of this regimen in their monthly surgical reports. To Colonel Cutler, it was a matter of waiting and seeing if the results bore out the contention of this directive, which opened with the statement: "Recent observations have suggested that the traditional duration of bed rest following surgical procedures can be shortened materially with benefit to the patient. This leads to a reduction in the patient's recovery period, a conservation in manpower, and a saving of hospital beds."

Curiously, the same proposition was brought up in a meeting of the British Army's consultant committee meeting, but Lt. Gen. Sir Alexander Hood and his consultant accepted Colonel Cutler's recommendation that the British Army await results of the American experience before committing themselves to such a program.

Recapitulation.—At the Chief Surgeon's meeting with his division chiefs on 2 June 1944, Colonel Cutler heard General Hawley close the meeting with these words:

> I don't know when D-day is, and if I did I couldn't tell you anyhow. But it is logical to assume that it is not too far off now; if we have left anything undone, the time is falling short. We must be ready to go. I think in the transit areas they are ready to go.

What had the Chief Consultant in Surgery done to be ready to go? In summing up, the following things stand out:

1. Everything possible from the professional side had been done to clear beds in anticipation of the expected casualties. Disposition boards had been trained, checked, and exhorted to carry out their functions rapidly and properly. A program of early ambulatory management had been instituted to get the patient on his feet more quickly. When it was discovered that administrative proceedings, rather than professional, were holding up the disposition of patients, the consultants had adamantly brought this to the attention of those in the position to do something about it. The rehabilitation program had been put in full force to clear hospital beds and return men to duty earlier and in better physical condition.

2. The blood bank was ready to go, and bleeding sets had been constructed and distributed to augment the distribution of whole blood. Last minute procedures had been completed to supply LST's with 10 pints of blood each. Marmite (Thermos) cans had been procured so that whole blood could be packed in them and taken along by the leading assault elements (fig. 71). Too late, possibly, it had been realized that the supply of whole blood available from local sources might be insufficient. It would be sufficient for the initial phases, however, and plans had been made for increasing blood-collecting facilities.

3. Penicillin for the initial assault had been assembled or was on its way. Quantities required to sustain subsequent operations had been calculated and requisitioned. Decisions had been made on how penicillin was to be used, and the command instructed accordingly.

4. LST's had been carefully studied and the lifesaving procedures necessary on shipboard had been agreed upon and were well understood by all concerned. Surgical instruments, scarce as they were, had been assembled into kits and placed on these ships. Linen was obtained and rolls of disposable rubberized sheeting had been supplied to be used for surgical drapes. Finally, a handpicked complement of 100 qualified surgeons was ready to board

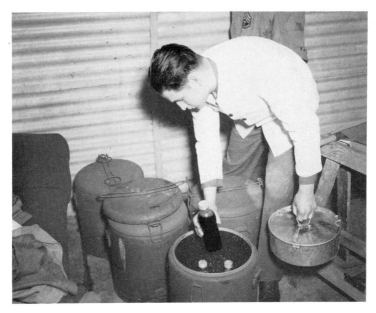

FIGURE 71.—Marmite cans adapted for transporting whole blood.
The tray in the soldier's left hand is filled with ice.

the ships—one to an LST. They had been briefed by Colonel Cutler and his assistant, Colonel Zollinger. They were also being briefed by the Navy.

5. Principles of triage on LST's had been formulated, and cards for tagging the casualties had been prepared. Surgeons of mature and sound judgment had been selected to act as triage officers at the hards and ports. The supervision of these triage officers and the control of surgical teams in the transit areas were in the able hands of Lt. Col. George K. Rhodes, MC, surgical consultant to Southern Base Section. He had also personally inspected the personnel and facilities at all the hospitals in his area to be sure that the work to be done at each facility was being supervised by a topnotch surgeon and that all understood just what was to be done and what was to be left undone.

6. Surgical teams had been picked, organized, briefed, and stationed at holding and transit hospitals to augment their regularly assigned staffs. Policies for the assignment and use of surgical teams in the field army and in other areas of the communications zone had been elaborated and announced.

7. Policies and procedures for the professional administration and management of battle casualties from the frontline areas to hospitals in the rear had been established and promulgated. A pocket-sized edition of the Manual of Therapy had been printed and distributed so that each medical officer caring for patients in the combat zone or in the communications zone would have a ready reference as to how injuries and diseases were to be cared for in the European theater.

8. A close and sympathetic understanding had been established between the British and the Americans as to the surgical plans each was following. They were ready to accept each other's casualties and care for them until they reached the base areas.

These were the preparations. Was there anything yet undone? There was.

Use of consultants during assault phase.—On Thursday, 1 June, the day before the 2 June meeting with the Chief Surgeon, Colonel Cutler had approached Colonel Mowrey and Colonel Liston as to what the professional men might do during the assault on the Continent. He had proposed that certain of the consultants might help out at the holding hospitals for the nontransportables, the orthopedic men could help out at the transit hospitals, and the remainder of the specialist consultants might work out of Cheltenham and be used wherever their services were required. Now some had been opposed to these thoughts, but on this occasion, both Colonel Mowrey and Colonel Liston were agreeable to the idea.

Earlier during the Chief Surgeon's meeting on Friday, 2 June, Colonel Cutler had managed to mention, in passing, his hopes for the use of consultants during the attack. "They may be used in transit hospitals best by pushing patients through," he said. And then, dwelling on General Hawley's favorite theme during this period, Colonel Cutler added: "Hospitals tend to keep patients too long."

"I agree with you," the general replied, "but those people down there have a responsibility, and if these consultants are used in that capacity only, that is fine, but none of us, short of an extreme emergency where the system will fall down, none of us can step in down there to operate the system. That is the function of SBS [Southern Base Section]."

To Colonel Cutler, this reply was noncommittal and discouraging. He took it to mean that General Hawley was against the proposal. So, he remained after the meeting and, in the afternoon, was able to see General Hawley with Colonel Liston. Both General Hawley and Colonel Liston were entirely in favor of the proposed use of consultants. Moreover, General Hawley asked Colonel Cutler to be with him, personally, during the early phases of the attack. To Colonel Cutler these reactions were wonderful. He was elated, but at the same time he was cautious. "So I laid it on in a memo," he wrote in his diary. The 4 June 1944 memorandum, the subject of which was the utilization of surgical consultants during operations, was addressed to the Chief Surgeon through the Chief of the Professional Services Division. It stated:

1. During periods of great activity, the function of *evacuation* must be the prime concern of the Medical Department.

2. The surgical consultants are senior officers with a long experience in this theater, and are fully cognizant of the importance of evacuation. They realize that to choke a hospital with more casualties than the surgical teams assigned there can handle in a 24-hour period means undesirable delay in the period before definitive surgery can be

carried out. If evacuation is prompt and efficient, casualties passing through transit hospitals without definitive surgery will actually have surgical care at an earlier period in some general hospital behind the transit hospital area.

3. There are two points at which evacuation may be unnecessarily delayed.—

a. By holding "transportable" casualties as "nontransportable" in *field hospitals*.

b. By attempting to hold too many casualties for elaborate surgical care at the "transit" hospitals.

4. To assist in facilitating evacuation and equally to hold in field and transit hospitals those who should be held there I recommend that the following officers be assigned as designated below during the first phase of the operation until a proper procedure is established.

a. To the field hospitals for "nontransportables" at each area as follows:

Hard A–S [Southampton area] (FH 46, FH 28, SH 110)—Lt. Col R. M. Zollinger.

Hard B–P [Portland-Weymouth area] (FH 12, FH 50, EH 109, EH 12)—Lt. Col. G. K. Rhodes.

Hard C–B [Torquay-Brixham area] (FH 7, FH 49)—Lt. Col. E. M. Bricker.

b. To the transit hospitals above A–S (GH 95, GH 48, SH 38)—Lt. Col. M. Cleveland.

To the transit hospitals above B–P (GH 28, SH 228, SH 315)—Lt. Col. W. Stewart.

To the transit hospitals above C–B (SH 316, SH 115)—Special assignment unnecessary.

5. The remaining senior consultants in the surgical specialties, Colonels Stout, Vail; Colonels Spurling, Allen, Canfield, and Tovell will remain at Headquarters, SOS, prepared to go where their services are required. Since definitive surgery will largely be done in the general hospitals behind the level of the transit hospital, their activities will be largely in that area.

The memorandum was returned quickly to Colonel Cutler with one word on it in General Hawley's bold scrawl, "Approved," followed by his initials. This document facilitated the procurement of necessary passes for the consultants to permit their entry into and egress from the staging area. It was difficult enough to enter the critical areas, but it was more difficult to get out, once a person was in. The actual date for the invasion was still obscure, but the surgical consultants were now ready.

NORMANDY

D-Day Week

On Tuesday, 6 June, Colonel Cutler was off on a trip with Colonel Kimbrough and Colonel Zollinger in the direction of the A–S hard to check on preparations made by holding and transit hospitals in the area. They first visited the 38th Station Hospital at Winchester, Hampshire, and found everything satisfactory. Next was the 110th Station Hospital at Netley, Hampshire. The Southern Base Section surgeon, Col. Robert E. Thomas, was there. He appeared surprised when three officers from headquarters appeared on a relatively routine visit. The invasion was on, he told them (fig. 72). Colonel Cutler could scarcely believe him. The radio was turned on, and, sure enough, the same story appeared. With renewed purpose, the three officers continued their tour. At the Royal Victoria Hospital, which had recently been turned

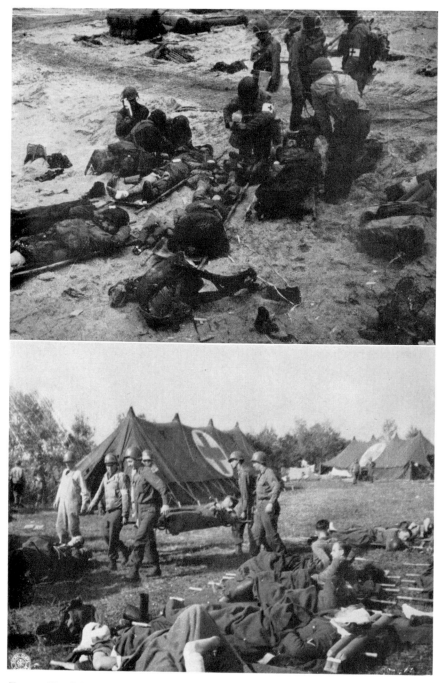

FIGURE 72.—Medical service on the Normandy beachhead, D-day, 6 June 1944. Upper view, an aid station of the 8th Infantry Regiment, 4th Infantry Division. Lower view, casualties being collected at a field hospital platoon.

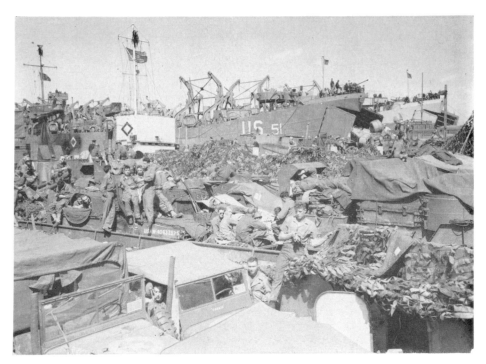

FIGURE 73.—American equipment, ships, and men at Plymouth, England, awaiting orders that will send them to the Normandy beachhead.

over to the Americans by the British, quantities of ammunition crates littered the beach where they had drifted in after being thrown overboard from combat ships of the Navy on their way out (fig. 73). The three officers completed their tour with visits to the 46th Field Hospital, a holding unit, and to the 48th General Hospital, one of the transit hospitals supporting the A–S hard, and returned to London.

Arriving at 9 North Audley Street the next morning, Colonel Cutler learned that General Hawley had packed and motored to Cheltenham. Colonel Cutler hastened to the 1st Medical General Laboratory at Salisbury, Wiltshire, which had been designated the command post for the Chief Surgeon during the assault phase. There, he learned that penicillin was a problem and that the fifty billion units ordered for June had not arrived. "Ordered 50 billion," he wrote in his diary, "only 600 million now here. Half on beaches 'far shore,' half on LST's and for distribution here. But it is a mess. All write lots of penicillin! We order and none comes." At midnight, he was still preparing a letter to Col. (later Brig. Gen.) John A. Rogers, MC, First U.S. Army surgeon, for General Hawley, saying there was no penicillin. Nevertheless, he did have time to note: "The continental invasion is on at last. All are excited; too much so. Here I am with General Hawley sleeping in next room to me. I wouldn't have believed it possible 2 weeks ago."

Thursday, 8 June, Colonel Cutler wrote, was a "wonderful day with PRH [General Hawley], all day." He was up at 0630, had breakfast at 0700, and embarked on the following:

1. Off with PRH at 8:00 a.m. * * *.

2. Southern Base Section and reports on wounded arriving and evacuated on.

3. 12th and 109th Evacuation Hospitals. In tents, pretty good—not too good—interesting femur and buttock at 109th. Bad jaw and chest at 12th. Sent jaw, chest, femur, and 1 other by ambulance to 67th General Hospital.

4. Lunch at 50th Field Hospital in Weymouth (two platoons) (fig. 74). George Rhodes there. Bad eye case; sent for D. Vail. Many cases were treated. GKR [Rhodes] had seen 3 abdominal cases all operated on LST's. Good work * * *.

5. To Bristol, hard. Other platoon of 50th Field Hospital close by. Did not visit and did not go to 12th Field Hospital. Roads full of LCP's; went on one. U.S.S. *Quincy* in harbor; 1 major general and 1 brigadier general [aboard]. Skipper told of tough time on beach. Many dead * * * underwater stuff.

6. To 305th. Interesting cases. Spleen, 36 hours. Eye and brain case.

7. To Sherborne to see train unload; late (fig. 75).

8. Visits to 3d Armored Division to Meet General Hawley's son-in-law, Captain Towsey. All in pup tents.

9. To Southern Base Section headquarters.

10. Here Salisbury. Thomas came to call. He said (a) Orders not to do surgery but evacuate means no evacuation 'till hospital fills; negative number of cases, therefore nothing doing. (b) No record if in hospitals under 48 hours—wrong. Field Medical Record (FMR) should start with first definitive procedure. (c) Thomas reported cases at various hospitals, including 60 PW's, largely at 110th Station Hospital.

11. Call in from First Army re penicillin. I said General Hawley had written letter to Colonel Rogers.

12. Now I must write something for Colonel Thomas.

At the end of the day, Colonel Cutler had these thoughts in mind:

The war is on here. Have been about, as one can see. * * * But is it going OK? Where are the LST's? They are not coming back and wounded are coming in on APA's; no good staff, poorly cared for. One femur with no splint. Stories from wounded: Left on beach between 6:00 and 8:00 a.m., lay on beach, no assistance * * * got wet as tide came up, crawled to rocks (one with fractured femur), help to one at 4:00 p.m.

The next day, 9 June, was D+3. Colonel Cutler arrived at Southern Base Section headquarters at 0830 for a long talk with Colonel Thomas. They discussed further the problem of hospitals erroneously assuming that they were to do no surgery and just wait until enough patients accumulated to be evacuated by train. They also spoke of means to rectify the situation with respect to initiating field medical records at the time of first definitive treatment. Later, Colonel Cutler visited Maj. Gen. Eric Barnsley, RAMC, the surgeon of the British Southern Command. General Barnsley said that the British had had 400 wounded on D+1 and 1,200 on D+2. Next, Colonel Cutler went on to the 109th Evacuation Hospital, where he had lunch and spent the remainder of the day at the beach at Portland (fig. 76). It was a great day and experience. Some 19 to 22 LST's came in with about 2,000 wounded (fig. 77). Care on the LST's had been good, but Colonel Cutler noticed considerable crowding and disorganization on some of them. Ships with casualties were waiting an inordinately long time in the harbor in order to come in and unload their precious cargo.

The next day, Saturday, 10 June, was spent in catching up with the events of the past week and reflection upon what he had observed. In the morning Colonel Kimbrough held a meeting of the Professional Services Division, and the remainder of the day was spent by Colonel Cutler in writing letters, preparing reports, and putting some order into the data being assembled. The following recommendations were submitted to Colonel Kimbrough in a memorandum, dated 11 June 1944, as a result of the observations made during the first week:

1. *Medical record.* In all hospitals visited found F.M.R. was not started following surgical therapy for fear of staff that this was not allowed (see SOP). Because of this feeling, and with the desire for some record, most hospitals had mimeographed a form of their own with a clinical chart, so that some record could be kept of surgical cases.

Recommendation: The F.M.R. shall begin at the time any definitive medical or surgical care starts.

2. *Surgical care.* At all hospitals visited I found that the staff and the commanding officer had interpreted the SOP to mean that only the first aid care could be given in transit hospitals. This had led to men being given first aid care and then, since there were few admissions, the staff sitting around waiting for the patients to be evacuated, but, as only a trainload could dictate when a hospital was to be evacuated, casualties were not being evacuated and were sitting around with nothing but first aid care, when a surgical procedure might have greatly increased their opportunity for rapid restoration to duty and survival with better function.

Recommendation: a. Surgical procedures shall be carried out in transit hospitals as indicated by the nature of the casualties and in relation to the pressure exerted by the number of casualties admitted. Thus, when there are only a few casualties, most of them could have definitive surgery in a transit hospital. When there are large numbers of admissions, only those urgently requiring surgical care should have it at the transit hospital level.

b. In special instances where ambulances are available and the condition of the patient justifies travel and the treatment of the condition can best be done at a neighboring hospital, then that patient shall be transferred by ambulance to the appropriate hospital where the facility is available.

3. In observing the unloading of LST's at Portland, it is clear that only 5 LST's can unload at one time, 2 on the hard and 3 at the pier. It did not appear to us that more than 6 LST's would be unloaded and loaded in a 24-hour period, for the loading of an LST after the wounded are evacuated takes 6 to 8 hours. This delay is injurious to the condition of casualties, and another method must be found for unloading critically ill people.

Recommendation: When the hards and the pier are filled with LST's and more are waiting in the roads than can be unloaded in the next 12 hours, smaller crafts, such as LCT's (fig. 78) shall go out to the LST's, take off the casualties and land at the many beach areas where such smaller craft can unload.

The "SOP" Colonel Cutler was referring to in his recommendations was, as the reader may have realized, Administrative Memorandum No. 62, which is discussed on pp. 173, 175. To Colonel Cutler, his fears had been realized. The arbitrary changes which had been made on his recommendations had resulted in a situation where patients who could and should have received definitive care were being neglected, and proper records were not being prepared.

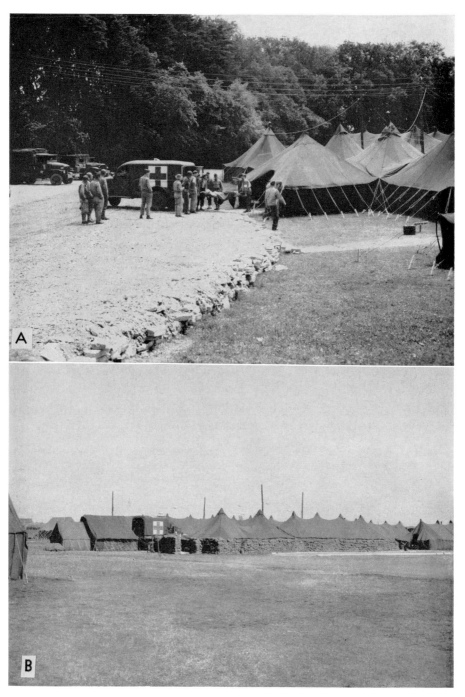

FIGURE 74.—The 50th Field Hospital at Weymouth, England, during the Normandy invasion. A. The admissions area. B. A sandbagged surgical area with a mobile X-ray unit set up nearby (the truck and two adjoining tents on the left).

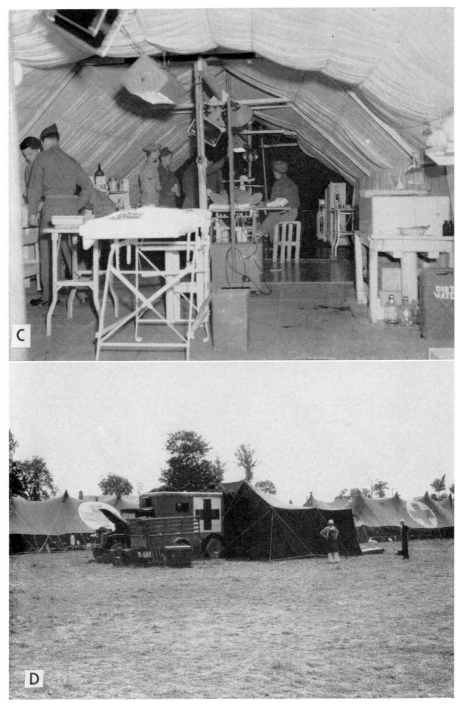

FIGURE 74.—Continued. C. An operating pavilion. D. A surgical truck with attached operating tent.

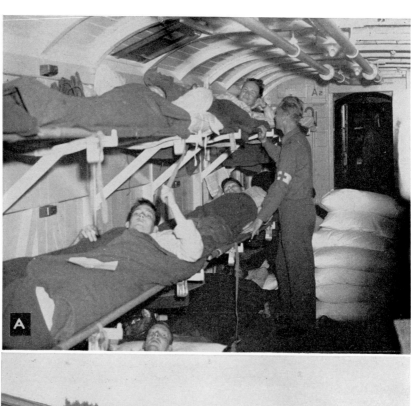

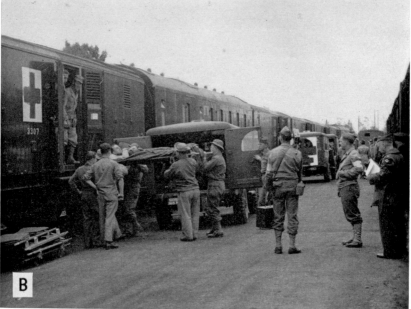

FIGURE 75.—Unloading of a hospital train at Sherborne. A. The interior of a war car (a converted box car). B. Ambulances stand by to take patients to the 305th Station Hospital at Warden Hill, St. Quintin, Dorset.

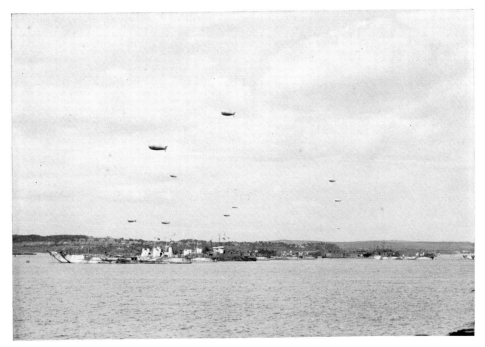

FIGURE 76.—A view of the Portland area and Weymouth, South Dorset, England.

Second Week, D+5 to D+11

The second week after D-day was pretty much a resumption of the first few days. On Monday, 12 June, Colonel Cutler accompanied General Hawley, Col. Howard W. Doan, MC, Colonel Humphrey, and Mr. Littell, war correspondent for *The Reader's Digest*, on a field trip to the Portland area. Concerning a visit to the 109th Evacuation Hospital during this trip, Colonel Cutler recorded: "* * * saw bad case blown up on ship; left foot gone, open fracture on right leg into knee joint. Very ill; not yet dressed; 6 days. Bad Rx, but not yet infectious. Suggested blood and then dress under ether." In connection with the visit to the 50th Field Hospital, he recorded: "* * * have had five or six cases of gas gangrene; not all amputations, yet 6 days old! Why no more infection? Sulfonamide and penicillin? Saw German with right lower-quarter abdominal wound. Prisoner said: 'We Germans have no chance—replacements not allowed.'" At the Portland hard, Colonel Cutler was shocked to see many prisoners of war with wounded hands being taken off LCT's as litter patients.

Colonel Cutler was most pleased to see that LCT's were going out to the LST's to unload patients as he had suggested the week before (fig. 79). The entourage went out on a Higgins boat to watch the procedure. At LST 59, they found: "Bob White aboard as triage [officer]. Captain Steward of 85th

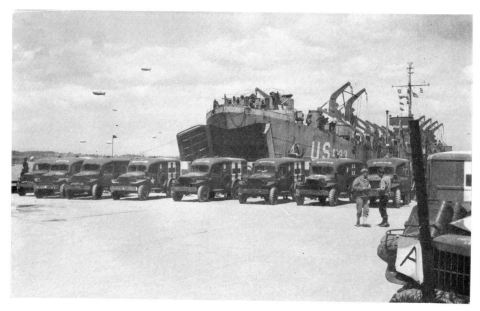

FIGURE 77.—Ambulances on a dock at Weymouth awaiting the unloading of casualties.

General Hospital in charge. 85-plus Germans (fig. 80) ; 266 casualties picked up wounded on D+2, 3, 4 but convoy [was] slow in returning." And then: "To LST No. 501. (Should have seen General Hawley go over side!) Captain Keleher, 16th General Hospital, in charge. He had done one abdominal wound on LST; OK; and one tracheotomy—died from multiple wounds [of the] chest. Needs blood and more penicillin; needs Atabrine for malaria and Levin tubes. Major Wilcox, 2d General Hospital, aboard as triage officer. Saw *women snipers* in civilian clothes as wounded PW's. American boys had thought they had come to help French, yet French women had shot them."

It was a busy day at Portland. By 1400, 715 casualties had been taken off LST's, and by 1500, the total had risen to 1,052. The joy of seeing LCT's unloading LST's was short-lived, for, as the party returned to the 50th Field Hospital, they were informed that LCT's could no longer be used for this purpose. Back at the 1st General Medical Laboratory that night, there was more talk about women snipers and, Colonel Cutler wrote, "PRH said you (ECC) and I go [to] France next week—goody !"

But, before going to France, Colonel Cutler was able to observe the reception of casualties evacuated by air. Air evacuation had started early in the campaign, perhaps as early as D+4. A platoon of the 6th Field Hospital was at Ramsbury, East Wiltshire, and a platoon of the 28th Field Hospital, at Membury to receive air-evacuated casualties (fig. 81). Colonel Cutler visited these facilities on 14 June. He saw three planes unloaded in 20 minutes, and thought: "A-1. This is the secret for future good care, but cases must be se-

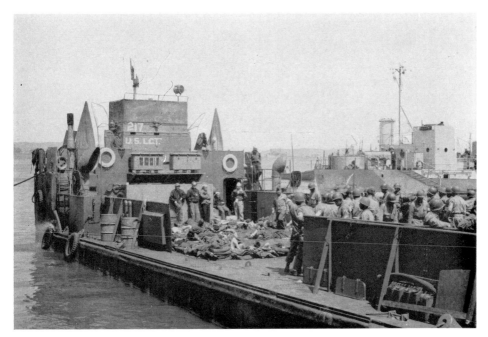

FIGURE 78.—U.S.S. LCT 217, beached at Weymouth, England.

lected: no post-operative abdominal cases. Almost killed Lt. Col. [William D.] McKinley."

On Friday, 16 June, Colonel Cutler worked in the morning at the Cheltenham office. He was back at the Salisbury "CP" by noon, where General Hawley had said he would meet Colonel Cutler.

The *Prague* and Normandy

The period from 17 through 22 June was spent on the hospital carrier, *Prague*. The *Prague* was one of four hospital carriers loaned by the British to the Americans during last-minute preparations for Operation OVERLORD. It was a 4,100-ton vessel with British crew and a complement of U.S. Army medical personnel. These hospital carriers were protected by the Geneva Convention, and were painted white with prominent markings using the Geneva Cross. The *Prague* was the largest of the four vessels loaned to the Americans and could carry 194 litter and 228 ambulatory patients at one time. Its complement of medical personnel included female nurses and attached American Red Cross workers. The record is notable for the absence of any information concerning this period on the *Prague*. But, in thanking the ship's captain on behalf of General Hawley and himself, Colonel Cutler wrote: "It was pleasant and the enforced rest did us much good." It also gave Colonel Cutler the opportunity to observe the evacuation of a group of casualties from the time they were loaded on the continental shores until they disembarked in England.

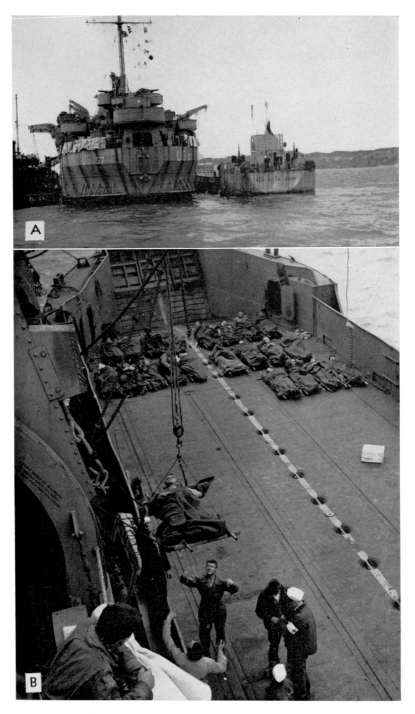

FIGURE 79.—(*See opposite page for legend.*)

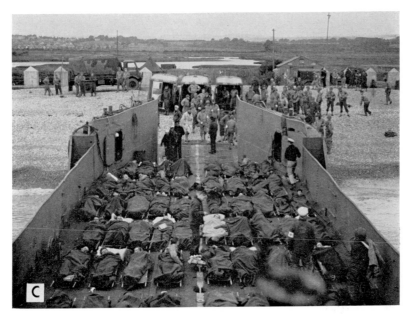

FIGURE 79.—The unloading of LST's by transfer to an LCT and direct beaching of the LCT, Weymouth, England. A. An LCT tied alongside an LST. B. A patient being lowered to an LCT. C. An LCT being beached where ambulances and trucks await.

General Hawley and Colonel Cutler returned to Salisbury for the night of 23 June (fig. 82) but left early the next morning by air for the Normandy beachhead, arriving at the Utah air strip at 0845 on 24 June. They departed from Omaha airstrip at 2000 the next day, but in the interim Colonel Cutler was able to visit the three platoons of the 45th Field Hospital, the 3d Platoon of the 13th Field Hospital, the 621st Clearing Company at the Utah airstrip, and the 5th, 24th, 41st, 44th, 45th, 67th, and 97th Evacuation Hospitals. In addition, he had the opportunity for lengthy conferences with the First U.S. Army surgical consultant, Colonel Crisler, and also Colonel MacFee. Upon returning, the Chief Consultant in Surgery reported to General Hawley in a memorandum, dated 28 June 1944, as follows:

*　　　*　　　*　　　*　　　*　　　*　　　*

4. It is unnecessary here to take up individual professional comments which were made directly to Colonel Crisler and many of which were embodied in the memo for the First U.S. Army Medical Bulletin which he was preparing at the time we were there for Colonel Rogers' study and signature, but the following comments may be of value:—

a. *Blood.*

A large quantity of blood is being used by the First U.S. Army (fig. 83). I saw no instances, however, where I felt it was not helpful and indeed desirable for the treatment of casualties. Should pressure decrease, perhaps more plasma can be used in proportion to blood. I could not judge from statistical data the exact relation between

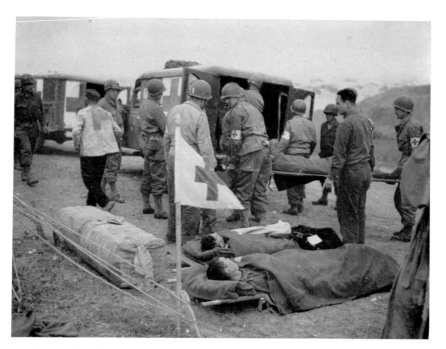

FIGURE 80.—Wounded German prisoners being unloaded at a collecting point on the Normandy beachhead (Omaha Beach) near Vierville-sur-Mer, France, 10 June 1944.

blood and plasma but I had the impression it was being used almost as frequently as plasma; that is, in the ratio of 1 : 1, whereas one has some justification for the hope that a smaller amount of blood, backed up by plasma might yield almost as beneficial results, i.e. in the proportion of 1 of blood to 3 of plasma. * * *

There were numerous complaints about the "set" not working well. Some thought it was the filter, some the size of the giving needle in the vein, which was a part of the plasma set, and some thought it was the needle which let air into the bottle as the blood ran out. * * * I am of the opinion that a chief difficulty lies in the method by which air enters the bottle, * * * or if the blood is not shaken and carefully mixed it becomes clogged by the buffy coat and coagulum which always settles out on top. This matter was discussed in detail with Major Hardin on my return, and he hopes to make a trip immediately to the First U.S. Army and see if the difficulties cannot be smoothed out. Not all officers made complaints, so that the difficulty certainly is not insurmountable.

b. *Penicillin.*

I believe the theater stocks will be able to keep up to the demand for 500 million units of penicillin daily. * * * 500 million units will treat only a little better than 2,000 casualties a day. * * * if the casualties are of a less serious type, the dose is halved and therefore 500 million units would suffice for 4,000 casualties a day. I am of the opinion that as pressure decreases and the hospitals become well stocked, 500 million units of penicillin will be ample for the present. Also, during my visit I found one surgeon who was giving 100,000 units per injection instead of the 40,000 prescribed. This is neither proper nor scientific and * * * I warned him it was unwise for individual surgeons to experiment with doses at this time.

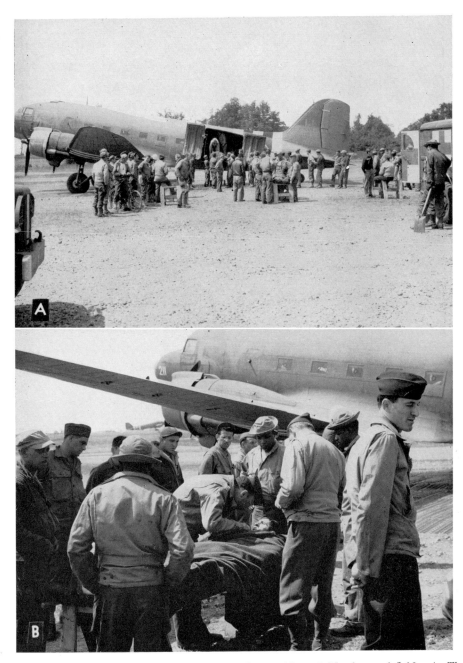

FIGURE 81.—The reception of air-evacuated casualties at Membury airfield. A. The unloading and triage of patients. B. A closeup view of a medical officer examining a casualty. Note the use of simple sawhorses to hold litters.

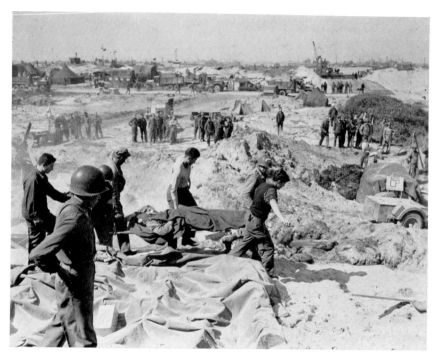

FIGURE 82.—Omaha Beach, 23 June 1944.

c. *Wound debridement.*

This, on the whole, was being well carried out, but Colonel Crisler and I did see some assistant team surgeons operating while their chiefs were resting who were not sufficiently well trained for this purpose, and it would be wiser for the assistant to go off duty while his chief is resting, and the casualty shipped by air to the United Kingdom, where there are hundreds of capable surgeons waiting, than to do inadequate debridement under the circumstances imposed. In commenting on surgery as a whole, I thought it was a little better in the field hospital platoons than in the evacuation hospitals, but my visit was very short and perhaps some brilliant surgeon's work in one of the platoons of the 45th Field Hospital and one platoon of the 13th Field Hospital overweights my judgment, or it may be that Colonel Crisler has wisely placed his best surgeons with the field hospitals, where the nontransportables are being cared for.

d. *Plaster of paris.*

I thought the general level of plaster work excellent but I did notice a tendency for all femurs to be put in double spicas with a good deal of abduction. It must be recalled that plaster is used to immobilize the fracture in the period between the evacuation and general hospital and that this period should be short. In the general hospitals, plaster would invariably be removed and replaced by skeletal-suspension traction. This merely requires temporary immobilization and low-waisted single spicas should be sufficient for transport. If double spicas are to be applied, the abduction must not exceed litter-width, else transport becomes difficult.

e. *Abdominal surgery.*

I found four eviscerations in two days. This was due to failure to use retention sutures. Colonel Crisler has called attention to this in his professional memo for Colonel

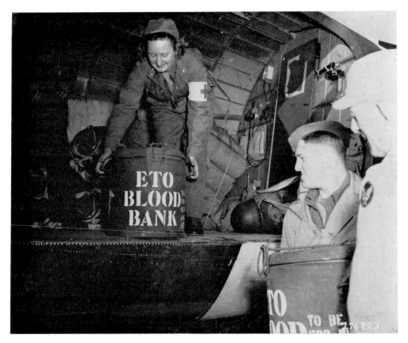

FIGURE 83.—Whole blood for the First U.S. Army being loaded on evacuation aircraft returning to the Normandy beachhead from the Membury airfield, 14 June 1944.

Rogers. I also saw two cases in which the surgeon did not exteriorize large bowel wounds but closed them without a colostomy. I believe this to be an unfortunate mistake and if frequently occurring would surely bring disaster.

f. *Thoracic and thoraco-abdominal wounds.*

The wounds I saw done at field hospitals bring forth my most sincere appreciation. I still recollect a very difficult case of this type being done by Partington at a 45th [Field Hospital] platoon which had every element of perfect surgical performance.

g. *P.O.W.'s.*

At one hospital, where some 300 preoperative cases had accumulated, I found three prisoners being operated upon ahead of our own soldiers.

h. *General comment.*

It is my overall opinion that the level of professional care is very high, certainly better than in the last war. The fact that members of the 3rd Auxiliary Surgical Group, who are well trained and thoroughly instructed in battle casualty care are doing much better work than the 4th Group as a whole, who had little in the way of orientation and instruction, emphasizes again the importance of Army instruction even in professional work. The low incidence of serious infection was striking and must be related to the bacteriostatic agents, penicillin and the sulfonamides, now employed in military surgery. The incidence of amputations seemed happily low, the incidence of gas gangrene also much lower than was expected or was present in the European War, 1914–18.

In closing his report, Colonel Cutler recommended that medical elements of the First U.S. Army, at this time, should direct their energies to providing first aid care for the wounded and surgery only for those in which it would save life or limb. These priorities should be adopted, he explained, for the following reasons:

Casualties given expert first aid care arrived in the United Kingdom even two or three days later in excellent condition, but a good many did not have this. Many wounds had lost their dressings because they were improperly applied, many were improperly splinted, and some, even compound femurs (personally observed), reached the United Kingdom totally unsplinted. If every medical officer in the first week devoted himself to the control of hemorrhage, adequate dressing, adequate treatment of shock with plasma and blood, and perfect immobilization, a perfect task would have been performed. When surgery is permitted early, many hands treat but a few, and many others must go carelessly dressed or improperly splinted.

Even at the present time I would suggest less emphasis on immediate surgery for all and more emphasis on properly evacuating those who can travel safely. This must be a large number, and it seems most unwise to allow any evacuation hospital to carry a backlog of unoperated cases of much over fifty cases.

Major Hardin Visits Normandy

On 28 June 1944, when Colonel Cutler submitted his report, Major Hardin was already on his way to Normandy to determine whether whole blood was being used in excess and what difficulties were being encountered in its administration. In the 3 days that he was there, he contacted members of the Medical Section, Headquarters, First U.S. Army; 1st Medical Depot; Advanced Blood Bank, ETOUSA, Detachment A, 152d Station Hospital; and the 45th, 67th, and 128th Evacuation Hospitals (fig. 84).

He informed Colonel Cutler, on his return, as follows:

*   *   *   *   *   *   *

3. The problems encountered in the use of stored blood were first discussed with Colonel Crisler, Consultant in Surgery, First U.S. Army. The difficulties were mainly in administration of the blood in that the speed of flow was inadequate. The general opinion seemed to be that the filter was at fault.

*   *   *   *   *   *   *

Other errors in the use of the equipment which when corrected will help increase the speed of flow were failure to thoroughly mix the blood by shaking and improper use of the filter. * * *

In the three hospitals visited the ratio of blood to casualties was one (1) pint to four and seven tenths (4.7) casualties. The ratio of plasma to casualties was one (1) unit to three and two tenths (3.2) casualties.

The ratio of blood to plasma was one (1) pint to one and four tenths (1.4) units plasma. Many casualties receive plasma before admission to hospitals, so that these figures do not present a wholly accurate picture of the ratio of plasma to blood.

Reactions to blood as reported are extremely low. It is not believed that this paucity of reactions is possible. Undoubtedly, minor febrile reactions are being overlooked in the rush of caring for numerous casualties. No serious hemolytic reactions were encountered and consequently no deaths from transfusion have been reported. A few instances of jaundice have been encountered in patients who have received large amounts of blood (3,500–5,000 cc's). In each case complicating factors were present such as hepatic injury, sulphonamide therapy, and collections of blood in body cavities or muscles. There was no case in which the jaundice could be attributed solely to blood transfusion. However, * * * all stored blood, regardless of age, contains some free hemoglobin and * * * with massive

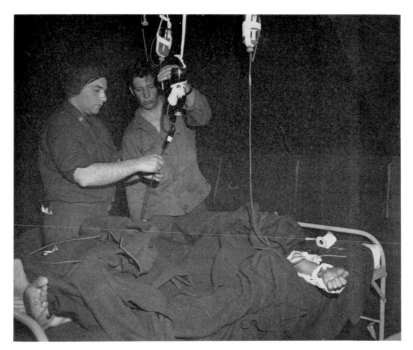

FIGURE 84.—Blood from the Blood Bank, ETOUSA, being administered at the 128th Evacuation Hospital, Normandy, 12 June 1944.

transfusion there is a possibility of exceeding the renal threshold for hemoglobin with consequent kidney damage * * *.

An excess of recipient sets was found in hospitals and in the Advanced Blood Depot. * * * It is estimated that approximately two thousand (2,000) sets were lost in the first few days of operation. Fewer sets are being returned to the Blood Bank daily than are being shipped.

Significantly, Major Hardin, Senior Consultant in Transfusion and Shock, observed: "It does not appear that blood is being used in excess. It is administered not only for treatment of shock but to combat gas gangrene and other infections and to quickly build up the hemoglobin level in exsanguinated patients."

As a result of his visit to the Continent, Major Hardin recommended that:

*   *   *   *   *   *   *

4. * * *

a. Blood be shaken vigorously before administration.

b. The filter chamber be completely filled by inverting when transfusion is started.

c. No. 15 needles be used when rapid transfusion is desired.

d. Hospitals keep the same number of giving sets and bottles of blood on hand thus avoiding tieing up of sets needed elsewhere.

e. Patients receiving more than fifteen hundred (1500) cubic centimeters of blood in twenty-four hours be alkalinized by the same procedure as used when administering sulphonamides.[84]

---

[84] Essential Technical Medical Data, European Theater of Operations, U.S. Army, for June 1944, dated 22 July 1944. Inclosure 4, subject: Report of Visit to Combat Zone, by Maj. R. C. Hardin, MC.

Activities of Surgical Consultants During Invasion Phase

By the end of June, a fairly clear picture could be obtained of the initial activities of the U.S. Army Medical Department during the Normandy campaign, and it was possible to assess trends and contemplate future actions. In reflecting on the activities of the consultants during this invasion phase,[85] the Chief Consultant in Surgery made the following observations concerning his activities during the first week:

(1) Col. E. C. Cutler was permitted to remain with General Hawley, with headquarters at the 1st General Medical Laboratory, and from that point visualize the reception of casualties at both the Southampton and Portland hards and their distribution through the subsidiary transit hospital areas and final evacuation to the base area by hospital train. This permitted a full evaluation of the system used to evacuate casualties from the far to the near shore, the limits and advantages of professional care as given whilst casualties were on craft in the Channel, received at the hards and cared for in holding and transit hospitals.

He described the activities of the other consultants during the first week, as follows:

(2) Lt. Col. G. K. Rhodes was assigned to the holding hospitals at the Portland-Weymouth hards, Lt. Col. R. M. Zollinger was assigned to the holding hospitals in the Southampton area, and Lt. Col. E. M. Bricker was assigned to the hards in the Torquay-Brixham area.

These men were of the greatest assistance in advising regarding the professional care of the serious, nontransportable wounded in their respective areas and in designating what cases could be reclassified as transportables and therefore removed from the nontransportable hospitals to the transit hospitals.

(3) The surgical consultants in the specialties confined their work for the first week largely to the area of the transit hospitals. Here, they were able to assist greatly in the professional care of casualties, the proper choice of priorities for surgical procedures and the evacuability or transfer of patients from transit hospitals to the base area and on occasions directly to special hospitals, where competent specialists were present. Indeed, on more than one occasion they were able to advise in the proper location of specialist teams at hospitals in the transit area, such as the moving of a neurosurgical team (a) to the 28th General Hospital, and (b) to the 217th General Hospital, where neurological cases tended to concentrate and where it seemed wise to provide expert professional care.

The characteristics of the activities and assignments of the surgical consultants, after the first week, were described by Colonel Cutler as follows:

*   *   *   *   *   *   *

b. * * * By this time it was clear that the advice of the surgical consultants could wisely be used in the area of the holding or nontransportable hospitals as well as in the transit hospital areas, and from time to time the surgical consultants visited these institutions. Colonel Vail's advice was necessary regarding certain difficult items and [that of] Colonel Tovell to help with anesthesia supply and administration. On the whole the surgical consultants continued to confine their work to the transit hospitals and continued increasingly to visit these institutions and to assist in establishing a high level of professional care. At the same time, the surgical consultants began to follow the cases back

---

[85] Memorandum, Chief Consultant in Surgery to Chief Surgeon, ETOUSA (through Chief, Professional Services Division), 30 June 1944, subject: Synopsis of Activities and Reports of Surgical Consultant Group During the First Two Weeks of the "Liberation Invasion."

into the general hospitals which, unused to the sudden influx of a large convoy, were at first thrown into some confusion, but gradually straightened their organization out and on the whole functioned in a highly satisfactory fashion, * * *. By this second week also air evacuation began to flourish and visits to the 217th General Hospital, which bore the brunt of air evacuation at first, assisted this hospital in the proper care of large numbers of casualties.

In his synopsis of activities during the first month of the operations, Colonel Cutler gathered professional comment from each of the senior consultants on his specialty and showed how their help and observations were contributing to the success of the medical support of the invasion. He ventured to hope that "this brief citation of the work of the surgical consultants in the first weeks of the 'Liberation Invasion' will justify the request that they be permitted as soon as accessible to visualize the problem on the far shore, that they in turn may benefit the professional care there as well as that they in turn may learn more and benefit the casualties returning to this shore." And his hope was to be fulfilled, for, as has been noted, Major Hardin was already in Normandy, and Colonel Cutler was instructed to establish priorities and schedules for each of his other senior consultants to visit the Continent at an early date.

Observations, recommendations, and actions

By the end of June 1944, as previously mentioned, a fairly clear picture could be obtained of the initial operations. As combat on the Continent changed from the area of the immediate beachhead to hedgerow fighting further inland, trends became more clearly established, and patterns for the immediate future became manifest. The Normandy campaign ended on 24 July, and the Northern France Campaign began. The Third U.S. Army officially engaged in combat a few days later on 1 August 1944.

Colonel Cutler and his surgical consultant group made the following observations of surgical activities during the Normandy campaign.

Evacuation by sea.—The LST and hospital carrier operations during the invasion were described by Colonel Cutler as follows:

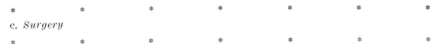

c. *Surgery*

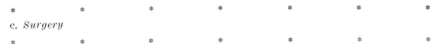

The care on ships during the Channel crossing was carefully coordinated and worked out with the Navy and perfect collaboration was obtained. LST's had two Navy medical officers and one qualified Army surgeon, were equipped with small operating rooms and liberally supplied with surgical instruments, surgical supplies, penicillin, and refrigerated whole blood. All of this equipment and personnel proved valuable. Only life- and limb-saving surgical measures were carried out on LST's, but probably some ten abdomens were operated upon and a similar number of sucking chest wounds closed in the first few days, thereby possibly saving life. Moreover, adjusting splints, reapplying and reinforcing dressings and the giving of plasma and blood kept the entire medical personnel on both ships and LST's busy without let-up from embarkation to debarkation. Members of the Professional Services Division boarded many LST's and hospital carriers, discussed problems with the medical staff and were able to evaluate the care given on such ships. It

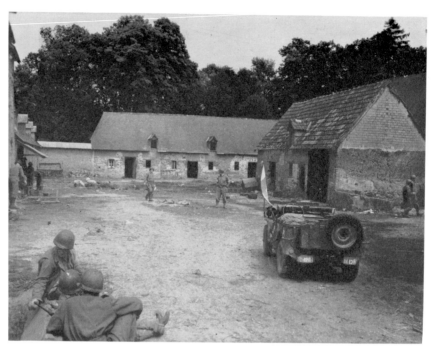

Figure 85.—An aid station and rest point in a captured farmhouse, during the battle of the hedgerows, 14 July 1944.

was universally noted that LST's were easy to load and unload. At the same time, they were dark, often cold, sanitary facilities were extremely difficult, and feeding anything more than a "quick lunch" and a hot drink was out of the question. LST's carried as many as 350 casualties at the maximum, though sometimes as few as 60 to 70 casualties. When the larger numbers were aboard, the number of personnel assigned was scarcely sufficient to give even routine sanitary care and food, let alone professional skilled care. There was general agreement that the hospital carriers were unsuitable for stretcher cases because of difficulty in carrying litter patients down narrow stairways, et cetera. More-over, the double decker system of beds on some carriers was inappropriate for litter cases on the top bunk (fig. 85).[86]

The hospital carrier had its advantages over an LST in other respects (fig. 86). For one thing, it had better feeding and sanitary facilities. Colonel Cutler advised, moreover, as follows:

* * * in arguments as between hospital carriers and LST's one must consider the safety of the casualty once aboard a hospital carrier, [painted] white and properly marked as per the Geneva Convention with its green strip and its Red Cross. Should we have an LST sunk with 300 wounded men aboard and at the same time have a hospital ship we could with justification be bitterly criticized. It appears to us that, with greater air evacuation and a more rapid turnabout of hospital carriers which could at least take care of the prisoners of war and the lightly wounded, we would have an optimum evacuation system for this kind of a cross-Channel effort. Moreover we must recall the hospital ship

had nurses, Red Cross workers and a chaplain. It is warm compared to an LST and these arguments in its favor counterbalance in our minds the ease with which the LST is loaded and unloaded.[87]

"On the whole," the Chief Consultant in Surgery said in summary, "the professional work accomplished during the trans-Channel crossing was highly creditable and very beneficial to the casualties." [88]

Air evacuation.—"Air evacuation proved excellent from the beginning and should be enlarged," Colonel Cutler said. Elsewhere, he noted that the reception and holding facilities were not ideal at the terminals for air evacuation. But, the important point, as Colonel Cutler later observed, was as follows:

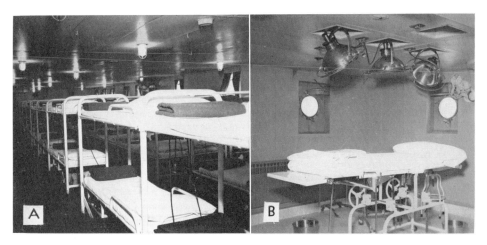

FIGURE 86.—Facilities aboard a converted hospital carrier. A. A ward with double-decked beds. B. An operating room.

What lessons have we learned from the Normandy experience? It early became apparent that definitive surgery for all could not be performed in our forward units because of the load. At one 400-bed evacuation hospital, for example, I saw 250 men waiting for surgery, when empty planes were going to the United Kingdom the same day. Had these casualties been lifted at once their first surgical treatment would have come earlier. The policy was then changed so that only nontransportable cases were given definitive surgery on the Continent.[89]

"Near shore" medical service.—Colonel Cutler's first comment on the near shore operations follows:

The S.O.P. is laid out in Administrative Memorandum #62, 3 May 1944. It worked well as a whole. A comment might be made that its rigidity in the first few days had some unhappy results in that at certain transit hospitals definitive surgery was not being done and men were being held several days until enough casualties accumulated for a train

[87] See footnote 85, p. 224.
[88] See footnote 86, p. 226.
[89] Tidy, Sir Henry (ed.). Inter-Allied Conferences on War Medicine, 1942–1945, Convened by the Royal Society of Medicine. New York, Toronto, London: Staples Press, Ltd., 1947, p. 426.

evacuation. Also the rule that the FMR should not start [with] anyone who is not kept over 48 hours was unfortunate when definitive surgery had to be done at a transit hospital, for the paucity of information that went on with the casualty mitigated against his proper care. A further suggestion arose in the early days, that possibly neurosurgical and maxillo-facial specialists should be in transit hospitals near hards so that cases with this type of damage could early be placed under specialists for care.[90]

Otherwise, Colonel Cutler was satisfied with the overall results of the hospitalization and evacuation procedures that were carried out on the near shore. His account of his views follows:

The reception on this shore, whether from planes or ships, was organized on a similar basis; i.e., close to the unloading points field hospitals were set up, to which were attached surgical teams who were to care for the heavily damaged, nontransportable casualties. These field hospitals were of the greatest value during the first few days of the invasion, when surgery on the far shore was at a minimum, or nonexistent. Later, when an evacuation hospital was set up with the Army on the far shore and a larger percentage of the cases arrived already having had definitive surgery, the pressure on the holding hospitals for nontransportables decreased. These holding hospitals were adequately sup-plied with whole blood and penicillin daily, had a generous allotment of expert surgical teams and proved themselves to be a highly desirable part of such an undertaking.

The less seriously damaged patient passed by these holding hospitals for nontransport-ables to "transit hospitals," which were either station or general hospitals within a radius of 30 miles of the beachhead where, according to the pressure exerted by the numbers being evacuated, either definitive surgery was carried out or the patient was dressed, his splints readjusted, blood and penicillin given, and he passed from these transit hospitals into the rear areas either to a hospital center or to an available general hospital by train. The number of casualties passing through some transit hospitals was very high, perhaps the heaviest service being at the 110th Station Hospital, where some two thousand casualties were received in a period of 24 hours. At these transit hospitals were also located attached surgical teams, but the major function of the transit hospital was to properly sort cases and only allow those to go on who were in a suitable condition for further travel. The dispatching of patients from the transit hospitals to the back areas by hospital train worked well. The medical personnel aboard such trains worked well, were able to give hot drinks, sandwiches, and see that where dressings had slipped or splints needed to be readjusted suitable care was given (fig. 87).[91]

General surgery and wounds.—The following thoughts were recorded as of the end of June by the Chief Consultant in Surgery:

It is our overall opinion that the level of the professional care is very high, certainly better than in the last war. The evaluation of early and good surgery and of the sulfona-mides and penicillin in combatting infection cannot now be stated. Both undoubtedly con-tribute to this happy result. There may be a relation between controlling ordinary pyogenic infection and the low incidence of gas gangrene and subsequent low incidence of amputa-tion. The surgeon is certainly pushed nearer to the wounder soldier and the decreased interval of time between wounding and surgery may be a dominant factor in the unusually satisfactory results. In addition, the early application of secondary suture is going to restore a large body of men to active duty within a period of a few weeks.[92]

---

[90] See footnote 85, p. 224.
[91] See footnote 86, p. 226.
[92] See footnote 86, p. 226.

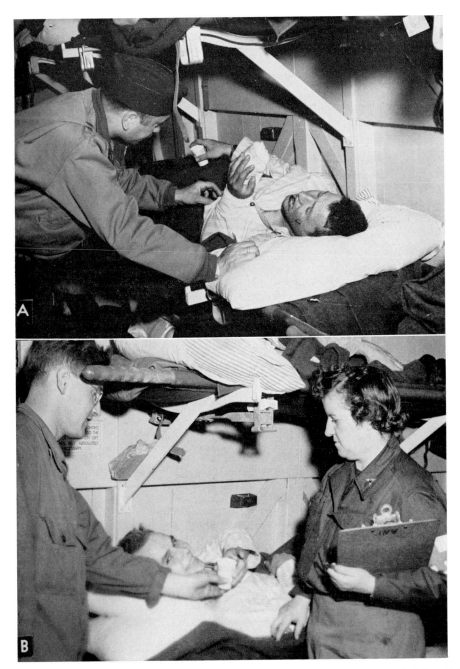

FIGURE 87.—Care aboard hospital trains during the Normandy campaign.   A. A hospital train medical officer checking the condition of a patient.   B. An attendant giving a patient liquid while a nurse observes.

Essential Technical Medical Data, ETOUSA, for June 1944 reflected his views substantially as follows:

The percentage of infection was surprisingly low, even at 4 or 5 days after injury and without surgery. Indeed, some surgeons with experience thought it wiser not to explore battle casualty wounds that looked well. It is in a way unfortunate because eventually practically all of these wounds need debridement, since the sulfonamides and penicillin tend to prevent widespread cellulitis but leave an abscess above bits of cloth which are carried in with the missile. There can be no question whatsoever but that spreading cellulitis as seen in the last war is now a rarity, and one must feel that the sulfonamides and penicillin play a definite role in this betterment. Gas gangrene was present in but few cases. We have at this time no final figure, but the impression of all surgical consultants is that it is not a major problem at this time. Moreover, the separation of cases infected with the clostridia into those with simple cellulitis and into those with widespread myositis resulted in the saving of many extremities, for the simple cellulitis cases do not need amputation and do well with widespread incision and debridement. Abdomens usually reached this shore having had surgery. Sometimes this had been done on the far shore, sometimes on the LST carriers or APA's (transports, attack). Many of these cases did surprisingly well and proved again that early surgery in abdominal injury is the important factor. One case arrived by air 3 days after operation and was in a critical condition on arrival. This patient was seen shortly afterward by Colonel Cutler, and he was of the definite impression that it was not the air transport that caused the trouble but moving the patient and that had he come on an LST his condition might well have been worse.

In July, Colonel Cutler reported, the load of surgical work was extremely heavy. In May, the total number of surgical admissions to fixed hospitals of the communications zone had been 23,375, as revealed by the monthly surgical reports. In June, there had been 53,124 surgical admissions. For July, the figure had risen to 71,623. Colonel Cutler further reported, as follows:

We have maintained the closest liaison with the combat forces on the Continent so that what we have learned here concerning bettering the care of casualties might be implemented by the Army. The most cordial and happy relations exist and have certainly led to great benefit for the soldier. This liaison has been particularly useful in improving the treatment of shock, by the segregation of the seriously injured from the less seriously injured and in the proper utilization of whole blood and plasma. It has led to an extension of air evacuation particularly involving the special groups such as neurosurgery, maxillofacial surgery and thoracic surgery. We have attempted as a principle to push the early closure of battle wounds, and from large spot surveys are content that some 75 percent of our wounds are being closed by early secondary suture between the fourth and the fifteenth day. Many of the hospital and hospital center reports show an extremely high percentage of primary union after secondary suture. Thus, at the 15th General Hospital primary union occurred in 93.4 percent after secondary suture. The 82d General Hospital shows primary union in 94.1 percent after secondary suture. The 83d General Hospital had primary union in 83.7 percent of 93 wounds. These are merely samples of information which will be amassed later and submitted in tabulated form.

It is interesting that, though great attempt has been made to use penicillin liberally, many wounds have been closed in which no chemotherapy was practised, either sulfonamides or penicillin, with equally satisfactory results. The major difficulty with secondary closure has been where too great tension was put on the lips of the wound by trying perhaps to pull together the area which should have been grafted rather than closed with sutures. Out of a mass of material is slowly merging what was known early, that the earlier a wound is closed the more easily it closes and the less apt it is to break down, also that wounds which are too large to close should be immediately grafted. As a part of this effort we have begun to close compound fractures, utilizing penicillin therapy in all cases in which this is done. It is too early to report results, but at least we have no bad consequences to speak of. Again, in relation to wounds we have a large number of patients in whom *Bacillus welchii* and *Bacillus pyocyaneus* have been cultured from wounds healed without difficulty when submitted to secondary closure. In relation to this, our report from last month should be noted, [p. 87 ff.], which included the study of wounds with the 8th Air Force in which a high percentage of the wounds showed clostridia, but almost none showed any clinical evidence of invasion by these anaerobes.[93]

As a result of these and previous observations, the need to revise and add to certain clinical policies contained in the Manual of Therapy and Circular Letter No. 71 was apparent. Circular Letter No. 101, Office of the Chief Surgeon, ETOUSA, was therefore published on 30 July 1944. It included the following instructions under the heading of wounds:

a. Wounds will not be plugged or packed with Vaseline gauze. Only sufficient gauze should be used to keep the wound temporarily open.

b. Sulfonamides are being dumped in excessive quantities in wounds, and this makes subsequent repair difficult.

c. Wounds *must not be closed by sutures* at the time of the first debridement, except for the following :—

(1) Neurosurgical injuries.

(2) Thoracic injuries.

(3) Wounds of eyelids.

(4) Certain maxillofacial injuries, as outlined in the Manual of Therapy, ETO.

d. Penetrating wounds of the paranasal sinuses should be thoroughly explored, foreign bodies and blood removed and external drainage provided at the original operation. Drainage of the antrum into the nose is the method of choice unless the wound has destroyed so much tissue that external closure is not possible. The frontal sinuses should be drained through the wound or through an incision to allow opening in the floor of the sinuses.

e. The routine culture of wounds is unnecessary, and wasteful of time and materials. Cultures should be limited to those wounds where there is clinical evidence of infection and where they may contribute to its subsequent clinical management.

f. Wounds seen late, after wounding, without debridement, may be debrided in the usual manner.

g. Wounds can usually be closed within 3 to 5 days after debridement. A satisfactory preparation of the wound for secondary closure has been the application of warm saline dressings. Chemotherapy locally in the wound at the time of secondary closure is not necessary; penicillin therapy should be resumed before and after secondary closure in all large wounds.

h. As a rule, foreign bodies which interfere with function or wound healing should be removed. Modern chemotherapy obscures the signs of local infection only *temporarily* and

[93] Essential Technical Medical Data, European Theater of Operations, U.S. Army, for July 1944, dated 17 August 1944.

many times delayed infection, with breakdown of the wound, may result after a long interval.

i. Continued local and excessive applications of sulfonamides in wounds are detrimental to wound healing, produce dermatological lesions, often increase blood levels above safety limit, and are unsupported scientifically as the proper therapy.

Gas gangrene.—While some mention was made in the foregoing of the occurrence of gas gangrene in battle casualties being received, Colonel Cutler noted the following:

An attempt has been made to gather in all the cases of true gas gangrene. Up to the present we have been able to collect 198 cases in whom there were 14 deaths, a mortality of 7.07 percent. These figures must not be considered final, for some of these 198 cases may not be true gas gangrene, for one must distinguish between simple anaerobic invasion of an avascular extremity, or simple anaerobic cellulitis and true clostridial myositis. Bacteriology is of no assistance here, for, as pointed out above, many wounds without the slightest evidence of gas gangrene contain the Welch bacillus, and many of these have been closed by early secondary suture with primary union. Of the above 198 cases, 76 (38.3 percent) had amputations. Thirty-one percent of the amputations were done in the forward area and twenty-five percent of those cases amputated in the forward area were reamputated in SOS units later.[94]

The "gas gangrene" portion of Circular Letter No. 101 was extensive and informative as well as instructive. It read:

a. Incidence of serious infection with clostridia is fortunately low up to the present time, and surgeons have shown a wise discrimination between diffuse myositis and cellulitis. This has restricted amputation, led to recovery by simple incision, excision of involved muscle and adequate drainage.

b. Routine culture of wounds is unnecessary unless there is clinical suspicion of gas bacillus infection. Gas-forming organisms can commonly be cultured from a wound, and such findings should not influence the surgical treatment unless consistent with the clinical diagnosis. Only in clinical cases of gas gangrene infection should cultures be taken and sent to the First Medical General Laboratory for final identification of the organisms.

c. Amputations have in some cases been too radical. Always demand a consultation and always explore locally in wound before amputation. In many cases the apparent diffuse involvement, as shown by a swelling, crepitation and discoloration of the skin, has extended far above the actual muscle involvement. Failure to appreciate that amputation or muscle excision can be carried out at a much lower level has at times resulted in the needless high amputation of the thigh or upper arm. Extensive incision and drainage above the level of amputation is commonly required in such instances.

d. Following amputation for widespread clostridial myositis, skin traction should not be applied for the first 24–48 hours, since some cases thus treated have had unfortunate results because of restricting dressings. Such cases should be held as nontransportable until skin traction is applied.

e. In performing the circular amputation, the skin should always, if possible, be longer than the underlying soft tissue and bone. Except in amputations following clostridial infection skin traction should in every instance be applied immediately. * * *

f. There has been an unfortunate waste of both material and effort in applying to clostridial infected wounds the hospital precautions usually applied to virulent and easily transmissible organisms. There is no reason for special isolation for ward care of gas gangrene cases other than simple hospital routine and cleanliness. However, the group-

---

[94] See footnote 93, p. 231.

ing of such cases may be desirable as a matter of efficiency in their management. It is wise to have special dressing sets prepared for gas gangrene cases, since these instruments should be sterilized by autoclaving. These should not be mixed with other instruments on the surgical cart which may not require autoclaving. Linens and blankets *directly* in contact with discharges from wounds infected with clostridia should be autoclaved before laundering.

g. Radiographic depiction of gas in the tissues, regardless of its distribution, does not necessarily indicate gas gangrene, and, unless other clinical signs and symptoms are present, should be disregarded.

Use of penicillin and sulfonamides.—Colonel Cutler reported at the end of June that 500,000,000 units of penicillin were being supplied to the First U.S. Army daily, an amount which he said should be sufficient for the present and immediate future, and a quantity which could be supplied with reasonable assurance. The buildup to this daily maintenance supply was described as follows:

The demands for this drug increase daily in spite of heavy deliveries earlier. Far shore deliveries were 300,000,000 units by carrier, early, 100,000,000 twice by air up to 17 June. Since 25 June we have been delivering 500,000,000 by air daily. Some of this may not have been properly used, but we are convinced from observations here and on the far shore that the casualties are receiving all of it and observations make us believe it is beneficial.[95]

Colonel Cutler's views with regard to the part played by penicillin and the sulfonamides in the control of wound infections, as witnessed in these early days, are set forth in Essential Technical Medical Data, ETOUSA, for July 1944, as follows:

It may be said that the low incidence of serious infection in the present campaign is still a source of wonder to those who were in the last war. The fact that the wounds of those who have never had sulfonamides or penicillin are not to a great extent more infected than in those who had penicillin seems to point out that other factors than just chemotherapy must be studied. We must not forget that the American soldier today is far better fed than in 1917–18, that he is physically in a great deal better condition, that he individually knows much more about looking after himself, including first-aid, that the [Medical Department] soldiers * * * are far better trained than they were in the last war, and that the resistance of the individual himself may be so much greater that even without chemotherapy his wounds do well. Moreover, plasma and whole blood are given liberally and must be weighed in the scales when one discusses immunity and infection.

With reference to the penicillin section of the new directive, Circular Letter No. 101, Essential Technical Medical Data, ETOUSA, for July, states:

Circular Letter #101, which is the followup on Circular * * * Letter #71, contains further data regarding penicillin in wounds and fills in what we have already learned from our brief experience. It is fair to point out that sulfonamides are liberally utilized, and penicillin also. Perhaps we would have liked to give penicillin to one army and not to another, if this [had been] just a scientific question, but, there being evidence that penicillin benefits infection, we felt forced to give every American soldier the benefit of penicillin. This is going to modify and make difficult suitable controls, but an attempt

---

[95] See footnote 85, p. 224.

is being made to find enough wounds amongst our own troops, or in prisoners-of-war, who did not get penicillin or sulfonamides, that these cases may be used as controls against the remainder.

The penicillin instructions in Circular Letter No. 101 were simple and explicit. The earlier "penicillin circular," intended for the instruction of those using penicillin in the fixed hospitals of the communications zone (p. 142), was rescinded. The new circular stated that dosages as given in Circular Letter No. 71 should be adhered to. It warned that some medical officers have on occasion tripled the dosage without scientific justification, and the supply would be imperiled if such experimentation is carried out. The newer directive also took cognizance of the fact that no special forms for reporting casualties treated with penicillin existed. Consequently, medical officers were instructed to record the words "Penicillin Treated" after the diagnosis on the emergency medical tag or field medical record as required by Circular Letter No. 71.

Whole blood.—Colonel Cutler was immensely pleased with the work of the blood bank and, at the end of June, reported the following:

> The tremendous demand for blood completely justifies the establishment of the blood bank and from reports and observations it is clear we must have saved life by the establishment of an ETO blood bank. 2,000 pints with sets went over by hospital carrier or air. About 1,000 pints have been given up by medical officers on LST's to far-shore medical groups. Landing troops took in 240 pints and sets on landing. Lt. Riordan of the blood bank is now on the far shore. He has a large Navy-type refrigerator buried in the ground at the Omaha air strip, and [8] trucks (each taking 80 pints) are well working with the First Army delivering blood at this time (fig. 88). Almost all LST's and hospital carriers either gave up their blood to people on the far shore or used it up on casualties on the trip back.[96] Little was actually wasted. The major difficulty about blood has been the return of kits and sets and marmite jars.[97]

As the Third U.S. Army joined the fray, and it was evident that the conflict in Europe was to expand ever larger, there were ominous and unmistakable signs that the European theater blood bank could not come close to providing the demands which would be made. The First U.S. Army required 500 pints per day. The Third U.S. Army insisted upon a daily supply of 550 pints. Moreover, the First U.S. Army had been borrowing 200 pints per day from the British with no possible way of ever replacing this loan. But, this is a story which highlights the period of the next campaign in Europe. At the close of the Normandy campaign, there was a comment to the effect that whether or not blood was being wasted or used without adequate reason had been carefully considered, and that there was a firm opinion in the whole European theater that the Army needed blood.

The instructions in Circular Letter No. 101 pertained to the mechanical difficulties which had been encountered in using the whole blood supplied from

---

[96] "Medical supply dumps were established at each port of embarkation in the Southern Base Section. LST's were supplied from them, and unloaded them on the far beach. Each outbound LST carried twice the amount of blood estimated to be needed on the return trip. The excess was unloaded on the far beach. This was the way in which blood was supplied on the early beachhead." (Letter, Paul R. Hawley, M.D., to Col. John Boyd Coates, Jr., MC, 17 Sept. 1958.)

[97] See footnote 85, p. 224.

the European theater blood bank and the alkalinizing of patients who had been given massive transfusions. This circular letter stated:

*   *   *   *   *   *   *

14. * * * The following instructions should be observed in the use of blood obtained from the ETO Blood Bank:—

a. Return of sets. All used sets must be returned at the first opportunity to the drivers of the delivery trucks. Sets should not be kept on hand in excess of a level of one (1) per pint of blood.

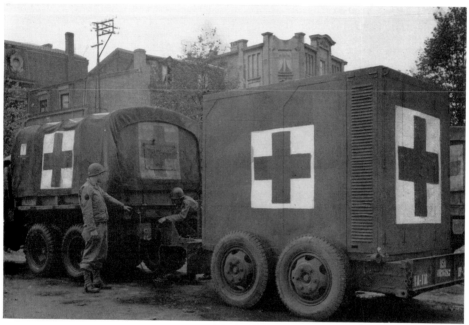

FIGURE 88.—A unit of the Blood Bank, ETOUSA, with the First U.S. Army, hitching a storage refrigerator, mounted on an artillery carrier, to a cargo truck.

b. Observance of the following will facilitate the administration of blood:

(1) Plasma should be given first except in exceptional circumstances (exsanguination).

(2) The blood must be vigorously shaken before administration.

(3) The filter (both steel and gas mantle) chamber must be completely filled to utilize all of the filtering surface. This is accomplished by inverting and filling the chamber before starting the transfusion.

(4) When a transfusion must be given rapidly, a No. 15 needle should be used.

(5) When the transfusion is started the air vent should be checked and, if necessary, cleared by positive pressure.

c. Any patient receiving more than 1,500 cc. of blood or exhibiting evidence of intravascular hemolysis including hemoglobinuria as shown by chemical test, will be alkalinized according to one of the following procedures:

Oral.

(1) Initially: 8 gms. sodium citrate, dissolved in water.

(2) Maintenance: 2 gms. sodium bicarbonate by mouth every two hours.

(3) Fluid intake to be 3,000 cc. per 24 hours.

Intravenous.

(1) Initially: 4 gms. sodium citrate in twenty-four hours by intravenous drip, or 1½ gms. every two hours intravenously.

(2) Maintenance: 16 gms. sodium citrate in twenty-four hours by intravenous drip, or 1½ gms. every two hours intravenously.

(3) 3,000 cc. fluid intake.

The urine will be tested chemically for hemoglobin and with litmus or other suitable indicator for pH. Alkalis may be discontinued when hemoglobin disappears from the urine which in the average case will occur in less than twenty-four hours.

Sorting.—Circular Letter No. 101 also presented the following advice and instructions on sorting—triage:

*   *   *   *   *   *   *

15. *Sorting.* On the perfection with which *sorting* is accomplished, will depend the proper care of many soldiers, and lives may be lost if improper sorting under pressure occurs. Sorting (triage) should separate into at least three categories.

a. Those in shock and critically ill, possibly moribund.

b. Those awaiting their turn at the operating table in preoperative ward (and not necessarily in shock).

c. Lightly wounded individuals who may be evacuated with nothing more than a fresh dressing. In this group may be placed, unless the Commanding Officer desires separate wards, the medically sick, if they are evacuable. Observations have revealed that the division of seriously ill and shocked people and those merely awaiting their turn has been poorly accomplished. This has resulted in men with simple injuries being unnecessarily damaged psychologically by being placed in beds next to dying or critically ill individuals. Also, this mixture of critically ill and lightly wounded had taken up the time of those working in the shock wards, who should devote all their energy to the critically ill.

Other instructions.—Circular Letter No. 101 also warned that evisceration had resulted in cases where retention sutures had not been used in abdominal wounds. It directed that all abdominal wounds should be liberally supported with retention sutures. In addition, it stated that small bowel enterostomies should not be performed unless this was the only possible procedure in a special case and that colostomy should always accompany the repair of injuries to the large bowel with exteriorization, when possible, through a separate incision.

The circular letter stated that plaster splints were being applied too thick and that, if bilateral spicas were applied, they had to be litter width and reinforced with a strut placed posteriorly. All initial circular plaster of paris dressings, the directive went on to say, following trauma, manipulation, or operation had to be split to the skin and slightly spread.

There were also instructions with regard to thoracic surgery, vascular surgery, spinal cord damage, ocular injuries, blast ears, radiographs, laboratory procedures, prophylactic tetanus antitoxin, sterilization of ampules, and the coloring of cocaine to insure ready identification.

Joy and tragedy.—On 19 July, Colonel Cutler learned that some 60,000 German prisoners had been taken since D-day, and he was most elated (fig. 89). "Pretty good. We're on our way!" he wrote. There was no doubt but that

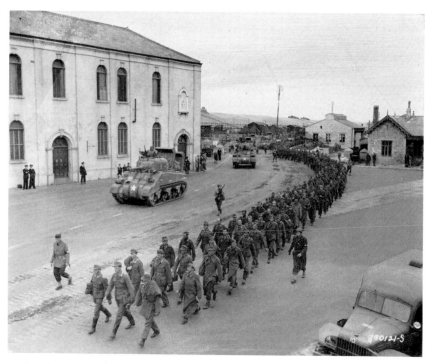

FIGURE 89.—A long line of German prisoners of war being marched ashore at Weymouth, England, on 10 June 1944.

a good start had been made in Normandy. But at the same time, the "Buzz Bombs" were beginning to fall on England, and over 3,500 had been counted (fig. 90). A Britisher had been killed for nearly every bomb counted, and the total killed and injured was over 25,000. At about the same time, Colonel Kimbrough became sick and was hospitalized with pneumonia. Colonel Zollinger had been sent to the Continent for temporary duty with the Advance Section, Communications Zone. Colonel Cutler had to do the work of both. And then, on 23 July, Lt. Col. George K. Rhodes, MC, who had been of immeasurable help, passed away.

It was Sunday morning, 23 July. Colonel Rhodes had not felt well at breakfast, and Lt. Col. (later Col.) Yale Kneeland, Jr., MC, medical consultant for the Southern Base Section, had persuaded Colonel Rhodes to rest. When Colonel Kneeland came back to see him in 1300, he was dead, the body was still warm, there was no disturbance of the clothing, and it appeared that he might have died in his sleep. Autopsy later proved the diagnosis, coronary occlusion. His body was taken to the Cambridge Cemetery by Colonel Kneeland, and there he was buried.

At various times Colonel Cutler had said that the sacrifice a medical officer makes in war cannot compare to that of the infantryman or airman

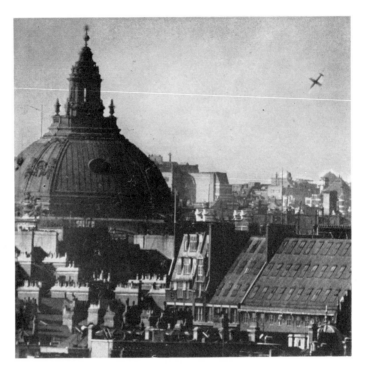

FIGURE 90.—A "Buzz Bomb" (German V–1 rocket) cutting its motor
and diving into the Picadilly section of London.

who must constantly expose himself to direct enemy fire.   But, in this instance,
there was no doubt that Colonel Rhodes had made the supreme sacrifice.   In
his characteristic brevity on such occasions, Colonel Cutler stated in his diary
merely: "G. K. Rhodes died of a coronary today; my age.   Hell, Terrific
pressure."   To the Chief Surgeon, he wrote in a memorandum, dated 24 July
1944, as follows:

1. Lt. Col. G. K. Rhodes arrived in this theater as chief of the surgical service of
the 30th General Hospital, of which he was the original organizer and civilian director,
and which was one of the earliest general hospitals to reach the ETO.   This hospital
was comprised largely of University of California Medical School people with a smattering
from Leland Stanford University Medical School.   It proved to be staffed with personnel
of high professional caliber.

Because of his maturity, excellent clinical judgment, ability to get on well with
people, he was moved to the important post of Consulting Surgeon, Southern Base
Section, when that base section became large and active.   In that capacity he proved
himself an ideal candidate for the position.   The Surgeon of the Southern Base Section
and the Commander of the Southern Base Section were unanimous, as were other officers
in that section, in their praise of his work and abilities.   During the early days of the
invasion his judgment at the nontransportable hospitals serving the hards in the Portland-
Weymouth Area undoubtedly saved some lives and several amputations.   He never spared
himself, and was always available for duty wherever and whenever called.   His relations
with the Headquarters Group, Professional Services Division, of your office, were of the
most amicable and satisfactory type.   The immense load of properly vetting new insti-

tutions and moving candidates of proven quality to weak institutions, etc., was an onerous one in which Colonel Rhodes played a major and beneficial role.

*   *   *   *   *   *   *

5. I know of no officer in your command who has better performed his duties than Lt. Col. G. K. Rhodes. * * * His example of devoted service and his abilities professionally were of the highest order, and your Command has profited by his having served within it.

At the next meeting of the Chief Surgeon's Consultants' Committee, General Hawley, in closing the meeting, said:

The only thing I have is to express to you what we all feel about the great loss that we have suffered in Colonel Rhodes. He worked very hard during this push, and this, I have no doubt, hastened his leaving us in the manner he did, by death.

I was very impressed with his work and his approach to it. You could never get him excited or worried, and he had the keen affection as well as the respect of the young surgeons he advised. He is very difficult to replace. We are very fortunate in having Colonel Morton to replace him. Colonel Morton has done outstanding work with casualties. I welcome him in this group of consultants.

NORTHERN FRANCE

The Northern France Campaign was short-lived, beginning on 25 July and ending 14 September 1944. In that period, the Third U.S. Army broke out from the Normandy beachhead and immediately threatened German positions in northern France. The Seventh U.S. Army landed in southern France on 15 August with relatively light resistance. On 25 August, the Allies liberated Paris. In early September, most of the area of the Benelux countries had been freed, and abortive attempts had been made to establish a bridgehead across the northern Rhine at Aachen. By mid-September, the fight for Germany itself was beginning.

Trip Home

Blood.—From the outset, the supply of sufficient quantities of whole blood was a critical problem. "A trying thing that came up is blood," Colonel Cutler reported at the Chief Surgeon's Consultants' Committee meeting of 28 July, "Everybody who has been to the Continent says that blood is being used improperly. I was asked to ask you [General Hawley] to make one more try to obtain blood from the United States by sending a cable to The Surgeon General requesting the shipment of blood by air to the ETO Blood Bank."

General Hawley was concerned about the time it would take to get the blood to England, making the project futile if the blood did not have sufficient life after arriving in Europe. "There will be a minimum of 72 hours before the blood leaves the U.S.," he maintained. But, after discussion of procedures which would probably be implemented in the United States, Colonel Cutler convinced the Chief Surgeon that whole blood could leave the Zone of Interior within 24 hours after drawing. Major Hardin then assured the general that the life of the blood, after receipt, would be a good two weeks.

"We all believe in this," Colonel Cutler said, "We think it can be gotten from the U.S. It should be given precedence."

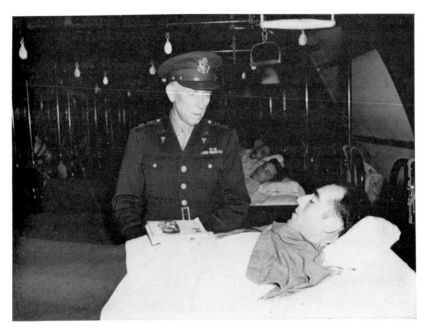

FIGURE 91.—Maj. Gen. Norman T. Kirk visiting the 160th General Hospital, Cirencester, England, during his quick visit to the European theater in July 1944.

General Hawley, however, had another condition which he wanted clarified. And that was the arrangement for air shipment from the United States to England and thence to the Continent. "If," he said, "we arrange a special service all the way there with the ATC and the TCC to get it to the Continent, it would be all right."

General Hawley concluded the discussion with the promise in the following statement: "The Surgeon General is definitely opposed to it, but I am willing to put it up to him." And well could he say this, because General Kirk had just completed a quick visit with General Hawley at which time the shortage of whole blood had been briefly discussed (fig. 91).

The Air Transport Command, when approached with the request, signified willingness to provide the necessary special service for flying whole blood from the United States to the United Kingdom, and the Troop Carrier Command assured that the blood would be flown to the Continent daily, weather conditions permitting. To insure that proper arrangements would be made, and made quickly, General Hawley decided that Colonel Cutler and Major Hardin should go to Washington. Upon Colonel Cutler's request, Colonel MacFee, who was working with First U.S. Army and the Advance Section, Communications Zone, was also added to the list of those to go.

Key personnel.—Before leaving, however, certain other matters were brought to Colonel Cutler's attention to be discussed in Washington. One of these was the lack of qualified professional personnel in units arriving in the

United Kingdom. At a London conference held by the Chief Surgeon on 4 August 1944, Colonel Kimbrough inquired: "Since you are sending such high-powered speakers back, why can't they take up with General Kirk this proposition of stripping key personnel from the hospitals coming over here from the States?"

"You're absolutely right," replied General Hawley, "and they will do that."

"Another hospital came in without a chief of medical service," Colonel Kimbrough warned, "We are running out of key personnel."

Evacuation to Zone of Interior.—When General Kirk had visited the theater, he had mentioned the fact that the air evacuation of patients was not as good as it could be. He said this with particular reference to the condition of patients being returned from the European terminal, Prestwick, Scotland, to the receiving hospital, Halloran General Hospital, Staten Island, New York (fig. 92). Well, this was not news. Among other inadequacies in the prevailing evacuation system, many had recognized the problem which existed at Prestwick, and steps had been taken to correct the situation. At this time, only a detachment from the 25th Hospital Train was there. Momentarily, the 57th Field Hospital was expected to move in and take over the holding and evacuation function at Prestwick. Later, when the British would be able to turn over certain buildings at the airport to the Americans, plans called for setting up a station hospital at Prestwick to provide local hospitalization service in addition to acting as the air evacuation hospital. Colonel Cutler had asked for the opportunity to investigate thoroughly the receiving and holding of patients at Prestwick and subsequent steps in their evacuation to the Zone of Interior. This opportunity was now his.

Colonel Zollinger fills in.—Fortunately, Colonel Zollinger had returned from the Continent, where he had been of inestimable value in organizing surgical and shock teams from general hospitals in transit to augment hospitals of the First U.S. Army and the Advance Section, Communications Zone. During this period, Colonel Cutler had sorely lamented the fact that the best general hospitals with topnotch people could not be used because they had been closed and earmarked for early movement to the Continent. Colonel Zollinger's efforts had attenuated the loss when he was able to put many of these officers to good use where they were sorely needed. And now he was present in England to fill in for the Chief Consultant in Surgery during his absence. There were many items which required his immediate attention. Certain station hospitals, selected to function as general hospitals, required review and augmentation of their personnel; 16 general hospitals had recently arrived, and all required extensive bolstering of professional personnel with qualified individuals, including chiefs of services; the newer auxiliary surgical groups, the 5th and 6th, needed reshuffling of personnel in the component teams and augmentation with temporary-duty personnel from general hospitals before they could be profitably employed; and a list of those LST medical officers meriting commendation was due in the immediate future.

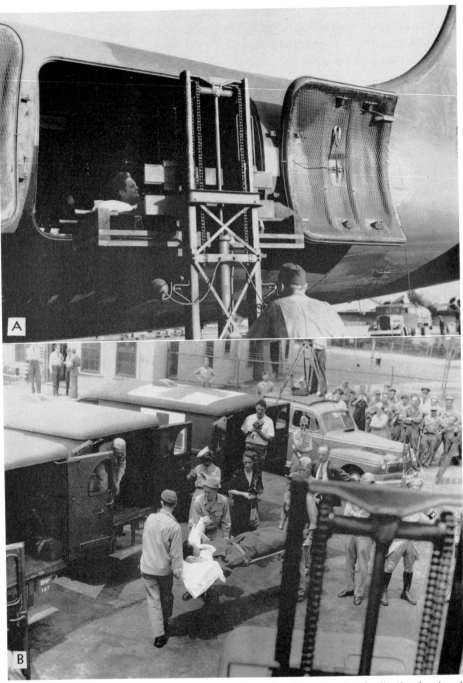

FIGURE 92.—Air evacuation to the Zone of Interior from Prestwick, Scotland. A. A hydraulic lift being used to raise litter patients to the hatch of a huge 4-motored C–54 evacuation aircraft. B. Patients arriving at Mitchel Field, N.Y., the initial stop in the Zone of Interior.

Prestwick, Scotland, "Very Sloppy Place."—At the last minute, on Saturday, 12 August, a cable from Washington was received which said that The Surgeon General had agreed to send 250 pints of blood per day beginning on 21 August and that the amount would be increased later. In view of this response, General Hawley was asked whether all three of the officers now had to return to the Zone of Interior. General Hawley replied that they did, and he insisted that they try to get off that night or the next day, Sunday. Colonel MacFee had not even arrived from the Continent at this time. Colonel Cutler and Major Hardin proceeded immediately with their plans. They were ready to leave Sunday morning. Colonel Cutler's account of the first day follows:

Left London by plane 9:30 a.m. Arrived at Prestwick 12:30 p.m. Visited "holding hospital". Commanding Officer, Major Roth of the 25th Hospital Train. Comment: Very sloppy place. No good doctors. 124 patients in 132 empty beds but patients arriving constantly. Very little professional care or supervision. Critically ill patients sent by mistake for evacuation to Zone of Interior sent to 112th General Hospital by officers at "holding hospital". Feel they have no right to reverse decision of disposition [boards] and *they must be given this right*. When the new field hospital takes over, an A.1 orthopedic surgeon and a competent physician must be on its staff to review all cases and have full right to reverse disposition board proceedings. While reviewing cases on ward, found a batch from 79th General Hospital that seemed inappropriately boarded to Zone of Interior, including five N.P.'s; 1 broken metacarpal. Wrote Colonel Kimbrough re this. Sent one maxillofacial wound with abscess to the 112th General Hospital. Visited 112th General Hospital, just giving over to 316th Station Hospital.

My interpretation of the whole matter at Prestwick is that we need a 750 bed station hospital, at the airport. We need nothing at Cowglen and the hospital at Prestwick must have the right to study and reboard people, to change disposition and to hold or return to duty or turn over to another hospital anyone they wish. Boarded ship at 11 p.m. 16 ambulatory patients with us, including one with rheumatic fever; one G.S.W., forearm left, with nerve damage; one F.C.C. radius and ulnar left (nerve damage); two tumors testicle; one arthritis of knee; two N.P.; one osteochondritis; one penetrating wound, left thigh; one cancer of the tongue; one G.S.W. humerus left; one compound fracture, left lower leg; one epilepsy; one [patient] * * * diagnosis: constitutional psychopathic state; * * * one fracture, left humerus; one chronic tenosynovitis muscle, right leg.

One of the patients, an Air Corps captain, appeared fit for duty. His wound had been skin-grafted and seemed satisfactory. Colonel Cutler believed that he was not a neuropsychiatric casualty but was bordering on it. The psychopath sat immediately in front of Colonel Cutler. His complaint was a headache. Colonel Cutler believed that he probably had the mental age of a 10 year old. "If these are a sample of soldiers returning to the Zone of Interior," Colonel Cutler noted in his record of the trip, "it is not good and should be studied in the light of my arguments above."

The plane took off at 2330 and arrived at La Guardia Airport, New York, N.Y., at 1700 the next day, 14 August. Stops had been made at Iceland and Newfoundland. An hour after arrival at La Guardia, they were on their way and reached Washington 2 hours later.

Washington.—Tuesday, 15 August, was spent in the Office of The Surgeon General. At a conference held in the offices of the chief consultant in surgery, the business of providing whole blood to the European theater was discussed. General Rankin, Col. B. Noland Carter, MC, Lt. Col. Roger G. Prentiss, Jr., MC, Colonel Kendrick, Dr. Bates (American Red Cross), Maj. (later Lt. Col.) Frederic N. Schwartz, MAC, and several others were present in addition to the two individuals from Europe. Colonel Cutler's account of the conference was substantially as follows:

In putting up the proposition, I explained that we had secured the airlift for one thousand pints, refrigerated, each day from the Zone of Interior to the United Kingdom, the United Kingdom to the Continent. It was proposed that blood preserved in Alsever's diluent be used. I immediately questioned this, stating that it was no time to experiment on the American soldier, that the airlift was ready for refrigerated blood, and that Alsever's diluent diluted blood 50 percent. I was assured that the National Research Council approved the transportation of blood preserved in Alsever's solution unrefrigerated, that they had carried blood to Hawaii and back, to Bermuda and back, and to Scotland and back, unrefrigerated, and had transfused American soldiers entirely satisfactorily.

This matter of unrefrigerated blood was new to us and seemed experimental, and we constantly repeated our desire for refrigerated blood. We were told every time that unrefrigerated blood and Alsever's solution was entirely satisfactory. As this would make the airlift simpler, we accepted unrefrigerated blood. (Since that meeting, further discussion with experts not in the Army has brought to light the fact that the cells preserved in Alsever's solution (tagged and studied) live but a little while in the recipient's circulation, and I shall take this up again in Washington.)

Deliveries promised: Beginning 21 August, 250 pints a day; beginning 28 August, 500 pints; beginning 4 September, 750 pints; and from 11 September on, 1,000 pints.

It is our understanding that this blood will be delivered in carts—liter bottles containing 500 cc. blood and 500 cc. Alsever's solution; that there will be a recipient-giving set, sterile, in the package with each bottle. We shall refrigerate this at Prestwick; when chilled, it will be shipped by air to the Continent; it will be refrigerated again at the airport on the Continent and then delivered by our trucks as usual.

In addition to the above, they will give us "re-suspended" O red blood cells in 10 percent corn syrup in 600 cc. Baxter intravenous bottles, this again to go unrefrigerated to Scotland. Afterwards, we shall refrigerate it. (The first of these cells will go over with Major Hardin who shall see that a proper distribution of these cells is made to hospitals in which the personnel is suitably trained for the use of such blood.)

During the day, the following items were reviewed with The Surgeon General, General Kirk:

a. The matter of utilization of experts for special jobs and the fact that if these experts are so detached from their fixed units their opportunities for promotion vanish (cited the case of William Sandusky). I was informed by The Surgeon General that nothing can be done about this. Men will have to suffer for their country!

b. The Surgeon General suggested "N.P." cases be used in labor battalion in SOS and should not be called malingerers and used up front by Army. I explained our "recovery" center and The Surgeon General was satisfied.[98]

c. Long discussion of medical education. It appears that Procurement practically prevents intelligent, healthy young men from entering medicine. All must go in the Army. A study of this would seem to show that the medical schools in the Fall of 1944–45 will contain only women and physical crocks which would seem to be a terrible blunder in regard to the future care of the American people.

d. No more hospital ships for the United Kingdom. Must use "troopships" and begin at once. (The Surgeon General says put patients in hospital beds in troopships.)

e. The Surgeon General would like to have us use the rubber traction material sent to the United Kingdom for amputation stumps. Will see that in the future elastic is less powerful. Suggested using ring splints and litter bars for traction to fasten to.

f. Evacuation from the Continent to the United Kingdom. (The Surgeon General hoped new general hospitals on the Continent would care for the majority returnable to duty.)

g. The Surgeon General also approves the attempt to send simple and compound femurs with skin traction (not in plaster) from the Continent to the United Kingdom.

h. Peripheral nerve surgery ought not be done in the United Kingdom but should be done in the Zone of Interior.

i. Stumps should be reoperated upon in the Zone of Interior, not in the United Kingdom. (Comment on h and i: Both these will save us beds.)

j. Long discussion concerning the availability of more specialists and expert surgeons for the United Kingdom. I was informed that we would get *absolutely no more competent people.*

k. Long discussion on history of the war. Apparently there is a quarrel between the Office of The Surgeon General and the National Research Council.

We have nothing to do with the National Research Council, and Lt. Col. Sanford V. Larkey, MC, is working for the Office of The Surgeon General and not for the National Research Council. I reviewed all of the topics with General Rankin and Col. B. Noland Carter and Major DeBakey. See my special notes on this topic. Should get all consultants working on this immediately. Send additional names with present notes to General Rankin.

---

[98] Medical Department, United States Army. Internal Medicine in World War II. Volume I. Activities of Medical Consultants. Washington: U.S. Government Printing Office, 1961, ch. IV, pt. III.

Long discussion on wound ballistics. Reviewed the excellent report by Colonel (Ashley W.) Oughterson of the Bougainville Campaign (copy to United Kingdom with me).[99]

Went to see Col. Robert Cutler, Pentagon. I got lost but finally found the intelligence officers to whom all incoming officers must report. News of landing near Marseilles just arrived.

The next day, Wednesday, 16 August, Colonel Cutler gave a short talk at The Surgeon General's weekly meeting with his staff. In the afternoon, he visited Brig. Gen. George R. Callender, MC, The Surgeon General's special representative for wound ballistics. General Callender pointed out that The Surgeon General would send a wound ballistics team to a particular theater if the theater commander so requested. General Callender urged that General Hawley take the matter up with General Eisenhower. When General Kirk had visited the European theater a short while before, he had given essentially the same information to General Hawley. But, later on this occasion, General Kirk informed Colonel Cutler that the original premise still applied, only there was nobody he knew of who could be sent. General Kirk suggested that Colonel Cutler feel out his friend, Dr. Moritz of Boston, for such an assignment.

On Thursday, there was more discussion with The Surgeon General on the matters discussed Tuesday, and there was a long discussion with Col. Augustus Thorndike, MC, concerning rehabilitation in the United States. Colonel Cutler was surprised and nonplused to learn that there were 140,000 patients currently in the rehabilitation system. In the afternoon he went by train to New York and on Friday, to Boston. On Saturday and Sunday, 19 and 20 August, he visited the Harvard Medical School and the Peter Bent Brigham Hospital. He also spoke with Dr. Diamond, an expert in hematology, concerning preservatives for whole blood. On Monday, Colonel Cutler was back in the Office of The Surgeon General with further discussions on blood, wound ballistics, history of the war, and photography which the Surgeon General's Office desired.

On Tuesday, 22 August, Colonel Cutler reported the following:

Conference with General Rankin and Major [Margaret D.] Craighill concerning new policies for care of officers and enlisted personnel, female, becoming pregnant in service. Conference with Major General [George F.] Lull, Colonel [Florence A.] Blanchfield and Major Craighill concerning the fact that women officers in Medical Corps are not given dependent allowances. All agreed this was wrong, that the bill had been loosely drawn for women in Medical Corps in that it did not specifically state that women medical officers could have dependent allowance because it was so specified in the bill setting forth the creation of these service officers. At the request of the above group, wrote a letter to Senator Walsh, Massachusetts Senator, and an old friend of mine, asking him to see that fair play and no class distinction occurred in this matter.

[99] Oughterson, Ashley W., Hull, Harry C., Sutherland, Francis A., and Greiner, Daniel J.: Study on Wound Ballistics—Bougainville Campaign. In Medical Department, United States Army. Wound Ballistics. Washington: U.S. Government Printing Office, 1962, pp. 281–436.

The next day, Colonel Cutler visited the National Research Council offices where he conferred with Professor Keefer and Dr. Guest, experts on blood. The National Research Council group promised to report to The Surgeon General of the Army what the best preservatives for whole blood were, refrigerated and nonrefrigerated. Later, on this Wednesday, 23 August, Colonel Cutler visited the Air Surgeon with reference to a matter of considerable concern to the Chief Consultant in Surgery from the European theater. His record for the visit states:

Conference at office of Air Surgeon regarding information from Mitchel Field forwarded to Surgeon General that cases arriving from ETO were improperly dressed and cared for. It appears that some of the cases specifically cited were Navy cases not coming through Army hospitals. Also it appears that the letter was written in an attempt to remedy defects in our system. General Grant was away and the conference was held with Brig. Gen. [Charles R.] Glenn, Lt. Col. [Alfred R.] Shands and Lt. Col. [Richard L.] Meiling. Colonel Shands is in charge of this work and will send me a weekly report on cases which arrived in bad condition or about which there may be criticism at Mitchel Field. The cases will be specific instances and will include not only the name of the patient but the hospital in the ETO where the patient was cared for. This should allow us to improve our care.

Prestwick again.—Colonel Cutler left the United States by air on 24 August. During the stop at Harmon Field, Stephenville, Newfoundland, he looked into the small 30-bed holding hospital there and found it quite satisfactory. Friday, 25 August, found him back again at Prestwick, Scotland, concerning which he recorded the following:

* * * had four hours at the 57th Field Hospital, and the blood bank set up. 350 pints of blood and Alsever's solution arrived in the plane I was on. These were still cool on arrival. Blood received at Prestwick as follows:
23 August: 258 bottles
24 August: 180 bottles
25 August: 336 bottles
Disposed as follows:
23 August, to Salisbury: 5
24 August, to France: 300
25 August, to France: 130
On hand, 25 August: 338
Capacity of present refrigeration at Prestwick: 222 boxes of 6 bottles each.
Went over the roster of 57th Field Hospital. It is not good. See full vetting in separate memo. Believe this hospital should have a physician and a surgeon so competent that they can be given the right to change disposition board findings in order that certain cases which arrive at this hospital may be returned to duty rather than sent to the Zone of Interior.

London.—Colonel Cutler arrived in London late Friday, 25 August. On Saturday, he telephoned Colonel Hays of the Medical Supply Division and requested that he cable the Zone of Interior immediately for donor sets. One expendable donor set was to be packed in each crate containing 6 bottles of the Zone of Interior blood. However, on opening a package at Prestwick, Colonel Cutler had found no donor set. At a conference with Colonel Spruit, Col. Joseph H. McNinch, MC, and Colonel Muckenfuss, the Chief Consultant in

Surgery explained the new procedure by which Zone of Interior whole blood would be supplied the European theater.

In a memorandum to the Chief Surgeon, dated 29 August 1944, he wrote the following concerning the subject:

*   *   *   *   *   *   *

3. * * * The blood will be brought to airports in the U.S.A. and held there refrigerated until the 'plane is ready to leave. It will then be flown unrefrigerated to Prestwick. There we will chill it again in our refrigerator, which means that it should be in the refrigerator at least 4 hours. The blood will then be flown to the Continent, where it can be immediately delivered in our refrigerated trucks or can be at the base in the large refrigerators. This would be safe to use up to 18 days; until we have further information from Washington, this is the method we will use.

*   *   *   *   *   *   *

The Surgeon General openly expressed the opinion at his staff conference that if the surgeons of E.T.O. wish for blood they should have it, and every effort would be made to provide us with what has been requested.

Evacuation

Immediately upon his return to London from the United States, Colonel Cutler was also embroiled in a conference on evacuation. Various aspects of evacuation from the Continent to the United Kingdom and from the United Kingdom to the Zone of Interior had been bandied about for some time, but it was now necessary to make some definite decisions—particularly in the light of the information Colonel Cutler had brought with him from The Surgeon General.

As for evacuation from the Continent to the United Kingdom, the consultants had objected to the lack of opportunities for using extensive air evacuation. More fields were needed to prevent one or two installations from receiving all the air-evacuated casualties. They were also of the opinion that it was no longer necessary or advisable to have transit hospitals in many cases. The same was true of water-evacuated casualties. The seriously injured requiring special care were of particular concern, since these patients were not getting to the right hospitals soon enough. At one time, Colonel Cutler had, by way of illustration, mentioned the case of a Private "S.", as follows:

* * * [He] was wounded through the right forehead on July 13th—cared for at 45th Field Hospital—crossed on LST. Admitted on 14 July to 50th Field Hospital—transferred from there to the 305th Station Hospital 17 July—transferred from there to the 314th Station Hospital 18th July—transferred from there to the 185th General Hospital 22 July— still unconscious with a cerebral leak.[100]

On that occasion, Colonel Cutler had said there were many such cases. He had also objected to the fact that good general hospitals were being used as transit hospitals or as holding hospitals for evacuation to the Zone of Interior. To him, this was a waste of talent and equipment, when a hospital with less able medical officers and more limited equipment could perform the mission adequately. Colonel Cutler had also suggested further evacuation to appro-

---

[100] Minutes, Twenty-First Conference of the Chief Surgeon's Consultants, London, 28 July 1944.

priate hospitals by light aircraft directly from planeside of evacuation aircraft arriving in the United Kingdom from the Continent.

As for evacuation to the Zone of Interior, Colonel Cutler, at this conference on 26 August 1944, said evacuation by air and by water had to be considered, priorities had to be set for air evacuation, and a determination made of cases to be evacuated by sea.

Fortunately, it was soon determined that patients could be evacuated directly from the Continent to the Zone of Interior and detailed instructions to implement the decision were issued by the Chief Surgeon to surgeons of all base sections on the Continent, and to commanding officers of all general hospitals on the Continent. In this instance, direct evacuation by air from the Continent to the Zone of Interior was to be provided patients for whom definitive treatment at special centers in the United States would be preferable to the treatment available in the European theater. The directive, dated 19 September 1944, stated that, normally, battle casualties should take precedence over nonbattle casualties. Particular priority for air evacuation was to be given to (1) peripheral nerve injuries, (2) maxillofacial injuries, (3) brain tumors, (4) patients requiring deep X-ray therapy, (5) patients requiring a series of plastic operations, (6) carcinoma, and (7) blindness. There was also a comprehensive list of conditions which were contraindicative of air evacuation.

These and other changes alleviated the evacuation situation somewhat, but the general situation on the Continent was so fluid and changing, that some decisions had to be held in abeyance. In fact, for a period, many of the activities of the Office of the Chief Surgeon came to a temporary halt.

Valognes and Paris

The occasion for disrupting the normal routine of the Chief Surgeon's Office was its move to the Continent. At an early date, the Forward Echelon, Communications Zone, had crossed to prepare the way for the eventual move of the Headquarters, SOS, ETOUSA, across the Channel. Each division of the Chief Surgeon's Office had plans to move its personnel on a staggered basis— a portion to go early, and the bulk to follow later. Some members of the Chief Surgeon's Office had been designated to remain in England until the move could be completed and the United Kingdom Base could be established with Colonel Spruit as its surgeon. The Medical Records Division was to remain permanently in England with Colonel McNinch as its chief.

The first move of the Chief Surgeon's Office was to Valognes, France. This followed a few days after Colonel Cutler's return to the European theater when he was extremely busy trying to catch up with unfinished business and the events which had transpired during his absence (fig. 93). The diary says little about the crossing: "Trip [from] Cheltenham to here—Wow! Wish I could write it in full. Trip with Ralph Tovell day after arrival here. Peninsular [base,] Caen * * * to Le Mans (2:00 AM). Next day beyond Chartres. Great destruction in British area and burned out tanks belittle talk Americans did it all!"

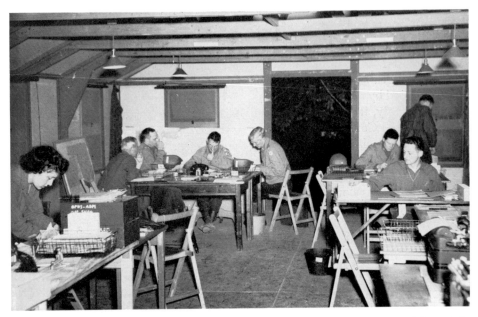

FIGURE 93.—The interior of the Operations and Administration Building, Office of the Chief Surgeon, ETOUSA, at Valognes, France. Colonel Cutler is seated in doorway. Lt. Col. John H. Voegtly, MC, is at table behind Colonel Cutler. With Colonel Cutler, from right to left, are Col. Robert E. Peyton, MC, and Col. James C. Kimbrough, MC.

Afterwards, Colonel Cutler flew back to England for one week where he spoke with Colonel Spruit and Colonel Morton about certain administrative and professional aspects of the medical service in the United Kingdom when the Chief Surgeon's Office had moved in its entirety to the Continent. Colonel Cutler advised the United Kingdom Base surgeon that Colonel Morton, the United Kingdom surgical consultant, was struggling with problems that had previously involved many consultants. Colonel Cutler suggested that there was a great deal of time-consuming work involved in the supervision of ortho- pedic care and that Lt. Col. (later Col.) Richard S. Farr, MC, would make an excellent assistant in orthopedics to Colonel Morton.

During this week in the United Kingdom, General Hawley also came over. He informed Colonel Cutler that he would like to sponsor a conference of Allied medical officers on the Continent as soon as things settled down a bit, and he instructed the Chief Consultant in Surgery to make the necessary arrangements.

When Colonel Cutler was ready to return to the Continent, the head- quarters was already moving to Paris. Colonel Cutler arrived in Paris on Thursday, 14 September 1944. He moved into the Hotel George V, his new "home," and the beginning of a new era in the fight against Nazi Germany. The War Department was later to designate 15 September 1944 as the date of the beginning of the Rhineland campaign.

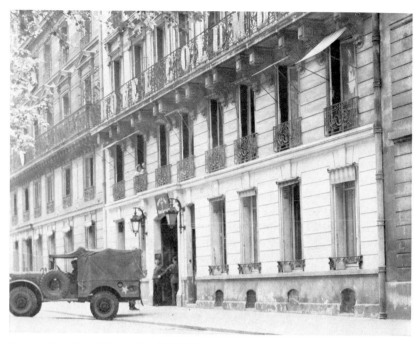

FIGURE 94.—The Office of the Chief Surgeon, ETOUSA, 16 Avenue Kleber, Paris, France.

THE RHINELAND

The Office of the Chief Surgeon was, to Colonel Cutler, in a continuous uproar when it opened at the Columbia Hotel, 16 Avenue Kleber, Paris (fig. 94). Desks and chairs continued to go up and down the stairs. The consultants were five to a room in small offices, on the seventh (top) floor, and there were no elevators. Many of the necessary working files were still packed away in boxes, as was the complete medical library which Colonel Cutler had assiduously assembled. Because all of the British civilian help could not accompany the move to the Continent, secretarial service was at a premium. While Colonel Cutler was fortunate enough to be billeted at the Hotel George V, he was sorry to discover that some of the senior consultants who came over did not fare as well, as they were placed in temporary billets 1 or 2 miles away. Fortunately, the weather was nice.

The move to the Continent heralded a new era in the war against Germany. For Colonel Cutler, there arose immediately the opportunity to renew old friendships with French surgical colleagues, including René Le Riche, Merle D'Aubigne, Marc Iselin, and Claude Béclere. There was resurgence of activity among French medical organizations, once again freed from German domination, and the Chief Consultant in Surgery was to be asked to participate frequently. Now no longer removed by an expanse of sea water, the proximity of the field armies was to foster an ever closer working relationship among those at theater headquarters, in the armies, and in the communications zone. The United Kingdom Base gradually took on a different character, acting, as it were, as an area for the Zone of Interior type of hospitalization of patients who were neither in the category of those to be cared for on the Continent nor in the category of those to be sent directly to the Zone of Interior, from the European mainland. To the south were a field army and support commands whose medical personnel were historically, professionally, and sentimentally rooted to the theater from which they had newly been transferred, but who now had to be integrated—professionally, insofar as Colonel Cutler was concerned— with the European theater.

Tactically, the swift progress of the Allies through France, which had raised hopes for an early end to hostilities, was to come to a standstill before the heavily fortified Siegfried Line in spite of vigorous assaults on these positions in the late fall. A bitter-cold winter—the coldest and wettest in many years—prevented the Allies on the Western Front from completely breaching at this time these advantageous German positions. And then, on 16 December, in frigid weather, the Nazi Wehrmacht struck suddenly and with great force through the forest of Ardennes to begin the "Battle of the Bulge." It was not to be until late winter or early spring that the Allies, after containing and repelling the German offensive, would generate enough momentum of their own for an all-out offensive on the German fatherland.

September-October: Orientation to Life on Continent

Inter-Allied meetings and conferences

With this as a background, one of the first specific tasks for the Chief Consultant in Surgery during this period was to carry out the desire of the Chief Surgeon to sponsor a meeting of Allied consultants on the Continent. At this time, many, apparently, were breathing more easily because there seemed no doubt that the Allies were on the Continent to stay, and progress had been quite satisfactory, once enemy resistance in Normandy had been crushed. It was second nature, then, to look back and reconsider what had been done, by whom it had been done, and how. There was also the desire to get together with those one might be associated with during the home stretch on the mainland. General Hawley had magnanimously thought of inviting consultants of all the Allied Armies on the Western Front, and particularly the French.

On further consideration, however, Colonel Cutler sensed that such a large meeting of consultants at this time might not be advisable. For one thing, the French really had not time to reorganize and reestablish themselves on firm footing. Besides, a meeting of representatives of many nations often became more concerned with social responsibilities and protocol rather than the conduct of business. And language problems, at such gatherings, were always a formidable barrier to both those sponsoring the meetings and the members of the audience. There was also the consideration that Sir Henry Tidy had laid the groundwork for a new series of Inter-Allied Conferences on War Medicine, sponsored by the Royal Society of Medicine, which had been so eminently successful in the past. In fact, Colonel Liston and Colonel Cutler had already accepted invitations to speak at the first meeting of the new series in October 1944, and permission had been requested to use Maj. Benjamin R. Reiter, MC, of the First U.S. Army as another speaker. Accordingly, Colonel Cutler proposed that the first meeting on the Continent be primarily with the British and Commonwealth consultants. Meetings with the French, he suggested, could easily be arranged at any time. And sure enough, U.S. and Allied medical officers soon received an invitation from the staff of the French Val de Grâce military hospital in Paris to join in a series of exchange clinics and meetings at monthly intervals, the first such meeting to be held at the Val de Grâce Hospital on 19 September.

Brussels and British 21 Army Group

On the morning of 23 September 1944, Colonel Cutler was preparing to motor to Brussels for a talk with Sir Percy Tomlinson and Brigadier Porritt, the DMS (Director, Medical Service), and surgical consultant, respectively, for the British 21 Army Group, when Colonel Kendrick, The Surgeon General's special representative on blood and resuscitation, returned from a visit to the First U.S. Army where he had been observing the administration and use of blood and plasma. Colonel Kendrick had come to the European theater shortly after Colonel Cutler's return from their meetings in Washington. While there was not time to discuss at length what he had observed, Colonel Kendrick said that he had contacted Colonel Crisler, as requested, and that arrangements had been made for Major Reiter to go to London and give a talk at the Inter-Allied Medical Conference to be held on 2 October. After receiving this welcome news from Colonel Kendrick, Colonel Cutler spoke briefly with the British Liaison Officer, Lt. Col. Brian Brennan, RAMC.

Equipped with the latest information from Colonel Brennan, Colonel Cutler departed for Brussels shortly after midday and arrived there at 1800. He was put up at the most comfortable Hotel Astoria, where Sir Percy Tomlinson and Brigadier Porritt were billeted. The next morning, after some discussion, it was decided that the various consultants should assemble in Paris by 1600 on 14 October. The Hotel George V was selected as the point at which to rendezvous. Suggestions for an agenda were received from Brigadier Porritt.

Eupen and First U.S. Army

After the meeting with these officers of the British 21 Army Group, Colonel Cutler traveled to Eupen, via Louvain and Liége, to visit Headquarters (Advance), First U.S. Army. Colonel Crisler, the surgical consultant, and Lt. Col. (later Col.) Neil L. Crone, MC, the medical consultant, were asked to

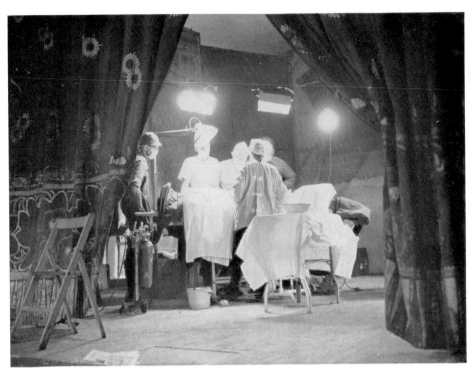

Figure 95.—The stage of an amusement hall in France being utilized by a surgical team
attached to a field hospital, 3 October 1944.

attend the meeting of consultants in Paris on 14, 15, and 16 October. They
accepted the invitation. Suggestions for an agendum were also received. In
addition, there was ample opportunity during the 4-hour visit to discuss many
other aspects of the prevailing situation of surgery in the First U.S. Army.
Colonel Crisler said that some 1,200 newly wounded were being treated daily.
He also informed Colonel Cutler that the truck and supplies comprising the unit
for the mobile surgical hospitals were excellent and had all been utilized.
But, he mentioned, the teams had very rarely found the need for or used the
tentage (fig. 95).

Coming back to Paris through driving rain, Colonel Cutler found that the
bridge across the Meuse at Givet was out. Consequently, he spent the night in
a small Belgian hotel at Dinant. Upon returning to Paris, he warned in his
résumé of the trip: "Those officers travelling Headquarters, First U.S. Army,
remember to turn sharp left at entering Eupen up a steep hill. There is no sign."

Back in Paris

108th General Hospital and blood for ETOUSA.—On Tuesday,
26 September, Colonel Cutler visited the 108th General Hospital in Paris (fig.

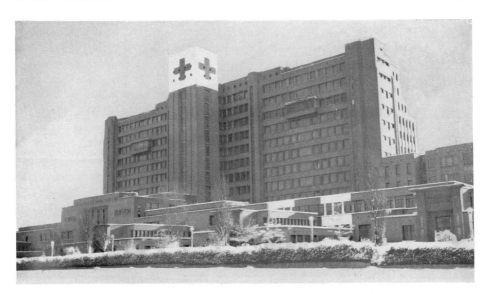

FIGURE 96.—The 108th General Hospital, Paris, France.

96), which was under the command of Lt. Col. (later Col.) Louis M. Rousselot, MC. This hospital was the site of the forthcoming meeting of consultants. Colonel Cutler inspected it completely and found its physical plant elegant and the personnel satisfactory, although professionally not up to the standards of some of the best general hospitals in the theater. Also visiting the hospital were Col. Silas B. Hays, MC, the theater medical supply officer, and Colonel Kendrick. They were experimenting with plasma tubing to replace Levin or Wangensteen tubes, which were scarce.

Colonel Cutler joined them and, during the afternoon, placed several of these tubes in patients, experimenting with the type of tip to be used. Six of these plastic tubes for intragastric decompression were placed in patients as a test of their efficiency.

Later that day, Colonel Cutler took the opportunity to discuss the whole-blood situation with Colonel Kendrick and Major Hardin. Colonel Kendrick had found the use of whole blood in the European theater entirely desirable and was anxious to bring the daily lift from the Zone of Interior up to 1,000 pints a day as promised. Major Hardin was concerning himself with the decision recently made to move the European theater blood bank to the Continent. He reported difficulty in finding a suitable facility for the blood bank, and he stressed the fact that it had to be relocated soon.

The next day, 27 September, Colonel Cutler checked on the efficiency of the plastic tubing, proceeded to write a proposed circular letter on the use of the tubing as a substitute item, and completed drawings to accompany the circular letter before leaving Paris for London.

Return to United Kingdom

Once again in England, Colonel Cutler visited the Operational Research Section and reviewed Major Palmer's progress on a casualty survey report which he was preparing on the accidental detonation of an M–41 fragmentation-type aerial bomb while it was being loaded on an aircraft at Deenethorpe, Northamptonshire, England. Later, in conference with Dr. Hamilton Southworth, U.S. Public Health Service, at the American Embassy, Colonel Cutler learned that the Intelligence Division in the Chief Surgeon's Office had a SHAEF report which detailed the scientific investigations which had been going on in France under the German occupation. Colonel Cutler was pleasantly surprised to learn also that the Rockefeller Institute and the American Library Association had jointly saved copies of American books and journals for distribution to the main libraries of the European countries as they were liberated. He planned to obtain copies for distribution from the Chief Surgeon's Office to the French Military Medical School at the Val de Grâce Hospital.

Medical statistics.—The Medical Records Division of the Chief Surgeon's Office had moved from Cheltenham to London, and Colonel Cutler met with its director, Colonel McNinch, and his assistant, Lt. Col. George D. Williams, MC, to plan on the type of statistical data the surgical consultants would find useful and necessary. Colonel Cutler requested casualty data from the field armies to include those for killed in action and wounded in action, with the latter divided into those dying in hospital, returned to duty from army facilities, and evacuated to the communications zone. He further requested statistics from field armies as to the anatomical distribution of wounds and identification of causative agents. For the communications zone, the Chief Consultant in Surgery requested statistics as to the number dying in hospitals, the number returned to full and limited duty, and the number returned to the Zone of Interior. In addition, he requested that the average length of stay in hospital per patient be calculated to accompany these communications zone statistics. Finally, he arranged for all gas infection records to be sent to himself, personally, for Colonel Cutler was convinced that, "the records, to be accurate, must be studied by surgeons themselves who can separate saprophytic infection from true clostridial myositis."

Colonel McNinch, in turn, gave Colonel Cutler a map of the United Kingdom Base Section which showed how all hospitals in that base section were being organized into seven groups with a central administration for each group of hospitals. Colonel Cutler was pleased to note that this new plan was doing away with the system of holding hospitals as previously contemplated.

Resumption of Inter-Allied Conferences on War Medicine.—One of Colonel Cutler's primary reasons for returning to England on this occasion was to participate in the first meeting of the new series of Inter-Allied Conferences on War Medicine. This meeting took place on Monday, 2 October 1944. As formerly, the location was the Royal Society of Medicine, 1 Wimpole Street, London, W. 1, and many American medical officers were guests.

Colonel Liston, the Deputy Chief Surgeon, gave a presentation on the organization and operations of American medical services on the "far shore" during the invasion of the Continent. Colonel Cutler gave a similar talk on the "near shore"—the handling of casualties in the United Kingdom during the assault on Normandy. Major Reiter presented the surgical experiences from D-day to D+7 of 16 teams from the 3d Auxiliary Surgical Group. These teams had been attached to engineer special brigades to function in medical battalion clearing stations which had been suitably modified for the amphibious operation.

Colonel Cutler later observed: "This meeting was as good as any we have had. Colonel Liston's talk was admirable and Major Reiter and a young Canadian, Captain Gosse, were the high points of the entire meeting. I was greatly interested in the fact that, after I had talked about disposition in the afternoon, some 20 officers came up and asked disposition questions, showing this is still not clearly understood in the United Kingdom."

At this time, Colonel Cutler also arranged for Colonel Morton and Colonel Kneeland to meet Sir Henry Tidy and to serve as representatives of the U.S. Forces on the editorial committee for the Inter-Allied Conferences in the event that the regular members, Colonel Cutler and Colonel Kimbrough, could not attend.

On Tuesday, 3 October, Colonel Cutler met with a Professor Loucks, formerly professor of surgery at Union Medical College, Peking, China. Professor Loucks, recently repatriated from a concentration camp in Japan, was being sent by the State Department to found a new medical school in southwestern China for the Chungking Government. Colonel Cutler made arrangements for him to be shown the U.S. Army facilities in England by Colonel Morton and then to be sent to the Continent for an orientation tour there. Afterwards, the Chief Consultant in Surgery returned to Paris by plane.

During his brief stay in Paris, Colonel Cutler attended the regular conference of General Hawley with his staff and the weekly meeting of the Professional Services Division. He worked, too, on arrangements for the Anglo-American consultants' meeting. And, on Thursday, 5 October, he had a most satisfying reunion with Dr. A. Brachot, president of the Académie de Chirurgie. Dr. Brachot told Colonel Cutler that the academy was to open again on 1 November and that it would be available to all members of the Office of the Chief Surgeon, ETOUSA. Dr. Brachot said the academy would be glad to sponsor international and inter-Allied medical meetings as seemed wisest.

Fresh warnings on trenchfoot.—Before returning to the United Kingdom, the Chief Consultant in Surgery again warned Colonel Kimbrough, in a memorandum dated 4 October 1944, of the problem which trenchfoot might be in the coming winter. This time, he called attention to word received from Colonel Crisler of the First U.S. Army, who said that he was fearful of trouble with cold injury in the coming weeks and months. "I agree with him," noted Colonel Cutler, "after having visualized the Italian Front, that we are in for trouble." He reminded Colonel Kimbrough: "I have written a memo to you and the Chief Surgeon and to the Quartermaster concerning this matter in the past." Colonel Cutler also informed Colonel Kimbrough as follows:

*   *   *   *   *   *   *

2. Colonel Crisler makes the suggestion that we set up in a forward general hospital, preferably in Liége, near the First Army (and this should also be done for the Third Army) a group of medical officers trained and interested in this particular field. In other words, we will have a hospital for specialized care of the cold foot in each Army.

After reiterating his previous statements on prevailing misconceptions and faulty footwear, Colonel Cutler wrote: "*These must be changed now else there will be disaster.*"

Thoracic and hand surgery centers in United Kingdom.—Sunday, 8 October, found the Chief Consultant in Surgery back again in England, where he participated in a round of conferences for the next 4 days. With Colonel Morton, he reviewed the provision for and progress of thoracic surgery, and the two agreed that Maj. (later Lt. Col.) John J. Cincotti, MC, of the 16th General Hospital should be ordered to assist Maj. (later Lt. Col.) Dwight E. Harken, MC, who was carrying a heavy load at the 160th General Hospital. With Lt. Col. George N. J. Sommer, Jr., MC, at the 140th General Hospital, Lt. Col. (later Col.) Arthur S. W. Touroff, MC, at the 155th General Hospital, Lt. Col. (later Col.) Laurence Miscall, MC, at the 137th General Hospital, and Major Harken at the 160th General Hospital, Colonel Cutler concluded: "It would seem that the United Kingdom Base Section has the four best thoracic surgeons * * * and is adequately covered from the point of view of thoracic surgery * * *. Thoracic surgery has made more advance than any other surgical specialty." It was also decided to establish special facilities for the care of badly damaged hands at each of the three original hospital centers in the United Kingdom in coordination with their commanding officers and surgical coordinators.

There was also an important conference with General Hawley, Colonel Spruit, and Colonel McNinch concerning evacuation to the United Kingdom and from the United Kingdom to the Zone of Interior (fig. 97), evacuation within the 30-day policy on the Continent directly to the Zone of Interior, and the necessity to clear out the many prisoner-of-war casualties that were creating great hardship at this time. Emphasis was placed on the urgent need to make better use of the "Queens" (the converted British liners, *Queen Mary* and *Queen Elizabeth*) and other surface water transportation. Colonel Spruit announced that plans were progressing well for the organization of all hospitalization facilities in his base under seven hospital-center headquarters.

During this week, the Chief Consultant in Surgery "vetted" the 150th Station Hospital, conferred with the commanding officer of the 6th Field Hospital on its defunct missions and lack of any workload in its holding facilities at the Southampton port and the Membury airfield, attended the regular monthly

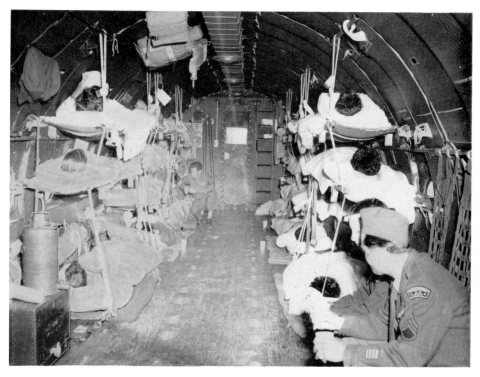

FIGURE 97.—The interior of a loaded C–54 aircraft evacuating casualties from Paris to the Zone of Interior. Note the canvas straps for holding the litters in place.

meeting of the British Army surgical consultants, and lectured at the Medical Field Service School, ETOUSA.

Conference with General Hood.—At 0930 on Thursday, 12 October, Colonel Cutler had the privilege of meeting with General Hood, DGMS, British Army, to confer on the coming meeting of consultants in Paris on 15 October. When Colonel Cutler had been in London a fortnight before, he had laid the groundwork for this meeting with the Director General by presenting Colonel Brennan, the British medical liaison officer, a copy of the agenda for the proposed conference of consultants and the desires of General Hawley for representatives from the British Army. On this Thursday morning, General Hood said that he would be glad to send over General Monro, consulting surgeon to the British Army, and Maj. Gen. Sir Alexander Biggam, consulting physician to the British Army. He thought that possibly Brigadier Sir Stewart Duke-Elder and Brigadier Rowley W. Bristow, Consultants in Ophthalmology and Orthopedic Surgery, respectively, could also attend. The general said that these British consultants would fly over on 14 October, Colonel Cutler was pleased. He informed the Director General that General Hawley planned to billet the two senior officers at the Hotel George V and the others at the 108th General Hospital. General Hood asked Colonel Cutler

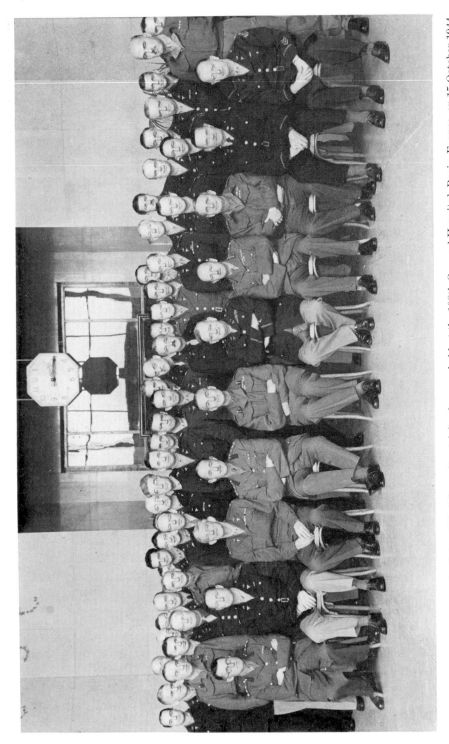

FIGURE 98.—Participants at the Inter-Allied Consultants' Conference, held at the 108th General Hospital, Paris, France, on 15 October 1944.

to inform General Hawley that he would be in Brussels in November, at which time he might come down to visit some of the medical facilities of the U.S. Army on the Continent.

After this meeting with General Hood, Colonel Cutler returned to Paris by air.

First Inter-Allied Consultants' Conference

The weekend of 14–15 October was a busy one for the Chief Consultant in Surgery. Saturday, 14 October, Colonel Cutler wrote, was devoted to the "hospitality of our guests!"

The conference (fig. 98) was opened on Sunday morning, 15 October 1944, with Colonel Kimbrough in the chair. He welcomed the delegates by saying:

This is the first meeting of the Inter-Allied Consultants' Conference. The principle of the plan was conceived by General Hawley, in order to get together the men who were responsible for making recommendations regarding the care of the troops in the field and who are really the consultants of the Armies. It was the idea to get them together to compare notes and discuss their problems.

General Hawley was first to be introduced. He officially opened the conference, welcomed the delegates, and thanked Colonel Rousselot and his staff at the 108th General Hospital for their hospitality. He then proceeded to comment on what the consultants in his headquarters had meant to him as a group, as follows:

I have given the matter a great deal of thought and I think, without any derogatory inferences to any other group, I am convinced * * * that the consultant group has contributed more, and continued to contribute more, to the success of the Medical Service than any other group of administrators, because they are, after all, administrators; that is, they have regulated, prescribed, and coordinated the professional services. This is tremendously important for the reason that one patient is treated by five, seven, eight different surgeons through the course of his illness and, right or wrong, in the long run, it is better that a patient follow through a regulated course of treatment than that each echelon through which he passes be permitted to exercise its own judgment in his basic care. I think that most of the surgeons doing the work are now reconciled to this point of view, although, and quite understandably so, it came sort of difficult to those who had been following their own particular pet ideas for a number of years. But that is, in my opinion, only one of the great services that the Professional Services Division of our army has rendered and is rendering. To me they are the most important eyes and ears that I have. These people get around. Their judgment is good in many things other than the care of the sick patient, and I have called upon them collectively and individually for advice upon many things not connected with the care of patients. I think, if they have not been exploited to their fullest value, it is because some divisions of the office have yet to learn of the tremendous potential value of this group. Some divisions have already learned that. The Chief of my Supply Division [Colonel Hays] sat and talked with me an hour the other night and told me of the great help this group is to him constantly, and that he would be unable to run his division without their help.

Then, for the benefit of the American consultants present, General Hawley continued with a subject which had been discussed at considerable length among the divisions of his office—the exchange of medical officers between the field

armies and communications zone. The reader may recall that a similar program
had been tried with considerable success during the preinvasion days in the
United Kingdom (p. 70). Obviously, such a program would now be a most
complex affair, but an endeavor which many thought would be more worthwhile
than ever before. Colonel Cutler was a proponent of the plan. General Hawley's explanation follows:

> While the consultants from the Armies are here, I would like very much to have
> you talk over with the chief consultant in your own specialty here in my office the
> question of rotating your people in the Armies with people in fixed hospitals. I feel
> that that should be done, not too fast, and probably at first on a temporary rotation
> basis. We may be in for a long winter of slugging it out or of lessened activity. Many
> of the people in the field units up with the armies have been working very hard and
> are tired. Maybe their morale has begun to waver a little. Nothing improves a person's
> morale as much as a change—a change of scenery. And, conversely, we have got a lot
> of people in these fixed hospitals who are just itching for a chance to get to the front
> and do some work there, and to get into some of the mud which the forward units must
> contend with all the time. I think it would be advantageous for both sides to let the
> people at the fixed hospitals learn of the conditions under which the forward surgeons
> work, and give them more understanding of the difficulties they encounter; and, con-
> versely, let the people who are doing the work forward come back and see how the patients
> are cared for after they leave them.

The conference then proceeded with the first item on the agenda, care
of the battle casualty up to the time of definitive surgery. As subtopics of
the item, there were the following: First aid in forward echelons, care during evacuation to the hospital where surgery is first carried out, sorting of
casualties, and preoperative preparation of the casualty to include blood transfusion, chemotherapy, and the like. There were no formal presentations, and
informal discussion was the keynote.

Lt. Col. R. K. Debenham, RAMC, surgical adviser to the British Second
Army, opened the discussion of the topic with these remarks:

> One of the problems of the Second British Army is whether to resuscitate in one
> place and operate in another place. That is to say, whether a patient should be resus-
> citated forward and operated at the first available surgical level. I feel quite strongly
> that you can't resuscitate in one place and operate in another. * * * your transfusion
> teams must be with your surgery. * * * The best level for surgery appears to be behind
> our guns. Sometimes we have had to operate forward of our guns and within shell
> fire from the enemy. I don't think patients do so well there; it may be heroic, but
> it isn't very satisfactory.

Colonel Debenham also explained that the British in general were of the
opinion that more than one-third grain of morphine was bad. He mentioned
certain other complicating factors in the use of morphine, and stated that
the British Second Army was finding it difficult to resuscitate anyone after
thiopental sodium had been given, some 6 to 7 hours being necessary to recover
from its effects. Colonel Debenham stated: "We like to treat all our femurs
in Thomas' splints and we find they travel far better in a 'Tobruk' plaster."
This was an interesting observation on a most controversial issue at the time.

In summation, he brought forth the following four points on which transfusion and early surgery were based:

It is very interesting—there are four points: First, extent of the wound. The
badly wounded patient is going to be shocked and must be reckoned as a shock case.
Second, time of wound; because, if he is recently wounded, his chances are better.
Third, the general condition of the patient. And fourthly, the pulse. And these four
points are taken into consideration by the transfusion officer. Blood pressure readings
are sometimes not very helpful. I feel in general that the forward surgeon should be
essentially conservative. Heroic surgery is not required. The surgeon forward must
know who will travel and who will not. If he can estimate that, it is very helpful.

Thanking Colonel Debenham for his remarks, Colonel Cutler asked that
the Army consultants, particularly, provide the conferees with information
relating to the first subtopic, first aid. "We hoped that the discussions would
deal with the soldiers as far forward as they are wounded," he said, "I had
hoped that the first part of the meeting this morning would devote itself
to first aid, * * * as a simple thing," he continued. As an example of the
type of information which might be desired, he asked: "Are your men trained
in first aid? How far does he go? Do you have any information on whether
your patients coming back have the original dressing? What are you doing
to prevent infection? * * * And in regard to splints * * * Who puts it on?
Where are they put on?" "It may be more important to put on a good dressing
than to give penicillin and sulfonamides," he observed.

Confessing that he didn't know just exactly who did what at the site of
the wounding, Colonel Debenham replied: "* * * From the point of view of
the casualty, I have seen the results and most of the dressings have been put on
extremely well. If the man himself doesn't know, someone near him does know
how, and most of those that I have seen have been 100 percent marvelous."

"What does the individual soldier take?" questioned Colonel Cutler.

"He carries a little field pack," replied General Monro, consulting surgeon
to the British Army, "The individual field dressing is an extraordinarily good
dressing."

Colonel Crisler, when asked about conditions of first aid treatment in the
First U.S. Army, maintained that, from a few spotty observations, he could
not say exactly what was being done for each patient or the percentage of well-
done dressings. He did comment, however, on early treatment in the First
U.S. Army, as follows:

Our treatment of casualties forward is taken from the "Manual of Therapy." It has
proved to be a splendid guide on all general principles of surgery and it has been followed
in general very closely. A few points need elaboration. Quite a few surgeons have
needed to be whipped into line about the policies. They have deviated from policies, but
after they had been treating casualties for a while, they conformed more or less throughout. * * * When we see them [casualties] come back, we judge them. At one time they
seem to be all handled well, and then again occasionally we see a patient come back who
perhaps has not been properly splinted; we see occasionally one who has been overlooked.
That varies with the number and the flow of casualties. Our percentage of approaching

perfection with which this is accomplished must be interpreted in the light of the number of casualties, and the tactical situation, and to sit back and criticize is a bit unfair. It seems to me that on the whole, they do a very good job.

"Have you any information as to how many dressings put on on the battle-field are changed?" asked Colonel Cutler.

"I think that most of them are not revised nor removed," answered Colonel Crisler. "They may find it necessary to determine the extent of the wound, but the dressing is not removed unless it is absolutely necessary in order to determine where that patient should go. It may be that it is drawn a little too tightly and in that case it is readjusted, but it stays on until the clearing station is reached."

Col. Frank B. Berry, MC, the Seventh U.S. Army surgical consultant, spoke in a similar vein. He stated: "* * * There is one thing that constantly comes to mind, and especially at this time of year and that is the morphine Syrette which I wish had never been invented—that is in that size [one-half grain]—because we have already seen cases of overdosage of morphine." Otherwise, he commented on the first aid type of treatment given in the Seventh U.S. Army in glowing terms, as follows:

I have only the highest praise for the work that is done in the first aid and battalion aid stations and by the aidmen going out in the field, as General Hawley and Colonel Cutler have mentioned (fig. 99).

As a rule the splint is pretty good. At times, of course, they slip. We have all been very much interested in the very good and judicious use of the splint by the first aidman in the field.

As to the dressings, I am happy to say that there is less change in them than there used to be, particularly in the Tunisian campaign, in the collecting station. There was a great tendency during the Tunisian days to do some surgery at the collecting station. I remember one particular clearing station which took pride in the major surgery that was done there. The changes of dressings is gradually lessening. It is interesting to check them, to see dressings inspected and changed, and I do think that there is more changing than necessary. I think they are very good in establishing their priority to get the urgent cases back to the hospitals. Very good judgment is being shown.

In his remarks, Col. Charles B. Odom, MC, Third U.S. Army surgical consultant, spoke of penicillin and sulfonamides:

One thing: Penicillin of course is not begun until we get back to a hospital; it is not used in the forward areas, and, from the number of infections that we have had, I don't think it is necessary to begin it forward. I think perhaps we would do well to stop using sulpha in the wounds forward. In checking a group of cases in the convalescent hospital, we have found some of these wounds well-healed and then when we begin to rehabilitate, the wound softens down and in the wound we are finding sulfonamides there because they have not been absorbed. In those that do break down, it increases the convalescence of those patients sometimes anywhere from 2 to 3 weeks.

Judging from the dressings that have been applied, I think our first aid men have been well trained and the effort that has been put forth has definitely shown results, because the patients arriving now in the field hospitals have been well cared for forward. The men know how to apply dressings and in most instances the dressings are well applied. However, there is a tendency in some cases to apply the dressings too tightly and, when swelling occurs, then they become a tourniquet.

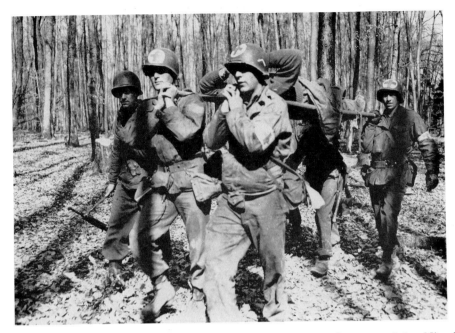

FIGURE 99.—Litter bearers of the Seventh U.S. Army bringing in a wounded soldier in southern France.

Brigadier Porritt, consulting surgeon to the British 21 Army Group, was asked to open the discussion on sorting. But before speaking of sorting, Brigadier Porritt commented on first aid treatment. He stated:

We feel about our stretcher bearers [aidmen] as you do about yours. Treatment at this level is not particularly skillful. It is a mixture of common sense and humanity—if they will only use common sense and stick to a routine treatment; simplification is what we want. They have to get the patients out, but they must get them out successfully treated so that nothing happens. They must give first aid medical treatment to get him back in at least no worse shape than he was when he started.

With respect to sorting in forward hospitals, Brigadier Porritt stated that the British had started the war with great ideas on classifying casualties for evacuation, resuscitation, and treatment. In actual practice, he remarked, these ideal-sounding plans do not work out. He made the following statement:

There is * * * no subdivision into classes, but there is again the essence of sound common sense. "Sorting" I much prefer to "triage." A man must learn the type of case he can treat at that surgical level or the type that he must send on. Anything he can send on saves effort. Surgery in forward areas should be very limited. Anything they do is merely to allow the patient to be taken back. A mediocre man may be much more valuable than a good surgeon who is going to complicate things by treating every case he sees.

General Monro was asked to say a few words as a representative of the consultant group for the Director General of Medical Services in the British Army. "I find myself in the same position as previous speakers representing the British service," he began. "This is rather a quick one," he commented wryly, "I came over here intending to enjoy myself and now I find my holiday is not going so well."

On the subject of consultants in general, the consulting surgeon to the British Army said:

If I may go back, sir, for a moment, I should like to state how closely all that General Hawley said appealed to me; how much he said about the contribution of the consultants coincided with our own. It is, as a matter of fact, within the last two years, I think, that our own senior directors in the field have come to realize what the advice of the consultants can mean. I am bound to state that actually in certain cases there was a little opposition to the work of the consultants to this all important supervision by the technical officer who is not only a technician but a born administrator.

On the subject of sorting, General Monro noted:

We have at the moment under discussion this question of the selection of cases. Under this new setup, this introduction of mobile surgical units undoubtedly gives us much greater flexibility and ability to concentrate surgery where it is wanted than was ever supposed before. The field dressings station idea was a sort of modified field ambulance made more mobile. It was quite obvious that we must have some sort of organization that would enable us to hold our cases further, so the field dressing station was evolved to take care of cases when distances prohibited evacuation. I think you will agree, our people will agree, that it is infinitely better than any other system we have had before. The word "triage" has been quite rightfully condemned. I think it is outlived and some much more sensible word such as grouping, or selection is the word of choice. I don't think it matters very much that we have three groups—a, b, and c, or one, two, and three. That, after all, is intended only as a guide for one who hasn't faced it before. It is, as Brigadier Porritt said, common sense that matters.

As an afterthought, General Monro added:

We also apply that [common sense] to our first aid. A paragraph in our little hygiene manual tells the soldier that first aid is simply common sense and then goes on to explain what the principles are and finally if he has any questions to ask the medical officer. Our men, when it is possible, are all trained in elementary first aid. I will agree with everything that has been said about first aid dressings and I would accentuate the fact that the main objective is to try to get the man back out of the field and keep that first original dressing in position.

On the topic of sorting, Colonel Crisler remarked:

I regard sorting as something that is in two categories. One sorts cases to decide which hospital they will be sent to, and then one sorts cases within the hospital. There are two different sets of criteria * * *. The sorting to decide which hospital they will be sent to is guided as much by policy, by the tactical situation, by the employment of the hospital at the particular moment, and under the particular phase of warfare, as it is determined by the condition of the patient. At the division clearing station the doctors become very proficient in the selection of the so-called "non-transportables" * * *. I do not feel that you must have your most experienced man for sorting at that level * * * [where they] may readily seek the consultation of the surgical teams (fig. 100) * * *. Then in the hospital, sorting is governed by professional policies and I think that the most important point about that is that the sorting be continuous. That is to say, one must not let a case become labeled and pin that label on him and make it permanent, but you should keep going around, because in a half an hour or an hour the priority may change. If you label him as a number two or three, in another one-half an hour he may be a number one.

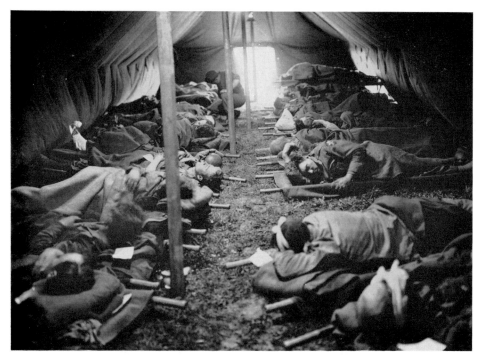

FIGURE 100.—Casualties being sorted at a clearing station in France.

The last subtopic on the agenda for the general session, transfusion and the preoperative management of the casualty, was opened by Col. J. S. K. Boyd, RAMC, consulting pathologist to the British 21 Army Group. He explained the evolution of the British system of resuscitation and transfusion and their use of wet and dry plasma and whole blood. Colonel Boyd explained that, to some of their divisions where there was a great enthusiasm for blood as opposed to plasma, the British were now shipping blood in small boxes holding three bottles and with a special compartment for ice to keep blood refrigerated for 24 hours. He went on to say:

The question of how much to transfuse is one that is very controversial. Transfusion is somewhat of a new toy and there is a great tendency to transfuse when it is quite unnecessary. * * * As to the level where it should start, I agree with the remarks made earlier in this morning's discussion. So far as possible, it should be minimal until the surgeon is prepared to operate on the patient. It has been found that, if a patient is transfused up to surgery level and then transported back from advance dressing station to casualty treating station, during that time he tends to go backwards, and, if he is allowed to recede, he is much more difficult to bring back. * * * As to the quantity required, that is a very variable factor. It depends very largely on what the patient has lost. The majority of severely wounded patients who arrive back at CCS have a hematocrit reading somewhere in the vicinity of thirty to thirty-five, taking the normal as forty-five. * * * But, in that, I think we must bear the scientific against the clinical, because, although many of the people who had a hematocrit reading under thirty were theoretically really ill, * * * in practice they weren't bad at all.

So far as the amount of blood or plasma used, I can't give you an exact figure. * * * The overall average is somewhere between one to two bottles of blood to a bottle of plasma. * * * Total quantities used might interest you. We find it very variable. Our budget in the early days was from 30 to 40 bottles for every 100 wounded men * * * but that has gone up very considerably, and at the present moment it is running somewhere on the far side—probably between 60 and 70 bottles per 100 wounded. Now, that does not mean that each man is getting between six and seven bottles, but means that a large number of patients are being transfused, and that is due partly to the different type of wounded we are getting in this campaign * * *. There is much blood lost, and there is more necessity for transfusion.

Speaking of the American experience with transfusion and resuscitation, Colonel Crisler stated, with reference to the First U.S. Army (fig. 101) :

Up to the present campaign, there was no such thing as shock teams. It was an idea gotten up in this theater, and I think Colonel Zollinger of General Hawley's office worked on that and that job has definitely turned out to be worthwhile. The shock team was originally with the auxiliary surgical group and there were only four teams in the auxiliary surgical group. Four shock teams for an army is just of no value whatsoever. It has been found that two shock teams per evacuation hospital and two per field hospital is the number that you should have. I have noted that with the Fifth Auxiliary Surgical Group which has just arrived there is a considerable increase in the number of shock teams in that particular organization. With the shock teams the patients have gotten better care than they did previously so far as treatment of shock is concerned.

Continuing with his discussion of resuscitation in the First U.S. Army, Colonel Crisler brought up a subject which was being noticed by many as a potentially serious problem. He commented :

There have been reactions to * * * stored blood and they are continuing to have reactions; we are trying to get some figures on it. They have increased in number and in severity as the date of expiration is approached. The unfortunate thing is that in our Army the expiration date is getting pretty close in the blood coming from the States. At the present time, there is not more than 3 days remaining when the blood arrives until the expiration date. * * * that expiration date is set only arbitrarily, and it is perfectly possible that the actual expiration date is past; and that is not a particularly good thing.

After General Hawley explained difficulties in providing whole blood— particularly with respect to forecasting needs and determining the amount to be kept on hand—Major Hardin gave his impressions of the situation, as follows :

We have received rather sketchy reports about reactions. There is no evidence in any large well-controlled number of cases that the number of the reactions increases with the age of the blood; and I do not believe that the answer to reactions is the age of the blood. It is some other reason. There are two possibilities that I can think of off hand. As you know, the blood from the States is flown across the Atlantic without refrigeration. It may be that there is some contamination, and perhaps enough to give a reaction. We have found so far no contaminated bottles. The other possibility, which I think is probably the answer, is that the sets through which the blood is given are dirty. * * * The other type of reaction which may be seen in stored blood is the hemogloblin reaction which does increase with the age of blood. That is the reason that hospitals have been asked to examine the blood, because all hemolized blood has its own degree of hemolysis. The blood coming from the States, no matter what the age is, has less hemolysis than that from the ETO Blood Bank. So far as the age of the blood

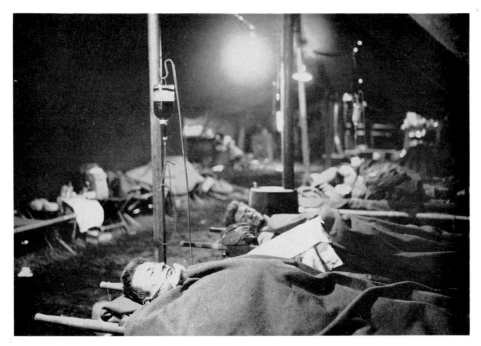

FIGURE 101.—A shock tent of a hospitalization unit of the 34th Field Hospital, First U.S. Army.

is concerned, you have got to get rid of your oldest blood first. As General Hawley said, we have had some difficulty in getting blood from the States. The blood from the States stops in the United Kingdom and then [is] flown here. Flying conditions have often been unfavorable.

This, the first general session of the meeting, was concluded with plans for a similar meeting at a later date. "I would like, before you break up," said General Hawley, "to have you discuss among yourselves how often these meetings should be held and perhaps fix a date for the next one. I am sure that, so long as we are in Paris, we will have a large turnout. Perhaps the next one should be in Twenty-One Army Group sector. I understand they are comfortably located up there."

Meeting of American surgical consultants.—The remainder of the day, after luncheon, and the morning following were devoted to smaller group sessions, the surgical and medical consultants going their separate ways (fig. 102). On Monday afternoon, the Chief Consultant in Surgery and the senior consultants met with consultants from the field armies and the surgical consultant from the United Kingdom Base, Colonel Morton.

Rotation of medical officers.—The consultants agreed that the exchange of medical officers between the armies and communications zone should begin immediately on an experimental basis. For this purpose, they thought it wisest to involve only the First U.S. Army initially, the Third U.S. Army to be

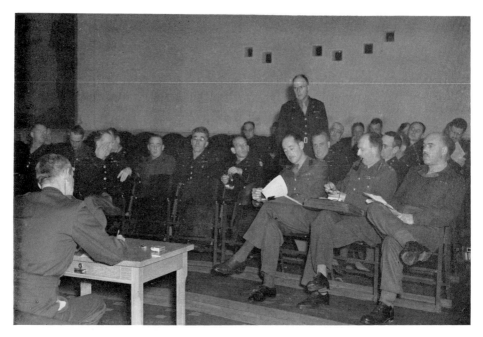

Figure 102.—Col. Frank B. Berry, MC, speaking at the meeting of surgical consultants during the Inter-Allied Consultants' Conference at the 108th General Hospital, Paris, France, 15 October 1944. Colonel Cutler, moderator, is seated at the table with his back to the camera.

brought into the plan soon thereafter. The consultants from theater headquarters promised highly trained and thoroughly competent surgeons from the best general hospitals for this interchange. It appeared also, from the conversation, that there were many highly competent surgeons in the field armies who, because of their age or long service in field army facilities, could now be better utilized as chiefs of services in general hospitals. Colonel Berry, particularly, said that there were highly trained men with a wealth of experience gained in 2 years of combat with the Seventh U.S. Army—men who would be much better off now if placed in general hospitals in the communications zone. And Colonel Berry was perfectly willing to give up these valuable men for such assignments to the rear.

Auxiliary surgical groups.—Another item of importance was the discussion on auxiliary surgical groups. At this time, the groups in the theater were assigned as follows:

Group	Assignment
1st	Theater reserve under operational control of Headquarters, SOS, ETOUSA
3d	First U.S. Army
4th	Third U.S. Army
5th (−)	Ninth U.S. Army

The 1st and 3d Auxiliary Surgical Groups were short of personnel. The 5th Auxiliary Surgical Group had only recently been assigned to the Ninth U.S. Army, and the Professional Services Division of the Chief Surgeon's Office had been busily bringing it up to strength. It now had 22 general surgical teams (6 of the team chiefs had been borrowed from general hospitals), 6 orthopedic teams, 1 neurosurgical team, 4 maxillofacial teams, 3 dental prosthetic teams, 3 X-ray teams, and 22 shock teams. However, many of these teams had been loaned to the Third U.S. Army, including those with chiefs borrowed from general hospitals. The 1st Auxiliary Surgical Group was being reassembled in Paris, but nine of the specialist teams were still in the United Kingdom pending the day when they could be replaced by teams formed from hospitals organic to that base section. There was a general shortage of competent chiefs of general surgical teams which prevailed throughout all the groups.

To bring all the groups up to their authorized strength and to return borrowed personnel and teams to their parent units were but typical examples of the personnel problems which continued to exist and required solution by the theater consultants (in coordination with the Personnel Division, Office of the Chief Surgeon). In this instance, Colonel Cutler elicited a promise from Colonel Odom of the Third U.S. Army that he would: (1) Return the six borrowed general surgeons on teams of the 5th Auxiliary Surgical Group to their hospitals, (2) fill their positions as chiefs of general surgical teams with second men from his 4th Auxiliary Surgical Group, (3) replace vacancies thus created in his 4th Auxiliary Surgical Group by competent junior officers on the shock teams borrowed from the 5th Auxiliary Surgical Group, (4) provide additional chiefs of general surgical teams for the 5th Auxiliary Surgical Group from assistants on general surgical teams of the 4th Auxiliary Surgical Group, and (5) return all teams of the 5th Auxiliary Surgical Group when they were required by the Ninth U.S. Army. If the Third U.S. Army should be caught short in an emergency as a result of these changes, teams were to be loaned to them from the 1st Auxiliary Surgical Group being reassembled in Paris. These and other steps necessary to bring the groups up to strength were coordinated on the spot with the senior consultants in their respective specialties and representatives from the Personnel Division of the Chief Surgeon's Office.

Another noteworthy development from this meeting was the fact that all the surgical consultants from the field armies were unanimous in pointing out that surgical instruments were beginning to wear out, particularly hemostats. They were being turned in for overhauling, but obviously this could only be carried so far. Colonel Cutler, after this meeting, alerted the Supply Division of the possibility that there might be a heavy demand for hemostatic forceps soon.

Meeting with French surgical consultants

On the day following this meeting with the consultants from the field armies, there was a meeting sponsored by the 217th General Hospital for medical officers in the Paris area with consultants from the French Army. In a memo-

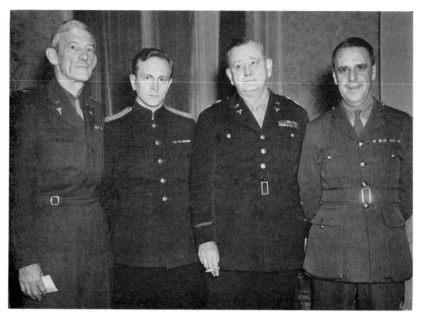

FIGURE 103.—Left to right, Colonel Cutler, Colonel Osipov, General Hawley, and Major Birch-Jones in General Hawley's office, Paris, France.

randum directed to the Chief Surgeon on 18 October 1944, Colonel Cutler reported that it had been a very pleasant and satisfactory occasion and that they had been warmly thanked by their French colleagues. He noted in his official diary: "An excellent program was provided at the hospital and in spite of language difficulties our French colleagues seemed greatly interested, and wish to give us a return meeting at the Val de Grâce hospital in 2 weeks."

Soviet visitor

On Thursday, 19 October, Colonel Cutler was again back in the United Kingdom. After conferences with Colonel Spruit and Colonel Morton, according to plan, Colonel Cutler met with Major Southworth who said that he had attended the recent international meeting at which the new penicillin unit had been established. Colonel Cutler was happy to note that it was almost one-to-one with the previously known Florey or Oxford unit, now so familiar to him.

On Monday, 23 October, Colonel Cutler returned to the Continent with Col. B. A. Osipov of the medical service of the Soviet Army and his attached British aide, Major Birch-Jones (fig. 103). Colonel Osipov had been visiting British medical activities and had now been invited and cleared to observe them in the U.S. Army. Upon arrival in Paris, Colonel Osipov was shown the 108th General Hospital, where he observed the reception of patients and their distribution to wards. He was taken through the surgical and orthopedic wards, and then he lunched with the hospital staff. In the early afternoon, he saw neuropsychiatric and malaria patients and then spent the remainder of the afternoon with various consultants in the Chief Surgeon's Office. The next day was also spent by Colonel Cutler in arranging the program for Colonel Osipov to see and talk with most of the consultants and the chiefs of the various divisions in the Office of the Chief Surgeon. Later there was a dinner given by General Hawley in honor of Colonel Osipov, at which another visitor, Brigadier J. R. Rees, Consultant in Neuropsychiatry to the British Army, was also a guest. The morning of 25 October was likewise spent with the guest from the Soviet Union, but, for Colonel Cutler, this day was memorable, too, for another reason.

Reopening of Académie de Chirurgie

In the afternoon of 25 October, Colonel Cutler attended the first meeting of the Académie de Chirurgie since the Germans had entered Paris years before. The meeting place was crowded with distinguished French surgeons, among them Professors Le Riche, Roux, Berget, Banzet, Quenu, Senec, Brocq, and the president, Professor Brachot. The first item was the reading of the obituary notice on Professor Gosse, following which was a speech welcoming officers of the U.S. Forces. Professor Le Riche insisted that Colonel Cutler reply to this address in French, which he did. Thereafter, Colonel Cutler had to sit next to the president on the rostrum and help conduct the meeting. The meeting, Colonel Cutler reported, proceeded as follows:

> The papers read were short, and during the presentation most of the members conversed with one another, paying little attention to the speaker but when this murmuring became too loud the President rang a great big bell such as one uses in our country to call in the cows with. No one seemed to pay any attention, but the President was relieved by the noise, and the murmuring continued.

Colonel Cutler discovered that this was not actually the first meeting since the occupation of France by the Germans, for there had been a planning meeting the week before, but it was indeed a noteworthy milestone heraldic of the peace and victory which was now surely destined to come.

Chief Surgeon's Consultants' Committee meeting, 27 October 1944

Evacuation.—The meeting on 27 October 1944 of the Chief Surgeon with his Consultants' Committee was devoted extensively to improving evacuation. Only the day before, Colonel Cutler had met with the chiefs of surgical services of hospitals in and around Paris on one aspect of this problem, the classifying of patients as transportables and nontransportables. Major Robinson, Senior Consultant in Urology, had made a trip by hospital train to review the condition and care of patients in transit by rail. Colonel Stout, Senior Consultant in Maxillofacial Surgery, had made a similar trip by evacuation aircraft to the Zone of Interior. There was a definite pinch on evacuation means, and General Hawley stated at this meeting of his Consultants' Committee: "The situation is really terrible." General Hawley exhorted his consultants, saying: "* * * I want to emphasize again here, keep checking on the care of patients in transit. It is just as important a part of our responsibility as is their care in hospitals, and I just can't keep on temporizing when people are not carrying out directives."

Long-bone fractures.—Casualties with fractures of the long bones provided a special problem of evacuation at this time. An analysis of the problem follows:

Skeletal traction to be used effectively had to be instituted within a maximum of a week or so after wounding, a requirement which sharply restricted the transportation period. It was often nip-and-tuck whether casualties with these injuries could be evacuated from the Continent to the United Kingdom within this limited time. If they could not be evacuated, there was the threat of Continental hospital beds' being occupied by many orthopedic patients in skeletal traction because The Surgeon General had directed that all fractures of the long bones must be firmly healed (frozen) before evacuation to the Zone of Interior was undertaken.

General Hawley's solution of this dual problem was to give casualties with fractures of the long bones maximum priority in evacuation. When this was not possible, they had to be held on the Continent in skeletal traction for the minimum of from 60 to 70 days required for the fractures to become firmly healed after which evacuation to the Zone of Interior could be undertaken without the risk of loss of position in the transportation cast.

Other significant matters.—There was a discussion on the Tobruk plaster with half-ring splint involving Colonel Cleveland and General Hawley in which the Senior Consultant in Orthopedic Surgery explained the mechanism of the Tobruk plaster and mentioned that the Ninth U.S. Army would give it an experimental trial.

Colonel Cutler reported that he had conferred with Major Hardin on transfusion reactions and that a new directive was being prepared which would identify transfusion reactions as allergic, pyrogenic, or hemolytic and would explain what to do in the face of such reactions.

Colonel Cutler mentioned that the exchange of medical officers had started off with eight elderly, poor-in-quality officers who would at best only do as ward officers.

Finally, Colonel Kimbrough announced the plans made by the surgical consultants for specialized treatment facilities on the Continent. It was necessary that these facilities be established to take care of difficult thoracic, neurosurgical, urological, and maxillofacial surgery cases which could not be evacuated to similar facilities in the United Kingdom owing to the condition of the patient or the temporary unavailability of evacuation means. At the present time, only the 48th and 108th General Hospitals in Paris had been named to handle these cases, but it was reported that similar facilities would need to be established at a later date which would be accessible to each of the field armies.

Notable guests.—Dr. Loucks, previously mentioned, gave a brief description of his activities in a Japanese prison camp as a "guest of the Imperial Government" in North China. He painted a dismal picture of conditions prevailing on the Asiatic mainland and in the concentration and prison camps. Colonel Osipov was also present and, when given an opportunity to speak, stated through an interpreter:

> The Colonel is very grateful for the warm reception he has received from all, and for his contact with these modern consultants. He especially wants to draw attention to the work in the evacuation hospitals, which he thought ideal examples of work done under field conditions. He noted with great satisfaction the excellent organization to bring home the wounded, and another thing, the very high level of cultural standing and education. He would welcome a discussion with a member of the organization or with General Hawley himself. Any questions which arise on his own medical service, he will be willing to discuss with your representatives. In conclusion, he thanks you very warmly and wishes everybody the greatest success.

General Hawley, replying for the consultants, said through the interpreter: "It has been a great pleasure to have him with us. He will be welcome in our service, not only as an ally, but as a member of the [consultant] group and we wish him to feel that he can come at any time and be quite welcome."

Immediately after this meeting, Colonel Cutler accompanied the Chief Surgeon to England, where he followed up further the reorganization of hospitalization in the United Kingdom under the seven groups of hospitals, the selection of personnel to staff the contemplated hand centers, and the studies on delayed early suture of wounds being conducted at the 91st and 158th General Hospitals. Colonel Cutler also planned with Major Palmer to turn over the facilities of the Operational Research Section to the Army Air Forces so that, the theater commander permitting, the personnel of the unit could be reorganized to conduct casualty surveys of battle casualties occurring during ground warfare.

An Extremely Busy November

Hospitals and hospitalization

On returning to the Continent, 2 November 1944, and for much of the entire month, Colonel Cutler and his surgical consultants were particularly busy on various aspects of hospitalization. New general hospitals were arriving in numbers—hospitals with a dearth of well-trained personnel. In the last week of October and the first of November, eight new general hospitals had been completely evaluated and oriented on the Continent. Major Robinson, Senior Consultant in Urology, and Lt. Col. Rudolph Schullinger, MC, borrowed from the 2d General Hospital, had to be used to go over some of these hospitals. Eleven new general hospitals had just arrived or were scheduled to arrive immediately in the United Kingdom and were destined to be employed on the Continent if and when their personnel could be strengthened to the required professional standards (fig. 104).

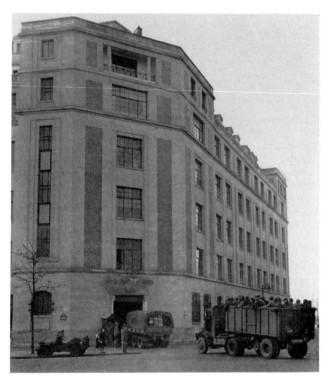

FIGURE 104.—The 194th General Hospital arriving in Paris, France, in January 1945 to establish facilities at Lycée Claude Bernard.

At the same time, a new table of organization and equipment had been published by the War Department which cut down medical officers in general hospitals by five, and all general hospitals in the theater had to be readjusted accordingly. Lt. Col. (later Col.) Norton Canfield, MC, Senior Consultant in Otolaryngology, immediately called attention to the fact that this new table of organization and equipment gave the rank of captain to the otolaryngologist in a general hospital. This was an impossible situation, for most of the theater's otolaryngologists were already majors, and it was soon to become painfully obvious that very few of the junior medical officers were willing to take on the position of the ENT (ear, nose, and throat) officer in a general hospital with the certain prospect of spending the remainder of the war as a captain while their associates could look for advancement in other areas.

Further to complicate matters was the fact that continued offensive actions against the Siegfried Line were now being felt in the form of over-crowded hospitals in the communications zone (fig. 105). Moreover, the uni-formly bad weather throughout November curtailed seriously all forms of evacuation, but particularly air evacuation in the United Kingdom.

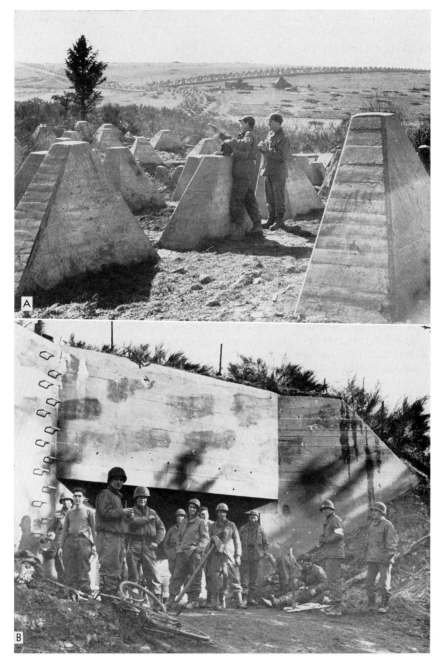

FIGURE 105.—The Siegfried Line. A. Miles of concrete antitank defense works. B. A heavily fortified pillbox taken over for an aid station by American troops.

Reestablishment of Blood Bank, ETOUSA.—On 3 November, the day following his return, the Chief Consultant in Surgery visited Vitry-sur-Seine where the 1st General Hospital was being established. He noted that it was going to be well housed and that the buildings would be quite satisfactory for a hospital. He recommended that one of the newly arrived hospitals, or a part thereof, be attached to the 1st General Hospital to operate a total combined bed capacity of from 1,500 to 1,800 beds. Colonel Cutler was most pleased to note that the 152d Station Hospital, the ETOUSA Blood Bank, was finally operational here. He noted:

* * * The Blood Bank is occupying a wing of a large building there and is admirably adapting these quarters to its purposes. This has meant a great deal of construction, plumbing work and other renovations, but all this has been accomplished by the personnel of the 152d Station Hospital, which is greatly to their credit. The first blood was drawn in Paris today, and it was being processed this afternoon when we were there.

Limitation of professional missions assigned to hospitals on Continent.—On 6 November 1944, the following words of caution and advice were given in a memorandum to Colonel Kimbrough by the Chief Consultant in Surgery:

It is clear, from our analysis of the hospitals which have recently arrived on the Continent * * * that these hospitals cannot be brought up to any reasonably professional standard so that they may act as general hospitals. We do not have qualified personnel to accomplish what is desired.

With this fact established, we must not use such hospitals as general hospitals, for we would then be responsible for both mortality and morbidity figures of which we would be ashamed.

This brings up a great principle, that hospitals should not be assigned to professional tasks beyond their competence, and that, when hospitals are assigned by Operations Division, that assignment should be coordinated with the Professional Services Division in order that reasonably safe care be given to the American soldier.

As to the eight new general hospitals, Colonel Cutler universally recommended that they be utilized to augment the bed capacity of an already existing and competent general hospital, thus making use of the superior officers in these older hospitals in supervising the work of the less able personnel of the new. The Chief Consultant in Surgery recommended that, if they could not be employed in this manner, these new general hospitals be used as holding hospitals or convalescent hospitals—missions within limits of their professional competence—to replace the more competent hospitals which, in spite of the protests of the consultants, were still being wasted in performing these missions when their abilities were sorely needed elsewhere.

Colonel Cutler spent the entire day of Tuesday, 7 November, as well as the previous afternoon, with each of the field army surgeons and members of the Supply Division, Office of the Chief Surgeon, in formulating recommendations for changes to the tables of organization and equipment of field hospitals and 400-bed evacuation hospitals.

Observations at the 62d General Hospital.—Colonel Cutler paid a routine visit to the 62d General Hospital the next day, Wednesday. He made the following two extremely significant observations:

At this hospital the first patient with a Blakemore tube had been admitted some days before. Apparently the femoral artery was severed, patient was seen first at the 8th Field Hospital, operated upon by Major [Charles A.] Rose of the 91st Evacuation Hospital and a Blakemore tube was put in the upper femoral region where some 2 inches of femoral artery had been removed. The patient arrived at the 62nd General Hospital in A 1 condition with perfect circulation in his feet, though no palpable pulse. This is the first instance of the proper and satisfactory use of this tube in the U.S. Forces.

A good many men are being admitted with "cold feet." All have about the same experience, that they have been in foxholes full of water for about 4 days, their feet feel sore, they take off their shoes and their feet swell so rapidly they cannot get the shoes on again. This is the condition I studied with the Fifth Army in Italy a year ago. At that time it was recommended that the American soldier be given socks with more wool in them, and that our soldiers should be encouraged to use larger shoes. This is going to be a heavy problem this winter unless very active steps are taken to prevent the disaster. In order to facilitate the studying of these soldiers with cold feet we must have thermocouples for registration of skin temperature. These have been ordered from Supply, and also it would be wiser if we set up a center at one of our general hospitals to concentrate on the problem. This is now being integrated in the Professional Services Division.

Newly arrived general hospitals in United Kingdom.—On Sunday, 12 November, Colonel Cutler flew again to the United Kingdom where, the next day, he held a conference with Colonel Morton, Colonel Tovell, Colonel Bricker, Colonel Cleveland, Colonel Kneeland, and Colonel Stout. He discussed with them the newly arrived general hospitals and the procedures which would be necessary to bring them up to usable standards. It was decided that Colonel Cleveland and Colonel Tovell would begin the very next day to "vet" each of them to determine first the numerical deficiency of these hospitals in professional personnel and to note the specific inadequacies from the professional point of view so that detailed recommendations could be made to Colonel Spruit as to: (1) the total number of medical officers necessary to bring the units up to strength and (2) the specific professional requirements to meet these deficiencies. They agreed also that all the operating general hospitals in the United Kingdom would have to be evaluated according to the new tables of organization and equipment so that the number and type of excess officers in these hospitals could be presented at the same time to Colonel Spruit with the requirements for the newly arrived units.

Sometime later, after all these new hospitals had been "vetted," there was the surprising revelation that their professional personnel were of a considerably higher caliber than had been experienced in newly arriving hospitals for a long time. Most of them were adequately covered in medicine and surgery, with only occasional shortages in pathologists, neuropsychiatrists, and X-ray personnel. None of these hospitals, just as it was true of those which had been "vetted" earlier on the Continent, had otolaryngologists.

Expedition of priority cases.—At the meeting of the Chief Surgeon's Consultants' Committee on 27 October (pp. 273–275), the need for specialized treatment facilities to care for severely damaged casualties had been discussed. Casualties in this category included neurosurgical, maxillofacial, thoracic surgical, urological (with neurological complications), and severely compounded fracture cases. Examination of a great number of seriously injured fracture cases during the time Colonel Cutler was in the United Kingdom, from 28 October to 2 November, had revealed that it was taking 10 days for them to reach the United Kingdom. These were the type of casualties who were supposedly being given the highest priority in evacuation to the United Kingdom, since skeletal traction for the reduction of fractures had to be initiated early. It was obvious, therefore, that the seriously damaged casualty was not reaching the United Kingdom soon enough for the initiation of reparative procedures. "We must not equivocate about this," Colonel Cutler had warned in a memorandum, dated 6 November, to Colonel Kimbrough, "Either we evacuate early * * * or we give up that hope * * *."

As a result of these warnings, a meeting was held on 17 November 1944 attended by Colonel Kimbrough, Colonel Mowrey (Chief, Evacuation Branch, Operations Division), Col. Robert E. Peyton (Chief, Operations Division), Colonel Cutler, and Col. William S. Middleton, MC. The meeting was called, as the Chief Consultant in Surgery reported later, to arrive at a decision on two questions: "Should we still hope for early rapid evacuation to the United Kingdom which would permit us to get patients to our centers for specialized care in the United Kingdom * * * within 5 days, or should we not struggle against the weather and set up some centers to cover periods of bad weather on the Continent?" [101]

It was agreed that centers for the care of craniocerebral, thoracic, and maxillofacial injuries should be set up on the Continent at each of the large concentrations of activities in the communications zone; that is, Paris, Liége, and Nancy. The Paris hospitals, of course, were already staffed to take care of patients in these categories. The conferees agreed, too, that airlift should continue to be used whenever it was possible to evacuate these casualties to the United Kingdom within 5 days following injury. They thought that criteria would have to be established as to what type of cases should be selected for admission to these continental centers for specialized treatment. Less seriously wounded patients could be cared for in other available hospitals. Colonel Cutler also thought that such a directive should specify how long patients could remain in these facilities for specialized treatment, and it was his impression that 14 days should be the limit.

Southern Lines of Communication becomes part of ETOUSA

Operational control of the Seventh U.S. Army, advancing through southern France for a link with ETOUSA forces to the north, had passed to the European theater in September (fig. 106). As of 20 November 1944, the

[101] Memorandum, Chief Consultant in Surgery, to Chief, Professional Services Division, 21 Nov. 1944, subject: Meeting re Care of Patients on Continent.

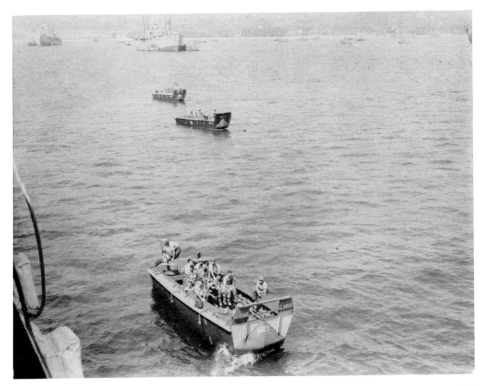

FIGURE 106.—Higgins boats bringing casualties of the Seventh U.S. Army to U.S. Army Hospital Ship *Shamrock* during the assault on beaches of southern France, 17 August 1944.

support areas in southern France for this force were to become a part of the Communications Zone, ETOUSA. The overall communications zone command for this area was called SOLOC (Southern Lines of Communication), and its surgeon was Col. Charles F. Shook, MC (fig. 107). Colonel Shook, with his deputy for administration and personnel, Lt. Col. James T. Richards, PhC, arrived for conferences with members of the Office of the Chief Surgeon, ETOUSA, on 15 November 1944 to effect a smooth changeover of command insofar as medical activities were concerned. Colonel Cutler, who was in England at the time arranging for the "vetting" of the 11 newly arrived general hospitals, also returned to the Continent on 15 November, and spent most of 16 November participating in conferences with the SOLOC surgeon. In a memorandum to the Deputy Chief Surgeon, dated 17 November 1944, Colonel Cutler stated that the following items were of pertinence to the Professional Services Division of the Office of the Chief Surgeon:

1. Technical correspondence with units in SOLOC was to be routed through the Surgeon, SOLOC.

2. The same evacuation policy was to apply to SOLOC as to the remainder of the Continent; namely, 30 days in SOLOC hospitals, patients requiring

more than 30 but not over 120 days to be evacuated to the United Kingdom. (The 120-day evacuation policy for the entire European theater had just been proclaimed in mid-October 1944.)

3. SOLOC had 14,000 beds, 5,000 of which were in Marseilles. With expansion, SOLOC bed capacity could be raised to 22,000 beds.

4. The Surgeon, SOLOC, stated that his hospitals expected to hold seriously injured casualties—neurosurgical, thoracic, and maxillofacial—until they could be evacuated to the Zone of Interior, but Colonel Cutler expressed his views in the matter as follows: "I am sure this will need elaboration by a personal visit of the Consultant Group to SOLOC."

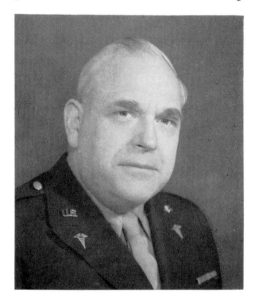

FIGURE 107.—Col. Charles F. Shook, M.C.

As for consultants, Colonel Shook assured Colonel Kimbrough and Colonel Cutler that he would like the advice of the consultants in European theater headquarters in setting up SOLOC consultants in medicine and surgery and any of the other specialties, as required, and also regional consultants according to the ultimate disposition of hospitals in SOLOC. Colonel Shook suggested that the qualifications of Col. Ira A. Ferguson, MC, be looked into for the position of surgical consultant to SOLOC. Colonel Ferguson was now at the 43d General Hospital as assistant chief of the surgical service, and Col. Edward D. Churchill, MC, had assured Colonel Cutler that he was qualified to be chief of surgery in a general hospital. Colonel Cutler did not want to commit himself on this item at the time, and Colonel Shook agreed to delay his appointment until Colonel Cutler could visit SOLOC. Finally, Colonel Shook stated that he would prefer not have any visit by European theater consultants until at least December, as they were just getting settled and could carry on until then with their existing service.

Cold injury studies

As cold injury continued to be a growing problem during November and it was apparent that knowledge of the conditions being observed was too scant even to estimate the degree of damage or possibilities of repair, the consultants agreed that a concerted effort to study the condition was needed. The Chief Surgeon agreed, and the 108th General Hospital was selected for the mission. Capt. (later Maj.) Octa C. Leigh, Jr., MC, who had considerable experience in the field, was reassigned from the 16th Station Hospital to the 190th General Hospital and then placed on temporary duty at the 108th General Hospital to take charge of the studies. About this time, Maj. Leiv Kreyberg, Royal Norwegian Medical Corps, joined Captain Leigh in this project. Colonel Cutler took it upon himself to arrange for the procurement of skin temperature thermocouples, Quinizarin, through Burroughs, Wellcome & Co., capillary microscope, Novocain (procaine hydrochloride) in oily solution for sympathetic blocks, and Diodrast (iodopyracet) to demonstrate vascular adequacy. Colonel Tovell promised to find a skilled anesthesiologist to perform the sympathetic blocks for the study group, and all the consultants were asked to contribute their ideas and knowledge toward solution of the problems which cold injury was presenting.[102]

Activities and Situation at Year's End

Second Inter-Allied Consultants' Conference

Colonel Cutler had met with Brigadier (later Maj. Gen.) E. Phillips, RAMC, and General Hawley on 6 November 1944 in the Chief Surgeon's Office to discuss the next meeting of British and American consultants. Brigadier Phillips represented the British 21 Army Group and was soon to become its DMS. It was decided that the next meeting would be held in Brussels at Rear Headquarters, British 21 Army Group. Because the number of guests would have to be limited, the Americans advised Brigadier Phillips that the essential people would be the consultants in medicine and surgery from each of the four U.S. field armies and those of Britain and Canada, the consultant group in the Office of the Chief Surgeon, ETOUSA, and representatives from the consultant group of the DGMS, British Army.

Plans for the meeting proceeded without complications, and Saturday, 9 December, found Colonel Cutler on the road to Brussels with Colonel Tovell, who was also scheduled to speak. They arrived in Brussels at 1830 hours.

The meeting of consultants was held at the British 8th General Hospital beginning on Sunday morning, 10 December. Major General Phillips opened the conference saying that he hoped the meetings would continue and that the

---

[102] Minutes, Twenty-Fifth Meeting, Chief Surgeon's Consultants' Committee, Paris, 24 Nov. 1944.

pooling of ideas by the Allies was essential to success.   Colonel Cutler's official
diary account of the first day's meetings follows:

The first professional topic was chest wounds, opened by Major Collis, RAMC. He
mentioned infection as a major item, a surprise to us, since at one of the chest centers in
the United Kingdom Major Harken has written that no cases of serious empyema have
occurred. Major Collis thought penicillin of little value except when instilled in the
pleural space. The next topic was "Penicillin," opened by Colonel Mitchell, RAMC. The
British use the intramuscular drip method, 100,000 units in 24 hours in 540 cc. of salt
solution. They believe this maintains a satisfactory bacteriostatic level. He asked for a
solution of a more satisfactory vehicle than sulfonamides, and he presented, as evidence
of the great value of penicillin in abdominal wounds, the following statistics :—

> 2,712 abdominal operations
> 2,307 with intraperitoneal damage
>   405 with extraperitoneal damage
>   759 deaths (27 percent)

There was a lively discussion of this matter.   Since the U.S. Army showed
similar or better statistics, and did not put penicillin in the abdomen, Colonel
Mitchell's suggestion that intraperitoneal penicillin was of value failed to find
general approval.

    Colonel Cutler continued :

In the afternoon the medical and surgical sections met separately. The first afternoon
topic was abdominal wounds, opened by Colonel Cutler. Colonel Cutler presented statistics
showing the frequency of abdominal wounds in the A.E.F. 1917–18 was 1.1 percent and
the fatality 66.8 percent. The figures for the First Army June 6–30, 1944, showed an
incidence of 4.3 and a mortality of 21.2 percent. The 5th U.S. Army, 9 September to 12
November 1944, showed an incidence of 4 percent and a mortality of 22 percent. Finally,
individual hospital reports were presented. 128th Evacuation Hospital, a mortality of
19.3 percent overall, but 10.7 percent postoperative mortality. 91st Evacuation Hospital,
October report, shows 20 percent mortality, overall, and 12 percent postoperative mortality.
Meanwhile, the Canadian I Corps Surgeon reported a mortality of 35 percent in August
and September 1944, and the French figures for the Italian Campaign showed a mortality
of 44.6 percent.

Obviously, more people with wounds of the abdomen are now reaching the surgeon,
and of those who reach the surgeon in the U.S. Army an overall mortality is somewhere
around 25 percent and the postoperative mortality somewhere around 12 to 15 percent.
This improvement is perhaps more largely due to the fact that the surgeon of the day
devotes more care to the general condition of his patient preliminary to the surgical
ordeal. Colonel Cutler reviewed the care of the abdominal case from the time he is
picked up in the field to his disposition in a general hospital. The low incidence of
infection, possibly due to chemotherapy, was mentioned. The better treatment of shock
was taken up in detail. The immobilization of abdomens after surgery was considered
highly important, and decompression by indwelling catheters thought a great step forward.
The separate treatment of small bowel and large bowel injuries was mentioned, and
the group was urged to see that all left large bowel colostomies were made complete
so that the faecal stream was entirely turned away from the buttocks. In the discussion,
Brigadier Porritt wondered whether all abdomens should not be subjected to surgery. In
rebuttal, it was stated that there was no point in operating upon hopeless cases, particularly when the surgeon's time might be better devoted to more important though less
seriously damaged soldiers.

The final paper was presented in the surgical section by Colonel Tovell, on Anesthetics
in the Field, and for this Colonel Tovell had prepared a mimeographed sheet revealing

the percentage of different types of anesthesia according to the hospital in which they were used. Thus, intravenous anesthesia is the predominant anesthetic in U.S. Army hospitals, reaching as high as 39.5 percent, whereas local anesthesia reaches 30.9 percent and inhalation anesthesia only 7.06 percent. However, when we consider the field for work we find the field hospitals doing chests and abdomens and using inhalation anesthesia for 41.4 percent of their cases.

During the second day, 11 December, the surgical and medical consultants again met separately. Again, there were morning and afternoon sessions, but Colonel Cutler attended only the morning session where the principal speaker was the surgical consultant for the Third U.S. Army. Colonel Cutler gave the following brief description of this meeting:

In the morning the surgical group considered "Vascular Injuries," which was opened by Colonel Odom, Third U.S. Army. He presented the overall figures for the Third Army and revealed that the number of cases in which arterial repair may be attempted is extremely small, sixteen out of 362 cases. He pointed out that 0.7 percent of 49,410 battle casualties had vascular damage to large vessels. 346 of these had simultaneous ligation of artery and vein and 50.7 percent of these came to amputation. The various vessels in which ligation had been carried out were specified, and again the grave danger of ligating the popliteal vessels was brought forward. The question arose as to whether the forward surgeon was not too conservative by not amputating limbs whose circulation was totally destroyed. It was pointed out that the figures for safe ligation in elective surgery might be entirely different in the arm where all the collaterals were blown out. No one said a good word for sympathetic block. The Canadians suggested that little glass tubes or a tube of plastic material might be utilized to recanalize injured vessels. All agreed that where a major vessel is ligated the patient must be held in the forward area for 4 to 6 days to see whether gangrene was to set in.[103]

After lunch, the delegates visited the British blood bank in Brussels where blood obtained from troops in and around Brussels was being processed for shipment forward. Colonel Cutler did not attend but spent the afternoon discussing the local situation with Professor Danis, professor of surgery at the university, and with Dr. Mayer, president of the Société Internationale de Chirurgie. There was particular concern about the future of the organization of which Dr. Mayer was president.

Trenchfoot was not an item on the agenda, for the British were having no great problem with ground-type cold injury, but there was considerable informal discussion concerning the matter. Colonel Cutler made the following entry in his diary concerning the discussion:

The total British figures were as follows:—21 British and 9 American soldiers have been treated in all of the British hospitals from the Invasion to December 1. General Phillips, commenting on this, spoke a) of the better footgear, noting that no constriction can occur because the two sides of the boot meet, so that the laces cannot make the shoe tight, and b) of better foot discipline as a command function. Brigadier Fenwick, who that night became Major General Fenwick and D.G.M.S. of the Canadian Forces, made the same comment.

---

[103] For a complete report on vascular injuries and vascular surgery in the Third U.S. Army, see the report entitled "Vascular Injuries in Battle Casualties" by Col. C. B. Odom. *In* Inter-Allied Conferences on War Medicine, 1942–1945, Convened by the Royal Society of Medicine (Sir Henry Tidy, Editor). New York, Toronto, London: Staples Press, Ltd., 1947, pp. 167–171.

The Second Inter-Allied Consultants' Conference came to a close after the second day's meetings with a dinner given by General Phillips which was characteristic of the traditional British hospitality and spirit of camaraderie. Colonel Cutler wrote in his journal:

> That night the D.M.S. gave a bounteous dinner for the Consultant Group. I had to sit between the DMS and Maj. Gen. Sir Miles Graham, Chief of Admin, 21 Army Group, and respond to General Phillips' kind words regarding the American Forces for General Hawley. I thanked General Phillips as best I could, intimating how much better General Hawley would have done it, and presented his deep regrets at being unable to attend. I then attempted to point out that this was the one time in the history of civilization when the English-speaking people should get together, since they are the only nations now functioning under free government.

Visit to Ninth U.S. Army

The next morning, Tuesday, 12 December 1944, Colonel Cutler and Colonel Tovell were joined by Lt. Col. (later Col.) Gordon K. Smith, MC, surgical consultant for the Ninth U.S. Army, in the drive to Ninth Army headquarters in Maestricht, The Netherlands. En route, they stopped at the 30th General Hospital in Antwerp, for lunch and a look at the installation. It was in nice buildings, but the utilities were deplorable and sewage was even running out onto the lawns. Colonel Cutler, Colonel Tovell, and Colonel Smith reached Ninth U.S. Army headquarters that evening. Col. William E. Shambora, MC, the surgeon, was away so they spent the evening discussing various professional matters—particularly necessary personnel shifts—with Lt. Col. Elmer D. Gay, MC, commanding officer of the 5th Auxiliary Surgical Group, and the other Ninth U.S. Army consultants. During the evening, buzz-bombs kept going over the headquarters, and Colonel Cutler surmised: "* * * Apparently they start on the German side of the line and on their way to Antwerp pass over Maestricht. They could not have been very high because the windows rattled every time they went over."

Colonel Cutler visited the Medical Section, Headquarters, Ninth U.S. Army, the next morning where he met some of the staff and learned that some 300 casualties had been admitted in the last 24 hours to Ninth U.S. Army hospitals. The remainder of the day was spent in visiting evacuation hospitals and one field hospital of the Ninth Army.

At the 108th Evacuation Hospital, Herzogenrath, Germany, Colonel Cutler learned that blood transfusion reactions were occurring about once in every ten transfusions. He recorded: "Initial chill, pressure fall, pulse becomes rapid, patient enters deeper shock, fever later. No haemolysis and no evidence of protein shock reactions. These are unquestionably pyrogenic reactions and probably due to improperly cleaned tubing. Plasma is giving the same type of reaction, again a pyrogenic reaction * * *." Tobruk splint experiments were being carried on at this hospital. The application of the splints seemed well done, and Colonel Cutler believed that Colonel Cleveland might be able to give an answer as to the efficacy of the Tobruk splint in another week or so.

At the 111th Evacuation Hospital, Heerlen, The Netherlands, the Chief Consultant in Surgery was pleased to meet again Maj. William R. Sandusky, MC, who was chief of the surgical service, doing the thoracic surgery there with the help of a Captain Johnson, and conducting an intimate study of gas gangrene. Major Sandusky, the reader will recall, had conducted the excellent studies on penicillin and gas gangrene in air casualties while he was attached as a captain to the 49th Station Hospital in East Anglia. "The hospital," Colonel Cutler noted, "has an A.1 professional service. Well organized, perfectly integrated and entirely competent."

The 91st Evacuation Hospital in Valkenburg, The Netherlands, Colonel Cutler found, was located in a beautiful Jesuit college which could well do for a general hospital some day. The chief of surgical service was Lt. Col. Charles S. Welch, MC. Colonel Cutler recorded: "This was the best hospital we visited. There is an excellent spirit of cooperation between the professional services, administration, and the chief of the surgical service; Colonel Welch is one of our best forward surgeons. This is the officer who is to speak at the next meeting of the Inter-Allied Medical Conference on thoracic surgery in the forward areas. I briefed him for his talk, told him and his commanding officer I would clear his orders * * * for January 4 for 8 or 10 days." In a discussion of blood and plasma reactions, the hospital personnel stated that plasma reactions occurred with chills followed by anuria on occasions. In further discussion of anuria, Colonel Welch agreed that crush syndrome might play a large role.

Colonel Cutler and Colonel Smith also visited the 105th Evacuation Hospital and a platoon of the 48th Field Hospital during the day. Back at their quarters, Colonel Cutler and Colonel Smith conferred on matters to be discussed with Colonel Shambora the next day. And again, Colonel Cutler uneasily noted: "Four buzz-bombs just missed the top of the house. Apparently these missiles start not very far away from Maestricht and scare people on the way up, whereas in Antwerp they scare them on the way down (fig. 108)!"

At 0800 the next morning, Colonel Cutler and Colonel Tovell joined in conference with Colonel Shambora, the Ninth U.S. Army surgeon, and his surgical consultant. Colonel Cutler asked and obtained permission to have Colonel Smith accompany him on a visit to the neighboring First U.S. Army so that Colonel Smith could participate in additional conferences on professional matters with the surgical consultant of the First Army. The many proposed personnel changes were also explained and discussed. Colonel Cutler emphasized that such changes had to be initiated as requests from the field Armies. There was discussion on the desirability for evacuation and field hospitals furnishing monthly hospital reports so that they could be consolidated at the field army level and distributed to the army units as a part of the educational program. Colonel Cutler advised the army surgeon on his impressions of the hospitals visited. They spoke of the unusual position occupied by Lt. Col. John Gilbert Manning, MC, the Ninth U.S. Army orthopedic con-

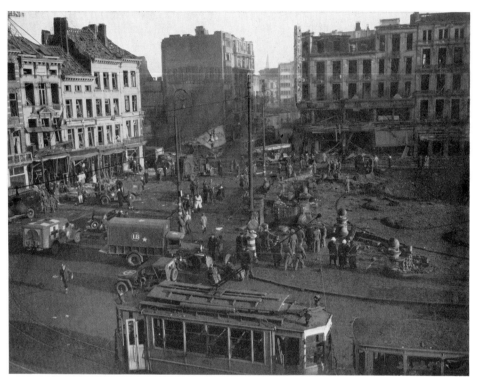

FIGURE 108.—Destruction in Antwerp, Belgium, following the detonation of a German V-1 rocket.   U.S. Army medical units helping to care for civilian casualties.

sultant, since this was the only field army with an orthopedic consultant. Colonel Shambora explained that Colonel Manning operated under Colonel Smith, that he was useful, and that he would be kept in his position for the time being.   Colonel Cutler promised to add Colonel Manning's name to the list of consultants so that he would be invited to attend and otherwise participate in activities of the theater's surgical consultants.   Pros and cons for uniting the position of surgical consultant and the commanding officer of an auxiliary surgical group under one officer, as was done in the First U.S. Army, were brought up.   The arrangement had worked well in the First U.S. Army.   "I did not urge this," Colonel Cutler later wrote, "as I am not sure this is a desirable situation, and I agreed with Colonel Shambora that he had a good commanding officer for his group, i.e. Colonel Gay, and a high grade consulting surgeon, and he might do well to continue as he was."   Colonel Cutler thanked the Ninth U.S. Army surgeon for the interesting and instructive visit to his units.

Following this meeting and before leaving the Ninth U.S. Army area, Colonel Cutler visited the 41st Evacuation Hospital where he had a pleasant visit on the wards and found a general feeling in the hospital that sympathetic procedures for vascular damage were of little value and that the Tobruk splint was not good.

Alleur, Belgium

En route to the First U.S. Army headquarters, Colonel Cutler and his party stopped by in Alleur, Belgium—several miles out of Liége—for visits to the 298th General Hospital and the 93d Medical Gas Treatment Battalion.

298th General Hospital.—Colonel Cutler was overjoyed at seeing many old friends from the days in England still with the 298th General Hospital, the affiliated unit from the University of Michigan and one of the first general hospitals to be sent to the European theater. Col. Walter G. Maddock, MC, the commanding officer, was on hand to greet the visitors and provide them lunch. The hospital was under tentage and Colonel Cutler noted: "* * * a general feeling in this unit that a good unit like this should be in permanent construction. I heartily agreed with this, and the same comment about too frequent moving of hospitals as came up in this hospital also came up at the 30th General Hospital in Antwerp and later at the 25th General Hospital in Liége."

In other discussions, it was brought out that 420 beds of this 1,000-bed hospital were set aside in a separate unit to be used as a holding hospital for air evacuation. The prevailing differences in opinion concerning the Tobruk splint were again evident here. Colonel Maddock thought it was more comfortable and easier to transport, but the orthopedic surgeon at the hospital felt the Tobruk splint was uncomfortable and that the half ring often rested on the perineum, causing difficulty. It was also said that gas gangrene had been very rare and that delayed primary suture was being accomplished on cases which, for some reason, had to be held for more than 5 days.

93d Medical Gas Treatment Battalion.—Colonel Cutler found the 93d Medical Gas Treatment Battalion a unique organization. It was located at a zinc mine about 2 miles from the 298th General Hospital. Detachment B of the 12th Field Hospital was attached to it. He described what he saw, thus:

Colonel Palmer, who was so efficient at the Southampton Hard, is commanding officer. He has 600 beds, 300 stretcher cases and 300 walking wounded. The patients come to him from the Liége general hospitals, and may be held for as long as 4 to 6 days, according to the air lift. The patients are all flown back to the United Kingdom. If any patient seems too ill and requires specific therapy, he is returned to the general hospital from which he came. In 3 weeks this hospital had returned 7,680 patients to the United Kingdom. Colonel Palmer made the comment that general hospitals are slow in sending patients to the holding hospitals. It was my impression that this holding group had done a bang-up job * * *.

First U.S. Army

Discussions with members of 3d Auxiliary Surgical Group.—Leaving Alleur, the party motored to Spa, Belgium, and the headquarters of the First U.S. Army. General Rogers, the army surgeon, was away for the day, but, while the visitors were speaking with members of the medical section, Colonel Crisler arrived. Colonel Crisler billeted the visitors with his 3d Auxiliary

Group and then took them to the group's mess. After dinner, Colonel Cutler
led a discussion on various professional matters—informally and openly, as was
his fashion.

One of the subjects discussed was trenchfoot. Statistically, the First U.S.
Army had no cases as of 27 September; by 8 October, there had been 140 cases;
and on 12 October, 320 cases had occurred. By that time, it had seemed wise
to organize to meet this problem, and the 91st Gas Treatment Battalion had
been set up as a center for the study of trenchfoot. Apparently, an ordinary
triage was being accomplished in evacuation hospitals, and 75 percent of the
patients were being evacuated out of the army area. The other 25 percent
were sent to the gas treatment battalion, where, the discussion revealed:

> Treatment was rest, repeated sympathetic blocks and later exercises. A summary
> of the sympathetic block work showed that the feet were more comfortable, but, using
> the other foot as a control, sympathectomy proved to give no additional benefit. Pressure
> bandages were tried with no benefit. Finally, exercises were tried, and these seemed to
> bring some benefit. After 10 days in this specialized hospital, troops were sent to the
> convalescent hospital, but only those with no evidence of disease. There they were
> refitted with larger shoes, given exercises, and by 20 days 80 percent were returned to
> duty. In anlyzing one thousand cases, the following occurs:—At the divisional level, 20
> percent, i.e. 200 cases, returned to duty as having had a mistaken diagnosis, i.e., just cold
> feet. Of the 800 left, 75 percent go to a general hospital and 25 percent to the Gas Treat-
> ment Battalion for specialized care and treatment. Of those who go there, 25 percent are
> returned to general hospitals and 75 percent via the 4th Convalescent Hospital to duty.
> This makes a total of about 30 percent of the originally diagnosed trenchfoot cases to duty.
> I brought up the matter, for insertion in their trenchfoot circular, that tetanus toxoid
> should be given when the skin is broken, as also penicillin or sulfonamide for infection.

There then followed a long discussion of the benefits which had accrued
in sending medical officers from combat units to hospitals in the base sections,
either on the 60-day temporary duty exchange program or on the short-visit
policy. Colonel Crisler pointed out that the greatest advantage had to do with
records, for the men in the forward areas had found out how poor the records
were which came down to the base areas and that it was not possible for
surgeons in communications zone hospitals to do intelligent work without adequate records. It was also asserted that these tours of duty in the communications zone revealed to the medical officers, who were characteristically initiating
reparative treatment of the battle casualty, the dangers involved when he failed
to split his cast or when he plugged wounds too tightly.

All were in agreement that new circular letters should be written stressing
the fact that abdominal retention sutures should not be removed until after
evacuation, explaining the difference in right and left colostomies, and detailing
the latest information on the surgery of major blood vessels. There was the
inevitable discussion on shortages of certain personnel and requirements for
changes in specialized personnel. Very satisfying to Colonel Cutler were remarks made by both Colonel Crisler and Colonel Smith that one of the greatest
boons to surgeons in medical facilities of the field army were the anesthesiologists supplied by Colonel Tovell. In his official journal of the visit, Colonel

Cutler remarked: "This may be taken as almost a personal triumph for Colonel Tovell, who has worked indefatigably in his special field and now is reaping a rich and well deserved harvest."

Hospital visits.—The next morning, 15 December, the Chief Consultant in Surgery was up early and visiting hospitals of the First U.S. Army. At the 2d Evacuation Hospital, he was happy to see again old acquaintances from the early days in England and had a long visit with Colonel MacFee. Colonel Cutler and Colonel MacFee were in complete agreement on the following points:

1. *Vascular surgery.*—Plastic tubes, over which suture could be done, might be better than the Blakemore tubes presently in use. If a vessel is ligated, it must be divided. All hospitals should make a definite assignment as to who should do the vascular surgery.

2. *Abdominal surgery.*—For left side procedures involving the large bowel, complete diversion of the fecal stream is desired; for the right side, an exteriorized opening is preferable. If the small intestine is damaged, it should be closed and not left as a separate opening. For combined head and abdomen casualties, the abdomen should be done first and the head later, by the 5th day, and preferably under local anesthesia.

3. Delayed suture should be practiced in evacuation hospitals if the patient must remain for an appreciable period of time before being further evacuated.

Colonel Cutler also asked Colonel MacFee if he would like an appointment as surgical consultant for the Fifteenth U.S. Army, a new field army, the headquarters of which had recently arrived in England. Colonel MacFee was favorably inclined toward such an assignment.

Elsewhere during the day, Colonel Cutler visited the 45th, 128th, and 96th Evacuation Hospitals and the 13th Field Hospital. On the whole, he found excellent work being done in these facilities and thoroughly competent surgical services. He found that a team from the 3d Auxiliary Surgical Group attached to a field hospital platoon consisted of one surgeon, two assistant surgeons (one for shock work), one anesthetist, and four corpsmen. The nurses, he found, were attached separately—four at a time—to a field hospital platoon from the group. This permitted two for night duty in the operating room and two for day duty. It had proved better than having nurses assigned directly to teams. There were reports that plasma reactions had been mild, and blood transfusion reactions were mostly of the pyrogenic type. It was the consensus in these hospitals that the European theater blood from England had given chills; the European theater Paris blood was full of clots; and the Zone of Interior blood was better, in that fewer reactions occurred, but contained too few red cells in relation to fluid for casualties in severe shock.

Meeting with First U.S. Army surgeon and departure.—On Saturday, 16 December, Colonel Cutler visited at length with General Rogers, the First U.S. Army surgeon, after earlier conferences with the chief of personnel in the Medical Section, Headquarters, First U.S. Army. General Rogers approved Colonel MacFee's transfer to the Fifteenth U.S. Army, if this were desired, and he favorably considered all of the personnel changes which had been conditionally agreed upon and coordinated with General Rogers' personnel officer. Finally, Colonel Cutler wrote: "I told General Rogers that such visits, particularly when two army consulting surgeons could be together with me, were of the most valuable and instructive type, and thanked him for the courtesies extended." Just as Colonel Cutler was concluding his meeting with General Rogers, reports arrived that Malmédy and Eupen in Belgium were being hard hit by what was supposedly a new weapon, and the decision was made to pull the 44th and 67th Evacuation Hospitals out of Malmédy.

On his return to Paris, Colonel Cutler visited the 25th General Hospital at Liége and Headquarters, Advance Section, Communications Zone, at Namur, Belgium. He reached Paris at 2300 hours that night.

Comments to Chief Surgeon on trip to Brussels and to First and Ninth U.S. Armies

Upon returning to Paris, Colonel Cutler provided the Chief Surgeon a copy of his journal describing his recent trip to Brussels and the First and Ninth U.S. Armies. The Chief Consultant in Surgery, in a cover memorandum, dated 19 December 1944, forwarding the journal of the trip, called certain important aspects of his visits to General Hawley's attention. One of the items which pertained to the Seventh U.S. Army, follows:

*   *   *   *   *   *   *

b. From the Seventh Army Consultants, while in Brussels, I found a sincere regret that members of the Professional Services Division, ETO, had not paid them more visits. I am afraid that we were scared off by a quotation from a letter from Colonel Rudolph (Seventh U.S. Army Surgeon) to Colonel Liston which Colonel Kimbrough circulated in the Professional Services Division, the following being quoted:—

"The commanding general issued instructions a long time ago to the effect that he expected potential visitors to be 'cleared' before their arrival in his area. On more than one occasion the chief of staff has personally questioned me as to the necessity and desirability of a proposed visit by some member of the medical section of a higher headquarters, and often inferring that the medical people were the worst offenders. In addition, the commanding general has severely pruned our headquarters throughout, and when he visits the section he always wants to know exactly who each one is and what they are doing."

Colonel Berry wanted to know whether we really were ETO consultants, which hurt a little bit. I had asked Colonel Kimbrough to run down the source of the quotation above, because no one from this office had visited the Seventh U.S. Army, except Colonel Middleton, and I am quite sure he gave no offence. This office took deep offence to the quotation from the letter, and therefore had not visited the Seventh Army. I expect to in the near future, unless Colonel Liston or you object to this.

Concerning Lt. Col. (later Col.) Gordon K. Smith of the Ninth U.S. Army, the Chief Consultant in Surgery advised the Chief Surgeon:

*   *   *   *   *   *   *

c. I would like to commend Lt. Col. Gordon Smith, Consultant to the Ninth U.S. Army. It is my impression that he knows more about the personnel in his field and evacuation hospitals than any of our army consultants. I told this to Colonel Shambora, and am in the hope that he will take steps to eventually elevate his rank to that held by the other army consultants.

Colonel Cutler reported the following concerning the general hospitals he visited:

*   *   *   *   *   *   *

3. Finally, and very important, I sensed in our general hospitals a deep sense of bitterness about the irrelative uselessness, as they put it. This turned up in the 30th, 298th, and 25th General Hospitals. Most of our good hospitals have the feeling that they have excellent personnel which has not been used. It is hard to counteract this, for they were stabled long before D-day, then acted as transit hospitals without a chance for real professional work, and are still acting as transit hospitals, or, as are the 25th, and 30th, stabling again. Apparently they are to act as transit hospitals again, and do not, therefore, have the opportunity to use their full professional talent. I have been consistently loyal in support of the movements dictated by this office. I find it extremely difficult to continuously support what from time to time seems to me not to be the best use of highly trained professional talent. Perhaps we can stabilize some of our good units soon and let them do high grade professional work for the good of the American soldier. I fully appreciate the flux and flow necessitated by the military situation, but I am equally sure that our good units could be put in places where they could carry on high grade professional work, and less good units could act as transit hospitals, under the present circumstances.

To Colonel Liston, Deputy Chief Surgeon, the Chief Consultant in Surgery addressed a terse and poignant note on 19 December, as follows:

In view of your interest in obtaining suitable transport for the consultants, you will be interested to know that the army consultants at Brussels arrived in nice big Packard Sedans, while the ETO consultants came in jeeps and command cars! [104]

New directives

During these first few months on the Continent, the consultants had been able to observe more directly and frequently a variety of medical treatment facilities, practices, and conditions. There had been many opportunities to discuss these observations with their fellow American medical officers and the medical officers in the services of the Allies. The initial implementation of new ideas or changes in thought concerning past practices had been carried out to considerable extent by personal contact with consultants in the subordinate echelons or through corrective action on the scene. But changes in policies and procedures could only be thoroughly implemented by directive, and many directives on professional matters were published toward the year's end as a direct result of earlier experiences during this period on the Continent.

Additions to directive on care of battle casualties.—One of the first directives to be published was Circular Letter No. 131, Office of the Chief Surgeon, ETOUSA, dated 8 November 1944, a supplement to Circular Letters No. 71 and 101, previously discussed, pertaining to the care of battle casualties. This was sorely needed, especially as it pertained to the care of fractures. Accordingly, the bulk of the directive concerned the treatment of wounds of bones and joints which was worked out by Colonel Cleveland working closely with the other senior consultants, the surgical consultant of the United

---

[104] Not all consultants arrived in Packard sedans. Col. Frank B. Berry, MC, Consultant in Surgery to the Seventh U.S. Army, arrived in an open command car. Consultants to the field armies routinely traveled in jeeps and command cars.—J. B. C., Jr.

Kingdom Base, and the Chief Consultant in Surgery. The portions pertaining strictly to orthopedic surgery have been reproduced elsewhere in this history.[105]

Under the section dealing with the treatment of wounds of bones and joints was also a subsection detailing policies and procedures to be observed in the care of injured hands. Earlier reference was made to efforts by Colonel Cutler and his subordinate consultants to establish special facilities for the adequate treatment of injuries to the hand. In this directive, emphasis was placed on early closure of fractured hands by secondary suture or skin graft and the insistence of active motion as early as possible. "Amputations of hands or fingers," the directive cautioned, "should be performed *only* where there is no possibility of restoring some useful function or when circulatory loss has resulted in complete necrosis of the part." The directive emphasized: "* * * an upper extremity prosthesis is not in any sense to be considered as an adequate substitute for a hand." As a measure further to implement these policies, a list of hand centers which had been established in the United Kingdom was prepared by Colonel Cutler, Colonel Morton, Colonel Cleveland, and Colonel Bricker for promulgation within the United Kingdom Base.

Circular Letter No. 131 also directed special measures to be observed in handling neurosurgical problems, in the care of the bladder in patients with spinal cord injury, in the care of injured nasal mucosa, in the management of colostomies, and in whole blood transfusions. In addition, this circular letter contained notes on radiology, and precautionary measures with respect to the condition of patients evacuated to the Zone of Interior. With respect to colostomies, the circular letter warned against a too short, approximated septum in the formation of a double-barreled Mikulicz colostomy and a too large initial opening in the loop type of colostomy. The directive also encouraged the closing of colostomies as soon as the wound was free from infection and the local edema of the bowel had subsided and before the patient was evacuated to the Zone of Interior. The directive called attention to the fact that many cases could be returned to duty in the theater.

Whole blood and transfusion.—Colonel Cutler, at the October meeting of the Chief Surgeon's Consultants' Committee, had mentioned that a new directive would be published defining transfusion reactions and stating what to do about them. This was accomplished by Administrative Memorandum No. 150, issued by the Office of the Chief Surgeon, under the dateline of 27 November 1944. The directive accepted the fact that reactions were bound to occur in the great number of transfusions being carried out. It dispelled major concern over allergic or pyrogenic reactions. For the relatively rare case in which bronchospasms occurred as an allergic reaction, the directive called for relief of the symptoms by subcutaneous injections of an Adrenalin (epinephrine) solution or intravenous administration of aminophylline. Hemolytic

---

[105] Medical Department, United States Army. Surgery in World War II. Orthopedic Surgery in the European Theater of Operations. Washington: U.S. Government Printing Office, 1956, Appendix A.

reactions, the directive recognized, were not common but were to be feared because death could result from hemolytic shock or uremia following renal damage. The administrative memorandum directed:

> Hemolytic reactions must be treated immediately and vigorously if survival of the patient is to be expected. Immediately upon the appearance of the symptoms of hemolytic shock the transfusion must be discontinued. Almost all patients will recover spontaneously when this is done. However, in patients with deep shock another transfusion of compatible blood should be started. All patients exhibiting hemolytic shock must be immediately alkalinized * * *.

The administrative memorandum also called for a report from each fixed hospital showing the total amount of blood given during any one week and the number of reactions encountered broken down into six subordinate categories. Fearing that the reporting provisions might be eliminated, Colonel Cutler, in forwarding the draft for publication, justified the reporting requirement on the basis that transfusion reactions were a prevailing problem and that good data were necessary if anything sound and constructive were to be done about the situation.

Equally important to the issuance of a directive is the followup to ensure compliance with it. With respect to the matter covered in the directive under discussion, Colonel Cutler, before the end of the year, was able to call attention to significant progress in following up the problem. At the Twenty-Sixth Meeting of the Chief Surgeon's Consultants' Committee in Paris on 30 December, he announced: "We have been quite disturbed about reports of reactions in patients who had received blood. Major Hardin has been up forward, and has come back with information on that." Major Hardin then explained:

> This report [the report called for by Admin. Memo. No. 150] that we have compiled has been very useful in making up our minds as to what is going on. Out of 3,741 transfusions that were given, 188 reactions of all types occurred. These were 3.7 percent pyrogenic and .48 percent hemolytic. That is high. It is four times as high as what we would like to see. I find that there is a lot of misinformation on how to distinguish between hemolytic and pyrogenic reaction. I pointed it out. It is very easy. All you do is draw 5 cc. of blood from the patient and spin it in the centrifuge. If the plasma is pink, you know the patient has had a hemolytic reaction. If not, you know he didn't. They were signing out a good many patients as hemoglobinuric nephrosis; patients who had died with anuria. When you go through their histories, you often find that anuria was present when they came to the hospital. Because the patient never put out any urine, they felt that the blood had killed the patient. The cause of this anuria has been discussed, and some think that in part it has been due to blast and in part to the shock and other people thought that there was something * * * due to alkalinization. The more we learn of patients not putting out urine, the more I am inclined to believe that it is not due to blood. There were some people who were giving patients 4,000 cc. of blood and then when they had a little febrile reaction, they read the directions and saw that they were supposed to have a 3,000 cc. intake, so they gave them 3,000 cc. of fluids more. This is particularly true in patients in whom anuria is found. Now, I am personally well satisfied with this reaction rate. I think it is pretty low, considering everything.
> I found errors in hospitals in handling blood. In the attempt to lower this rate more, there has been started a program to raise our own requirements about the handling of blood and sets. We are ready to go over that now.

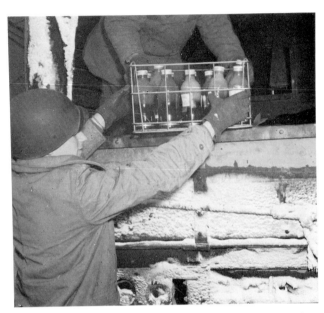

FIGURE 109.—A delivery of whole blood under freezing conditions, 16th Field Hospital, Boulaide, Luxembourg, 29 January 1945.

The other thing which we have done: we have learned that blood coming from the States is not inspected before it leaves the States. We have set up an inspection system here. It is inspected before it is distributed.

We warned all of the advanced blood banks about taking full care of the storage of blood, because we were running into danger of freezing of blood, even in refrigerators (fig. 109). We have asked for some ambulance heaters, and we are actually going to have to heat some of it. We found at least one unit that was warming blood before transfusion.

General Hawley was greatly pleased with this summary of the situation by Major Hardin. "That is all very enlightening, and it is very comforting," the Chief Surgeon said, "because these people howl, and I am glad we have something to howl back with. I suspected that this anuria point was due not to the blood itself." The Chief Surgeon then attributed to Stonewall Jackson, who, he said, was a man of very few words, the following statement: "I can guard against everything but the stupidity of my assistants." Paraphrasing this quotation, the Chief Surgeon alerted the consultants, saying: "You are in the same situation. You can guard your blood and use all precautions, but you can't guard against the stupidity of the people who are sometimes using the blood."

Professional care on hospital trains.—Supervision of professional care on hospital trains was effected by periodic checks at opportune moments. Since Major Robinson's trip on a hospital train movement, described earlier, there had been a notable incident wherein a general hospital had turned over to a hospital train a patient with dry gangrene of the hand because of a wound above the elbow. This was done with the expectation that it would be better professional care to let the line of demarcation be settled by time rather than to amputate early. To the consternation of everyone, the surgeon on the hospital train had proceeded immediately to amputate the extremity. On another occasion in mid-November, a hospital train had been loaded with serious casualties far up in the Third U.S. Army area. These casualties were to travel all the way to the port of Cherbourg through Paris for further evacuation to the United Kingdom. They were being sent by rail owing to the uncertain air evacuation situation. Colonel Cutler had sent Colonel Bricker and Colonel Canfield to "vet" the train when it arrived at Paris and had instructed them to use their judgment in supervising the removal of any casualties who could not reasonably continue through to Cherbourg. Colonel Cutler had gone to the 48th General Hospital the next day to inspect cases removed from the train, while Colonel Bricker had gone on with the train to Cherbourg.

Mindful of the dictum by the Chief Surgeon that professional care during transit was equally important with professional care of patients in hospitals, Colonel Cutler had conferred with members of the Evacuation Branch, Operations Division, Office of the Chief Surgeon, following Colonel Bricker's return from Cherbourg. As a result of this conference on care provided during hospital train movements, and in the light of observations that had been made from time to time, Colonel Cutler on 25 November submitted to the Office of the Chief Surgeon a memorandum containing a proposed circular letter concerning professional care on hospital trains. The proposed directive urged the continuous sorting on trains of the seriously ill from those who could travel further without detriment to their recovery. It described the types of casualties that would require special care and have to be removed at the first opportunity. It specified where certain categories of injuries would have to be detrained in order that they could obtain proper therapy. The proposed directive closed by giving suggestions on the care of immobilized patients in transit on hospital trains (fig. 110).

Since the scope of the directive pertained only to hospital train units, a limited portion of the theater's medical service, and since all hospital trains were directly under communications zone control, the directive was published, on 9 December 1944, as a command letter from the Office of the Surgeon, Headquarters, Communications Zone, ETOUSA, to commanding officers of all hospital trains on the Continent.

Guidance to disposition boards.—On 5 December 1944, Colonel Cutler submitted two directives for publication. One pertained to changes in a previous directive giving guidance to disposition boards and the other delineated hospitals established on the Continent for specialized treatment. Shortly before the invasion, Colonel Cutler had convinced the Chief Surgeon that some sort of a yardstick was necessary to serve as a guide to hospital disposition boards for the early determination and selection of patients to be evacuated to the Zone of Interior (p. 190). The previous directive had been published when the 180-day evacuation policy was in effect. But the evacuation policy had been dropped to 120 days in October 1944, and instructions had been given that a

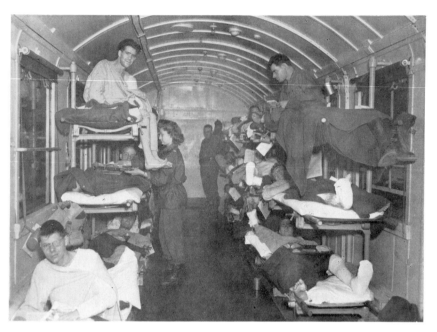

FIGURE 110.—Caring for immobilized casualties in a hospital train.

90-day policy would be in effect whenever crowding of facilities dictated it or when the available lift to the Zone of Interior could not be filled with cases selected under the 120-day policy.

Moreover, the many new general hospitals which had arrived since publication of the earlier directive were in a quandry over the disposition problem. In addition, certain station hospitals had from time to time been permitted to establish disposition boards and act as general hospitals in the selection of patients to be evacuated to the Zone of Interior. The situation was particularly acute in the United Kingdom where casualties destined for longer-term hospitalization had been evacuated from the Continent. On each occasion of his visits to the United Kingdom, Colonel Cutler had been advised by both Colonel Spruit and Colonel Morton that a revision of the outmoded directive was urgently required.

In view of these conditions, Colonel Cutler had obtained recommendations for changes and additions to the original directive from the senior consultants in surgery. He consolidated their recommendations and forwarded them to Colonel Kimbrough, on 5 December 1944, for any changes he desired to make with respect to genitourinary conditions. In forwarding the proposed modifications, Colonel Cutler noted that the situation made it clear that it was necessary to revise the conditions which automatically returned people to the Zone of Interior under the new hospitalization program.

By the time Colonel Cutler returned from his trip to Belgium and the First and Ninth U.S. Armies, the new directive (Circular Letter No. 142) had been promulgated. Portions of Circular Letter No. 142, issued by the Office of the Chief Surgeon, ETOUSA, on 8 December 1944, which pertained to surgical conditions making it advisable to evacuate a patient to the Zone of Interior under a 120- or 90-day evacuation policy, are contained in appendix C (p. 973). The list should become of increasing historic significance with the passage of years in view of the difficulty which always seems present when a decision must be made as to whether a soldier or officer remains in a theater of operations or goes home.

Hospitals for specialized treatment on the Continent.—Colonel Cutler's proposed directive for the establishment of hospitals for specialized treatment on the Continent had been worked out after careful and long planning. As of the time he had completed his draft (4 December) the hospitals designated to provide the specialized treatment were equipped and in a position to carry out their specialized mission, and the specialists necessary to provide the surgery were present. Colonel Cutler submitted his draft of the proposed directive on 5 December advising Colonel Kimbrough as follows:

1. Attached is a draft for a circular letter on specialized treatment, which has incorporated in it
   a. All the suggestions made by Operations Division, and
   b. Redesignation of certain hospitals after a more careful selection.
2. Recommend immediate publication of this circular.
3. When the matter of these specialized treatment centers was proposed, both the Hospitalization and the Operations Divisions proposed moving hospitals selected for such work into permanent buildings, if they are now in tented construction areas. Perhaps final approval of this letter should therefore pass through Hospitalization as well as Operations.

Colonel Cutler's proposed directive designated the following hospitals for the treatment of patients requiring specialized treatment:

	Hospital	*Area*
Neurosurgery units:		
	48th General Hospital	Paris
	298th General Hospital	Liége
	100th General Hospital	Toul
Thoracic surgery units:		
	48th General Hospital	Paris
	15th General Hospital	Liége
	5th General Hospital	Toul
Urological surgery units:		
	48th General Hospital	Paris
	298th General Hospital	Liége
	100th General Hospital	Toul
Units for plastic and maxillofacial surgery and surgical treatment of extensive burns:		
	108th General Hospital	Paris
	15th General Hospital	Liége
	5th General Hospital	Toul

The directive, in draft, specified: "Patients requiring treatment in neurosurgery, thoracic surgery, plastic and maxillofacial surgery, surgical treatment of extensive burns and urological surgery, when transfer to the United Kingdom is impracticable or inadvisable, will be sent without delay to the appropriate hospital designated * * *."

When Colonel Cutler returned from his extended trip in the field, he found that the directive had not been published. Investigating further, he learned that the heavy bombardment experienced just before leaving the First U.S. Army area had been in earnest and that the Germans had launched a large counteroffensive. He conferred with members of the Evacuation Branch and Operations Division of the Chief Surgeon's Office, who informed Colonel Cutler that the directive had to be held up in view of the fluid situation. They decided, however, that there would be no objection to the Seine Base Section surgeon's issuing a directive pertaining to the special facilities in the Paris area. General Hawley, later in the month, decided that the designation of the specialized facilities should be made but that there could not be the rigid enforcement of the distribution of patients as was exercised in the United Kingdom.

Christmas and year's end

Even during war in an active combat theater, a few days of idyllic peace may suddenly appear. Colonel Cutler's third Christmas in the European theater was one of these, a day far-removed from the routines of war. He was able to meet his son, Capt. Elliott C. Cutler, Jr., Inf., who had recently arrived in England with an infantry division. Colonel Cutler, doting parent for the day, toured London leisurely with his young West Point son. Later, the two joined Admiral and Mrs. Gordon-Taylor for Christmas dinner.

The year ended with the lengthy but most worthwhile meeting of the Chief Surgeon's Consultants' Committee on Saturday, 30 December. This time, Colonel Cutler was in the chair since Colonel Kimbrough had been returned to the Zone of Interior for a period of indefinite temporary duty. Among other things, Colonel Cutler arranged for Colonel Tovell to present to the Chief Surgeon a very comprehensive analysis of various anesthetics and procedures being used in the theater according to the type of medical facility. It had been mentioned by the other consultants, too, but it was after this report that General Hawley made the statement which perhaps more than ever impressed the consultants with the Chief Surgeon's true, fine mettle. General Hawley said:

This is a very splendid study here. It is very illuminating. It only to me emphasizes the splendid work that has been done in anesthesia in this theater. It is a reflection of the energy, the ability, and the aggressive, and I might say religious, application that Colonel Tovell has shown, and I would like to take this opportunity to say that, however much in the early days I might not have absorbed as much of his enthusiasm as he thought I should have absorbed, I have been converted, and I am quite convinced that the fine surgical results that have been gained in this theater are in no small way attributable to Colonel Tovell and the fine * * * service that he has brought here. I say that very sincerely.

The New Year

Need for a united theater

One of Colonel Cutler's utterances as the new year began was to the effect that the political implications of SOLOC were almost insurmountable, but a united theater was essential. The reader may recall that Colonel Cutler, following his return from Brussels, had given the Chief Surgeon due warning that he fully intended to visit the Seventh U.S. Army in spite of apparent reluctance by that Army to have visitors from theater headquarters. The Surgeon, SOLOC, had also requested that consultants from European theater headquarters refrain from visiting the SOLOC area until it could be established on firmer footing.

Meanwhile, the situation in the Ardennes and Alsace areas had tied down personnel of the Chief Surgeon's Office pretty much to the headquarters in Paris. While the theater surgical consultants were awaiting an opportunity to visit the units to the south and to observe the type of work being done, a letter from The Surgeon General questioned the Chief Surgeon, ETOUSA, on the numbers of orthopedic casualties with internal fixation who were arriving in the Zone of Interior from the European theater. It was quite obvious that most of these cases had been evacuated from Marseilles, and there was an urgent need for visits to the areas of southern France so that responsible persons at theater headquarters could speak intelligently on all aspects of the theater's medical responsibilities.

At the aforementioned 30 December meeting of the Chief Surgeon's Consultants' Committee, Colonel Cutler pointedly asked:

Some of the members of this group are going to visit SOLOC hospitals. There is one thing that has been brought up that we need clarification on. Hospitals there have been doing internal fixation of fractures. We wish to go with a clear mind as to what position we take. Shall we ask them to live up to ETO directives?

General Hawley replied:

Yes. I would like to stop at this point. I had to send that thing to the Surgeon General; I couldn't postpone it any more. I stated frankly that in that type of case where proper reduction could not be obtained by traction, which applied to only a very small amount of the cases that a certain amount of internal fixation of fractures has been done, but it is true that the number of that is from the Southern Line of Communications.

Further explaining General Hawley's answer, Colonel Cleveland commented:

It must be, General Hawley. After I wrote a little memo for that letter of yours in answer to General Kirk, I went over the disposition proceedings and I looked over fairly carefully those of the 21st and the 26th, but these hospitals are in SOLOC. The 21st had a very high percent of the internal fixation. It is often hard to get the information, but you know they are doing it, and I think it is only by going down there to find out what they are doing.

"Yes," General Hawley confirmed, "they have got to stop it." He continued: "Where proper reduction cannot be effected, then it is all right. I think even General Kirk agrees that we have got to do that." Then, in reply to Colonel Cutler's original question, the Chief Surgeon stated emphatically: "They are going to adhere to the policies of this office, or else."

On 31 December, the day after the meeting, Colonel Cutler hastened to write the following in a letter to Colonel Shook:

> I am frightfully sorry but I have been unable to get over to see you, and, now that I am holding down Colonel Kimbrough's desk as well as my own, it is impossible. Several of the officers on our staff will be over to see you shortly and I am giving this note to Colonel Spurling, the consultant in neurosurgery, who is traveling with Colonel Canfield, the consultant in otolaryngology and ophthalmology. These officers will see all your hospitals and, after a discussion with you, will also visit your southern area and study newly arrived hospitals. I am sure we all have the keenest desire to be of service to you, and please ask these officers to do anything you wish.
>
> Since I can not come myself, and since you and I have discussed the matter of your consultant in surgery, and after a long discussion with Colonel Berry, Consultant in Surgery, Seventh Army, who turned up at a meeting in Brussels, I am happy to recommend to you that Colonel Ira Ferguson become your consultant in general surgery. If this is in accordance with your desires, will you please take steps to implement this and move him to your headquarters. Perhaps by the time this is done I will be over to see you. Meanwhile, I hate to hold up anything important for better service in your area.

Colonel Canfield and Colonel Spurling returned from their visit to SOLOC and the Seventh U.S. Army and conferred with Colonel Cutler on 7 January 1945. Their visit had been most rewarding in respect to information gathered. General Hawley, himself, also planned to tour the SOLOC and Seventh U.S. Army areas, and asked Colonel Cutler to accompany him. After meeting with the Chief Surgeon on 9 January and obtaining a firm date for the proposed trip, Colonel Cutler telephoned Colonel Shook on 10 January and informed the SOLOC surgeon that General Hawley and Colonel Cutler would be visiting him on 14 January.

Visit to SOLOC and CONAD.—On Sunday, 14 January 1945, General Hawley and Colonel Cutler departed Paris at 0900 and arrived at Dijon at 1630. The Chief Surgeon contacted Colonel Shook by telephone and joined him, while Colonel Cutler proceeded to confer with Col. Ira Ferguson. The two quickly reviewed the professional status of all hospitals in CONAD (Continental Advance Section) and the Delta Base Section, the two base sections subordinate to SOLOC. They spoke especially of the problem of bringing up newly arrived general hospitals to a respectable professional standard, and it seemed to Colonel Cutler that the older established hospitals "had plenty of export material * * * for helping new institutions." Colonel Ferguson also informed Colonel Cutler that he would not particularly care for a full-time job as surgical consultant at SOLOC headquarters. He hoped that another officer could be found for the position, or that, with consultants at each of the two bases, a third at SOLOC headquarters would be unnecessary.

Later that evening, Colonel Cutler joined General Hawley, Colonel Shook, Col. Harry A. Bishop, MC, and Col. Crawford F. Sams, MC, for dinner at the

CONAD mess and conferences in Colonel Shook's quarters. They decided to defer the matter of appointing consultants until Colonel Cutler had completed his visit. Colonel Cutler promised to help obtain personnel from the field armies to "shore up" vacancies in the new SOLOC hospitals. Colonel Shook, in return, promised to distribute pertinent circular letters of the Office of the Chief Surgeon, ETOUSA, so that all medical treatment facilities in SOLOC could be apprised of European theater policy. While the visitors from Headquarters, ETOUSA, were most pleasantly entertained, General Hawley and Colonel Cutler could see that the SOLOC staff was not going to acquiesce to theater policies and procedures without some difficulty.

The next day, Colonel Cutler visited the 46th General Hospital at Besançon and was not impressed, although the orthopedic work and anesthesia were good. He thought the hospital was not closing wounds as early as should be done. After lunch at this hospital, Colonel Cutler returned to Dijon where he inspected the 36th General Hospital. The hospital and surgical service were excellent. The 36th General Hospital, with 2,000 beds available, had had a census of as many as 3,000 patients on occasion and had 2,873 patients on the day visited. After completing his hospital visit, Colonel Cutler took the night train to Marseilles with General Hawley and Colonel Ferguson.

Visit to Delta Base Section.—At Marseilles, the headquarters of Delta Base Section, the party was met by Col. Vinnie H. Jeffress, MC, base section surgeon. After breakfast at the headquarters mess, Colonel Cutler visited the 70th and 80th Station Hospitals which were acting as holding hospitals for evacuation to the Zone of Interior and were also providing local station hospital service. As expected, there were a good many cases with internal fixation. Soldiers with enucleations had been provided poorly fitted glass eyeballs not nearly as good as the acrylic eyes which were being made in the dental laboratories in the rest of the European theater. There were many patients earmarked for evacuation to the Zone of Interior who should have been retained in the theater. There then followed a visit to the 235th General Hospital. Here again, Colonel Cutler was not satisfied with the work being done, there was no clear idea of proper disposition procedures, and there was confusion because the hospital was operating partly under MTOUSA and partly under ETOUSA directives. Lunch at a hostel for nurses provided the opportunity to meet the commanding officers of the 69th and 78th Station Hospitals who had traveled from Cannes and Nice.

The afternoon visits were a revelation of another sort. Colonel Cutler found the 43d General Hospital affiliated with Emory University, Atlanta, Ga., and the 3d General Hospital, affiliated with Mount Sinai Hospital, New York, N.Y., excellent in their professional work. Colonel Ferguson was the chief of surgical service at the former, and there Colonel Cutler found the orthopedic work particularly good, although many cases were being bone plated. At the 3d General Hospital, Colonel Cutler was shown a ward for abdominal surgery run by Maj. (later Lt. Col.) Leon Ginzberg, MC. Colonel

Cutler considered this the most interesting and beautifully run ward seen on the whole trip.

Back to SOLOC headquarters and CONAD.—On the night train back to Dijon, Colonel Cutler was able to have a long discussion with Colonel Ferguson on the overall hospitalization plans for SOLOC. Colonel Cutler recorded that they were in general agreement on the following: "* * * The forward general hospitals at CONAD should absorb all the people who could go back to duty within 30 days, and have a high-powered reconditioning center. The rear hospitals, that is those in Delta Base, should take up the cases requiring long hospitalization, whether going to the Zone of Interior or not." In such a scheme, the station hospitals in and around the Marseilles area could act as holding hospitals for water evacuation to the Zone of Interior. Too, there would be a need for hospitals to provide specialized care. These should be in the Delta Base Section, and Colonel Cutler suggested that the 43d General Hospital could well take care of thoracic surgery and neurosurgery and the 3d General Hospital, of maxillofacial, abdominal, and hand surgery.

Back again in the Dijon area, Colonel Cutler visited the 23d General Hospital, the affiliated unit from Buffalo at Vittel, France. Here, he met Lt. Col. Baxter Brown, MC, chief of surgery, whom he described as "an excellent man." Colonel Brown was a urologist, but his services had been requested by the CONAD surgeon as surgical consultant for the command. Colonel Cutler also visited the Sixth Army Group headquarters where the surgeon, Col. Oscar L. Reeder, MC, explained the French medical service of the First French Army, a component of the Sixth Army Group.

In the afternoon, Colonel Cutler proceeded to the 21st General Hospital at Mirecourt, France, which he described as follows: "* * * an enormous new insane institution spread out over a mile, but well adapted." Commanding officers and chiefs of surgery from nearby hospitals assembled at the 21st General Hospital for meetings and dinner with the guests from up north. The hospitals represented included the 236th, 237th, and 238th General Hospitals, and the 23d, 35th, and 51st Station Hospitals. Colonel Berry from the Seventh U.S. Army, Colonel Ferguson, and Colonel Brown were also present. Colonel Cutler had the wonderful opportunity to have a long discussion with these chiefs of surgery and the surgical consultants—it was becoming quite obvious, now, that Colonel Ferguson would be the consultant for Delta Base and Colonel Brown, for CONAD. Colonel Cutler, as a result of his visits to the various facilities in SOLOC, urged the early restoration to duty of all patients and less use of internal fixation.

That evening, there were two meetings of great consequence for the fostering of close and cooperative relationships between those at Headquarters, ETOUSA, and the personnel of SOLOC. Of pertinence to the Chief Consultant in Surgery were the following, as recorded in his official diary:

Later in the evening we had a long meeting, attended by General Hawley, Colonels Bishop, Berry, Ferguson and Brown, regarding functions and duties of consultants. We agreed it was unnecessary for the moment to have free [full-time] consultants for SOLOC, but accepted the consultants chosen for CONAD and DELTA. These consultants will remain in their hospital posts, will feel free to go out and examine institutions when they desire, will not speak to Commanding Officers or members of units regarding any changes they may deem wise and will not make promises to Commanding Officers or people concerning new equipment, but when they have examined their unit will go back and give a complete report to the Surgeon, SOLOC. Further, all consultants will feel free to correspond directly with their consultant colleagues in any base section or at ETO headquarters without such letters going through the base surgeon. This facility of professional correspondence is fundamentally to better the professional care, and General Hawley urged this strongly as the very basis of the consultant group. Colonel Bishop is to distribute ETO circulars shortly. Colonel Shook will be given a report of all this, and then will establish any other policies which he deems wisest for SOLOC. At this discussion, the matter was brought up as to whether men fresh from hospital who might later be general assignment could go on limited duty for 3 months and then be reevaluated.

Still later in the evening there was a meeting of professional people at which there was a long discussion * * *[concerning] the reasons * * * [for] internal fixation. These would seem to be as follows:

1. Fractures into joints.

2. Multiple fractures, long bones.

3. Where fragments of fracture may possibly injure blood vessel, if reduction is not perfect.

Visit to Seventh U.S. Army.—The following day, Thursday, 18 January, General Hawley, Colonel Cutler, and Colonel Berry motored to Headquarters, Seventh U.S. Army, Lunéville, France, after making rounds at the 21st General Hospital. At Seventh U.S. Army headquarters, they were met by Maj. Gen. Arthur A. White, USA, Chief of Staff, and Col. Myron P. Rudolph, MC, army surgeon. General Hawley impressed on Colonel Rudolph the importance which was being placed on the rotation of medical officers between the field armies and communications zone facilities. The Chief Surgeon made it clear that requests for rotation had to be initiated within the field armies. He specifically instructed Colonel Rudolph that correspondence pertaining to such interchanges was to be made directly to his office and not with the base sections.

Privately with Colonel Berry, Colonel Cutler discussed the administration of the 2d Auxiliary Surgical Group and the availability of qualified surgeons. The Seventh U.S. Army had one-half of the 2d Auxiliary Surgical Group. The group's executive officer, Maj. (later Lt. Col.) James M. Sullivan, MC, customarily remained forward of army headquarters and, from this forward location, disposed and supervised the teams. He habitually maintained close liaison with Colonel Berry, who remained with the surgeon, Colonel Rudolph, at Seventh U.S. Army headquarters. This had worked well, and Colonel Berry told Colonel Cutler that it would be a mistake for the consulting surgeon of a field army to try to operate directly the auxiliary surgical group, as Colonel Crisler was doing in the First U.S. Army, in addition to his duties as the surgical consultant. Colonel Berry also confirmed his advice earlier offered that there were many surgeons in the evacuation hospitals and the auxiliary surgical group to the Seventh U.S. Army who could go to the new hospitals in SOLOC to strengthen their surgical services.

Return to Paris.—Before leaving the Seventh U.S. Army area, General Hawley and Colonel Cutler visited the 9th and 95th Evacuation Hospitals. After this, they proceeded to the 2d General Hospital which was just setting up at Nancy and spent the night of 18 January there. The next day, they went to Headquarters, 8th Armored Division, at Pont-à-Mousson, and were given a guide by the assistant division commander to take them to Raucourt, where General Hawley's son was located. After a pleasant reunion with the son of the Chief Surgeon, General Hawley and Colonel Cutler visited the 58th General Hospital in Commercy and, finally, arrived back in Paris at 1730 on 19 January.

Back in Paris, Colonel Cutler provided the Chief Surgeon with a summary of items which had been discussed, a draft of a letter to Colonel Shook confirming agreements made, and a draft of a letter for the Chief Surgeon to send to The Surgeon General explaining the three general circumstances when the internal fixation of fractures should be permitted. Colonel Cutler initiated necessary procedures in coordination with the Dental Division in the Chief Surgeon's Office to train dental personnel in SOLOC to fabricate acrylic artificial eyes. He also made the necessary arrangements to have shipped to the Seventh U.S. Army some units of the mobile surgical team assembly for use by attached French surgical teams which had been trained by the U.S. Army Medical Department.

It is interesting to note, in the letter on use of internal fixation under special conditions, Colonel Cutler wrote: "We have not utilized these procedures in ETOUSA, but we are always willing and eager to improve our service to the soldier, and I think we are convinced that under special circumstances these procedures are desirable." Certainly, these thoughts clearly indicate that, however strong Colonel Cutler personally felt about any matter, he always maintained an open mind to the suggestions and feelings of others. On this occasion, he had gone to SOLOC with a strong obligation to curtail the widespread use of internal fixation in the hospitals of that command, but, nevertheless, he had returned to vindicate their practices, where warranted.

Trenchfoot meeting

But a few days after Colonel Cutler's return from southern France, medical and surgical consultants from throughout the European theater began to assemble in Paris for a combined meeting and a coordinated assault on a major problem which the winter fighting in the Rhineland had fostered for the Medical Department—the problem of trenchfoot. Present also were representatives of the theater's preventive medicine activities and members of the trenchfoot study group (surgical) at the 108th General Hospital, Paris, and the medical group in England at the 7th General Hospital.

The proceedings of this meeting held at the 108th General Hospital on 24 January 1945 are more thoroughly covered in another volume of this history.[106]

---

[106] Medical Department, United States Army Cold Injury, Ground Type. Washington: U.S. Government Printing Office, 1958, pp. 179–184.

But, in summary, General Hawley opened the all-day sessions and expressed the hope that agreement on the means to prevent and treat trenchfoot might come from the meeting. Col. John E. Gordon, MC, chief of the Preventive Medicine Division, Office of the Chief Surgeon, demonstrated some intriguing rates in relation to smaller units of battalion size and showed the prevalence of trenchfoot with respect to the command of such units. By field armies, Colonel Gordon showed, in order of severity, rates for the Third, First, Seventh, and Ninth U.S. Armies. He recommended the rotation of combat troops and better foot discipline. Lt. Col. Richard P. Mason, MC, of the Preventive Medicine Division, Office of the Chief Surgeon, emphasized the value of discipline and dry socks and the proper use of the shoepac.

Captain Leigh from the study group at the 108th General Hospital presented proposals for classifying patients for sorting and evacuation. He suggested that a circular letter now be published on the type of treatment which would be beneficial in the army areas and the criteria under which patients would be evacuated to the communications zone and to the Zone of Interior. Colonel Kneeland, medical consultant for the United Kingdom Base, explained the benefits of active exercise in the treatment of patients restorable to duty. Maj. Laurence B. Ellis, MC, studying trenchfoot at the 7th General Hospital, called attention to the remarkable rapidity of the disappearance of edema with the use of a thoracic respirator. He pointed out that this result was more rapid with the use of the respirator than with exercise or position of the patient, but that an explanation was wanting. It was observed, however, that femoral vein pressures were definitely diminished.

Colonel Crisler explained procedures used in the First U.S. Army in the management of trenchfoot cases (p. 290). He spoke of recurrent trenchfoot, asked for the criteria to differentiate trenchfoot and frostbite, and warned of the importance of associated injuries. Colonel Odom and Lt. Col. Guy H. Gowen, MC, presented the experience of the Third and Seventh U.S. Armies, respectively. Others spoke of the frequent superficiality of lesions studied and of the finding of an intact nervous system in most cases.

During the general discussion, there was agreement that amputations should rarely be done for uncomplicated trenchfoot and that pain was an insufficient symptom for removing a soldier from duty. Cases to be evacuated to the Zone of Interior, it was generally observed, should either show obvious tissue damage or have associated combat exhaustion. Those who at the end of 5 or 6 weeks of treatment still evidenced disturbed physiology, it was recommended, should also be evacuated to the Zone of Interior. The conferees were convinced that sympathectomy was undesirable, except for late manifestations of Raynaud's disease.

Colonel Cutler recorded his opinion, as follows: "The remarks made by Colonel [Sterling A.] Wood, [Regimental Commander,] 313th Infantry * * * in both afternoon and evening were more effective than any of the professional discussion." Colonel Wood was an Infantry regimental commander. While a patient in a general hospital for other reasons, he had become personally interested in the tremendous wastage of manpower he had observed in the number of patients coming through with cold injury. He had personally acquainted himself with the facts then available and had studied the means by which a unit commander could curtail this great loss. Colonel Wood, before returning to duty, had spoken to Gen. Omar N. Bradley, the 12th Army Group commander, about what the line should do in preventing cold injury. At this trenchfoot meeting, he mentioned that directives to the line had to be brief and specific. He explained that new socks were now coming up at night with the rations and recommended that each soldier keep extra socks inside his shirt to keep them warm and dry. Colonel Wood emphasized the difficulty of keeping all company commanders apprised of the importance of preventive measures and of maintaining proper procedures in the prevention of cold injury because of heavy losses among his officers. Since D-day, he stated, the 313th Infantry had lost 200 officers and 4,800 men.

The occasion of this trenchfoot meeting also gave the Chief Consultant in Surgery the opportunity to speak with his surgical colleagues on many pressing matters of the moment. A dinner was given by General Hawley for all the participants at the meeting, and a period of lucid, informal discussions followed. Not a few of the visitors also attended the meeting of the Chief Surgeon's Consultants' Committee with General Hawley the following day. Further talks on items which were discussed in Paris at this time were taken up again after Colonel Cutler flew to the United Kingdom on Sunday, 28 January.

One of the factors which permitted Colonel Cutler to fly to England at this time was the return of Colonel Kimbrough from the United States one week previously.

United Kingdom revisited

Thoracic pulmotor.—One of the things Colonel Cutler looked into on this visit to the United Kingdom was the functioning of the thoracic pulmotor at the 7th General Hospital, as used for the treatment of trenchfoot. The Chief Surgeon had classified all activities at this hospital in the possibility that, if the experiments being conducted there were going to provide something truly constructive, the enemy should not have the benefit of our discoveries.

Colonel Cutler learned that the machine induced a negative pressure of 10 or 12 mm. of mercury and was being used 1 hour daily for from 7 to 15 days per patient. Studies showed that trenchfoot patients submitted to this treatment late did less well than those submitted early. Moreover, patients originally apparently relieved of symptoms by this treatment were experiencing recurrence of symptoms. Little scientific information had been gathered on the physiological correlates to the machine's actions—decrease in femoral vein pressure, elevation of diaphragm with inspiration rather than depression, and unchanging pulse rate and blood pressure throughout the course of the machine's action.

Since little information had been gathered on the unusual action of the diaphragm, Colonel Cutler suggested that fluoroscopy be carried out. He pointed out that the apparatus was aluminum and that aluminum would not obstruct the roentgen rays.

Finally, Colonel Cutler noted in his journal: "I was not greatly impressed with this machine."

The Chief Consultant in Surgery spent the remainder of the day individually checking cold injury cases on the wards in this hospital. He was appalled to learn of the indiscriminate awarding of the Purple Heart decoration to frostbite cases of very minor severity. Such actions were making a farce of the decoration, he declared.

Meeting of United Kingdom Base surgical consultants.—Colonel Morton had arranged for a meeting of all the surgical consultants in the United Kingdom Base Section. These consultants—coordinators in surgery at the hospital centers and specialist consultants strategically located at various hospital centers to act as regional consultants in their specialty—had assembled on Thursday, 1 February 1945, at the 7th General Hospital. Colonel Wright from the Air Forces and Col. Baxter Brown, MC, surgical consultant to CONAD, were also present. Colonel Brown had come to England with Colonel Cutler following the trenchfoot meetings in order to observe the organization for and care of patients in the United Kingdom Base Section. General Hawley, who had flown over to England, welcomed the group and pointed out the debt of the Army to the doctors. He asked them to try to assume fully the responsibility of the early restoration to duty of those who could be restored, pointing out the danger of trying to restore to duty those who could not be brought up to the standard. He mentioned that the alleged sending to replacement depots of those unfit for duty was currently a matter of joint investigation by the Chief Surgeon's Office and the theater Inspector General's Office.

Colonel Cutler then discussed with the group the overall system for the care of the wounded American soldier, beginning at the forward areas and ending up either with restoration to duty or evacuation to the Zone of Interior. He stressed particularly the importance of sorting and maintained that, if sorting was properly done all along the chain of evacuation, most of the problems to which those in the United Kingdom were heir would disappear.

"The next matter under discussion," Colonel Cutler later reported, "was early restoration to duty." He recorded:

I placed before the group the hope that within 2 weeks they could evacuate 5,000 beds in the United Kingdom of patients and bring some relief to our pressing need for beds. The matter of a more vigorous attack on the wounded soldier and a greater effort to make him exercise and move was brought forward as being the most important factor.

The rest of the morning was devoted to the improvement of current circular letters on the treatment of battle casualties. Particular stress was placed on the improvement of instructions concerning abdominal surgery, fractures, trenchfoot, hernia, and thoracic surgery.

The discussion on thoracic surgery was continued throughout the afternoon. First, it was brought out by the thoracic surgeons from the special treatment facilities that casualties were taking an extremely long time reaching them—an average of some 30 days after wounding. This fact, they stated, was completely nullifying the advantages of having special treatment facilities, since the patients reached them in bad condition and unsuitable for early primary treatment. Another difficulty, it was noted, was the reticence of individuals to accept thoracic cases as fit for duty even when they had been playing baseball and walking 4 or 5 miles a day. There seemed to be a prevailing psychological barrier that soldiers wounded in the thorax could not go back to duty. Facing this problem squarely, the Chief Consultant in Surgery was obliged to conclude: "I am afraid to do this whole thing properly we will have to re-educate all of the doctors in the FFRS (Field Force Replacement System)." Finally, Colonel Cutler received many sound ideas on specific items which would have to be included in a directive on thoracic surgery. Before returning to the Continent, Colonel Cutler was able to work up the data for the thoracic surgery directive in more or less final form with Colonel Morton and Colonel Miscall.

End of Long Winter Campaign

Another round of directives

Colonel Cutler crossed the Channel to France on 3 February 1945 with General Grow and Colonel Wright. In the afternoon, he spent his time preparing the new "professional circular" for publication. On 4 February, three new directives were ready to be submitted for publication in rapid fashion. One was the professional circular on the care of battle casualties, another dealt with changes to the list of conditions issued to disposition boards for guidance in selecting patients for return to the Zone of Interior, and the third was a paper on priorities for air evacuation to the Zone of Interior. Before going to the United Kingdom, in fact before the trenchfoot meeting, Colonel Cutler had submitted another directive, in draft, pertaining to information given to casualties. Immediately after, and as a result of, the trenchfoot meeting, the draft of a directive on trenchfoot had also been submitted.

Information to casualties.—Colonel Cutler had originally intended to include the item pertaining to information being given casualties in the new directive on care of battle casualties. Colonel Bricker, however, convinced him that the matter was so important that it should be published separately. Consequently, it was issued by the Office of the Chief Surgeon on 31 January 1945 as Circular Letter No. 11. The reader will note that this directive pertained but little to professional matters outwardly; nevertheless, it had much to do with the successful rehabilitation of a casualty to duty and without his returning again to the medical chain of evacuation for the same injury. The directive, as published, was terse and quite self-explanatory. It stated:

1. Under no circumstances will medical officers in forward hospitals, whether Army units or general or station hospitals, tell casualties that their injury is such as to necessarily take them to the Zone of Interior. Frequently, what appears to be an injury necessitating evacuation to the Zone of Interior turns out to be recoverable, and, if the soldier has been told that he is to go to the Zone of Interior, the reverse of this decision

leaves him disappointed and embittered, and lowers his usefulness to the Army in the future.

2. The practice of discussing the disposition of patients in hospital wards in the presence of the patient himself or of other patients must be stopped. All disposition board proceedings must be held confidential. Giving the patient strong implication that he may go to the Zone of Interior should be guarded against until final movement of patient commences.

Trenchfoot directive.—The trenchfoot directive was submitted on 28 January 1945 immediately following the meeting at the 108th General Hospital. It stated that TB MED (War Department Technical Bulletin) 81, which had been reproduced in the European theater, was the basic directive on the treatment of cold injury. However, the new directive, Circular Letter No. 18, Office of the Chief Surgeon, ETOUSA, dated 21 February 1945, gave additional advice on therapy based on current information gained in the theater. This guidance was in two parts—treatment in the forward area and treatment in fixed hospitals. The important part of the directive was a greatly simplified chart that attempted to show how to classify this type of casualty and to aid in the evaluation and disposition of these casualties. Dividing trenchfoot cases into mild (first degree), moderate (second degree), and severe (third degree), the directive showed under each of these categories what to expect in the way of history and physical findings and how the cases in the three categories were to be disposed of. The physical findings were further broken down into those observable during the hyperemic and posthyperemic stages and in the motor functions of the foot.

When Colonel Cutler was in England shortly after submitting this directive for publication, he discovered in no uncertain terms how necessary it was. During the meeting with the United Kingdom Base surgical consultants, Colonel Cutler was informed by the consultants that the routine care of cold injury was the responsibility of the medical service in the hospitals of that base as differentiated from the surgical service, and that the internists had not yet decided who could or could not be returned to duty.

Certain directives, however, by reason of the fact that they had been issued by higher headquarters, could not be changed or countermanded at the ETOUSA level. The directive pertaining to the awarding of the Purple Heart for frostbite was one of these. As it was seen, Colonel Cutler had found that the awarding of the Purple Heart decoration was being badly handled, but the basic directive permitting this had been issued by the War Department. Accordingly, the only action Colonel Cutler could take was to prepare for General Hawley's signature a letter to The Surgeon General requesting that he take action to correct the situation. The letter, as prepared in draft by Colonel Cutler, follows:

We are greatly troubled by War Department regulations stating that the Purple Heart is given for "Severe frostbite". We have qualified severe frostbite as follows:—

"The words 'severely frostbitten' will be interpreted to apply to only those cases of frostbite in which the lesion is so extensive and lasting that cells are killed and the result will show actual loss of substance; either loss of a digit or a slough which extends throughout the whole thickness of the corium."

The fact is that with the temperature just at freezing, one day above and one below, and with "cold injury" the pathological agent, it is almost impossible to make a distinguishing diagnosis. Thus, some soldiers get a Purple Heart and others do not. As a result our wards contain many embittered Infantry men. This is emphasized when the "trenchfoot" victim has a greater injury than the "frostbite" casualty. It would appear that the Medical Department is asked to apply a policy which it did not establish or suggest and which it finds impossible to administer fairly. Forward units confer the Purple Heart and under pressure from Line Commanders, who demand liberality in order to keep troops reasonably mollified, are naturally not too strict. The Purple Heart is gradually becoming worse than a joke.

I think this is going to give us all a headache, but, still worse, it has greatly disturbed combat soldiers. Men with simple blisters from frostbite are getting the Purple Heart and men with incapacitating lesions from trench foot get nothing!

If you agree in this, perhaps you will take this up with the War Department and see if there can be any change in the present regulations.[107]

Care of battle casualties.—Circular Letter No. 23, Care of Battle Casualties, 17 March 1945, issued by the Office of the Chief Surgeon, ETOUSA, was the last comprehensive directive on the surgical care of the wounded to be prepared under the direction of Colonel Cutler during the period of hostilities in the European theater. This directive, together with the Manual of Therapy, ETOUSA, Circular Letter No. 71, 15 May 1944, Circular Letter No. 101, 30 July 1944, and Circular Letter No. 131, 8 November 1944, all from the Office of the Chief Surgeon, ETOUSA, constituted the sum total of basic policies which prevailed during the period from D-day to V–E Day with reference to the surgical treatment of the wounded. The Manual of Therapy and the first circular letter, the reader will recall, were prepared before the invasion and stood in good stead—good enough to be still applicable in most respects at the war's end. The second letter published in July 1944 was a hurried affair to correct the mistakes which had been observed during the initial stages of the invasion. And, in November, with the difficult evacuation situation, Circular Letter No. 131 had been published, dealing extensively with the management of fractures, care of hand injuries, colostomies, and other items which were of immediate concern at the time and which required standardization.

And lastly, the new circular letter was the result of observations made by Colonel Cutler, the senior consultants in surgery, and the many consultants in subordinate commands—whether in field armies or base sections—throughout the course of this campaign in the Rhineland. This directive, together with its predecessors, tells a story which might well be entitled, "Surgery in the European Theater, World War II." The first of these circular letters has been reproduced as appendix B (p. 963), and, in like fashion, the last of the series, Circular Letter No. 23, Office of the Chief Surgeon, ETOUSA, of 1945, is reproduced as appendix D (p. 977).

---

[107] Memoradum, Professional Services Division (Col. E. C. Cutler, MC) to Chief Surgeon, ETOUSA, 4 Feb. 1945, subject: Letter to Surgeon General re Purple Heart Award for Frostbite and Trench Foot.

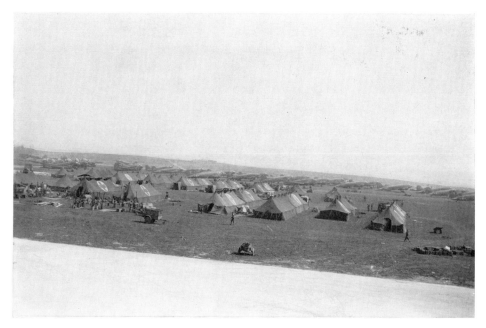

FIGURE 111.—The 91st Medical Gas Treatment Battalion operating as an air evacuation holding unit at Giessen, Germany. Note the great numbers of aircraft available.

Hospitals for specialized treatment on Continent.—Some time later, Colonel Cutler's directive, prepared in November 1944 and pertaining to hospitals for specialized treatment on the Continent, was approved for publication. Modified to bring it up to date, the directive eventually appeared as Circular Letter No. 32, Office of the Chief Surgeon, ETOUSA, dated 6 April 1945. Ironically, however, the field armies, by that time, had moved so rapidly that they had left the general hospitals in the forward sections of the communications zone far behind, and casualties were reaching hospitals in the Paris area by air more rapidly than they could be evacuated by land transportation to the intervening hospitals where some of the specialized treatment facilities had been established (fig. 111).

Visit to Third U.S. Army

After clearing the decks, as it were, of the staff work which was required after every period of visits to the field—including the submission of indicated directives for publication, Colonel Cutler next departed on a field trip to the Third U.S. Army where he had long conferences with Colonel Hurley, Surgeon, Third Army, and Colonel Odom. He was able to locate Captain Cutler, and on the evening of 6 February 1945 they dined with Lt. Gen. George S. Patton, Jr., Commanding General, Third U.S. Army, Maj. Gen. Hobart R. Gay, Chief of Staff, and others of the commanding general's staff (fig. 112).

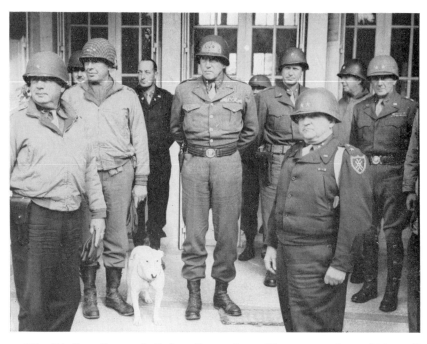

FIGURE 112.—Lt. Gen. George S. Patton, Jr., center, with some members of his staff, and other key officers in the Third U.S. Army.

The visit to the Third U.S. Army was most enlightening and encouraging in many respects. First, General Patton, himself, said that he would be delighted to have an operational research team work with the Third U.S. Army; next, Colonel Cutler discovered that a command letter had been issued to all units of the Third U.S. Army over the commanding general's personal signature forbidding the awarding of a Purple Heart for frostbite within the army area since the severity of this condition could only be determined late in the period of convalescence; and, finally, at the commanding general's briefing on the morning of 7 February 1945, Colonel Cutler was pleasantly surprised at the optimism which prevailed for an early crossing of the Rhine and the subjugation of Nazi Germany. But perhaps most satisfying to Colonel Cutler was the discovery that the mobile surgical teams—with tents and all—which he and Colonel Zollinger had so laboriously organized and established two years earlier were now finding great acceptance in the armored divisions of this field army. Colonel Cutler reported the following on his return:

Visits to Armies employing armored divisions in rapid tactical movements have revealed that PROCO units (the mobile surgical teams previously described in ETMD reports) have proved valuable with armored divisions. These PROCO units consist of a surgical team from an auxiliary group with organic transport and additional equipment. In this equipment is a tent used for the operating room and the supplies are adequate for approximately two hundred (200) surgical procedures. At first, divisions did not desire such assistance but after being employed one (1) or two (2) times, these units

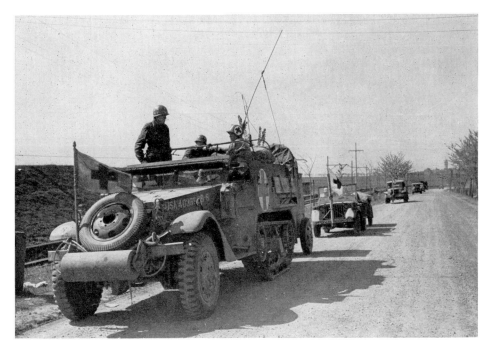

FIGURE 113.—Armored medical vehicles.

were attached to the armored train and have reached a point where the armored divisions are demanding that these units become an integral part of their medical support. In the field, the following use is made of this unit: when the collecto-clearing station of an armored division is set up, the mobile surgical team sets up next to it and is immediately available for definitive surgical care. If the armored division moves a day or even hours later, the team again moves with it. The use of such a unit should be further studied, and it may be discovered that a unit anticipated for general service and use, will find its most logical placement with armored or motorized infantry divisions (fig. 113).[108]

Colonel Kimbrough departs

At about that time, it became definitely known that Colonel Kimbrough was to return to the United States. After conferring with General Kenner on 10 February, as mentioned earlier, Colonel Cutler proceeded to a farewell dinner for Colonel Kimbrough, given by General Hawley on what, it turned out, was his eve of departure (fig. 114).

In addressing the dinner guests and toasting the departing chief of the Professional Services Division, Colonel Cutler said:

We meet to bid goodbye and to do honor to a colleague and a friend. It will be hard for Jim to listen to some of this because he is essentially a modest man, but he must bear with us and our encomiums, for we must be permitted this privilege.

In 2½ years that we in the Professional Services Division have been together, all have made friends with Colonel Kimbrough, not lightly, for in one's adult years friend-

---

[108] Essential Technical Medical Data, ETOUSA, for March 1945, 16 May 1945.

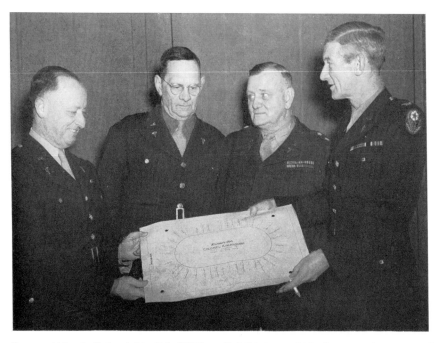

FIGURE 114.—Left to right, Col. William S. Middleton, MC, Colonel Kimbrough, General Hawley, and Colonel Cutler at Colonel Kimbrough's farewell dinner. Colonel Kimbrough being presented with an autographed seating plan for the dinner, held at Hotel George V.

ship is a sacred matter not given easily to each unfledged comrade but given only to those whom time and trial have proven worthy. Love and friendship are the greatest gifts within the possession of individuals, and that our Division has so universally welcomed Jim Kimbrough to this grade is our greatest possible compliment. We have literally taken him to our hearts.

And now, let us examine what type of man we honor. First let us speak of his constructive, organizing ability. The plan under which Professional Services has operated in the European theater is the plan set by Colonel Kimbrough, to guide the Chief Surgeon, before any of us were in the theater. It has been tested by time and found satisfactory. It provides specialists in all the major fields of medical practice. It makes full use of professional skills for the soldier. It bespeaks a "canny" imagination.

Next, let us examine his professional attributes. He is a specialist in urological surgery and we his colleagues are happy to testify to his complete competence. But, soon we learned he was more than a surgeon, for we watched him as a teacher helping his junior colleagues. Thus, he is admitted to the company of "surgeons," who sit above the "operations" in a world where humanity loves to use its hands.

And, finally, we've travelled far with Colonel Kimbrough, sometimes actually in trains and cars, but often, in his stories, to the afterdecks of steamers in the China Seas, to many strange places. It is then that Jim often reaches his greatest heights. In the warm evening, with dusk shutting out the greater world, men (and women) are driven to a closer communion, life is freely discussed with individuals and, untrammelled by too much sunlight, takes on an added significance. Thus are friends born. They cannot be won by money. Life without them is an empty shell. And always, in his perception of the important, the amusing has cropped up, for he has an uncanny flair for rapidly judging the meat and truth of any matter. He has always said it was hillbilly common sense, but many of us who have played at the game of life and success for years know that such intuition is not confined to Tennessee, and we have learned that Jim's prognostications and judgments are usually confirmed by subsequent happenings.

Our feelings of Jim have fortunately already been inscribed in the annals for posterity by Sir Henry Tidy, President of the Royal Society of Medicine. In conferring an honorary fellowship on Colonel Kimbrough, he spoke of one who had a suitable and kindly disposition proven by the fact that he directed a diversified and motley group of independent scholars who peculiarly, from the British point of view, spoke of him as "Uncle Jim"—Thus was his fellowship conferred!

Jim Kimbrough, we who are your friends wish that happiness may dog your footsteps and "Lady Luck" always sit on your shoulder and kiss your cheek.

I give you "Uncle Jim!"

Colonel Kimbrough left for the Zone of Interior on 11 February 1945 via the United Kingdom. Before leaving, however, he addressed the following undated note to Colonel Cutler which, obviously, was intended for all the consultants in the theater headquarters:

My duties with the Professional Services Division are terminated. I take this opportunity to convey my deep appreciation to each of the Consultant Group for your hearty cooperation during these many months. A more proficient and splendid group of physicians has never been on duty in any echelon with the United States Army. It has been a great privilege and pleasure to have had the opportunity to be associated with you in a personal and professional capacity.

Your efforts have assured the American soldier the best medical care that has ever been given to any army at any time. Whatever recognition may be given you for your great work, I am sure the greatest reward each of you has is the consciousness of having given the best of your efforts and talents to the care of the U.S. Army personnel in this emergency.

Best wishes.

On the day of Colonel Kimbrough's leaving, Colonel Liston, Deputy Chief Surgeon, informed Colonel Cutler that he was to assume the position of Chief, Professional Services Division. Colonel Cutler's private feelings on the change were: "If I succeed, I'll be tied down; if I don't, we're stalled." To be sure that he would be neither completely tied down nor stalled, Colonel Cutler asked for and received the assignment of Lt. Col. Bernard J. Pisani, MC, as his executive officer. Colonel Pisani was the officer who had so successfully administered the Medical Field Service School, ETOUSA, while it existed at Shrivenham Barracks in England. Capt. Wayne H. Jonson, MAC, who had been administrative assistant to the chief of the Professional Services Division, remained. It is said that a new broom sweeps clean, and, without exception, Colonel Cutler obtained concessions from Col. John C. Rucker, MC, of the Personnel Division and from Colonel Doan concerning the Administrative Division so that he could effect "office changes leading to greater comfort and efficiency of personnel."

Rhine is breached

In early February, a series of coordinated onslaughts against German positions west of the Rhine had begun. The announcement from Supreme

Headquarters, Allied Expeditionary Force, confidently stated that these attacks should mark the beginning of the destruction of German forces west of the Rhine. By the end of February, the First U.S. Army was besieging Cologne on the west bank. A few days later, this bastion city—a mass of ruins—had fallen to the First U.S. Army. On 7 February, a task force from the 9th Armored Division could hardly believe its eyes, for at Remagen a tre-

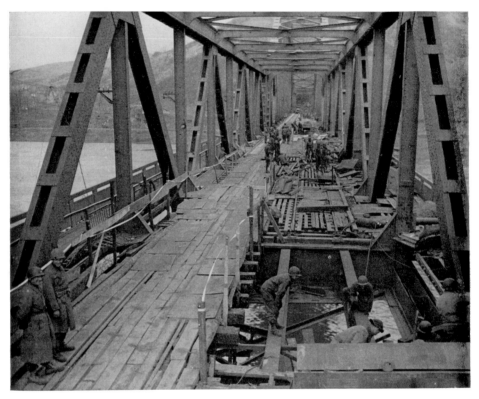

FIGURE 115.—First U.S. Army men and equipment pouring across the Remagen Bridge, 11 March 1945.

mendous bridge across the swollen river barrier remained intact. It has often been told how, through many fortuitous circumstances—drunkenness of the German demolitions officer, faulty fuses, alertness of the U.S. reconnaissance party commander, and so forth—the bridge was secured minutes before its scheduled demolition. The First U.S. Army commander, quick to seize this favorable turn of the fortunes of war, exploited rapidly this breakthrough and jeopardized the carefully planned German defenses along the Rhine River line (fig. 115).

Colonel Cutler said to himself: "War going well. I believe it will be over in two months. Then how do we get out?"

CAMPAIGN IN CENTRAL EUROPE

Collapse of Enemy

True to Colonel Cutler's private prognostication, the fight on German soil rapidly turned into a pursuit of demoralized German forces. To the extreme north the British 21 Army Group resorted to full-scale, amphibious operations to cross the Rhine, secure strongly held enemy islands in the Baltic, and advance across the Elbe River to occupy Wismar on the Baltic coast by the end of April. The First U.S. Army also neared the Elbe by the end of April and waited on the banks of the Fulda River for the Soviet Army, while the Soviets waited on the banks of the Elbe for the Americans. On 23 March, the Ninth U.S. Army crossed the Rhine in the vicinity of Düsseldorf and by the end of April, it too was on the Elbe-Mulde line to link up with the Soviet Army. The Third U.S. Army crossed the Rhine in March, drove rapidly through Bavaria and Hitler's "last redoubt" and was in Austria and Czechoslovakia by early May. The Seventh U.S. Army, in late March and early April, breached the upper Rhine defenses in the area of Worms and, by early May, a portion of the Army had made the complete circle and was back to its starting base, Italy. There, it linked up with the Fifth U.S. Army south of the Brenner Pass and received the surrender of all German forces in its area on 5 May 1945 (fig. 116). Fighting alongside the Seventh U.S. Army in the Sixth Army Group, were elements of the valiant First French Army.

Responsibilities of Chief, Professional Services Division

With this rapid collapse of the enemy's resistance, Colonel Cutler was extremely harried by the many responsibilities which befell him as the new chief of the Professional Services Division, Office of the Chief Surgeon. Some of these problems were inherited immediately upon Colonel Kimbrough's departure, and others came his way soon thereafter.

The first of these problems was the examining, evaluating, and profiling of the physical fitness of every enlisted man in the theater. The War Department had directed that a new PULHES system of physical profiling be accomplished rapidly so that the resulting profiles could be used in the redeployment of personnel in the European theater to other theaters of war when active hostilities in Europe ceased. Colonel Cutler could not help but recall with some dismay that he had participated in British talks on this system of profiling in January 1944 when it was devised by the Canadians. At that time, he had submitted complete notes on the Canadian system. He stated: "* * * for it is felt that perhaps some other division than The Professional Services Division would be interested in seeing this method of assessment." Even then, when ground hostilities had not yet begun in Europe, Colonel Cutler had stated:

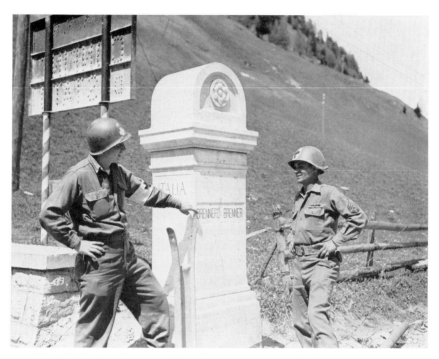

Figure 116.—Medical soldiers of the Fifth and Seventh U.S. Armies meeting at the Italian border at the Brenner Pass.

"It seemed to me that this is no time to establish such a system." [109]   Now, at this late date with an extremely fluid situation and the pursuit of the war at its peak, there was no choice but to take the matter in hand and fashion out plans which could be carried out with the minimum of disruption to the conduct of the war in Europe.   Eventually, it was necessary to establish a physical standards branch under Colonel Middleton's direction to plan, supervise, and coordinate matters in this area.

Brig. Gen. Hugh J. Morgan, Chief Consultant in Medicine to The Surgeon General, had arrived and presented preliminary plans and ideas on the redeployment of medical personnel and units, and this was to be an ever-increasing problem as the end of hostilities neared.

The evacuation policy for hospitals in the communications zone on the Continent had been raised to 60 days, effective 1 March 1945, except for Delta Base Section which was permitted to keep patients for the 90- or 120-day theater policy.   This necessitated changes in evacuation policies, for it meant that casualties who could be rehabilitated during that period now would be cared for in continental hospitals.   This also required changes in rehabilitation procedures themselves, for it placed added responsibilities on general hospitals in this

---

[109] Letter, Col. E. C. Cutler to Chief, Professional Services Division, 16 Jan. 1944, subject: Meeting, British Consultants' Surgical Sub-Committee, 12 Jan. 1944.

respect, concurrently taking some of the load off the rehabilitation centers. Obviously, this lengthened evacuation policy for the continental hospitals changed the complexion of the extent of treatment to be given therein.

Colonel Cutler had to coordinate activities aimed at establishing a "recovery center" on the Continent. The original recovery center in England had been established by Col. Lloyd J. Thompson, Senior Consultant in Neuropsychiatry. The recovery center set up in a strictly nonhospital atmosphere, had been extremely successful in salvaging manpower from borderline cases of adjustment, such as the mentally deficient and those with character and personality disorders. The success of the center in England led line officers on the staff of the communications zone headquarters to desire strongly the establishment of a similar facility on continental Europe.

The care and treatment of RAMP (recovered Allied military personnel), liberated civilian prisoners, and displaced German nationals grew into problems of monumental proportions as the subjugation of the Nazi forces permeated ever deeper into the fatherland. Providing for the care of prisoners of war had been a problem since the Northern France Campaign and continued to mount in complexity as ever-larger numbers of the enemy surrendered (fig. 117). Colonel Cutler was the writer of the basic directive regarding their medical care and treatment.

There was also the program for establishing extensive educational opportunities throughout the theater following the cessation of hostilities. The overall theaterwide program was being coordinated by ETOUSA headquarters and theaterwide medical education and training by the education and training branch of the Operations Division, Office of the Chief Surgeon, ETOUSA. But it was the responsibility of Colonel Cutler to make plans and arrange for the professional education of medical officers during the posthostilities period in the renowned civilian medical centers of France and England and in U.S. Army general hospitals with qualified instructor personnel.

These, and many other problems of lesser scope, were to occupy much of the time and energies of Colonel Cutler in his new position. To compensate for the resulting loss of time and attention to his other position as Chief Consultant in Surgery, Colonel Cutler made more and more use of his specialist consultants on general surgical matters. This was particularly true of Colonel Bricker and Colonel Robinson who, perhaps, were in narrower fields of specialization than the others. There were many direct dealings with Lt. Col. Theodore L. Badger, MC, the medical consultant in Normandy Base Section, on whose able shoulders fell the brunt of the work in planning and supervising the professional aspects for the initial reception and care of RAMP. Colonel Zollinger, now commanding officer of the 5th General Hospital, helped Colonel Cutler in the preparation of directives on rehabilitation in general hospitals and, later, was to become a key figure in certain phases of the relocation and selection of personnel for redeployment. Colonel Pisani, as mentioned earlier, was of invaluable help on administrative matters pertaining to the entire divi-

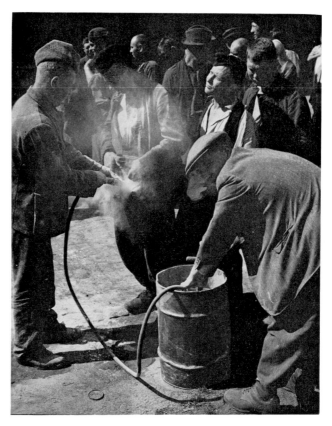

Figure 117.—Delousing Soviet-recovered prisoners at Prisoner of War Exchange Camp No. 17, Lippstadt, Germany, 1945.

sion, and also in formulating plans and taking care of the liaison involved in the preparation of a posthostilities educational program. Through these various means, Colonel Cutler maintained close touch with the surgical picture in the theater and assured himself that he would not be completely tied down.

Colonel Cutler Crosses Rhine

On 25 March, Colonel Cutler departed Paris by air for a visit to the First and Ninth U.S. Armies. Arriving at Euskirchen airport at 0915, he found that the 45th and 128th Evacuation Hospitals located near the airport were preparing to move across the Rhine (fig. 118).

Headquarters, First U.S. Army.—At Headquarters, First U.S. Army, Colonel Cutler greeted General Rogers and obtained his concurrence for releasing Colonel MacFee to go to the Fifteenth U.S. Army as its surgical consultant. Then, with Colonel MacFee, he motored to Cologne to look over the St. Eliza-

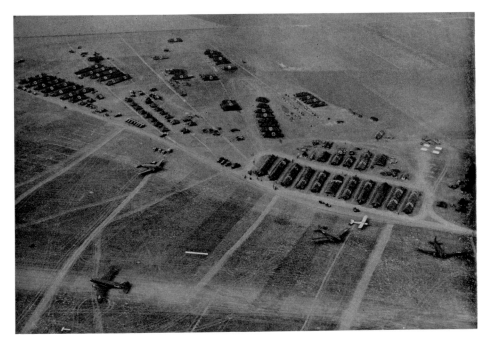

FIGURE 118.—The extensive holding and evacuation facilities of the 91st Medical Gas Treatment Battalion, Euskirchen airstrip, Euskirchen, Germany, 26 March 1945.

beth's Hospital. During the trip, Colonel Cutler was interested in the "delightfully complete" destruction of Cologne and the grimness of the people.

That evening, after messing with the 3d Auxiliary Surgical Group, Colonel Cutler engaged some of the surgical personnel of the First U.S. Army in his usual after-dinner free-for-all discussion. Later this same evening, Colonel Cutler discussed a proposed directive governing care of hand injuries with Colonel Crisler and Colonel MacFee. Colonel Cutler had already discussed this matter with Colonel MacFee, but one of the reasons for his having made this trip was further to discuss the topic with Colonel Crisler. Colonel Cutler was pleased to find, as expected, that the First U.S. Army surgical consultant had valuable ideas to offer.

Eventful Monday, 26 March.—Colonel Cutler was up early the next morning, 26 March 1945. With Colonel Crisler, he made his first crossing of the Rhine during his participation for the second time in a war against Germany. The crossing was by motor vehicle over a pontoon bridge. Once across, he found the 45th Evacuation Hospital, under the command of Col. Abner Zehm, MC, already setting up in a disbanded schoolhouse. This was a unit Colonel Cutler had visited many times previously and always with pleasure. The hospital was well run, and the superior vascular surgery being performed under the direction of its chief of surgical service, Col. Bert Bradford, Jr., MC, always shed new light on developments in that field.

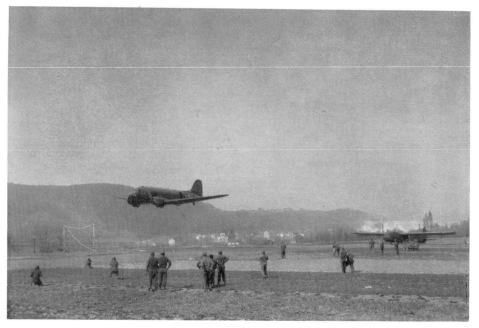

FIGURE 119.—Glider evacuation of wounded. The plane swooping low to hook up the gliders.

The present visit proved to be no exception, and a long discussion concerning vascular surgery ensued.

The next stop was the 42d Field Hospital, concerning which Colonel Cutler noted the following:

* * * The field hospital from which the gliders, loaded with patients, were jerked off the ground by a plane which did not stop. Reports from workers in this hospital indicated that the gliders worked well. Colonel Amspacher, who made a trip in one of them, thought they were very satisfactory, though it was frightening when the plane swooped low to hook up the gliders (fig. 119). Later, I heard that this type of evacuation had been called off.

A visit to the 13th Field Hospital completed Colonel Cutler's visit east of the Rhine. With Colonel Crisler, he recrossed the Rhine to the west bank over another pontoon bridge and visited the 102d Evacuation Hospital at Bad Neuenahr. Later that afternoon, Colonel Cutler drove to Headquarters, Ninth U.S. Army, with Major Hardin, who had accompanied him on this trip.

Ninth U.S. Army.—The visit to the Ninth U.S. Army at this time was occasioned by an allegation prevailing in the Office of the Chief Surgeon that, owing to reactions, the 91st Evacuation Hospital had absolutely discontinued the use of blood supplied by the European theater blood bank. This was why Major Hardin had been brought along.

Colonel Cutler and Major Hardin arrived at Ninth U.S. Army headquarters at 1830 hours and reported immediately to Colonel Shambora, Surgeon, Ninth Army. The diary record of subsequent events follows:

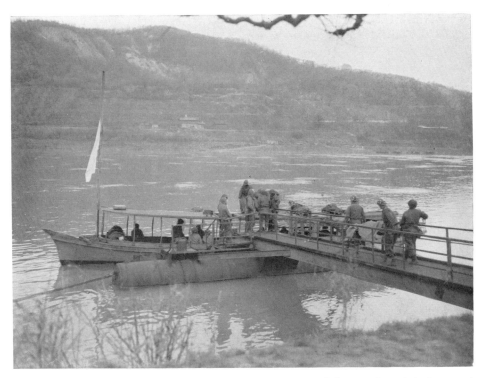

FIGURE 120.—First U.S. Army medical troops using a captured German launch to transport casualties across the Rhine, Unkel, Germany, March 1945.

After dinner we spent two hours with Colonel Shambora, his consultant group, the chief of the medical laboratory, and members of the 91st Evacuation Hospital, discussing transfusion reactions. We had learned at headquarters (SOS, ETOUSA) that the 91st Evacuation Hospital would no longer use ETO blood bank blood. This is not true. They would merely like to continue their study of blood transfusion reactions with (1) ZI blood; (2) ETO blood, and (3) freshly drawn citrated blood from a panel in their vicinity. They expressed an interest in the overall study of blood and I believe we should encourage this, so we offered to send them either Major Emerson or Major Ebert of the 5th General Hospital, both of whom are experts in blood work, and have had long experience with blood banks. I feel that we reached an amicable settlement on what could have been a serious problem. The desire to have Major Emerson and Major Ebert sent here was immediately telephoned to Colonel Pisani.

Twenty-seven hundred yards away, the enemy.—During the next four days, Colonel Cutler alternated between the First and Ninth U.S. Armies and crossed and recrossed the Rhine, all this having started with a telephone conversation with Colonel Doan and Colonel Pisani on the morning of 27 March, at which time he was informed that General Hawley wanted to see him at the First U.S. Army for lunch (fig. 120). After missing him on two occasions, Colonel Cutler was finally able to meet General Hawley late on 28 March for dinner at First U.S. Army headquarters and a night at the 102d Evacuation Hospital. The next morning, 29 March, he left with General Hawley to go back to the Ninth U.S. Army and visited Headquarters, XIII Corps, where he discussed the job of a corps surgeon with Colonel Shambora. On the morning of Friday, 30 March, Colonel Cutler and General Hawley discussed with Colonel Shambora certain aspects of the professional services in the Ninth U.S. Army and the blood situation. As there was no aircraft available for a return to Paris, General Hawley and Colonel Cutler borrowed Colonel Shambora's staff car and proceeded to the banks of the Rhine on the approaches to Dorsten. There they borrowed a jeep and proceeded up to General Hawley's son's unit, the 399th Field Artillery Battalion of the 8th Armored Division. Colonel Cutler recorded: "They were firing at targets twenty-seven hundred yards away! It was a very interesting day. The Germans are apparently short of artillery as well as air."

Colonel Cutler and General Hawley were finally able to fly back to Paris later that day, arriving at 1900 hours. The one overall impression which prevailed was the relative inactivity of the evacuation hospitals of both armies, most of which were either on the move or preparing to move.

Eminent Visitors

On Monday, 2 April, after his return from visits to the First and Ninth U.S. Armies, Colonel Cutler first entertained Colonel Jurash, surgical consultant to the Polish Army in Exile. After a long conference with him, Colonel Cutler took the Polish officer for an audience with the Chief Surgeon and then escorted him to the G–5 Division, ETOUSA, for further conferences.

Later that day, Maj. Gen. Morrison C. Stayer, MC, Chief Surgeon, MTOUSA (Mediterranean Theater of Operations, U.S. Army), and his surgical consultant, Col. Edward D. Churchill, MC, arrived for a liaison visit to the European theater. Colonel Cutler dined with them and had a long evening with these colleagues whom he had not seen since November–December 1943. He continued talks with Colonel Churchill the next morning and also spoke with Lt. Col. Michael E. DeBakey, MC, Consultant in General Surgery to The Surgeon General.

Colonel DeBakey had arrived in the theater for a liaison visit following a similar visit to the Mediterranean theater. On 9 March, after conferring with him, Colonel Cutler had sent Colonel DeBakey off for a visit to the First U.S. Army in the company of Colonel MacFee, who was opportunely in Paris helping Colonel Cutler on certain personnel shifts and being interviewed concerning his contemplated reassignment to the Fifteenth U.S. Army. After the First U.S. Army visit, Colonel DeBakey had visited the Ninth, Third, and Seventh U.S. Armies. His visits in the army areas had included conferences with the army surgeons and their surgical consultants and some corps surgeons. He had visited auxiliary surgical groups, evacuation hospitals, convalescent hospitals, field hospitals, and collecting and clearing stations, and, in the 75th Division area, he had visited a battalion aid station in action. He was at this time, 3 April, continuing visits to communications zone facilities in and around Paris.

In the afternoon, 3 April, Colonel Cutler left with the visitors from the Mediterranean theater for the United Kingdom.

In the United Kingdom, they met with General Spruit and Colonel McNinch and planned an itinerary for the officers from MTOUSA. The tour included a visit, on the first day, to the showpiece of rehabilitation facilities, the 327th Station Hospital; hospitals of the Cirencester hospital center the second day, with special attention on the specialized treatment facilities of the center; and, on the third day, a trip to Oxford University to visit with Professor Florey and, later, visits to the 97th and 91st General Hospitals nearby. Colonel Spurling and Colonel Morton were sent out to escort the visitors while Colonel Cutler remained behind to arrange for their meeting with members of the staff of the DGMS, British Army, and for a continuation of their tour by visits to the First U.S. Army.

On Thursday, 5 April, however, Colonel Cutler learned during a telephone conversation with Colonel Pisani on the Continent that General Hawley wanted to see Colonel DeBakey soon. Colonel Cutler instructed Colonel Pisani to ask General Hawley to defer any meeting with Colonel DeBakey until he, Colonel Cutler, could get back, which would be the next day. Colonel Cutler returned to the Continent on 6 April. Before taking his hasty departure from England, Colonel Cutler had spoken by telephone with Colonel Spurling and Colonel Morton on the trip being taken by General Stayer and Colonel Churchill. He was pleased to note: "Reports were highly satisfactory."

Back in Paris, Colonel Cutler joined in conference with General Hawley and Colonel DeBakey on Saturday, 7 April. In the conference, Colonel Cutler emphasized the fact that the Army in the European theater, and the medical service in support of that Army, were extremely busy. He stressed the point that the professional care of patients must be planned and executed with the single thought in mind of the influence of tremendous numbers of casualties on professional activities.

On his return to the Zone of Interior, Colonel DeBakey reported to The Surgeon General in a letter, dated 17 April 1945, as follows:

The therapeutic adjuncts and basic surgical principles utilized in the program of wound management developed by the theater surgical consultant and his consultant staff and presented in various publications of the Office of the Chief Surgeon are being effectively applied by the surgeons in the Army hospitals. The Army surgical consultants have contributed immeasurably in the implementation of this program. In general, the policies established by this program of wound management conform closely with those presented in the recently published War Department Technical Bulletin (TB MED 147, March 1945). The development of this rational program of wound management and its successful application have been largely achieved through the profound influence of the theater surgical consultant and his staff. The attainment of such a high standard of surgical practice and the gratifying results achieved form a signal tribute to his broad vision, his untiring educational efforts, and his trenchant surgical judgment. The admirable manner in which he has performed his function is further reflected by the fine spirits of cooperation that exist between his staff and the Army surgical consultants and the respect and loyalty manifested by the surgeons in the hospitals toward him.

That same evening, after the conference with Colonel DeBakey and General Hawley, a telephone call came in to the Chief Surgeon's Office from the Third U.S. Army—General Patton urgently requested Colonel Cutler's presence and was sending an airplane for him. Colonel Cutler was instructed to be ready to leave the first thing the next morning.

At 0800 hours on Sunday morning, 8 April 1945, Colonel Cutler left Paris by air, taking Colonel Pisani with him. Some 2 hours later, they arrived at Headquarters, Third U.S. Army, where General Gay, Chief of Staff, and Colonel Odom met them. From the headquarters, they went to the 34th Evacuation Hospital to look at the officer for whom consultation had been requested.

This officer, a Colonel "W." of Armor, had been captured by the Germans in North Africa more than 2 years earlier at the battle of the Kasserine Pass, where he had distinguished himself by bravery and exemplary action. He had been shunted through various prison camps by the Germans and had recently arrived at the camp at Hammelburg, east of Kassel. General Patton, learning that there were American prisoners at the camp, in characteristic fashion sent a special armored task force knifing through the enemy defenses to liberate them. Colonel "W.," the ranking officer among the Americans in the camp, accompanied the German camp commander out of the compound under a flag of truce to surrender the camp to the oncoming Third U.S. Army task force. As he did so, a sniper shot Colonel "W." from very close range, and he was taken back to the camp for treatment. Meanwhile, the Germans surrendered the camp, and some of the liberated prisoners were loaded on the tanks for evacuation back to the Third U.S. Army lines. Strong and persistent pressure from a retreating German Division, however, forced the task force to withdraw under perilous circumstances. It was not until some 4 days later that Colonel Odom was able to fly to Kassel, join a combat patrol, and, skirting the fighting still going on around Hammelburg, enter the camp. During the night, he gave Colonel "W." what emergency treatment he could, including a transfusion of whole blood. The next morning, he called back to Third U.S. Army headquarters and requested that light aircraft be sent up. Two such aircraft were sent; Colonel "W." was evacuated to the 34th Evacuation Hospital in one, and Colonel Odom returned in the other.

Colonel Cutler found the officer's wound most unusual. The sniper's bullet had entered just below the right groin externally to the great vessels, must have passed under the neck of the femur, and emerged through the anus and buttock area, blowing out a considerable amount of tissue and the coccyx. A Serbian doctor in the prison camp had debrided the wound as well as he could with the limited facilities available to him and had sewed the sphincter, which was now intact. The wounded officer was having his second transfusion. He obviously required proctoscopy in order to determine the extent of damage to the rectum. Proctoscopy might reveal that a temporary colostomy was indicated until the rectum could heal. To Colonel Cutler, he looked well enough to transport.

Back at Third U.S. Army headquarters, Colonel Cutler advised General Patton that the officer should be taken back to the 1st General Hospital in Paris to carry out the necessary examinations and operations. The General agreed to follow any advice the consultants gave him and expressed his gratitude.

After lunch, General Patton loaned the consultants his personal staff car so that they could go to Heidelberg to visit Dr. Richard Kuhn, the winner of the 1938 Nobel Prize in Chemistry. Dr. Kuhn, up to the time of the war, had been the director of the Max Planck Institute for Medical Research at the University of Heidelberg. He was one of the first to describe the constitution of riboflavin, vitamin B_2. It was Dr. Kuhn who had first isolated 1 gram of riboflavin, vitamin B_2, from 53,000 liters of skimmed milk. Dr. Kuhn had also isolated pyridoxine, vitamin B_6.

Dr. Kuhn mentioned to the visitors, Colonel Cutler, Colonel Odom, and Colonel Pisani, that he had placed himself in considerable jeopardy by having spoken openly against the Nazi party. He said that an SS trooper lived in the institute and knew everything that went on. He informed the visitors that Dr. Martin Kirschner had passed away 3 years earlier (1942) and had been succeeded by Dr. K. H. Bauer, formerly of the University of Breslau.

Reviewing his wartime work, Dr. Kuhn first corrected a prevailing misconception that he had created a substance that acted as insulin and could be taken by mouth. He mentioned a complex unsaturated hydrocarbon that he had isolated which was similar to some of his other discoveries among the long-chain compounds containing conjugate double bonds. This deep-blue liquid had been found to be an effective bacteriostatic agent in experiments conducted in vitro against gram negative organisms. It had also been proved very useful against mustard gas injuries of the skin, although it had not been developed for general issue in the German Army. He also mentioned a product, "3065," that had been synthesized by a Professor Kahn. This product acted like penicillin and had been used extensively in experiments involving man and animals. It appeared especially efficacious against *Staphylococcus aureus* and gonococcus. With respect to the latter, it had proved particularly useful in genital infections of women proved to be sulfonamide resistant.

At dinner that night, at the Third U.S. Army headquarters mess, Colonel Cutler was pleased to meet John J. McCloy, Assistant Secretary of War, who was inspecting in the area. Among other items, the Assistant Secretary declared, during a discussion on the difficulties in paying troops in the European theater, that his chief difficulty with the Finance Department was having sufficient money printed! General Patton singled out, as one of his difficulties, getting decorations for acts of valor occurring in the Third U.S. Army. He stated that he had been able to obtain only two Congressional Medals of Honor for members of the Third U.S. Army, one of which had been given to a medical aidman.

The next morning, the consultants were up early to attend the departure of Assistant Secretary McCloy. Later, they went to the 34th Evacuation

Hospital with General Patton where they dressed Colonel "W." They then put him in an ambulance, took him to the airplane, flew him to Paris, took him to the 1st General Hospital, and arranged details for the proctoscopy to be done the next day. Colonel "W." was eventually evacuated to the Zone of Interior where he recovered completely from his wounds and continued to serve on active duty, becoming a general officer in the U.S. Army.

Later that month, Colonel Cutler also met with a neuropsychiatric mission of distinguished civilian consultants headed by Dr. Karl Menninger to study the changes occurring in neuropsychiatric casualties during their evacuation from the front to the rear. There were conferences with Col. Esmond R. Long, MC, Consultant in Tuberculosis in the Office of The Surgeon General, concerning the care of recovered Allied military personnel. Colonel Cutler was also pleased to renew his friendship and talk with U.S. Senator Leverett Saltonstall, when he visited the theater late in the month.

"A Piece of Sadistic Thinking"

As more and more of German soil was conquered, the peoples of the Allied nations were shocked to learn of the horror which had been perpetrated by Nazi fanatics in their prison camps. In a way, too, they were humbled at the extremes to which man's inhumanity to man could be carried. The stories of these camps—Buchenwald, Pilsen, and many others—have oft been told by the soldier, statesman, and journalist. Each has contributed from his particular frame of observation in the telling of the complete story, and the doctor at war may tell his story, too, in a slightly different light from the others. Colonel Cutler visited Buchenwald on Saturday, 28 April 1945. The following account of his observations—unpolished and hastily written immediate recollections of his visit—were taken from his official journal:

We were given a 'plane and were lifted by air from Paris to a field near Weimar at 9 a.m. The party included Colonel Shook, Colonel Tovell, Colonel Long (from SGO), Maj. [Sarah] Bowditch, Major Loizeaux, Major [Malcolm E.] Beckham and Corporal Sansone. Rough ride under low clouds, just above trees, for 2¾ hours. At the airport near Weimar, I believe R–7, found an ambulance company, No. 429, who were working for the evacuation hospitals in that area; set up and had lunch; it was raining.

We were given two ambulances to take us to the camp, and took with us the crew of the aircraft, who were anxious to see the camp, and three correspondents who attached themselves to us. Found the 45th Evacuation Hospital set up next to the gate of the camp, but Colonel Zehm was away for the moment. Went to the gate and it was obvious that great restrictions had now been placed upon visiting this camp. Our orders were sufficient authority for us to enter but the newspaper correspondents were not allowed, though I did get permission to take in the crew of the aircraft, who were grateful for the opportunity.

We were shown around by two guides, one of whom was a doctor, a Slovak from Prague, captured in 1939. He told us that the original camp was built in 1937 for 7,000 people, and that in 1939 the first Czechs came in, the camp having been used for political prisoners, not war prisoners, precedingly. We were shown the crematorium, with the beating room beneath it. Wards, rooms off wards, where so many patients a day—usually 30 or 40—were taken out for an injection, died and never returned to the ward. We were

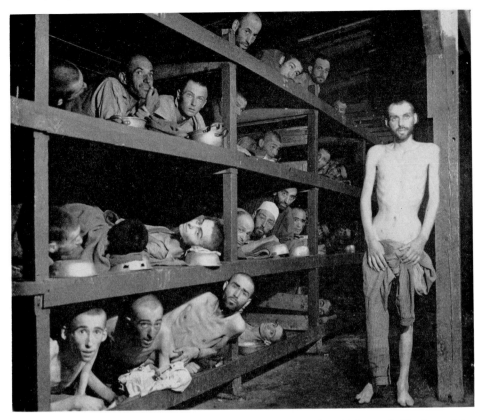

FIGURE 121.—Four-tiered compartments in a so-called hospital ward, Buchenwald Concentration Camp.

shown a ward, at the end of which operations were done, which housed children as well as men. In this ward there were four tiers of bunks, each compartment about 6 feet wide, and six lay in these compartments (fig. 121). The guide told us that 3,400 died in the hospital section alone, many of them with tuberculosis. We were told there were still 20,000 there, that only 2,000 French had been removed.

At a laboratory building, we saw tatooed sections of human skin, which apparently was a pet hobby of the former commanding officer, and we went through the tuberculosis ward and other wards in detail. In all, we were told, 51,000 people had died in this camp.

Comment: The fact that they used a crematorium to get rid of the hundreds that died daily is no criticism; it is the most intelligent and the best way to keep sanitation adequate. The beating room beneath the crematorium, where there were hooks on the walls where men were strangled, and where they had a noise machine so that the cries of those dying could not be heard elsewhere, was unpleasant. Also, the rooms off wards where men were taken for injections, and subsequently died, was a piece of sadistic thinking in line with the German attitude. They might say in defense that this was euthanasia, that all these people were suffering and about to die. We were told, however, that sometimes young people died under similar circumstances, whether because their skins with tatoos were desirable, or whether because they were political agitators, no one will ever know.

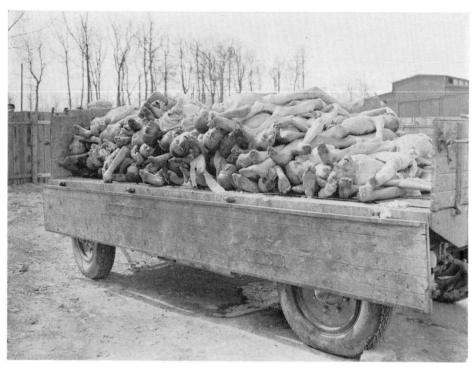

FIGURE 122.—Evidence of the starvation policy found at Buchenwald Concentration Camp.

The crowding, the placement of children on benches and in cubicles off an operating theater, the filthiness of the whole place, was something that cannot be denied.

The obvious starvation policy was pictured everywhere (fig. 122). I saw many men breathing with difficulty, sitting in bed and obviously soon to die, but whether with tuberculosis or other disorders, I did not determine. I talked to a young Pole, who said he was 17 and had been a prisoner three years; and I talked to many Russians, Jews and Poles, whose only release can be a kind and rapid death, for recovery appears impossible in such people.

The hospital section had really been well cleaned up. Floors had been scrubbed; it smelt and looked clean, but the bed linen was nasty and the whole thing looked hopeless. In the tuberculosis ward two men with tuberculosis were practically in bed together, coughing with each other. They all said they were much better and that the food was vastly improved, but such a mass of sick and starved humanity left a bad impression.

We were told that the Germans of the population nearby felt no responsibility; said they did not know it was going on, though on frequent occasions they were turned out to watch hangings of prisoners. Moreover, a renovated stables where some 7,000 Russian soldiers were shot in the neck when ostensibly backed naked against a wall for measuring, was just another part of the whole picture.

Colonel Cutler's journal entry for the same day, 28 April 1945, continues with details of conferences held with members of the Army surgeon's staff, Headquarters, First U.S. Army. The questions discussed were more-or-less characteristic of the entire front at this time—what to do about German military personnel and civilians requiring care; the problem of Soviet nationals, Poles, Czechoslovaks, Yugoslavs, and others liberated from the prison camps; idle specialists in the First U.S. Army's medical service; and so forth, as follows:

After leaving the camp, we had a talk with the commanding officer of the 45th Evacuation Hospital and then went to headquarters of the First Army in Weimar, where we discussed the care of these people with Colonel Snyder, Colonel Amspacher, Colonel Crone and Colonel Crisler. The First Army have adopted the following system:— they have a captured Major General of the German Army, Medical Corps, who has seen 33 years' service, and seemed to be able. They are giving him the responsibility of caring for all Germans, whether Army personnel, wounded in their hospitals or the civilian population. The First Army area has been broken up into districts under this German General and they have attached certain Medical Corps officers to him and in his district for overseeing the care of these people. The only difficulty that remains, since all the German Army casualties will be kept where they are, is what to do with them when they are ready for discharge from hospital (this matter was discussed in detail with Colonel Fancher this morning and a paper submitted to him regarding it).

The care of RAMP is difficult and will be looked after by the teams of medical officers set up by the Army for this purpose. Insofar as possible, the RAMP will be kept where they are, their food improved and as much care as possible given to them. Every attempt will be made to utilize their own medical personnel. The only exceptions to be made will be that all tuberculous people will be screened, removed from the RAMP hospitals and taken to Bad Berka a few miles out, for improved care.

Conference with Colonel Crone [medical consultant]. If he is not to return to the ZI he desires to take a course in tropical medicine to improve his usefulness in CBI. Colonel Middleton is implementing this.

Conference with Colonel Crisler. The First Auxiliary Surgical Group, attached to the First Army, are being returned to the headquarters. His own Auxiliary Surgical Group, the 3d, is being pulled in and he would like to send them to our Communications Zone hospitals soon. I approved this and hope he will send in recommendations so that we may use this valuable professional personnel in our busy Com Z hospitals.

Brought down a load of guns and swords for Colonel Doan.

Left by 'plane at 4:30, having picked up a full load of officers and newspaper men trying to get out of the First Army area, back to Paris. The trip back took three hours; it was by far the worst air trip I have ever taken, in spite of the fact that I have flown, since I have been in the Army, some 25,000 miles, including the great trip to Russia and back. It snowed hard while crossing the Rhine area, one could scarcely see the wing tips and, barely visible a few feet below us, tree-tops, while mountains were about us on all sides. I shall send a note of commendation to the commanding officer of the unit to which the pilots who took us there belong, expressing our appreciation for their excellent services.

V–E DAY

Victory in Europe, V–E Day, came as no surprise to anyone. For days, its imminence had been the headline news. When it did come, there was some conjecture as to whether it was 7 or 8 May; it was 8 May. Colonel Cutler was in London at the time. Whether this was by coincidence or choice, his diaries do not say, but it is not difficult to conjecture that it was the latter.

AFTER V–E DAY: GETTING OUT

The period after V–E Day settled down into a routine uninspired but still full of pressing items. All realized, with various feelings and motivations, that there was still a war on, but there was very little enthusiasm left.

Miscellaneous Activities

Physical standards and redeployment.—The projects of physically profiling all enlisted men and redeployment went hand in hand, for the second could not be accomplished without the first. Accordingly, the making out of the physical profile serials became a problem of extreme urgency in the post-hostilities period. Colonel Cutler, himself, was more personally involved, however, in the selection of professionally qualified surgical personnel for redeployment and the organization of professionally balanced and qualified units to be shipped to the Pacific and Asiatic areas. This eventually became a nightmarish activity. "What a life," the diary states, "Redeployment a terrific headache." Then, later: "It has all been a jumble. We're all exhausted and probably don't make sense, but I think there will be a Congressional investigation of redeployment—there should be. I've told Hawley so. Asked him to exonerate Professional Services Division as we have no authority, therefore no responsibility." Officially, in his semiannual report to the Chief Surgeon for the first half of 1945, Colonel Cutler stated:

Following V–E Day, redeployment began rapidly and pushed the Professional Services Division into greater activities, at a time when it was exhausted. While the theater was feverishly searching for a critical score system, and even before it was available, we had to assemble balanced professional units for immediate redeployment. During the phase of redeploying the first * * * units direct to the Pacific, urgent cables from Washington instructed us to send home about 1,000 doctors. Lists of certain critical specialists in fixed numbers were included. These were rapidly gathered and were ready for transshipment to the Zone of Interior by early July. This further depleted the supply of specialists to a critical point, since this theater never had a sufficient quota for adequate T/O coverage. Redeployment demanded the greatest co-operation between the Personnel and Professional Service Divisions. The Personnel Division drew up plans and, although every attempt was made to assist them, the result has not always been satisfactory. Redeployment of professional personnel has not been on a strictly professional basis, and only irregularly submitted to this Division. Although the point score may seem fairer than any other, it has definitely compromised the setup of these units. In disregarding longevity of service, it has worked hardship on a group of highly trained professional people. The Army has lost many of its best and critically needed officers, who are more tired and worn out than the general lack of battle stars, points and decorations might indicate.

Battle casualty survey team.—The Operational Research Section, Office of the Chief Surgeon, under Maj. Allan Palmer, MC, had been reconstituted as the 250th Medical Detachment, and, after 10 weeks of feverish activity, the necessary personnel and equipment had been assembled and authority had been obtained for independent action in the Third U.S. Army area. Colonel

Cutler had great hopes for the collection of significant data by the team—an expectation which was the culmination of Colonel Cutler's efforts since his first days in the European theater. He had personally arranged with the Third U.S. Army commander, General Patton, and his chief of staff, General Gay, that every consideration would be given for the efficient employment of the team. But, even after the team was prepared to move into action, there were many administrative obstacles to be overcome before such an unusual unit could be moved from Cambridge Cemetery, England, to the Third U.S. Army front in Bavaria and Bohemia.

When the unit finally reached its destination, but 2 days of fighting remained before the surrender and the total number of casualties sustained during the period in the area in which the survey team was to operate turned out to be 21—12 killed in action and 9 wounded in action.

Colonel Cutler was disappointed that the casualty survey team could not have functioned sooner. It was small recompense for his work, but, in the period after V–E Day, the 250th Medical Detachment was singled out by Washington as a unit to be retained intact for possible redeployment to the Asiatic areas. At least, it seemed, someone else might obtain some use from his work.[110]

Transfusion reactions.—Maj. Charles P. Emerson, MC, who had been sent to the Ninth U.S. Army to study transfusion reactions, completed his studies and submitted a preliminary, but extensive, report on his findings. Other studies on the problem, notably that by the 43d General Hospital, were also consummated to contribute to the pool of overall knowledge on transfusion reactions. In a memorandum, dated 19 May 1945, bringing the Emerson report to the attention of General Hawley, who was personally greatly interested, Colonel Cutler stated:

2. * * *

a. Investigations point that there is a case against old or aged blood. Apparently a certain amount of blood becomes hemolyzed through the packing of red cells at the bottom away from the diluent. This is always more extensive when the diluent is a small quantity, such as the 160 cc. amount rather than the 500 cc. amount. The agent causing the reaction is stroma of the red cells, not of the free hemoglobin.

b. Transfused cells disappear slowly.

c. There is a definite danger from old ["O"] blood whether from the blood itself or O plasma. This is a relatively new contribution and points out that the universal donor is not without danger.

The renal failure cases seem to be largely due to anoxia, i.e., the period of low blood pressure preceding the transfusion. Thus, it is not the transfusion but primary injury of the cells through anoxia.

---

110 (1) Palmer, A.: Report of a Ground Force Battle Casualty Survey Initiated Two Days Prior to V–E Day, With Appendix II, Diary of the 250th Medical Detachment. [Official record.] (2) Medical Department, United States Army. Wound Ballistics. Washington: U.S. Government Printing Office, 1962.

Major Emerson, in his report, laid great emphasis on the point briefly mentioned by Colonel Cutler, the danger of the concept of the universal donor. The report stated:

The importance of these findings, from the practical point of view, lies in the following inferences:—

1) *Repeated injection of group O blood into other than group O patients may be an ineffectual and uneconomic procedure,* except in emergency replacement therapy.

2) *The transfusion of very large amounts of group O blood, and even of pooled plasma, into recipients of other blood groups may result in serious hemolytic disease, as has been noted in certain cases with severe burns requiring massive plasma transfusions.*

3) It is possible that irreversible organic changes involving the kidneys, liver, central nervous system, and other organs, could occur as a result of prolonged and diffuse intracapillary agglutination.

The implication is strong that, whenever feasible, *strictly compatible blood, of the same group as the patient, should be used;* and that, under conditions that render the exclusive use of group O blood advisable, only blood of low titer should be supplied. *There are strong reasons to suspect that even pooled human plasma,* with low agglutinin titer, when administered in very large amounts to individuals of blood groups other than group O, *may have undesirable or even dangerous effects,* and that the use of fractionated human albumin would be far preferable in such cases.[111]

Tobruk splint studies.—Studies on the efficacy of the Tobruk splint, so popular with the British, were completed under the direction of Colonel Manning, orthopedic consultant to the Ninth U.S. Army. The results of his studies were read at the last grand meeting of American and British consultants to be described below.

Rank and promotion.—As the years passed during the war, Colonel Cutler became more and more incensed at the inequalities of the promotion system in a theater of operations that was inexplicably tied to tables of organization and seemed to give the higher ranks to those in command and administrative positions at the expense of those in professional positions. For the last 2 years of the war, Colonel Cutler made the correction of these seeming inequalities a personal battle which he fought at every opportunity. The discussion at the meeting of the Chief Surgeon's Consultants' Committee on 30 December 1944 brought out well the facets which made the problem so difficult of solution. The following minutes show that Colonel Cutler brought up the matter by mentioning the inequality of the rank of otolaryngologists, previously referred to, and the discussion which ensued:

Col. Cutler: It has been brought up repeatedly that there are discrepancies in rank that we find difficulty in correcting. One in the new T/O, for instance, where the otolaryngologist is listed as captain. We happen to have some otolaryngologists who are lieutenant colonels and majors. It does present a problem. We also have many expert people who have served their country three years as captains, but it will be difficult for them to be promoted, unless we move them out into an administrative post. Then they will be promoted, but we don't want to lose them. What are we to say about the future of those cases?

---

[111] (1) Essential Technical Medical Data, European Theater of Operations, U.S. Army, for June 1945, dated 13 August 1945. Inclosure 9, subject: Investigation of Transfusion Therapy, Ninth U.S. Army. (2) Emerson, C. P., Jr., and Ebert, R. V.: Study of Shock in Battle Casualties; Measurements of Blood Volume Changes Occurring in Response to Therapy. Ann. Surg. 122: 745–772, November 1945.

Gen. Hawley: Everything you say is true. In so far as the specific case you mention as the otolaryngologist being a captain, I think that we can make strong presentations to the War Department to have things like that corrected. I don't know whether the War Department will do anything about it. It is a very difficult thing. Everything you can say that these people deserve rank can't be refuted. When you compare their ability, their training, their value to the government, when you compare them with officers of other branches, or even to other officers within the Medical Department, it is obviously unfair and unjust. There is no question about it. I agree with that wholeheartedly.

Col. Cutler: Would it be proper for us to write this up in the technical data report?

Gen. Hawley: Yes, it is really irrefutable argument.

Col. Cutler: It might be good for the next war.

Gen. Hawley: Yes, it might. You come into the question of a military organization. Now, there has got to be in every organization—it may be a necessary nuisance, but there has got to be a commander, and the wide experience—I am not talking about the Medical Department now; I am talking about the Army in general—many, many years of experience has shown that it is always essential that the commander be of at least one grade higher than anybody else in his organization. All right then, we come down, and nobody could defend in a one-thousand bed general hospital, I think, of rating the commander as a general officer. I think that colonel is all we can defend in a one-thousand bed hospital. Now, we come down to the chiefs of services. They are more or less specialized; their training may be, and usually is, much better, much more comprehensive than that of the hospital commander. Then when we come down to the chiefs of services, we have got to have section chiefs under them. When you analyze the ratings of our officers, and compare the other branches of service with the ratings in the Medical Department, you find that there is a much higher proportion of high rank than in any other branch of the service, with the exception, possibly, of The Judge Advocate General's Department.

I don't believe that we are ever going to solve this problem on the basis of military rank, because I think you run into that formidable thing of weakening the entire military structure when you get into it. Now, if there is any other approach to the problem, some other way—if we can discard rank from pay, for example, or any other way to give recognition to these people, we may be able to get them, but when we get right back into those things which were tried for 74 years in our army, and it worked awful. It didn't make for a very smooth staff, and particularly in the Medical Department, so they fought for years and years and finally they got general military rank instead of rank within their own branch, and I don't think that anybody who knows the history of those 75 years would want to go back to that system. I think that the thing that we have got to foster—this may sound silly to you; I realize that I am talking from a different point of view. I am trying to take into consideration your point of view. I know it is easy for me to talk and pat you on the back, because it was only through the channels of chance that I got much more than I deserved.

I was down in Nicaragua with Dan Sultan, who is now in the India Theater * * * That is separate from China-Burma now. He showed me several reports from some young Engineer officers. I knew about what the second lieutenants out of the academy were like, and these men were at the top of their class. Some of them were rated very, very low, and yet they were better officers than those in the same grade in any other service, and I said to him, "My God, man, what are you doing to these people? Compared to some other branches of the Service, these lads are superior plus. They have got everything." He said, "Yes, but that isn't the point. I am not rating them according to the other services; I am rating them with Engineer officers. They may be superior plus compared to the rest of the Army, but I am rating them within the Corps of Engineers."

That is one point of view. I think we are going to have to go back to that old-fashioned hillbilly religion, where they take the attitude that we are not going to set our rewards on earth, but in Heaven. I don't know of any way of recognizing by military rank the high professionally qualified experts and at the same time preserving the military structure. If anybody can work out a more feasible plan, that will fit both of those requirements, I will go along with it. On the other hand, I think it is quite correct to put that in a report, and I will send it to The Surgeon General.

Col. Cutler: In the last war, it was felt that this terrible matter of rank consciousness which is doing so much injury now is due to the fact that there has been too much rank given. I was up in the Ninth U.S. Army, and I saw four evacuation hospitals with young colonels commanding. I don't see why the commanding officer of a 400-bed evacuation hospital should be a full colonel. If they had left it down to a lower grade, there wouldn't be this problem. There is certainly a lot more trouble in this war than in the last war.

Gen. Hawley: I think that it is a good point to take up with The Surgeon General. I think they are overrated. Well, all I can do is to say that I am terribly sympathetic, and I will support any program that will solve this problem.

The first result of this discussion, and the General's promise to do anything he could about it, was that, whenever necessary, hospitals were exhorted to carry specially qualified professional personnel as overstrength to be absorbed by the total number in various grades regardless of the position for which these grades were specified. This permitted the placing of well-qualified specialists wherever they were needed, regardless of vacancies, but it certainly did not enhance their popularity. Moreover, this procedure had merely permitted the unrestricted placement of "over in rank" professional medical officers, but did not, per se, clear a path for their promotion.

The alternative, within the existing system to provide positions calling for higher rank was to obtain tables of organization for larger hospitals. Quite fortuitously, at about that time, the War Department informed the European theater that no more hospital units could be provided from the Zone of Interior, and, if more beds were needed, some of the 1,000-bed units presently in the European theater would have to be expanded.

When General Hawley received this information, he called Colonel Cutler and Colonel Middleton into his office and instructed each to give him the names of the twelve best chiefs of surgery and of medicine in the European theater. He told them that the hospitals to be expanded had to be selected on the basis of the adaptability of present plants and facilities to expansion, and that it was unfair to afford the opportunity for increased rank upon any such basis. Therefore, he said, before announcing the hospitals to be expanded, he would transfer the best chiefs of surgery and medicine into them so that these men would get the promotions.[112]

Colonel Cutler selected the surgical individuals personally with the advice and recommendations of the other consultants. He interviewed each individual selected as to whether he would leave close friends and working associates for the dubious reward of recognition by an advance in rank at a strange hospital. It so happened that most of those deserving promotion to the rank of colonel were in hospitals in the United Kingdom, while the hospitals with

---

[112] Letter, Paul R. Hawley, M.D., to Col. John Boyd Coates, Jr., MC, 17 Sept. 1958.

expanded tables of organization were on the Continent. Now, these individuals singled out for the new promotion positions were superior officers, and everyone knew it. Hospital commanders and General Spruit, the United Kingdom Base surgeon, were not inclined to release them. Again, through the persuasive efforts of Colonel Cutler, and eventually, by the positive actions of General Hawley, these objections were overcome. Meanwhile, individuals in these hospitals with expanded tables of organization who thought they were deserving of the promotion had to be pacified, and the hospital commanders, from whose hands the requests for promotion had to emanate, required close scrutiny so that they would not give the rank called for by the professional position to some other officer.

After these herculean efforts, recommendations for promotion had finally been submitted for the selected few. Periodically, Colonel Cutler was obliged to ask what was happening to the promotion requests and to exhort their rapid promulgation. For instance, on 19 May 1945, he wrote, in a memorandum to the Chief Surgeon, the following:

1. At your request we brought over to the Continent the seven best surgeons we could find. This was done after considerable difficulty with General Spruit and all the Hospital Commanders who were affected.

2. It was my understanding that these officers would be promoted to the T/O vacancies of Colonel.

3. None of them have been promoted, and I have serious misgivings about their being promoted, for at the 203rd I understand the Commanding Officer has put in the Executive Officer for one of the colonelcy vacancies.

4. I believe failure to promote these men will be highly destructive of morale and broaden the chasm between the Regular Army Medical Corps and civilian doctors which it will be extremely difficult to heal.

5. Perhaps you feel this is important enough to take action personally.

The ultimate result was that, by theater policy, all promotions in a wide category of units were suddenly frozen before these selected officers could be promoted, although the necessary requests had been submitted a long time previously. The Chief Consultant in Surgery, on this untoward turn of events, asked whether exceptions could not be made in the case of those whose promotion recommendations had been submitted prior to the restriction. He was asked to cite specific examples as basis for pressing the case. Citing the case of three officers on 22 July 1945 in a memorandum addressed to the Deputy Chief Surgeon, General Cutler wrote:

1. * * *
Note that the original promotion request went in in February 1945 and was just kicked around by the worst kind of red tape.

2. General Hawley asked me to submit individual instances of this kind and said that some relief could be had. It would, in my opinion, be a far better solution to have G–1 draw up a general recommendation, stating that officers whose request for promotion was submitted in good faith and approved at all levels preceding V–E Day, but whose promotion did not go through because of red tape, should now be permitted the channels for promotion. If this cannot be done, something should be done to wipe out the most regrettable situation which has occurred because of Army red tape and favoritism.

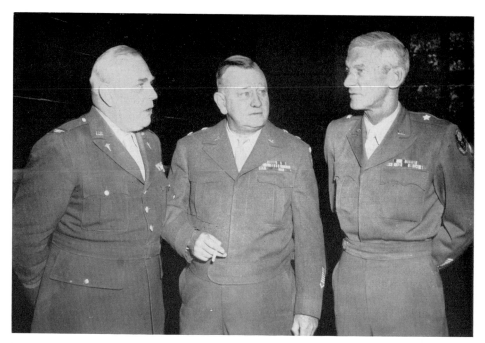

FIGURE 123.—Colonel Shook, General Hawley, and newly promoted Brig. Gen. Elliot C. Cutler.

On 11 August 1945, the day before his departure home and, possibly in the last paragraph of the last piece of official action correspondence to be prepared by Brigadier General Cutler, he bitterly and plaintively wrote:

5. I should inform you also that General Hawley and I submitted to General Lee the names of those surgeons who were brought to hospitals with increased T/O's in March, for promotion to full colonelcy. General Lee promised he would see these things through, and I hope the matter will not be forgotten. These men were brought here in good faith, they have filled a T/O vacancy for the required time, and Army red tape should not jeopardize their greatly deserved promotion.[113]

The U.S. Senate, when asked to consent to his promotion to temporary brigadier general rank, among others, was quick to comply (fig. 123). But General Cutler could not budge what he called the "red tape" in the theater with respect to the promotion of a mere handful of deserving, outstanding surgeons—lieutenant colonels—to full colonels.

Professional services for the occupation army.—From time to time during the posthostilities period, General Cutler, by request, made recommendations for the organization of professional services in the occupation army. It was planned to have a system of hospital centers to administer the farflung network of hospitals which would be required for the occupation forces. The

---

[113] Memorandum, Professional Services Division (Brig. Gen. E. C. Cutler) to Deputy Chief Surgeon, 11 Aug. 1945, subject: Status of Professional Service Division, 11 Aug. 45.

prevailing system of appointing qualified specialists in hospitals of a particular center as consultants in their specialties for the hospitals of the center and the surrounding area was quite applicable for the contemplated centers of the occupation force. Likewise, the system of surgical coordinators to coordinate the surgical activities within a hospital center was quite appropriate. Thus, new directives outlining the functions and operations of hospital centers included these plans just as they had been operating for some time.

In a memorandum, dated 6 July 1945, General Cutler advised the Deputy Chief Surgeon concerning the plan for the constitution of the Professional Services Division as it was to serve USFET (the U.S. Forces in the European Theater), the posthostilities command. General Kenner, who had relieved General Hawley as Chief Surgeon, accepted in principle the concept expressed in the following excerpt from this memorandum:

2. I spent five hours on 5 July with General Kenner, discussing matters relating to Professional Services Division, ETO, and redeployment. This conference resulted in the following plan for the Division of Professional Services, ETO, being approved by General Kenner:—

a. There are to remain in Professional Services Division the following officers:—

One Colonel, Chief of Division.
One Colonel, Chief Consultant in Surgery.
One Colonel, Chief Consultant in Medicine.
One Field grade officer, Psychiatry.
One Field grade officer, Orthopedic surgery.
One Field grade officer, Consultant to WAC.
One Executive officer.

b. In addition to these officers permanently assigned to the Office of the Surgeon, ETO-Com Z at this time, and later to move to U.S. Forces Headquarters, Frankfurt, there must be in the Paris hospitals thoroughly competent specialists in the following fields: Radiology; Otolaryngology; Neurosurgery; Maxillofacial surgery; Anesthesiology; Ophthalmology; Urology; and Burns. These officers should be of high caliber, competent to act as consultants, and holding the respect of their fellow officers for their professional abilities. They in turn, or substitutes for them to be provided later, must be moved to hospitals near Frankfurt when Professional Services Division moves to Frankfurt from Paris—Versailles.

3. The group of consultants in Paris will be the only consultant group in ETO, other than Army consultants, and they will continue to function to set proper professional standards and policies for the optimum care of the American soldier. In particular, during the period of redeployment, when confusion exists, visits to hospitals must continue in order that there be no relaxation in the care rendered by the Medical Department.

4. In order that this program be implemented immediately, it is now requested that orders be issued moving Lt. Col. Hall G. Holder, Lt. Col. Wm. Field and Lt. Col. Currier McEwen on D/S into the Office of the Chief Surgeon, so that they may become acquainted with the duties that they must shortly assume in their entirety.

In the interim before General Cutler was ready to leave the European theater, there were several minor changes to the original recommendations, and General Kenner decided that a director of professional services was not required. Lt. Col. Hall G. Holder, MC, had, however, been ordered to Headquarters, ETOUSA, to understudy the position of Chief, Professional Services

Division, and was still filling the job on 11 August 1945 when General Cutler advised:

1. I hope to be flying from the Continent on 12 August.

2. Arrangements have been made for Colonel Pisani and Major Loizeaux to leave the theater within a month.

3. By the end of this month, Professional Services Division will consist of the following officers:

Chief of the Division—Lt. Col. Hall G. Holder
Chief Consultant in Medicine—Lt. Col. O. C. McEwen
Chief Consultant in Surgery—Lt. Col. L. Miscall
Senior Consultant in Orthopedic Surgery—Maj. G. T. Aitken
Consultant to the WAC—Capt. Martha Howe

And, for a period of a few weeks, 1st Lt. Jean L. Beatty, PTO [Physical Therapy Officer].

4. The enlisted personnel remaining will consist of 3 EM and 3 WAC, together with 3 or 4 British secretaries.[114]

Third Anglo-American Consultants' Conference

The long-drawn-out period after V–E Day had its bright moments, too. One of these was the continuation of the conferences between British and American consultants. The first had been held under American auspices in Paris, the second was in Brussels under sponsorship of the British 21 Army Group, and the third reverted to Paris again. The site was the same, the 108th General Hospital; the dates, 25 and 26 May 1945. On each successive occasion of these conferences, consultants who should have been invited to previous meetings, and were not, had been added to the list and, by the time of this third and final conference, there were American consultants from the field armies, base sections, and theater headquarters plus Dr. Karl A. Meninger, Dr. Romano, and Dr. Kubie from the visiting commission of civilian neuropsychiatric consultants to The Surgeon General. From the British side, there were consultants from the headquarters of the British Army, the Royal Navy, and the Royal Air Force and from the 21 Army Group. There were representatives from the Canadian Forces. In addition, as observers, there were Colonel Osipov representing the Soviet Armed Forces and guests from the French Army (fig. 124).

The discussions were lively and the points made were vigorously indorsed or opposed. Coming as they did so shortly after the cessation of hostilities, the meetings were very much a review of thinking on the professional highlights of the war—the failures, the successes, and the unresolved problems. It is most unfortunate that space does not permit the reproduction of the complete transcript of the meetings, for, together, the thoughts expressed represent the combined and individual thinking of the officers who were the leaders in professional medical matters throughout the war in Europe and elsewhere in their respective services and commands.

---

[114] See footnote 113, p. 340.

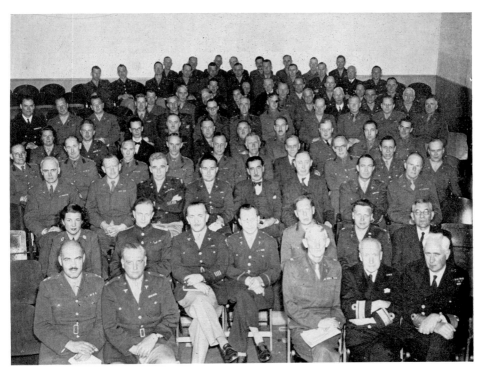

FIGURE 124.—Participants at the Inter-Allied Consultants' Conference on 25 and 26 May 1945 at the 108th General Hospital, Paris, France.

Medical manpower.—The topic for the general session on 25 May 1945 was medical manpower. General Hawley was chairman of the session and opened the proceedings with the following remarks:

Gentlemen. I have a very happy memory of the last meeting of this group in this room. One of the happiest is that the discussion was full, fluid and often forceful. I hold that up to you as an example and I hope that this meeting repeats. I want to remind you of the famous remark made by Duke-Elder when the inclusion of other people in the membership of this club was the topic under discussion at a dinner meeting. Duke settled the discussion by saying to us Americans: "I can tell you that you don't know what you are talking about, but we can't tell that to some of the other nationalities." So I ask, if anyone disagrees with anything that is said here, that he take exception to it. I assure you I shall be a qualified and unprejudiced referee of all bouts here. The subject for this morning's discussion was selected by Colonel Cutler who talked to me about it at length before the program was made. It is a subject which has been very close to his heart for a long time. It is a subject which didn't concern the Americans very much at the outset of the war but has been of increasing concern to us as the war has gone on. Never has it been more critical than it is now with the necessity of redeployment to the Pacific. This is especially true in the field of specialties. It is a subject which has concerned the British from the outset of the war. When I first came to Britain in 1941, I remember meeting with your Medical Manpower Board. They wanted information on our use of medical manpower, and told me at that time of the critical shortage. For these reasons we think that this is a very vital subject. We have all had experience in the campaign here. Now do we need more medical manpower or can we do without some that we have? The subject has been divided into echelons of service because obviously the problem varies with the different echelons of the fighting forces.

Accepting General Hawley's suggestion that the meeting pick up the full, fluid, and forceful discussions of previous meetings, the conference proceeded at a lively pace on the discussion of medical manpower as it affected the division medical service, medical service in the field army, and finally the communications zone. Fortunately, the transcript of the meeting contains a summarization written by Colonel Cutler at a later date. His synthesis of the opinions expressed was as follows:

1. The major matter brought up by all speakers, and approved by all, was that highly-trained professional personnel must be kept mobile. This principle referred to the personnel not only in "Army" installations but also in Com Z institutions.

2. The division personnel. It would appear that no cut could be had in the medical battalion personnel attached to the division per se, which numbers about twenty-six (26), but some further cut might be made in the attached personnel which brings the total medical officers in [U.S.] divisions to around forty-four (44), as compared with the British number of thirty (30).

3. Army. All but Colonel MacFee thought the surgical teams should be kept mobile and there was even a suggestion that evacuation hospitals, as well as field hospitals, be largely housekeeping units, though the evacuation hospital should have a medical and surgical chief and a few officers to enable it to give competent assistance when acting as a station hospital.

4. A suggestion was made that the surgical teams should be cut down to one (1) surgeon, one (1) anesthetist, and two (2) enlisted men.

5. The final suggestion was that difficulties of mobility, and thus saving manpower, were more wrapped up in:—
    a. Transportation, or
    b. Red tape,
which prevented easy interchange between the Army and the Com Z units.

Few of the comments made can here be quoted; however, using Colonel Cutler's summary as a jumping off point, the following excerpts from the transcript were typical of the thoughts expressed.

Colonel Berry, Consultant in Surgery, Seventh U.S. Army, and with experience in North Africa, Italy, and the campaigns in the European theater, said of medical manpower in the field army:

General Hawley and guests. The [types of] Army medical installations of the second echelon, as you know, in our army consist of the field hospital with the auxiliary teams and two evacuation hospitals; a semimobile one of four hundred (400) beds and one of seven hundred and fifty (750) beds. We also have a neuropsychiatric center, a venereal disease center, a convalescent hospital of three thousand (3,000) beds, a mobile army laboratory, an optical unit, and a blood bank detachment. It seems to me our function in the army is twofold: First aid medical care to the patient and retention of the maximum number of ill or wounded soldiers within the army area. The field hospital has been a godsend to us. It was first used in the Sicilian campaign in its present type. It was easy to adapt and carry over and it has been used essentially in the same manner by the various armies conforming to a standard that was finally developed by the Fifth Army where it was perfected. It has operated largely as a housekeeping unit. It has a small headquarters detachment and it has three (3) platoons each commanded by a major with three (3) medical officers. All of the professional work, all of the casualties, have been handled by the auxiliary surgical teams. The three (3) officers have been used to help out in resuscitation, assisting in the operating room and postoperative care. Immediately behind that was the four hundred (400) bed semimobile hospital on the basis of one (1) per division. Now discussion has centered particularly on this unit and the seven hundred and fifty (750) bed evacuation hospital, which we have used on the basis of one (1) per two (2) divisions or one (1) per three (3) divisions. The personnel of the four hundred (400) bed evacuation hospital has twenty-seven (27) medical officers. The seven hundred and fifty (750) bed evacuation hospital has thirty-five (35) medical officers, including two chiefs of services. Now, if you ration patient beds, you will find that the medical officers in the seven hundred and fifty (750) bed unit have about five (5) or six (6) more patients per officer. The seven hundred and fifty (750) bed unit is so styled that it is capable of expansion up to double the number with the same number of doctors and enlisted men. It creaks and groans when it gets over twelve hundred (1,200) beds, but it will go over. The four hundred (400) bed is so streamlined in personnel that it is incapable of going over fifty (50) or one hundred (100) beds more than its table of organization and equipment. The four hundred (400) bed has been made more mobile than the seven hundred and fifty (750) bed. One argument that has been advanced for the four hundred (400) bed evacuation hospital is that it is mobile. Well, the difference is not in the size of the hospital but in the fact that the four hundred (400) bed evacuation hospital is equipped with twenty (20) trucks and eighteen (18) trailers and the seven hundred and fifty (750) bed evacuation hospital until recently has been equipped with two (2) trucks and no trailers. It wasn't the size that made the difference in mobility. That has been overcome by arranging headquarters transportation. Now, the question of saving manpower comes on various stages and it seems to me first from the professional standpoint that these large staffs in the evacuation hospitals could be cut down somewhat. How much I am not prepared to say and the auxiliary teams could be greatly expanded to include groups of other specialists. Let's take the neurosurgical team. That is a highly skilled group. They are needed badly. Having them permanently assigned as the staff of an evacuation hospital ties them up because it is very difficult to move them from one evacuation hospital to another. It is far less difficult to call up or send a message to the commanding officer of an auxiliary group and say that the neurosurgical team is needed and as soon as it is finished it could return to group headquarters. One evacuation hospital has had the same neurosurgical team since August. It became part of the staff. Two others have had theirs for two (2) or three (3) months; one throughout the winter. It seems to me that the same type of team could be greatly expanded. On the latest T/O of the seven hundred and fifty (750) bed evacuation hospital there are at least eighteen (18) on the surgical side and thirteen (13) on the medical side and included in that number are specialists—neurologists, thoracic surgeons, to say nothing of plastic, oral, eye, ear, nose and throat, and other surgeons. It has been very difficult to get all the specialists and yet an army should have that within the army area. All of them should be used where necessary. It is a waste of manpower to send a soldier back to the communications zone for those specialist services * * *.

Col. J. P. Ross of the RAMC, Consultant in Neurosurgery, to the EMS, spoke also, as follows, of the problem of moving medical officers to where they are needed when they are needed:

* * * The difficulty with medical manpower is this. It is exemplified in this chart very well. You have three (3) divisions [echelons] perhaps four (4) and you have communications zone, and these, medically speaking, are all water tight compartments. You give to each of those regiments, divisions, corps, armies, etc., a number of medical men and they think that they own them. They hesitate to allow them to shift, because they

fear they will not get them back again. In any army or in any campaign a battle lasts only so long and that must always be so. There may be a great many casualties or there may be a few casualties, but the battle can only last a certain length of time because of other factors. If you have an organization which will allow you to move medical men from the front and back again without too much red tape, you can save medical manpower. When you set up forward medical installations with certain skeletal staffs, then you require a pool or a series of pools with medical officers who can be attached. The difficulty we have had in our army, and I think it is the same in other armies, is that of movement of officers. We decide there may be a fair number of casualties in this area and we want to get some medical personnel from the back area. We have had the battle, we have had the casualties, they have been evacuated, and the medical officers are needed in the rear. The necessity is to have skeleton staffs on hospitals, on CCS [Casualty Clearing Stations], and on teams and add to them. You see, what happens is that when a commanding officer of twelve hundred (1,200) bed hospital thinks that he has thirty (30) or forty (40) medical officers and he is quite convinced that he owns them and that if they get away he will never get them back, he will not release them.

Brigadier H. C. Edwards spoke of the tremendous potential usefulness of the British FSU (Field Surgical Unit).

General Hawley, the moderator, asked Colonel Bricker to say a few words as Consultant in Plastic Surgery because most of the discussion had been monopolized by the general surgeons. An earlier speaker had said that specialists were not needed up front and that the more specialized a doctor became, the further to the rear was his place of business. At any rate, Colonel Bricker confined his comments to the specialist in the communications zone, without arguing the point made earlier, as follows:

What I have to say * * * [concerns] * * * the efficient use of specialists in communications zone hospitals. We have a large number of one thousand (1,000) bed general hospitals in the communications zone. It has obviously been impossible to make them self-sufficient. The solution has been the obvious one of putting the specialty in the designated hospitals and placing them in a strategical location and seeing that the patients get to them. This has had serious difficulties because of our T/O in certain hospitals. We need thoracic surgeons, neurosurgeons and plastic surgeons. They have filled the jobs of the assistant chief of the surgical and chief of septic surgery and ward officer. We have had to use them. This means that once they are in the hospital they are assigned. If the situation changes as it can change, we have to change the personnel, that means making the [trade] between hospital center, commanding officer and finding replacement and it takes time and in some cases it has taken weeks. In an emergency we can make a trade quickly. Routine changes have taken a tremendous amount of time * * *. In England we had time to get our plan set up. It has worked very well. On the Continent, it hasn't worked so well because the hospitals were coming in rapidly. The solution, I am quite convinced, is the one mentioned by Colonel Seeley. It is putting specialist personnel in cellular units * * *.

Surgical meeting.—The surgical meeting took place the following morning, Saturday, 26 May 1945. Colonel Cutler was the chairman and moderator. The initial topic was the management of combined bone and nerve injury, procedures which had seen considerable improvement during World War II with the realization and acceptance of the fact that a flail limb was a useless one, regardless of the condition of bone, and that repair of the nerve in these cases had to take precedence over the fracture. It was mentioned that asepsis of the wounds seen in World War II was a great factor in permitting the early repair of nerve injuries. Colonel Spurling and Colonel Cleveland were very much in evidence throughout the discussion, which was opened by the reading of a report by Colonel Spurling on the experience of the U.S. Army in the European theater in the management of combined bone and nerve injury. From the British side, Mr. Geoffrey Jefferson, EMS Consultant in Neurosurgery; Brigadier Rowley W. Bristow, British Army Consultant in Orthopedics; and Air Commodore Osmond Clark, RAF Consultant in Orthopedics, carried the discussion. Brigadier Porritt, surgical consultant to the 21 Army Group also spoke at length.

The second subject for discussion was the Tobruk splint. Colonel Manning, orthopedic consultant to the Ninth U.S. Army, opened the topic by reading his paper on the studies conducted in that Army. He explained:

During the months of November and December 1944 five evacuation hospitals assigned to Ninth U.S. Army applied the Tobruk splint to every fracture of the femur treated, with the exception of those cases in which the ring of the splint would cause pressure on a wound of the upper thigh or buttock and those in which skin traction could not be applied because of wounds or fractures of the leg.

Every effort possible was made to obtain a supply of full ring leg splints so that the British technique of application could be followed. However, this was found to be impossible. A technique of application was standardized * * *.

After giving detailed data on the results of the study, Colonel Manning, in his summary, said that 19 percent of the total number of 63 splints were considered to be superior to the spica cast as a transportation splint, 78 percent were inferior, and 2 percent were not recorded on the questionnaires returned. He also mentioned that the comfort of the splint and the opinion as to its superiority did not coincide because 32 percent of the splints were considered to have been comfortable, but only 19 percent were recorded as being superior to the spica cast. His conclusions follow:

The Tobruk type splint requires less plaster, time and work to apply than does the spica cast, but it cannot be applied universally to all fractures of the femur, and does not provide adequate splinting or comfort. The results of the study are conclusive that the Tobruk splint is inferior to the spica cast as a transportation splint for fractures of the femur.

The barrage of opinion from the British side, following this report was pretty much one sided. The minutes describe Brigadier Bristow's comments on the British experience as follows:

He would like it to be clearly understood that he was not going to try to sell the Americans anything, he was not competing with Colonel Cleveland! He was just trying to tell the experience they had had with this splint. The name "Tobruk" was perhaps almost unfortunate because it appeared as if this was something tremendously new and some great invention. It was simply Hugh Owen Thomas' splint, designed in the year 1870, reinforced with a bit of plaster of paris around the outside to keep it snug on the limb while the patient was on his journey. It was a transport appliance and nothing else. The British experience had been that this splint, properly applied, helped patients on the whole to travel back extremely well. The experience now was fairly large; they had seen them return from long distances from the Western desert, had seen many in Italy and Africa, and had had over 2,000 femurs back to the United Kingdom out of this theater. We were speaking of a considerably large section, and the experience was not that of any individual man. * * *

As regarded ease of application, he noted that the Americans were now in agreement with the British that this method of splintage did save time and material. He had had a report only a week or two ago from one of the hospital ships, from the surgical specialist, who remarked that he wished people would not send the patients with spicas because he very often had to change them en route and it was difficult to change spicas on a hospital ship. The meeting could take it that it was a considered opinion in Britain, by all types of surgeons who had seen these patients return, that they were satisfied that they do travel home pretty well, and they all thought this a good and useful appliance.

Colonel Eyre-Brook, orthopedic consultant, 21 Army Group, mentioned that the result of finding 19 percent who were of the opinion that the Tobruk plaster had been superior to the spica was very good as a start, considering the difficulties involved in training people to put on the Tobruk as it should be put on, and allowing for various technical difficulties which must have been weighty. Colonel Eyre-Brook had come to the European theater from the Mediterranean completely uninfluenced and stated that he had been quite convinced that the Tobruk splint, properly applied, effectively immobilized the limb and gave comfort.

There were other opinions from the British which generally coincided with these. Colonel Cleveland said that this splint of the Americans was not the Tobruk splint. They had not the same material and had not been able to put it on as well. He stated that this was the Maastricht splint, and it had not been as satisfactory as the spica. General Hawley said that this topic was the "piece de resistance" which had brought him to that particular session. Colonel Cutler closed this subject with the remark that this slight difference over the Tobruk splint served to put in very considerable relief the fact that this was about the only thing concerning which they had had any controversy in the past 3 years.

The meeting then continued on to similarly detailed discussions on anesthesia in war and thoracic surgery with active participation in the discussions on the part of both the British and the Americans. Colonel Cutler, at the close of the meeting, made the following speech:

I wish to take a moment before we part to speak about consultants in general and this group in particular. The life of a consultant is difficult; more difficult in the American Army than in the British Army because consultants are not on a regular T/O and are not a part of our Army in peace time. I know also, as a background to these remarks, that the United States Army Consultant Group in the last war did not have a very happy relation with the officers of the Regular Army. As a result, officers of the Medical Corps were in fact warned of the difficulties that might arise if consultants were used. Thus, officers now acting as consultants started under a certain cloud. Those who had been through the last war and knew of this were able to discount some of their difficulties. The life of a consultant is difficult for many reasons. It is difficult physically and difficult intellectually. It is difficult physically because to be a good consultant one should be steadily moving; it is a peripatetic existence. It is the Hippocratic method of teaching. It necessitates continual visits to hospitals, ward rounds, conferences with medical officers, all of whom have a differing point of view. And in each place and with each officer advice must be given so that treatment is of a high order and standardized. It is difficult intellectually because you are always meeting new people, always having to convince others by persuasion rather than force, which is a very real strain. In addition, as deficiencies show up new standards must be set; and where personnel are inadequate transfers must be brought about. To move continuously, with inadequate transport, shift your bed each night, eat field rations—to do this day after day and talk to new people day after day is difficult and it is a life of strain. I congratulate the United States Army officers here for having lived through it so well. I know you have done a good job and I know that your Chief feels that way. I wish to add my own deep conviction of satisfaction that you have done your job well; that is all that any man should ask for. You have served your country well and you will be satisfied in that service.

To our British and Russian colleagues I have a different message. We are under a very deep debt of gratitude to each of you individually, and to the group as a whole. You have offered us every facility, and you have offered us the kindest and most generous personal hospitality. It is something we will probably never be able to repay. You all cannot come to our homes, and we cannot thank you individually, and we cannot entertain you in the way we should like. But I know I can speak for all the United States Army officers in this room when I say that if there are any of you who ever do come to the United States of America, each officer here in this room will be happy to entertain you, he will be grateful to see you again, and he will be privileged that you came.

General Hawley then addressed the meeting in the following words:

I think that from my point of view I realize that everything Colonel Cutler has said is true. I was very young and unimportant in the last war, but I have heard handed down to me by the older men who were in responsible positions that the situation in our services in France was not always completely happy with the consultants. Well, I think that the consultants perhaps may have exaggerated that feeling here. Certainly, no group around me has been more essential and more welcome at all times. It takes a lot of adjustment on both sides, and I separate the sides into administrative and professional. It takes most of the adjustment on the administrative side. It takes some little adjustment for the professional men to realize not that things cannot be done, but to realize that we are treating hundreds of thousands of patients instead of one patient, and that all methods and all procedures must be adjusted to that point of view. The policy in our office has been that the only reason for the existence of the medical service has been the care of patients, and there are no administrative reasons why a thing cannot be done professionally for 100,000 patients.

The American soldier, in my considered opinion, has received better care than he has ever received in his life, in former wars or in civilian life. There is only one reason for this, because this Consultant Group of mine have completely directed and administered the care of the soldier, and to them all credit for this is due. Wherever this, in a few cases, has not been achieved, the reason usually is an administrative one, where we have not been able to get that patient and that doctor together at the proper time, and so I say, without any effort at flattery, but most sincerely, that all the good in the care of patients in this theater has come from this group of consultants, and all the bad has come from the administrative side.

I am awfully happy to have had all of you here and, while I shall probably not be having the privilege of meeting with this group again, these meetings we have had will always stand out in all my life as very high spots. Thank you all.

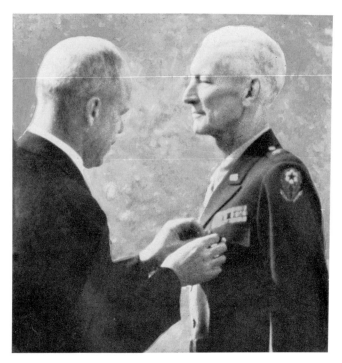

FIGURE 125.—General Cutler being decorated with the Distinguished Service Medal by Robert P. Patterson, Secretary of War, at Boston, Mass., in 1947.

Military Surgery, ETOUSA, 1944–45

Perhaps, to General Cutler, the greatest honor which was bestowed on him as a result of his wartime activities in the United Kingdom and on the Continent was the invitation from the Royal College of Surgeons of England to give the Hunterian Lecture for 1945. He humbly accepted the invitation, and at a time when he was close to exhaustion, placed all his faculties into an effort to make a worthy contribution to the first resumption of this traditional lecture following the peace in Europe. No more fitting ending could be given to this account of a great chapter in General Cutler's life, which except for 2 short years that followed was his final chapter (fig. 125), than to quote from his Hunterian Lecture.

The topic was "Military Surgery—United States Army—European Theater of Operations, 1944–45." The date was 14 June 1945. General Cutler began his lecture by saying that the mission of the Medical Department, U.S. Army (as far as military surgery was concerned), was threefold: (1) Evacuation of the wounded from the battlefield where their presence jeopardizes morale, and from army hospitals where their care infringes upon the mobility and supply of combat forces, (2) provision of professional medical care wherein the battle casualty, medical officer, and proper facilities must all be brought together, and (3) restoration of the injured man to combat. He then proceeded:

To accomplish this threefold mission, there must be a carefully integrated organization, and some understanding of this is desirable if one is to appreciate the results which it has achieved. A primary consideration is the complete interdependence of administration and professional care, on which depends its effectiveness. The civilian doctor is prepared to expend every ounce of energy and all of his time on a single patient, knowing that others can be found to care for additional injured or sick people who might present themselves at the same time. This policy, when one is confronted with thousands and not individuals, must be forgotten in the greater good for the larger number. This change of outlook from the individual to the mass is the chief difficulty confronting the civilian doctor when he enters military service. Moreover, if the three functions of the Medical Department are to be fulfilled—evacuation, medical and surgical care, and restoration to combat fighting— attention must be focused more and more on those who can be returned to duty. By so doing, eventually a greater good for humanity will be achieved, for, if large numbers of men can be restored to the fighting forces, war will end sooner and thus humanity suffer less. This need not result in neglect of the severely damaged soldiers.

After explaining in detail the complete accepted organization of the medical service of a theater of operations, he continued:

* * * only the perfect interdigitation of administrative and professional personnel can lead to a happy solution when thousands of wounded men are handled daily. Professional personnel must be informed where the load is to be borne, how long casualties can remain in one hospital, and what methods of evacuation are to be used if proper care is to be given. And personalities must be forgotten. In spite of difficulties, the professional group always attempted to carry out the policies set by the Chief Surgeon, both those which placed a time limit on professional care and that which demanded of us that the American soldier be given the best care possible under the conditions imposed by the military situation. Administration must set evacuation and hospitalization policies, but these policies and the burden they impose are borne by others. Good results will accrue only when both are completely informed of the labor and responsibility of the other. Directives are no substitute for good briefing, whether the goal be tactical or medical.

Next, General Cutler presented statistical data showing the load carried in the European theater and comparing it with the other theaters of war with respect to total numbers of casualties and the types of wounds received. He began his discussion of professional care provided in the European theater by referring to the Manual of Therapy and the various circular letters on professional policies and procedures. He said:

* * * the Medical Corps, scattered throughout the entire theater, have been willing to assimilate these standardized methods and have greatly improved the original directives by suggestions and additions as experience hardened our opinion or showed flaws and defects in the original methods outlined.

This willingness to accept standardization, the thirst for education in military surgery, and the ability to improve on original standards has characterized our professional colleagues from the very beginning.

Further, on professional care, the general pointed out:

The one item in professional care which distinguishes care in this war from care in World War I, as well as the single factor most directly contributing to the improvement of morbidity and mortality statistics, is the resuscitation of the wounded man. This transcends in importance any single method of therapy, such as our ability to procure and deliver blood and plasma to casualties, for it betokens that the American surgeon has at last appreciated the importance of the complete evaluation of his patients before therapy. He has learned to care for the whole of man and not for any fragment or any particular wound. * * *

* * * It is this overall appreciation of diminution in the amount of circulating blood, and this overall desire to look at the whole man, and not the wound alone, that has led to our greatest advance in this war.

Following the discussion of professional care, General Cutler then described the various surgical specialties and their contribution to the war effort. He made a particular point of the importance of delayed wound closure in the restoration of the fighting man to early duty, emphasizing that delayed closure had to be attempted at the first safe moment, that delayed closure did not mean a secondarily closed wound because it had never been closed before, and that delayed closure was not delayed primary closure because there had been no primary closure. General Cutler then attempted to outline the reasons for improved statistics in World War II in the following words:

It would be impossible, at this time, to evaluate and put in proper perspective the reasons why the mortality rates in the United States Army in World War II are one-half as great as those in World War I, but there is every reason to believe that the following have each played a role:

1. *Resuscitation.* The proper treatment of the patient in shock, chiefly by the use of plasma and blood.

2. *Better first aid* by the Company Aid man on the battlefield.

3. *Penicillin and sulfonamides*, which have vastly reduced the horror of infection.

4. *Improved methods of transport and evacuation*, which allow earlier meeting of surgeon and casualty, and more comfortable travel.

5. *Good general physical condition of the soldier.* This may be partly diet, or it may relate to the physical training to which he has been subjected before battle.

6. *Standardization of therapy* and the great medical and surgical educational programs emanating from the Office of the Chief Surgeon, European Theater of Operations. This did not exist in World War I.

7. *Better surgery*, through better anesthesia, better development of specialists and better training of the young surgeon in the Army.

The surgical technique has been put last to give full credit to obvious new advances that did not exist in World War I, and because no amount of good surgery could play such a major role in freeing the wounded from terrible infection. However, the great debt of every wounded soldier to his surgeon remains a hard fact.

And, finally, General Cutler paid his respects to the civilian doctor in uniform without whose efforts the fine results in the European theater could never have been achieved:

In conclusion, it is fitting to pay a tribute to the civilian doctors of the United States. Of the 16,055 Medical Corps officers in the European Theater of Operations, over 97 percent are civilian doctors who have been but recently commissioned. These civilian doctors have shown a willingness to conform to a standardized method of therapy that does them great credit. At the same time, they have revealed an immense capacity to learn from experience, and it is suggestions from the workers in the field, in all installations, both in the forward and in the rear areas, which have permitted us to improve consistently the methods of therapy originally outlined. Their ability to withstand great physical hardship, to subordinate themselves for the good of the Army, their ability to learn in the face of the conditions which have been imposed upon them in the forward areas, all show how very real are the personal attributes of these doctors.[115]

EPILOGUE I

Elliott Carr Cutler's contribution toward the physical care of the men in the European Theater of Operations is difficult to overestimate. The preceding medical history documents this fact only too well. It seems fitting to enlarge upon some of the personal attributes of this man who bore the principal responsibility of setting the level of professional surgical care in the European theater which he believed, by the end of the war, surpassed that in other theaters.

General Cutler was an individualist, a forceful man tempered by experience and endowed with great charm. He was not readily adaptable to the standardization required by a great war, but he made it his primary mission to cooperate, obey, and implement orders which served the medical betterment of the soldier. Cutler could become volubly indignant over what appeared to him stupidity, negligence, or lack of foresight; on the other hand, he was relentless in his efforts to gain promotion or reward for the men he considered deserving. The observations he had made during World War I had given him a good concept of military procedures which often enabled him to accomplish worthwhile objectives that might otherwise have been missed.

It is difficult to write an estimate of the person who was Elliott Cutler because he had so many facets to his personality. In retrospect, those qualities that stand foremost are dedication, intelligence, and practicality. He had a great sense of and feeling for history. He was in fact a man of parts, with a background in no way confined to medical and surgical knowledge. Extremely well read, and with more than a nodding acquaintance with art, he was a fine sportsman, and, in everything he did, his curiosity, competence, and enthusiasm were boundless. He could, and would, discuss at length anything from cattle raising to sailing to vintage wines. Cutler was not a visionary by any means, but neither were his thoughts confined to present or personal problems. In 1942, he was already considering the eventual victory over Germany, which to him was inevitable, and remarked that he thought the Allies should take over all teaching after the war. In other words, the man whom all knew as an outstanding surgeon was also one of the most interesting and rewarding friends a man could hope to have.

Whether on philosophic matters or with the more practical concern of supplying the front with blood and plasma, Cutler's mind was always active, inquiring, and inventive. No task was too small; no mission, unimportant. His efforts were unending, and, in view of what we now know about his increas-

---

[115] Cutler, E. C.: Military Surgery—United States Army—European Theater of Operations, 1944–1945. Surg. Gynec. & Obst. 28 : 261–274, March 1946.

ingly poor health, it is the more amazing to realize what he accomplished. He
never spoke of himself but confided in his diary about sleepless nights, persistent cough, headache, and loss of weight. He fought this personal battle alone,
although it was in all probability the prelude to the disease that finally killed
him. In the presence of others he was all energy, and wherever he went, which
was everywhere, he left the inspiration and heightened morale of his own great
spirit.

One thing the war availed him was the opportunity to teach, which he loved
to do and which no one could do better. His schedule was crowded with conferences at the Air Force School, at the American School Center, and with the
staffs of hospitals or field units. So high a priority did he place on teaching and
so great was his power of persuasion that he had little difficulty in prevailing
on his British colleagues to help. He arranged for men like Grey Turner,
Gordon Gordon-Taylor, Lionel Whitby, Willie Anderson, Tudor Edwards,
and many others to address groups of U.S. Army medical officers.

Cutler undoubtedly made enemies, just as every purposeful man does; but,
he would never compromise with his own high standards, and most of the
quarrels involved the maintenance of these standards for everyone. Of far
greater importance are the friends he made for all of us. Some of these friends
he had met 25 years earlier during service abroad in the First World War, and
others knew of him through his own professional attainments. No man tried so
hard and so successfully to unite the efforts of the Allied medical forces. The
following eulogy written by Sir Gordon Gordon-Taylor in 1947 after Cutler's
death gives eloquent expression to this:

"The death of Elliott Cutler * * * will occasion deep sorrow in the
hearts of his many friends in the United Kingdom. Perhaps no surgeon of the
United States ever yearned or strove more earnestly to forge lasting bonds of
friendship, not only between the surgeons, but between the peoples of the great
English-speaking countries on either side of the North Atlantic, and to this end
he directed both written and spoken word."

Despite his sophistication, Cutler was delighted at being made an Honorary
Fellow of the Royal College of Surgeons of England and the Royal Society
of Medicine. He was similarly honored by the Royal College of Surgeons of
Edinburgh, and, as a final, unique award, he was placed on the Editorial Committee of the *British Journal of Surgery*. No other "outsider" had ever
attained such a position. Small wonder that, after the end of the war in 1945
when he had been roundly applauded for his Hunterian Lecture, he recorded:
"Certainly the British make me feel they appreciate my services more than
my own people. It's rather sad when one has worked one's heart out. But I
am satisfied we have done a good job."

But Cutler probably took greatest pride in the Inter-Allied Conferences
on War Medicine, held within the precincts of the Royal Society of Medicine.
He had been a main figure in the accomplishment of these meetings. As Sir
Gordon Gordon-Taylor wrote: "Elliott's wonderful tact and diplomacy at these

Inter-Allied Conferences will long be remembered by those privileged to attend." Cutler was never happier than when the evidence submitted at these conferences bore out his belief and pride in American primacy and efficiency. At the same time, he held in great respect the British medical tradition, and he admired the individual ability of many of the men in surgery who, like himself, were devoting their skill to the war effort.

It was to Cutler's great advantage that he had on his side Maj. Gen. Paul R. Hawley, Chief Surgeon, ETOUSA, an exceptional soldier-physician, who dared to make operative a division of his office that in the past had been mostly consultive and advisory. Cutler speaks of Hawley thus: "* * * Though demanding standardization, you have always been willing to allow changes in our form for practice, once a better way has been demonstrated. This openmindedness and the backing of new ventures * * * are evidence of an unusual perspective and critical appreciation in science. We believe in you, we acknowledge you as a stimulating and exemplary leader and we are happy that we have been privileged to serve with you."

Cutler, for his part, ably fulfilled his own description of the task of the consultant, and this fact was recognized by his chief, General Hawley, in the following encomium:

"Obviously, the complexity of the functions of a Professional Services Division, the peculiarity of its organization which makes necessary both action as a whole and much individual action on the part of its members—these characteristics require the very highest type of leadership at its head. Its leader must be a man of force; otherwise, individual differences among its members may create serious dissentions. He must be a man of courage because he risks his personal standing among his colleagues in the profession when he admonishes them or rules against them. And he must be a man of kindness and understanding because he must keep discord out of his division and all of his men happy and contented.

"These qualifications are not often found in one man. But it meant more to the sick and injured soldier in the European theater than he, or any of the rest of us, can tell—that my Chief of Professional Services had all those qualifications."

Because he did consider the future and all its implications so thoughtfully, forgetting his own increasing fatigue and ill health in his enthusiasm, he became interested in General Hawley's urgent plea to help with a reorganization of the Department of Medicine and Surgery within the Veterans' Administration. He helped formulate some of the basic criteria by which the medical service of the Veterans' Administration is being run today.

This was Elliott Carr Cutler, who died before he could realize all of his objectives but had accomplished far more than most of us even dream of. In conclusion, let us be generous enough to quote again from the British who said of him: "* * * Perhaps the finest ambassador in surgery the world has known."

And, for ourselves, we might reflect on this man of extraordinary caliber and stature. Many of us have our own personal feelings of bereavement, but far more important is our sure knowledge of what his vision and statesmanship could have accomplished today.

BERNARD J. PISANI, M.D.
February 1959

EPILOGUE II

The rugged individualism of the American physician was never more apparent than after his indoctrination into the Armed Services. His antagonism to what he believed was the unnecessary regimentation of the military tended all too frequently to interfere with his peace of mind and at times his professional efficiency. While the consultants were usually older and more seasoned in administrative, professional, and military experience, they too were not immune to the same human emotions, especially during the early part of World War II. They tended to be discouraged by the interest of the administrative planners in supply and evacuation during the early years of the war. This, in the opinion of the consultants, did not provide adequate consideration for the professional care of patients. Furthermore, they were frustrated by their prolonged absence from heavy professional responsibilities, irked by the lack of suitable transportation, aggravated by the discipline of military red tape, and depressed by slow promotions which rarely approximated their counterpart in the Allied armies.

On the other hand, the administrative planners were impatient with the consultants' "impossible" demands, their intentional ignorance on occasion of military channels, the difficulties arising from a sympathetic ear lent to a disgruntled medical officer who could think of nothing but a promotion, memorandums prepared without due regard for the problems of evacuation and theater policies, and, finally, the problem of pacifying commanding officers who on occasion angrily objected to the consultants' raids on their personnel.

History must record these problems, although it is doubtful if the Chief Consultant in Surgery, European Theater of Operations, Brig. Gen. Elliott Carr Cutler, would have mentioned them had he lived personally to record his own activities. There was, however, no doubt that he was very disturbed in the early days when he encountered some of the same problems he had known as a medical officer in World War I. Yet, his intense patriotism and keen desire to prepare young medical officers for things to come maintained his spirit. Like his chief, Maj. Gen. Paul R. Hawley, to whom he was devoted, he was dedicated to the ideal that American medicine must and would provide the best surgical care in the quickest possible time, starting in the forward areas, which was ever offered a soldier in time of war.

The lack of medical challenge to the consultant group by the Army in the European theater during the early planning days was compensated for by the medical problems presented by the Eighth Air Force, the problems of medical supply, lectures at the Medical Field Service School, ETOUSA, and the organization of medical meetings for the exchange of ideas with the consultants and medical officers of the British and other Allied armies. Later on, they eagerly welcomed a trip to the Mediterranean theater to gain firsthand information of the problems to come on a much larger scale to their theater. By this time, it was "their theater" in thinking and loyalty. As the time of the invasion grew nearer, the consultants became more indoctrinated into the Army and the Army in turn became more convinced of the value of the consultants. It was very soul-satisfying to General Cutler to observe the ever-increasing usefulness of the consultant group. He was freed to give his energies to projects more suitable to his background and capabilities. Few experiences made as great an impression on him as his membership in the medical mission to the Soviet Union. He was tremendously impressed, and some believed so much enthusiasm was not warranted. Subsequent events attest to his astuteness in predicting the Russian people were a major force to be reckoned with in the future.

The consultants came to their own with the invasion of Normandy. These "nomads" of the Chief Surgeon were familiar with the professional background and location of thousands of medical officers who could be used to meet the constantly shifting needs of combat. Their mobility tended to overcome one of the great weaknesses of military medicine by providing a followup system on the effectiveness of treatment from clearing station to general hospital. Despite failing health, General Cutler continued an aggressive interest in all of the problems associated with the care of the wounded soldier. His spirits were maintained in part by the active participation of two sons who were on active duty in the European theater and the thousands of medical officers who looked to him as their chief link with civilian surgery. This Master Surgeon, Inspiring Teacher, Peppery Patriot, and Intense Anglophile, who had few equals in personal charm and natural ability, assumed this responsibility with enthusiasm and determination. His natural talents toward the dramatic and idealistic invariably lifted the morale of the individual medical officer, not only during but in the hectic days after the war. His dream and active participation in the Veterans' Administration to insure better care for the wounded veteran and opportunities for the returning veteran medical officer were typical of his complete devotion to his country and profession. Perhaps, his greatest contribution was to plant the seeds for the active participation of civilian medicine in military medicine long after the war ended. The loyalty and continued interest of the consultants to the Army Medical Corps since their return to busy civilian life is ample proof of the fine esprit de corps that has continued, thanks to leaders like General Cutler.

It was his hope and dream that military medicine would make adequate provisions for the active participation of civilian consultants during peacetime as well as in wartime. To some, this may be hard to justify, since the role of the consultant was so frequently of such an individual effort without documented evidence that history may find it difficult to evaluate the consultant's true worth. Testimonials of thousands of individual medical officers would be required to ferret out their greatest contribution to the war effort. None will be remembered longer or with more warmth and affection by American and Allied physicians than the late Elliott Carr Cutler, Brigadier General, MC; Chief Consultant in Surgery, European Theater of Operations; Moseley Professor of Surgery of the Harvard Medical School; and Surgeon-in-Chief of the Peter Bent Brigham Hospital.

ROBERT M. ZOLLINGER, M.D.
February 1959

CHAPTER III

General Surgery

Robert M. Zollinger, M.D.

By the fall of 1943, Lt. Col. (later Col.) Robert M. Zollinger, MC, had been serving for approximately 15 months as chief of the surgical service in the 5th General Hospital, ETOUSA (European Theater of Operations, U.S. Army). This was a unit affiliated with Harvard University and was the first general hospital to be shipped overseas. The 5th General Hospital was established in Northern Ireland early in the spring of 1942.

The incumbent Senior Consultant in General Surgery became ill, necessitating his return to the Zone of Interior (fig. 126). The possibility of Colonel Zollinger's replacing him was first broached to the author by Col. (later Brig. Gen.) Elliott C. Cutler, MC, Chief Consultant in Surgery in the European theater. At first, this new assignment seemed quite acceptable, since the author had worked with Colonel Cutler for many years during his surgical training and as a member of Dr. Cutler's immediate staff before the war. The author conferred with Col. Maxwell G. Keeler, MC, the commanding officer of the 5th General Hospital, concerning this proposed reassignment (fig. 127). He was then sent to Cheltenham, England, to meet with Col. James C. Kimbrough, MC, Director of Professional Services in the Office of the Chief Surgeon, ETOUSA, in order that the actual appointment might be submitted for formal consideration by the Chief Surgeon.

APPOINTMENT AS SENIOR CONSULTANT

There were both advantages and disadvantages inherent in an appointment as a senior consultant at the theater headquarters level at that particular time. These were graphically pointed out by Colonel Kimbrough, who was both a Regular Army officer and a urologist enjoying national reputation. He discussed the advantages of taking care of patients as compared to those of administering their professional care. He pointed out, however, that the consultant could be of utmost value in the long run by coordinating the utilization of personnel and standardizing therapy so as to provide optimum surgical care. He also warned that a "desk job" incorporating the difficulties of amalgamating the talents of various rugged individualists in the surgical world could be particularly harassing.

Although, according to the letter of the protocol, the author had the privilege of refusing the appointment, it became obvious that it was incumbent

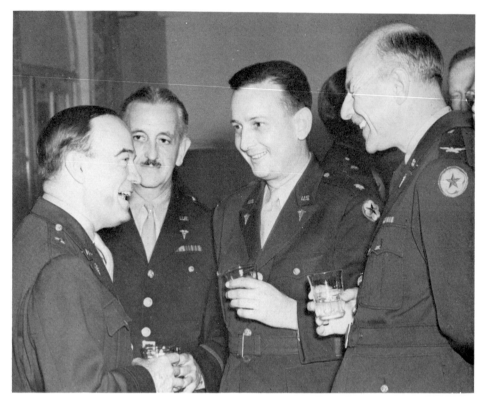

FIGURE 126.—Lt. Col. Ambrose H. Storck, MC, first Senior Consultant in General Surgery (third from left), at a reception given for Brig. Gen. Fred W. Rankin (left). Also in the group are Col. Lloyd J. Thompson, MC (between General Rankin and Colonel Storck), and Col. Rex L. Diveley, MC.

upon him to accept the appointment with good grace—much as he was disinclined to leave the Harvard unit. Members of the unit had been promised, when it was organized, that it woud be left intact; however, this was not the case. In addition, although living conditions at a higher headquarters were usually exceptionally good, there was no particular sense of unit pride, and the junior officers were conscious of the presence of "brass." The most imposing deterrent was the knowledge that 50 percent of the senior consultants had developed poor health as a result of their service and had been sent back to the Zone of Interior. Several of these men were nationally known in their respective surgical fields. Any replacement, therefore, took a 50 percent chance on physical grounds alone.

One of the desirable features was that reportedly there was a good chance that senior consultants would be promoted from the rank of lieutenant colonel to that of colonel. The advantage of this became so striking that most medical officers, after a year or two overseas, would have led the Charge of the Light

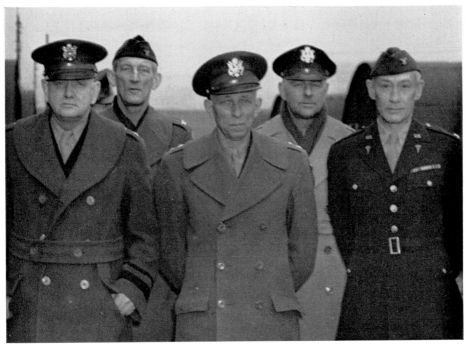

FIGURE 127.—Col. Maxwell G. Keeler, MC, extreme right, on the occasion of The Surgeon General's visit to the 5th General Hospital. Left to right, Brig. Gen. Paul R. Hawley, Col. Elliott C. Cutler, MC, Maj. Gen. Norman T. Kirk, and Colonel Diveley.

Brigade if the reward for survival had been promotion to a full colonel. A medical officer acting in an advisory capacity, rather than participating purely in the professional care of patients, would need to have this much rank, at least. Without it, he could not expect his recommendations for changes in procedure or personnel or his efforts to commandeer transportation to carry any weight, nor could he expect cooperation in other endeavors.

The author accepted and was appointed to the position of Senior Consultant in General Surgery in September 1943.

ORGANIZATION, FUNCTIONS, AND ACTIVITIES

The director of the group of consultants was the previously mentioned Colonel Kimbrough. The Chief Consultant in Medicine was Col. William S. Middleton, MC, of Madison, Wis., professor of medicine and dean of the University of Wisconsin Medical School. He headed the consultants who covered the various medical specialties. Colonel Cutler was the Chief Consultant in Surgery. The surgical group was larger than the medical group and included representatives of ophthalmology, otolaryngology, plastic surgery, neurosurgery, orthopedics, roentgenology, anesthesiology, maxillofacial surgery, and general surgery—the position to which this writer had been appointed.

Colonel Kimbrough's office was one room about 12 feet square. The Chief Consultant in Surgery and the Chief Consultant in Medicine had desks side by side in an adjacent room of similar size. Opposite them was a room about 12 by 20 feet, which was used for a common meeting place. Activities of the week were reviewed, and policies were formulated at meetings held each Saturday morning in this room. Beyond this was a rather large room with desks around the periphery. These desks were placed back to back. In other words, there were groups of two consultants sitting face to face around the sides of the room. At one end of the room and in the middle were British civilian secretaries and several enlisted men who were used as messengers and file clerks. As one might expect, the main room was quite noisy and inefficient for ordinary working conditions. It was in many ways reminiscent of a boiler factory.

The amount of work done, therefore, depended a great deal upon how many of the consultants were present in the room at the time, how many were dictating, how many were holding conferences, how many were trying to make themselves heard over the telephone, how many were arguing with the personnel officer, the supply officer, or the motor pool or trying to interview new hospital personnel. These poor working conditions accounted in no small measure for the high mortality which had existed among consultants up to this time. In one room, gloom spreads rapidly. Certainly, these were working conditions quite dissimilar to any these surgeons had previously encountered. This does not imply that they needed more comfort than the surgeons in the field, but the nature of their work required a lot of planning and discussion, which was virtually impossible in the peculiar offices assigned to them.

Responsibilities of Senior Consultant in General Surgery

Although the specialty consultant ordinarily handled only those problems in his field, the Senior Consultant in General Surgery served more or less as a coordinator of the surgical group. This difference in responsibility was in some respects due to the fact that the Chief Consultant in Surgery was a general surgeon who had a wide experience in practically all fields of surgery and one who did not hesitate to make decisions upon professional or administrative matters in these particular fields. At times, however, the specialty consultants felt that this was an infringement upon their province; thus, perhaps, the situation was responsible for the creation of discord.

The specialty consultants were in close liaison with their counterparts in the British Army. In the field of general surgery, however, the entire group was represented by Colonel Cutler, who maintained living quarters in London. During the fall of 1943 and the winter of 1943–44, Colonel Cutler devoted considerable time to liaison work with the British and to the study of the care of wounded air force casualties who were being treated in the U.S. hospitals in East Anglia. The hospitals in East Anglia were, at that time, the only hospitals taking care of fresh casualties, since they were responsible for the reception and care of casualties from the U.S. Eighth Air Force.

Evaluation of Surgical Service in New Hospitals

One of the chief assignments of every consultant was to visit the various hospitals as they came into the theater, in order to evaluate their professional personnel in his particular field. If at all possible, the incoming hospitals were visited in the staging area. In general surgery, each man on the surgical service was interviewed and a record of his professional background was maintained. Special attention was given to the evaluation of the chief and assistant chief of the surgical service, since the quality of professional care of any particular hospital was closely related to the training background of the chief of the surgical service.

The value of the intensive Halsted type of resident training was never so clearly demonstrated as in those surgeons working in oversea hospitals. Although they were far away from their ivory towers, they were never far away from the surgical principles they had been taught.

After each hospital service had been visited, the entire surgical complement was reviewed and annotations were made with regard to the qualifications of each surgeon. The probable efficiency and competency of the surgical service was discussed and assessed. In the fall of 1943, the quality of the surgical services in the theater's hospitals was quite good, and evaluation was not difficult. Eventually, however, as the theater began to be flooded with new hospitals, the quality of the surgical services became more of a problem. Also, at that time, many medical officers were transferred from the Army Air Forces to the Army Service Forces, and a number of officers of high rank but limited professional ability began to appear—distributed here and there—in the roster of almost all of the new hospitals in the European theater.

The visiting of hospitals by the consultant was important, since it gave each hospital's medical officers contact with men who were interested only in the professional care of patients. Frequently, the new medical officers felt that the Army was interested only in a type of surgical and medical care of which they disapproved. It was essential that the army directives and methods be explained to them by men who had been in the European theater for some time—men who had some idea of their possible future problems and of the reasons for differences between military and civilian practices. The medical officers in the hospitals did not hesitate to talk freely with the consultants on a "doctor to doctor" basis, and the consultants' visits were very beneficial in bolstering the morale of medical officers. On the other hand, the consultants occasionally might have been a little too sympathetic with a man desiring to make a change to further his own promotion.

Of greatest importance was the fact that at all times there were consultants who had on record and also personally knew the professional qualifications of all the medical officers of the hospitals in the European theater. In case illness incapacitated a key surgeon, or if a particular hospital experienced an increased professional load, the consultants knew whether or not the particular hospital involved was adequate and, if it was not adequate, where to find men who had the qualifications to assume this additional load. In order to make the most efficient use of this detailed knowledge of personnel, it was important that the senior consultants be appointed for a long period of time. This knowledge was invaluable, since the consultants could very readily supply the personnel officer with the names of additional, trained men to speed up the organization of new surgical services when the need arose among the many hospitals which eventually entered the theater without surgical personnel of the requisite high caliber.

The consultants, however, could only evaluate the professional personnel of the service as a whole and act as advisers to the personnel officer. Only the personnel officer at the appropriate headquarters could initiate orders for the transfer of a surgeon from one place to another. The consultant could recommend such a transfer, but this did not make it automatic. It was important, therefore, that the consultant be in close liaison with the personnel officer in the Office of the Chief Surgeon as well as with personnel officers in the base sections; and it was equally important that a spirit of complete confidence and cooperation exist between them.

Preparation of Manual of Therapy, ETOUSA

The Senior Consultant in General Surgery was also intimately associated with the preparation of memorandums and directives. Information regarding the efficacy of treatment being given casualties in England, Ireland, and Wales was discussed as it was gained. Considerable time was taken to review previous directives and to prepare directives incorporating the new information. Every effort was made to promulgate directives that would be clearly understood by the surgeons and that would adhere to the best surgical standards yet be in accordance with the tradition of military directives and objectives.

This led to the realization of a need for developing a standard manual of therapy, including the medical and surgical aspects of care of the wounded soldier. Colonel Zollinger's predecessor had obviously encountered many obstacles in the preparation of such a manual, and practically no utilizable material had been compiled. After considerable discussion, it was decided that such a manual of therapy should (1) be small and compact so that it could be easily carried by the medical officer far into the forward area, (2) be up to date and consistent with the directives of The Surgeon General and the Chief Surgeon, ETOUSA, (3) contain the most recent information gained by experiences of the Medical Corps during the Italian campaigns as well as information from the British and French Allies, and (4) serve medical officers in the forward area as well as those carrying out definitive treatment in the base areas. It was finally decided, therefore, that each chapter should be divided into two parts—the first to deal with emergency treatment, and the second to be concerned with definitive treatment.

In order to restrict the manual to pocket size, each chapter had to be very concise and more or less in outline form. The medical consultants apparently had very little disagreement in the preparation of their chapters. The various surgical specialists, however, submitted long chapters and were loath to endorse the requirements of emergency therapy so vital in the most forward areas. It took considerable time and experience gained from their visits to the North African theater to persuade them that evacuation must take precedence over definitive treatment. It was extremely difficult to convince the medical officer, newly commissioned from civilian practice, that only the simplest things possible should be done in the forward areas; that is, cover the wound and then evacuate the patient to a place where definitive treatment could be carried out under more satisfactory conditions. The desire to do too much and therefore delay evacuation was a constant problem.

Since there was no consultant in thoracic surgery, this consultant was responsible for the chapters on the treatment of abdominal wounds and thoracic wounds. The directives issued from the Office of The Surgeon General were utilized, but, for the most part, the material was gleaned from experience gained in visits to various hospitals caring for Air Force casualties as well as for those casualties returning from Africa to the United Kingdom. Information was also gained from the North African theater and from talking with Colonel Cutler and others who had visited the North African theater and the eastern front of the Soviet Army.

There was little disagreement regarding the general care of the wound. Some of the major problems at that time were the use of chemotherapy and antibiotics—whether to use them locally or systemically, how much to use, and whether to use them simultaneously or separately. The use of gas gangrene sera and tetanus antitoxin and toxoid was also thoroughly discussed, and decisions were made as to their use.

It was this consultant's impression that the European theater had very little in the way of directives or information from the Zone of Interior regarding the treatment of casualties. However, it was frequently reemphasized through channels from the Office of The Surgeon General that all wounds were to be left open. Before the proofs for the Manual of Therapy, European Theater of Operations, were sent away, Colonel Kimbrough again called the author's attention to a recent cablegram stating that all amputations were to be left open. These instructions were, of course, contrary to everyday experience in civilian life, when wounds had been seen early and under ideal conditions. Furthermore, Col. William F. MacFee, MC, had carried out primary debridement and closure in a number of casualties in East Anglia which had occurred in the Army Forces, and he had apparently obtained excellent results. Men in the Army Air Forces, however, returned to their bases every day and had baths and clean clothing. The surroundings of an aircraft were not apt to be so contaminated as were those of the foot soldier who might be wounded on soil which had been tilled over a period of centuries.

A great deal of space was taken to describe the debridement of a wound. In order to demonstrate debridement with a simple sketch, a sergeant who had been interested in drawing was transferred from the author's old unit, the 5th

General Hospital, to Cheltenham. He made some very helpful pen-and-ink sketches illustrating various principles of first aid treatment.

This consultant's experience in preparing the Manual of Therapy convinced him that the most recent well-substantiated methods and principles of treatment of war casualties should be taught to all medical students and become a part of the indoctrination of each medical officer. It seemed a great waste of time and energy for surgeons to indoctrinate thousands of medical officers scattered throughout the hospitals and bases in principles which could have been given better during medical school or at least during their basic training.

In May 1944, Maj. Gen. Paul R. Hawley, the Chief Surgeon, and Colonel Cutler presented the Manual of Therapy at a conference with Lt. Gen. John C. H. Lee, Commanding General, SOS (Services of Supply), in the British Isles. They were very proud of this booklet which could be carried in the medical officer's pocket. General Lee noted that it had not been dated and asked for which war the booklet had been prepared. This omission was remedied by handstamping the date on the front of each booklet. It was the first U.S. Army manual printed without having been officially dated.

Lectures at Medical Field Service School

One of the responsibilities of the consultants was to lecture at the Medical Field Service School. Each man was assigned to lecture in his particular field to a group of medical officers brought there from time to time for indoctrination (fig. 128). The Medical Field Service School was under the direction of Capt. (later Lt. Col.) Bernard J. Pisani, MC, an excellent director who cooperated extremely well with the consultants, making the trip a most enjoyable one.

This was one of the functions of the consultant group which was always pleasant, since it involved teaching younger men. Perhaps the teachers would not have been so enthusiastic had they realized that many of their students had been sent there for disciplinary indoctrination rather than for purely professional instruction. This consultant suspected that the mediocre medical officers from many of the units were given a better medical education thereby than the men who adhered to the line. This was not altogether true, however, since many of the superior officers were originally sent to this school (fig. 129).

PREPARATIONS FOR NORMANDY INVASION

Planning LST Operations

In the latter part of February 1944, Maj. Gen. Albert W. Kenner, Chief Medical Officer in General Eisenhower's Headquarters, SHAEF, held a meeting with General Hawley, Col. David E. Liston, MC (Deputy Chief Surgeon), and representatives of the First U.S. Army, the British Army, the British Navy, and the U.S. Navy concerning the professional care to be provided on an LST (landing ship, tank). The Chief Surgeon's Office had made recommendations concerning the policies to be carried out on these ships.

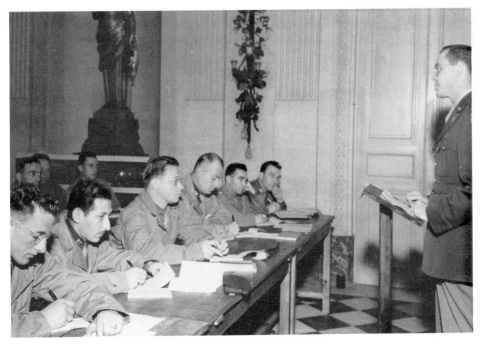

FIGURE 128.—Lt. Col. William A. Howard, MC, Chief, Intelligence Section, Operations Division, Office of the Chief Surgeon, ETOUSA, lecturing to a class of medical officers at the Medical Field Service School, ETOUSA, upon its reopening at the Chateau Du Marais, near Paris, France.

Planning for the treatment of casualties to be evacuated on LST's during the initial invasion of Normandy became one of Colonel Zollinger's responsibilities. He thus became a liaison officer to the U.S. Navy for this preinvasion planning. The number of LST's available, which was then, of course, secret information, was 110.

Preparing these plans involved the following problems. First, what treatment could be carried out on the LST after it was loaded with casualties on the far shore and directed back to the three unloading points in southern England? Second, what medical personnel would be needed in addition to the personnel of the LST? Third, what medical and surgical supplies would be needed?

LST's converted to provide an operating-room platform were discussed. Other proposed minor changes were to be made to assist the moving of casualties about the ship through the narrow passageways. It was planned that the casualties would be loaded on stretchers and placed on the floor of the inside deck after the tanks and trucks transported to France had been landed. This would provide a huge, readymade, one-room hospital ward.

The type and amount of surgery to be performed would depend upon how soon functioning hospitals could be set up on the far shore. It was apparent that, in the initial stages of the invasion, many fresh casualties would have

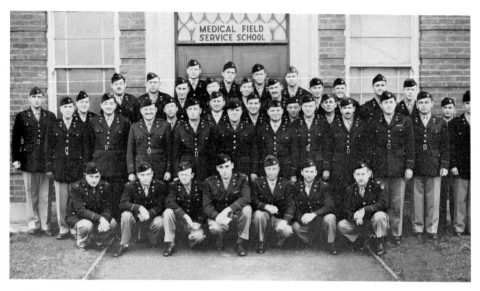

FIGURE 129.—One of the first classes to graduate from the Medical Field Service School,
ETOUSA, at Shrivenham Barracks, England. Capt. Bernard J. Pisani, MC, commandant
of the school, kneeling in the center of the front row.

to be loaded on LST's and treated by the personnel aboard. It was then agreed
and promulgated in a directive that conservatism would be the policy with
respect to major surgery in the treatment of casualties being returned to England in the LST's.

Since the Navy had the primary responsibility, planning for supplies and
personnel to be placed aboard LST's involved close coordination with the
Navy. The author, acting as liaison officer to the Navy, required frequent
conferences to find out details concerning medical supplies already available
on LST's and what was needed from the Army to complement them. A
pharmacist's mate in naval headquarters in London seemed to be the most
thoroughly informed concerning the medical complement of every class of
ship in the U.S. Navy. These supply lists had to be reviewed, and, so far
as possible, necessary additions had to be furnished by the Navy. Any further
supplies would have to be provided by the U.S. Army. A means of accomplishing this was the cause of considerable concern.

A problem which seemed almost insurmountable was how to provide sterile
dry goods for the performance of any surgery on the LST. There was no room
to store a large supply. Furthermore, since the LST was to return to the far
shore immediately upon delivering the casualties to England, how were sterile
dry goods to be laundered and replaced promptly at the end of each trip?
Although there was some sterilizing equipment aboard an LST, the amount
of dry goods was almost insignificant.

The previous year, while the author was assigned to the 5th General
Hospital, he had been instrumental in developing a mobile surgical unit. At

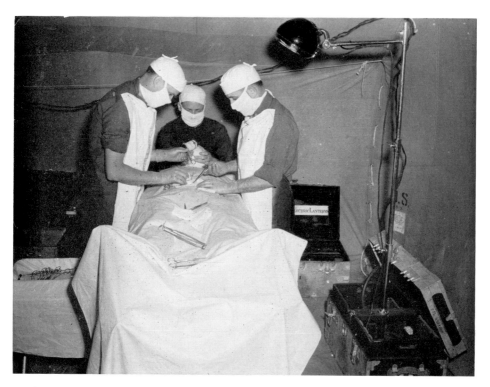

FIGURE 130.—Rubberized sheets replacing cloth drapes in a mobile surgical unit.

that time, it was learned that rubberized material supplied by the British could be made available in place of the dry goods. The material came in bolts, and given lengths could be cut with a hole in the middle to be used as laparotomy sheets. Similar sizes could be utilized for towels and drapes for tables and sterile instruments. The material, weighted down with clamps, could be boiled at the same time as the instruments. It could be boiled repeatedly without deterioration. It was decided that 25 yards of this material would be made available to each LST (fig. 130).

Each surgeon to serve aboard an LST was given a copy of the Manual of Therapy, a dozen pairs of rubber gloves, and the 25 yards of rubberized material to prepare for operating drapes and gowns. The army kit of surgical instruments was also given to each surgeon. Chemotherapy was made available to each LST in a larger supply than its usual complement. All these supplies were delivered to the three collecting points where the personnel selected for LST duty were to be gathered for instructions.

The Navy was ready to supply, for each LST, one medical officer who had been brought into the Armed Forces immediately upon finishing a 9-month internship. One surgeon and two surgical technicians were to be supplied by the Army for each LST.

Discussions were held with the medical officer of the 1st Medical General Laboratory, who was in charge of meeting the demand for whole blood on each LST, and adequate plans were made.

Toward the middle of May 1944, recommendations were made for the actual selection and assignment of surgeons and surgical technicians for the LST's. One-third of the group was to come from theater SOS units, one-third from the Third U.S. Army which was staging at that time, and one-third from the Army Air Forces. These men were ordered to various places in southern England for indoctrination preliminary to being ordered to a particular LST.

It was part of this consultant's responsibility to coordinate the indoctrination of these groups of men. They had not been aware, up to this time, that they were to comprise the medical complement of the LST's. When the medical personnel assigned to these LST's were apprised of their mission, they were quite shocked. Most of them regarded it as being more or less a suicide assignment. They believed that the shores of France were loaded with heavy artillery, mines, and multiple German divisions, and that poison gas would probably be used. They had no way of knowing how poorly the coastline of France was defended, compared to their expectations. Most of the line officers had already been reassured.

Discussions as to procedure were started about 16 May 1944. On that day, this writer visited the 28th General Hospital, at Trowbridge, and reemphasized conservatism in the care of the wounded aboard LST's. At this late date, only 16 of the 34 men ordered to report to this collecting point had arrived, and some of these were without proper clothing. It was essential to supply the physicians and their technicians with additional clothing, especially underwear.

The group at the 316th Station Hospital at Newton Abbot was also interviewed and briefed, and the men seemed well qualified and confident of their capabilities to do major abdominal surgery, if necessary.

On 17 May 1944, a discussion was held with the group assembled at the 115th Station Hospital, near Plymouth. The majority of these men had been taken from the Army Air Forces. One officer disclaimed his ability to perform general surgery because he was a proctologist. Arrangements were made for his replacement.

In discussions with the physicians assigned to these LST's, it was amazing to find that they invariably expressed concern over the qualifications of their so-called surgical technicians. Since the true nature of the technicians' assignments was not known, many of them were, in reality, anything or everything but surgical technicians. The officers evidenced real panic and attempted in every way possible to contact their parent units to effect a return of the untrained enlisted men and to have them replaced with well-trained technicians. Necessary steps were taken to facilitate these transfers.

Considering the operation with the aid of hindsight, it would seem that the commanding officer of a hospital dispatching a medical officer to serve on an LST should have known the importance of the assignment. On the other hand, his consideration of the possible hazards involved might have made his decision more difficult.

Planning Special Studies

Lt. Col. (later Col.) Joseph A. Crisler, Jr., MC, surgical consultant to the First U.S. Army, visited Cheltenham rather regularly at the time of the surgical consultant's Saturday morning meetings. In addition, other conferences were held concerning his estimated requirements for penicillin, medical supplies, specially trained personnel, and so forth. Plans were also made for gathering data on abdominal wounds, thoracic wounds, and cases of gas gangrene, as they were treated on the far shore by the First U.S. Army.

Several forms were proposed in an attempt to gain some statistical information regarding the treatment and outcome of these wounds. It was hoped that these reporting requirements could be printed and distributed to surgical teams and that each unit in the hospital could be made responsible for collecting such information. Actually, each form required too much information to be practical, and, although such information would have been invaluable, there was no way that it could be secured easily. Certainly, it was regrettable that there was no table of organization to provide for study groups which could have developed special studies for the cases carrying a high mortality.

Distinguished scientists were present and available in the European theater, who could have constituted a research study group, had an appropriate table of organization been available. Such a group should have been assigned not only to theater headquarters but also to each base section and each hospital center.

It probably would have been most desirable to have had an officer in every hospital, regardless of its size, designated as the responsible individual for collecting such professional data or for the maintenance of an appropriate and official diary concerning the treatment of patients—a diary which could have been submitted to the Office of the Chief Surgeon at regular intervals for study and appropriate action.

Provision of Whole Blood

Several months before the invasion, there was considerable discussion concerning the use of proportions of plasma and whole blood in the treatment of casualties. This aspect of planning has been thoroughly covered elsewhere. It should be mentioned, however, that Maj. (later Lt. Col.) Charles P. Emerson, MC, and Maj. (later Lt. Col.) Richard V. Ebert, MC, of the 5th General Hospital, devoted a great deal of time to the development of a mobile field transfusion kit. Their kit could be stored in a wooden box used in the shipment of 50-caliber ammunition. It consisted of material for typing and cross-matching and all other material necessary for collecting and giving blood. These very thoughtful, sincere individuals proved to their own satisfaction that it was possible to wash out transfusion bottles with distilled water and sterilize them with alcohol. Actually, they took blood from each other under these circumstances and readministered it to themselves without ill effects. This was, to be sure, a very crude arrangement, but it would have made available whole blood transfusions in any area, should it have become necessary as a lifesaving measure.

At that time, it was not clearly understood how sufficient amounts of whole blood could be delivered to the far shore, especially to forward areas. The Signal Corps, in cooperation with these two officers of the 5th General Hospital, developed a teaching film on the use of the field transfusion kit. It eventually became apparent that blood would be flown from the United States, and these kits would not be necessary; but it did show that, despite great handicaps of equipment and supply shortages, the ingenuity of the U.S. Army officer could provide the best possible care for the American soldier.

Preparing for Reception of Casualties

In addition to attending conferences with the First U.S. Army consultants, this consultant took part in several meetings in the Southern Base Section, at which time the surgical chiefs of the various hospitals were gathered together. At these meetings, emphasis was placed on the rehabilitation of patients and their early return to duty. It took constant surveillance by the consultants to make certain that patients were not held for definitive surgery which would prevent their being returned to duty within a period of 60 days. This became increasingly important, for, as the time of the Normandy invasion drew near, the necessity for providing empty beds in the transient hospitals, especially in the southern part of England, became more acute.

The surgical consultants visited hospitals in the Southern Base Section rather frequently during May 1944, urging clearance of all possible beds in preparation for the reception of casualties. In addition, plans were drawn up to provide surgical teams to the hospitals that were concentrated around the reception zones for casualties returning from the LST's. Detailed plans were made for the reception of these casualties and for the triaging of these cases in order that specialty care would be made available as soon as possible, depending upon the type of wound.

Last-Minute Activities, May 1944

Late in May 1944, there were constant changes in the maxima of demands upon the consultants. The First U.S. Army had raised the requirements for whole blood, and new transfusion sets had arrived which were being made available for the Third U.S. Army. This occasioned changes in the supplies to be provided LST's.

There was also considerable discussion regarding the proper use of sulfanilamide, as well as penicillin. The feasibility of providing the First U.S. Army alone with sulfanilamide, to be taken by mouth as well as dusted on wounds, and providing the Third U.S. Army only with penicillin was considered, in that it would afford a well-controlled experiment to determine which was the more effective in the control of infections in war wounds. It was the consensus, however, that the American public would not approve such a study and that the U.S. soldier was entitled to everything that was available for his care. The

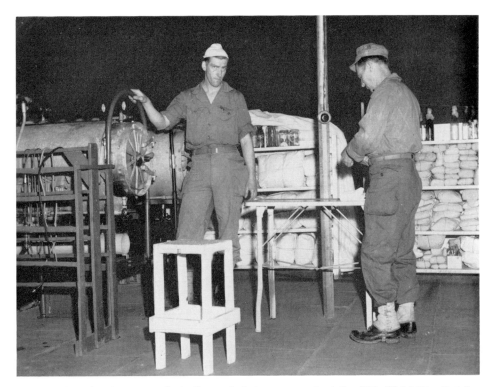

FIGURE 131.—Ample stores of sterile goods being prepared at the 50th Field Hospital for the Normandy invasion.

U.S. soldier seemed to feel psychologically secure when he had sulfanilamide available for his own protection. The uniformed soldier or technician had more confidence in these drugs as far as their ability to save life was concerned than had the experienced medical personnel responsible for the details of administration of the drugs.

Some time was spent visiting the various hospital centers, which had now become organized for the mass reception of casualties. A consultant in surgery was to be assigned in each of these hospital centers, or the best qualified chief of surgical service in one of the center's hospitals was to be nominated as a senior consultant for the center. Everywhere the hospitals were well organized for the reception of casualties. They had improved their central supply, and ample stores of sterile dressings and so forth had been prepared in anticipation of a great inflow of casualties (fig. 131).

This consultant was not apprised of the date of the invasion, nor did he meet anyone who appeared to want to know the date. All were afraid that they might violate security in an accidental way. As far as could be ascertained, the hospitals were empty, the supplies were adequate, the staffs were well balanced, and the hospitals were supplemented by members of the 1st Auxiliary Surgical Group until such time as they were needed on the far shore.

ACTIVITIES DURING NORMANDY INVASION

A conference was held with LST surgeons at Southampton on 8 June 1944 concerning observations on the unloading of casualties. This procedure was carried out quite smoothly, but the triaging officer was unable to carry out the plan to sort the patients at that point because of insufficient time. The LST's had to be reloaded quickly with fighting equipment.

Several LST surgeons were interviewed. One of these men stated that he had brought back 46 casualties on his LST. He had been able to debride some wounds and utilize his rubber sheeting, had given blood transfusions, and had carried out penicillin therapy. He seemed quite convinced that his supplies were adequate and that he would be able to do the necessary surgery in a satisfactory manner. When the casualties were received, those who needed it were given a large amount of plasma and some were given whole blood and prepared for early evacuation.

The surgeons who served on the LST's were required to submit a report of their experiences. One of these reports may be found in appendix E (p. 985).

Observations on Treatment of Casualties

One of the functions of the consultants was to observe and report on the treatment of casualties from the time they were received from the LST's to the time they were admitted to the various hospitals, including observations on the methods of transportation used (fig. 132). The consultants were the only ones who could provide any followup information and then report back to the surgeon responsible for the initial treatment regarding his successes or failures. The lack of adequate followup observations was one of the most disappointing experiences of the military surgeon.

Treatment by these physicians was quite good, and the few cases of gas gangrene seen during the everyday reception of casualties were usually in prisoners of war. Scanty records, failure to continue penicillin therapy, inadequate immobilization, improperly made colostomies, and failure to evacuate patients when the patient load became excessive were some of the mistakes most commonly made.

Directives were quickly prepared by the consultant group in the Office of the Chief Surgeon to point out the common and more serious mistakes. These directives were disseminated to all hospitals and surgical tams. For example, some of the transient hospitals noted that abdominal cases were given fruit juices quite early, and this, combined with early evacuation, resulted in considerable distention of the abdomen.

Study of Gas Gangrene and Wound Closure

There was hope that an extensive study of gas gangrene could be carried out and that facilities available at the 1st Medical General Laboratory could be used to develop a training film in gas gangrene. For example, it was observed that many patients with so-called cases of gas gangrene had received the customary 18 ampules of gas gangrene serum but actually had never had this dreaded infection. Some of these diagnoses were based on the smear taken of the wound, while others were based on inexperience—failure to appreciate the fact that most gunshot wounds contained air in the tissues and that crepitus was a common finding. Several illustrative cases were found, and motion pictures were made of these particular patients, including their treatment.

Another function of the surgical consultant in the early days following the invasion was to urge the principle of early secondary closure of wounds. By 18 June, some hospitals were already taking cultures of wounds, with the idea of making intensive studies in the proper method of treating such wounds. Information gained regarding the proper debridement of wounds and proper principles to be followed in secondary closure was taken to each hospital by frequent consultant visits. This was the only way that such information could be rapidly disseminated. Any directive issued would have lagged far behind in the promotion of better care for thousands of patients.

Practically every hospital center began its own study, trying to determine the best principle of carrying out secondary closures. Some of the questions in the minds of the surgeon follow:

1. How extensively should the wound be debrided before secondary closure?

2. Could the wound including the skin be closed?

3. How soon after injury should the secondary closure be carried out?

4. Should local chemotherapy or antibiotics have any place in the management of the secondary closure?

5. Did the adminstration of these drugs systemically before and following the procedure enhance the chance of success of the closures?

6. How long should the wounds closed secondarily be immobilized?

7. How soon could rehabilitation exercises be started without danger of disruption of the secondary closure?

It soon became apparent that it was the thoroughness and care of the surgeon carrying out the debridement in secondary closure more than the type of chemotherapy or antibiotic which was used that determined the result. If the surgical service of a hospital was in the charge of a very well-trained surgeon—especially one who believed in attention to the fine details in technique in care of patients—then the results in the hospital were good.

Regional Wounds

Eventually, thoracic wounds began to be concentrated in the various hospital centers, and the principles of early closed drainage and early decortication were followed. The principles had been developed in Italy, and it was the duty of all surgical consultants to impart this information wherever thoracic surgery was being performed.

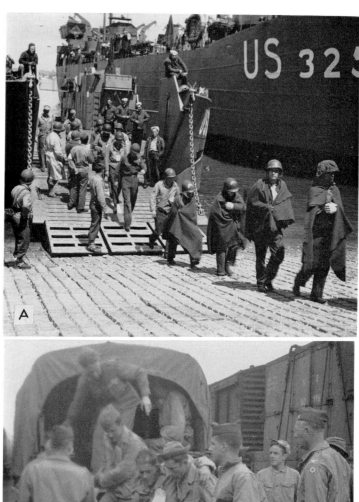

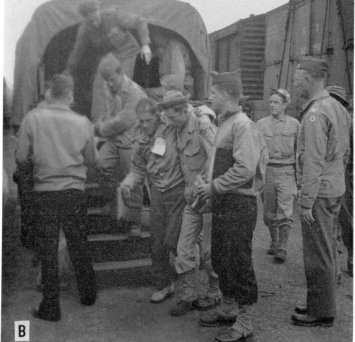

FIGURE 132.—The reception and transportation of casualties from the Normandy invasion. A. Ambulatory patients walking off an LCT. B. Transportation by cargo truck to a train loading point.

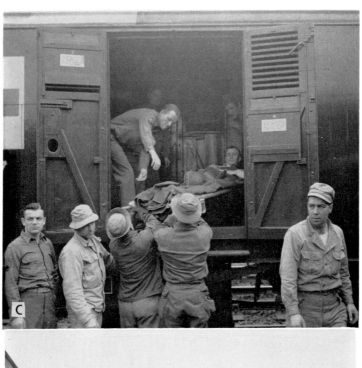

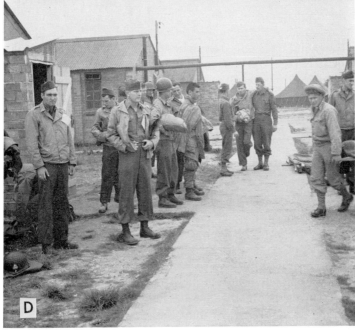

FIGURE 132.—Continued. C. Transportation inland by a hospital train. D. Patients arriving finally at the 305th Station Hospital on 15 June 1944.

Although the treatment of abdominal wounds was good and the majority of these cases were kept on the far shore within a few days after the onset of the invasion, the problem of the management of high intestinal fistulae was not satisfactorily solved. Small bowel fistulae were noted for their poor response to transportation. The surgeons were urged to avoid ileostomies or jejunostomies either by tube or exteriorization, if at all possible. They were further urged to administer sufficient fluids to bring these patients into fluid and electrolyte balance and to make every attempt at early surgical closure of the fistulae.

The management of vascular injuries of the extremities was also a problem. There was a tendency at times to incorporate the extremity in a lot of padding and a plaster case, which resulted in overheating as well as in covering the tissues and making it impossible to appraise the viability of the tissues during the hours of evacuation. The closeness of the cast to the heel enhanced the possibility of necrosis and infection. It was urged that these extremities be covered with sterile towels and that the patients be evacuated from the transit hospital in traction.

Before the end of June, many casualties were being received by air, and the majority were in good condition.

ACTIVITIES ON THE CONTINENT

As Senior Consultant in General Surgery, the author was informed that he would be assigned to the advance section of the communications zone, under the overall command of Col. (later Brig. Gen.) Charles B. Spruit, MC, as soon as this headquarters was established on the far shore. After spending some time in the staging area, this consultant finally arrived on the far shore on 16 July 1944. Reporting to the surgeon of the communications zone, he was advised to report to Col. Charles H. Beasley, MC, surgeon of the advance section headquarters, to work in the Professional Services Division of that headquarters and on 19 July, he first contacted Colonel Crisler, surgical consultant to the First U.S. Army.

Surgical and Shock Teams From Base Hospitals

After 19 July, the author met almost daily with the consultants of the First and Third U.S. Armies. During these evening meetings, the needs for surgical teams and other needs were discussed.

As soon as general hospitals had been set up in the staging area in France, Colonel Zollinger contacted them and asked them to organize their professional personnel into surgical teams. These teams were to consist of two surgeons, one anesthesiologist, one surgical nurse, and two surgical technicians. Each team was given the designation "A," and each was to be ordered out by number.

The First U.S. Army was to keep by number and name the chief of each team. It was planned that, insofar as possible, these teams would be assigned to evacuation hospitals to facilitate their relocation and eventual return to their parent units. In many instances, these men in general hospitals had been in the staging area in England for a considerable time and were more than eager to get into active work as members of a surgical team. They were instructed to report to a particular hospital, as designated by the army surgical consultant. No official orders were ever issued for these teams, and probably no official record was ever made of the fact that between 60 and 70 of these teams were used to supplement the surgical care of patients within the First U.S. Army during the middle of July 1944.

When the flow of casualties was quite heavy, it was obvious that mortality, especially in field hospital platoons receiving nontransportable wounded, could be lowered if sufficient personnel were available to administer whole blood to casualties awaiting operation. Accordingly, shock teams from the medical service of these same general hospitals in staging were formed to consist of one officer, one nurse, and one enlisted man. Two such shock teams were to be attached to each of the three platoons of a field hospital. These teams were to take along with them a form to record the amount of whole blood and plasma given in a clearing station both preoperatively and postoperatively. It was believed that in this way valuable information could be obtained as to the actual needs for whole blood and plasma in the forward areas. These data were to be gathered and correlated each week.

It was necessary for the author to visit the various field hospitals and explain the setup and function of the shock teams, since the newly formed teams were very much overworked. It was estimated that one surgical team could do about 7 or 8 abdominal operations or 12 chest cases within 12 hours (fig. 133). There were not enough personnel with the surgical teams to provide preoperative and postoperative care, and for that reason the shock team performed a valuable service. After these shock teams were assigned, they were so busy and engrossed in their work that records were inadequately kept. It was necessary, therefore, for this consultant to suggest that the nurse be made responsible for keeping these records. A report of the activities of these teams was submitted to communications zone headquarters for transmission to the Chief Surgeon.

Approximately 104 surgical and shock teams were drawn from the various general hospitals in the staging areas. These teams were returned to their own units within a relatively short time after the breakthrough at Saint-Lo, France. The experience demonstrated that each hospital, regardless of its size, should be subdivided and organized into surgical teams as well as shock teams. In this way, all professional personnel, including both surgeons and medical officers, could be assigned a useful function. Certainly, a shock team should be available to support each surgical team during the time of reception of heavy casualties. These shock teams, previously organized and set up, probably served as great a function in saving lives as did the surgical teams.

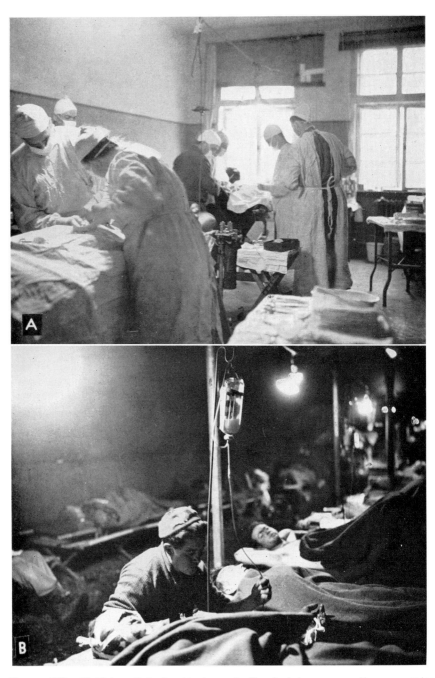

FIGURE 133.—Field hospitals functioning. A. Surgical teams operating on nontransportable, seriously wounded patients at the 45th Field Hospital. B. A shock ward at the 34th Field Hospital.

Evacuation and Sorting

This consultant visited various evacuation hospitals largely to maintain contact with the surgical and shock teams on temporary duty from the general hospitals and to make an effort to obtain data concerning the most efficient use of whole blood and plasma (fig. 134). On occasion, the consultants were also directed to visit holding units to assist in the triage of patients. For example, as many as 600 casualties awaiting air evacuation might be held by a medical battalion. Patients with large wounds, casts, or wounds of the abdomen and chest and those with complications were carefully checked before air evacuation. Chemotherapy was not attempted unless these casualties were to be held overnight. Surgical teams from the 1st Auxiliary Surgical Group were assigned to these units. Occasionally, surgery was necessary, especially when bad weather prevented evacuation by either air or sea. Hospitals did not find it difficult to supply auxiliary mobile surgical teams that had their own equipment. The parent hospitals were all in need of additional help, and a great spirit of cooperation existed among them.

The problem of triaging patients from holding units to advance section hospitals consumed increasing amounts of time. At first, those cases were selected that had a reasonable chance of returning to duty within 10 days after admission to hospitals in the advance section area. Allegedly, the first time abdominal cases were kept 10 days instead of 7, the patient load in the field hospitals was increased. The rapid forward advance of friendly armies after 1 August, however, resulted in a marked decrease in the number of casualties.

On 4 August, members of the Advance Section, Communications Zone, visited the holding unit at Omaha Beach. There were 1,100 patients in the particular unit, and 300 were selected for transportation on the first ambulance train from Lison Junction to Cherbourg. The visitors attempted to select cases that might have a reasonable chance of getting back to duty within 10 days or 2 weeks. Therefore, soft-tissue wounds, acute sprains, medical complaints, and similar cases, for the most part, were chosen. No fractures, nerve, tendon, or major blood vessel injuries, or wounds of the palm of the hand, the sole of the feet, the scrotum, the peritoneum, or the buttock were selected unless they were quite small.

Officers were instructed as a group and as individuals in triaging these cases. Two hundred and twenty-one were sent by the first train. The author accompanied this group to observe how well patients could tolerate transportation in the 40 *hommes et* 8 *chevaux boxcars*, which had been converted into an ambulance train (fig. 135).

There were three tiers of litters, with the wounds of the patients positioned toward the aisle in order that they could be inspected frequently by the medical officer. Several No. 2 medical chests were on the train, as were plasma and tourniquets. Fruit juice, K-rations, urinals, water, and so forth, were available in each car. The train ride was extremely slow, the train fairly crept to Cherbourg, and the entire trip took about 5 hours. The patients, however, withstood it quite well and were delivered to the 298th General Hospital.

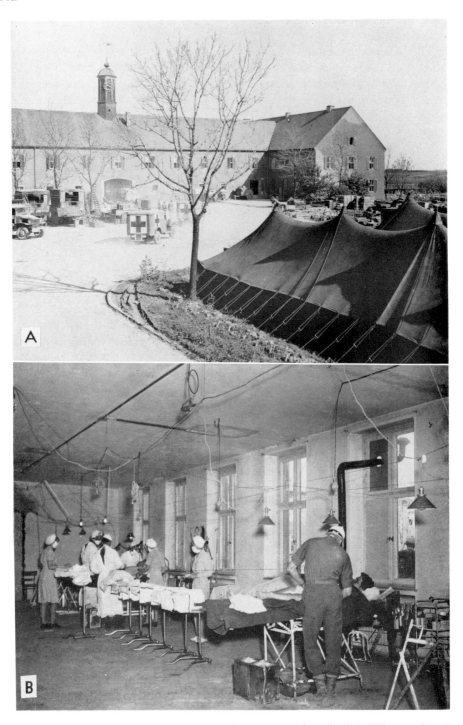

FIGURE 134.—The 9th Evacuation Hospital. A. A general view (both buildings and tentage
were utilized). B. Operating room.

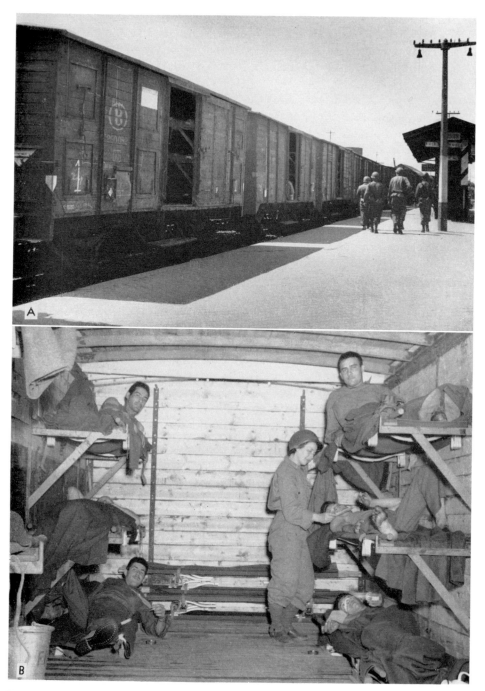

FIGURE 135.—The first hospital train movement on the Continent. A. *Chevaux* boxcars at Lison Junction. B. The interior of a boxcar fitted with brackets to hold litters.

Evaluation of patients with hernias, varicose veins, and similar disorders determined whether they should be operated upon at that time or should be transferred to another type of unit. The entire policy of necessity changed rather rapidly, depending upon the bed space available in the advance section hospitals.

On 5 August, the author visited the 5th General Hospital, which was functioning in Carenton, France, at the base of the peninsula. The hospital staff estimated that no more than 10 or 20 percent of its cases could be returned to duty within 10 days. The period of rehabilitation then had to be extended, and it was suggested that triage be more rigid in order to make more beds available for minor casualties that had a good chance of returning to duty within 2 weeks. These types of cases usually included soft-tissue wounds under 3 inches in length without associated damage to nerves, tendons, and major blood vessels.

From time to time, the consultants returned to England or other parts of the United Kingdom to visit the various hospitals and hospital centers. On these visits, they made rounds with the chiefs of surgery in order to discover any mistakes made on the far shore. It was worthwhile to point out to these men the difficulties under which the surgeons on the far shore labored. It was also necessary to check upon how well the patients were withstanding transportation by air, because there was some question as to how well thoracic and abdominal patients would tolerate the airlift. When the consultants returned again to France, they could report to the surgeons in the forward area concerning the good work that they had done as well as note errors which might be rectified with benefit to the patients.

In addition to visiting hospitals, consultants reviewed articles for inclusion in the monthly medical bulletin which was prepared for the information of all officers. Several meetings were held with the various thoracic surgeons in order to develop general principles of thoracic surgery to be included in the medical bulletin. Similar notations were made concerning the treatment of arteriovenous aneurysms.

The consultants shuttled back and forth between the United Kingdom and France as the occasion demanded. Toward the latter part of August 1944, a fair amount of the consultants' time was concerned with changes in policy. More and more patients were being held in the general hospitals, which became more completely established in France as the army moved eastward.

As patients were evacuated, it became necessary to mark on the outside jacket or record whether or not they were to go to communications zone facilities on the Continent or to the United Kingdom. As a general policy, it was suggested that all patients with fractures of the long bones and those with hernias be sent to the United Kingdom. On the other hand, patients with soft-tissue wounds were to be held for as long as 30 days and then be sent to convalescent hospitals located in areas near the general hospitals in Normandy. It was also planned that any patient whose condition would permit transfer to the Zone of the Interior at the end of 1 month would be treated in a general hospital on the Continent. The same rule was to apply to prisoners of war.

It was necessary to arrange for the indoctrination of triaging officers at the various field hospitals near airstrips. These triaging officers were selected from general hospital personnel because they played a very important role in the conservation of manpower and in keeping patients in France who might be quickly rehabilitated and returned to duty.

Miscellaneous Activities and Observations

During the latter part of August, a circular instructed all general hospitals to compile lists of various types of surgical shock teams, according to the new table of organization that had been sent over from the Zone of Interior, for assignment to the 12th Army Group, which in turn would determine their distribution.

Arrangements were made to assign Major Ebert and Major Emerson of the 5th General Hospital to a forward field hospital to study shock. They carried their own laboratory equipment. These men ultimately gathered very significant data which were later published in *Annals of Surgery*. One of their most significant findings was the fact that, by actual measurement, many of the compound fractures of the femur had lost as much as 40 percent of thier total blood volume. These medical officers were impressed by the great need for whole blood replacement and emphasized that plasma was not an adequate substitute for whole blood in a severely wounded soldier.

As the armies began to move forward farther and farther into Europe, distances became so great that the role of the consultant became less effective. Furthermore, the consultants in the United Kingdom had been well organized and were quite capable of functioning independently. More and more attention could be devoted to the development of principles regarding definitive treatment of casualties. For example, some hospitals began to segregate all their hand cases into a separate ward.

A number of surgical principles seemed to be violated from time to time. Such errors as the inadequate exteriorization of the colon for a temporary colostomy were studied, and corrective measures were then written up as an editorial in the European theater *Medical Bulletin*. Some difficulty was encountered in the evaluation of casualties in holding units before they were finally sent back to the Zone of Interior. The holding units apparently were too busy and did not assume the responsibility of continued treatment before the patients were evacuated. It was obvious that more experienced surgeons were needed to evaluate these cases and screen them before the patients were evacuated, whether by sea or air.

Toward the end of August, this consultant visited various army areas and continued a close relationship with the very cooperative consultants in the armies. Toward the end of September, the consultants were directed to visit the 16th Field Hospital which had received a number of wounded French from the 2d Armored Division. The question arose why this hospital should encounter such a high mortality. Upon visiting it, the consultants learned that these patients were severely wounded because, like many brave Frenchmen, they had left their tanks and walked directly into the line of enemy fire. Their distaste for taking cover, as practiced by other types of troops, accounted for the very extensive wounds.

As a matter of fact, a platoon of this hospital received 60 severely wounded during this specific period, 34 of whom came from the 2d Armored Division. Four of the thirty-four patients had been operated upon in the clearing station of the French division. All four died within 2 days.

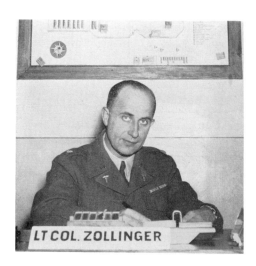

FIGURE 136.—Lt. Col. Robert M. Zollinger, MC, Commanding Officer, 5th General Hospital, Carentan, France.

The average delay from admission to operation was 10 or 12 hours. This was due to the fact that, during the first 24 hours, the platoon had but one surgical team. This time interval was consistent with the delay observed in many other field hospitals during the study on shock. Actually, when receiving casualties, the field hospitals needed both surgical and shock teams.

About the first of October 1944, it became a policy that affiliated units which had been overseas for a long time should be commanded by members of their own units. Accordingly, Lt. Col. (later Col.) Louis M. Rousselot, MC, of Columbia University, was assigned as commanding officer of the 2d General Hospital, and, on 9 October 1944, the author replaced Col. Maxwell G. Keeler, MC, as commanding officer of the 5th General Hospital (figs. 136 and 137). Such a change was welcome, since the great distances involved made the role of the consultant increasingly difficult. Furthermore, the various armies were well organized with their own consultant staffs, and the principles of treatment were by then well understood by all. Professional care in the army areas was excellent, and the theater was filled with highly skilled men. Base sections had been set up in France as well as in the United Kingdom. At this time, it would have been invaluable had research teams been

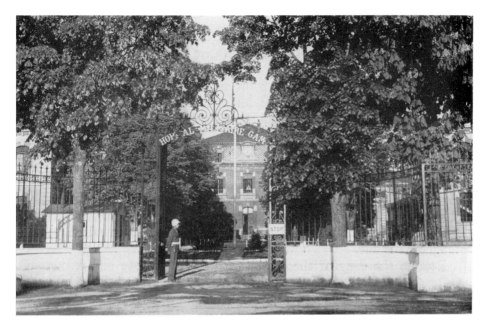

FIGURE 137.—The entrance to the 5th General Hospital.

organized to gather and record data regarding the professional care of these patients, returning such data to the Zone of Interior.

The author was in command of the 5th General Hospital until it returned to the United States in October 1945. The unit was disbanded at Fort Dix, N.J., that same month.

CONCLUSIONS

The position of a consultant in a theater of operations is hard to define, since there was no tangible table of organization and no precedent as to authority and responsibility. It might be said that the consultant had the same relationship to the regular medical officers as the regular medical officers had to the line officers. In other words, under ordinary circumstances they were a necessary nuisance, especially when they justifiably sought promotion to the rank of colonel; but they were absolutely essential when casualties were high, when morale of the soldier was low, and when morbidity and mortality were unsatisfactory.

Provision should be made to insure sufficient rank up to and including brigadier general for nationally known men who serve in oversea theaters as consultants. High rank is most essential in order to command the same authority as consultants of similar capacity in Allied armies and to add weight to the consultant's recommendations to hospital commanders.

Since the professional care of patients is not limited to any particular army or base section, and since casualties must invariably be evacuated from the field army back through the communications zone and finally to the Zone of Interior, the nomad consultant should be welcome in any area. He is, after all, concerned with the professional care of patients and functions primarily as a doctor.

There was too great a barrier between the consultants in the headquarters of the Office of the Chief Surgeon and those in the various field armies. There was no friction between the consultants themselves, but limitations did exist, since each army was independently responsible for its own internal administration and resented any outside interference.

The consultants in the European theater were concerned especially with their inability to requisition transportation. Perhaps it would have been better, however, had they moved more as a group. When several consultants, each in a special car, arrived simultaneously at a hospital, it was disturbing to the officers of the hospital and tended to create a friction which persisted throughout the war.

Because the duty of the consultant was to "observe and recommend," he often lacked the authority to achieve his goal. It may have been due partially to the fact that he was not thoroughly informed as to the overall program of the theater. Consultants should have been better briefed by administrative officers concerning their problems of supplies, men, and equipment.

Both the regular and the reserve medical officers who served as consultants point to the fact that the morbidity and mortality rates were lower than those of any previous war, despite the great mass of casualties. These low rates are attributed to many factors, among which are planning, training, evacuation, and indoctrination in the professional care of patients. Each group, therefore, played a vital role and should have made every attempt to understand the goals and problems of the other group. By the end of the war, a much clearer understanding had developed among them.

RECOMMENDATIONS

Under the system which prevailed in the European theater during World War II, consultants could only recommend the transfer of individual medical officers. The rapport attained with the personnel officer, therefore, became a matter of utmost importance. It should have been incumbent upon the personnel officer to accept without reservation the consultant's recommendations for the transfer of professional personnel.

The tables of organization of headquarters of all levels should include authorized positions for the entire group of consultants and provide for their ranks. Sufficient authority should be given consultants to carry out their recommendations. This, of necessity, includes the granting of sufficiently high rank, commensurate with the authority desired. Furthermore, promotion or appointment of one of the consultants in a table of organization headquarters should not preclude the promotion of another because there is only one vacancy in that particular rank. This situation could be alleviated by the creation of a separate table that provides for the positions and ranks of consultants.

In order to assure the most efficient application of their time and energies, consultants should have permanently assigned transportation on call, as does a physician in civil practice. To enable consultants to visit various facilities at will and coordinate professional activities by personal conferences would greatly aid the standardization of procedures, bolster the morale of surgeons, and improve the professional care of patients. The consultant should not have to waste time trying to wrangle transportation from the motor pool.

The theater surgeon, the army surgeon, the base section surgeon, and even the commanding officer of a hospital center should have a table of organization and manpower allocations for research and observation teams. Such teams should be accepted, in principle, as being just as essential for good surgical care as are logistics, evacuation, and the like. These teams could then observe and record the type of professional care casualties receive as they pass from first echelon medical services all the way to the installations for definitive treatment and rehabilitation.

CHAPTER IV

Neurological Surgery

Loyal Davis, M.D.

At the Arcadia Conference, held in Washington from 24 December 1941 to 14 January 1942, a broad policy was decided upon for offensive actions against Germany. It was decided that, during 1942, Germany's resistance would be worn down by increasing air bombardment by British and U.S. Forces, giving assistance to the Soviet offensive, and gaining possession of the entire North African coast. This policy was examined many times, so that it is not surprising that many changes were made in the program. For example, the J.P.S. (U.S. Joint Staff Planners) believed that a considerable land attack could be launched across the English Channel in 1942. This was to be accomplished largely by British troops in the beginning, but participation of U.S. Forces, it was believed, could be built up rapidly. In fact, the planners outlined a possible cross-Channel operation which would take place in the summer of 1942 with a D-day between 15 July and 1 August.

With this background, it is not difficult to understand why The Surgeon General of the U.S. Army hastened to implement his share of planning in this proposed operation and attempted to build up his medical forces rapidly. A part of this planning was to supply the Chief Surgeon, ETOUSA (European Theater of Operations, U.S. Army) with a staff of consultants in the fields of medicine, surgery, neurological surgery, plastic surgery, ophthalmology, radiology, anesthesiology, orthopedic surgery, and otolaryngology.

On 2 July 1942, Col. (later Brig. Gen.) Fred W. Rankin, MC, chief surgical consultant to The Surgeon General, telephoned the author and arranged for a conference in Washington on 5 July. Col. (later Brig. Gen.) Elliott C. Cutler, MC, professor of surgery at Harvard Medical School; Lt. Col. (later Col.) William S. Middleton, MC, professor of medicine and dean of the University of Wisconsin Medical School; Maj. (later Col.) James B. Brown, MC, professor of plastic surgery at Washington University; Maj. (later Col.) Rex L. Diveley, MC, of Kansas City, Mo.; and Maj. (later Col.) Lloyd J. Thompson, MC, of Yale University School of Medicine, were either in England or on their way to join the Chief Surgeon's consultant group. To the specialties of surgery, medicine, plastic surgery, orthopedic surgery, and psychiatry, Colonel Rankin explained, would be added neurological surgery. Though it was never at any time during the conference so stated, the impression was gained that there were several general hospitals in the European theater (and this meant the British Isles) and that several would be added very rapidly. It is obvious that there was an immediate urgency to speed up Operation BOLERO, the buildup operation for invasion of the Continent.

Col. (later Maj. Gen.) Paul R. Hawley, MC, had been named as Chief Surgeon, ETOUSA, by Maj. Gen. (later Lt. Gen.) John C. H. Lee, who had been sent to England as the commanding general of SOS (Services of Supply), ETOUSA. Colonel Hawley had been a member of the London Committee which had been made up of representatives of various British supply ministries and representatives of the U.S. Army who had functioned in mufti in London during the entire year preceding the attack on Pearl Harbor. General Lee had arrived in England, however, with another medical officer designated as his Chief Surgeon, and it was a fortuitous circumstance which made him appoint Colonel Hawley on the spot.

GETTING ACQUAINTED

Obviously, none of these circumstances were known to Lt. Col. (later Col.) Loyal Davis, MC, the newly appointed Senior Consultant in Neurological Surgery (fig. 138), when he arirved in England by air on 6 September 1942, after having been commissioned on 20 August. Soon after his arrival at Headquarters, SOS, in Cheltenham, Gloucestershire, the author was formally introduced to the Chief Surgeon. Then the neurological surgical consultant joined the staff of Col. James C. Kimbrough, MC, Chief of Professional Services, a urologist, who had been on duty at Walter Reed General Hospital, and whose good humor and patience were exemplified in his statement and belief that the war spoiled the Army Medical Service.

It became evident immediately that for some reason, unknown, the speed of action had slowed considerably. There was one U.S. Army general hospital in southern England, at Oxford, the 2d General Hospital, staffed by medical officers from Columbia University College of Physicians and Surgeons, New York, and Presbyterian Hospital, New York. There was one in the Midlands, at Mansfield, the 30th General Hospital, comprised of doctors from the University of California School of Medicine, San Francisco. Another, the 5th General Hospital, had been for some time in Northern Ireland; the staff of this hospital was composed of members of the Harvard Medical School faculty. There was one neurological surgeon on the staff of the hospital at Oxford, Maj. (later Lt. Col.) John E. Scarff, MC, who needed no help from the Senior Consultant.

It had become the custom, and certainly it was logical, for each consultant to make a tour of the theater and get acquainted with the U.S. hospital units as well as the English and Canadian groups. Mr. Hugh W. B. Cairns, Nuffield Professor of Surgery at Oxford, and an old friend who had studied at the Peter Bent Brigham Hospital, Boston, had become a brigadier and Consultant for

Neurological Surgery to the RAMC (Royal Army Medical Corps). There was one important difference, however, in the respective posts of the British and U.S. consultants. Brigadier Cairns was responsible for advice in neurological surgery wherever the British Army was fighting, and his mobility and responsibility created a unity which produced results in treatment and policies far surpassing anything which the U.S. Army attained.

On 17 September, this consultant submitted a memorandum describing his initial tour of inspection, and it was approved and returned by the Chief Surgeon with a request that the recommendations be implemented.

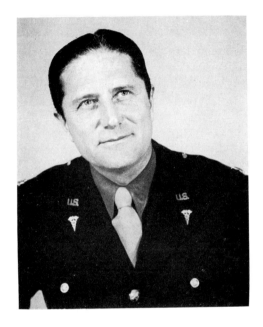

FIGURE 138.—Lt. Col. Loyal Davis, MC, at his desk in the Office of the Chief Surgeon, ETOUSA, Cheltenham, England.

Review of British Activities

A Military Hospital for Head Injuries was located in the buildings of St. Hugh's College for Women in Oxford. This British hospital received only patients who had received craniocerebral injuries of all degrees of severity, and, as a result of the careful and scientifically professional service which was given there, they demonstrated conclusively that a high percentage of men so injured could be returned to their military units for duty. One of the most reliable symptoms upon which they prognosticated the ability of the soldier to return to military duty, particularly in blunt craniocerebral injuries, was the length of the period of post-traumatic amnesia. Brigadier Cairns instituted the policy of treating open craniocerebral injuries by shaving the hair, cleansing the wound carefully with soap and water, applying a sterile dressing, and transporting the wounded soldier as quickly as possible to a hospital where he could receive definitive treatment. The patients' records were carefully made and kept so that they would provide a basis after the war for a study of the immediate and prophylactic treatment of craniocerebral injuries.

The Middleton Park Convalescent Hospital, near Bicester, Oxfordshire, was situated 10 miles from the head injury hospital in Oxford and to it patients were sent from the latter hospital for convalescent care and rehabilitation. The care at Middleton Park had been planned and was supervised by Brigadier Cairns, and not by a student of physical medicine who knew nothing of the residuals of head injuries. Even Radcliffe Infirmary, a hospital of Oxford University, was utilized for the study of compound fractures of the extremities and severe burns.

Within the environs of Oxford was the Wingfield Morris Orthopaedic Emergency Hospital under the direction of Herbert J. Seddon, an orthopedic surgeon who had received a considerable amount of surgical training at the University of Michigan Medical School, Ann Arbor. The RAMC found it possible to make use of Professor Seddon without insisting that he be in uniform. To this hospital were sent all of the peripheral nerve injuries from the British military forces and the civilian population. It was immediately obvious that one of the most important contributions to peripheral nerve surgery would one day come from this well-planned and well-organized hospital for study and treatment.

In the aforementioned 17 September memorandum it was emphasized that the U.S. Army records of examination, diagnosis, and treatment of the peripheral nerve injuries in World War I were totally inadequate, were incomplete, and were rarely available for study or for use in following up the few patients who made their appearance from time to time in Veterans' Administration hospitals. It was emphasized repeatedly that this should not obtain during World War II and that the records at the Wingfield Morris Orthopaedic Emergency Hospital could be used as models. Colonel Davis emphasized the point that neurosurgical records need not be so elaborate that they would obstruct the care of the wounded but that they should be complete so that future military surgery would benefit from their study. This required unified direction which was never obtained.[1]

Brigadier Cairns, through his friendship with Lord Nuffield, had initiated a project at the Morris Garage in Oxford for the construction of mobile surgical units for the RCAMC (Royal Canadian Army Medical Corps). These units were 3-ton motor vehicles with 4-wheel drives and contained an electric generator so that the unit could pull up beside a church or schoolhouse and go to work to help a forward hospital. Each unit carried two folding instrument and operating tables, head rests, sterile drums of supplies, sterile basins, and a water tank but were not as elaborately equipped as were those originally designed by Brigadier Cairns, one of which was lost at Dunkirk.

---

[1] The recent five-center study of peripheral nerve injuries conducted by the Veterans' Administration with moneys made available through the National Research Council has pointed up this glaring error of organization repeated through two world wars.

Other projects were underway at Oxford. Prof. S. (later Sir Solly) Zuckerman was working upon the effects of blast as observed during the Battle of Britain. In his opinion, blast did not produce cerebral damage but for the most part affected the lungs. He was given the opportunity by Brigadier Cairns of doing actual fieldwork. Professor Zuckerman accurately plotted the scene of a bombing, the number and position of the individuals affected, the exact character of the agent, and whether the injured individual was stationary or moving, in an effort to determine eventually what prophylactic measure might be worked out. By photographing and measuring the body in all conceivable positions assumed during combat, Professor Zuckerman determined that the head and neck offered a target equal to about 12 percent of the entire body. Interestingly, a checkup on the actual location and nature of injuries which he had investigated showed a remarkable percentage of correlation with Professor Zuckerman's calculations on the projection of various body areas as targets. While he worked under the auspices of the British Medical Research Council, cooperation with the military was maintained through Brigadier Cairns.

In the laboratories of the Department of Anatomy at Oxford, Graham Weddell and Prof. John Z. Young were investigating the degeneration and regeneration of nerve fibers to the skin and muscles following peripheral nerve injuries. They found that any method of treatment which increased the blood supply to the involved muscles was very important in the rehabilitation of these patients. By recording the degree of muscle fibrillation following injury, Weddell believed he could determine whether or not a given paralyzed muscle could regain its function.

Canadian Activities in United Kingdom

The Canadian Neurological (1st General) Hospital was situated at Basingstoke, Southampton, and was built around Hackwood House in 1940. From the beginning, it was designed and equipped as a neurological surgical installation. It was superbly organized and administered. In addition to giving excellent care to the wounded, it served as a training place for young general surgeons who could be taught the fundamentals of the immediate care of neurosurgical injuries in forward hospitals. Personnel of this hospital had called attention to the following important facts: (1) Small, apparently trivial, scalp wounds often hid serious underlying comminuted fractures of the skull with destruction of brain tissue; (2) injuries of the head had been treated as long as 36 hours after receipt of the wound in the Dieppe raid and after careful surgery, aided by the use of sulfanilamide; (3) no infections had been observed when the craniocerebral injury had been cleaned carefully, the head shaved, sulfanilamide placed in the wound, a sterile dressing applied, and the wounded man sent back immediately to the Canadian Neurological Hospital for definitive treatment; and (4) in the presence of a defect in the skull, in a patient who has recovered function, repair of the defects by the use of a prosthesis could result in the return of the soldier to active military duty. This viewpoint upon the use of the sulfonamides was prior to the demonstration that their general administration with determination of the blood level was as effective as, and less destructive to tissue than, their local administration.

Observed at this hospital were several patients who had been operated upon for herniated nucleus pulposus and returned to duty. This experience resulted in a memorandum, which was adopted as U.S. Army policy in the European theater, to the effect that these patients should be operated upon by neurological surgeons, but only when the clinical syndrome pathognomonic of this condition existed and when careful X-ray studies using the new myelographic material, Pantopaque, corroborated the diagnosis. Finally, it was emphasized that intensive and supervised physical rehabilitation exercises should be carried out upon each patient.

Inadequate Facilities in U.S. Hospitals

This get-acquainted tour emphasized the complete lack of instruments and equipment on hand in the 2d General Hospital for neurological surgery. In company with the Senior Consultant for Plastic Surgery, this consultant visited the British surgical instrument houses of Allen & Hanburys Ltd., and Down Bros., Ltd., and a representative of the British Ministry of Supply, in order to determine whether there were any instruments upon their shelves or in their stocks which could be supplied to U.S. Army general hospitals. This was an unproductive day because those instruments available were completely outmoded; the field of neurological surgery and its appliances and instruments had been developed in the United States. It was, however, a demonstration, many times repeated, of the facts that the Army could put supplies into a depot but could not get them out; that, because an officer was a doctor, it did not follow that he was capable of getting the right supplies where they belonged; that a good stock manager from a mail-order house would have served far better; and, finally, that the principle of ordering a stipulated supply of a particular item for a given number of men every 90 days would result in enough thermometers to roadblock an invading force and enough hypertonic glucose solution to float the British Navy.

ANALYSIS OF THE SITUATION AND RECOMMENDATIONS

As a result of this tour, this consultant wrote a detailed memorandum of the principles learned by the British for the care of neurosurgical injuries and requested that it be sent to the Office of The Surgeon General in Washington for dissemination among military and civilian neurological surgeons in the United States. He hoped that thus might be started a method of communication which would make it obvious that a unified method of care and handling was essential for obtaining results which later could be studied to the advantage of the injured man. Whether this memorandum was ever sent to Washington, this consultant never knew; if it was, nothing came from it because, throughout the war, it seemed to the author that the European theater remained a distinct, isolated entity instead of having a close liaison with the Office of The Surgeon General. It became evident, more and more, that a Consultant in Neurological Surgery should have been responsible, through the Chief Consultant in Surgery to The Surgeon General, for the proper organization of the care of neurosurgical injuries in whatever theater of war they occurred. Such a consultant could have been mobile enough to have spent the time necessary in each theater to have provided methods and means of obtaining results which could later have been the basis for valuable contributions to this field of surgery. In the Mediterranean theater, there was no senior consultant in neurological surgery. In the European theater, during Colonel Davis' tour of duty, there were never more than two qualified neurological surgeons with whom one could consult.

It was apparent on 19 September 1942 that the 1st Infantry Division was preparing to leave for a combat zone (Africa). The author gave the medical officers of this division an hour's talk on neurosurgery in war. They had had no previous instruction on this subject during the 18 months to 2 years they had been on active service. Perhaps it was just as well, considering that they lacked morphine Syrettes, blood pressure apparatus, anesthetic agents, and sulfonamides, to name a few glaring shortages. Medical officers were being used as transportation officers and in other capacities; the division surgeon did not attend the meeting and had never attended a medical meeting of the division. The morale of the division's medical officers was low.

St. Bartholomew's Hospital, which had been badly bombed, had its neurosurgical unit, under Mr. John E. A. O'Connell, at Hill End Emergency Hospital, St. Albans, London, and was visited on 28 September, as was the Canadian 15th General Hospital. On the same tour, this consultant visited the 30th General Hospital. The Canadians presented a series of papers relating their experiences in the treatment of casualties received following the Dieppe fiasco. They emphasized the use of surgical teams consisting of two surgeons, two nurses, an anesthetist, and an orderly. The records of their examinations and operations were dictated to, and kept in order by, ambulatory patients and enlisted men. Their data were uniform and provided excellent material for future studies.

A young captain with some training in general surgery and with no aspirations to be a neurological surgeon had been assigned to care for neurosurgical injuries, when and if they occurred, at the 30th General Hospital. Colonel Davis recommended that a census of the number of neurosurgical injuries in each of the U.S. hospitals in the theater be provided the Professional Services Division because there was no way of knowing where such cases were or how they were being treated. It became known that many American soldiers, injured severely in jeep accidents in the blackout, were scattered through British EMS (Emergency Medical Service) hospitals and were receiving treatment for their craniocerebral injuries which was below American standards of treatment. On 1 October, an example of an American soldier taken to an EMS hospital instead of to the 2d General Hospital at Oxford was cited as a reason for seeking a method to transport such injured American soldiers to a U.S. hospital. As a corollary to this, and as a result of a line officer's refusing to move one of his men from a British hospital even after the British doctor and an American medical officer directed his transfer, authority was also requested for the recognition of the American medical officer's orders in such instances.

As a result of many conferences with Brigadier Cairns, Mr. Geoffrey Jefferson, and Dr. George Riddoch, as well as with various members of Canadian hospital units, Colonel Davis recommended on 5 October 1942 that all general hospitals have a qualified neurological surgeon assigned to their staff; that instruction in the primary surgical treatment of neurosurgical injuries should be given, in a teaching course, to battalion aid station, collecting station, clearing station, and evacuation hospital medical officers, since the final results of the definitive treatment of those injuries depended upon the accuracy and effectiveness of the early treatment. It was recommended that this be done without removing the officers from their units and before they reached the combat theater where such periods of instruction might interfere with more immediately urgent activities. Thus, another attempt was made to bring about some sort of unity of effort in the care of neurosurgical injuries.

On 13 October, this consultant wrote the first of seven memorandums to govern the general principles of the treatment of craniocerebral, spinal cord, and peripheral nerve injuries. Six of these memorandums were criticized on the grounds of poor English, and the seventh was accepted and disposed of most effectively by one of the Chief Surgeon's staff officers when he filed it away among his effects.

On 15 October 1942, the author submitted a detailed memorandum about the transfer of injured American soldiers from EMS hospitals throughout the British Isles to U.S. Army hospitals. With reference to neurosurgical patients (and it would have applied easily to other types of injuries), it was recommended that:

1. All EMS hospitals be requested through the director of their service to notify immediately the Division of Professional Services, Office of the Chief Surgeon, ETOUSA, of the admission of American soldiers with craniocerebral, spinal cord, and peripheral nerve injuries.

2. The Director, EMS, be requested to supply to the Division of Professional Services, Office of the Chief Surgeon, a list of the neurological surgeons and the name and location of the EMS hospitals in which they are located.

3. In the absence at this time of an adequate number of qualified and certified neurological surgeons in the American Forces, the Senior Consultant in Neurological Surgery be given authority to contact the EMS neurological surgeon of the region nearest the EMS hospital to which the soldier has been taken and request that he assume responsibility for removal of the soldier to his

own facility and there treat him, or direct his treatment if in his judgment transportation is inadvisable.

4. An American soldier so injured be moved to a U.S. general hospital where a qualified and certified neurological surgeon is available, just as quickly as the condition of the patient warrants, in the judgment of the EMS neurological surgeon.

5. The treatment of American injured by EMS neurological surgeons be discontinued as soon as neurological surgeons in U.S. general hospitals are available in sufficient numbers to render this service themselves.

6. Authority be granted to employ indigenous ambulance service to remove a patient to a U.S. hospital in the event that the employment of American ambulances is impossible or would involve unnecessary delay in the treatment of the soldier in the judgment of the Senior Consultant in Neurological Surgery or an individual to whom he delegates the responsibility for such judgment.

On 19 October 1942, this consultant wrote directly to General Rankin in Washington and asked that he assign neurological surgeons to the 5th and 30th General Hospitals. Evidently, this gentleman quickly recognized the failure of this memorandum to stay within "channels" and by not answering it saved the author momentarily from his ultimate difficulty.

On 22 October, a visit to the 30th General Hospital revealed that no suction apparatus was available to the surgeons and that operations upon one patient with a rupture of the spleen and upon another with a rupture of the kidney had nearly resulted in fatalities, although the surgeons had improvised with two bicycle pumps and the strength of an orderly. The first of a series of requests for such a suction apparatus was written immediately and was followed by several others containing minute descriptions of a suction pump available from a supply company in Reading, England, for fifty dollars. The size of valves, the overall size and weight, and minute specifications were given; in fact, a pump for each of the general hospitals in the European theater was available and could have been delivered by hand by this consultant, if necessary. The requests ended up without action in the Supply Division, Office of the Chief Surgeon, ETOUSA, which was at that time the most persistent of General Hawley's problems.

On 26 October, in answer to a query from the personnel officer, Office of the Chief Surgeon, ETOUSA, this consultant emphasized the facts that (1) the neurological surgeons suggested for the 5th and 30th General Hospitals were already commissioned in the Medical Corps, AUS, and would not, therefore, be taken from civil life, (2) there was only one neurological surgeon in the European theater, and therefore the need could not be supplied from the European theater, (3) the request was not for consultants but for experienced neurological surgeons capable of assuming responsibility for the treatment of craniocerebral, spinal cord, and peripheral nerve injuries and, finally, (4) dependence upon the British EMS head centers for the treatment and care of neurosurgical cases in the European theater should not be continued.

Many memorandums later, it was evident that the Chief Surgeon had never seen any of the many recommendations made by the Senior Consultant in Neurological Surgery. They were passed back and forth or conveniently filed by a personally hostile medical officer who openly boasted that he would put the new lieutenant colonel specialist consultants in their place. Soon, thereafter, a roster of officers was issued for allnight duty to answer the telephone to receive reports of deaths of soldiers in the theater. The roster began with the lieutenant colonel consultants to the Chief Surgeon, and the duty was served, at least by one consultant, until the roster and duty were canceled by General Hawley when it was called to his attention.

On 3 November 1942, accompanied by the Senior Consultant in Plastic Surgery, the author gave the first of a series of lectures at the Eighth Air Force Provisional Medical Field Service School to young air force medical officers. At this time, it was not apparent that a schism existed between the Army Air Forces and the rest of the Army, based upon the Air Forces' attempts to establish a medical service quite separate and distinct from that of the remainder of the Army. At this same time, the 92d Bomber Group Combat Crew Replacement Center at Bovingdon was visited. This tour also included the East Grinstead Royal Victoria RAF Plastic Center, which was under the direction of Mr. A. H. McIndoe, Chief Consultant in Plastic Surgery to the RAF. Mr. McIndoe made it possible to visit Group Captain Atcherly of the RAF, who was in command of a fighter group, and who personally conducted the two U.S. Army consultants over his station. Following these visits, comprehensive memorandums were written which recommended the placement of well-staffed, completely equipped, smaller types of hospitals, strategically located within rapid evacuation distance by ambulance from bomber and fighter airdromes, and the assignment of a liaison medical officer from the U.S. Army Air Forces stationed in the United Kingdom to the Office of the Chief Surgeon to advise in the eventual disposition of injured air force personnel. It is now clear that, at the time of the writing of these memorandums, the struggle for independence in medical organization was taking place, and these memorandums could not have been more timely, though they were completely ineffective.

On 9 November 1942, Colonel Davis wrote a detailed memorandum to the Chief Surgeon, ETOUSA. The author was quite unaware of the organization of the Army and the relationship of a theater of operations to the War Department in Washington as far as the Medical Department was concerned. It was becoming more and more apparent that the Medical Department was completely subservient to the SOS command and that the Chief Surgeon had access to the Commanding General, ETOUSA, only through the Commanding General, SOS, ETOUSA. This fact, learned by diligent study of the volumes depicting the history of World War I, during which the same struggle for direct responsibility of the Medical Department to the commanding general occurred, made it obvious that the Air Forces eventually would have their separate medical service. If they were not to succeed immediately in such a division, at least it appeared they would conduct their affairs in such a manner. The memorandum to the Chief Surgeon read:

1. The Consultant in Neurological Surgery in the European Theater of Operations held the following views, which were expressed, when he accepted the post offered by the Surgeon General's Office:

(a) Military neurological surgery differs in many of its technical aspects from the neurological surgery of intracranial tumors and other common civilian neurosurgical conditions.

(b) There is no place for the trained, experienced neurological surgeon in forward areas of combat.

(c) Only careful, well-directed immediate general surgical treatment should be given to neurosurgical injuries in forward combat areas.

(d) Properly instructed and trained younger medical officers should have the responsibility of giving the type of immediate surgical treatment in forward areas necessary to obtain good definitive results.

(e) Meticulous, definitive surgical treatment should be given to neurosurgical injuries in general hospitals only, located within reasonably rapid evacuation distance of a combat area.

(f) Experienced, well-trained and recognized neurological surgeons should direct definitive treatment for neurosurgical injuries in a general hospital.

(g) Neurological surgery should be a service in a general hospital and special neurosurgical hospitals have no place in an Army.

2. With the statement contained in Paragraph 1b, the Chief Surgeon of the E.T.O. has expressed complete agreement.

(a) This viewpoint is supported by the experience of the Royal Army Medical Corps at Dunkirk and the Middle East and by the Royal Australian Medical Corps.

3. The Consultant in Neurological Surgery has (a) completed personal investigations and observations of facilities, equipment and personnel of the U.S. Army Medical Corps in the E.T.O., as they apply to neurological surgery and (b) has visited and observed the British and Canadian Army neurosurgical service in the U.K. and (c) the neurosurgical services in the E.M.S. and the Scottish E.M.S.

4. As a result of the statement contained in Paragraph 3, the following facts are evident:

(a) Competent, experienced and self-reliant neurological surgeons are now assigned to two of the four U.S. General Hospitals in this theater (#2 and #298).

(b) Ground and air force combat neurosurgical injuries in British hospitals in the United Kingdom, both military and E.M.S., are comparatively small in number. The majority of such cases have been the result of blitz or ordinary civilian accidents.

(c) Only one neurological surgeon in Great Britain and one from Canada are in Army service.

(d) The overwhelming remainder of the neurological surgeons in the United Kingdom are in the Emergency Medical Service.

(e) Very few, if any, peripheral nerve, spinal cord and compounded craniocerebral injuries can be returned to military duty within the 180 day evacuation period established by the Chief Surgeon of the E.T.O. Only relatively minor closed cranio-cerebral injuries can meet the requirement of this evacuation period.

(f) Based upon neurosurgical casualty figures in World War I, on the figures available from British services thus far, and upon the combat casualties which can be projected in the immediate future in this theater, four neurological surgeons will meet all the needs for the highest type of surgical treatment for neurosurgical injuries.

(g) Equipment and supplies, for obtaining the best possible results for the soldier suffering from neurosurgical injuries, are lacking in completeness in U.S. General Hospitals in the E.T.O. This equipment cannot be obtained from English surgical instrument firms.

(h) Younger medical officers in the division who have been observed in this theater are poorly prepared by training and equipment to give proper immediate surgical treatment to neurosurgical injuries in forward combat areas.

5. The function of the Consultant in Neurological Surgery is to act in an advisory professional capacity to the Chief Surgeon of the E.T.O. and to establish and correlate the highest type of neurosurgical service in this theater to the end that eventually it will be possible for the Medical Corps of the U.S. Army to make a significant and substantial contribution to the surgical care of the injured soldier.

6. As a contribution to this desired result, the Consultant in Neurological Surgery with the fullest sympathy of understanding on the part of the Chief Surgeon, has recommended:

(a) That experienced, competent and self-reliant neurological surgeons be assigned to U.S. General Hospitals #5 and #30 in the E.T.O.

(b) That medical clinical records, supplemental to the F.M.R., together with the necessary clerical aid, be made available to U.S. General Hospitals in E.T.O. The purpose of this recommendation was to afford the opportunity of compiling a record of the end results of neurological surgery in this War which would surpass that of World War I.

(c) That a course of instruction to division medical officers be given in training camps on the principles of the immediate surgical treatment of neurosurgical injuries.

(d) That neurosurgical injuries be transferred as soon as practical from station hospitals in the E.T.O., and be evacuated as rapidly as possible from forward combat areas, to general hospitals in the E.T.O. for definitive surgical treatment.

(e) That all equipment and supplies necessary to obtain the highest type of neurosurgical end results be furnished U.S. General Hospitals without delay so that these hospitals would be able by their work to represent the highest type of American medicine and surgery.

(f) That a general directive governing the principles of the treatment of neurosurgical injuries be issued to general hospitals in the E.T.O.

(g) That a fixed general hospital with a neurological surgeon assigned be strategically located within rapid evacuation distance of the present dispositions of the American Air Force installations in this theater.

7. The Consultant in Neurological Surgery has been able to effect the following service to injured American soldiers:

(a) Through personal contact with the Chiefs of the neurosurgical service in E.M.S. and Scottish E.M.S., American soldiers with neurosurgical injuries taken to E.M.S. hospitals receive the immediate services of the regional neurological surgeons and are evacuated as rapidly as possible to U.S. General Hospitals.

8. The Consultant in Neurological Surgery finds himself in disagreement with the Table of Organization for U.S. General Hospitals, issued in April 1942, which does not provide for a competent, experienced neurological surgeon.

9. The Consultant in Neurological Surgery is in entire agreement as to his function as a professional advisor to the Chief Surgeon of the E.T.O. and if the theater of warfare was contained within the United States, it is reasonable to assume that he would act as liaison between the Chief Surgeon of the forces and the Surgeon General's Office. The intervening distance which exists under the present conditions, and can be rapidly bridged, should not be a deterrent to that function.

10. The Consultant in Neurological Surgery, therefore, is firmly of the opinion that to accomplish his function to the best interests of the injured soldier, the Chief Surgeon and the Army Medical Corps and because of the significance of the facts cited above, he should be given the opportunities inherent in a liaison officer, representing the Chief Surgeon in neurosurgical matters only, between this theater and the United States, particularly during the present period of comparative combat inactivity.

Recommendations:

1. The Consultant in Neurological Surgery should be given the opportunities of liaison between this theater and the United States, in matters pertaining solely to neurological surgery, to accomplish better the functions of his appointment.[2]

On 17 November 1942, four circular letters were prepared by Colonel Davis for the signature of the Chief Surgeon, ETOUSA, to be sent to the commanding officers of U.S. general and station hospitals in the United Kingdom, covering the subjects of the treatment of: (1) Craniocerebral injuries, (2) spinal cord injuries, (3) peripheral nerve injuries, and (4) ruptured intervertebral disks (herniated nucleus pulposus). On 21 November, these circulars were included in one, entitled "The Disposition and Treatment of Neurosurgical Injuries," which was included in Circular Letter No. 75, Office of the Chief Surgeon, ETOUSA, issued 4 December 1942.

On 18 November 1942, this consultant visited the 298th General Hospital, the University of Michigan Medical School unit, at Frenchay Park. Arriving in England with the 26th and 29th General Hospitals, the units affiliated with the Washington University School of Medicine, St. Louis, Mo., and the University of Minnesota Medical School, Minneapolis, respectively, the 298th General Hospital had been kept in England while the other two had been sent on to North Africa. The 298th General Hospital was sadly lacking in equipment and supplies, and much time elapsed before this hospital became effective. A quotation from the memorandum report of the visit written by the author will make evident these difficulties: "The professional staff is working hard, and because of their own efforts they will rectify many of the difficulties which now exist, but they need prompt and sympathetic understanding, and implementation of their needs, none of which are extravagant."

THE SURGEON GENERAL'S VISIT

About this time, Maj. Gen. James C. Magee, The Surgeon General of the U.S. Army, visited the European theater, and the consultants were asked by Colonel Kimbrough to prepare a list of questions which might be propounded to him. The naive assumption was expressed that they would be presented to The Surgeon General at the time of his visit and would be answered. Neither part of the assumption proved to be correct. However, the questions prepared and submitted by the Senior Consultant in Neurological Surgery show the difficulties which existed in connection with the attempt to establish a medical organization patterned on the Office of The Surgeon General but without any relation to it whatever. They were:

1. Is neurological surgery recognized by the Office of The Surgeon General as a surgical specialty in the Medical Corps?

2. If so, why has a neurological surgeon been removed from the latest published table of organization of general hospitals?

---

[2] Memorandum, Lt. Col. Loyal Davis, MC, for Chief Surgeon, European Theater of Operations, U.S. Army, 9 Nov. 1942, subject: Consultant in Neurological Surgery, ETO.

3. If it is not recognized, why should a consultant in neurological surgery be considered essential in this theater?

4. In view of the latest table of organization of general hospitals, why have neurological surgeons been assigned to general hospitals in the United States?

5. Does The Surgeon General agree that the standards of professional work in general hospitals in the United Kingdom should represent the highest type of medical and surgical care that can be given American soldiers?

6. Should not the professional care given the soldiers in general hospitals in the United Kingdom compare favorably with that of U.S. civilian practice and with neurosurgical practice in British and Canadian military hospitals of a similar type?

7. If The Surgeon General's answers to questions 5 and 6 are in the affirmative, would he agree that the supplemental list of instruments plus a portable Bovie electrical surgical apparatus, necessary to do neurological surgery properly, should be made available immediately to each of the general hospitals in the United Kingdom?

8. Is The Surgeon General aware that such a supplemental list of neurosurgical instruments plus a portable Bovie electrical surgical apparatus was inspected in Washington at the Walter Reed Hospital by Colonel Davis on or about 1 September?

9. Does The Surgeon General agree that the greatest compensation for the loss of life in any war is whatever contribution the Medical Corps can make from a humanitarian standpoint?

10. If he agrees, could not one contribution to military surgery and to the art and science of surgery in general come from the compilation of the results of neurological surgery in this war?

11. Would The Surgeon General agree that this would be a significant contribution from his office, and, also, could not the Consultant in Neurological Surgery be more effective in bringing this about if he had liaison privileges between this theater and the Zone of Interior in order to correlate, to the highest degree, neurological surgery that is being done in general hospitals in both places?

12. Would The Surgeon General agree that the Consultant in Neurological Surgery would be of more service to the effort if, in this period of inactivity in the United Kingdom while the consultant has a total of 30 patients upon which to consult, he was given this opportunity of liaison?

By 1 December 1942, the consultants were still attempting to get proper records for the general hospitals, and the senior consultant in neurological surgery was still pursuing the suction apparatus for the 30th and 298th General Hospitals. The harassed supply division was still denying an understanding of Colonel Davis' requests for "all-day suckers," even though one had been purchased and installed in the 2d General Hospital and was performing efficiently.

ATTEMPTS TO IMPROVE THE CONSULTANT GROUP

With the coming of the 3d Auxiliary Surgical Group to the European theater, the consultants were asked to evaluate and advise about the assignment of the group's personnel. The Chief Surgeon's Office had been told to expect the 2d Auxiliary Surgical Group, which was to be staged in England and reorganized, and the majority of whose members were to be reassigned to North Africa where fighting had begun. One of the consultants, Colonel Brown, volunteered to go to Glasgow to meet this contingent as a representative of the Chief Surgeon. He hurried there and waited 2 weeks to greet the commanding officer of the 2d Auxiliary Group by name, only to be told on the dock that he, the commanding officer, was Col. John F. Blatt, MC, and that the group was the 3d.

The mud around Oxford, where the group was eventually billeted, was ankle deep, and it was cold and rainy. They had no instruments and no other equipment worth discussing. Attempts were made to give them temporary assignments according to their surgical interests to relieve the frustrated sense of having been hurried from their surgical practices in many instances to meet an emergency which turned out to be a field of mud 2 miles from Oxford. There was difficulty because the Personnel Division of the Chief Surgeon's Office had no idea whatever of the character of the Military Hospital (Head Injuries), Oxford. So, without advice, two officers who had no fundamental training or interest in neurological surgery were assigned to that fine head injury hospital. This brought a protest from Brigadier Cairns and required placing the matter before General Hawley to effect a solution, which he accomplished swiftly.

On 4 December 1942, the Senior Consultant in Neurological Surgery called attention to the fact that the majority of craniocerebral injuries among U.S. soldiers in the United Kingdom were due to accidents they met with while driving jeeps at night under circumstances which were not strictly military missions. The author recommended that the activities of enlisted men in jeeps be restricted to purely military missions. This resulted in an immediate lowering of the incidence of these compound head injuries and a commendation for the consultant, apparently for the complex solution which had been suggested.

It was obvious to anyone who gave it thought that the consultants were being thwarted at every turn by some of the Chief Surgeon's staff and without General Hawley's knowledge. He had instituted dinner meetings with medical officers from other countries, principally from the Royal Army Medical Corps, and the group of consultants properly acted at his invitation as his aides to entertain his guests. This was only one of the many incidents which, at this time, led some of the Regular Army medical officers to resent the consultant group. For a time even Colonel Kimbrough, under whom the consultants served, appeared suspicious of their motives until he was assured that no one of them sought his post and that each consultant desired only to get the job done and to bring to him whatever credit was due.

This situation caused the Senior Consultant in Neurological Surgery to attempt to express a critical evaluation of the surgical consultant group in the Chief Surgeon's Office to The Surgeon General of the U.S. Army through the Chief Surgeon, ETOUSA.[3] The following three reasons were assumed to have been the basis for the creation of the consultant group: (1) The Chief Surgeon's need for a professional advisory body in order to maintain the highest type of surgical service to the U.S. soldier in the European theater, (2) the need to perfect liaison in professional service between the U.S. Army, British, and Canadian medical services, and (3) the need to establish liaison between the European theater and the surgical profession of the United States and the Office of The Surgeon General. The author reiterated the point that the majority of the consultants did not seek their appointments but were told they were chosen because of their professional attainments and standing in their particular surgical field and because of their potential ability to organize and correlate the activities of their surgical specialty in the Medical Corps. General Hawley knew none of the consultants before he arrived in his command and had no voice in his choice. The Senior Consultant in Neurological Surgery was told that he alone would be responsible directly to the Chief Surgeon for the policies governing the professional activities in neurological surgery. At the creation of the post of Chief Consultant in Surgery, it became necessary to pass recommendations through three channels before the Chief Surgeon could be reached by the consultants in the surgical specialties.

It was pointed out that the Chief Consultant in Surgery, Colonel Cutler, was speaking for and establishing policies for surgical specialties about which he had only a smattering of general knowledge. The surgical consultant group had not been included in the plans for medical care of the casualties which would result from military operations in North Africa and which at that time were a responsibility of the European theater. It appeared illogical that the majority of the surgical specialties represented by consultants were not recognized by the Office of The Surgeon General officially in the tables of organization of general hospitals.

Suggestions to improve the effectiveness of the surgical consultants group included:

1. Implement the recommendations of the surgical consultants that are designed to raise the standards of professional service in U.S. hospitals in the United Kingdom.

2. Make it possible for the surgical consultants to observe, correlate, and give advice concerning the surgical treatment being given U.S. soldiers in the North African operations.

---

[3] Letter, Lt. Col. Loyal Davis, MC, Consultant in Neurological Surgery, to The Surgeon General, U.S. Army, through the Chief Surgeon, European Theater of Operations, U.S. Army, 9 Dec. 1942, subject : Critical Evaluation of the Surgical Consultant Group.

3. Improve the operations of the several divisions in the Office of the Chief Surgeon by changing personnel if necessary.

4. Change the organizational plan of the surgical consultants group and restrict the duties and responsibilities of the chief surgical consultant to the field of surgery exclusive of the surgical specialties.

5. Remove restrictions from the surgical consultants that limit their activities to the United Kingdom.

6. Make the surgical consultants more mobile by extending to them controlled liaison privileges in their own field of surgery with the Zone of Interior, the United Kingdom, and the North African theater.

7. Extend the functions of the consultant group to the general hospitals situated in service commands in the Zone of Interior.

8. Allow surgical consultants to establish contacts between the Office of The Surgeon General and the civilian surgical profession to effect:

   a. Better understanding of the problems of the Office of The Surgeon General.

   b. Support of the policies of The Surgeon General before the medical profession and the American public.

9. Establish immediately the principle of advisory function to the Office of The Surgeon General so that in peacetime the consultants' services as civilian advisers may be utilized.

Whether these suggestions were passed on to General Hawley is open to question; but, there is some reason to think that, without fanfare, the consultants began to reach his attention directly. This consultant had written a long memorandum to the Chief Surgeon on 22 December after a thorough study of the neurosurgical aspects of injuries to tank crews. The investigation was made at Tidworth Barracks with Capt. Thomas M. Mar, MC, medical officer for the 751st Tank Battalion attached to the 29th Infantry Division (fig. 139). The memorandum concerned recommended changes in the helmet worn for head protection, certain aspects of armored tank construction to minimize the occurrence of vertebral and other injuries, the evacuation hatch, first aid equipment, armored ambulances for tank battalions, and the contents of the field chest for use by the medical officer of an armored tank battalion. Promptly, a reply came from the Chief Surgeon, signed by him and dated 26 December, stating that the report had been forwarded to the Chief Ordnance Officer and expressing his interest in the comments and recommendations made concerning the use of an armored halftrack personnel carrier as an ambulance since he had first proposed such an adaptation. A date was made to visit the battalion together on 5 January, but unfortunately the joint trip never materialized.

Had the above correspondence occurred sooner, it would undoubtedly have prevented the author from sending copies of the memorandums he had written for 3 months, arranged in chronological order and with the addressee's name removed, as separate letters, to Brig. Gen. Fred W. Rankin, Chief Consultant in Surgery to The Surgeon General; Dr. Irving S. Cutter, dean of Northwestern University Medical School, Chicago; and Dr. Howard C. Naffziger, chairman

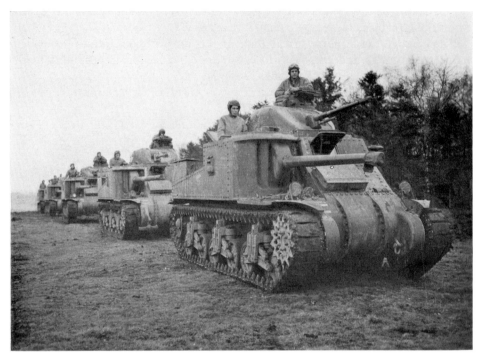

FIGURE 139.—Tanks of the 29th Infantry Division on maneuvers in southern England on
5 December 1942.

of the Department of Neurological Surgery of the University of California.
An unwise attempt to bring to the attention of men who, it was believed, might
accomplish small changes which would make an organization more effective
was stopped when censors opened the three envelopes and charged this consultant with going outside channels of military communication and violating
the rules that gave him the right to censor his own mail. The information that
he was to be court-martialed was telephoned to him by a fellow consultant on
the day before Christmas 1942 when the author was visiting the 2d Evacuation
Hospital, which had reached its destination in Huntingdon just 12 hours earlier.

The timing of events is almost always more significant than the event itself.
The author learned later that, in anticipation of the result of pressing the
charges against him, a successor had already been selected, put into uniform,
and informed of his mission. However, General Hawley was still to be reckoned with, and Colonel Davis' interview with him was calm, frank, and direct.

The method of procedure was admittedly an improper one, but this consultant pointed out the motivating reasons which could be found clearly explained in the memorandums. They concerned the care of the U.S. soldier
fundamentally and were not being made effective in any field. There was no
desire to serve elsewhere, and all difficulties could be solved by a more direct
access to the Chief Surgeon on matters that concerned the treatment of injured

men. The Chief Surgeon assured the author that there would be no court-martial of one of his men, and he was sure organizational changes could be made which would accomplish results more smoothly. The discussion made it obvious to this consultant that the Chief Surgeon, on the one hand, and his consultants, on the other, were separated by the chief surgical consultant, the chief of the Professional Services Division, and the remainder of the Chief Surgeon's staff.

This interview with General Hawley put at rest the worries over arrest, court-martial, and disgrace which had caused two sleepless nights. It also formed the basis for the beginning of a close friendship and association which exists at the present. It made possible contributions to the care of the injured soldier which will be described and which required the authority of the Chief Surgeon to effect.

YEAR'S END

By the end of December 1942, the 298th General Hospital, the University of Michigan Medical School unit, was functioning, and it was arranged to have all of the peripheral nerve injuries from the North African combat zone sent to that hospital where they could be cared for by Maj. (later Lt. Col.) Edgar A. Kahn, MC, a qualified neurological surgeon. Among the first group of patients, the majority of whom were German prisoners and injured British Army personnel, were four patients with extensive soft-tissue injuries of the upper extremity, comminuted fractures of the humerus at the junction of the lower third and upper two-thirds, and a paralysis of the radial nerve. The wounds had been packed open with petrolatum-impregnated gauze, and a plaster cast had been applied without support of the wrist. Attention was called to the desirability of better immediate care for these patients, the use of the sulfonamide drugs, and proper dressings. These recommendations were based upon the experiences observed in the Wingfield Morris Orthopaedic Emergency Hospital, which was devoted exclusively to the care of peripheral nerve injuries under the direction of Professor Seddon.

There was considerable discussion and certainly no unanimity of opinion about the method of using the sulfonamides. A large number of observations upon experimentally produced peripheral nerve injuries had been made in the surgical laboratory at Northwestern University Medical School prior to 1942 under a grant from the National Research Council. It had been shown that sulfonamides used locally in potentially infected, severely lacerated soft-tissue wounds which involved nerves did not affect the results of nerve repair. However, it was believed that administration of the drugs by mouth, raising the blood level of the sulfonamides, would be equally or more effective. At this time, however, it was a moot question, and the colored photomicrographs which recorded the results of the controlled experiments provided some basis for opposing the prohibition of the sulfonamides locally in the wounds. There were other psychological factors surrounding the use of the "wonder" drugs which affected the injured men and were not easily evaluated.

The Senior Consultant in Neurological Surgery attempted to establish the 298th General Hospital as a peripheral nerve injury center, similar to that existing at Wingfield Morris, and recommended that this be accomplished. It was possible through Mr. Seddon's cooperation to have Major Kahn assigned for temporary duty at that British hospital to assume Mr. Seddon's duties during his absence in Malta to investigate an outbreak of poliomyelitis. However, this effort to establish special facilities at the 298th General Hospital did not come about because of the rule to hold the injured in general hospitals in the United Kingdom not longer than 180 days after admission. They were then to be returned to the United States. Thus, one of the functions of a qualified neurological surgeon in the European theater, that of properly treating a peripheral nerve injury definitely, was made impossible, and peripheral nerve centers in general hospitals in the United States assumed an importance which should have been planned for in the beginning.

The qualified neurological surgeon belongs in the place where definitive treatment can be given and postoperative and rehabilitation care can be properly supervised. This plan was effectively carried out by the British with the assistance of Brigadier Hugh Cairns, the Consultant for Neurological Surgery to the DGMS (Director General of Medical Services) of the British Army. Well-trained and instructed young general surgeons can give the finest immediate treatment for neurosurgical injuries, and their activities could be supervised by a Consultant in Neurological Surgery who would also advise The Surgeon General about policies in this field of surgery in the combat zone and the Zone of Interior.

Another method of approach to the Chief Surgeon, ETOUSA, was initiated by Colonel Cutler in the form of one memorandum which would include all of the suggestions from each consultant. These "Reports of the Surgical Sub-committee" failed, in the opinion of the author, because the chief surgical consultant frequently vetoed suggestions and recommendations made by the senior consultants in their specialty.

1943: FIRST HALF

By the first part of January 1943, a new supply officer in the Chief Surgeon's Office had improved the flow of material and equipment to the hospitals, and good clinical records were made available to the hospitals in the theater. A letter, dated 13 January 1943, from this author to Colonel Kimbrough contained a report for the period 7 September 1942–15 January 1943, chronologically summarizing the author's opinions concerning the functions and utilization of the consultants. At all times, General Hawley had the greatest sympathy with and understanding of the aims, desires, and ideals of the consultant group; this he proved by word and deed on many occasions.

Head Protection for Aircrews

On 13 January 1943, this consultant wrote the first of several communications upon the subject of protection of the heads of airmen. The regular issue steel helmet worn by the U.S. soldier admittedly furnished excellent protection against craniocerebral injuries and (sometimes more important to the soldier) had many other utilitarian advantages. However, it was not designed for the use of the crews of aircraft or tanks and could not be used to advantage by them, mainly because of its size, shape, and weight. Nevertheless, the desire of a particular copilot for protection to his head from bursting 20–mm. Oerlikon shells led him to remove the liner of his helmet and pull on the outer steel shell over his regulation leather flying helmet. The effectiveness of this protection was emphasized when his pilot, wearing only a leather helmet, was struck in the head by the fragments of an Oerlikon shell which burst between them. The pilot immediately lost consciousness, developed a left hemiplegia, and a complete left homonymous hemianopsia. While the copilot's helmet was punctured in several places by the high velocity fragments, it afforded complete protection from even a scalp laceration.

It became obvious that members of an aircrew needed adequate protection from craniocerebral injuries. However, any helmet designed for their use had to meet certain specifications. First, it had to be close fitting and comfortable so that it would simulate as closely as possible an ordinary leather flying helmet and be considered a personal possession which might gather "good luck" like a favorite, battered felt hat; second, it had to allow free and unrestricted movements of the head in all directions and not interfere in any way with the field of vision; third, it had to be light in weight and afford protection from the heat and cold; and fourth, it had to afford protection, at least equal to that afforded by the regular issue steel helmet, against craniocerebral injuries produced by fragmenting Oerlikon shells, antiaircraft flak, or concussion due to direct, blunt trauma.

The percentage of wounds to the head, comparing the head's surface area to that of the body, was found to be approximately 12 percent. It was also found that the largest number of craniocerebral injuries in airmen resulted from the fragmentation of 20–mm. Oerlikon shells. Craniocerebral injuries next most common were injuries from the largest pieces of antiaircraft flak and concussion due to direct trauma, in that order. When an Oerlikon shell burst, it fragmented into thousands of pieces which varied in weight from less than 1 mg. to 20 gm. (fig. 140). However, the largest number of "effective" Oerlikon shell fragments bursting in an area 5 feet in diameter and capable of causing incapacitation to the person exposed was 260. The majority of those 260 fragments weighed between 10 and 50 mg., and their velocity varied between 400 and 600 m.p.s. (meters per second).

Many materials were subjected to accurate ballistic and other tests at the ballistics laboratory of Oxford University which was made available by Briga-

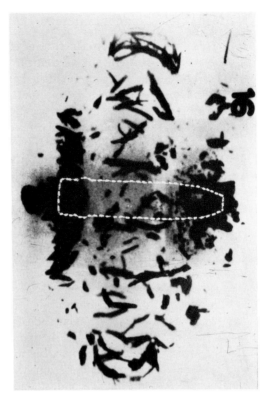

FIGURE 140.—A flash radiograph of a German
20-mm. HEI (high-explosive, incendiary) shell,
Mk. 1, showing the fragmentation pattern. The
broken line gives the reference position of the
shell before static detonation.

dier Cairns.   It was finally concluded that an acrylic resin, methyl methacrylate, properly manufactured, offered the largest number of advantages for the
purpose and most closely met the specifications laid down.   This material was
obtained, through the friendship which existed between this consultant and a
civilian in England, from a plastics firm which had begun to make artificial
dentures.   There are, of course, almost unending variations of the stages which
can be reached in the manufacture of the products of an acrylic resin.   The
properties of the final product may vary within extremely wide limits so that
one may think of it as a substitute for glass, a denture, a surgical suture, or a
puttylike material.   By modifying the amount or character of the plasticizer
added, the flexibility, resiliency, hardness, water and weather resistance, flam-
mability, and ballistic-protective properties of the material can be varied at
will between wide limits.

The material tested was 4 mm. in thickness and had a velocity resistance, in
relation to its weight per unit area, of 440 m.p.s. when tested with a 52-mg. steel

ball fired and photographed electrically. The velocity resistance per unit weight area of the same material of 8-mm. thickness, similarly tested, was 700 m.p.s. Velocity resistance per unit weight area of 1-mm. thickness manganese steel, tested under identical circumstances, varied from 500 to 600 m.p.s.

The acrylic resin studied had a tensile strength of from 9,000 to 12,000 p.s.i. (pounds per square inch); a flexural strength of from 12,000 to 14,000 p.s.i.; an impact resistance of 0.1 to 0.3 ft.-lb., and a Brinell hardness greater than gold. It had a specific gravity of 1.10, so that it almost floated on water, and it absorbed less than 0.5 percent of water by weight upon immersion for 7 days. It was resistant to the rays of the sun and would not soften until a temperature of between 190° and 240° had been reached. It was a good non-conductor of heat and cold. It smoldered if a flame was applied to it, but it would not burn with an explosion; if it flamed, the slightest movement extinguished it. When the material was hit directly, the lines of shatter were at right angles to the force and not directly forward as in steel.

The consultant was able to mold pieces of the acrylic resin over a wooden hat mold so that they would conform to the frontal, temporal, occipital, and vertex portions of the skull (fig. 141). These segments were hinged together snugly so that protection would not be lost and yet so that a certain pliability would be gained and a sense of a solid, bucketlike structure would be avoided. The helmet was then covered with the commonly used regulation leather flying helmet and lined with chamois skin or fleece. Portions of the protective material were brought down over the ears, and openings were left into which the earphones could be fitted. This afforded further protection and added the distinct advantage of the property of acrylic resin to exclude ambient noises.

Such a helmet allowed for complete movement of the head in all directions, provided complete protection over the skull, and in no way interfered with the field of vision. As one molds a derby hat which may impinge slightly upon the parietal eminences and be uncomfortable, so the individual flyer could mold this helmet by applying heat to the protective liner so that it became an integral and comfortable part of him. The pieces of molded plastic could be fitted into pockets of the leather helmet and be removed when it was not being worn in combat. The completed helmet, made of 4-mm. methyl methacrylate covered and lined, weighed 18 ounces, and, if material 8 mm. thick was used, affording more protection per unit weight area, the total weight was 27 ounces. The steel body of the regulation helmet weighed 35.84 ounces.

It was also suggested that similar plastic panels could be inserted into the regular-issue flying suit for protection against chest, abdominal, and extremity injuries.

Several flights were made in a B–17 bomber on practice missions with Maj. Daniel Wheeler, AC, and his crew, during which the model protective helmet was adjusted and revised until it suited the entire crew.

At this time, Brig. Gen. (later Maj. Gen.) Malcolm C. Grow, Surgeon, Eighth Air Force, had engaged the services of an armorer in England to devise

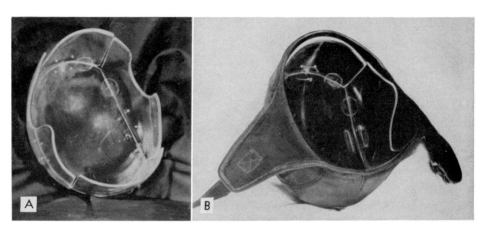

FIGURE 141.—A protective helmet for flyers. A. A fabricated and segmented acrylic resin protective liner. B. A protective liner within an ordinary leather flying helmet.

a metal protective suit of armor for airmen. Ignoring the ballistics test, he rejected the use of plastic material on the ground that he had shattered a piece of the plastic material with his own .45-caliber pistol. The obvious answer was, of course, that if one got close enough to a heavily armored battleship with a large enough shell, the battleship could be sunk. Under actual flying combat conditions, however, it was evident that the acrylic resin would afford real protection.

The difficulty with the metal armor was its weight and awkwardness, against which all of the bomber crews reacted unanimously. It was their consensus that General Grow should put it on himself, fly with them, and be asked to bail out over the North Sea, an action which they were allowed 10 seconds to perform successfully. Moreover, the pilot, the last to leave the plane, was required to leave through a small window at his side through which he had to propel himself from a sitting position.

Actually, the Senior Consultant in Neurological Surgery could progress no further in spite of the support and enthusiasm of his Chief Surgeon. It was not until late in 1943 that the Quartermaster General's Office in Washington accepted all of the work performed and the suggestions made. Col. (later Brig. Gen.) Georges F. Doriot and his colleagues were working on a material named Doron, similar in many respects to the material tested. Later, in the surgical laboratory at Northwestern University, the author assisted General Doriot in making studies of tissue reaction to the implantation of Doron in subcutaneous tissue, muscle, and brain.

High-Altitude Frostbite

During the period when work was being done on the flyer's helmet, the Senior Consultant in Neurological Surgery had his attention called to the problem of the results of cold injuries, in a lecture given by Maj. C. C. Ungley, RAMC, at the British Post-Graduate Medical School.

In a memorandum dated 13 January 1943, the subject matter of this lecture on immersion foot was summarized and the symptoms of the prehyperemic, hyperemic, and posthyperemic stages were described in detail. However, the most important portion of the memorandum called attention to the advantage of sending these patients to one general hospital where they could be studied as a group and stated that severe injuries from cold would produce similar symptoms. In other words, immersion foot was only one type of cold injury, and the cold injury received on the ground or in the air would differ only as to the time and temperature of the exposure.

It was not long after that the first airman was seen at the 2d General Hospital with tremendous bullae upon the dorsum of his hands. It was believed at first that these were burns, since his aircraft had crashed on landing and burned. Careful questioning elicited the fact that he had been at a waist gun position in a B–17 bomber, which at that time was an open window (fig. 142). He had worn his electrically heated flying suit at the time but had taken off his gloves to urinate. The parts of the suits, it was found, were wired in series, and thus the entire suit was turned off completely if one portion was disconnected. The aircraft had been at an altitude of considerably over 20,000 feet, and the temperature, $-30°$. Instances of cold injuries to the hands, occasionally to the feet, in isolated instances to the buttocks, and only once to the cheeks and ears, multiplied rapidly through April and May and early in June of 1943. Exposure to low temperatures and airblasts at high altitudes with failures of oxygen supply and, most important of all, failure of, or lack of, electrically heated clothing were the important etiological factors.

Colored photographs were made of the striking lesions, which were resulting in the complete disability of the airmen, and studies were begun to devise the proper treatment and to prevent these injuries. This consultant was ordered by General Hawley to present his data upon 25 patients to General Grow, the surgeon of the Eighth Air Force. An appointment was made, and the author was allowed to stand for 15 minutes while General Grow carried on a discussion with Lt. Col. (later Col.) Herbert B. Wright, MC, of his office about his own experiences with frostbite when he was in Russia following World War I. General Grow did not, at this time, take the problem seriously. He was inclined to believe that cold injury in airmen was the result of carelessness.

The author placed on General Grow's desk copies of the patients' own stories and color photographs of their lesions, which included complete casts of the skin of the fingers which had been shed, dry gangrene amputation stumps, and bullae of all degrees of severity.[4] Colonel Davis stated that he had been instructed by General Hawley to deliver this material and turned to leave. When he reached the door, he was called back, asked to take off his

---

[4] For examples of these photographs and for additional discussion of high-altitude frostbite, see Medical Department, United States Army. Cold Injury, Group Type. Washington: U.S. Government Printing Office, 1958.

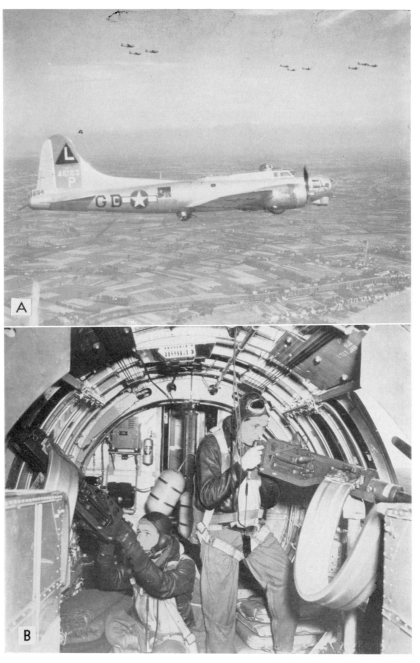

FIGURE 142.—The waist gun position in the B–17 bomber. A. A B–17 on a tactical mission over The Netherlands, showing the open waist gun position with protruding muzzle of a flexible machinegun, September 1944. B. Waist gunners of the Invader II model of the B–17 bomber, March 1943.

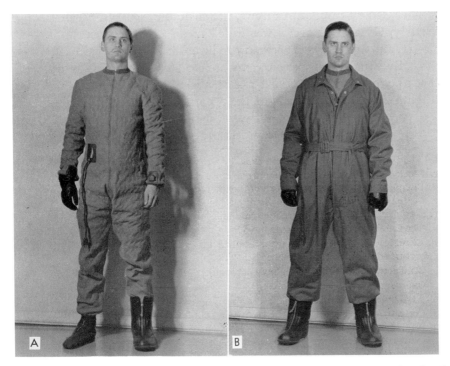

FIGURE 143.—Flyers' clothing. A. An electrically heated suit. Note the sockets for plugging in gloves. B. Flying clothing worn over an electrically heated suit.

overcoat and sit down. A lengthy discussion followed with an antagonistic attitude prevailing on the part of General Grow. He doubted that the electrically heated clothing was wired in series, and Col. Harry G. Armstrong, MC, director of the Eighth Air Force Central Medical Establishment, was called into the discussion. Colonel Armstrong said quite frankly that he had no idea how they were wired (fig. 143).

Following this experience, permission was granted by General Hawley to designate the 2d General Hospital as the center to receive patients with cold injuries and to establish a laboratory and special wards for their study. By 9 May 1943, capillary microscopic studies were under way, and mildly injured patients who had recovered without loss of digits were being studied at fixed low temperatures to see if they could be returned to flying duty with safety.

Requests were initiated for investigators to go to operational Eighth Air Force fields to make capillary microscopic studies upon airmen immediately upon landing. Many methods were investigated in an effort to prevent the injuries, and it was recommended that the clothing be wired differently and that the open waist gun positions be protected. All requests to visit airfields were denied by the Eighth Air Force, and finally, these patients became so numerous as the activities of the Eighth Air Force increased during May and June 1943 that the Chief Surgeon discussed the situation directly with Lt.

Gen. (later Gen.) Frank M. Andrews, Commanding General, ETOUSA. Unfortunately, General Andrews was killed in an airplane accident in Iceland soon after, and again it was necessary to brief his successor, Lt. Gen. Jacob L. Devers. Eventually, permission was obtained, and observations were made over a 2-week period by Major Scarff and this consultant at a bomber station of the Eighth Air Force. A part of the report on these observations follows: [5]

*   *   *   *   *   *   *

2. The observations and studies have included:

a. Skin temperature readings.

b. Microscopic capillary observations.

c. Black and white and colored photographs.

d. Complete physical examinations of the affected parts.

e. Personal observations of the Senior Consultant in Neurological Surgery upon the effects of cold at 13,000 feet on a practice raid mission.

3. The following types of patients have been studied:

a. Chronic cases (2) previously treated in the acute stages at U.S. General Hospital #2 and returned to duty at this Bomber Station.

b. Mild acute cases (12) which have not required hospitalization.

c. One severe acute case involving both hands removed to Evacuation Hospital #2 complicated by a severe intra-abdominal injury.

4. Certain facts should be noted from the result of these studies to date:

a. Mild acute cases continue to occur in spite of the rise in ground temperature because, at this altitude of the operational missions, the temperature has ranged at —30 degrees C.

b. The mild acute cases warm up rather promptly at room or free air temperatures without serious damage to the digits; but, the symptoms of tingling, stiffness and numbness continue for two or three days and require that the patients be grounded temporarily.

c. There is no demonstrable microscopic damage to, or change in, the capillaries in these mild acute cases.

d. Microscopic capillary studies of the severely frozen digits in the one patient show a complete obliteration of the capillaries and extravasation of blood into the subcutaneous tissue within three hours of the trauma.

e. Capillary loops disappear with severe cold damage to the skin and in chronic cases, three months after injury, have not regenerated.

f. Defective clothing equipment and other technical defects pointed out in the first memorandum on this subject continue to play an important role in etiology.

g. The new type of "demand" oxygen mask provided is a distinct improvement and answers the suggestions raised in the first memorandum written which would prevent the injurious effect of anoxia common to all the cases observed early in the study.

h. Progress is being made to the end that an accurate, scientific method of treatment can be outlined but this cannot be done at this time.

Cases continued to occur, and, during the 2-week period at the bomber station where observations were made, 30 patients had cold injuries requiring hospitalization for varying periods of time. One medical officer at a bomber station denied that any of his personnel had received such injuries, until their names, ranks, and serial numbers were supplied to him during the discussion.

---

[5] Letter, Lt. Col. Loyal Davis, MC, Senior Consultant in Neurological Surgery, to Brig. Gen. Paul R. Hawley, Chief Surgeon, European Theater of Operations, U.S. Army, 14 June 1943, subject: Cold Damage to Extremities.

Proposal for Acrylic Helmet

In the meantime, a detailed report upon the number of craniocerebral injuries that had occurred in the European theater from 1 September to 1 May 1943 was reviewed for the Chief Surgeon. The number of patients returned to duty, the number returned to the Zone of Interior, and the average number of days in hospital were furnished to him. On 26 May 1943, another proposal of a helmet for the protection of aircraft and tank personnel was sent to the Chief Surgeon by the author, listing the following 16 advantages of the helmet.

*   *   *   *   *   *   *

3. The proposed helmet consists of segments of an acrylic resin product moulded to fit the head snugly, covered by soft leather and lined with chamois skin.

The advantages of this helmet are:

(1) Compared with manganese steel per unit weight, acrylic resin affords one third more protection against the penetration of metal fragments.

(2) Acrylic resin of 8 mm. thickness has a velocity resistance to a 52 mgm. steel ball of between 700 and 800 meters per second (2,100 to 2,400 ft./sec.).

(3) The model helmet made of 4 mm. thick acrylic resin weighs 18 ounces and has a velocity resistance to a 52 mgm. steel ball of 500 meters per second. If 8 mm. thick material is used, the weight of the helmet would be 27 ounces.

(4) Acrylic resin is one of the best non-conductors of heat and cold known to science.

(5) Acrylic resin can be moulded by heating so that this helmet will fit comfortably and becomes an integral part of the soldier's head.

(6) The proposed helmet allows unrestricted movements of the head in every direction and does not obstruct the field of vision of the wearer.

(7) Acrylic resin has a tensile strength of from 9,000 to 12,000 lbs. per square inch; a flexual strength of 12,000 to 14,000 lbs. per square inch; an impact resistance of 0.1 to 0.3 ft. lbs., and a Brinell hardness greater than gold (500 kilograms on a 10 mm. gold ball, 17–20).

(8) Acrylic resin has a specific gravity of 1.10, so that it almost floats on water. It will absorb less than 0.5% of water by weight upon immersion for 7 days. It is resistant to the rays of the sun and will not soften until a temperature of between 190 and 240 degrees F has been reached.

(9) If driven into or buried in the brain or soft tissues, acrylic resin is absolutely inert and there is no tissue reaction.

(10) The lines of shatter of acrylic resin are at right angles to the force, and not directly forward, as in steel.

(11) Acrylic resin smoulders if a flame is applied but will not burn with an explosion, and if it flames the slightest movement extinguishes it.

(12) Shatter proof goggles can be made from the same material which can be so attached to the helmet that the present use of elastic bands to support goggles can be eliminated.

(13) Pieces of spring steel can be set into the acrylic resin which will catch the elastic bands of the oxygen mask and will obviate the necessity for an airman to take off electrically heated gloves to fasten the small clips now used to keep the elastic bands secure.

(14) This helmet can be worn constantly by tankmen and need not be removed when the head is thrust through the tank turret, or when using a periscopic sight, as is true with the helmet for tankmen now in use.

(15) Acrylic resin can be used in making a solid complete helmet similar to the present steel helmet, if desired. It would afford one-third more protection for the same unit weight against penetration and would not dent or cave in from rough usage. It could have an inner lining made of softer acrylic resin which can be moulded to the head by the soldier him-

self. The inner softer acrylic resin will fuse inseparably with the harder material. The proposed helmet would afford greater protection against penetration and impact resistance than the present steel helmet even if it was desired to have it weigh less.

(16) This material can be manufactured cheaply, easily and quickly into helmets, and the use of high priority steel is eliminated. The number of manufacturers now necessary for the production of steel helmets can be reduced.

Immediately, General Hawley indicated that upon return from a surgical mission to the U.S.S.R., Colonel Davis would be sent to the Zone of Interior to present the proposed helmet and its advantages to The Surgeon General.

Professional Activities in June 1943

On 14 June 1943, a request was made for additional suction units for the 2d Evacuation Hospital to which injured airmen were being taken. A portable unit had become a part of the table of equipment of evacuation and general hospitals, but one was insufficient. On the same date, further data were submitted concerning patients with cold damage to the extremities. On 21 June 1943, information obtained in experiments in the surgical laboratory of Northwestern University Medical School about the local use of the sulfonamides in experimental gunshot injuries in animals was presented to the Chief Surgeon in a memorandum. Even at this date, it had not been completely established that the systematic administration of the sulfonamides would offer the patient sufficient protection from infection.

Policies for the surgical treatment of herniated nucleus pulposus were established in a directive that required examination and consultation upon these patients by the Senior Consultant in Neurological Surgery, the performance of a myelogram, and performance of the operation by a qualified neurological surgeon in a general hospital. Pantopaque had just been prepared and was sent to the theater for use before it had become available on the open market.

SURGICAL MISSION TO THE U.S.S.R.

In the latter part of April 1943, General Hawley asked the author if he would be interested in a trip to the U.S.S.R. Nothing further was added after an affirmative answer, and it was assumed that a well-laid plan undoubtedly had gone astray. However, on 6 May 1943, the Public Relations Division of G-2 (Intelligence), Headquarters, SOS, ETOUSA, requested of the author that an interview on a proposed trip to the U.S.S.R. be granted to Mr. Frederic Kuh, the London correspondent of the Chicago Daily Sun. After verifying the fact that all the proper channels had been cleared and permission had been granted, Mr. Kuh experienced a great disappointment. He was in complete possession of all the facts regarding a surgical mission to the U.S.S.R., upon which Col. Elliott Cutler was also to be included with four British surgeons, at least one of whom belonged to the RAMC. Mr. Kuh must have thought the interviewee was an excellent security risk; the fact was that this consultant was ignorant of all the information which Mr. Kuh gave him. He went on to say that this was the first mission of its kind ever to go to the Soviet Union, that Sir Archibald Clarke-Kerr (later Lord Inverchapel), British Ambassador to Russia, had arranged for it, and that the Soviet officials had insisted upon professors of surgery. This explained why Colonel Cutler and the author were invited to go because they were the only two professors of surgery in the U.S. Army Medical Corps then in the European theater. Thus, this consultant first learned that Mr. Reginald Watson-Jones (later knighted), Mr. Ernest Rock Carling, Surgeon Rear Admiral Gordon Gordon-Taylor, and Maj. Gen. D. C. Monro would be on the surgical mission representing the British. Following this, there began a series of episodes confusing to the Chief Surgeon no doubt, as well as to his neurosurgical consultant. It was the latter's first personal experience in a joint effort between one of the armed services and the State Department.

About the middle of May, the members of the mission had luncheon with Prof. Semon Sarkisov,[6] recently arrived from the U.S.S.R., and Sir Henry Dale, representing the Medical Research Council of Great Britain. On the same afternoon, the mission had tea with Ambassador Ivan M. Maisky at the Soviet Embassy. Before going to tea, Colonel Cutler and this consultant had a 10-minute chat with John G. Winant, the U.S. Ambassador to the Court of St. James's, who told them that Wilder G. Penfield would represent Canada on the mission. Ambassador Winant indicated at that time that the mission would leave London on 12 June.

Later, Ambassador Winant requested the author to call upon him at the Embassy. General Hawley was informed of the request and acquiesced. Ambassador Winant asked this consultant to represent the National Research Council while on the mission to the U.S.S.R. He also insisted that the author travel as a civilian throughout the trip, and not as one of the representatives of the U.S. Army Medical Corps. The reasons for making this unusual request were not explained by the Ambassador. After consulting General Hawley, this consultant decided to retain those advantages which could be obtained by being in uniform if by slight chance the aircraft was forced down over enemy territory.

Finally, the two members of the surgical mission to the U.S.S.R. from the United States were given informal instruction by Ambassador Winant, General Lee, and General Hawley, and travel orders were issued.

On 28 June 1943 the members of the mission were loaded into a bus at the Swindon railroad station and driven about the countryside until it became dark. They were given dinner at Marlborough and taken to the airfield which was recognized as the one at Lyneham. The four-engine British aircraft carried the members of the mission and two Soviet nationals, who remained grim and uncommunicative throughout the entire trip. The mission members were informed that these two men were diplomatic-pouch couriers, but also members of the NKVD, the Soviet secret police. The takeoff was at midnight, and,

---

[6] The variation in the spelling of the names of Russian individuals in this volume is due to the fact that there are two systems of transliteration in use.

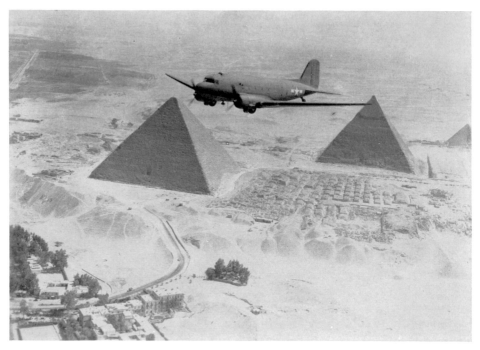

FIGURE 144.—Mena House Hotel at Al Jizah, Egypt, at the foot of the Pyramids.

flying well out beyond the Bay of Biscay (where a plane carrying Leslie Howard, the famous British actor, had been shot down by the Germans 2 weeks before), the mission landed at Gibraltar at 0830 hours the following morning, 29 June. After breakfast, the military hospital, a 200-bed unit built in a tunnel which had been drilled out of the rock, was visited. This hospital served also as a bomb shelter if the "Rock" was bombed.

The mission was off again at noon and flew over the U.S. 12th General Hospital at Oran, Algeria, and on to Castel Benito, the airport at Tripoli, Libya. From the altitude of 8,000 feet, the country appeared a solid brown color with only occasional green spots to break the monotony. The flight followed the route of the advance of the British Eighth Army, and damaged, abandoned material was visible along the road. The British 48th General Hospital was visited in Tripoli, and it proved to be one which they had taken over from the Italians. After tea in a setting of desert sand, flies, bougainvillaea, and heat at an RAF (Royal Air Force) staging area, the flight was continued at midnight to arrive at Cairo at 0830 hours on the morning of 30 June.

Barefooted Egyptians, with long wrappers and fezzes on their heads, were working on the airfield and the roads. Arrangements had been made for the mission to stay at Mena House, a clean, cool, well-staffed hotel on the outskirts of Cairo and at the foot of the Pyramids (Al Jizah) (fig. 144). The military members of the mission (Gordon-Taylor, Monro, Cutler, and Davis) went to

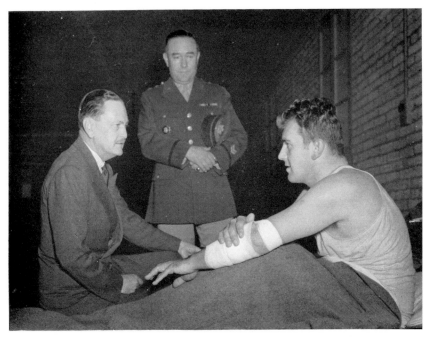

FIGURE 145.—Hon. Alexander C. Kirk, U.S. Minister to Egypt, on the occasion of a visit to the 38th General Hospital, Heliopolis, Egypt, with Maj. Gen. Russell L. Maxwell, Commanding General, Services of Supply, U.S. Army Forces in the Middle East.

the British Embassy to register their presence. The various headquarters were grouped around the Embassy buildings that had been requisitioned, and the entire area in the center of Cairo was fenced off with barbed wire.

A similar visit to Mr. Alexander C. Kirk, U.S. Minister to Egypt, disclosed a tall, impressive, well-dressed man who complained discouragingly and with a real nostalgia that diplomacy had died in 1918 and that he would be glad when it was all over so he could go back home, sit down, and not be bothered (fig. 145). A representative of the British Medical Research Council gave a luncheon, at which there were several representatives of the medical profession of Egypt, in the famous and exclusive Mohammed Ali Club. Cold meats, watermelon, strawberries and cream, and an American beer constituted the luncheon in a private dining room adjacent to a large, ornate gambling room.

Two British hospitals were visited; the one in a newly constructed modern hospital which the Egyptians had to close because they could not make it support itself and the other in the building of a former beautiful hotel. The U.S. 38th General Hospital, staffed principally by the faculty of Jefferson Medical College of Philadelphia, was located at Heliopolis, but a visit there had to be postponed until the return trip.

On the morning of 1 July, after considerable delay while the plane's fuel and cargo were being redistributed at the insistence of the RAF pilot

on a desert airfield which became hotter and hotter, the leg of the trip from
Cairo to Teheran, Iran, began. Without oxygen and at 13,000 feet, one of the
mission became cyanotic, another had periods of apnea, and a third developed
scintillating scotoma, could not remember names, and had a homonymous
hemianopsia. All of these symptoms disappeared, and the mission presented
a unified front upon landing at Teheran late in the afternoon. A representative of the British Embassy met the mission but had been notified of the arrival
only 2 hours previously by the Soviet Embassy. There were no U.S.
representatives.

It was hot and dusty on the airfield, which was surrounded by high mountains with snow on their peaks. There were many American soldiers to be
seen, and a station hospital was under construction. Water was running in a
small gutter along the side of the street, and people were washing their bodies
and clothes in it, watering horses in it, sweeping street cleanings into it, and
putting it into pails which they were carrying away. The Palace Hotel provided two iron beds, a wooden washstand with a flowered china bowl, and one
water faucet. The guests sprinkled insect powder on the mattress and pillow
in liberal quantities.

A visit was paid by the Americans to Maj. Gen. Donald H. Connolly,
Commanding General, Persian Gulf Command, an engineer who was accomplishing the project of supplying the Soviet Union through the Persian Gulf
and Basra, Iraq (fig. 146). General Connolly inquired about the purpose
of the visit to the Soviet Union, since he knew nothing of the mission. When
the purpose was explained, he expressed his doubts of the mission's learning
any more than what the Soviet hosts would specifically designate. From this
conversation, the author received the distinct impression that it would have
been more advantageous for the U.S. representatives to make this trip alone
because of the Soviet distrust of the postwar intentions of the British.

Sandfly fever, characterized by a high fever for 2 or 3 days and no fatalities, was a common disease amongst the natives. A form of malaria was
described as occurring in places where the *Anopheles* mosquito could not be
found. Typhus had been prevalent during the previous winter, and typhoid
fever had caused an unheard of number of deaths in the spring and summer
months. Trachoma was abundant, as was syphilis.

The following morning there was another delay on the hot, dusty Teheran
airfield while petrol was removed from the tanks so that the Liberator would
be able to gain altitude quickly enough to clear the mountains surrounding
the field. After a bumpy, rough trip, the mission landed in Moscow late
on the afternoon of 2 July at a field about 30 miles from the city. They
were met by Vice Commissar Vasillii Vassilievich Pairin, Vice-Commissariat
of Public Health, and Leonid Aleksandrovich Koreisha, Secretary of the Medical Scientific Council, and a woman interpreter. Two U.S. Army Air Forces
officers, who, Colonel Cutler believed, would be their aides while the two
colonels were in the U.S.S.R., accompanied them to a cottage in a woods adjacent to the airfield where they were served tea, bread and butter, sausages,

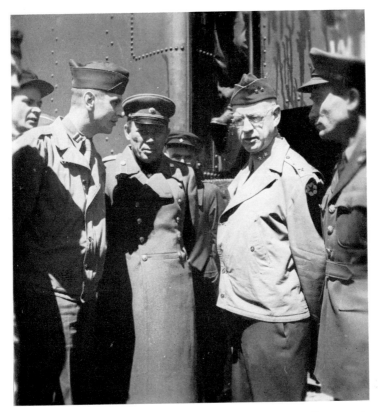

FIGURE 146.—Maj. Gen. Donald H. Connolly and Soviet officers meeting, at the Soviet acceptance point, the first all-American supply train from the Persian Gulf, in March 1943.

white caviar, and strawberries. On the trip to the National Hotel where the mission was to be quartered, it was learned that the Army Air Forces officers were in Moscow with Capt. "Eddie" Rickenbacker on a mission which he was attempting to carry out for Secretary of War Stimson (fig. 147). Captain Rickenbacker's mission concerned the complaints which the Soviet Union was making about the Airacobra (P–39) planes that the United States was furnishing them on lend-lease agreement. The complaint was to the effect that they would not stand up in combat. It developed later that the Soviet military had no concept of ground crews to service the aircraft and keep the intricate mechanisms in good working order. It was their idea to fly them, discard them if they broke down, and ask for new ones. The complaint was that the planes did not stand this type of treatment long enough, and they were put to considerable trouble in asking for replacements.

After an assignment of rooms, the mission members found they had a large common sitting room which had a ceiling-to-floor mirror on one wall. The mirror was decorated with gold-painted birds and angels concealing a

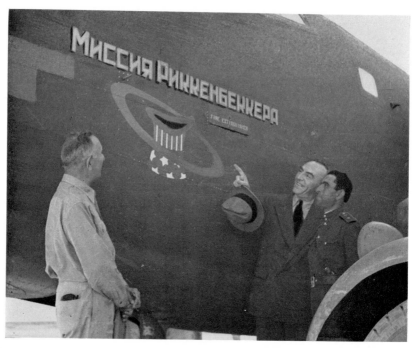

FIGURE 147.—Capt. "Eddie" Rickenbacker, in Teheran, Iran, in July 1943, proudly pointing to the inscription, "Mission Rickenbacker," painted on his Liberator bomber by Soviet pilots in Moscow. Maj. Jacob Popov, U.S.S.R. air officer, is on the right.

microphone. To the credit of the members of the mission, there was no one who lowered his voice or changed the frank expression of his opinions at any time. On one occasion when Prof. Serge Yudin visited the members furtively at midnight, he kept up a constant tapping of the table with his pencil during the 2-hour visit to interfere with a clear pickup of his voice.

After a cold-water bath (and this did not vary at any time during the mission's stay), they had a breakfast of tea, cherry jam, cheese, caviar, and bread. Neither did this menu vary, except as they could vary it with instant coffee and hot water heated over a Sterno can which they had brought along. The business office of the U.S. Embassy was only a door or two from the National Hotel, and both faced Red Square, across which they could see the Kremlin and the new, gaudy, heavily built, yellow-stone Moskva Hotel. The entire mission called upon Adm. William H. Standley, U.S. Ambassador to the U.S.S.R., who was charming and interested in learning each man's name and his particular field of surgery. Leaving the British for a moment, they called upon Brig. Gen. Philip R. Faymonville who had been in the U.S.S.R., on four tours of duty, for 10 years. General Faymonville was the Lend-Lease Administrator and, in a frank talk with them, made his position perfectly clear. He was under direct instructions and orders from President Roosevelt, delivered by Mr. Harry Hopkins, to supply everything possible to the U.S.S.R., regardless and without thought of getting something in return. He stated that other branches of the U.S. Government wished to barter with the Soviet Union, using lend-lease material as leverage, on the grounds of protecting the United States. It became obvious quickly that the military attaché and embassy officials were in direct conflict with General Faymonville and believed him personally responsible for a situation which was intolerable to them in dealing with the Soviet nationals, without accepting the fact that General Faymonville was carrying out specific orders from the President, and failing to consider that his own personal views might be entirely different. General Faymonville's knowledge of the Russian language, his long residence in the U.S.S.R., and his familiarity with the Soviets' music and customs made them friendly to him, and this was obvious at the social gatherings which were given for the mission and at which he was present. However, this made him all the more suspect by his colleagues of favoritism when the war had finished and when the relationship between the United States and its former ally was changed.

British Ambassador Clarke-Kerr met the mission formally and indicated that it had been made possible by his friendship with Serge Yudin who had suggested such a visit by U.S. and British surgeons. This version of the origin of the mission was at variance with the one which emanated from the U.S. Embassy in London—that it had been arranged by the U.S. Ambassador to Great Britain as the result of discussions between members of the National Research Council and the Medical Research Council of Great Britain. The truth probably is that all had a hand in the project and that priority of ideas would be difficult to establish. Each member of the mission received 1,000 rubles from the British Embassy, but they could use them only for gratuities to hotel employees, since there were no shops or stores where one could purchase any kind of article without a ration card.

In the afternoon of 3 July, Monro, Cutler, Watson-Jones, Penfield, and the author, with Brimelow, who was attached to them from the British Embassy, visited VOKS—the Soviet society to promote cultural relations with foreign countries. Large posters of Churchill, Stalin, and Roosevelt hung side by side in the large museumlike room of the building to which they were taken by Pairin and Koreisha. Oil paintings of Soviet soldiers in various units, cartoons, and large photographs of Charlie Chaplin and Paul Robeson completed the display. On the return to the hotel, a stop was made at a park where there were pictures of the party leaders lining the walk, a Ferris wheel and various airplane rides for the children, an area for dancing to the music coming from the loudspeakers distributed through the park, and a children's library. The orthopedist in the group remarked that it was much like saying: "Come into the park and we'll give you culture, damn you."

At dinner, the mission members discussed when and how they would get their visit underway, and Admiral Standley's admonition to be patient was agreed upon to be the line to follow. After dinner, they walked around Red Square, Lenin's tomb, the Kremlin, and the Church of St. Basil, a Byzantine structure, highly colored and resembling a gingerbread cake. This was their first unaccompanied trip of any distance on the streets, and they noted that guards, walking along the top of the walls of the Kremlin, were either curious about them or were very alert to their duties. There were no taxicabs, and only the Intourist organization could supply transportation.

There were several discussions about drawing up their own agenda for procedure and discussions with the People's Commissariat for Health. The mission wished to see surgery of the war wounded in the forward areas and at the bases and to see and discuss the Soviet research projects and ways of exchanging information. These were pleasant periods of conversation with each other but were like shadowboxing in a gymnasium.

During this interval while the mission waited for the date of a meeting with Soviet authorities, a memorandum was written to be left with the People's Commissar for Public Health, which would explain the desires of the mission (pp. 97–99).

So, July 4 was spent in viewing a large collection of captured German war material—guns, planes, trucks, and medical supplies—gathered together on the bank of the Moscow River and looking much like a World's Fair. Groups of soldiers were taken through and given lectures on the material displayed. Large crowds of civilians were at the exhibition, and clothes and uniforms of the visitors from the Western World were the center of close, unabashed, personal inspection. The afternoon was spent at Spasso House, the official home of Ambassador Standley, which had been occupied also by his predecessors, U.S. Ambassadors Bullitt, Davies, and Steinhardt. Capt. "Eddie" Rickenbacker was present and brought up the question of the damage airmen were receiving from high-altitude frostbite, interesting the Ambassador in the discussion.

The evening was spent watching the ballet "The Swan Lake" with Dudinskya, the première danseuse. The audience that evening consisted of workers from factories who had purchased tickets from allotments given to their factory. When the mission members went into the lobby between acts and returned, they had difficulty in regaining their seats from individuals who had moved into them from less desirable ones.

Eventually, at 1500 hours on 5 July, the mission was received in the office of the People's Commissar for Public Health, Georgii Andreevich Miterev. There were seven mission members and seven Russians; there were three of the mission in uniform and three of them in mufti. The Soviet military included Lt. Gen. Efim Ivanovich Smirnov of the Soviet Army Medical Service, who was 38 years of age and corresponded to The Surgeon General, and Nicolai Nilovich Burdenko, the chief surgical consultant to the Soviet Army, not a regular medical officer and with the added great distinction of being a member of the Academy of Sciences. The meeting got underway with a formal speech by the Commissar, who described the existing organization for the treatment of battle casualties and provided a typewritten program of activities for the week. The care of the injured and sick in the army was directed from two departments, the People's Commissariat for Defense and the People's Commissariat for Public Health. General Smirnov's medical organization was responsible for the care of the soldier in combat units, in army hospitals, and through all evacuation steps to the base area. The care of the wounded soldier in the base area, as well as the care of all civilians, was the responsibility of the People's Commissariat for Public Health. It was stated that the methods of treatment were identical in both organizations in order to insure continuity in the patient's care when he was transferred from the combat zone to the rear. The line of demarcation between these two areas was never unchangeably fixed. When a patient received a certificate of fitness from the civilian doctors, he was transferred back to the military authorities for reassignment. Patients requiring long convalescent care remained under the jurisdiction of the civilian authorities in hospitals which were required to devote their chief attention to the treatment of the war wounded. The People's Commissar for Public Health stated that 70 percent of all wounded were returned to the combat zone for duty, and he was obviously proud of the small incidence of tetanus and gas gangrene.

A detailed description was given of the organization for care of the wounded on the field at battalion, regiment, and division aid stations and in the sorting-evacuation hospitals, placed 30 to 50 km. from the front, and from 1,000 to 4,000 beds in size. An explanation was provided of the methods of evacuation by train, automobile, and plane. The percentage distribution of beds was described, and it was emphasized strongly that 0.2 percent were devoted to neuropsychiatry at the front and 0.1 percent, at the base area.

On 6 July, the members of the mission began their tour of the facilities which the Soviet hosts wished them to see, and nothing beyond that was possible. The Botkin Hospital, the Sklifossowsky Institute headed by Serge Yudin, the Central Institute for Traumatology and Orthopedy, the Institute of Neurological Surgery (Burdenko's Hospital), a clearing hospital of the People's Commissariat for Public Health, two frontline hospitals near Vyazma, a hospital for the "lightly wounded," the first Medical Institute, the Pirogoff Clinic, the Balneological Institute, the Central Institute for Blood Transfusion, the Central Institute for Medical Research, and a final meeting with the People's Commissar for Public Health fulfilled the agenda provided by the hosts. At no time was any member of the surgical mission asked to present his opinions about any surgical or research problem or to relate experiences of the British or U.S. Army Medical Corps in treating the wounded.

In summary, the principles of Soviet surgical practice in the care of the war wounded, as shown and explained to the mission, were: [7]

Wounds were debrided as far forward as possible, usually in the sorting-evacuation hospitals, although also in base hospitals. Excision, even in com-

---

[7] See also appendix A, p. 953.

pound fractures, was carried out as late as 10 or 15 days after wounding, and the sulfonamides and immobilization were relied upon to prevent generalized sepsis.

Large soft-tissue injuries, as well as fractures, were immobilized by wooden splints of the Thomas type for evacuation to the place of first definitive surgical treatment, after which plaster of paris was applied. This was put directly over the wound, "skin tight" without padding.

Active immunization was obtained with tetanus toxoid. The booster dose was given at the regimental aid station.

A potent antiserum was used in all serious wounds against the development of gas gangrene. It was usually given intravenously. Several surgeons admitted privately that the antiserum was not effective.

Sulfanilamide was used in both forward and base hospitals locally in the wounds, by mouth, and intravenously. A small supply of sulfapyridine was in existence at that time. A special form of sulfanilamide in which the drug was broken down into small particles by subjecting it to ultrasonic waves was used as a cream and applied to gauze dressings. The latter product was in an experimental stage, it was said, and was not in mass production.

Secondary suture of wounds was practiced whenever possible, even more than 7 to 12 days after injury.

Inhalant anesthetics were commonly used, especially ether. Spinal anesthesia was used only in base hospitals, but no nitrous-oxide or oxygen machines were seen.

Sucking chest wounds were closed in forward areas; empyema was treated by drainage for 3 weeks, following which two or three rib fragments were removed and the wound was packed. Only large foreign bodies were removed from the chest cavity.

Tannic acid and silver nitrate were used in the treatment of burns, but the Soviets preferred an open method in which a powder containing an analgesic agent and an antiseptic was dusted on the burned area.

The best impressions of the Soviet methods of treatment were obtained in their treatment of fractures. From the time of Pirogoff, in the Crimean War, they had become masters in the use of plaster of paris. They had a line of continuity in the treatment between surgeons at the front and in base hospitals which represented the same institution and methods. Yudin at the Sklifossowsky Institute had cared for over 2,000 fractures during the war with Finland. They preferred to splint the limb in the field with wooden, wire, or Thomas' splints at the place of the first definitive treatment. The wound was widely excised and sulfanilamide was placed in it. Often the wound was sutured open by uniting the skin edges to the deep fascia. "Skin tight" plaster was then applied directly to the wound and skin. Casts were not split and they never used windows.

An interesting sidelight resulted from the discussion which developed between Dr. Serge Yudin, who was not a member of the Communist Party, and the mission, particularly Mr. Watson-Jones, about the results of their methods of treating fractures.   It was a give-and-take friendly exchange of opinions until Watson-Jones indicated that it was difficult to believe the successes claimed.   Yudin, whereupon, inquired if Watson-Jones had ever treated 2,000 compounded fractures, and, when the reply was in the negative, Yudin stated again that he and his associates had and these were the methods and results.

The Soviet Army Medical Service used large amounts of citrated whole blood and little or no plasma.   An excellent technique was employed to collect the blood in the larger cities, but chiefly in Moscow, where 2,000 pints a day were obtained.   Donors were given a special food ration and a small amount of money, but 85 percent of the latter was returned through gifts to the Government for airplanes and other military purposes.   The name of each donor was placed on each container, and the name of the recipient was given to each donor. The blood was refrigerated at 6° C. and flown to a point near the front, from which it was distributed in refrigerated vehicles to frontline hospitals.   The use of plasma was confined to regimental aid stations.   Much time was taken to describe many other fluids used, but it was obvious that this was done only to indicate the extent of their knowledge.

Amputations, prostheses, and plastic surgery were well done in special hospital centers.   One plastic surgeon, Frumkin, had received publicity in the Allied press for a series of patients upon whom he had operated to create a tubular graft which would simulate a penis through which the bladder could be emptied.

When the mission gave a dinner at the National Hotel where they were billeted, the guestlist included Frumkin, a genial, intelligent, capable surgeon, who spoke English well.   Frumkin's name was removed from the list, as well as several others, and other names were substituted, none of whom the mission had met.   This was done without asking the mission's approval, and no reason was ever given for the action.

Lt. Gen. S. S. Guirgolave lectured to the mission at some length about cold injuries received on the ground and in water but dismissed questions about high-altitude cold injuries in flyers by denying their existence, an attitude which appeared to be common among air force medical officers, Soviet or American, who were in positions of responsibility.   It was their opinion that treatment should be guided by rapid heating of the individual and the injured part.   Longitudinal incisions were made in necrotic tissue within 5 or 6 days to promote the rapid development of dry gangrene.

All of the neurological surgeons in the U.S.S.R. had been trained under the supervision of General Burdenko, who also was a member of the Academy of Sciences.   The latter conferred far more distinction and privileges than any other classification with which we came in contact.   It was said that Academicians ranked in these respects just below the Politburo.

General Burdenko had established an Institute for Neurological Surgery, and it was claimed that 16 neurological surgeons at the front had 3,200 beds at their disposal and that there were 3,700 beds in the rear.

In brief, the neurosurgical techniques shown were those which developed from World War I, without the subsequent refinements which were being practiced in the United States. In no area could Soviet surgery make any contribution to this surgical specialty.

An incident occurred while the mission visited the Institute for Neurological Surgery which revealed more of the Soviet mind than was being disclosed surgically. General Burdenko demonstrated a microscopic slide which purported to show the excellent regeneration which had occurred as the result of the experimental use of a formalin-fixed nerve graft in the repair of a peripheral nerve injury. The specimen was poorly stained and showed nothing conclusive, and one of the mission turned away without comment. Brudenko, through the interpretress, insisted upon a comment about the demonstration, stating that he had a copy of the American's book on peripheral nerve injuries. He indicated that an opinion would be highly appreciated. The answer was, of course, that it had been proved during World War I, and subsequently many times, that such formalin-fixed grafts were completely useless. General Burdenko was asked to indicate how many patients had been operated on and to demonstrate one who showed a return of sensation or motion in any area in which overlap did not occur. General Burdenko replied with a smile that 25 patients had been so operated on, that all had recovered, and that they were unavailable for demonstration because they were at the front in combat.

The other members of the mission, and, in particular, the other member from the United States, were not hesitant in indicating that such a doubting attitude might well impair the entire success of the mission and, if carried into other fields, might even destroy the alliance between the Western nations and the Soviet Union and allow Germany to win the war. The sequel to the incident occurred later at the dinner given by the mission in the National Hotel. During the cocktail hour, General Burdenko was observed rearranging the placecards. It was protocol to have a lieutenant colonel sit at the foot of the table and certainly not on the left of General Burdenko. However, this is what occurred—much to the embarrassment of the senior ranking officers on the mission who believed it must be due to the ignorance of the lieutenant colonel or else his persistence in attempting to offend the Soviet officials. However, the placecard was authenticated by Ambassador Standley who viewed the incident with amusement. During the dinner, General Burdenko summoned the interpretress and asked again the neurosurgical consultant's opinion of the formalin-fixed nerve grafts and again was informed that they had been proved to be unsuccessful beyond any doubt. Whereupon, General Burdenko said he agreed completely but then inquired why the other members of the mission, particularly the British, had been so complimentary in their praise of the experiment. He went on to say that this was an example of how difficult it was to trust and negotiate with people who did not always bluntly state their views and position. Ending by a firm, pumping handclasp, he stated that henceforth there would be no difficulty in understanding opinions expressed by the American neurological surgeon.

Several clinical methods were under study which were emphasized as being completely new and original ideas. These included the injection of 70 percent alcohol with 2 percent Novocain (procaine hydrochloride) solution about fractures in the early days following injury to increase the blood supply and to stimulate callous formation; the use of placental extract to stimulate healing in chronic wounds or the growth of skin in severe burns; the use of a cytotoxin made by injecting mesenchymal tissue into a horse and using the antiserum to stimulate the healing of ulcers of the stomach, the healing of bone, and the loosening of scars and stiffness in joints; the use of the smoke from burning pinewood to stimulate healing; the use of naphthalene broken down by ultrasonic methods to stimulate healing; and the treatment of shock by the suboccipital cistern injection of potassium phosphate solution to stimulate the vasomotor centers in the medulla.

The mission visited Dr. Lena Stern's laboratory to observe an experimental animal tested for shock by this method of cisternal injection. Allowing for all of the difficulties which are inherent in the demonstration of any experiment to a group, the basic technical methods employed were so crude and inaccurate as to throw complete doubt upon any conclusion which had been expressed. Dr. Stern was one of the few women Academicians, and her apartment, automobile, food, and gasoline rations could not be compared with those of the average citizen.

One of the outstanding demonstrations to the mission was that of the organization which had been effected, without recourse to the more democratic method of employing committees, to hospitalize the emergency injuries to the civilian population of Moscow. In fact, when organization alone was considered, the Soviet plans were efficient and superior.

It was apparent that women held equality with men in the U.S.S.R. as members of the street-repairing gangs and of other construction groups on the country roads and as soldiers and officers in the Army. In the line, the mission was informed that there was no woman with a higher rank than colonel; several junior officers were seen with artillery and infantry insignia. In the medical service, the Inspector General, Brigadier Surgeon Valentina Gorinovskaya, was a woman.

On 11 July 1943, the mission began a trip to the frontline hospitals near Vyazma. It will be remembered that, during the following month, the Soviet Army opened an extensive and decisive campaign along the Orel-Kursk-Belgorod Line which extended directly south of Moscow. Vyazma was about 125 miles southwest of Moscow and represented a point to which the Soviet Army had driven the Germans back from their advance on Moscow.

The entourage consisted of several automobiles containing the members of the mission and their hosts. But there were two additional cars which served to transport the mission when the cars in which they were riding broke down, and this occurred four times going and coming. Extra cans of gasoline were carried with the passengers, and the rugged, jolting ride was only a part of the rigors which it is said every doctor-soldier should be trained to expect. All of the traffic officers on the way to Vyazma were women, armed with rifles, whose demeanor and expression left no doubt as to their ability and willingness to use them.

At about 1700 hours, the mission arrived at a casualty clearing station, well camouflaged in a thick forest. After the mission was shown through the wards, vodka, strawberries, caviar, and smoked fish were served in a fine example of a Mongolian tent. General Faymonville had briefed one of the U.S. delegates on the drinking of toasts in vodka in the Russian fashion. It consisted of making up one's own mind about how many vodka toasts could be tolerated and then going through the motions, substituting wine or water if possible, or otherwise simply raising the glass. It became obvious at this first stop that, if one accepted the Soviet rules, defeat was inevitable.

The mission arrived at a large evacuation hospital at about 2200 hours that same night. It was raining and pitch dark, but the hospital too was obviously placed in a thick forest and seemed to be constructed of logs. A sumptuous dinner had been prepared with an exact protocol of seating arrangement along one side of an enormous table which occupied a large dining hall. The senior military member of the mission sat in the center of the table, and on his left was a young, blonde, Amazon-like woman with the rank of major of infantry. Lower ranks and civilian representatives graduated downward to the ends of the table. Vodka, wine, champagne, and enormous quantities of all types of food were served while representatives of various Republics of the Soviet Union, dressed in their native costumes, entertained the guests with folk music and dances.

The toasts came thick and fast and, as was customary, by the time it came to a lieutenant colonel, there was little left to toast. The ruling heads of governments, the Soviet Army, and the women of the Soviet Union had been honored, and a few well-delivered mumbled words with the correct emphasis and gestures now sufficed. It was evident that the young woman major had considerable capacity for vodka and a technique of eating large pieces of bread between toasts. It was also apparent that her table companions were slowly but surely becoming unable to accept her challenges. It did not help for one of the mission to invite her to dance to the Ukrainian music in the hope that the exercise might slow down her vodka-consuming abilities. As a matter of fact, her vigorous dancing probably burned up the alcohol more rapidly and only exhausted her partner. She was physically superior to any one of the mission and probably was devoting herself single-mindedly to carrying out an order.

The dinner was terminated abruptly, and the members of the mission were guided to their billets by their Soviet hosts. They were bedded in one of the wards of the hospital which was cleaned and had comfortable beds. During the night, one of the mission had the first attack of severe renal colic and experienced the nursing technique of Soviet nurses whose calloused and rough hands were nonetheless gentle and reassuring. The following morning the log and plank structure could be admired. It had been erected by officers, nurses, and enlisted personnel, and the nurse who had been on night duty was observed using a hand ax as she, with others, worked on a window frame in a recently added portion of the hospital.

A breakfast of tea, smoked meats, and bread was followed by a visit to Colonel Davis from the previous night's table companion, a Soviet medical officer of the same rank. The Soviet officer apologized for attempting to embarrass a member of the mission by publicly calling attention to the fact that he had not drunk each toast in vodka. He conceded as quite correct this consultant's direct, frank answer that if he (the Soviet colonel) was a guest in the United States he would be permitted to drink as often and as he pleased, and on that basis the American guest to the Soviet Union would conduct himself. The Soviet officer went on to say that there was no real necessity for accepting the Russian rules about drinking toasts, but, if they were accepted, then the Soviet people went all out to drink their guests under the table. A Russian salutation on both cheeks ended the apology and appeared to cement a friendship between at least two of the Allies.

The return to Moscow was completed late that night and the next day was spent in rest and at a symphony concert. The following day the mission visited a hospital for lightly wounded who were able to be quickly rehabilitated and returned to the combat zone. On 15 July, the British and Americans conferred honorary Fellowships upon Burdenko and Yudin in the office of the People's Commissar for Public Health with as many Soviet officials as members of the mission present and no other guests. The British and U.S. Ambassadors were not present, and both Soviet recipients prominently displayed their stars of the Order of Stalin. It was a ceremony completely unworthy, in its setting, of the Fellowships from the distinguished Colleges of Surgeons of England and America, both of which had broken a precedent in conferring their Fellowship away from the home of the College.

The following activities occupied the remainder of the mission's stay in Russia: A return visit to the Sklifossowsky Institute; visits to the Pirogoff Clinic and to the Balneological Institute, where it was claimed that a pine-oil water and Odessa mud were miraculous curing agents; a visit to the Central Institute for Blood Transfusion where, accidentally, it was learned that the mission's constant Soviet companion, physiologist Pairin, understood English perfectly, though he had never uttered one audible word of English; attendance at a performance of the ballet from Otto Nicolai's opera, "The Merry Wives of Windsor," and at a performance of Tschaikovsky's opera, "The Queen of Spades;" a meeting at the Central Institute for Medical Research, at which Mr. Carling, Professor Penfield, and this consultant recited that Great Britain, Canada, and the United States freely exchanged research information, without eliciting the slightest sign of encouragement that the Soviet Union would join in.

On 23 July, the mission finally took off on their return flight. The last week had been difficult for the hosts as well as the members of the mission, and it had been hard to keep occupied. The time allotted to the mission had been overstayed. It had been impossible to walk about alone, because the ever-present NKVD representatives had been nearby; there were no shops in which

to purchase mementos of the trip, and the members of the mission had become
slightly weary of one another's frailties.

The obstacle, however, was the fact that no airplane was available to take
the mission back to their starting place. The British and Soviet authorities
had been negotiating an agreement whereby, in the summer months, one route
would be flown by way of the Mediterranean, Cairo, and Teheran, as the mission
had come, and another directly across Europe from London to Moscow. One
aircraft by each route each week was the schedule. In the winter months,
two planes would fly the southern route. The British believed the agreement
to be firm, but flew two planes in one week in July via the southern route,
instead of one directly across Europe, because of operational difficulties, which
would quickly straighten out. The Soviet authorities considered this a violation of the agreement and refused to allow any plane to enter Soviet territory
by any route.

The week passed with the British Ambassador frankly admitting that he
could get nowhere with the Soviet Foreign Office. The U.S. Ambassador
finally demanded passage out of the U.S.S.R. for the two U.S. citizens and,
on 23 July, all of the members of the mission arose at 0300 hours and arrived
at an airfield near Moscow at 0545 hours. They could see the two-motored
U.S.-built plane sitting on the field. A large red star decorated its side.
After waiting 2 hours for Walter Citrine, a British labor leader and his
companions who had also been in the U.S.S.R. studying Soviet labor relations,
they boarded the plane whose motors were still idle. The motors were started,
and, without preliminary revving of the motors, the plane taxied to the end of
the field and took off. The flight was never above 1,000 feet because, recently,
an order had been issued to the antiaircraft crews to shoot at any plane above
that height, without attempting to identify it. Stalingrad was circled at
500 feet and all that could be seen standing was one stone chimney. At 1730
that evening, the pilot dove the field at Teheran, and, with the smell of
scorched rubber tires in their nostrils, the members of the mission were un-
ceremoniously deposited on the airstrip. They were out of the U.S.S.R.

The unceremonious delivery of the members of the mission in Teheran
left the Americans stranded at the airport, while the British left by an automobile provided by Sir Reader W. Bullard, British Minister to Iran. A car
was commandeered, and, after a great deal of shouting and gesticulating, the
billet of General Connolly was reached. Hot, dirty, and tired, Colonel Cutler
and the author burst in upon the general and his staff who were having a
cocktail before dinner. The general quickly grasped their predicament and
sent an orderly outside to silence the Persian driver who was honking the
automobile horn and screaming Iranian curses on his passengers.

After hearing their story and realizing that they had no means of transportation from Teheran to Cairo, General Connolly arranged for hotel accommodations overnight, removed two passengers from a U.S. freight-passenger plane
that was leaving in the morning for Cairo via Basra, and said he would send
a car to pick them up early in the morning and put them on the airfield. With

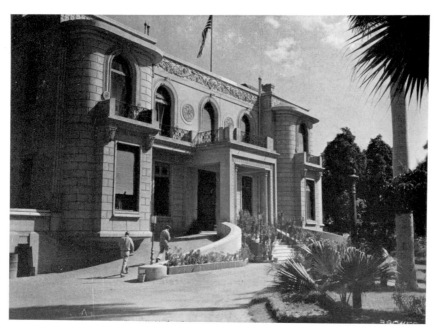

FIGURE 148.—The headquarters of the U.S. Army Forces in the Middle East.

many sighs of relief, they arrived at the hotel with the general's aide, cleaned up, and answered a telephone call from the British Minister to come to dinner at his home. There was some tension after dinner when methods of transportation to Cairo were compared. The British were being flown directly to Cairo in the commanding general's comfortable plane.

The U.S. plane had two motors, and its aisle was filled with engines, crated to be returned to Cairo. Its bucket seats were filled with officers and enlisted men, all of whom had one goal in common—to be able successfully to crawl on their hands and knees across the engine crates to and from the toilet, since all were suffering from diarrhea. Basra's temperature was 120° that morning at about 1000 hours, and griddlecakes and thick molasses was not an appetizing menu. It was not long, however, before the plane took off again and landed in Cairo at about 1730 hours that evening, 24 July.

Colonel Cutler and the author were unsuccessful in obtaining a room at Shepheard's Hotel and eventually got to Mena House where they found the other members of the mission. The next 3 days were spent in talking with Mr. Kirk, U.S. Minister to Egypt, the members of the U.S. Typhus Commission, and Col. Crawford F. Sams, Surgeon, U.S. Army Forces in the Middle East (fig. 148); visiting the U.S. 38th General Hospital; sightseeing among the Pyramids and the Sphinx at Al Jizah; lunching with Ali Pasha Ibrahim, Dean, Faculty of Medicine, Egyptian University (Cairo); and listening in on a critique of the British-American landings in Sicily.

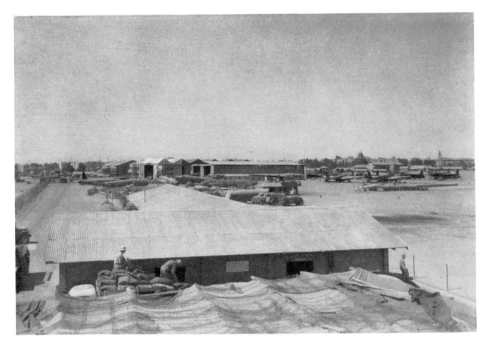

FIGURE 149.—A parting look at the airfield at Heliopolis, Egypt, July 1943.

The DMS of the British Eighth Army in Cairo at that time was Maj. Gen. William H. (later Sir Heneage) Ogilvie. Colonel Cutler and the author were warned by him that the critique would be highly critical of the American air forces and paratroopers. After they had sat down and after Gen. Henry Maitland Wilson had arrived, the Americans were given the opportunity to leave if they chose. The critique lost all of its objectiveness and value, even to the British Armed Forces, when the colonel who conducted the critique became highly emotional and delivered a sarcastic diatribe about the favorable publicity that the U.S. Armed Forces had received and their popularity with the female population of the British Isles.

At midnight on 28 July, the mission was driven to the airfield at Heliopolis (fig. 149). It was stifling hot on the desert, and the sand was blowing as they sat in a small brightly lighted room without ventilation. The young RAF wing commander who had been delegated to fly the mission back to England had been one of the heroes of the Battle of Britain. It was as if he had been an engineer on the Twentieth Century Limited and now was hauling an express milk train. Each of the members of the mission was asked to demonstrate his proficiencies in getting into a life preserver and a parachute and in adjusting an oxygen mask.

Again, they landed at Gibraltar and the Americans found a small room in a barracks. One iron bed without a mattress was hardly a place for two men to sleep or rest, and so the day was spent sightseeing and having dinner in the hotel. At midnight, off they went, but it was with great difficulty that their wing commander managed to get the plane off the short runway. Early the next morning, 30 July, the plane sat down on the airfield at Swindon. As they were getting their bags off, the pilot discovered that the flight had been particularly difficult for him because a cargo, placed beneath the floorboards of the passenger cabin and sent from London to Cairo, had never been unloaded. He had carried it all the way back to England again. This explained the difficulty with which his plane became airborne.

The mission had learned little about new advances in surgery, but each member had formed his own opinion of Soviet practices from observation of the individuals with whom he had come in contact. The Soviet people appeared to be like 10-year-old American boys who brag about the size of their houses and chimneys and recklessly claim that their fathers can lick anyone. They were unsure of themselves and suspicious and could understand only directness, frankness, and the show of confidence which comes from strength, both physical and intellectual.

It was learned that medical education, formerly under the control of the universities, was put under the Commissariat for Public Health in 1930. There were, then, 72 institutes (schools) of medicine with 107,000 medical students. Students were admitted after 10 years in secondary schools, and the medical course was 5 years. The first 2 years were spent in scientific studies, and the last 3 years were clinical. During a part of the clinical years, the students were farmed out to village and town clinics for practical experience. There was specialization with training for industrial surgery, military surgery, hygiene, and bacteriology. Upon their passing a required state examination, a diploma was issued which conferred the right to practice medicine. Higher degrees, those of bachelor or doctor of medicine, were given after 2 or 3 additional years of postgraduate work, which could be clinical practice or continued work in the institute. A thesis was required which determined whether or not additional examinations were to be given. The percentage of students who become bachelors or doctors of medicine was small. From 1935 to 1940, there were 140 doctor's degrees given at the First Medical Institute and 284 bachelor's degrees. From this group came the professors and teachers. When a chair was vacant, anyone could apply, but a commission chose and appointed the individual. It was said that they had a Research Council, also under the Commissariat for Public Health, and that into that organization flowed problems from the army, navy, industry, and the faculties of the medical institutes. This council then assigned special problems to certain faculties or individuals.

WASHINGTON AND RELEASE FROM SERVICE

Colonel Davis spent the month of August 1943 preparing reports [8] and accompanying General Hawley to the wards of the 2d General Hospital where Major Scarff and his associates had been caring for the high-altitude frostbite

---

[8] See pp. 92–106, and appendix A for additional chronicling of the mission to the Soviet Union and appendix A for a report on the mission prepared jointly by Colonel Cutler and Colonel Davis.

cases. Gen. Henry H. Arnold, Commanding General of the Army Air Forces, Maj. Gen. David N. W. Grant, the Air Surgeon, and General Grow were also present on that Sunday morning when General Arnold visited the men at their beds and heard their stories of failure of clothing and equipment.

General Grow accompanied General Grant and General Arnold back to Washington. Colonel Davis received orders the following week to go to Washington and present the colored photographs of high-altitude frostbite injuries, the clinical histories, and all other data which had been developed during the study of these patients. He was also instructed to present the data on the protective helmet.

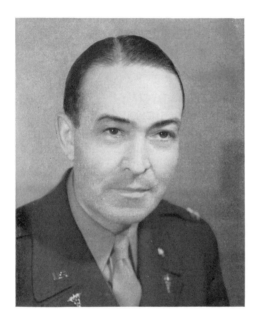

FIGURE 150.—Col. R. Glen Spurling, MC.

Maj. Gen. Norman T. Kirk, The Surgeon General, and his staff were greatly interested in the high-altitude cold injuries. General Kirk took the author to the Pentagon and arranged a presentation of the material to the Air Surgeon's executive officer, Col. Walter S. Jensen, MC, and a group of other Army Air Forces medical officers. General Grow appeared during the presentation. He objected strenuously to any implications that he and his staff had missed the injuries in the first place, had continued to disregard them, and had failed at any time to study them. The facts, not the implications, needed no defense.

Mr. Henry Field, a friend from Chicago, was in Washington engaged in governmental work which made use of his great knowledge of the Middle East and his abilities to bring important matters to the attention of those in high places, who otherwise had to rely upon the complex lines of communication between bureaus and departments. He was greatly interested in the story of the high-altitude cold injuries and in the possibilities of the protective helmet.

Thus it was that contacts were made with Colonel Doriot and Mr. Bradford Washburn [9] of the Quartermaster Corps. These men had been working energetically to develop clothing for airmen which would protect them against extreme cold. Mr. Washburn had had considerable experience in mountain climbing and exposure to severe cold. Unfortunately, this research group had been ordered to stop working further on protective clothing for airmen. Colonel Doriot's group was also working on a new protective material—Doron—named for Colonel Doriot, and it was possible for the author to help at length on the medical aspects of its development (p. 414).

After a tour as a patient through three general hospitals ended on 30 March 1944, Colonel Davis was released from active duty and returned to his duties as chairman of the Department of Surgery, Northwestern University.

On 12 March 1944, Lt. Col. (later Col.) R. Glen Spurling, MC (fig. 150), was appointed Senior Consultant in Neurosurgery in the Office of the Chief Surgeon, ETOUSA.[10]

The Army Air Forces eventually requested the author's colored photographs of high-altitude frostbite and made educational posters designed to instruct the airman on proper protective measures. Properly wired clothing was issued, and the sidegun apertures on aircraft were closed in.

The plastic material for protective armor was field tested by the Marine Corps and the Navy, and finally, on 15 September 1951, Maj. Gen. Edgar E. Hume of the Army Medical Corps announced that a plastic-protected vest would stop a .45-caliber bullet fired from a distance of 3 feet. In an article published in 1944, this consultant had suggested that the plastic material designed for use in aviators' helmets could also be adapted for protective clothing.[11] Such armored protective clothing was finally used in the field during the Korean War with great success. At the time of this writing, the plastic material forms the basic principle of protection for the jet pilot's acrosonic helmet.

---

[9] Director, Boston Science Museum, Boston, Mass., in 1959.

[10] For accounts of Dr. Spurling's activities, see: (1) Medical Department, United States Army. Surgery in World War II. Neurosurgery. Volume I. Washington: U.S. Government Printing Office, 1958, chapters III and VII; (2) Medical Department, United States Army. Surgery in World War II. Neurosurgery. Volume II. Washington: U.S. Government Printing Office, 1959, chapters IV, VIII, and XII.

[11] Davis, L.: Helmet for Protection Against Craniocerebral Injuries. Surg., Gynec. & Obst., 79: 89–91, July 1944.

CHAPTER V

Ophthalmology

James N. Greear, Jr., M.D.

The first Senior Consultant in Ophthalmology in ETOUSA (European Theater of Operations, U.S. Army) was Col. Derrick T. Vail, MC, (fig. 151). Colonel Vail returned to the Zone of Interior on 26 December 1944 for a period of temporary duty in the Office of The Surgeon General. His presence in the Zone of Interior at that time permitted a desirable and indicated exchange of certain key ophthalmologists. Colonel Vail was reassigned permanently to the Office of The Surgeon General as consultant in ophthalmology, relieving the incumbent, Maj. (later Lt. Col.) M. Elliott Randolph, MC. Major Randolph, in turn, relieved Lt. Col. James N. Greear, Jr., MC (fig. 152), as the officer in charge of the rehabilitation program for the blind at Valley Forge General Hospital, thus freeing the author for assignment to the European theater as Senior Consultant in Ophthalmology. Colonel Vail has recorded his experiences and activities as the first Senior Consultant in Ophthalmology in the European theater in the volume, "Ophthalmology and Otolaryngology," of the history of the Army Medical Department in World War II.[1]

During Colonel Vail's absence, Col. Norton Canfield, MC, the Senior Consultant in Otolaryngology in the European theater, took care of problems in ophthalmology that demanded attention at the theater headquarters. When Colonel Vail had not returned to the European theater by the end of January 1945, Colonel Canfield recommended that Maj. Byron C. Smith, MC, of the 1st General Hospital be assigned temporarily as Senior Consultant in Ophthalmology in addition to his other duties. The recommendation was approved. Major Smith was in charge of an active service in ophthalmology at his own hospital; therefore, he was unable to make extensive visits to medical units in the theater. He did keep in touch, however, with the activities concerning the Senior Consultant in Ophthalmology and gave valuable assistance and advice relative to problems of a specific nature which were constantly arising.

Colonel Greear reported for duty at the Office of the Chief Surgeon, ETOUSA, on 29 March 1945 and began his tour as Senior Consultant in Oph-

---

[1] Medical Department, United States Army. Surgery in World War II. Ophthalmology and Otolaryngology. Washington: U.S. Government Printing Office, 1957, Chapter V, "Administrative Aspects of Ophthalmology in the European Theater of Operations," and Chapter VI, "Clinical Policies in Ophthalmology, European Theater of Operations."

thalmology in the European theater. He devoted the first few days after his arrival to searching the files of Colonel Vail in an effort to determine the established policies of the theater and to familiarize himself with the many problems to be considered.

ORGANIZATION

The original plan for the organization of the Professional Services Division, Office of the Chief Surgeon, as set up early in 1942 by Col. James C. Kimbrough, MC, Director of Professional Services, was still in effect. In brief, the division consisted of a Chief Consultant in Medicine with subordinate senior

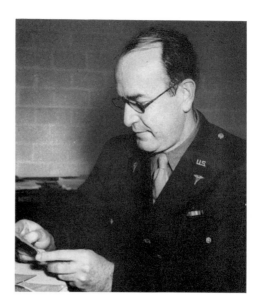

FIGURE 151.—Col. Derrick T. Vail, MC.

consultants in neuropsychiatry, tuberculosis, dermatology, and infectious diseases and a Chief Consultant in Surgery with subordinate senior consultants in the specialties of orthopedic surgery, plastic surgery and burns, neurosurgery, anesthesia, transfusion and shock, ophthalmology, radiology, urology, otolaryngology, and maxillofacial surgery.

By January 1945, decentralization of all activities had occurred owing to the great number of wounded and the presence in the theater of some 200 hospitals. The larger base sections had consultants in medicine and surgery, who reported on purely professional matters to the Chief, Professional Services Division, Office of the Chief Surgeon, through either the Chief Consultant in Medicine or the Chief Consultant in Surgery. This plan, alone, did not provide adequate coverage of professional activity within the theater. Therefore, in order to maintain close contact with professional work, consultants in medicine and surgery were set up in the hospital centers. These officers in turn re-

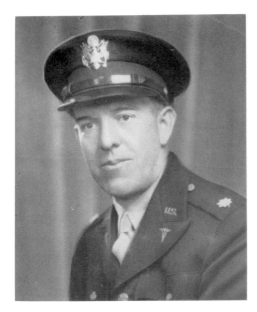

FIGURE 152.—Lt. Col. James N. Greear, Jr., MC.

ported on professional matters through the base section surgeons to the Chief Consultant in Medicine or the Chief Consultant in Surgery. Consultations in the medical and surgical specialties were also decentralized. In each hospital center, officers selected for their superior ability acted as regional or hospital center consultants while carrying on their regular duties. At a high level, and separate from this intimate organization for the supervision of professional work in communications zone hospitals, there always existed a close liaison with the consultants of the various field armies and the air forces. This close liaison with the tactical elements was essential, for it was believed that in any single theater there should be but one professional policy if the soldier, whether sick or wounded, was to receive proper therapy.

POLICIES AND PROCEDURES

The policies of the Professional Services Division as established in 1942 were designed to implement measures whereby personnel of the U.S. Forces would receive promptly the highest standard of medical and surgical care. The condition of all patients reported seriously ill in U.S. Army hospitals as well as British hospitals could be easily and quickly determined. In order to stimulate and maintain professional morale and disseminate recent medical information, it was considered advisable that medical meetings be held regularly at general and station hospitals. The type and frequency of these meetings depended on local conditions at each hospital and on the general situation.

The specialty senior consultants in medicine and surgery submitted written daily reports of their activities to Colonel Kimbrough through their respective chief consultants, Col. William S. Middleton, MC, in medicine, or Col. (later Brig. Gen.) Elliott C. Cutler, MC, in surgery. These reports were consolidated by Colonel Middleton, Colonel Cutler, and Colonel Kimbrough for transmission to the Chief Surgeon. It was the policy of the Professional Services Division to have consultation service immediately available at all times. Senior consultants for the various specialties in the Office of the Chief Surgeon coordinated the activities relating to their respective areas. They made such recommendations to the appropriate chief consultant as were considered necessary for the instruction of subordinate consultants and specialists in hospitals and other units. Under the guidance of the senior consultants, the consultants for field armies and base sections supervised and coordinated the work of specialists functioned under the direction of the Chief, Professional Services Division, and its members were the responsible advisers to the Chief Surgeon on all professional and technical medical matters.

The specialist senior consultants visited all Medical Department units for the purpose of giving their guidance and assistance with regard to technical and professional matters falling within their fields of activity. They advised on the selection and assignment of junior consultants and specialists and reported from time to time on the standard of professional efficiency maintained by such officers. They collaborated with members of the Operations Division, Office of the Chief Surgeon, in arranging courses of instruction, medical meetings, and training schools and in other measures designed to keep the officers of the Medical Department in touch with the latest developments in medical science. It was their duty to initiate and carry out research and investigations with a view to conserving manpower in the field and restoring to health the sick and wounded. It was their responsibility also to maintain liaison with the consultants and specialists in all branches of medicine of the British Armed Forces and civilian practice. They advised as to the suitability of drugs, instruments, and equipment of a specific nature and made recommendations on other matters pertaining to the health of the U.S. Army in the European theater.

The most important function of the Senior Consultant in Ophthalmology was to see that every U.S. soldier requiring eye care, in the European theater, received the highest possible standard of medical care (fig. 153). The best method of accomplishing this was to determine the capabilities of the ophthalmologists assigned to the general and station hospitals. This information was obtained by personal contact and through the hospital center consultant in ophthalmology. On several occasions, groups of ophthalmologists from both station and general hospitals were invited to meet with the Senior Consultant in Ophthalmology. The meetings were very satisfactory, and many important phases of the handling of patients were discussed. Following the general discussion, individual interviews were held with most of the men who had attended the meeting.

It was impossible for the Senior Consultant in Ophthalmology to cover the entire area and to see the work that was being done in each individual hospital. Nevertheless, he made every effort to visit hospitals where the larger number of eye cases were being treated. These hospitals were primarily those treating large numbers of neurosurgical patients and maxillofacial injuries where, naturally, many eye cases would be located. On several occasions, groups of hospital center consultants met at some centrally located hospital or at a base section headquarters, and informal discussions were carried on among these consultants and the Senior Consultant in Ophthalmology. These discussions proved of great benefit to all concerned insofar as the care of patients was concerned. Not infrequently, it was necessary for the center consultant in ophthalmology to have patients transferred from another hospital to his own to assure adequate medical care, and this could be carried out without too much difficulty. The hospital center consultant had no authority to initiate transfers of personnel from one hospital to another; however, it was his duty to report to the Senior Consultant in Ophthalmology when he felt that such transfer was necessary, and the transfer could then be initiated from the Senior Consultant's level.

Regular monthly reports were received by the Senior Consultant in Ophthalmology from most of the ophthalmologists in station and general hospitals in the theater. These reports were informal, but they contained information pertinent to both the type and the number of ophthalmic lesions being dealt with in each particular hospital. This information was valuable to the author in that it kept him acquainted with the needs for personnel and equipment in various units as conditions changed. A monthly report was not received from some of the newer units.

Early policy in the European theater had dictated that newly blinded casualties be sent to St. Dunstan's Institute for the Blind near Shrewsbury, Shropshire, England, for a period of training before evacuation to the Zone of Interior (fig. 154). Since September 1944, however, the established policy in the European theater was to evacuate all blinded patients to the Zone of Interior, at the earliest possible moment after they were transportable. Before his transfer to the European theater, this consultant had learned that patients who had been sent to St. Dunstan's in England for initial rehabilitation before returning to the Zone of Interior were usually critical of the training they received at special rehabilitation centers in the Zone of Interior. They constantly compared procedures carried out in the two places. Therefore, personnel dealing with blinded casualties in the theater were instructed as to the proper psychological approach. The necessity for these blinded patients to become independent as quickly as possible in order to regain confidence in themselves was emphasized.

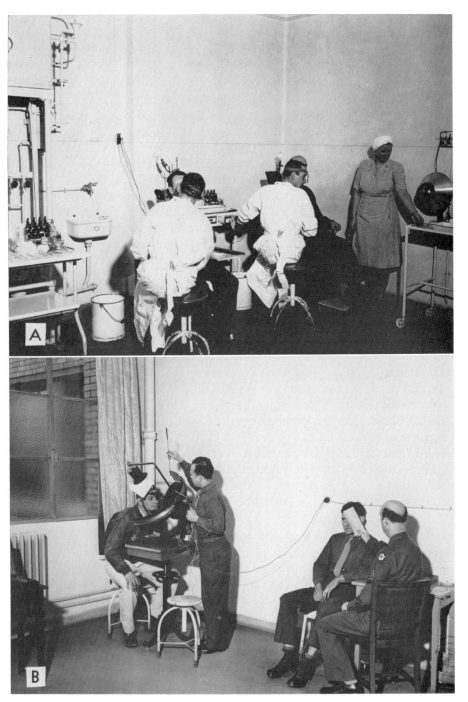

FIGURE 153.—Ophthalmological service in a general hospital. A. Examining facilities.
B. Perimetry and the determination of distant visual acuity.

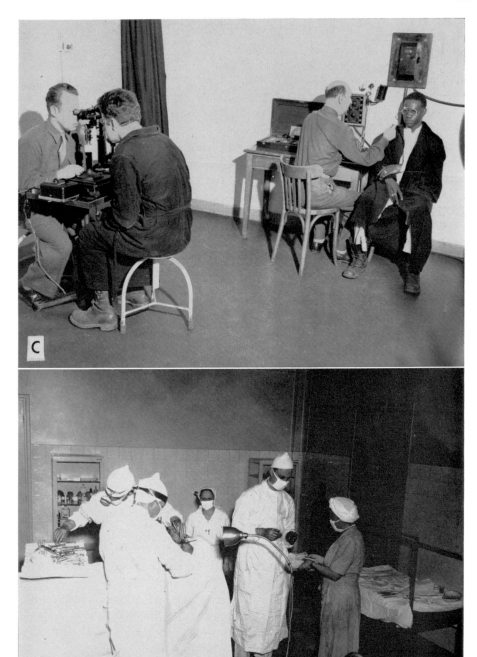

FIGURE 153.—Continued. C. Optometry. D. An eye operation in progress.

HOSPITAL CENTERS

During November and December of 1944 and the early months of 1945, thirty 1,000-bed general hospitals had arrived in the European theater. In addition, there were 10 new 400-bed evacuation hospitals and 1 new 750-bed evacuation hospital (fig. 155). In some of these hospitals there was no ophthalmologist, and in others the ophthalmologist had received meager training in his specialty. The rapid movement of the armies had necessitated an increased dispersion of hospitals and had thus made the author's personal contacts with the ophthalmologists in the theater much more difficult. This greatly increased the importance of competent and active subordinate consultants.

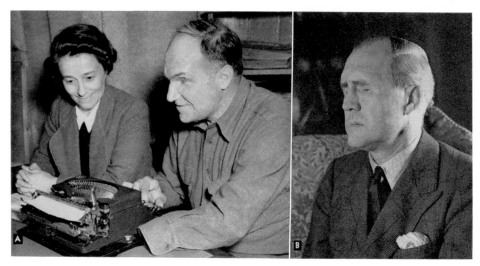

FIGURE 154.—St. Dunstan's Institute for the Blind, Shropshire, England. A. A blinded amputee learning to type. B. Sir Ian Fraser, founder and director.

Hospital centers were well established in the United Kingdom Base and were well organized. In each center, there was a very competent consultant in ophthalmology who made regular visits to hospitals in the center and who worked, in most instances, in close cooperation with the commanding officer of the center. Thus, the commanding officer was kept advised concerning the care of ophthalmological patients in his center. Shifts in personnel were recommended through the center consultant in ophthalmology wherever it was deemed necessary. The more serious eye problems were concentrated in hospitals where more capable ophthalmological officers were assigned.

On the Continent, hospital centers generally were less well organized, and, while consultants in ophthalmology had been assigned in a few instances, they had not had their functions well defined and were of the opinion that they should not visit hospitals until they were invited. An effort was made to clarify this situation in order that this consultant might be kept informed as to the ophthalmic care of patients in widely scattered hospitals. Additional consultants were appointed to new centers which had been organized on the Continent and every effort was made to acquaint them with their duties and responsibilities. An able center or regional consultant was of inestimable value in coordinating the functions of his specialty in his area.

The majority of the hospital center consultants in the European theater were captains. This was a great handicap to them in carrying out their duties, since a great many of the eye, ear, nose, and throat men assigned to general and station hospitals were majors and resented an officer of a lower grade in

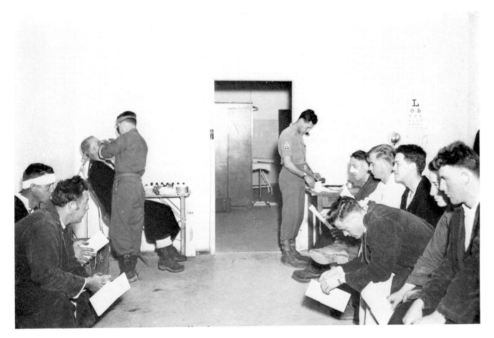

FIGURE 155.—An eye clinic in an evacuation hospital.

specting their services and making recommendations as to the care of patients. This situation was common throughout the entire theater. The hospital center consultant had important responsibilities. It was his duty to visit the hospitals in the center at least monthly and oftener if necessary; he certainly had to visit them often enough to ascertain that the patients in the hospitals of his center were receiving the best possible eye care. It was important that he gain the confidence and respect of the ophthalmologists assigned to the hospitals in his center in order that they would freely seek the center consultant's advice on problem patients. A higher rank would have made it easier for him to carry out his responsibilities.

Geographic dispersion of hospitals in each hospital center rarely offered any real problem since most of the hospitals in the centers were situated within a relatively small radius and in most instances could easily be reached within less than an hour. The question of transportation was never a serious problem. Most hospital center consultants could obtain transportation from their own units; if not, transportation was available from the hospital center headquarters.

SUPPLIES AND EQUIPMENT

The standard equipment supplied to general and station hospitals in the European theater was extremely deficient in certain items which were essential to accurate diagnosis of many eye disorders. Because of the inability of the medical officer to make early and accurate diagnoses as a result of a lack of diagnostic instruments or because of inadequate equipment, alleviative measures were not instituted until the patient reached another hospital where such equipment was available.

The slit lamp and corneal microscope are indispensable to the accurate diagnosis and treatment of injuries or diseases of the anterior segment of the globe. A good many of these instruments were distributed to hospitals in the United Kingdom Base, but very few ever reached the hospitals on the Continent. In one hospital center, there was not one single such item, and, in another center, there was only one such item—and that was in a rather isolated hospital.

Abnormal fields of vision could be accurately determined only by plotting such changes with the use of a perimeter or tangent screen. Neither of these items was on the standard table of equipment for general or station hospitals. In some instances, through the ingenuity of some medical officers or their technical assistants, both tangent screen and perimeters were constructed. These proved to be very satisfactory and most useful.

It was the opinion of all concerned that every general hospital should have been supplied with a giant magnet as standard equipment since the hand magnet was found to be not sufficiently powerful to remove many of the smaller intraocular magnetic foreign bodies.

OPTICAL SUPPLY

Full credit was given to Colonel Vail for establishing the optical program in the European theater. This program had worked and was thoroughly organized at the time the author arrived in the theater. Late in 1944, one section of the issue branch of the ETOUSA Base Optical Shop was moved from Blackpool, England, to Paris. Col. Silas B. Hays, MC, Chief of the Supply Division, Office of the Chief Surgeon, ETOUSA, was most cooperative in instituting this transfer to the Continent. This unit was designed as the Base Optical Shop and located at the 7th General Dispensary to service the optical requirements of the U.S. Army on the Continent. This facility not only filled prescriptions for glasses arising from the immediate area but also provided all optical supplies to mobile units, both Services of Supply

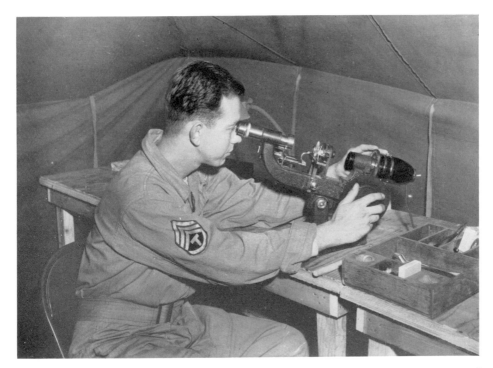

FIGURE 156.—A technician in a mobile optical repair unit checking a lens for accuracy of grinding.

and field army, on the Continent. Initially, requisitions were drawn on the Blackpool Base Optical Shop in England to maintain stock levels. Special jobs could be expedited with the use of air courier service to the United Kingdom.

By 1945, there were 2 base optical shops, 27 mobile optical repair units (fig. 156), and 54 portable optical repair units employed on the Continent. In the first 6 months of 1945, 186,000 spectacle requisitions were processed by these units, of which more than 99 percent were processed immediately from available materials. Mobile units processed 102,000 prescriptions, portable units processed 66,000 prescriptions, and 82,000 of the total number of prescriptions were processed by optical units operating in the army areas. Without these units, approximately 10,000 troops each month would have been evacuated because they were visually unfit for duty. Capt. Chester E. Rorie, SnC, commanding officer of the Base Optical Shop, also had the responsibility for compiling information and requisitioning, receiving, storing, and issuing all optical supplies and equipment for all echelons. His work in this field was outstanding.

Soon after plans for redeployment had been announced, a letter was received from Colonel Vail, then Consultant in Ophthalmology to The Surgeon General, outlining the necessity for equipping troops being redeployed with spectacles and gas mask inserts. On 18 May 1945, the author was in conference with Colonel Cutler; Colonel Hays; Col. Angvald Vickoren, MC, Chief, Troops and Training Branch, Operations Division; Col. John E. Gordon, MC, Chief, Preventive Medicine Division; Lt. Col. Bernard J. Pisani, MC, Executive Officer, Professional Services Division; and Captain Rorie. The question of supply of eyeglass gas mask inserts and spectacles was the chief topic under discussion. It was proposed that an ETOUSA directive be sent to all unit commanders concerned with the medical processing of troops for redeployment. The following day, a proposed directive dealing with spectacles and gas mask inserts was transmitted to the Deputy Chief Surgeon. The directive was never published on the basis that items covered by the proposed directive were already adequately covered in published ETOUSA command directives on redeployment. On 29 June 1945, this consultant submitted a letter to the Chief Surgeon pointing out the necessity for more specific instructions relative to this phase of redeployment because there was so much misunderstanding.

Accompanied by Major Smith and Captain Rorie, the author visited Twelfth Army Group headquarters and then the headquarters of the Third, Seventh, and Fifteenth U.S. Armies and discussed with the army surgeons the eyeglass and spectacle requirements for troops being redeployed. This information was well received and the army surgeons were quite willing to cooperate.

Despite early planning, after V–E Day (8 May 1945), some critical problems developed which demanded immediate action. Some 2 million troops were to be redeployed either directly or indirectly just as quickly as transportation facilities would permit. All troops having visual error were to be redeployed with their maximum spectacle requirements of two pairs of issue spectacles and, if visual acuity was less than 20/70, one pair of gas mask inserts. Service troops were to be redeployed first, and this was the category that most optical units came under. In practically no time at all, 65 percent of optical facilities had ceased operations in preparation for redeployment. The personnel on temporary duty in the Base Optical Shop had dwindled down to four.

The Commanding General, Assembly Area Command, had demanded six mobile units to serve the assembly area alone. The commanding general of the Le Havre area had requested an extra unit, the Marseilles Port had requested an additional unit there, the armies were demanding additional units to replace those that had ceased operations for redeployment, the Bremen Port had requested a unit, and a unit was requested for Berlin. In short, the requirements had increased to about 20 percent more than they ever had been at any time during the war, and about 65 percent of the optical supply units had ceased operations. This, of course, created temporarily a serious condition and "Immediate Action" was stamped on practically every requisition placed on the operating optical supply units.

This problem was solved in the following manner. A teletype message was sent to all prisoner-of-war stockades directing that prisoners be screened immediately for experienced opticians. Between 50 and 75 opticians were located and allocated to various units. A 24-hour shift was put in operation in the assembly area, and additional equipment was set up. The stocks of supplies were doubled in all units having a large demand. Nine Belgian civilians were employed in Liége. Twenty-seven French civilians were employed in Paris. A unit was sent to Bremen Port. Two portable units were sent to Berlin. In the last month of operations prior to V–J Day (14 August), 37,000 pairs of glasses were processed. Again, Captain Rorie cannot be too highly commended for the splendid job he did in supplying the entire Army in Europe with instant service on optical supplies under the most difficult circumstances.

TRAINING

Early in May 1945, the Medical Field Service School, ETOUSA, was reestablished near Paris. The Senior Consultant in Ophthalmology, assisted by Maj. Kenneth Fairfax, MC, and Maj. Byron C. Smith, MC, gave lectures on war ophthalmology to the medical officers attending the school. These lectures and demonstrations were designed to impress upon the general medical officers the need to handle patients with injured eyes carefully, particularly patients with perforating wounds of the globe. Lectures were also given to nurses attending the school (fig. 157). These talks emphasized the necessity for nursing care in patients with severe eye injuries. Procedures pertaining to the nursing of newly blinded soldiers were discussed.

During 1944, it was anticipated that there would be a period following hostilities in which some type of training program or refresher courses in the various medical specialties would be of tremendous value to the men in various fields of medicine, either in continued service activities or in civilian practice. Before reporting for duty in the Office of the Chief Surgeon, ETOUSA, the author had conferred with Colonel Vail relative to posthostilities training for the ophthalmologists in the European theater. Colonel Vail had given the subject considerable thought, but no definite action had been taken. Prior to the cessation of hostilities, this subject was discussed with center consultants and with individual ophthalmologists throughout the theater. It was decided that a didactic program in ophthalomology would be inaugurated at Oxford University under the direction of Prof. Ida Caroline Mann, Head of the Department of Ophthalmology at the university.

A conference was held with Professor Mann, and plans were completed for such a program to begin on 17 July and extend through 14 August 1945. This course was to consist of lectures and demonstrations by Professor Mann and her staff, supplemented by a number of invited lecturers from the United Kingdom. Following this lecture course, ophthalmologists who were available were to be assigned to various civilian ophthalmological services in the United Kingdom for a period of 2 weeks. This consultant visited several of these

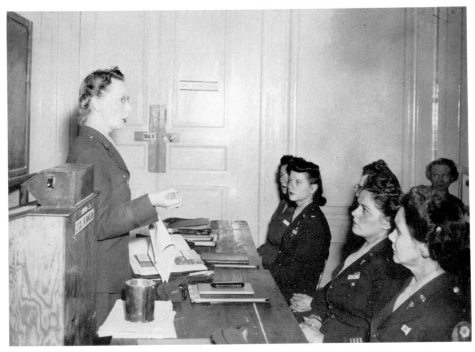

FIGURE 157.—Nurses receiving instruction at the Medical Field Service School, ETOUSA,
at Chateau du Maurais near Paris, France.

hospitals, and, in each instance, they were willing to have U.S. Army officers
attend clinics and observe the activities of the hospital generally. Lt. Col.
(later Col.) Einar C. Andreassen, MC, Chief of the Operations Division, Medical Section, Headquarters, United Kingdom Base, assured the author that the
91st General Hospital would be available for billeting and messing the officers
attending the course at Oxford University. All financial arrangements for
the course were completed with the authorities of Oxford University, utilizing
theater information and education funds. Maj. Ferdinand P. Calhoun, MC,
of the 2d General Hospital was appointed coordinator of the course and,
from 13 June to 30 June, was attached to the Office of the Surgeon, United
Kingdom Base. With the cooperation of Professor Mann, eminent British
ophthalmologists throughout the United Kingdom were interviewed and
worked into a lecture timetable. The coordinator found that the lecturers,
all prominent in ophthalmology, were most eager and willing to do all they
could, despite the inconvenience of preparing a lecture and of traveling to
Oxford from their homes throughout England. Except for Sir Stewart Duke-
Elder, who was prevented by his important military duties, every British
ophthalmologist who was asked to participate accepted the invitation. This
spirit was a great tribute to the friendly and cooperative relationship between
the U.S. and British ophthalmologists, established during the war by Colonel
Vail.

The course was eminently successful in providing a taste of academic ophthalmology to men who had been doing military ophthalmology for varying periods of time. The men were unusually and uniformly appreciative and eager to take advantage of the opportunity afforded them and were repeatedly impressed by the education, poise, and affability of the British lecturers, many of whom were internationally known. The scope and duration of the course did not in any way qualify an officer for a certificate, diploma, or degree. The intention of the course was merely to give the officer who had been doing military ophthalmology a review of academic ophthalmology, to refresh and broaden him, and to stimulate his future serious study of ophthalmology. Owing to unavoidable redeployment requirements at this particular time, only about half the number of students originally scheduled to attend could attend.

SUMMARY AND CONCLUSIONS

The consultant system made possible the high type of medical and surgical care that was available to the U.S. soldier in the European theater in World War II. A consultant in ophthalmology was always available in the hospital center, and, if it was his belief that the Senior Consultant in Ophthalmology should be called to see any individual patient, the latter could be reached through the base section headquarters. The consultant system was essential for the best surgical care of the Army in the European theater. It did not work perfectly; however, in the event of any future conflict it should work far more smoothly than it did in World War II.

No general or station hospital should have been sent to an oversea theater without adequate equipment to render all the specialized services for which the hospital was formed. Certainly, they should have had the essential equipment for specialties such as ophthalmology. The equipment should have included a perimeter, a giant magnet, slit lamp and corneal microscope, a first-rate ophthalmoscope, and a tangent screen. These items are mentioned because they were not included in the standard equipment of ophthalmolgical departments in the hospitals of World War II.

In a theater of war, hospital centers should be organized and hospital center consultants should be given very explicit instructions as to their duties and responsibilities. One of the chief responsibilities of the hospital center consultant should be to apprise his senior consultant in ophthalmology of any hospital in which a low grade of ophthalmology is being practiced.

The sole purpose of any system is to provide the U.S. soldier with the very best medical and surgical care, and this purpose certainly was accomplished in World War II. It is believed that the system could be improved in any future conflict with only minor changes. Perhaps the most important advance would be to commission ophthalmologists in ranks in keeping with their professional attainments and previous training. This applies particulary to men who have been selected as regional or hospital center consultants.

CHAPTER VI

Orthopedic Surgery and Rehabilitation[1]

Rex L. Diveley, M.D., and Mather Cleveland, M.D., Sc.D.

ORTHOPEDIC SURGERY, AUGUST 1942–MAY 1944

Maj. (later Col.) Rex L. Diveley, MC (fig. 158), was offered and accepted the position of Senior Consultant in Orthopedic Surgery, ETOUSA (European Theater of Operations, U.S. Army), on 4 July 1942. He reported to the Office of The Surgeon General, Washington, D.C., on 24 July 1942, where he was indoctrinated for the oversea mission. On 3 August, he was promoted to the rank of lieutenant colonel, and, on 12 August 1942, he received orders to proceed overseas. Colonel Diveley arrived at Headquarters, ETOUSA, on 26 August 1942, where he reported to Col. (later Maj. Gen.) Paul R. Hawley, MC, Chief Surgeon, ETOUSA.

Early Observations and Recommendations

The Professional Services Division in the Office of the Chief Surgeon was headed by a Director of Professional Services who supervised the professional activities of the Medical Department in the European theater and coordinated the work of consultants and specialists. There was a Chief Consultant in Surgery and a Chief Consultant in Medicine immediately subordinate to the Director of Professional Services. The senior consultant of each surgical specialty was, in turn, accountable to the Chief Consultant in Surgery.

As Senior Consultant in Orthopedic Surgery, the author's mission was to organize and supervise the conduct of orthopedic services and activities in the theater.

In September 1942, there were very few U.S. Army hospitals in the theater. Therefore, the first task was to ascertain the experiences of the British and Canadian Allies, as their organizations had been functioning many months. This consultant immediately contacted Brigadier Rowley W. Bristow, orthopedic consultant to the British Army; Mr. Reginald Watson-Jones, honorary orthopedic consultant to the RAF (Royal Air Force); Group Captain (later Air Commodore) Osmond Clark, orthopedic consultant to the RAF; Mr. H. A. T. Fairbank and Prof. Harry Platt, orthopedic consultants to EMS (Emergency Medical Service) hospitals; Mr. G. R. Girdlestone, orthopedic consultant to the Ministry of Pensions; and Prof. T. P. McMurray and Mr.

---

[1] For detailed discussions of the administrative and clinical policies and practices in orthopedic surgery in the European theater during World War II, see: Medical Department, United States Army. Surgery in World War II. Orthopedic Surgery in the European Theater of Operations. Washington: U.S. Government Printing Office, 1956.

S. L. Higgs, regional orthopedic consultants to EMS hospitals. The EMS hospitals, while civilian institutions, were receiving and treating service cases in the various outlying sections of England.

The medical sections of the various headquarters of the Allied forces in the theater were visited, to include headquarters of the RAF, the British Army, and the Canadian Army. All of these offices were in London.

The principal British and Canadian hospitals and rehabilitation depots were visited, and several of the larger EMS hospitals which were receiving service cases were surveyed and studied. This consultant was very much impressed with the type of orthopedic work being accomplished in the British Army, Canadian, and RAF hospitals. These units had had several years of experience,

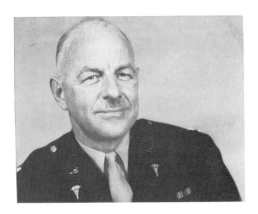

FIGURE 158.—Lt. Col. Rex L. Diveley, MC.

and this study gave the Americans a basis for the organization of the U.S. Army orthopedic services.

At this time (October 1942), there were some 10 or 12 U.S. hospitals, and all of these units were inspected as to supplies, personnel, and type of work being accomplished. The medical and surgical supply situation was quite acute, and there was an alarming shortage of materials and surgical supplies available to the U.S. Forces. To investigate further the supply situation, the author visited the British medical supply depot at Ludgershall, the U.S. Army medical supply depot at Thatcham, and various medical and surgical supply houses in London.

As a result of the observations made and the information gained from these tours and a general survey of the theater, the author recommended to the Chief Surgeon that:

1. The medical and surgical supply situation in this theater being inadequate, the quantity of supplies should be increased, and a more efficient supply service should be rendered to the various hospital units.

2. Photographic records should be made and retained in each major hospital in the theater. A photographic department should be established in the Office of the Chief Surgeon for the making and filing of medical pictorial records and for the production of motion-picture training films.

3. If hospital records and/or X-ray films were to be retained as permanent records, they should be preserved and stored by mass photography (microfilming). This would give a permanent record and conserve storage space.

4. An intensive program of military orthopedic training should be instituted and given to surgeons in the European theater, especially to those in station hospitals. This training should stress the techniques of immobilization and transportation of fractures in the forward areas as well as the definitive treatment at the base areas.

5. A rehabilitation depot should be established in the theater to care for the convalescent patient and to recondition the underdeveloped soldier who had broken in training.

6. Certain specialized bone and joint injuries and conditions should only be operated upon by the orthopedic surgeon or the especially trained traumatic surgeon.

7. More study and care should be given the problem of foot and march injuries in combat troops undergoing training. This supervised care would save many man-days lost to divisions in training.

This consultant spent the remaining few months of 1942 attempting to implement the foregoing recommendations. First, he immediately contacted British military and private surgical supply sources and was able to obtain a limited quantity of instruments and supplies which would suffice the U.S. Army until standard U.S. Army types could be obtained from the United States or be manufactured in the United Kingdom. The author contacted the Signal Corps for the procurement of photographic supplies, but this branch was unable to furnish supplies or personnel to the Office of the Chief Surgeon or to the hospital units. Therefore, through Kodak, Ltd., Harrow on the Hill, this consultant was able to procure sufficient photographic materials to activate a central laboratory in the Office of the Chief Surgeon and to equip photographic laboratories in six general hospitals. To train personnel, Kodak, Ltd., established a medical photographic school in London. Medical Department personnel were trained at this school and then assigned to the central photographic laboratory or to the general hospitals.

No equipment was available in the United Kingdom suitable for photographing records. Conferences were held with Kodak, Ltd., and, through its research department, the company developed a photographic apparatus which would photograph transparencies (such as X-ray film), hospital records, and charts as large as 14 by 17 inches. Records were photographed on 35-mm. film and could be viewed on a Recordak film reader and be reproduced to any size by photographic enlargement. This machine, after perfection, was turned over to the Medical Records Division in the Office of the Chief Surgeon.

The author presented orthopedic lectures and demonstrations in the major hospitals and to medical personnel in the smaller units and the combat divisions.

In November 1942, approval was received to train personnel in rehabilitation. Negotiations were started to establish a rehabilitation depot. This rehabilitation program as planned was to (1) provide care for the convalescent,

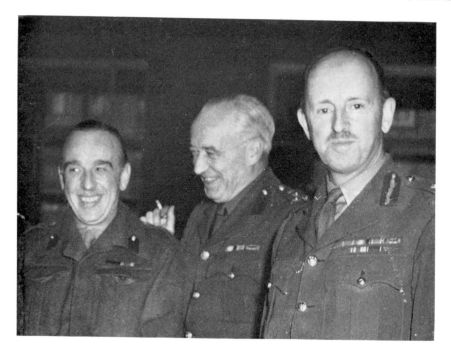

FIGURE 159.—Left to right, Brigadier L. E. J. Whitby, RAMC, Brigadier Rowley W. Bristow, and Maj. Gen. D. C. Monro, Consulting Surgeon, RAMC, at a reception given by Maj. Gen. Paul R. Hawley and consultants, Cheltenham, England, 30 April 1943.

sick, or wounded personnel to reduce their period of hospitalization and return them to their units in a fit condition for regular duty and (2) redevelop personnel who had broken down in training, in order that they might be salvaged for full duty. (Further details concerning the rehabilitation program are presented later in this chapter.)

A study of march injuries and foot conditions was made in the 29th Infantry Division. It was found that 5 percent of a company would fall out when a forced march exceeded 15 miles. It was noted also that about 1 percent of the foot troops sent overseas would need reclassification, that 2 percent of the troops in the 29th Division needed special training to overcome abnormalities of the feet and legs, and that an additional 10 percent would definitely benefit by such treatment. After this study, certain troop-training regulations were altered which very materially cut down on the number of troops lost to the Division by training injuries. Also, several bulletins of instruction on the care of the feet were issued and distributed to line officers and troops.

Activities in 1943

In the early part of 1943, this consultant worked very closely with Brigadier Bristow (fig. 159), orthopedic consultant to the British Forces, and correlated U.S. and British teaching programs and the handling of the sick and wounded in the two armies. This was accomplished both by conferences and by touring and inspecting line and hospital units in both the U.S. and the British Forces. In the latter part of January, Brigadier Bristow toured the United States, giving lectures on the operations of the Allied armies overseas with special reference to their orthopedic services.

Maj. (later Lt. Col.) William J. Stewart, MC (fig. 160), joined the Senior Consultant in Orthopedic Surgery as Associate Consultant in Orthopedic Surgery. Major Stewart spent most of his time giving lectures and demonstrations on orthopedic surgery to various active and staging hospitals. Four regional consultants in orthopedic surgery had also been appointed. These consultants handled orthopedic problems in their particular locality.

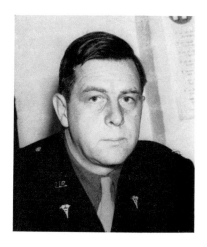

FIGURE 160.—Maj. William J. Stewart, MC.

In order to demonstrate and teach plaster of paris technique to the medical officers of the command and especially to those in combat units, schools were established in key positions throughout the theater. Medical officers and their corpsmen were ordered to these schools for a 3-day course in the handling and application of plaster of paris, splints, and casts for the immobilization of fractures and extensive wounds prior to transportation.

In the latter part of February 1943, the author was ordered on temporary duty to the North African theater to inspect hospitals and line units there and to study methods being used in the transportation and treatment of orthopedic casualties (fig. 161). This consultant returned to the European theater in the latter part of March 1943. During this trip, he obtained much information for the Chief Surgeon, ETOUSA, relative to medical supplies, field medical service, casualties, and various aspects of professional services. For orthopedic surgery, the author obtained considerable information of value relative to the training and instruction of European theater medical personnel in the transportation of fractures, plaster of paris technique in forward units, first aid treatment in the forward areas—especially in the handling of fractures, and initial orthopedic surgery in the forward areas.

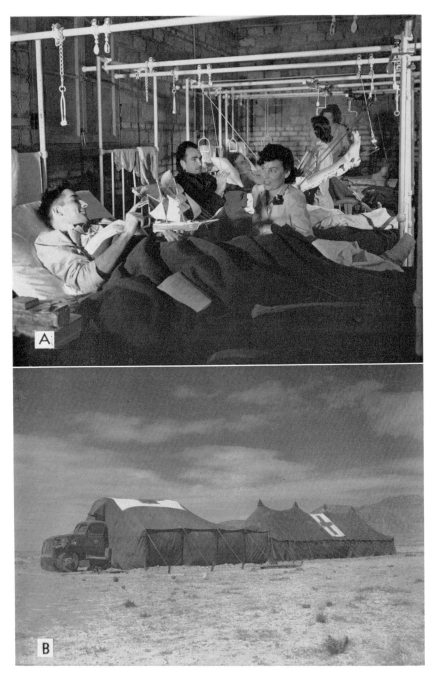

FIGURE 161.—Surgery in the North African theater approximately at the time of Colonel Diveley's visit. A. An orthopedic ward in the 38th General Hospital, Heliopolis, Egypt. B. A mobile surgical truck and tentage permitting the simultaneous operation of three surgical teams.

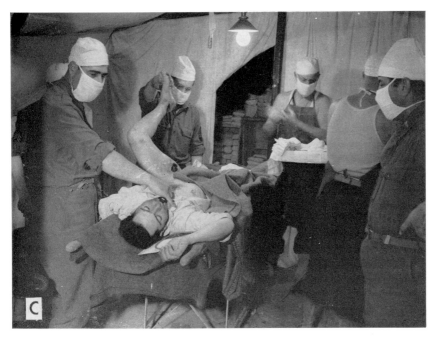

FIGURE 161.—Continued.   C. The operating room of a surgical hospital.

As this consultant toured the entire North African theater, a photographic unit from the Signal Corps traveled with him and was most helpful in obtaining thousands of feet of motion picture films. The footage was assembled into a tour report which was shown to the Chief Surgeon's staff and to various units in the European theater upon the author's return.

Much time was spent at the Queen Elizabeth Hospital and the British Amputation Center at Roehampton, England, in correlating the fitting of artificial prostheses to U.S. personnel and in making motion pictures for training films on amputation technique.   Eventually, the following training films were produced in color and with sound track:

"Rehabilitation," which provided a complete description of the program of rehabilitation and reconditioning in the theater;

"Forward Plaster Technique," which was made and used in collaboration with the British and Canadian orthopedic services and demonstrated the transportation plaster of paris technique then in use in the forward areas;

"Medical Service in the Air Force," which showed medical activities in the Eighth Air Force;

"Amputation Technique," which demonstrated the technique of the emergency amputation and the manufacture and fitting of a prosthesis for a below-knee amputation; and

"Medical Service in the North African Theater," which depicted the medical services in the various echelons of the Medical Department in the North African theater.

The Eighth Air Force was especially active with its daily bombing runs, and most of the American casualties in the European theater during 1943 originated as a result of air combat. Therefore, this author spent increased amounts of time with the Eighth Air Force units. Practical demonstrations and lectures were given in the handling of fractures, gunshot, and fragment wounds, and especially in the transportation of casualties from aircraft to the airfield first aid station and thence to the hospital for definitive treatment.

The Senior Consultant in Orthopedic Surgery and his associates spent considerable time in the investigation of the possible use of resins and plastics in the treatment of fractures. After considerable research, it was believed that there were neither time nor facilities in the European theater even for carrying out a preliminary investigation. It was considered, however, that the use of plastic splints for external as well as internal fixation was a most important subject and should be studied at some future time.

The European theater Medical Field Service School at Shrivenham was activated and the Senior Consultant in Orthopedic Surgery was responsible for several lectures and demonstrations each week, especially in the use of splints and dressings in the field.

This consultant was appointed a member of the EMS consultant group on orthopedic surgery of the British Ministry of Health. Since the EMS hospitals cared for service personnel locally, this gave the author an excellent opportunity to work out a close liaison for the handling and exchange of U.S. sick-and-wounded personnel. Monthly meetings of the consultant group were held in London.

There was some difference of opinion between general and orthopedic surgeons as to who should handle certain bone and joint conditions and fractures. General Hawley issued orders that these bone and joint conditions and all fractures would be handled by the orthopedic surgeon when available.

The orthopedic surgeons in U.S. Army hospitals had been organized, and plans were made for monthly meetings. The first meeting of the command's orthopedic surgeons was held at the 2d General Hospital near Oxford on 27 April 1943. Brigadier Bristow and Mr. Girdlestone were the guest lecturers on orthopedic subjects. The Inter-Allied Conferences on War Medicine, held monthly under the auspices of the Royal Society of Medicine, gave an opportunity for the interchange of ideas among the medical members of the Allied forces in the United Kingdom.

The author worked closely with Col. Lloyd J. Thompson, MC, Senior Consultant in Neuropsychiatry, to correlate the rehabilitation program which had been activated for convalescent neuropsychiatric patients.

General Hawley appointed a committee of three theater consultants to inspect each new hospital unit as it arrived in the theater. After a thorough study, this committee was to report to the Chief Surgeon any deficiencies in supplies or personnel and to outline a course of indoctrination for the unit in the theater.

On 23 and 24 July 1943, a combined conference of orthopedic specialists of the British Military Forces, the British Ministry of Health, and the U.S. Forces was held in London. Two of the previously mentioned motion picture training films, "Medical Service in the North African Theater" and "Forward Plaster Technique," were shown. These films were then made available to the British Forces for showing and instruction.

The American Medical Society, ETOUSA, held its first meeting on 23 June. The majority of papers and addresses were given by the orthopedic personnel of the theater.

The author returned to the Zone of Interior for a period of temporary duty extending from 20 September 1943 to 1 January 1944. Major Stewart assumed the duties of Senior Consultant in Orthopedic Surgery during the author's absence. During this temporary duty, this consultant presented many lectures and the European theater motion picture training films throughout most of the United States. He visited a majority of the rehabilitation centers in the Zone of Interior. At the request of The Surgeon General, the author helped to activate and equip a model rehabilitation center at England General Hospital, Atlantic City, N.J.

In October, during this consultant's sojourn in the United States, an orthopedic shoe repair program was instituted at the Disciplinary Training Center No. 2912, Shepton Mallet, Somersetshire. At this institution, corrective shoe repairing services could be provided. This program not only gave service to the Medical Department but was very valuable in the rehabilitation of the inmates of the disciplinary training center.

Activities Early in 1944

In 1944, after he returned to the European theater, the author placed great stress on the rehabilitation program and devoted much time to future planning for expansion of the program.

In February, this consultant was appointed Director of Rehabilitation in addition to his other duties. Therefore, a request was made for Lt. Col. (later Col.) Mather Cleveland, MC, to come to the European theater and assume the duties of Senior Consultant in Orthopedic Surgery.

Much pressure was being exerted on General Hawley by Lt. Gen. John C. H. Lee, Commanding General, SOS in The British Isles, to use osteopaths in the Medical Department. General Lee asked that they be commissioned in the Sanitary or Medical Administrative Corps and be used in the Medical Department, especially in rehabilitation activities. General Lee held the opinion that the osteopath could treat the back case better and more efficiently than could the orthopedic surgeons. General Hawley suggested a plan of assigning a group of osteopaths to the rehabilitation center at Stoneleigh where an osteopathic manipulative department was activated. As the cases were admitted to this unit complaining of low-back pain and disability, they were assigned for treatment alternately, one to the manipulative department and one to the orthopedic section. General Lee also required the assignment of orthopedic surgeons who were staying in the theater and were not busy to observe this test of talent in the treatment of low-back pain and disability. After several months of competitive treatment, the osteopathic department was discontinued in complete vindication of the Medical Department's treatment.

During the spring months of 1944, the author continued with his routine duties as Senior Consultant in Orthopedic Surgery (fig. 162). Finally, in May 1944, Colonel Cleveland arrived to relieve Colonel Diveley as orthopedic consultant. Thence, Colonel Diveley's entire time could be devoted to rehabilitation activities (pp. 477–501).

REX L. DIVELEY, M.D.

ORTHOPEDIC SURGERY, MAY 1944–JULY 1945

Chronology

As Senior Consultant in Orthopedic Surgery for the European theater, Col. Mather Cleveland, MC (fig. 163), arrived 20 days before D-day and was completely unfamiliar with the hospitals and orthopedic personnel of the theater. During a period of initiation from 20 May to 6 June 1944, he visited 42 of the hospitals in the United Kingdom in the company of Lt. Col. William J. Stewart, MC. Colonel Stewart was thoroughly familiar with all hospitals and orthopedic surgeons assigned to the theater, having served under Col. Rex L. Diveley, MC, for considerably over a year. His evaluation of the orthopedic officers and orthopedic sections of hospitals was accurate and stood up well. During this pre-D-day period, everybody was tensely awaiting the invasion of the Continent. Most of the orthopedic sections of the hospitals visited had a very low patient census in anticipation of battle casualties due to arrive.

With the invasion on 6 June, the author was assigned to consult at the 38th and 110th Station Hospitals and the 48th and 95th General Hospitals in the Southampton area. These hospitals were serving on a so-called transit basis—really as near-shore evacuation hospitals whose function was to perform essential emergency surgery and then evacuate the casualties by hospital train to the general hospitals to the north. For the most part, these hospitals received their first casualties on 8 or 9 June, gradually and in small numbers. The 110th Station Hospital, however, did an excellent job in receiving and sorting 1,000 battle casualties in 20 hours. By 12 June, the transit hospitals were busy and the chain of evacuation was filled with casualties. There were many blast injuries due to explosion of mines at sea. These casualties had profound vascular damage, with fractures or dislocations of the knee, and the like, and amputation was usually necessary.

The author's duties next led him to the Normandy beachhead in July at the time of the Saint-Lô breakout. At the time of this visit, the necessity for

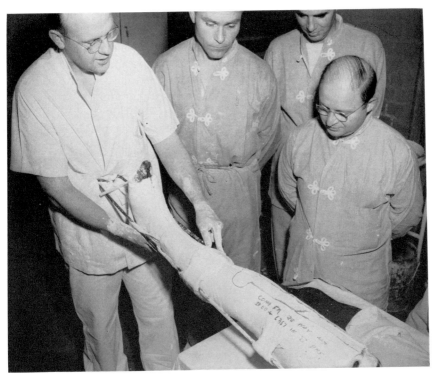

FIGURE 162.—Instruction in plaster technique being carried out under Colonel Diveley's overall supervision at the 298th General Hospital, Bristol, England, on 24 February 1944.

increased supplies of whole blood was obvious. Plasma was not an effective substitute. Soon thereafter, at the urgent request of the Chief Surgeon, whole blood began to arrive from the Zone of Interior.

This consultant then devoted much of his time to a continuous round of visits to the various medical activities of the theater, 232 altogether in the 6 months following D-day. General, station, evacuation, and field hospitals and three army headquarters were visited, consultations were held, and reports on the visits were rendered to the Chief Surgeon. In the following 5 months, the author made 107 hospital visits and visited three army headquarters as well. During the 11 months that active hostilities lasted on the Continent, approximately 340 visits were made to various medical activities by the Senior Consultant in Orthopedic Surgery.

Professional Care of Wounded

During the 6-month period after the invasion, the chief preoccupation was on setting and maintaining an optimum standard of professional care for the constant and heavy stream of battle casualties that flowed from the main line of resistance back through the field and evacuation hospitals to the general hospitals (fig. 164). While the Manual of Therapy for the European theater, published on 5 May 1944, dealt with the treatment of bone and joint casualties in general terms along fundamental lines, it soon became apparent that more specific instructions were necessary. These instructions, based on experience gained by consultants and surgeons who were caring for the wounded, were formulated in Circular Letters No. 101 (dated 30 July 1944) and No. 131 (dated 8 November 1944) issued by the Chief Surgeon, ETOUSA. These instructions dealt with circular amputation, debridement of the wound, im-

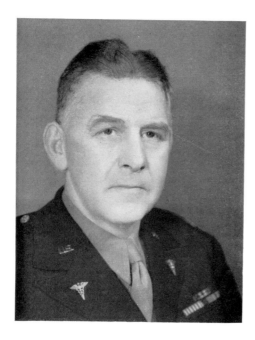

FIGURE 163.—Col. Mather Cleveland, MC.

mobilization of fractures for transportation, treatment of wounds over bones and joints in general hospitals, delayed primary closure of wounds over compound fractures (then called secondary closure), and injuries of the hands. The instructions in the circular letters were very specific and, in general, were strictly adhered to. By this means, the function of each hospital in the chain of evacuation was defined and thereby each medical echelon knew what treatment it was expected to perform, what had been done forward, and what would be done in the rear.[2]

The hand wounds were under the care of orthopedic and plastic surgeons. Hand centers were established both on the Continent and in the United Kingdom Base. Outstanding salvage work was performed in many of these centers.

---

[2] See footnote 1, p. 459.

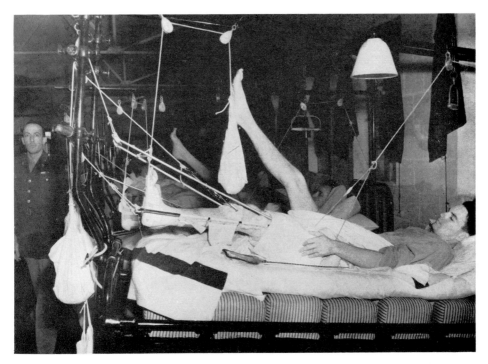

FIGURE 164.—Orthopedic casualties in a general hospital (55th General Hospital).

Problems arising from combined neurosurgical and bone and joint injuries were resolved by the Senior Consultant in Neurosurgery and the Senior Consultant in Orthopedic Surgery. Such casualties were treated at neurosurgical centers. These two activities have been described elsewhere in this history.[3]

Delayed closure of wounds over compound fractures.—Delayed closure of wounds over compound fractures was the most important single accomplishment in the care of bone and joint casualties. Some of the older surgeons were at first reluctant to try delayed closure, but younger surgeons readily acquiesced in the attempt. Successful delayed primary closure in general hospitals depended on complete or adequate debridement performed in evacuation hospitals. The failures, with breakdown of the wounds and resulting bone infection, could be traced to early technical failure or delay, sometimes unavoidable, in the debridement. This delayed primary or immediate primary closure of wounds over fractures was not new. It had been done in World War I, in small numbers to be sure, but it had been forgotten or ignored. The effort to reestablish the idea of closure of wounds over compound fractures reemphasized the saying: "They who forget the past are condemned to repeat it."

---

[3] See footnote 1, p. 459.

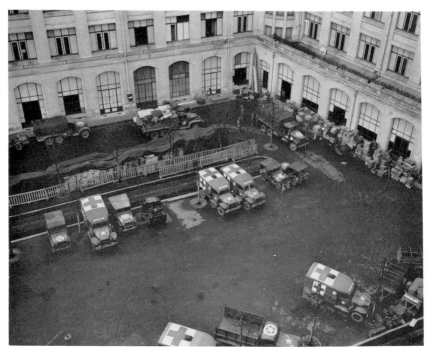

FIGURE 165.—The 198th General Hospital arriving in Paris in January 1945.

Orthopedic Surgeons in the European Theater

The European theater, at the close of hostilities, had a total of 281 hospitals of which 146 were general hospitals. Among these general hospitals, only slightly over 10 percent were affiliated units. These affiliated hospitals arrived very adequately staffed with actually an overabundance of trained personnel. The orthopedic sections of these affiliated hospitals which arrived in 1942 and 1943 were plundered to obtain chiefs of orthopedic sections for other hospitals arriving later with no trained orthopedic personnel.

By the end of 1944 and early 1945, general hospitals were reaching the theater "staffed with bodies," as the saying was, but with little or no trained personnel. The problem of finding chiefs for orthopedic sections (and other chiefs also) became almost impossible to solve (fig. 165).

Of the 16,000 civilian doctors of medicine who served in uniform in the European theater, there were only 63 diplomates of the American Board of Orthopaedic Surgery. In addition to these, there were 95 partially trained orthopedic surgeons and 85 young general surgeons with training in the handling of fractures. This hard core of about 240 medical officers was responsible for the professional care of approximately 250,000 bone-and-joint casualties and injuries among U.S. Army troops and, in addition, of many thousands of prisoners of war.

The tables of organization of the various hospitals in the theater called for a total of almost 450 trained orthopedic specialists, Military Occupational Specialty 3153, B or C rating or better. There were only 217 medical officers who could possibly be considered as possessing these skills. The proper utilization of available orthopedic surgeons was, and in the future will be, a matter of great moment, since at least 40 or 45 percent of battle casualties and injuries will invariably involve bones and joints.

It was the author's considered opinion that each field army should have had as consultant a highly trained orthopedic surgeon with the rank of colonel. Such a consultant could have supervised and trained younger surgeons in evacuation or other army hospitals where the bone and joint casualties were received for debridement and applications of proper splints for evacuation to hospitals in the communications zone. The general hospitals needed one or, if available, two orthopedic surgeons to treat compound or simple fractures and amputations and to handle other bone and joint problems that were received. Large station hospitals, if serving large bodies of troops in training or if acting as general hospitals, also needed a trained orthopedic surgeon.

There will never be an oversupply of these officers in the event of another great national emergency, and therefore careful planning will be required to see that all are effectively used.

Proper Utilization of Experienced General Hospitals

The utilization and proper location of experienced, affiliated hospitals was of the utmost importance. At the time of the invasion, most of the affiliated general hospitals in the European theater during World War II (12 to 14 in number) had been in the theater for from a year to 18 months. They were given priority for movement to the Continent. This was a reward for service, but unfortunately it meant that during the first 6 or 8 weeks after D-day, the "first team" was sitting on the bench. That is, they were staging, crossing the Channel, and in the process of being set up. A good many of the personnel of these hospitals were used on temporary duty to augment other hospitals, to be sure, but the smooth operation of well-established hospitals was missing. At the beginning, most of these hospitals were first set up on the beachland and later moved to other parts of France or Belgium (fig. 166). In planning their second moves, it would have been ideal if they could have been dispersed in such a way as to serve as parent hospitals for the hospital centers and base sections later established on the Continent. At times, two or more of these affiliated general hospitals were assigned to a single center and, at the close of hostilities, there were two hospital centers at Reims with some 17 new and inexperienced general hospitals and with no older experienced hospital within call. These older affiliated general hospitals furnished the junior consultants in all branches of medicine and surgery.

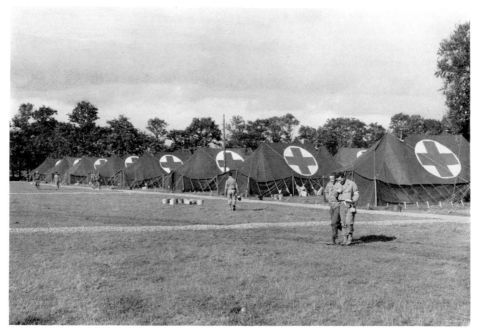

FIGURE 166.—The 25th General Hospital, affiliated unit of the Cincinnati General Hospital and the University of Cincinnati, Ohio, in temporary location at Lison, France, September 1944.

Junior Consultants

It was impossible for a single senior orthopedic consultant, in spite of his making more than 30 visits a month to various medical installations and traveling thousands of miles, to cover the theater adequately. The young surgeons needed professional advice and supervision, in many instances, at frequent intervals.

In late November or December 1944, seven junior (regional) consultants in orthopedic surgery were appointed in the United Kingdom Base—each to cover one of the seven hospital centers in addition to their duties as chiefs of orthopedic sections at their own general hospitals. Most of these junior consultants performed very valuable service in helping their colleagues to maintain a high standard of professional care for the wounded and injured soldiers. At that time, and in fact during most of the campaign on the Continent, those with fractures of the long bones were all evacuated to the United Kingdom, where the holding period before evacuation to the Zone of Interior was 120 days.

Most general hospitals on the Continent were serving on a transit basis, with a holding period of only 30 days. During a good part of the winter of

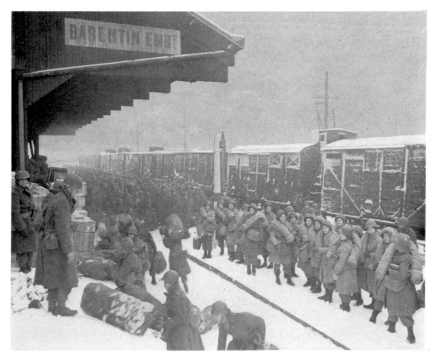

FIGURE 167.—The 221st General Hospital on the move in the dead of winter, 26 January 1945.

1944–45, many of the continental general hospitals were moving from a first to a second location (fig. 167); consequently, junior consultants in orthopedic surgery on the Continent were not appointed until the spring of 1945, when nine such appointments were made. The cessation of hostilities supervened so shortly thereafter that only a little over half of these appointees actually served effectively. If these continental junior consultants could have been appointed earlier, they would have helped materially in enhancing and standardizing the care of the wounded with bone and joint problems.

The reports of the junior consultants had to travel a long road through channels before a few of them eventually reached Colonel Cleveland. Some of these reports never arrived. The junior and senior consultants should have ready access to each other.

The Senior Consultant in Orthopedic Surgery held two meetings in London with the United Kingdom junior consultants in December of 1944 and June of 1945. The continental junior consultants met with him in Paris in June 1945. Out of these conferences came the revision of the orthopedic portion of the Manual of Therapy.[4]

---

[4] See footnote 1, p. 459.

Rank for Orthopedic Surgeons

For the responsibility which the orthopedic surgeon carried, there was no provision made for commensurate rank. There was actually no provision in the tables of organization for theater consultants, and any promotion to the grade of colonel had to be borrowed from some new hospital or hospital center that entered the theater with vacancies in these higher grades.

There were approximately 12 outstanding orthopedic surgeons who had served as many as 3 years in the grade of major in various general hospitals of the theater. It was the firm conviction of the Senior Consultant in Orthopedic Surgery that each of these officers should have been promoted to the grade of lieutenant colonel, and such recommendations were made. Of the 12 orthopedic surgeons recommended for such promotion, only one reached that grade while in the European theater.

It was difficult to explain to an orthopedic surgeon why the dental officer, the roentgenologist, the psychiatrist, the chief of laboratory, the chief nurse, and so on, in a 1,000-bed general hospital should, by table of organization, be advanced to the grade of lieutenant colonel, while the orthopedic surgeon, who was responsible for the professional care of 40 or 45 percent of the wounded, could not advance beyond a majority. Such discrepancies should be remedied so that responsible and outstanding officers can be given rank commensurate with services rendered.

Meetings of Senior Consultants

The position of senior consultant in the European theater carried great responsibility and afforded endless possibilities for improving the professional care of the sick and wounded and maintaining a high level of such care.

When possible, the senior consultants met weekly at headquarters in Cheltenham, London, Valognes, and Paris as the Office of the Chief Surgeon moved forward, and once a month the Chief Surgeon met with his consultants. The most inspiring meetings to this consultant were the informal weekly gatherings presided over by Col. (later Brig. Gen.) Elliott C. Cutler, MC. These were high level discussions of all prevailing problems, in which suggestions were freely offered and were usually well received by all 12 or 13 surgical specialists present.

During active hostilities, two meetings were held with British and Canadian consultants and one with all the Allied consultants. With the exception of the polylingual meeting with translations into and out of French and Russian, which instantaneous translation would have helped, these meetings were extremely helpful.

The Chief Surgeon supported the consultants to the hilt if he thought they were correct and did not hesitate to correct or reprimand them if they were wrong. The writer will always consider it a great privilege to have served with the senior consultants in the European theater during World War II.

MATHER CLEVELAND, M.D.

REHABILITATION

Activities Centered in the United Kingdom, 1942–44

Soon after arriving in England in August 1942, Lt. Col. (later Col.) Rex. L. Diveley surveyed all U.S. Army Hospitals that were then functioning. During this survey, he observed that a significant percentage of military personnel was being readmitted to hospitals because the men were unable to carry on the physical rigors of their former duties. An examination of a sampling of these patients revealed that their prolonged stay in hospitals had definitely deteriorated them mentally as well as physically. No attempt was being made to bring these hospitalized personnel to their former physical capacity before discharge from the hospital. The result was a great loss of man-days to the Army.

Colonel Diveley immediately undertook to ascertain how the British services had solved this problem. It was found that the RAF, the British Army, and the Royal Navy had established special convalescent depots to which convalescent, sick-and-wounded personnel, after hospitalization, were being sent for rehabilitation or reconditioning. In these depots, a complete and comprehensive program of exercises was given to restore these men to their former physical capacity.

In the fall of 1942, Colonel Diveley outlined for the Chief Surgeon a plan for the establishment of a convalescent rehabilitation center in the European theater. He proposed the establishment of a center where sick or wounded military personnel could be sent as soon as they became convalescent and no longer needed active surgical and medical attention in a hospital. At these centers, he suggested a complete and supervised physical, educational, military, and recreational program which could be given to restore patients to their former physical and mental capacity.

This plan, in general, was approved by the Chief Surgeon. He issued orders to select a site, to prepare a provisional T/O&E (table of organization and equipment), and to train personnel who would be required to operate such a convalescent center.

Rehabilitation and reconditioning facilities

Rehabilitation Center No. 1.—After the author had inspected several available sites, the All-Saints Hospital, Bromsgrove, Worcestershire, was selected and procured. A provisional T/O&E was prepared by the Operations Division, Office of the Chief Surgeon, based upon the personnel and equipment of a 150-bed station hospital. Five officers and six enlisted men with proper qualifications were trained at the British 102d Convalescent Depot at Kingston and the British Army School of Physical Training at Aldershot. On 7 April 1943, the 16th Station Hospital, augmented by specially trained personnel, opened Rehabilitation Center No. 1 in the All-Saints Hospital. The essential staff consisted of Maj. (later Lt. Col.) Clayton H. Hixson, MC, Commanding

Officer; Captain Gullingrud, Executive Officer; Maj. (later Col.) Frank E. Stinchfield, MC (fig. 168), Chief of Professional Services; Capt. (later Lt. Col.) Marcus J. Stewart, MC (fig. 169), orthopedic service; 2d Lt. (later Capt.) Gerald F. Seeders, Inf., Director of Physical Training; and 2d Lt. Paul E. Hall, MAC, Director of Military Training. Under the efficient professional guidance of Major Stinchfield, a well-balanced physical and military program was developed (fig. 170). Patients were admitted from station and general hospitals as soon as they became convalescent, were able to be up and around, and could care for their own toilet. Although the hospital load of the theater was very light, the census of the center had rapidly increased to 431 by 1 September 1943.

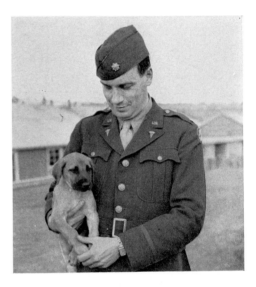

FIGURE 168.—Maj. Frank E. Stinchfield, MC, at All-Saints Hospital, Bromsgrove, Worcestershire, England.

It soon became evident that the facilities at Bromsgrove and the staff of the 150-bed station hospital were insufficient to handle the anticipated convalescent patient load of the theater. Consequently, a general hospital site at Stoneleigh Park, near Kenilworth, Warwickshire, was secured, and the 8th Convalescent Hospital replaced the 16th Station Hospital as the operating unit of Rehabilitation Center No. 1. Key personnel of the 16th Station Hospital were transferred to and retained in the 8th Convalescent Hospital, which opened the center at Stoneleigh on 5 October 1943. Major Stinchfield assumed command of the center at the new location.

By December 1943, the census of trainees at the rehabilitation center had reached 1,300 (fig. 171). At this time, it was necessary to release the 8th Convalescent Hospital for assignment to a field army. This unit was replaced by the 307th Station Hospital (750 beds). Key personnel of the 8th Convalescent Hospital were retained for assignment to the 307th Station Hospital, and Major Stinchfield continued in command. This exchange of units was consummated on 5 December 1943. In January 1944, the census at Rehabilitation Center No. 1 showed over 1,700 officers and enlisted trainees.

By the time D-day, 6 June 1944, arrived, the patient load at Rehabilitation Center No. 1 had increased tremendously and, with the assault on the Continent, further expansion of its facilities became extremely necessary. After many unsuccessful attempts to obtain the Irish Labor Camp (Ministry of Works), adjoining the center, the Camp was made available on 19 June 1944. This allowed for an expansion of 700 patients and increased the overall capacity at Rehabilitation Center No. 1 to approximately 3,700 (fig. 172).

Rehabilitation Center No. 2 (Officers).—Early during the operation of Rehabilitation Center No. 1, it became evident that officers and enlisted men

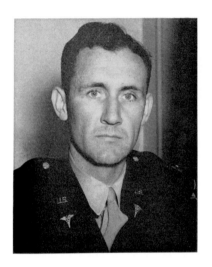

Figure 169.—Capt. Marcus J. Stewart, MC.

should be segregated when undergoing a program of convalescent rehabilitation. Accordingly, a rehabilitation center for officers, Rehabilitation Center No. 2, was activated at All-Saints Hospital, the original site of Rehabilitation Center No. 1. A detachment of trained personnel from the 307th Station Hospital was assigned to operate this facility by working with members of the 1st Auxiliary Surgical Group, which was now temporarily quartered at Bromsgrove. Later, when the 77th Station Hospital had been made available for the rehabilitation program, Detachment B of this hospital relieved the detachment of personnel from the 307th Station Hospital in the operation of Rehabilitation Center No. 2. This change took place on 23 February 1944. Still later, the 123d Station Hospital was assigned the mission of operating the rehabilitation center for officers.

Reconditioning Center No. 1.—As the patient load of the theater continued to increase, and additional centers became necessary, experiences indicated that certain convalescent patients needed only general exercises or body hardening to bring them to their former physical capacity (reconditioning), as contrasted to others who required certain specific remedial exercises in addi-

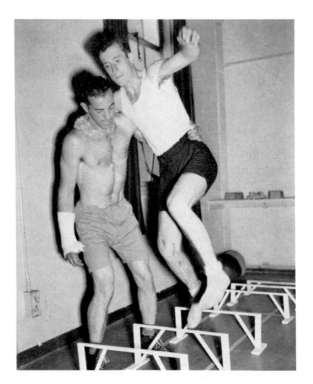

FIGURE 170.—Remedial exercises at Rehabilitation
Center No. 1 (16th Station Hospital), All-Saints
Hospital.

tion to general body hardening (rehabilitation). Accordingly, an additional
unit was requisitioned to establish a reconditioning center. A general hospital
site was secured at Erlestoke Park, near Devizes, Wiltshire. This site had
accommodations for about 1,500 convalescent patient-trainees. The 77th Station Hospital (750 beds) was designated the operating unit for this new center.
The staff of the 77th Station Hospital was ordered to Rehabilitation Center
No. 1 (307th Station Hospital) for indoctrination and orientation. Since
the entire unit would not be required to operate Reconditioning Center No.
1, a detachment of the 77th Station Hospital, as mentioned earlier, was ordered
to operate Rehabiltation Center No. 2 for officers. The remaining unit personnel
of the 77th Station Hospital, having completed their training and indoctrination at Rehabilitation Center No. 1, moved to Erlestoke Park, and during
March 1944 began to operate Reconditioning Center No. 1.

The facilities of Reconditioning Center No. 1 at Erlestoke Park, however,
were limited, and this plant was needed for a general hospital. It was necessary
to procure an additional site. A military campsite was secured at Packington
Park, near Coventry. The advance party of the 77th Station Hospital moved
into this site on 5 July.

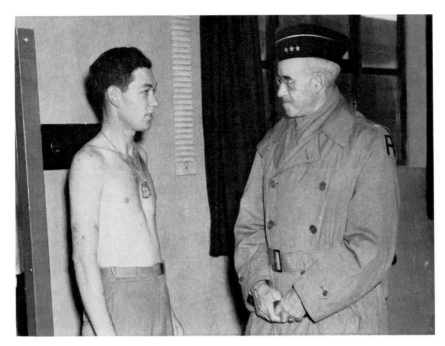

FIGURE 171.—Lt. Gen. Omar N. Bradley, chatting with a patient at the 307th Station Hospital, 3 December 1943.

At the request of the British War Office, arrangements were made for an interchange of convalescent soldiers undergoing rehabilitation. The purpose of this exchange was to further Anglo-American relationships. The interchange was started during the first week in June 1944, and a party of British convalescent patients was continually maintained at Reconditioning Center No. 1 throughout the year, except during the change in location of the center.

Rehabilitation Center No. 3.—With the increase of the patient census following D-day, it became apparent that an additional number of rehabilitation beds would be needed. The 313th Station Hospital was selected for conversion into a 3,000-bed rehabilitation center. This unit was operating a station hospital at Fremington, Devonshire. The site was not suitable for a 3,000-bed center as its capacity was limited to about 2,000 patients. It was decided, however, to use this plant temporarily. The staff was indoctrinated at Rehabilitation Center No. 1, and, on 20 July 1944, this unit started to receive patients for rehabilitation. Physical training instructors, as well as military and physical training officers, were assigned to augment the regular staff.

Not long after activation of Rehabilitation Center No. 3, a suitable site was obtained at Warminster Barracks, Warminster, Wiltshire. After appropriate adaptation of the site, Rehabilitation Center No. 3 was moved to Warminster and began operations there on 21 December 1944.

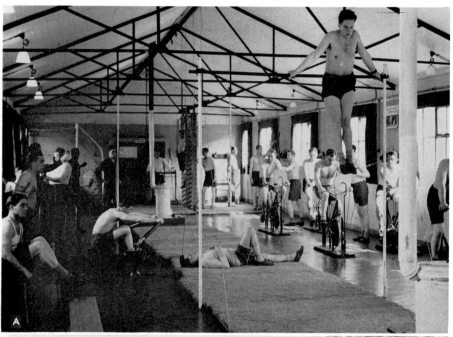

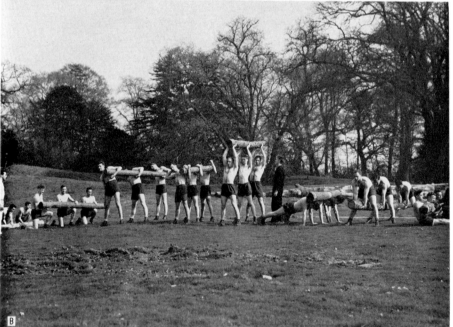

FIGURE 172.—Full-scale rehabilitation activities at Rehabilitation Center No. 1, 307th Station Hospital, Stoneleigh Park.   A. A remedial gymnasium.   B. A log drill.

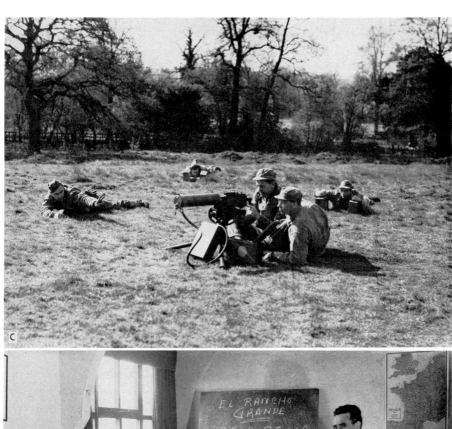

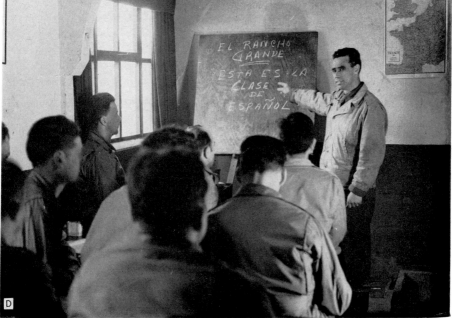

FIGURE 172.—Continued.   C. Military training .   D. Educational training.

Rehabilitation Center No. 4.—By the latter part of August 1944, the facilities of the three rehabilitation centers and the Reconditioning Center were about filled, and a unit and a site for an additional center were requested. The 314th Station Hospital was committed to the mission. The staff, then operating a tented hospital at Truro, Devonshire, was ordered to Rehabilitation Center No. 1 for indoctrination. A site was selected at Honiton-Heathfield which would accommodate some 2,300 trainees and which, with tented expansion, could handle a total of 3,000 patients. On 13 September 1944, the unit was activated as Rehabilitation Center No. 4 and began to receive convalescent patients.

Conversion to convalescent centers.—As the first rehabilitation and reconditioning centers began operations, it was very apparent that the standard T/O&E for a 750-bed station hospital did not provide for sufficient personnel with appropriate qualifications to operate a large rehabilitation center. General Hawley, when the difficulty was brought to his attention, directed that the Operations Division of his office make a study of the conversion of the T/O&E of a 750-bed station hospital to that appropriate for a 3,000-bed rehabilitation center and the conversion of a 250-bed station hospital to a 1,000-bed reconditioning center. Colonel Diveley and Colonel Stinchfield collaborated in this study. With concurrences from the ETOUSA G–1 (personnel and administration) and G–3 (operations and training), special tables of distribution and allowances were created for 1,000-bed reconditioning centers and 3,000-bed rehabilitation centers. These tables were sent to the War Department, which, the author learned on 23 June 1944, had approved them for publication as T/O&E's for 1,000-bed and 3,000-bed convalescent centers. Early in December 1944, the War Department ordered conversion of five hospitals on the theater troop list to convalescent centers in accordance with the new T/O&E's. This was accomplished by converting four station hospitals (750 beds) to 3,000-bed convalescent centers and one station hospital to a convalescent center of 1,000 beds. The convalescent centers thus activated were designated as follows:

New designation	Old designation	Bed capacity
825th Convalescent Center__	77th Station Hospital (Reconditioning Center No. 1)__	3,000
826th Convalescent Center__	307th Station Hospital (Rehabilitation Center No. 1)__	3,700
827th Convalescent Center__	313th Station Hospital (Rehabilitation Center No. 3)__	3,000
828th Convalescent Center__	314th Station Hospital (Rehabilitation Center No. 4)__	2,300
833d Convalescent Camp____	123d Station Hospital (Rehabilitation Center No. 2)__	400

Convalescent hospitals on the Continent.—Upon the request of the Chief Surgeon, the author proceeded to the Continent in August 1944 to survey the requirements for reconditioning and rehabilitation and to examine the conduct of the convalescent training program within such station and general hospitals as were operating. This consultant recommended that, because of the short evacuation policy in effect on the Continent, it would be impracticable to conduct a full rehabilitation program there at this time.

On 12 September 1944, upon request of the Chief Surgeon, the writer made a second trip to the Continent. He inspected the 7th and 8th Convalescent Hospitals, which were operating under the communications zone. After this visit, he recommended that additional physical- and military-training personnel be assigned for the more efficient operation of these units, if they were to continue functioning as communications zone units. This recommendation was concurred in by the Chief Surgeon. Cadres were selected from among trainees at the training school at Rehabilitation Center No. 1 and were sent to these units. This consultant followed up these actions with frequent visits to the Continent to survey and maintain contact with the 7th and 8th Convalescent Hospitals.

The 7th Convalescent Hospital was established at Étampes and had facilities for handling approximately 1,700 convalescent patients. With the addition of military- and physical-training personnel, it established a commendable convalescent training program. The unit was handicapped by the added function of operating as a station hospital to care for personnel of the 19th Reinforcement Depot, which was adjacent.

The 8th Convalescent Hospital had its initial location at Barneville, on the Channel, later moving to Valognes, near Cherbourg. The Valognes site was not ideal and was capable of housing only some 2,000 convalescent patients. But, with the addition of a cadre of military- and physical-training personnel, this unit operated a fair convalescent training program.

Organization for supervision

Rehabilitation activities in the Office of the Chief Surgeon were begun on the initiative of Colonel Diveley and incidental to his primary duties as Senior Consultant in Orthopedic Surgery. On 25 February 1944, Colonel Diveley was appointed Director of Rehabilitation in addition to his other duties as Senior Consultant in Orthopedic Surgery, and Major Stewart, who had just reported to the Office of the Chief Surgeon, was named as his assistant. As a result of a special conference attended by General Hawley, Colonel Eyster of the G-3 Section, ETOUSA, and Colonel Diveley, it was deemed advisable to have a representative of the Chief Surgeon on the G-3 staff section in order to correlate the rehabilitation program. This was accomplished by the appointment of Maj. (later Lt. Col.) Milton S. Thompson, MC, to this duty on 15 February 1944.

As the rehabilitation work in the office increased, Capt. (later Maj.) Julian A. Sterling, MC, from Rehabilitation Center No. 1, was assigned to duty as an assistant. Several clerks, artists, secretaries, and a physical training instructor were also added to the staff. Capt. (later Maj.) Blaise P. Salatich, MC, Medical Liaison Officer from Headquarters, U.S. Strategic Air Forces, ETOUSA, to the Rehabilitation Division, Office of the Chief Surgeon, reported for duty on 18 April 1944.

On 3 June 1944, by Office Order No. 32, Office of the Chief Surgeon, the Rehabilitation Division was formally established as an independent division within the Office of the Chief Surgeon. Colonel Diveley was appointed chief of the division. The functions of the division were listed as follows:

1. To direct and conduct research in rehabilitation procedures.

2. To control rehabilitation technical operations.

3. To direct the training of personnel for implementation of the rehabilitation program.

4. To formulate policies on rehabilitation.

5. To consult on matters relating to the conservation of manpower. All these functions had been inaugurated during the previous 6 months by Colonel Diveley, the Director of Rehabilitation.

On 16 June 1944, a conference was held with members of the ETOUSA G–1 and G–3 staffs and the Field Force Replacement System at which Col. David E. Liston, MC, Deputy Chief Surgeon, ETOUSA, clarified the obligations of the Chief Surgeon in carrying out the program of rehabilitation in the theater, as follows:

1. The Chief Surgeon would expand the convalescent training program as the need arose and insofar as such expansion would not jeopardize availability of beds for hospitalization. Hospital personnel would in each instance be supplemented by branch immaterial personnel to supervise military training coincident with physical reconditioning. Such personnel would not be charged to the Medical Department.

2. The Chief Surgeon would discharge patients to the Field Force Replacement System when conditioning had proceeded to that point where the individual would not be physically harmed by normal physical exertion and would be capable of returning to his former or new occupation after 2 or 3 weeks further hardening in the Field Force Replacement System.

By the latter part of June, base section surgeons had appointed rehabilitation officers to their staffs. Maj. William N. Brewer, MC, was appointed in the Western Base Section, and 2d Lt. (later 1st Lt.) Robert S. Rice, MAC, was appointed in the Southern Base Section.

On 12 July 1944, the forward echelon of the Office of the Chief Surgeon moved from the United Kingdom to the far shore. By decision of the Chief Surgeon, the Rehabilitation Division remained in the United Kingdom and was attached to the Office of the Surgeon, United Kingdom Base.

In August 1944, a request was made that a rehabilitation division be established in the Office of the Surgeon, United Kingdom Base. Major Brewer, who had previously been the rehabilitation officer for Western Base Section, was appointed chief of this subdivision of rehabilitation in the Office of the Surgeon, United Kingdom Base. He selected a staff of officers and enlisted assistants.

Later in 1944, Maj. (later Lt. Col.) Richard F. Kelsey, MC, a staff member of Rehabilitation Center No. 2, was added to the staff of the Rehabilitation Division, Office of the Chief Surgeon. Maj. H. Heim, Ord, was assigned to duty with the Rehabilitation Division, Office of the Chief Surgeon, to coordinate the information and education work within the convalescent training program.

In the latter part of December, word was received from the Office of the Chief Surgeon, then at Paris, that the Rehabilitation Division would move from its location with the Office of the Surgeon, United Kingdom Base, to Paris. At that time, the Rehabilitation Division, Office of the Chief Surgeon, in addition to an artist-statistician and clerks, consisted of the following officers: Colonel Diveley, chief of the Division; Colonel Thompson, Rehabilitation Liaison Officer from the Office of the Chief Surgeon to the G–3 Section, Headquarters, ETOUSA; Major Sterling, assistant chief of the Division; Major Kelsey, Consultant in Rehabilitation and Hospital and Convalescent Center Inspector; Major Salatich, Rehabilitation Liaison Officer from Headquarters, U.S. Strategic Air Forces, ETOUSA; and Major Heim, Coordinator for Information and Education Activities.

Similarly, in the Office of the Surgeon, United Kingdom Base, Major Brewer, was Chief, Division of Rehabilitation; Capt. Herzl M. Daskal, MC, was Hospital Inspector and Consultant in Rehabilitation; and 1st Lt. Andrew M. Gould, MAC, was Administrative Assistant.

Special programs

Convalescent training program in hospitals.—With the guidance of experience in the European theater and instructions from the Office of The Surgeon General in Washington, a general program of convalescent training and education was initiated for each station and general hospital in the theater (fig. 173). Much opposition was evidenced by hospital staffs to the introduction of such a program. This was due for the most part to a lack of understanding on the part of professional men in the concepts of convalescent rehabilitation. The program at the rehabilitation centers progressed most satisfactorily, but the program within the station and general hospitals was very sluggish, and little interest was evidenced. It became necessary to undertake special indoctrination and training activities to encourage more active convalescent training programs in hospitals (pp. 492–494).

A constant check was maintained on the convalescent program in hospital units. Two or three representatives of the Rehabilitation Division continuously inspected the programs and gave indoctrination lectures. Ward surgeons were made aware of their responsibilities in the conservation of manpower through an adequate convalescent program and through the proper reclassification of sick-and-wounded military personnel to duty.

Reclassification.—Considerable difficulty was evidenced in both rehabilitation centers and hospitals in the proper reclassification of personnel being returned to duty. Through the efforts of the Rehabilitation Division and the Ground Force Replacement System (formerly the Field Force Replacement System), classification teams were selected and trained. These teams were placed in special hospitals, hospital centers, and rehabilitation centers to orient personnel in the proper reclassification of sick-and-wounded personnel.

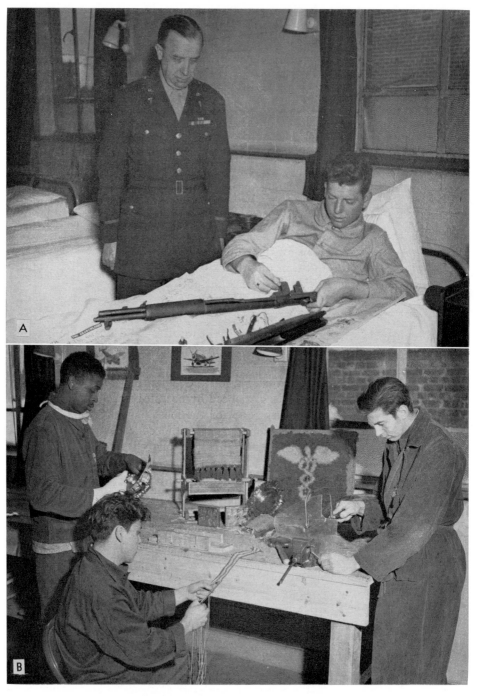

FIGURE 173.—Rehabilitation in hospitals.   A. Rehabilitation in a general hospital ward.
B. Occupational therapy in a general hospital.

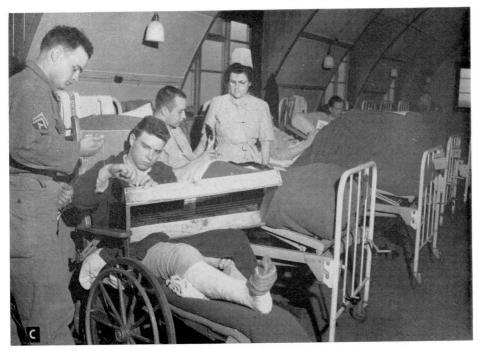

FIGURE 173.—Continued.   C. Rehabilitation in a station hospital ward.

Rehabilitation in station hospitals acting as general hospitals.—By 1 August 1944, the general hospitals were filled to capacity. Many convalescent patients in the general hospitals still needed surgical dressings or followup medical care. These patients could not be sent to rehabilitation centers but should have been evacuated from general hospitals to make bed space for casualties who required definitive medical or surgical care and treatment. The situation was alleviated by the designation of certain station hospitals to act as general hospitals in the care of the slightly wounded and those convalescent patients still requiring some active medical or surgical care. The Rehabilitation Division, appreciating the fact that over half of the patients in these station hospitals would be in the convalescent training program, took steps to upgrade their rehabilitation programs. Special supplies and training aids were furnished, and special training personnel were attached to each hospital.

Army Air Forces participation.—Initially, about 10 or 15 percent of the trainees in the rehabilitation centers were patients from the Army Air Forces. It was believed that more specialized training should be given to these trainees. Brig. Gen. (later Maj. Gen.) Malcolm C. Grow, Surgeon, Eighth Air Force, was contacted through Col. Herbert B. Wright, MC, in regard to obtaining specialized personnel to carry on this mission. However, cooperation of the Air Forces at this time was very meager.

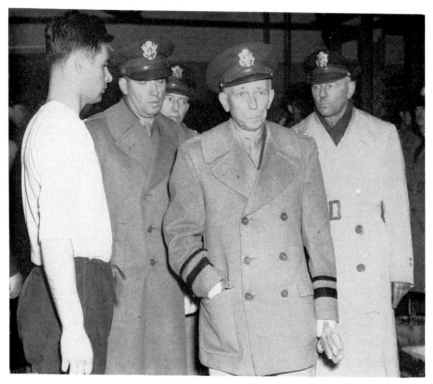

FIGURE 174.—Maj. Gen. Norman T. Kirk inspecting the 307th Station Hospital. Others pictured are, left to right, Colonel Stinchfield, Brig. Gen. Malcolm C. Grow (partially obstructed by Colonel Stinchfield), and Colonel Diveley.

In February 1944, following a special visit and inspection of hospitals and rehabilitation centers by Maj. Gen. Norman T. Kirk, The Surgeon General, Maj. Gen. David N. W. Grant, the Air Surgeon, General Hawley, and General Grow (fig. 174), a coordinated program of rehabilitation training for Air Force personnel was outlined, and the Office of the Chief Surgeon, ETOUSA, was assured the cooperation of the Army Air Forces in the theater. An Air Force liaison officer to the Rehabilitation Division, Office of the Chief Surgeon, was requested and obtained. Special surveys were made to determine needs of the program, and training aids and equipment were supplied as required, not only to all convalescent centers but also to the program in each station and general hospital.

General Grow, now Surgeon, U.S. Strategic Air Forces, assigned flight surgeons to duty with the six general hospitals that were caring for most of the Air Forces personnel. These flight surgeons supervised the convalescent care and rehabilitation of Air Forces personnel in accordance with directives of the Chief Surgeon. The Air Forces provided excellent cooperation in supplying personnel and training equipment for the rehabilitation program. Rehabilita-

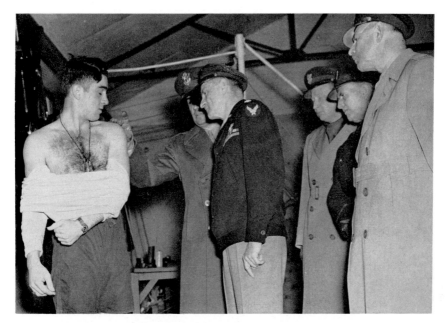

Figure 175.—Lt. Gen. Carl Spaatz, Commanding General, U.S. Strategic Air Forces in Europe, listens to an explanation by Colonel Stinchfield of treatment being provided.

tion Center No. 1 was designated as the center for Air Force enlisted men, while officers were sent to Rehabilitation Center No. 2 (fig. 175).

Amputee morale team.—At the request of the Chief Surgeon, an "amputee morale team" was organized in the early part of November 1944 to visit all hospitals. The team demonstrated the use of prostheses and showed a motion picture film on what could be accomplished by a man who had lost his arms. This aided greatly in lifting the morale of those personnel who had lost a limb.

Personnel and training

Special rehabilitation and reconditioning personnel.—With the steady growth of the rehabilitation and reconditioning programs, it was found necessary to train a large number of officers and enlisted men to be used in the activation of other centers and to be assigned to hospitals for the convalescent training program (fig. 176). An initial allotment of 50 officers and 100 enlisted men was made available for this training and subsequent assignment to specialized positions. With the continued growth of the rehabilitation program and as requirements for trained personnel became greater, the Ground Force Replacement System, ETOUSA, G-1, was asked to provide additional officers and enlisted men of either general- or limited-assignment status for training as physical education instructors and directors of other

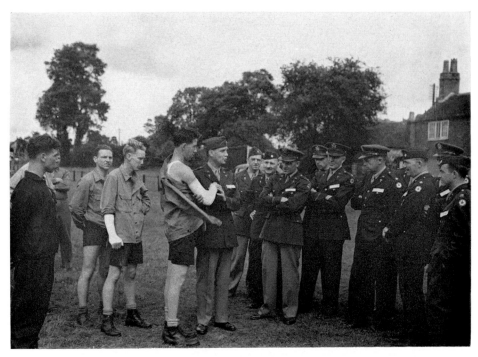

FIGURE 176.—Major Stinchfield at a demonstration for student officers at Bromsgrove, Worcestershire, during July 1943.

duties pertinent to the rehabilitation (convalescent training) program. On 6 July 1944, an additional 100 officers and 300 enlisted men were allotted to the rehabilitation program for training purposes. This made a total of 150 officers and 400 men available for use in the rehabilitation program.

Training and indoctrination of personnel engaged in the hospital convalescent training program.—To overcome initial resistance to the hospital convalescent training program and to orient the staffs of the various hospital units involved, indoctrination lectures were given, and a motion picture film on rehabilitation was shown. There was also a lack of trained personnel to implement the convalescent training program in hospitals. To obviate this, a special school was established at the rehabilitation center where wardmasters from various station and general hospitals were sent for a course of training in the conduct of a convalescent training program (fig. 177). Upon returning to their units, these trained men were able to indoctrinate the hospital staff as well as other wardmasters and enlisted personnel in the proper principles of the convalescent training program.

Later, in order to encourage a more active hospital program several conferences were held with the hospital personnel. In May 1944, the commanding officer, rehabilitation officer, and orthopedic surgeon of each station and general hospital were ordered to Rehabilitation Center No. 1 for an orienta-

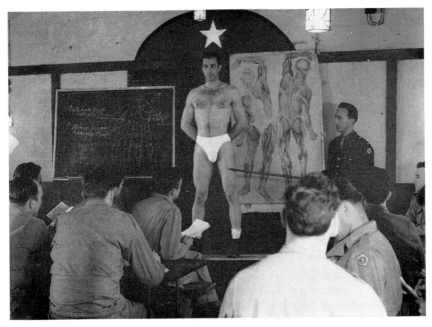

FIGURE 177.—A class in anatomy for physical training instructors at the 307th Station
Hospital, Rehabilitation Center No. 1, Stoneleigh Park, Warwickshire.

tion conference. This meeting was addressed by General Hawley. Following his address, indoctrination papers on representative activities and results
of rehabilitation were given. A model program was inspected during the
afternoon. In addition to this meeting, two regional conferences were held
later in the month with rehabilitation officers from hospitals in the various
base sections.

To assist in the conduct of the hospital convalescent program, several
additional publications were issued by the Rehabilitation Division. One, titled
"Bed Exercises for the Convalescent Patient," described and illustrated many
essential and valuable exercises and was used as a guide by patients and wardmasters. A second publication, in the form of a mimeographed pamphlet, described and illustrated various types of remedial apparatus that could be
improvised for use by the convalescent patients. A third publication, in mimeographed form, listed, by subjects, the training films and filmstrips available
for use in the convalescent training program.

On 31 August 1944, a regional conference on the conduct of the convalescent training program was held at the 55th General Hospital and was
attended by all rehabilitation officers of the 12th Hospital Center. On 1
September 1944, a similar meeting and demonstration was held at the 160th
General Hospital for rehabilitation officers of the 15th Hospital Center. On
11 October 1944, a regional conference was held at the 160th Station Hospital
for all rehabilitation officers from hospitals in the Southern Base Section. On

12 October 1944, a conference was held at the 160th General Hospital for all rehabilitation officers from hospitals in the Western and Eastern Base Sections. The meetings were attended also by representatives from staging hospitals. These conferences provided an excellent medium for interchange of ideas, indoctrination, and the demonstration of a model convalescent training program.

Training films.—During the summer of 1943, a documentary motion picture film was produced in sound and color depicting the program and activities of a rehabilitation center. The author took this documentary film to the Zone of Interior, and, after a showing to The Surgeon General, and following his request, the film was screened for various hospital units throughout the country with accompanying indoctrination lectures. This tour covered a 3-month period, which gave ample time for all to study the reconditioning program that had been activated at Bromsgrove. A model convalescent rehabilitation unit, based on experiences in the European theater, was set up by this consultant at England General Hospital in Atlantic City, N.J.

By the end of August 1944, two additional motion picture films on activities of the program had been completed and distribution had been started. One, an orientation film, titled "The Convalescent Training Program," was shown to the staffs of all hospitals. The other, titled "Physical Training Instructors," was used in the Physical Training Instructors' School at Rehabilitation Center No. 1, for indoctrination and training.

On 24 August 1944, a group of visual aid coordinators arrived and were immediately oriented in the conduct of the rehabilitation program. Their mission was to establish film libraries, to screen films, to repair projection apparatus, and to give other assistance to the conduct of the convalescent training program throughout the theater.

Supplies and equipment

In anticipation of an expanded program in the theater, sufficient gymnastic supplies, remedial apparatus, training films, and other training aids were requisitioned and secured early in the program. Supplies, special equipment, and training aids for use in the convalescent training program in hospitals were secured for each hospital and distributed. Also, in May 1944, through arrangements with Special Services, additional stocks of athletic, recreational, and educational equipment were set aside for requisition and use within the convalescent training program. Through special arrangements with the Army Pictorial Service, 16 mm. motion picture and 35 mm. filmstrip projectors were obtained for the rehabilitation program. The Rehabilitation Division placed and distributed the projectors. The limited supply of remedial apparatus and gymnastic equipment that had been obtained was exhausted. Requirements were computed for the ensuing 12 months, and sufficient apparatus was secured through the General Procurement Authority from Spencer, Heath and George, Ltd., Enfield, England, to meet immediate needs. Close liaison was maintained with the American Red Cross, which was responsible for many of the recreational and diversional activities. The latter organization was most cooperative at all times and provided personnel and supplies to the centers and hospitals unstintingly.

Maximum use was made of improvised aids to physical rehabilitation in which both construction (or fabrication) and use provided a means for augmented physical reconditioning. Such apparatus included shoulder wheels, knee pulleys, finger grips, and steps.

Statistics

December 1943.—At the end of the year 1943, Rehabilitation Center No. 1 had been in operation for 9 months, since April, at its two locations, Bromsgrove and Stoneleigh. During this period, there were 3,089 admissions and 1,808 dispositions. Of the dispositions, 83 percent were discharged back to duty and 17 percent were sent back to hospitals for further treatment. The caseload was divided approximately into: Orthopedic, 80 percent; general surgery, 10 percent; and medicine, 10 percent.

On 31 December 1944, approximately 31,500 beds were available for convalescent patients in the European theater. In addition to the 12,400 beds in the convalescent facilities in the United Kingdom, general and station hospitals had set aside areas for the use of 11,500 convalescent patients. Nine station hospitals had been completely set aside to handle approximately 3,600 convalescent patients. The 7th Convalescent Hospital at Étampes, Seine Base Section, France, and the 8th Convalescent Hospital at Valognes, Normandy Base Section, France, were each rated at 2,000 beds for a combined total of 4,000 beds on the Continent.

Convalescent trainees actually in the five centers in the United Kingdom and two convalescent hospitals on the Continent totaled 13,600 at the end of 1944. The total number of convalescent patients discharged from all rehabilitation and reconditioning centers in the United Kingdom from 7 April 1943 through 31 December 1944 was 34,761. Of these, 88.0 percent had been returned to duty in the European theater (chart 3). Among the aforementioned 34,761 patients discharged in the United Kingdom during this period, there were 14,247 battle casualties, 82.7 percent of whom were returned to duty in the theater (chart 4). Overall dispositions from all convalescent facilities (five in the United Kingdom and two on the Continent) during the period from April 1943 through December 1944 totaled 40,440, of whom 86.5 percent had been returned to duty in the European theater. A greater number of days was required for rehabilitation than for reconditioning; rehabilitation required an average of 49 days per patient, and reconditioning, an average of 39 days. A total of 1,637 officer patients had been discharged from the 833d Convalescent Center during the period, of which 78.7 percent were returned to duty in the European theater (chart 5).

CHART 3.—*Disposition of 34,761 conval-*
escent patients discharged from all reha-
bilitation and reconditioning centers in the
United Kingdom during the period 7 April
1943–31 December 1944

CHART 4.—*Disposition of 14,247 battle*
casualties discharged from all rehabilita-
tion and reconditioning centers in the
United Kingdom during the period 7 April
1943–31 December 1944

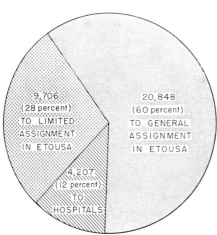

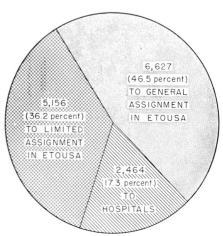

CHART 5.—*Disposition of 1,637 officer*
patients (classified as disease, battle, and
nonbattle injuries), discharged from the
833d Convalescent Camp (Officers) during
the period 7 April 1943–31 December 1944

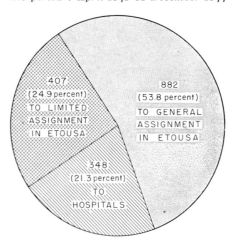

Activities Centered on the Continent, 1945

During final operations

On 8 January 1945, the Rehabilitation Division, Office of the Chief Surgeon, moved from London to Paris, leaving an adequate and competent staff with the Office of the Surgeon, United Kingdom Base, London, and established its officers at 127 Champs Élysées. On 9 January, two veterans of World War II who had suffered limb amputations and who had been fitted with prosthetic appliances at Walter Reed General Hospital reported for duty with the Rehabilitation Division. These veterans visited hospitals in the theater to meet personnel who had lost limbs and to indoctrinate them as to their expected normalcy in future activities. The two veterans were great morale builders to these unfortunate patients.

During January, the hospitals of the European theater were operating at fullest capacity due to the large numbers of battle casualties. This naturally curtailed rehabilitation activities in hospitals but made for more efficient early transfer of patients to the rehabilitation and convalescent centers. Particularly efficient convalescent reconditioning was being accomplished at the 7th and 8th Convalescent Hospitals operating in the communications zone on the Continent. The economy of centralized convalescent care was never more strikingly emphasized than during this critical phase of military operations in the European theater.

Two officers were assigned to the Rehabilitation Division from the Special Services and Information Services of the theater to coordinate the procurement of supplies and to advise in educational reconditioning. Arrangements were made with the cinema branch of Special Services for the distribution of recreational movies to hospitals and with the library section of Special Services for the acquisition of additional books and magazines for the use of the convalescent patients.

Additional rehabilitation personnel were being trained at the school conducted by the 826th Convalescent Center in the United Kingdom. These personnel were greatly needed in the hospital programs. In early February, an allotment of 150 officers and 400 enlisted men was made available for training in the rehabilitation program and for subsequent assignment to hospitals and convalescent centers.

During this period, a 30-day evacuation policy was operating on the Continent; therefore, the conduct of a convalescent program was not universally required. With the 60-day evacuation policy, beginning late in February, the program of convalescent training was reinstituted within the hospitals in France and Belgium. On 21 February 1945, at a special conference of hospital center commanders and base surgeons, plans for convalescent rehabilitation on the Continent were outlined. Tentatively, a convalescent facility was to be established within each hospital center. It was also announced at this conference that trained rehabilitation personnel would be assigned to each hospital. Later, conferences were held with surgeons of base sections and with the commanding officers of hospital centers to assist in the reorganization of the convalescent training program on the Continent. A series of lectures was given by members of the Rehabilitation Division to the personnel of all the hospitals.

Frequent indoctrination visits were being made to the convalescent hospitals within the field armies. The purpose of these trips was to recommend methods of improving the program of convalescent activities for patients retained in the army area. It was difficult, however, to activate definite programs due to the rapid advances being made. It was noted, however, that patients in army convalescent hospitals had little or no problem of physical or morale reconditioning and that patients were anxious to return to their units as soon as possible.

On 25 February, Colonel Stinchfield was appointed supervisor of convalescent rehabilitation in the United Kingdom, in addition to his other duties. He retained command of the 826th Convalescent Center.

In March, Colonel Thompson was relieved of his liaison duties with the G-3 Section, Headquarters, ETOUSA, and assigned to the Rehabilitation Division, Office of the Chief Surgeon.

A continuing search was being made throughout this period for suitable sites for convalescent rehabilitation facilities in France and Belgium. The Rehabilitation Division, in coordination with the Supply, Operations, Hospitalization, and Personnel Divisions, Office of the Chief Surgeon, completed plans for the activation of six convalescent centers on the Continent. Selected locations and bed capacities were as follows:

		Number *of beds*
Area		
Mourmelon_____		3, 000
Toul-Nancy-Verdun_____		3, 000
Paris_____		3, 000
Namur_____		3, 000
Liége-Aachen_____		3, 000
Suippes-Soissons_____		3, 000

Plans were also made to move the 828th Convalescent Center and several selected station hospital units from the United Kingdom to the Continent. Selected personnel from various rehabilitation units in the United Kingdom were ordered to the Continent for use in the activation of new units.

Since there were no true rehabilitation centers functioning on the Continent, and since, after 1 April 1945, patients were transferred to the Zone of Interior when they required more than 60 days of hospitalization, the burden for convalescent management was placed on each hospital (fig. 178). Medical officers in busy hospitals were not too favorably disposed toward their part in the program unless they had a clear concept of the relationship of rehabilitation and reconditioning to the principles and practice of scientific medicine.

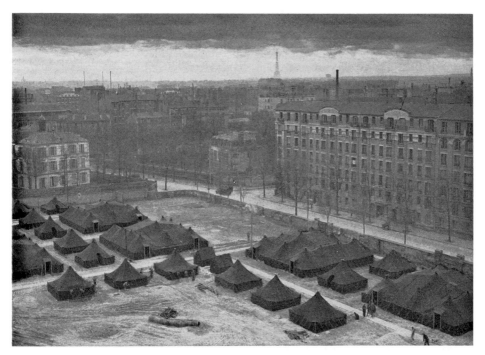

FIGURE 178.—Construction of a tented rehabilitation area at 108th General Hospital, Paris, France.

Therefore, complete and thorough indoctrination of the medical officers was constantly being carried out.

During the latter part of April, many conferences were held with the Chief Surgeon and his officers in regard to the redeployment of convalescent centers and personnel to the Zone of Interior.

V–E Day and phasing out

On 8 May, V–E Day was announced, and immediate plans were made for the redeployment of the 826th Convalescent Center to the Zone of Interior.

On 15 May 1945, Colonel Diveley proceeded to the Zone of Interior in order to coordinate the redeployment of the convalescent center and the rehabilitation personnel. Colonel Thompson was appointed acting chief of the Rehabilitation Division.

The major emphasis in the hospital convalescent training program was shifted to the augmentation of educational reconditioning.

Toward the end of May, arrangements were made to return all air force specialized-training equipment and all other surplus supplies. Many rehabilitation personnel were made available to the Zone of Interior.

Sites in Germany for use as convalescent centers were surveyed, but the selection of these was dependent upon the policy of occupation.

As of the end of June 1945, the Rehabilitation Division consisted of 10 officers, 2 stenographers, and 2 clerks. During the period from December 1944 through June 1945, 138 officers and 585 enlisted men had been trained as rehabilitation training personnel. The convalescent centers had discontinued operations and had disposed of all patients as of 6 June 1945. In the United Kingdom, convalescent centers were in staging areas preparatory to movement to the Zone of Interior. Supplies and personnel were being prepared to maintain a convalescent facility in occupied Europe (U.S. Military Zone) when required. The 7th and 8th Convalescent Hospitals had been recalled to the armies. A convalescent training program was being conducted in all operating general and station hospitals. The activities for the convalescent patient were adapted to the local situation and the patient's requirements.

Statistics

Dispositions for the period from January through June 1945 indicate that 35,597 patients were discharged from the convalescent centers in the United Kingdom. Of the 28,846 patients returned to duty, 55 percent were returned to general assignment and 27 percent to limited assignment. During the total period of operations of convalescent centers from April 1943 through June 1945, there were 70,358 dispositions reported, of whom 84.5 percent were returned to duty after an average total period of hospitalization and convalescence of 95.7 days (table 2).

TABLE 2.—*Average duration of hospitalization and convalescence, during period from April 1943 through June 1945, of trainees returned to duty from convalescent centers*

Category of trainee	Average number of days in hospital	Average number of days in convalescent center	Average number of days of hospitalization and convalescence
Battle casualties_____	57. 2	50. 9	108. 1
Disease and nonbattle injuries_____	44. 7	36. 9	81. 6
Aggregate_____	51. 0	44. 7	95. 7

The general and station hospitals in the United Kingdom, for the first 4 months of 1945, reported that 259,834 patients were discharged, of whom 197,846 were ultimate dispositions. Of the latter, 29 percent were returned to general duty, 17.5 percent were sent to limited assignments, and 53.5 percent were transferred to the Zone of Interior. During the first 4 months of 1945, these hospitals transferred for advanced rehabilitation in their convalescent sections 63,269 patients, of which 49,949 were ultimate dispositions. Of these, 53.8 percent were returned to general duty, 39.2 percent were given limited assignments, and 7 percent were transferred to the Zone of Interior. The average duration of stay for a convalescent patient admitted to the convalescent section in these general and station hospitals was 46.1 days in the hospital and 18.5 days in the convalescent section for a total of 64.6 days.

Summary

The convalescent activities program in the European theater was conducted most successfully during World War II with adherence to the following principles which were developed early in the program.

1. Each convalescent patient was graded periodically by his medical officer upon the basis of objective as well as subjective findings. The patient's activities were prescribed in accordance with his rate of recovery and his military occupational specialty. The activities program was adapted to local requirements and was generally proportioned among physical and military reconditioning and recreational diversion.

2. The entire program was based on the fact that the mission of the Medical Department was the conservation of manpower and the preservation of the fighting strength of the military forces. This was accomplished by furnishing those who had become disabled with such hospitalization facilities as would speedily restore them to health and finally to fighting efficiency. It was not enough that the patient be cured of his disease, or that his wounds be healed, but it was necessary that treatment cover the entire period from the time he became a casualty until he was physically and mentally normal and could return to take his former place in his unit. Specifically, the rehabilitation program covered that phase from the time he became a convalescent patient and could leave the hospital until he had completely recovered and could return to his unit.

3. The rehabilitation center was a military unit that prepared convalescent military personnel for further military service or for discharge to useful civil life. The scope of a rehabilitation center included the acceptance of the patient from the hospital as soon as possible after he had reached the convalescent stage. He was then treated with specific physical therapy or remedial exercises, as well as general reconditioning and hardening exercises, which cut the period of convalescent days to a minimum and prepared the soldier to return to duty in a strong, able physical condition. The rehabilitation center had as its aim mental as well as physical rehabilitation. With these goals achieved, the soldier, when discharged to duty, had not only the physical ability to carry on his task, but also the proper mental attitude to carry the task to completion.

The reconditioning center had none of the hospital atmosphere. Mental and physical deterioration occurred while the soldier was in the hospital, and the longer he was hospitalized, the more permanent this deterioration became. He was, therefore, removed as soon as possible from the hospital to an atmosphere of appropriate military and physical training.

REX L. DIVELEY, M.D.

CHAPTER VII

Otolaryngology [1]

Norton Canfield, M.D.

Otolaryngology in the Office of The Surgeon General at the beginning of
the war was a division of general surgery, and so it remained both in the Office
of The Surgeon General and in most military hospitals, except in a few where
the administration wisely saw fit to make it a separate service. Where there
was a separate otolaryngology service, the specialty made its greatest progress
because the service was usually under the direction of professional talent which
was also responsible for separate services in the civilian teaching hospitals
associated with large medical centers. In a rapidly expanding medical service,
such as the Army was obliged to manage from 1941 to 1945, the administrative
wisdom of surgical specialties' being professionally responsible to the chief of
general surgery was undeniable in many instances. But the inflexibility of
this policy as interpreted by some commanding officers led to patient care
which was often unfortunate. So rapid and frequent was the shifting of personnel in many medical units that a set professional "chain of command" was
deemed of major importance. Indoctrination of newly commissioned medical
officers was, however, often insufficient to make Army policies for the administration of professional services completely acceptable to many civilian-trained
specialists during their military service.

THE CHIEF SURGEON

In mid-1942 the European Theater of Operations, U.S. Army, was expanding, and the medical service was under the direction of the theater Chief
Surgeon, Col. (later Maj. Gen.) Paul R. Hawley, MC, whose military career
had been of long standing. His preliminary close association with the British
which was so manifestly the result of his professional knowledge, human understanding, and military acumen, coupled with his absolute respect for professional integrity wherever it appeared, made him a superb "chief" in every
respect. In addition to his excellent, but understandably not perfect, ability
to select men for important posts and his willingness to replace officers who
did not meet his expectations, General Hawley was so often correct in his decisions that even the professional consulting staff was hard put to it to substantiate recommendations when they ran counter to his ideas.

---

[1] For amplification of matters briefly reviewed in this chapter, see: Medical Department, United
States Army. Surgery in World War II. Ophthalmology and Otolaryngology. Washington: U.S.
Government Printing Office, 1957.

Those consultants who were on duty in the Office of the Chief Surgeon, ETOUSA (European Theater of Operations, U.S. Army), for the period 1942–45 can never forget the "battle of the anesthetists" under the amazing leadership of Col. Ralph M. Tovell, MC. Colonel Tovell's strategy was based on solid professional polices and execution and was so keen that it took General Hawley by surprise, which he did not fancy. The general took special pains to make his displeasure emphatically obvious. The outcome, however, under the guidance of Colonel Tovell was so beneficial to the troops who needed professional medical care that the Chief Surgeon, in the presence of his professional advisers and his administrative staff, accepted completely Colonel Tovell's magnificent work, thereby demonstrating his stature (p. 300). General Hawley did this in a manner which was worthy of the finest of human character, and he let it be known that he was mistaken in his previous emphatic opposition to policies which eventually made anesthesia one of the great services during the war. This was but an example of the many instances in which he acceded to the high-grade professional advice from the men whom he preferred to have associated with him.

ACTIVITIES AND OBSERVATIONS

Appointment of Consultant in Otolaryngology, ETOUSA.—In mid-1942, Col. (later Brig. Gen.) Elliott C. Cutler, MC, Chief Consultant in Surgery, ETOUSA, initiated a request to The Surgeon General for an otolaryngologic consultant for the European theater. The Surgeon General responded by requesting Dr. Lyman Richards of Boston and, later, Dr. Albert C. Furstenberg of Ann Arbor, neither of whom, because of their important civilian posts, could accept the position. By the gracious recommendation of Dr. Furstenberg, the post was offered to Dr. Norton Canfield (fig. 179). At that time, Dr. Canfield was a full-time head of the Division of Otolaryngology, Yale University School of Medicine. Earlier, he had been designated as essential for medical school teaching, but, when this position became available, the dean of the Medical School, Dr. Francis G. Blake, agreed to remove his name from the essential list. Thus, on 28 November 1942, the author entered the Army as a lieutenant colonel and was placed on temporary duty in Washington in the Office of The Surgeon General to prepare for his duties in the European theater.

At that time Col. (later Brig. Gen.) Fred W. Rankin, MC, was Chief Consultant in Surgery to The Surgeon General. Colonel Rankin outlined the functions that the otolaryngologic consultant in the European theater might be called upon to carry out. Arrangements were then made for the author's prompt transport to England. Within one week of landing in England in January 1943, he reported to the Chief Surgeon and was assigned as Senior Consultant in Otolaryngology, Office of the Chief Surgeon, ETOUSA. The author held this position from then until his return to the United States in 1945, after V–J Day. Before this consultant's arrival in the European theater, duties of the otolaryngologic consultant were performed by Maj. (later Lt. Col.) Frank D. Lathrop, MC, formerly associated with the Lahey Clinic in Boston, and by Capt. (later Maj.) Edmond P. Fowler, Jr., MC, Chief, Otolaryngological Section, 2d General Hospital, then at Oxford, England. The preliminary work of these two officers was of great assistance, especially in the procurement of special surgical instruments from British sources during the early part of 1943.

Chief Consultant in Surgery.—Under the wise counsel and able advice of Elliott Cutler, the otolaryngologic consultant during his entire tour of duty was given full professional authority. As he looks back upon the experience,

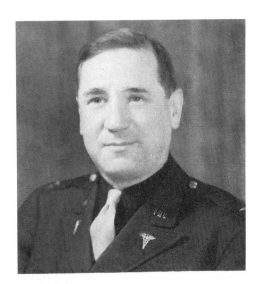

FIGURE 179.—Col. Norton Canfield, MC.

it would be hard for this consultant to believe that any superior could have been more thoughtful and helpful in the execution of his duties. General Cutler's experience in World War I as a medical officer with combat forces admirably fitted him for the much more important post which he held as Chief Consultant in Surgery for the European theater in World War II. His military knowledge, high professional integrity, consummate geniality, and untiring efforts were largely responsible for the success in the handling of surgical problems in the European theater.

Associations with British.—Immediately upon the assumption of his position in England, the author was placed in touch with the British authorities in his specialty. His association throughout the rest of the time in Europe with Brigadier Myles L. Formby, RAMC, was entirely satisfactory. Not only were many professional ideas exchanged, but the actual surgical care of members of both armies was at all times a matter of closest cooperation. One of the most pleasant and beneficial associations of the specialty officers in Europe during the period 1943–45 was the association with both British military and civilian specialists. The meetings of the Royal Society of Medicine in London were open to all medical officers of the U.S. Army, and it was the pleasant duty of the Senior Consultant in Otolaryngology to arrange for specialists in the theater to attend these meetings. On their own initiative, U.S. Army otolaryngologists attended meetings, both Army and civilian, at British installations near their own stations.

Administrative considerations.—It was the policy in the European theater not to train otolarygologists, although there were available men capable of conducting such training in several of the large general hospitals. As the theater expanded, no one consultant could cover all of the hospitals; consequently, a system of regional consultants was initiated by General Hawley. The outstanding men in any one locality were assigned as regional consultants with orders to travel, if necessary, to nearby hospitals for consultation on individual difficult cases. The transfer of patients from one hospital to another was permitted under certain circumstances, always with the idea that the injured or sick soldier would receive the best possible professional care. It was the express policy of General Hawley that the administrative side of military medicine justified itself only when it could make the best possible professional care available to the sick and wounded (p. 349). Military considerations sometimes seemed to make this policy ineffective, but it never assumed this flavor by any design of the Chief Surgeon whose professional qualifications were of an exceedingly high order.

Relations with Army Air Forces.—The Army Air Forces in Europe had their own unit medical service to which no otolaryngologic consultant was assigned during the war. At the operational airfields, much of the medical support found to be necessary for the pilots and aircrews was in the field of otolaryngology, and a number of qualified otolaryngologists were assigned to the various airbases. The U.S. Army hospitals in the area of East Anglia, where Army Air Forces activities were the greatest, provided most of the medical service for the Army Air Forces, and capable otolaryngologists were always assigned to these hospitals. Before D-day, battle casualties were confined largely to bomber crews flying between East Anglia and the European mainland. These casualties were given preliminary medical attention at airfields and were then quickly transferred to Services of Supply hospitals for definitive care. Much credit is due Captain Fowler for his initiation in the theater of special attention to aero-otitis and for his direction of the subsequent care given to aircrews by otolaryngologists assigned to those medical units which directly supported the Air Forces. The Senior Consultant in Otolaryngology and other highly qualified specialists were active in medical training courses given at Eighth Air Force headquarters for flight surgeons assigned to individual airfields.

Manual of Therapy.—The training of otolaryngologists before their Army service had been largely directed toward providing definitive care to an individual needing medical attention. In a theater of operations, however,

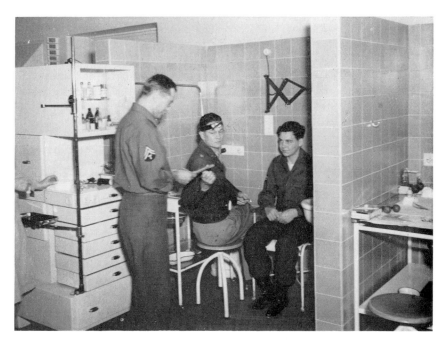

FIGURE 180.—An otolaryngologic clinic in a general hospital.

it was not always possible for the original specialist to give final care. There-fore, practices which at times seemed contradictory to the civilian training of medical officers were necessary because of troop movements on the one hand and the need to concentrate special surgical ability on the other. It was one of the duties of the senior consultant group to formulate policies to comply with such exigencies, and the Manual of Therapy, ETOUSA, setting forth these policies, was written and distributed in 1944.

Otolaryngologic service prior to D-day.—During the time of the troop buildup before D-day, otolaryngologic service in the various hospitals was largely similar to that rendered to any fairly healthy civilian group (fig. 180). Outpatient clinics were, in general, very busy with routine respiratory infec-tions, tonsillitis, otitis media, and sinusitis. The problem of hearing loss was not great, but many soldiers were sent to the European theater with hearing defects which required their assignment to special duties in order not to en-danger them and their comrades unduly in combat (fig. 181). As the war progressed, a system for issuing hearing aids was instituted with considerable success.

Otolaryngologic service after D-day.—After D-day, the nature of pro-fessional service from otolaryngologists necessarily changed, although as a group these specialists were rather busy before D-day. Thereafter, how-ever, their activities were directed toward the wounded in their specialty, and, in general, they were well prepared for the onslaught of casualties as they

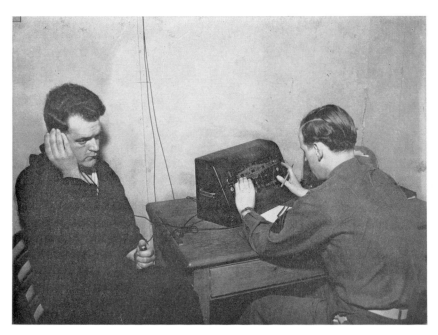

FIGURE 181.—Audiometric testing for hearing acuity.

poured into the hospitals. Let it be known that many medical officers were on duty before D-day without much professional activity. These included the plastic surgeons and the oral surgeons who immediately assumed much more importance when the wounded began to appear. This naturally led to some conflict of ideas concerning the responsibility for certain types of cases, and expected controversies were encountered. Wounds of the head and neck were frequent, and professional policies of treatment had been carefully enumerated by medical officers of World War I, whose writings were well documented but not widely distributed for use in World War II. Again, the Manual of Therapy referred to earlier was extremely useful. As the fighting proceeded, hospitals were quickly transferred to the European mainland, and specialty services were established along the chain of evacuation of the wounded. Medical records noted previous treatments in sequence, but of course they were in many cases too briefly or incompletely prepared because of the tactical situation.

Relations with French.—After the liberation of Paris by the Allies, large hospitals in the vicinity were used by the U.S. Army. Again, association with French surgical specialists and attendance at their meetings were sources of professional interest which continued during the years following the final victory.

Redeployment.—After V–E Day, the selection of medical officers for redeployment to the Pacific was a difficult and unpleasant task for the professional consultants. Although most of the men in Europe had had more than 2 years of duty, it was necessary to assign many of them to duty in the Pacific. V–J Day, however, came so soon after V–E Day that much of this work was fortunately found to be unnecessary, and most of the specialists from the European theater were returned directly to the United States.

REASSIGNMENT IN THE UNITED STATES

Following the duty in Europe, this author was assigned as Consultant in Otolaryngology to The Surgeon General at his offices in Washington, D.C. Upon his return, he found Maj. (later Lt. Col.) Leslie E. Morrissett, MC, who had so ably directed the program for hearing rehabilitation centers in the Zone of Interior. After the war, prompt demobilization was a source of satisfaction to many of the specialists, but there was much more work to be done in the Office of The Surgeon General. The author remained on active duty until May 1946 attending to administrative matters and collecting data for the history of the Medical Department of the U.S. Army in World War II. His recommendations for the initiation of several clinical research projects which might have been carried out by officers remaining on duty were not acted upon by The Surgeon General, although it would have been possible to arrange for a very excellent facial nerve surgery service under the direction of Colonel Lathrop at Cushing General Hospital, Framingham, Mass. In addition, this consultant inspected the three aural rehabilitation centers and found them to be of the highest possible order. These centers were gradually closed, but The Surgeon General saw the wisdom of this extraordinarily fine program and established a permanent aural rehabilitation center at the Forest Glen Section of Walter Reed General Hospital, Forest Glen, Md. This involved a construction program in an old building, but a permanent hearing and speech center with a highly qualified staff was established. So effective was the program for aural rehabilitation that later the Veterans' Administration, also under the leadership of General Hawley, established a program for those servicemen who were discharged and were found to have service-connected hearing impairment. That story is still being written and will constitute one of the brightest spots in the annals of military and Veterans' Administration medicine.

SUMMARY

In looking back on his experiences as Senior Consultant in Otolaryngology in the European theater during World War II, this author is convinced that, if knowledge and experience in any way can be carried forward into future years, much grief will be prevented.

One of the civilian medical profession's main objections to military medicine is the fact that professional ability does not necessarily lead to a commensurate advance in military rank. The history of this problem in the U.S. Army was reviewed on several occasions by General Hawley, and he, at various times, admitted that a solution was difficult to find (pp. 336–338).

It is the belief of this writer, whose experience can be said to have been extremely gratifying from his standpoint, that a small corps of well-trained otolaryngologists with every opportunity for professional advancement as well as advancement in military rank should be the solid policy of The Surgeon General during peacetime.

The consultants' program fully justified the high importance placed upon it during World War II, and the civilian organization which existed following the war, namely the Association of Medical Consultants of World War II (later The Society of Medical Consultants to The Armed Forces), attested to this fact.

CHAPTER VIII

Plastic Surgery

Eugene M. Bricker, M.D.

INTRODUCTION

In a description of the activities of a surgical specialty consultant in a theater of operations, the subject divides naturally into two main headings: Administrative and professional. While, in fact, the functions of administration and professional care were inseparably related, they were so completely different in nature that it appears justifiable to separate them in this account for purposes of clarity. Two admissions are readily made: (1) The history will be biased in that the author is convinced of the importance of plastic surgery in a theater of operations if the best care is to be available to all casualties; (2) any suggestions concerning the organization and use of personnel are made with an operation such as that in the European theater in mind, and with the realization that a future war may be entirely different.

At the beginning of World War II, plastic surgery could still be considered as a relatively new specialty. It was adolescent during World War I, when it was practiced by few surgeons who approached it from various other fields of primary interest, including dentistry, otorhinolaryngology, and general surgery. Following World War I, plastic surgery grew to maturity, as a well-defined specialty, in very few clinics throughout the country. Its function in a theater of operations was incompletely realized at the outbreak of World War II, though the need for adequate coverage in plastic surgery was recognized by Maj. Gen. Paul R. Hawley, Chief Surgeon, ETOUSA (European Theater of Operations, U.S. Army), and a full-time consultant in this specialty was present in the theater throughout the campaign. It could be said that the specialty, as applicable to a theater of operations, approached full maturity during the war in Europe.

In the development of the Professional Services Division, Office of the Chief Surgeon, ETOUSA, a consultant in plastic surgery was one of the first to be named. The value of adequate organization of this specialty had been impressed upon members of the U.S. Armed Forces in the British Isles by the great number of casualties resulting from the Battle of Britain that required reconstructive plastic surgery. Lt. Col. (later Col.) James B. Brown, MC (fig.182), arrived in England on 2 July 1942 in response to a specific request for a plastic surgery consultant. Colonel Brown was accompanied by Lt. Col. Eugene M. Bricker, MC (fig. 183), who succeeded him as Senior Consultant in

Plastic Surgery, ETOUSA, on 12 June 1943, after Colonel Brown had returned to the Zone of Interior to organize and direct a plastic surgery center at Valley Forge General Hospital, Phoenixville, Pa. Throughout the entire campaign until the dissolution of the Professional Services Division of the Chief Surgeon's Office in July 1945, the author worked in close cooperation with the consultants in the other surgical specialties. The work of the Senior Consultant in Plastic Surgery was closely associated with that of Col. Roy A. Stout, DC, Senior Consultant in Maxillofacial Surgery of the Dental Corps (fig. 184). This relationship was maintained on a completely cooperative basis, the function of the two specialties being determined by the fundamental consideration of surgical training and experience.

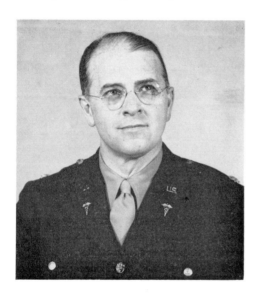

FIGURE 182.—Lt. Col. James B. Brown, MC.

ADMINISTRATION

The administrative duties of all consultants were concerned with the provision of a high standard of professional care for casualties at all echelons. This responsibility became intimately involved with tables of organization, tables of supply, professional qualifications of personnel, evacuation of casualties, and the establishment of professional policies. At the time of this writing, and for the purpose at hand, it seems best to cover the subjects briefly and in a general way as they concern the specialty of plastic surgery. The consultant found himself continually traveling from hospital center to hospital center and from hospital to hospital out of headquarters based successively in London, Cheltenham, Normandy, and Paris. This was a remarkable experience for a consultant out of civilian life. The enormity of the buildup in England for the invasion of Normandy will probably never be equaled in the future. Indeed, if future wars are to occur, it is doubtful that such an enormous land force poised for invasion will be necessary. The magnitude of the Channel crossing and the problems presented in caring for and evacuating the wounded were unique in the annals of military medicine.

Tables of Organization

At the termination of the conflict, it was believed that the tables of organization should be brought abreast of the recent advances in the development of surgical specialties, and that they should particularly allow for the possible

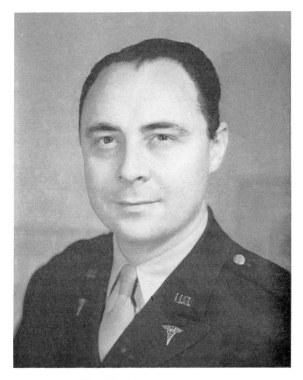

FIGURE 183.—Lt. Col. Eugene M. Bricker, MC.

limitation of the number of qualified specialists. There was a constant conflict throughout the campaign between the location of plastic surgeons according to the tables of organization and the actual location of plastic surgeons in line with logical developments based on need. Thus, as a result of the size of this operation and the number of hospital units involved, it was never practical or possible to supply each 750-bed and 400-bed evacuation hospital with a qualified plastic surgeon as required by the tables of organization. The placing of plastic surgeons on field army unit tables of organization was founded on the principle that a very important period for surgery of maxillofacial wounds is early after injury. The progress of the campaign proved this concept to be correct, but the planning that called for an impossibly large number of plastic surgeons to be in army areas was in error.

Plastic surgery in a theater of operations plays its major role at two levels: (1) At the evacuation hospital level in army areas where definitive therapy is required for compound facial injuries, and (2) in the general hospitals of the communications zone where later definitive therapy can be given to massive soft-tissue wounds, burns, and definitive therapy can be continued for maxillo-facial wounds. The placement of plastic surgeons in the communications zone general hospitals was accomplished without table of organization provision for them. This difficulty was not insurmountable, and it was one of the responsi-

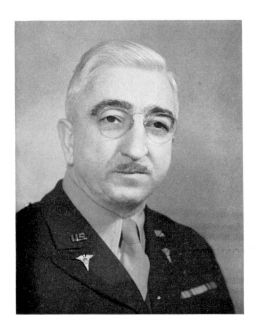

FIGURE 184.—Col. Roy A. Stout, DC.

bilities of the consultant to overcome it. However, the problem seemed to be of some magnitude at the time, both to the consultant who was trying to manipulate hospitals and personnel, and to the personnel being manipulated into tables of organization with no provision for them. The simple human characteristic of desiring earned advance in rank was frequently thwarted as a result of these administrative difficulties. It is recognized that some of these difficulties were unique to the specialty which was still developing and the role of which in a theater of operations was still not clearly understood.

Personnel

As the preceding discussion suggests, the problems of personnel were chiefly precipitated by the tables of organization. During the 2-year preparation for the invasion of France, the need for qualified plastic surgeons to care for the injuries occurring among thousands of staging and training troops was repeatedly demonstrated. During part of this period, there were only two plastic surgeons in England who could be designated as qualified for the care of complicated cases. The situation was relieved in the latter part of 1943 by the arrival of several plastic surgeons with incoming general hospitals and by the return of army units from North Africa. During this long period before D-day, active combat was being carried on by the Eighth Air Force in East Anglia. The Eighth Air Force was served by a group of station hospitals, into certain ones of which specialist personnel were placed. The whole experience of providing specialist care for tremendous numbers of staging troops, and for an active air force based in the communications zone, demonstrated again and again the urgent need for highly qualified surgeons in all the specialties. In the specialties in which there was a shortage of qualified surgeons, it became imperative that those who were qualified be placed in such a position that they could cover a geographical area, and not have their activities confined entirely to the unit in which they were assigned.

At the end of the war, there were present in the theater 70 medical officers with the MOS (military occupational specialty) classification of Specialist in Plastic Surgery. As 9 of the 70 were in administrative or other types of positions, it was impossible to use them in active clinical work in plastic surgery. Of the remaining 61 surgeons, 24 had a "D" classification; the majority of the 24 were general surgeons or specialists in some other branch of surgery. A much more accurate appreciation of the supply of plastic surgeons in the theater than is afforded by a survey of the 70 so listed can be obtained by realization of the fact that only 15 of the 70 were classified as "B" or above, and only 8 of the 15 were available for use in clinical plastic surgery. The total number of plastic surgeons available for clinical use with classifications of "C" or above was only 27. It seemed obvious that the place for the more experienced plastic surgeons was in the hospitals located to the rear where a large number of patients could be funneled to them, where the holding period was longer, and where they would have an opportunity to cover a broader field of surgery than was possible in the forward units. Accordingly, insofar as possible, the more capable surgeons were retained in the rear, and the excessive demands of army unit tables of organization were met with the surgeons in the lower classifications. Of the 24 surgeons in the "D" category, 13 were with evacuation hospitals. This consultant received wonderful cooperation from these men along with the remarkable patience and courtesy with which they accepted his own limitations.

The training of additional plastic surgeons within the theater proved to be a completely impractical task. The very nature of the work made it mandatory that a relatively long period be devoted completely to the specialty before any degree of proficiency could be attained. During the long, quiet period in England, there were not enough casualties accumulated in any one area or location to offer training material of any value. The medical officers who would benefit most from short periods of training were those who already had an extensive background in surgery. Such officers in most instances were loath to give up their chosen field of surgery which, in many instances, would have resulted in forfeiture of chance for advancement in rank. There were a multitude of officers who were anxious to get into plastic surgery, but almost invariably the meager surgical background of these men eliminated them from being anything other than assistants. Advantage was taken of the presence of established British plastic surgery centers for training of U.S. Army surgeons during the long periods of relative inactivity. The surgeons ordered to these units were those with previous training in plastic surgery who would be most benefited. The most extensively used British unit was that at the Queen Victoria Cottage Hospital, East Grinstead, Sussex East. Approximately 50 officers were sent there for 10 days of lectures and demonstrations by Mr. Archibald McIndoe (later knighted). Other units at which American officers were placed on temporary duty were the Hill End Hospital at St. Albans under Mr. Rainsford Mowlem and the Emergency Medical Service Hospital at Park Prewett, Basingstoke, under Sir Harold Gillies. These British surgeons and many others showed a marked degree of cooperation and courtesy throughout the period of close association in England.

It would be impossible to pay individual tribute to the various surgeons who did so much in this specialty during this phase of the war in Britain and Europe. To mention a few would be unfair to others. Much of the clinical work was quite outstanding, and many of the surgeons had an opportunity to demonstrate originality and imagination in their approach to the various complicated clinical problems. Furthermore, the administrative ability that, of necessity, accompanied the clinical work of setting up a plastic surgery service in a hospital and hospital center was enough to deserve special recognition.

Supplies

Problems of supply were a rather minor but a constant source of concern for each consultant. The Supply Division of the Chief Surgeon's Office was always found to be very cooperative in the procurement and distribution of nonstandard items. Tables of equipment and basic allowances were found to be inadequate for the needs of the hospitals for special treatment that were developed as the campaign progressed. The items concerned pertained to the specialized types of surgery on large volumes of casualties. Detailed comments regarding deficiencies of supply were made in a report to The Surgeon General completed shortly after the war. It was believed that, since the use of hospitals for special treatment had reached such a degree of development and recognition in the European theater, in addition to the changes in organization aimed at facilitating the establishment of these hospitals, consideration should be given to the need for supplementary tables of equipment to furnish such units. The items concerned were such things as suction apparatus, needles and suture material, needle holders, tissue forceps, skin hooks, small hemostatic forceps, cotton-waste dressing material, dental arch bars, and dental elevators, all of which, it can be seen, are instruments of a specialty nature.

The complete absence of photographic equipment as an item of medical supply to both communications zone and combat zone hospitals was keenly felt as a handicap throughout the campaign. The need for such equipment was partially relieved by procurement from the British. "Photographic units" were placed with most of the hospital centers. In most instances, the equipment was placed in a hospital performing plastic surgery. It was found that reliance on the Signal Corps for clinical photography was completely unsatisfactory. There always seemed to be plenty of photographs of British nobility visiting the hospitals, but, when an overworked operating surgeon wanted a photograph of some important clinical condition at an irregular hour or on an offday, it was often next to impossible to get it. Clinical photography in the U.S. Army Medical Department was a sorely neglected field that cannot adequately be discussed here. A single detachment of artists and photographers from the Army Medical Museum, such as was supplied in the European theater, was not a satisfactory solution.

Evacuation

Careful supervision of the policies regarding evacuation and constant observation of the flow of casualties to insure that those which were an exception to the general rule were promptly and adequately provided for proved to be among the most important duties and responsibilities of a consultant. The general picture of evacuation varied from day to day and was influenced by the tactical situation, the number of casualties, and the weather. Maxillofacial injuries were considered to travel well. Their early evacuation from army areas was urged, and provisions had to be made in the communications zone to insure against their being lost and not being transferred promptly into the hospitals for special treatment. Burn casualties were also evacuated into specialty hospitals as soon as possible. No special provision was made for the large number of extremity wounds which would require plastic surgery. These cases were picked out of the hospitals in the communications zone and transferred to hospitals providing plastic surgery service as soon as the need for this type of surgery was recognized. Transit and holding hospitals played a very important part of the evacuation of specialty type casualties. The following paragraphs from the Semi-Annual Report, Plastic and Maxillofacial Sections, Professional Services Division, Office of the Chief Surgeon, U.S. Forces European Theater, for the period 1 January–30 June 1945, indicate the main features of the evacuation problem presented by casualties with severe facial injuries:

The care of maxillofacial casualties is directly related to the efficiency and speed of evacuation, since continuity of treatment must be maintained. Throughout the campaign, one of the chief duties of the Senior Consultants in Plastic and Maxillofacial Surgery has been to enforce priority of evacuation for maxillofacial casualties, to brief air holding units in the preparation of casualties for air evacuation, and to see that patients were properly dispersed from landing areas in which a high concentration of cases accumulated. Train and boat evacuation also presented the problem of making Hospital Train crews and Hospital Ship Platoons aware of the special problems involved in caring for and feeding the severe maxillofacial casualties. Arrangements were finally made with Evacuation Divisions of the various Commands to have those maxillofacial casualties going to the Zone of Interior by water to go only on Hospital Ships, where care by properly instructed medical personnel could be depended upon.

1. *Air Evacuation:* a. Front to Paris: Maxillofacial casualties were given a high priority of evacuation directly from the front to Paris, where they were accumulated in the 108th and the 1st General Hospitals. This relieved the load on the forward transit general hospitals and placed the casualties early in the hands of specialists, where they could remain until ready for evacuation to the Zone of Interior.

b. Front to England: Any available air lift to England was taken advantage of by priority maxillofacial casualties. There were periods when casualties were admitted to the special hospitals in England within 36 to 48 hours of the time of injury. This proved to be a tremendous advantage in securing the quality of specialist care desired at an early date and making it unnecessary for the case to go through repeated stages of evacuation.

c. Liége to England: The 15th General Hospital at Liége, Belgium, functioned as a special maxillofacial hospital for the 820th Hospital Center and as a holding transit unit for air evacuation to England. This arrangement functioned very well during the heavy Ardennes fighting and served to decrease the load arriving in the Paris area, as well as to keep the casualties in the hands of specialists. Major Carroll Stuart, MC, and Major Leo La Dage's team of the 5th Auxiliary Surgical Group did a very commendable job at this unit while the casualties were heavy and Liége was being bombed. In England the air evacuated casualties were passed through the 154th General Hospital near Swindon. Personnel were added to this unit to care for the load of casualties. From the 154th General Hospital, the cases were dispersed to the 117th, the 91st, the 192nd, and the 158th General Hospitals by ambulance, and to other hospitals by train or hospital car.

d. Paris to Zone of Interior: Maxillofacial casualties were given first priority for air evacuation to the Zone of the Interior. Paris was the departure point from the Continent. The 1st General Hospital functioned as air holding unit where the adequacy of preparation for air evacuation was checked.

e. England to Zone of Interior: From all special hospitals in England cases were evacuated to the Zone of the Interior by air as air lift was available.

2. *Train and Boat:* Insofar as possible, all maxillofacial casualties were evacuated by air. Evacuation to the Zone of the Interior by boat was confined to Hospital Ships during the latter part of the campaign.

3. *Function of Transit Hospitals at Liége and Swindon:* The designation of such specialty transit hospitals was found to be a very necessary step to control the direction of evacuation and to insure patients falling to the hands of surgeons and dentists with special training and interest. Approximately 3,000 maxillofacial casualties passed through the 154th General Hospital at Swindon from D-day to V–E Day.

Plastic or Maxillofacial Surgery Centers

The establishment of hospitals for special treatment, or "plastic and maxillofacial surgery centers" presented problems that were inseparable from those described in preceding paragraphs on tables of organization and personnel. As a matter of fact, the establishment of these specialty hospitals was the solution to the tables of organization and personnel problems. On 30 March 1943, in a letter on the subject of patients requiring plastic surgery, the Office of the Chief Surgeon, ETOUSA, designated the 298th General Hospital, at Bristol, and the 30th General Hospital, at Mansfield, as centers for plastic surgery. During the following year eight more specialty hospitals for plastic surgery were developed in England. On 10 June 1944, Circular Letter No. 81, concerning hospitals with facilities for specialized treatment, was issued by the Office of the Chief Surgeon, ETOUSA, and designated hospitals for special treatment and plastic surgery, neurosurgery, thoracic surgery, and urological surgery. Thus 10 hospitals, scattered geographically to cover all areas of hospitalization in England, were designated as plastic and maxillofacial surgery centers. Subsequently, one more general hospital was so designated in England. This arrangement provided one plastic surgeon to approximately 10,000 hospital beds. If specialist care was to be made available to all casualties arriving in England, it would be necessary to scatter the available surgeons geographically rather than to place them in a smaller number of hospitals and thus allow each hospital a larger staff. Previous experience warned, and it was later vividly demonstrated, that during the heavy flow of casualties long ambulance hauls of patients to specialized hospitals would not be possible. Plastic surgery could not have served the mass of casualties in England through two or three ideally setup and ideally staffed plastic surgery services.

Preparation for the designation of a hospital as a so-called specialty center usually consisted of moving a qualified specialist into the hospital chosen. This move was preceded in eight of the centers by the installation of additional facilities in the hospital plant for the late treatment of burns by saline baths. From here on, development of the specialty section became largely the responsibility of the specialist himself. In the case of plastic surgery in 1,000-bed communications zone general hospitals, the difficulties encountered resulted directly from the tables of organization. A new surgical section requiring nurses, ward officers, trained technicians, and some items of special equipment had to be fitted into a hospital which was considered to be already organizationally complete. In some instances, weeks or months transpired before a section could be sufficiently developed to be considered possibly to be running efficiently. The plastic surgeon became an integral part of the hospital to which he was assigned. This was an advantage so far as cooperation from other members of the hospital was concerned, but it proved to be a great disadvantage when movement of the surgeons became necessary. Replacements were always necessary or wanted when a surgeon was to be moved. The finding of a replacement and the prolonged administrative details of changing the surgeon's assignment from one hospital to another resulted, in some instances, in defeating the object of getting the surgeon quickly transferred to a place in which he was more urgently needed.

In England, the plastic surgery centers had the most favorable opportunities to develop and to work efficiently. The administrative decentralization that started very early after the influx of large numbers of troops favored the efficient function of specialty hospitals. The breaking up of England into base sections made it possible for certain hospitals to be designated for the coverage of a base section. The desires and recommendations of the Chief Surgeon's senior consultants were enforced through a base section directive, and the base section consultants were of inestimable value in seeing that such directives were followed. Later, when England became designated as the United Kingdom

Base Section, the division of the hospitals into hospital groups again facilitated the use of special hospitals. The most efficient organization prevailed at the end of the campaign when all hospitals in England were included administratively under seven hospital center headquarters. The areas covered by the hospital centers were smaller, the hospitals were usually fairly well concentrated, and the contact between the surgeon of the hospital center and the commanding officers of various hospitals was direct. By the time this administrative organization had developed, the plastic surgery centers were established and their functions understood. Transfer of patients from other hospitals to the plastic surgery centers was carried out with a satisfactory degree of efficiency. The plastic surgeons in the designated hospitals acted as consultants for the hospital centers, thereby furthering the good relationship between the various hospitals and the specialty surgical services.

The situation as it existed in England during the terminal months of the campaign could be considered as being almost ideal, with one exception: The plastic surgery services in the individual chosen hospitals still had to be developed on an entirely improvised basis. The additional help that was necessary was not provided in the hospital organization. It was necessary to beg, borrow, or steal it. The same often was true of adequate ward, dressing room, and operation room space. In addition, with the shortage of qualified plastic surgeons, it eventually semed advisable to close a service in one of the hospitals and to depend for coverage of the area on transfer of patients to a hospital in an adjoining hospital center. Withdrawal of the specialist from a hospital nearly always met with opposition from the commanding officer of the hospital as well as from the commanding officer of the hospital center involved. This opposition was understandable, since it was the duty of the hospital center commanding officer to insure adequate professional coverage for his command. Nevertheless, it was often difficult to fit the supply of plastic surgeons to the obvious needs and at the same time supply the supposed needs of individual administrative subdivisions that were not acquainted with the overall picture of supply and demand in surgical specialists. These difficulties are enumerated not because they were insurmountable administrative obstacles but because they appeared to be unnecessary; that is, they could have been avoided by better planning for the distribution of specialist personnel.

Professional Policies

Professional policies for the theater emanated from the consultants in the Professional Services Division of the Office of the Chief Surgeon. The formulation of professional policies was influenced by many factors that required serious consideration in planning for the care of casualties falling into a surgical specialty. The factors of greatest significance were (1) the expected numerical flow of casualties, (2) the average professional ability of the personnel that were to handle the casualties, (3) the specific needs of the particular types of injuries, and (4) the hospitalization policy for the theater (which was gradually shortened as the reserve of hospital beds decreased). Policies were made known from the Office of the Chief Surgeon by circular letters, administrative memorandum, subject letters, and contact of the Chief Surgeon's consultants with the medical personnel in the various hospitals. The Manual of Therapy, ETOUSA, compiled by the consultants and published in May 1944, served as a guide to the general medical and surgical officers and to the various specialists. With the reception of large numbers of casualties, certain policies were changed and the changes made known in subsequent circular letters on professional care.

The very close contact it was possible for the Senior Consultant in Plastic Surgery to maintain with the plastic surgeons throughout the various centers in England and France proved to be of enormous value. Current professional problems could be discussed in this way and ideas of the various surgeons interchanged. In addition, frequent visits between the surgeons of the different plastic surgery centers were encouraged. It was thus possible to define the limits of plastic surgery to be carried out in the theater and to see that these policies were uniformly adhered to. It was always the aim to do only what was urgently indicated and to prepare the patients for evacuation to the Zone of Interior as soon as possible. The *Medical Bulletin, ETOUSA*, published monthly, served as a very valuable unofficial means of getting information to medical officers throughout the theater. This publication was used to advertise the specialty centers, to explain their function, and to encourage the transfer of patients to these hospitals. The administrative professional policies pertaining to the various types of casualties falling to plastic surgery are discussed in subsequent paragraphs devoted to professional care.

PROFESSIONAL RESPONSIBILITIES AND PROBLEMS

It was the responsibility of a surgical consultant to see that, so far as possible, each casualty was directed to the hands of a physician qualified to provide the necessary care as rapidly as this could be accomplished after injury. As indicated in the foregoing discussion of administration, this responsibility concerned the consultant with all phases of the tactical situation, but chiefly with the evacuation of casualties and the placement of professional personnel. Since plastic surgery was coming of age and was represented by a consultant in the Office of the Chief Surgeon, it seemed advisable to establish a definition of what plastic surgery should entail. Accordingly, plastic surgery was defined, in Circular Letter No. 5, Office of the Chief Surgeon, Headquarters, ETOUSA, by the Chief Surgeon on 12 January 1943, while Colonel Brown was still in the theater, as follows:

1. *Definition:* Plastic surgery includes maxillofacial surgery and is defined as the care and treatment, in all stages of:

   a. Injuries of the face and jaws that may alter the shape of the bony structure or leave disfiguring scars.

   b. Injuries of any part of the body which require skin grafts or flaps, scar adjustments or surface tissue readjustment.

c. Serious burns which may not be regarded initially as falling within the classes in subparagraphs a and b above.

2. *Technical Supervision:* The Senior Consultant in Plastic Surgery is the adviser of the Chief Surgeon and will, under the direction of the latter, exercise technical supervision of all plastic surgery in ETOUSA, regardless of echelon.

The definition was a good one and served a very useful purpose in clarifying responsibility in matters of professional policy. The inclusion of maxillofacial surgery under plastic surgery is difficult to justify completely since the fundamental sources of training are quite different for each, and the two fields, though closely associated in many ways, are quite divergent in others. Except in the case of a few surgeons, qualified in both surgery and dentistry, it was always necessary for the two specialists to work as a team if the highest standard of care was to be maintained. Patients were admitted to hospitals on the surgical service under the responsibility of the chief of surgical service. The dental officers were used to the fullest extent and furnished constant and invaluable assistance in caring for all cases of fractures and injuries about the mouth. Without the dental officers to help with such cases, the surgical services would have been crippled. Subsequent comments on the treatment of maxillofacial casualties in this chapter step considerably into the field of the dental officer with maxillofacial training. Colonel Stout, Senior Consultant in Maxillofacial Surgery, worked side by side with the Senior Consultant in Plastic Surgery in the care and supervision of maxillofacial injuries, and many of the views expressed on this subject stem directly from him.

This author, having been drafted into the position of Senior Consultant in Plastic Surgery, has long had mixed feelings about the advisability of a man who is basically a general surgeon acting as consultant in such a specialty. However, the professional policies and decisions that were required in this theater of operations were of such basic commonsense and general surgical nature that the situation was not as incongruous as it might have been. It was found that, in addition to bedside consultation, the consultant could provide an important professional service by the rapid word-of-mouth dissemination of information during his travels. He was in excellent position to observe and to utilize the knowledge and experience of many first-class surgeons and thus crystallize ideas and policies that were generally beneficial. It was most important that the natural process of learning by experience be speeded up as much as possible in order that the good in professional policies be separated from the bad and promptly put into general practice. The consultant was in a key position to facilitate this process and to appreciate the necessity for altering professional policies in accordance with the dictates of the tactical situation.

Maxillofacial Injuries

Before World War II, the only definite knowledge available concerning treatment of the severe facial wounds of war was that which resulted from World War I. The basic principle of treatment of severe facial wounds emanating from World War I was that such wounds should be closed, or partially closed, and that massive displacements of tissue were to be replaced as soon as possible, with primary healing as the aim. This basic principle had been supplemented because of two very important factors by the time the active phase of World War II approached: (1) Twenty years of civilian experience had been acquired in handling the severe injuries resulting from the speedup and increase in motor transportation; (2) chemotherapy had established an important place as a method of prophylaxis and treatment of infections. It was believed that these two factors would allow aggressive extension of the basic principles emanating from World War I. Thus, it was concluded that the time for complete definitive surgery was immediately in the hands of the first qualified specialist who received the patient, providing that the procedure was feasible and not complicated by such loss of tissue as to make it impossible. Even the latter cases should be treated definitively as far as possible, leaving only replacement and reconstructive procedures to be done at a later date. The object was to produce definitive treatment that would make it necessary, in many cases, for later surgery to consist only of superficial wound revision or excision. The proper treatment of fractures was an integral part of the procedure. In order to approach as nearly as possible the theoretical ideal, definitive surgery at the evacuation hospital level was urged to the limit of the professional talent available there. So far as possible, the most highly qualified plastic surgeons were retained in the rear medical installations where they could handle a greater volume of casualties through triage and where their talents could be used on a broader scope of surgery than at the front. The system produced results that were quite gratifying, considering the tremendous geographical area covered and the mass of casualties handled.

A section of the Manual of Therapy, ETOUSA (app. F, p. 989), indicates the policies pertaining to the treatment of maxillofacial injuries that were in effect at the time of the Normandy invasion.

The sources of severe facial injuries were multiple. Civilian-type injuries resulting from vehicle accidents and fist fights were always common, and, during the period before the invasion of France, provided the majority of maxillofacial injuries. Casualties from the Air Forces presented no notably characteristic features. Landing and takeoff accidents resulted in a number of blunt-force facial injuries, many of them complicated by associated burns. Flak wounds varied from massive shearing injuries caused by large shell fragments to small perforating ones resulting from small missiles. Some of the small missiles from flak were of exceedingly high velocity and produced considerable comminution and "blowing out" of the face. During the hedgerow fighting in Normandy, there was an unusually high incidence of maxillofacial injuries resulting from the close type of combat and the necessity for the men to expose their heads to see the enemy. These wounds were predominantly caused by small arms fire and were characterized by being exceedingly severe and not

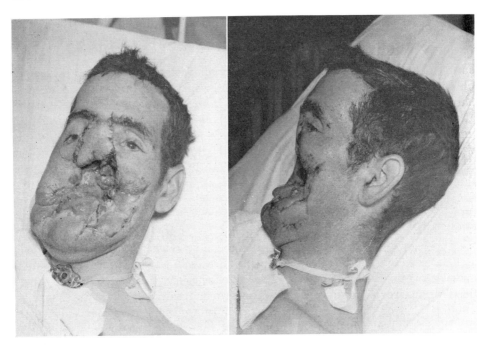

FIGURE 185.—Anterior and lateral views of very extensive injury, associated with extensive loss of tissue. Note the tracheostomy which was absolutely essential for the survival of this patient. Such casualties also presented extremely difficult feeding problems, and a gastrostomy was occasionally justified. Little of a truly restorative or a reconstructive nature can be done for such an injury during the early phase of care. The problem is one of keeping the patient alive and getting him ready for evacuation to the Zone of Interior.

being associated with wounds elsewhere in the body (fig. 185). This is the type of injury that lends itself to extensive early definitive treatment since associated wounds do not influence the patient's condition or have to be considered.

Also, during certain periods of the Normandy campaign, there was a high incidence of a virulent type of wound from "tree bursts" of mortar fire and high-explosive shellfire. In wooded sections, the shells would explode in the air upon striking a tree. This not only decreased the time in which a soldier could drop to the ground for protection but changed the dispersion of the shell fragments so that dropping to the ground gave no added protection. These wounds were very often associated with other wounds of the trunk or extremity which complicated treatment of the maxillofacial injury. Landmines produced a characteristic injury that often was extremely severe. During the fighting around Aachen and the crossing of the Siegfried Line, landmine casualties were especially numerous. They were usually accompanied by shattered feet or legs which made the patient's general condition so critical that little could be done for the face. The facial injury consisted of "tattooing" with multiple

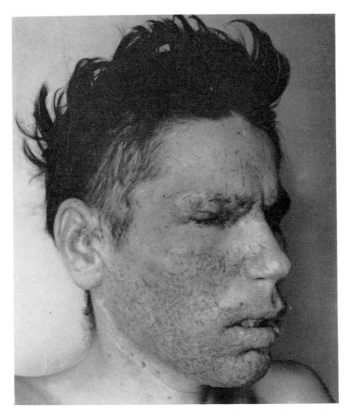

FIGURE 186.—Powder "tattooing" as illustrated by this casualty was almost invariably associated with blindness in one or both eyes. The aftereffects of this "tattooing" could be greatly lessened by vigorous early treatment. It was possible in some instances for the anesthesiologist to scrub and debride the powder marks of the face while the surgical team was taking care of other injuries. It was unfortunate that the insignificance of this particular phase of the patient's injury understandably led to its early neglect in so many instances.

small perforating wounds which usually involved both eyes (figs. 186 and 187).

Evacuation hospital.—Planning for the management of facial injuries was based on the belief that the time for the most effective definitive treatment was at the evacuation hospital level. This concept was proved to be correct, particularly for those casualties without massive soft-tissue loss. Maxillofacial surgical teams of the auxiliary surgical units were effectively used by being placed in evacuation hospitals. At this level, the casualty was treated for shock, all bleeding was controlled, the airway was insured, the extent of the injury was surveyed, and the patient was rested and prepared for operation. If the condition of the patient permitted and the tactical situation allowed, a complete definitive operation was then done (fig. 188). The bony skeleton

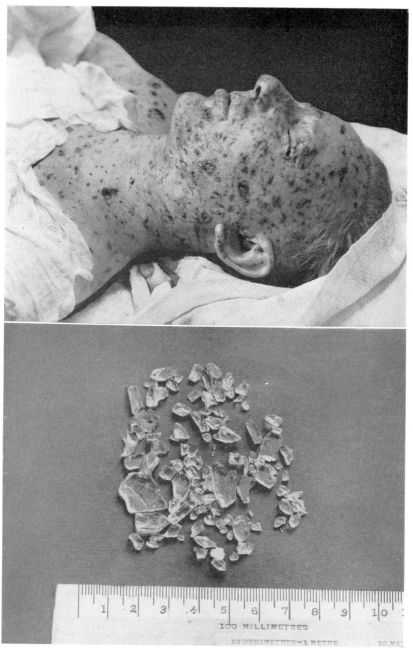

FIGURE 187.—A blast injury, resulting from a mine explosion, somewhat different from the usual in that the foreign particles were larger and were easily removed. Blast "tattooing" as illustrated by this case could be greatly benefited by prolonged and fastidious curettage and soap and water cleaning of the thousands of small punctate wounds. (Case of Maj. Byron C. Smith, MC, 1st General Hospital.)

was reduced and the initial fixation applied. The wound was debrided and, if advisable, closed in layers. The patient was continued on penicillin, which was started upon arrival at the hospital, and held until he had passed the critical period before being evacuated. Tracheotomized patients were held for a minimum of 4 days to become accustomed to the tracheotomy and to develop some degree of self-reliance in case of emergency. Feeding problems were held at least until the more acute problem of maintaining fluid intake had subsided. The object was to get these casualties back as quickly as possible to a specialty center in the communications zone as soon as they could be transported safely (fig. 189).

General hospital.—In the United Kingdom Base Section, there were 10 general hospitals, staffed and equipped as treatment centers for patients with maxillofacial injuries as well as for burn casualties and casualties with massive soft-tissue loss of the trunk or extremities. These specialty hospitals were geographically dispersed over England, one such hospital being designated in each hospital center. From the evacuation hospital where the initial definitive treatment had been given, the casualty was transferred to the communications zone and, if it was severe enough to warrant it, directly into one of the specialty hospitals. The severe facial injuries were continued on a logical regimen aimed at anatomical replacement of tissues, the promotion of healing as rapidly as possible, the reduction and fixation of skeletal derangements and through it all, the maintenance of morale and the nutritional state.

It is obvious that this effort involved many more people than those primarily concerned with plastic surgery or the treatment of maxillofacial injuries. Consultation with the general surgeons, the ophthalmologist, and the otorhinolaryngologist was an integral part of the conduct of such a service. Dental officers of the hospital staff became a part of the plastic and maxillofacial team. The Senior Consultant in Plastic Surgery was almost invariably accompanied by Colonel Stout of the Dental Corps during his inspection of these centers. The suggestions of Colonel Stout concerning the management of complicated jaw and facial fractures furnished an invaluable and indispensible supplement to the author's own inadequate experience in this field. However, it was found that the application of basic surgical principles and commonsense would usually point the way to a solution for most of the complicated injuries.

The degree to which early facial reconstruction and repair could be accomplished was a continual source of amazement and stemmed directly from the availability of antibiotics coupled with good surgical care. An effort was made to take full advantage of the opportunity afforded to obtain early tissue replacement and healing. Much of this was definitive plastic surgery at its best. However, the majority of the surgery in the European theater was aimed at preparing the facial casualty for evacuation to the Zone of Interior in the very best condition for travel with the wound in the very best condition for a continuation of whatever subsequent reconstruction might be necessary (fig. 190). Many things were learned, only a few of the most important and obvious of

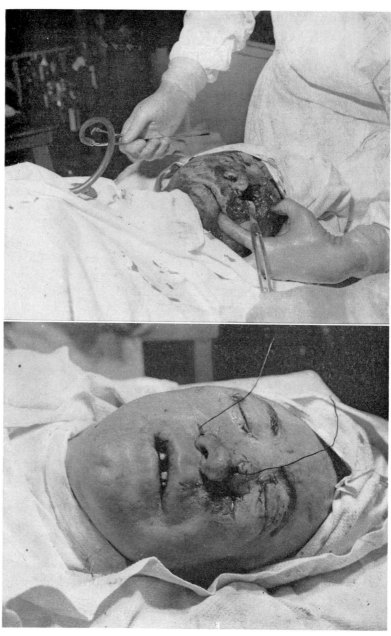

FIGURE 188.—The treatment of a compound facial wound at the evacuation hospital level. The wound illustrated is associated with fracture of the maxilla and loss of tissue about the nose. The maxilla was supported by an arch bar to which wires were attached and brought out through the wound for superior traction. The wound was then closed as much as possible after conservative debridement. No attempt was made to reconstruct features associated with loss of tissue. These areas were left open for later reconstructive surgery. (Case of Maj. Vilray P. Blair, Jr., MC, 45th Evacuation Hospital.)

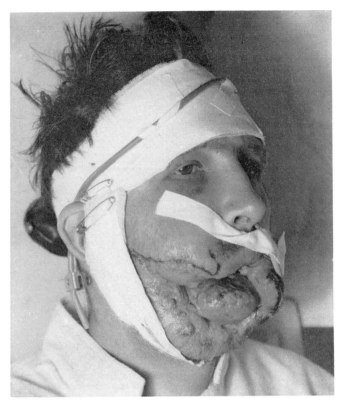

FIGURE 189.—A casualty with a severe wound of the chin and mandible as he arrived in the communications zone. Note the nasal feeding tube which had been of vital importance. In this case, superior traction and support was supplied to the mandible and tongue through elastic bands and a circumferential head bandage. The circumferential head bandage was found to be just about as reliable during evacuation as was the plastic head cap.

which can be mentioned in the following paragraphs. To discuss the treatment of maxillofacial injuries of war in detail would require a separate volume.

Hemorrhage.—When active intervention for the control of hemorrhage became necessary, it was found preferable, and in the majority of cases possible, to expose the bleeding point and ligate the vessel. Remarkably few cases were seen in which trunk vessels had been ligated for uncontrollable hemorrhage. The majority of these cases were secondary hemorrhage associated with infection, and the results of trunk vessel ligation was not the most satisfactory.

Airway.—By the end of the war, it was realized that tracheotomy was a much more vitally important procedure than had been anticipated. It was found to have a place for the critical patient who was near suffocation. In addition, it was found useful for the patient who had an adequate airway, but whose wounds made breathing difficult, messy, and a cause of continued anxiety

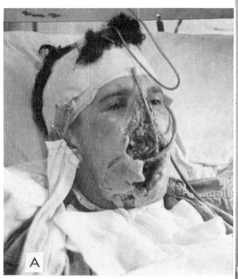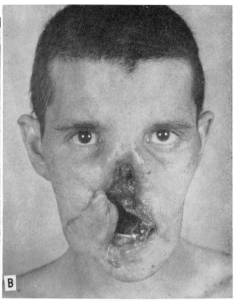

FIGURE 190.—A major facial wound with loss of nose, maxilla, and mandible, representing a composite of the problems presented by these casualties. The problem at first seems to be almost an insurmountable one of maintaining the patient's airway, nutritional state, and morale. A. The patient during his critical stage in an evacuation hospital. B. The man ready for evacuation to the Zone of Interior. The posterior mandibular fragments are stabilized by metal cap splints and a connecting bar. (Case of Maj. Leo H. La Dage, MC, 5th Auxiliary Surgical Group.)

on the part of the patient and his attendants (fig. 185). In such cases, tracheotomy relieved the anxiety, put both the patient and the wound at rest, and simplified nursing care, subsequent anesthesia, and operative procedures.

Debridement.—In the preparation of facial wounds for closure, the procedure of debridement was found to be as important as it was for wounds elsewhere in the body. However, it was completely different because it was necessary that it be conservative and at the same time thorough. Debridement and closure had to be judiciously associated with adequate dependent drainage for wounds involving the buccal mucosa, the floor of mouth, and the paranasal sinuses. Debridement and closure could not be practiced on facial wounds with massive soft-tissue loss. In such cases, the procedure was altered to provide for as early healing as possible without gross displacement of features (fig. 188). The suture of skin to buccal mucosa was a procedure frequently practiced (fig. 191).

Primary closure.—The success of primary closure of facial wounds was directly dependent upon the skill with which the debridement and closure were done and upon the extent and location of the wound. A surprising percentage

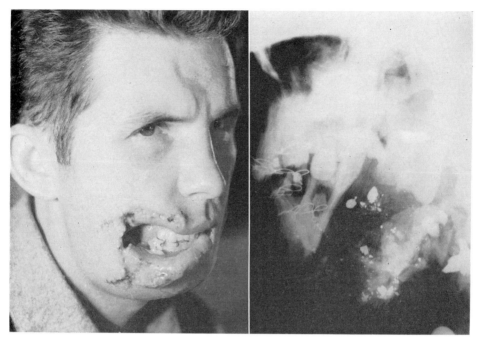

FIGURE 191.—This compound injury is associated with fracture and loss of bone and loss of overlying soft tissue. The skin to buccal mucosa suture provides early healing and at the same time simplifies the care of the fracture and floor of the mouth by making these areas more accessible. Any attempt at early closure and reconstruction of this facial defect would have been a serious error. Notice the multiple wire loops for control of the bone fragments by elastic traction. (Case of Lt. Col. B. Eugene Boyer, MC, 53d General Hospital.)

of them were successful (fig. 192). Those that were unsuccessful were subjected to secondary closure in the communications zone hospitals after the wounds had been cleaned up and the associated skeletal derangements stabilized.

Infection.—Routine antibiotic therapy had a definite role in the low incidence of spreading infections. It is of great interest that, in his travels, the Senior Consultant in Plastic Surgery did not see one case of Ludwig's angina. Spreading cellulitis and erysipeloid infections were practically nonexistent. The infections observed were localized and, for the most part, due to poor debridement or lack of provision for adequate drainage of wounds in which drainage was indicated (fig. 193).

Reduction and fixation of fractures.—Before a compound facial wound was closed, the initial reduction and fixation of fractures was accomplished with the following ends in mind: (1) Restoration of normal anatomical position and contour, (2) restoration of normal occlusal relationship between the maxilla and mandible, (3) maintenance of the dental arch and prevention of collapse

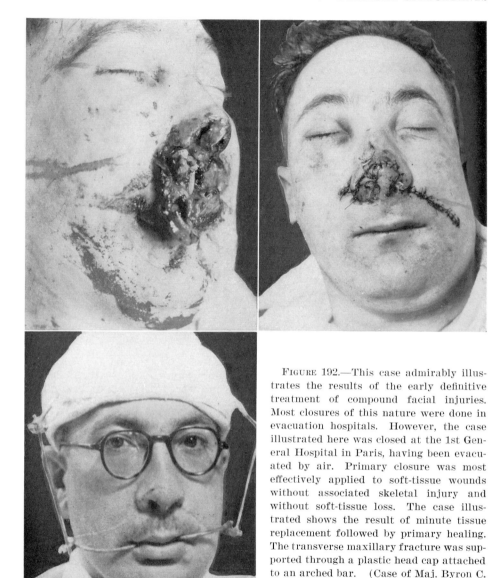

FIGURE 192.—This case admirably illustrates the results of the early definitive treatment of compound facial injuries. Most closures of this nature were done in evacuation hospitals. However, the case illustrated here was closed at the 1st General Hospital in Paris, having been evacuated by air. Primary closure was most effectively applied to soft-tissue wounds without associated skeletal injury and without soft-tissue loss. The case illustrated shows the result of minute tissue replacement followed by primary healing. The transverse maxillary fracture was supported through a plastic head cap attached to an arched bar. (Case of Maj. Byron C. Smith, MC, 1st General Hospital.)

(figs. 191 and 194). The multiplicity of means of fixation of facial and jaw fractures cannot be discussed in detail here. Suffice it to say that the problem was chiefly a mechanical one and was influenced by many factors. If the patient was seen early enough and if the anesthesia was adequate, reduction could usually be accomplished manually. If impaction or swelling and fixation prevented manual reduction, a plan for traction reduction had to be formulated.

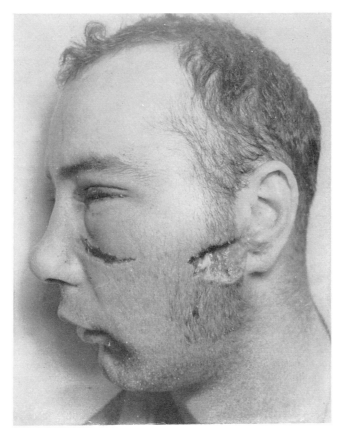

FIGURE 193.—This case illustrates a penetrating wound of the antrum with infection. Most infections observed were due to inadequate debridement or lack of provision for adequate drainage. Infection in the above case could have been prevented by debridement of the maxillary antrum and the provision of adequate drainage through the buccal fornix.

The mechanical means were multiple and those used would vary with the individual surgeon and the individual case. Certain principles, however, were considered in the application of these mechanical means. These principles were: (1) To strive for simplicity; (2) to take advantage of every favorable factor offered by the peculiarities of the case (that is, the presence of key teeth for application of apparatus, the holding of one fragment in place by impacting it against another, or the holding of a posterior mandibular fragment in position by a retained molar); and (3) to avoid external applications and plaster head caps when possible. It was in this phase of care that the "multiple loop" wiring method of Colonel Stout was used most extensively (fig. 191). Intermaxillary rubberband fixation, applied to multiple loop wires, served a great purpose in the European theater both for the early care of maxillofacial casualties and for the later definitive support of mandibular and maxillary fractures during the final healing phase.

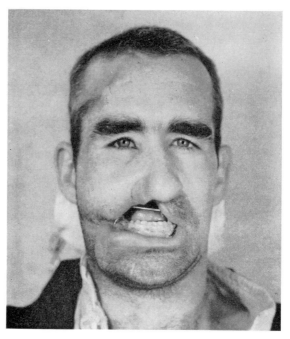

FIGURE 194.—Compound facial wound associated with loss of the maxillary alveolus and overlying soft tissue and a fracture of the mandible. Good early care with an acrylic resin splint to mandible and stabilization of the remaining maxillary fragments.

Drainage.—At the time of closure, the indications for establishing adequate drainage had always to be kept in mind. This was a principle that was well understood during World War I when infection after closure was much more likely to be a critical complication than at the time of the present conflict when spreading infection could, to a great extent, be controlled by sulfonamide or penicillin therapy. Failure to provide adequate drainage was a not uncommon error in the treatment of the first casualties following the invasion of Normandy. It was believed that drainage should be instituted routinely for the following types of wounds:

1. Wounds involving the floor of the mouth. The floor of the mouth should be closed, and dependent external drainage provided. This could usually be done through an external portion of the wound.

2. Severe wounds associated with the comminuted fracture of the mandible. The drained area should include the fracture site.

3. Deep wounds of the upper neck. Such wounds were subject to accumulation of blood and serum because of the unavoidable motion following swallowing and breathing.

4. Wounds involving the maxillary sinus were drained into the nose or buccal fornix.

5. Wounds which resulted in the turning of a large flap. Accumulation of serum and blood was guarded against by the insertion of a small drain after replacing the flap.

6. Compound wounds of the frontal sinus were drained externally (provided the wound did not involve the posterior wall and dura).

7. Extensive comminuted fractures of the mandible, compounded into the mouth, but not associated with external wounds through which drainage could easily occur. Such wounds were treated by a properly placed incision and the insertion of a drain.

Delayed primary and secondary closure.—Primary closure of facial wounds at the evacuation hospital was the general practice when possible. However, there were cases that for various reasons were found inadvisable to close in the evacuation hospitals. For instance, an evacuation hospital group swamped with casualties might be in a position to bypass maxillofacial injuries that were considered transportable through an air evacuation unit directly to hospital centers in England where they would arrive in only a few hours (fig. 192). Many facial injuries were then subjected to debridement and closure with successful results from a few hours to as long as 72 hours following injury. Without question, penicillin therapy had an important bearing on the fact that comparatively late, radical, definitive procedures were possible. The absence of invasive infection was the clinical finding supporting the rationale of late closure. Technically, delayed primary closure did not differ from early closure.

The cases requiring secondary closure might be classified in two categories, as follows: (1) Those that had previously been closed with unsuccessful results; (2) those that were not closed previously and in which delayed primary closure had been advisable. Both of these types became characterized by surface infection, sloughing of devitalized tissue, and abscess formation if drainage was inadequate. The problem resolved itself into one of nursing care, care of the wound, maintenance of the nutritional state, and control of infection in preparation for secondary closure. Reduction and fixation of skeletal parts proceeded concomitantly, and in these cases the procedure frequently became one of gradual traction reduction.

Secondary closure was done judiciously, with the realization that the results could not be accepted as final and with the understanding that the procedure was never strongly indicated unless it would increase the comfort of the patient or result in producing a healed wound that would terminate pathological processes detrimental if allowed to proceed (fig. 195). An effort was made not to lose sight of the fact that the normal healing process of an open wound produces results that are frequently difficult to surpass by surgical intervention. If the wound was not resulting in loss of bone or important loss of function, it was realized that closure or revision by experienced hands many weeks later, after the tissues had healed and softened, might be expected to offer the best results (figs. 196 and 197).

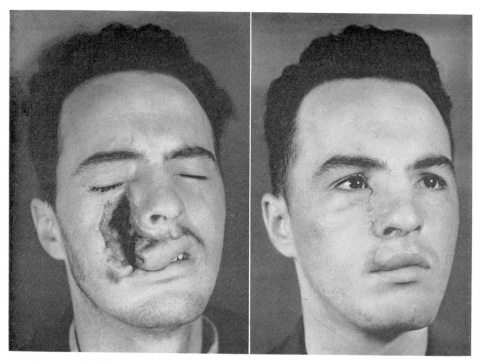

FIGURE 195.—This case illustrates the secondary closure of a compound facial wound. Some casualties were so severely injured and the circumstances of their treatment so complicated that early definitive care could not be accomplished before evacuation became necessary. The case illustrated here shows the condition of a casualty upon arriving at a general hospital 5 or 6 days following injury. There is an extensive defect of the maxilla. In such cases in which there was no extensive loss of tissue, the soft-tissue parts could be replaced as soon as possible. This case illustrates the results of such an early secondary closure. (Case of Maj. Douglas W. Macomber, MC, 91st General Hospital.)

Rotation flaps, pedicle grafts, free skin grafts.—With the exception of the free skin graft, none of the procedures listed in the title of this paragraph were considered to have a role in the early treatment of maxillofacial wounds. If there was massive loss of tissue requiring replacement, it was believed that this was better done at a later stage in the Zone of Interior. An occasional wound lent itself to free skin graft as a means of promoting a healed surface, though it was rather surprising how infrequently such wounds were encountered.

Feeding and maintenance of nutritional state.—In any hospital in which maxillofacial casualties were accumulated, the problem of their feeding soon became an acute one. In the specialty hospital in the European theater, it became the habit, as soon as the load of patients warranted it, of setting up special feeding facilities for these casualties. The American soldier, almost regardless of the handicap, will get enough to eat if he is given the opportunity. A few of the casualties were definitely reticent about feeding themselves before

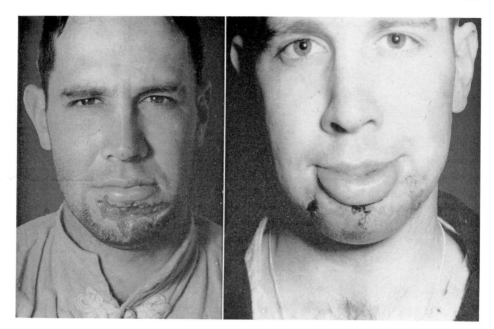

FIGURE 196.—This case illustrates a poorly advised secondary closure of a soft-tissue wound of the face. This wound obviously needed skin replacement rather than secondary closure since the wound was not causing disability and nothing was to be gained by closing it. If free skin-grafting was inadvisable at the time, such wounds were much better left for secondary healing and subsequent plastic revision.

others when this procedure involved the messy use of fingers or feeding tubes. If they were segregated with other patients suffering from the same handicap, this embarrassment disappeared, and a spirit of rivalry could be stimulated to see which could get the most food down and gain the most weight. Feeding of severe maxillofacial casualties in the late stage became a matter of simply supplying the soldier with suitable food in the right environment. Feeding in the earlier stages of care of such casualties provided a much more serious problem and frequently had to be solved by the insertion of a nasogastric tube for this purpose (fig. 190). Gastrostomy was not infrequently indicated in those severe types of casualties which could be expected to experience great difficulty in the ingestion of food over a long period of time and in whom a nasal tube could not be expected to be tolerated sufficiently long.

Blast injuries.—Blast injuries from landmines presented a most distressing problem. It was seldom the case that these patients were in good condition and without other associated severe injuries. Had this not been the case, it would have been possible to have given more of the blast injuries complete definitive treatment at an early hour. When it could be done, this treatment consisted of very careful, complete, meticulous cleansing of the face with removal of all embedded particles (fig. 187). Obviously, if thoroughly done, the procedure could be expected to require hours of operating time, and for this

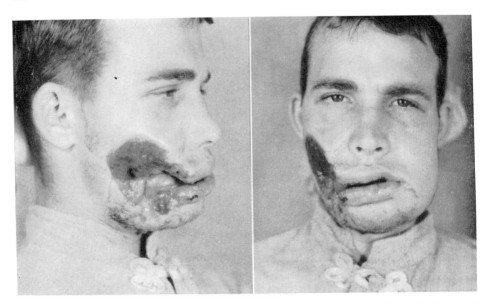

Figure 197.—This case illustrates a major facial defect at the time the patient arrived at a general hospital in England. Buccal mucosa to skin suture often is not possible in the extensive cheek defects. All efforts should be bent toward promoting bony replacement and union, in controlling sepsis, and in maintaining the patient's nutritional state. This type of patient is one requiring extensive nursing care and oral hygiene. Reparative or reconstructive surgery is not feasible at an early date. It is possible that an occasional wound of this nature might be speeded in healing by an early free skin graft, although occasions when this procedure could be used are not frequent.

reason it was frequently impractical because of other priority casualties or because of other associated more severe injuries. The condition resulted in very disfiguring scarring and "tattooing," and, when possible, complete early care was administered.

Summary.—The concept that certain types of injuries could best be managed by triage and evacuation to specialty centers in the communications zone was amply verified during World War II. The time and effort expended in establishing plastic and maxillofacial centers certainly proved to be justified. The same could be said for the specialties of neurosurgery and thoracic surgery. So far as facial reconstruction was concerned, it was of the greatest importance that proper judgment be exercised in determining just what and how much should be done in a communications zone. The policy of providing skeletal replacement and stabilization plus soft-tissue healing in as good an anatomical position as possible was a sound one. Such a policy made it possible to evacuate the casualties to the plastic surgery centers in the Zone of Interior in the best possible condition for final definitive surgical correction. The advent of the chemotherapeutic drugs and antibiotics had a profound impact upon the successful management of maxillofacial casualties as well as of all others.

Burns

By direction of the Chief Surgeon, ETOUSA, the treatment of burns that might require skin-grafting was made the responsibility of the Senior Consultant in Plastic Surgery. In view of the fact that so many burn casualties were expected to fall into this category, the Chief Surgeon and Col. Elliott C. Cutler, MC, Chief Consultant in Surgery, ETOUSA, asked the Senior Consultant in Plastic Surgery to formulate the policies for the treatment and evacuation of all burn casualties. At the time Colonel Brown, the first Senior Consultant in Plastic Surgery, ETOUSA, and this author arrived overseas in July 1942, there was still considerable debate within the National Research Council and the Surgeon General's Office over the problem of "closed" and "open" treatment of burns. At this time, "closed" and "open" methods referred to treatment by eschar-forming protein precipitants such as tannic acid, and non-eschar-forming dressings such as bland ointment or plain gauze.

Since Colonel Brown had always been an advocate of open methods of treatment, there was never any question in the European theater about which would be used. At the outbreak of the war, the use of tannic acid for the surface treatment of burns was still the official policy of the Army. By late 1942, this policy was changed by directives from the Surgeon General's Office, and 5 percent sulfadiazine in a water soluble cream base was advised. Tannic acid was taken off the tables of supply, and 5-percent-sulfadiazine cream was inserted. Early in 1943, the Cocoanut Grove disaster occurred in Boston and the voluminous writing following the treatment and study of these burn casualties, along with further studies by the National Research Council, led to the withdrawal of sulfadiazine for local treatment of burns by the Office of The Surgeon General because of the danger of toxic absorption of the drug from the burn surface. These various occurrences led to complete confusion in the minds of the individual medical officers who were to have the responsibility of treating burn casualties under combat conditions. Studies emanating from treatment of the Cocoanut Grove fire casualties led to the widespread belief that not only should treatment of the burn surface be restricted to the application of a bland ointment but any preliminary cleansing and debridement of the burn could be dispensed with.

The Senior Consultant in Plastic Surgery disagreed with both of these concepts in the treatment of war burns. A program was then instituted in the European theater to brief all incoming medical units concerning a standardized method of treating burns and to insure that each hospital unit had a well-defined plan of admitting, sorting, and treating these casualties if they should arrive in large numbers. In all planning at that time, thought had to be given to the possibility of mass civilian as well as military casualties. It was believed to be possible that many civilian casualties might result from enemy bombing, as in the Battle of Britain. It was believed mandatory that some semblance of standardization of treatment of burn casualties be established. This was not accomplished without some difficulty. Many first aid kits, particularly those kits supplied to the armored divisions, were still arriving in the theater containing tannic acid jelly. It was also of interest that, during the height of this educational program, a prominent visiting surgeon from the United States gave several very important lectures in which he not only deprecated the use of local antibacterial agents and of local cleansing and debridement but also created doubt and confusion concerning the efficacy of plasma replacement therapy in resuscitation. With the endorsement of Colonel Cutler, Senior Consultant in Surgery, and General Hawley, the Chief Surgeon, the policy was established in the European theater that burns would be treated by gentle and careful debridement and cleansing when possible, and the burn surface would be covered with a thin layer of fine-mesh gauze impregnated with 5-percent-sulfadiazine cream over which would be placed a pressure dressing. The policies concerning the treatment of burns, as crystallized in the Manual of Therapy, ETOUSA, appear in appendix G (p. 993) of this volume.

An interesting facet of this story was precipitated by the withdrawal from the tables of supply of the 5-percent-sulfadiazine cream by direction of the Office of The Surgeon General and upon the advice of the National Research Council. Again, with the backing of the senior medical officers of the European theater, it remained the policy that sulfadiazine cream would be used, and an attempt was made to procure the drug from local British sources. Unfortunately, the British could not produce sulfadiazine in adequate quantities at that time. A substantial quantity of sulfadiazine powder was therefore ordered from the United States, and arrangements were made for its incorporation in a cream base by British drug firms. However, when the sulfadiazine powder arrived (almost 2 years later) it was well past D-day, and the matter of local chemotherapy in the treatment of burns had faded into insignificance with the advent of unexpectedly adequate supplies of penicillin. It was suggested by the Senior Consultant in Plastic Surgery that the sulfadiazine powder residing in a warehouse in London be turned over to the British on reverse lend-lease. Two weeks after this was accomplished, the Eighth Air Force had traced this supply of the drug and requested it for use on their bomber crew personnel as a prophylactic to reduce the incidence of upper respiratory infections and otitis media which were exacting such a toll from the crew members. What became of the ton of sulfadiazine powder is not known, but this consultant was immensely relieved to have heard no more about it.

In retrospect, the advocacy of 5-percent-sulfadiazine cream in fine-mesh gauze for the treatment of all burns was probably poorly advised. It was used extensively during the early part of the war and, so far as this author is aware, there were no deaths directly attributable to overdosage from absorption of the drug from the burned surface. However, it was recognized that this danger did exist. There is no doubt in this author's mind that this was an effective way of controlling infection of the burned surface in the early postburn period. However, when penicillin became available in adequate amounts, it was quite logical to dispense with local chemotherapy and whatever hazard it may have entailed. It was this consultant's strong clinical impression that sulfadiazine cream was most effectively used in the treatment of hand burns. Here, there was no danger of overabsorption, and surface infection seemed to be better controlled than by other methods. It is unfortunate that there were no reliable controlled studies made on this subject.

Etiology.—Accidents accounted for a large portion of the burn casualties, and, as might be expected, they occurred most frequently in the wintertime. Command directives were issued forbidding the use of gasoline and other flammable materials for starting fires, for cleaning clothes, and for cleaning garage floors. In spite of these efforts, high octane gasoline continued to be used for such purposes, and some of the most severe burns occurred as a result. Because of the experiences of the British during the Battle of Britain, a high incidence of burns from the Eighth Air Force was expected. However, burn casualties from this source were never received in the numbers anticipated. It was believed that the low incidence of Air Force burns in the early days resulted from the fact that active air combat was carried out only across the Channel. Fighter pilots fell in France or Germany; and bomber crews most likely to have been subjected to burns did not get back to the bases in England. Burns from the Air Force as a result of active combat were limited almost completely to those received during takeoff and landing accidents in England. After the liberation of prisoners at the end of the war, a large number of the Air Force casualties were found to have suffered from burns and had been treated in enemy prisoner-of-war hospitals.

The landing on the shores of Normandy did not produce the large number of burns that might have been expected from closely packed troops in flammable vessels landing on a hostile shore. The incidence of burn casualties increased after the breakthrough at Saint-Lô when troops practically lived in traveling tanks and armored vehicles. These vehicles almost invariably burned upon being hit, and, in the case of the tanks which were hard to get out of, the resulting burns among the crew were very severe. Flash burns from bazooka fire were occasionally seen but were not common. Burns from white phosphorus and chemicals were comparatively rare. An unexpected and not infrequent type of burn was that occurring in paratroopers when they struck high tension wires during descent, with resulting limited but deep electrical burns.

An estimated 90 percent of all burns involved only the hands and face. A majority of the hand and face burns were superficial and could have been completely eliminated by the slightest degree of protection. In spite of continued efforts, it was impossible to get air force personnel to wear gloves as a precautionary measure against burns. The attitude of the young flier was that, while flying in combat, protection against burns was the least of his worries. He would not hamper himself by wearing gloves, nor would he consider any face protection that would restrict motion or limit the field of vision. Essentially the same philosophy was characteristic of the tank crewmen. Ordinary clothing was adequate protection against flash burns elsewhere on the body.

Evacuation hospital.—During combat, the evacuation hospital provided the first opportunity for the effective treatment of burn casualties. For resuscitation, reliance was placed on plasma and on saline and glucose solutions in adequate amounts. After resuscitation, the burn casualty was taken to the operating room and the burn surface was cleansed of dirt, clothing, and hanging devitalized skin. The dirt and filth that covered many of these wounds made it seem inadvisable to apply dressings without some effort at cleansing and debridement. Frequently, a mild soap or detergent was used gently on the burn if the condition of the patient permitted it. A good many burns were of limited surface extent and were not associated with other injuries. Under these circumstances, a meticulous debridement and cleansing seemed advisable. Burn surfaces were covered with 5-percent-sulfadiazine cream, petrolatum-impregnated gauze, or boric acid ointment gauze, and a pressure dressing was applied. Often, plaster splints would be added for immobilization. The casualty was then held, and resuscitation therapy was continued until his condition was considered satisfactory for evacuation. Patients with severe burns traveled poorly and often had to be held for several days before they could be safely moved. Evacuation was through regular channels by hospital train or air.

General hospital.—Upon reaching the communications zone, the bad burns were transported to hospitals designated for their care within a hospital center. In the United Kingdom Base Section, there were always hospitals that had been designated for plastic and maxillofacial surgery and had been prepared with adequate physical facilities for the management of complicated burn casualties. The plastic surgeon and his team in these hospitals worked with members of the general surgical service and medical service in preparing the burn casualties for the necessary skin-grafting operations. The 10 specialty hospitals in England treated the great majority of burn casualties occurring in the European theater, and the standard of professional management was uniformly high. The casualties were cared for by nurses, orderlies, and medical officers with a special and detailed appreciation of their needs. Saline bath units had been provided in eight of the specialty hospitals in England, and they were used extensively to make the changes of dressing as painless as possible and to promote hygiene of the wound (fig. 198). During the period of preparation of the wound for grafting, the general care of the patient was of utmost importance. His feeding and his state of morale were factors demanding constant attention. Corpsmen placed in charge of these patients were often combat soldiers on limited duty after having been burned in combat and having gone through treatment similar to that which they were now overseeing. The morale factor provided by these corpsmen as well as the enormous physical effort they expended in caring for the casualties in these burn centers was tremendous and cannot be acknowledged adequately. During the heaviest phase of the war, the burn centers were uniformly filled to capacity, and several

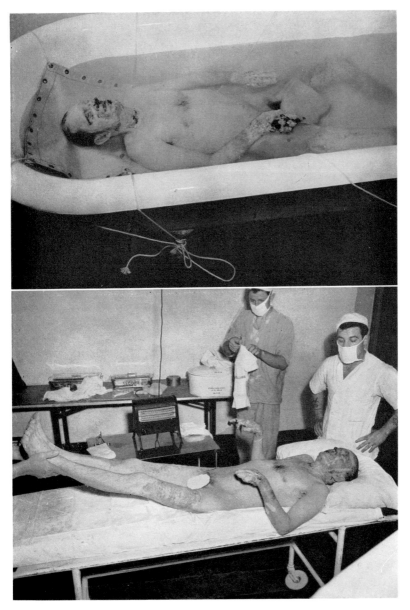

FIGURE 198.—There were 10 burn centers in England, scattered from the south coast to Liverpool and Nottingham. These centers proved invaluable for the accumulation of severe burn casualties requiring prolonged dressings and grafting. Large porcelain tubs for saline baths were provided in these centers and were used practically around the clock for the changing of dressings, debridement, exercise of extremities, and so on. The personnel of these centers, in addition to the doctors and nurses, consisted of corpsmen, many of whom were combat soldiers who themselves had suffered from burns. These men were trained to handle the patients in the baths and to do the debridement and dressings, and they proved to be ideal for the job.

of them worked on a 24-hour basis in keeping up with the resuscitation, dressing, debridement, saline tubing, and skin-grafting of these badly injured soldiers.

The saline bath units consisted of from one to four large tubs placed in rooms provided with adequate heat in the hospital selected and designated for the handling of burn cases. Some of these hospitals were selected before and during construction, and the burn units were incorporated in the hospital plan. In other completed hospital plants, or in those taken over from the British, an existing ward was modified and the saline bath units were added. The tubs were obtained from a firm in Scotland and were large and of cast iron with a thick, high-grade porcelain that would permit satisfactory cleansing and sterilization. The units were used during the late stages of treatment of burns and were considered particularly necessary for those burns involving the trunk, buttocks, and lower extremities. The first burn dressing in the general hospital was usually done in the operating room under light general anesthesia. This first dressing was usually from 2 to 6 days, or longer, after the initial application of the dressing in an evacuation hospital. Subsequent dressings were usually done in the saline bath units, at which time debridement of sloughing, devitalized tissue could be done most advantageously. This procedure greatly decreased the pain of dressings and facilitated the rapid healing of the wound surface and its preparation for grafting if this was going to be necessary. The bathrooms were supervised by medical officers and nurses.

Much of the actual work was done by corpsmen who were trained to do the dressing, cleansing, and debridement of wounds and the filling, emptying, and cleaning of the tubs. These were the enlisted men, a good many of whom had suffered severe burns themselves and had been through one of the treatment centers. The possibility of cross infection received careful study and consideration. Casualties with active hemolytic streptococcal infections were either not subjected to saline baths or were submitted to the procedure in a bath reserved for their use. Other organisms presented no difficulty from cross infection if the tubs were properly cleansed. Cleansing of the tubs was done with hot water and soap, followed by an antiseptic detergent. Cetyltrimethylammonium bromide, a British preparation, was the detergent most frequently used. This detergent was also found to be very good for the primary cleansing of the burned surfaces and for the subsequent cleansing of the wound and the surrounding skin. Submission of patients to saline baths had to be done with some caution. Reactions were not uncommon, and occasionally a sick patient had to have the baths discontinued. An effort was made to keep the temperature constant at about 105° F. and to keep the degree of salinity at normal by manual manipulation of the inflow of water and the addition of salt. It was not believed to be of great importance that these factors be absolutely controlled so long as the patient was comfortable and the solution was not allowed to become hypertonic. The baths offered an excellent opportunity for exercise of muscles and joints, and, with the minimum of effort, it was possible to prevent the marked deformities that so often have a tendency to occur before skin-grafting can be done. The baths were a very great factor in maintaining the morale of the patient, particularly if the patient had been unfortunate enough to have undergone a series of changes of dressings without baths before admission to the specialty hospital.

With the professional talent available and the physical facilities provided, it seemed advisable to establish the policy that all burns would be held until they were healed or grafted. These same intensive efforts that were aimed at getting the burn wound ready for grafting were equally effective in promoting healing. Care had to be exercised not to graft unnecessarily. It was to the credit of the medical officers taking care of these patients that hundreds of them were successfully grafted at an early date with resultant restriction in disability and loss of function. Immediate burn excision and grafting was not practiced except in an occasional case of electrical burn. The general practice was that of repeated debridement and dressings until the wound was clean enough for graft. If, by that time, the remaining third-degree loss was great enough and appeared to warrant it, a split graft was applied. The advent of penicillin to help control infection contributed greatly to the success of early grafting. The manually operated Padgett dermatome was available in the theater but was not an unmixed blessing. Good blades were available for those surgeons capable of cutting free hand grafts. So-called stamp grafts and pinch grafts were used occasionally in special situations.

Burns of various parts of the body presented different problems, but two areas in particular warrant special comment. Eyelid burns were very frequently observed. If these were severe enough, the problem of management in a communications zone hospital in preparation for evacuation to the Zone of Interior was a very trying one. The concern was primarily one of protection of the globe and preservation of sight. Almost invariably, patients with severe eyelid burns would have severe burns of the hands and could not be depended upon to take care of themselves during evacuation. In those cases in which lid eversion made it evident that the cornea was endangered, it seemed advisable to make some effort to decrease the danger by promoting lid adhesions or by grafting the lids (fig. 199). A decision as to just what to do for an individual casualty was frequently very difficult. It is beyond the scope of this presentation to go into this matter in detail. Suffice it to say, grafting of lids should not be done in a theater of operations if it can be avoided without endangering the cornea (fig. 200). It can be said also that the promotion of lid adhesions is not an entirely effective method of protecting the cornea since, in the severely burned lid, the contracting force is great enough to cause the adhesions to stretch and reexpose the cornea to ulceration (fig. 201). The situation is one demanding the most stringent nursing care and the closest collaboration between ophthalmologist and plastic surgeon.

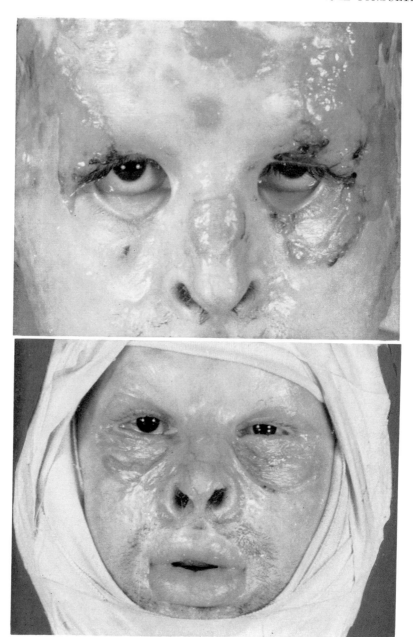

FIGURE 199.—This case illustrates ectropion from burns and is the type of case which, it is believed, urgently required correction by grafting before evacuation from the theater of operations. The danger of resulting corneal ulceration was considered to be too great to allow such patients to go through the chain of evacuation without being able to close their eyes. This case illustrates an extreme situation in which an early graft was done with very acceptable results. (Case of Maj. Dean W. Tanner, MC, 158th General Hospital.)

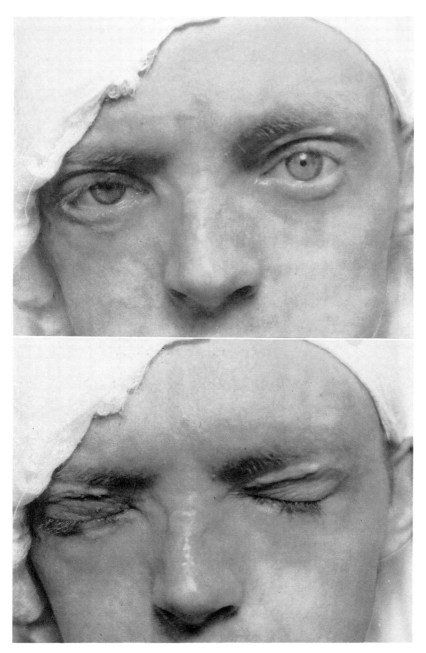

FIGURE 200.—This case is an excellent example of a needlessly applied eyelid graft. Obviously, there would have been no ectropion if the lids had been left to heal spontaneously. It was sometimes extremely difficult to determine whether grafting was indicated or not. Usually, if there was any question about it, it was better to postpone the procedure until it could be done by competent plastic surgeons in the Zone of Interior.

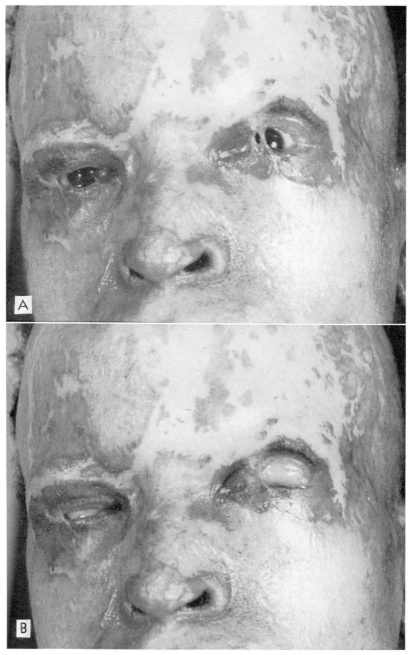

FIGURE 201.—Illustration of the futility of controlling lid contraction after burns by formation of interpalpebral adhesions. If adhesions appeared effective they were not necessary. Where protection was most needed because of contraction, the adhesions usually stretched and required protection did not result. This patient probably required grafting before evacuation. A satisfactory result was obtained. A and B. Views of eyelids, with eyes open and closed, before grafting.

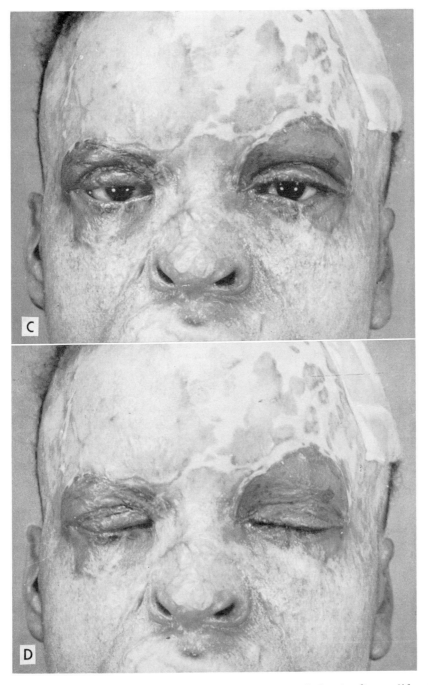

FIGURE 201.—Continued. C and D. Views, with eyes open and closed, after eyelid grafts were applied. (Case of Maj. Dean W. Tanner, MC, 158th General Hospital.)

Burns of hands were obviously of very great importance from both the numerical and functional standpoint. It was with hand burns that the prevention of edema and early control of infection were found to be of such great practical value, since the ultimate loss of full thickness of skin was as dependent on these factors as on the initial thermal injury. A burned hand allowed to develop uncontrolled edema not only resulted in embarrassing the circulation of the tightly stretched skin of the dorsum but made this skin more susceptible to infection. In this way, large areas of skin that were not destroyed by the initial thermal injury could be converted into third-degree burns. Therefore, it was the aim to make hands surgically clean as early as possible and to control edema by effective pressure dressings and elevation. The position of the hand and fingers during this period of immobilization was, of course, considered to be of great importance. The initial hand dressing was left on for from 6 to 8 days, following which exercise of the hand in saline baths and careful daily debridement was started. From this time on, supervised active exercise was emphasized in maintaining flexibility of the joint capsules. The burn was made clean and debrided of eschar as rapidly as possible. When the hand was clean enough for graft, it was carefully evaluated to determine whether the overall function of the hand could be more benefited by grafting with its attendant period of immobilization, or by continued exercises while spontaneous healing progressed (figs. 202 and 203). A decision was made upon the merit of each individual case, with the realization that preservation of function depended upon early grafting when it was really necessary but that function could be lost by unnecessary grafting and its associated period of immobilization.

Summary.—During the buildup phase before the invasion of Normandy, this author had rather grandiose plans for detailed study of burn casualties. He was even successful in having the Chief Surgeon's Office approve certain directives and statistical forms and charts which he hoped to accumulate by the thousands and from which it was anticipated valuable information might be secured. Needless to say, from D-day until the end of the war, this type of research was out of the question and all efforts were simply bent toward adequate care of the injured and the maintenance of lines of medical evacuation. The author had a feeling of guilt that more positive information did not result from this tremendous experience. At the same time, he had a feeling of admiration and respect for the medical officers who performed the terrific task of taking care of the burn casualties in the various centers. In retrospect, it can be stated without equivocation that the establishment of the burn centers was good planning and paid off tremendously in the results which were achieved. Regardless of later concepts of burn treatment and cross infection, the saline baths, as used, were effective in the handling of mass casualties during

World War II, and the writer would still want such facilities. The European theater was well supplied with highly qualified personnel and, after combat began, they were utilized to the very highest degree possible. Some perfectly superb work was done by various medical officers in the management of burn casualties, particularly in the management of the severely burned hands, and it is to be regretted that the patients involved were not subsequently followed and the results of this experience properly recorded. For those readers who may wish to be critical, the foregoing account is admitted to be an extremely superficial exposition of the management of this important type of casualty during World War II in the European theater.

Wounds Other Than Head Wounds

If one examines the medical history of World War I, it will be found that the possibility of delayed primary and secondary closure of wounds was recognized and practiced to a limited extent near the termination of that conflict. However, the chief impression left by the First World War was that wounds should be debrided and left open for secondary healing. This impression was strengthened by the intervening experience of the Spanish Civil War and the widely publicized plaster immobilization of wounds after debridement. The wounds treated by this manner were those of the extremities, and after adequate debridement the wound was dressed open, usually with petrolatum-impregnated gauze pack, and a plaster encasement dressing was applied. The plaster was not changed for many days. The wounds did well and, if debridement had been adequate, usually at the time of first inspection of the wound the base was found to be covered by healthy granulations and there was no evidence of invasive infection. The transportation of casualties was simplified by this procedure as was the nursing care. The disabling effects of prolonged immobilization and healing by secondary intention were minimized.

World War II was entered not only with the background of knowledge from World War I and the Spanish Civil War, but also with more of an appreciation of the methods whereby function of an extremity could be preserved after a severe wound. Furthermore, the day of the wonder drugs had arrived and the sulfonamides and antibiotics were ready for exploitation. Another factor of very great importance was that surgeons interested in reconstructive and plastic surgery had been demonstrating for the past several years what could be accomplished with various types of grafts in the healing of wounds, and the importance of healing extensive burn wounds by early grafts was generally recognized. It was natural that these background factors led immediately to a more aggressive method of war wound management as soon as the medical officers had an opportunity to start taking care of casualties.

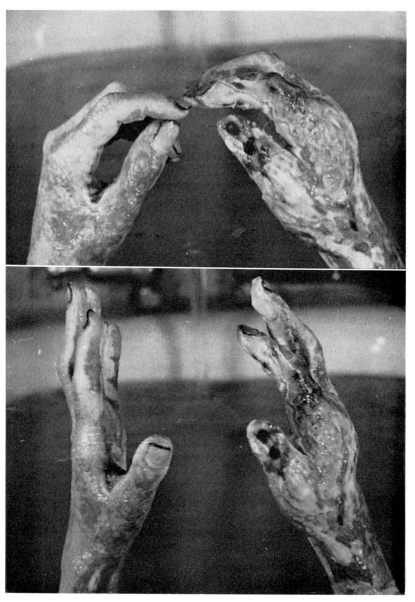

FIGURE 202.—This case ideally illustrates the principle of active motion and early grafting for the burned hand. Active motion can only be accomplished with all dressings removed. It was found to be most easily accomplished with the patient reclining in a saline bath so that the hands could be held in elevation and submerged at intervals as the exercise progressed. Smaller arm saline baths proved to be more practical when the burn was limited to the hand and arm.

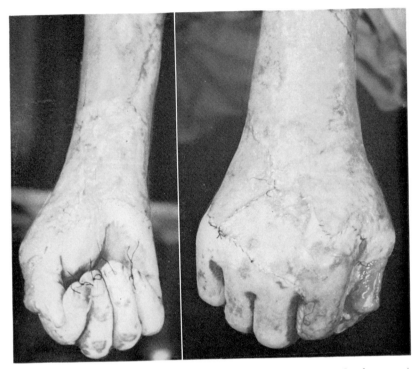

FIGURE 202.—Continued. The left hand, in the case illustrated, shows extensive persistent deep epithelial islands surrounding small areas of third-degree skin loss. This type of hand should not be grafted; instead, motion should be maintained and spontaneous healing encouraged. If grafting is indicated, eventually it may be done as a late, clean definitive operation. The right hand in this case obviously presents a deep third-degree burn with sloughing tissue and is the type of burn that should be grafted at the earliest possible date. The result of early grafting of the right hand in this patient was excellent. Some of the grafts were placed over small areas of exposed tendon. This type of work had to be done in the theater of operations. If the patient had been returned to the Zone of Interior, in spite of air evacuation, 1 or 2 weeks' time would have been lost before graft could be applied. (Case of Maj. Dean W. Tanner, MC, 158th General Hospital.)

Early in 1943, this consultant was attached to the 298th General Hospital from the University of Michigan Medical School which was stationed just outside Bristol, England. Shortly after he joined the hospital, it was filled with a boatload of casualties from the North African invasion. These patients had received what amounted to evacuation hospital care and arrived in England 2 or 3 weeks after having been injured. A remarkable opportunity was provided to study war wounds of varied extent and to crystallize opinions

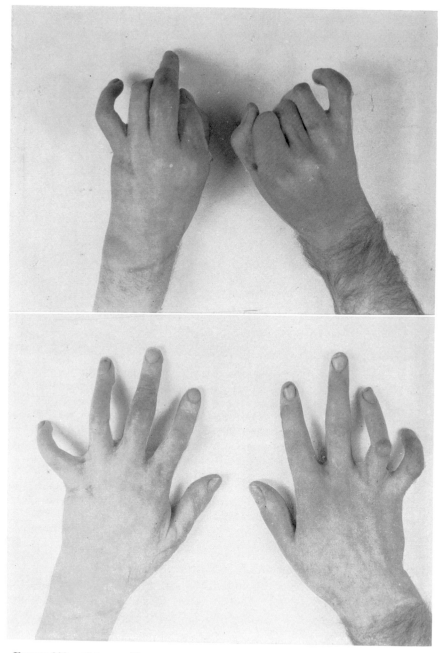

FIGURE 203.—This case illustrates the result that can be obtained by early radical graft to the dorsum of severely burned hands. The entire dorsum of each hand has been covered by an early graft. The flexibility and motion of the fingers are a direct result of the early application of skin covering. (Case of Maj. Byron C. Smith, MC, 1st General Hospital.)

regarding their treatment.   It was perfectly obvious that the provision of early healing by secondary closure would limit scarring, fibrosis, edema, and disability.   It was also perfectly obvious that the same results could be achieved with much larger and more extensive wounds, not amenable to secondary closure, by healing the wound with split graft.   Many such wounds were grafted very soon after the patients arrived in the hospital.   The results of these procedures were most gratifying.   The plastic surgery service at the 298th General Hospital pushed the principles of early closure and grafting.   This principle was extended subsequently to include pedicle grafting for compound injuries with exposed joints, tendon, and bone.   At the first ETOUSA Medical Society meeting held at the 298th General Hospital in June 1943, the results of an extensive grafting and secondary closure of war wounds were demonstrated, and it was predicted that such surgical procedures would play a very great role in the treatment of war casualties to be expected when the Continent was invaded.   The conception of excluding infection from the body by making the body surface intact was promulgated.   Just exactly when and on what type of casualties this conception could be successfully practiced was not completely realized at that time.   Early in 1943, a soldier was admitted to the 298th General Hospital after receiving an accidental explosive wound of the hand with exposure of bone and tendon.   This man was successfully treated with an immediate undelayed pedicle graft 24 hours following his injury.   In the light of this success and of the experience gained in treating casualties from North Africa, it was believed that secondary closure and free and pedicle grafting would be possible of application to war casualties on a large scale during the approaching invasion.   The plastic surgery centers throughout England were set up with this as one of the important functions in mind.   It later proved to be a very major portion of the work done in these hospitals.

The wounds under discussion were almost all confined to the extremities. A few of them were wounds of the shoulders and buttocks (fig. 204).   They were the result of small arms fire or shell fragments which had been treated by debridement at the evacuation hospital level.   The condition which had to be treated at the general hospital could be considered as due to the primary missile wound and its resultant necessary debridement.   When received in the general hospital, these wounds varied in age from 3 days to 2 weeks.   Many of them were associated with compound fractures.   Since secondary closure of such wounds can be considered as a general surgical procedure, the subject is not discussed in detail in this presentation.   However, the role played by the plastic surgery centers in the treatment of the complicated soft tissue and extremity wounds is briefly outlined.

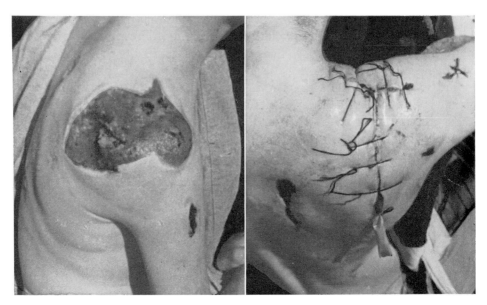

FIGURE 204.—This case illustrates the possibility of secondary closure of large, soft-tissue defects by extensive undermining and direct wound approximation. It was important that a proper balance be maintained between the possibility of closure by this method and the need for tissue surface replacement in the form of a free graft. (Case of Lt. Col. Thomas O. Otto, MC, 305th Station Hospital.)

Free skin grafts.—The type of wounds most frequently suitable for healing by the use of free grafts was those which presented extensive loss of skin with exposed muscle or fascia which could be expected to take a graft. If bone or tendon presented themselves within the depth of the wound, free graft was usually unsuitable, a pedicle graft being indicated if simple secondary closure was impossible. Wounds suitable for free graft were usually confined to the massive fleshy part of the extremities or of the trunk (fig. 205). Extensive wounds of the feet, ankles, lower leg, knee, and corresponding areas in the upper extremity usually required covering by use of the pedicle graft.

The wound was prepared for free skin graft in essentially the same manner that it was prepared for secondary closure. It was necessary that it be free of sloughing tissue and free of localized collections of pus. It was not necessary to wait until a granulation tissue bed had developed. It was found that a free graft could be applied satisfactorily at any time interval after debridement, provided the wound fulfilled the qualifications of being free of sloughing tissue and growth of surface organism. Repeated debridement and wet dressings played an important role in the preparation of the "dirty" wound. Dakin's solution was very prominent by its almost complete absence from the surgical armamentarium.

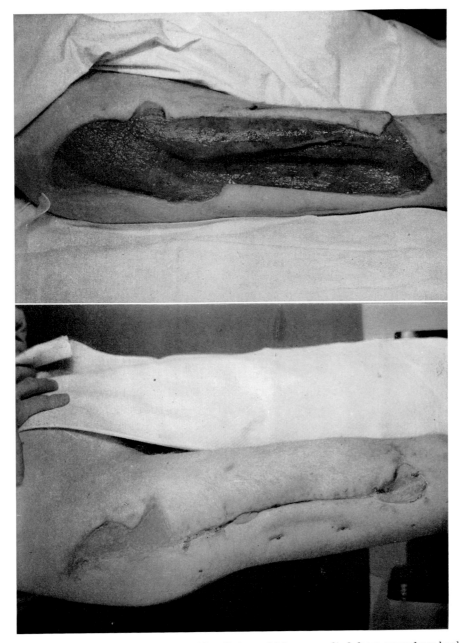

FIGURE 205.—The extensive disability that would have resulted from secondary healing of this wound is obvious. The postoperative illustration shows the admirable result obtained by closure of the large defect by mobilizing the skin edges and by free skin-grafting that portion of the wound which could not be closed. (Case of Maj. Douglas W. Macomber, MC, 91st General Hospital.)

The free grafts were applied in a fairly standardized manner which usually involved immobilization of the extremity and some type of pressure dressing. It was of some importance that proper judgment be exercised and that insignificant wounds not be grafted. Many wounds which appeared almost certainly to need a graft were found to be not worthy of a graft by the time they were clean enough for this procedure. Needless to say, a few instances were seen in which a small wound had been successfully grafted but the soldier remained disabled as a result of an unhealed donor area. It has been mentioned previously that the dermatome was not an unmixed blessing.

Pedicle grafts.—The wounds suitable for covering by use of a pedicle graft were those of the extremities in which important structures (bone, tendon, and nerve) are normally covered by a relatively thin layer of superficial tissue and skin. This situation exists in the feet, ankles, anterior portion of the lower legs, knees, hands, wrists, forearms, and elbows. These are all vitally important functional areas. A good many wounds involving these parts were of the avulsed type which, following adequate debridement, presented exposed bone and tendon and often open joints, impossible of closure by any other means than the use of a pedicle graft. If these important exposed structures were to be preserved, the pedicle graft must be applied at an early date. This was considered to be one condition in which a definitive plastic surgery procedure in a theater of operations was urgently indicated. If the procedure was postponed until the casualty arrived in the Zone of Interior, important function and structures would be lost. The recognition of the need for the procedure of pedicle grafting and its effective application in a theater of operations was a new development in war surgery. By effective application it is meant that the conditions requiring pedicle grafts were widely recognized and the casualties were accumulated into plastic surgery centers where the procedure could be properly controlled and well done. There were recorded 700 pedicle grafts of this nature, done in the plastic surgery centers in England alone. During the tour of the Senior Consultant in Plastic Surgery through the plastic surgery centers in the Zone of Interior in March of 1945, the evaluation of the procedure of pedicle graft by the Zone of Interior's surgeons was carefully sought. It was found to be held in very high regard and to be considered in many cases to have greatly simplified later reconstructive procedures.

The preparation of the wound for pedicle graft differed slightly from the preparation of a wound for secondary closure, or for covering by skin graft, in that it did not have to be nearly so complete. All gross sloughing tissue obviously needed to be removed. However, the covering of a wound by tissue which was viable, and which did not have to rely for continued viability on nourishment from the wound itself, offered possibilities which had never been exploited to the fullest. Not only was this covering self-sustaining in that it carried nourishing blood supply, but it served as a viable vascular dressing for the surface of the wound where it could actually contribute to the natural processes of overcoming infection and healing. It was felt that pedicle grafting to accomplish secondary covering of the wound was even more physiologically sound than was secondary closure in that there was no embarrassment of the circulation of the wound margin by tension or deep sutures, and the wound, always a contaminated one, was not closed in the true sense of the word, since complete drainage was afforded the entire wound through the wide margin to which the graft was not sutured.

Since the only reason for holding a casualty long enough in a theater of operations for the application of a pedicle graft was the early performance of the procedure to preserve function, the technique had to be developed for this purpose. If the peculiarities of the case were such that the graft could not be applied to the wound for 2 or 3 weeks or longer, there was no point in holding the patient in the European theater for the procedure. It was presumed that the medical organization in the Zone of Interior would be able to accomplish the procedure within that period of time. If the case was such that important structures and function would not be lost if a temporary free skin graft was applied, it was better that the free graft be done and the patient be evacuated to the Zone of Interior. The procedure was, therefore, reserved for those cases in which the graft could be applied without delay and in which early application was mandatory. The technique of application of the pedicle graft was consequently modified in order that it might be extended to as large a number of cases falling into this category as possible.

The great majority of pedicle grafts were done as direct undelayed flap grafts, elevated and attached to the recipient area at one sitting. The direct abdominal wall (fig. 206) and thoracic (figs. 207 and 208) flap grafts were the simplest to use. In the beginning, direct grafts from the lower leg were done with some trepidation. As experience and ingenuity increased, it was discovered that there were few wounds from the knee down that could not be covered with a direct graft from the other leg. It can be stated that the direct crossed leg pedicle grafts proved to be much better than attempts to close lower leg defects by the use of local rotation flaps. When the defect required coverage by skin and subcutaneous tissue, the results of pedicle grafts early in the war surpassed those of local methods of closure and the latter were discarded.

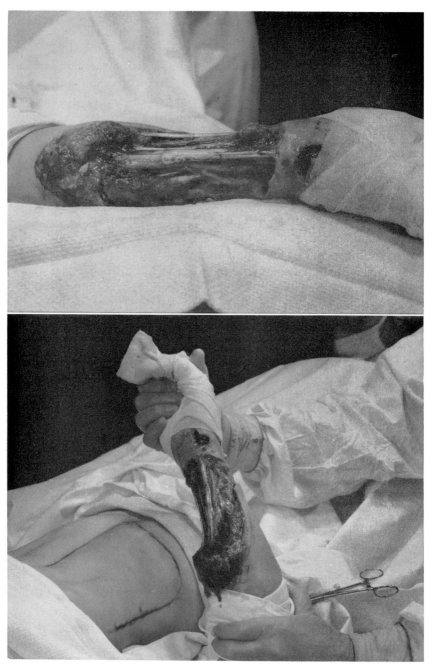

FIGURE 206.—This case is an ideal illustration of the type of injury in which pedicle grafting should be done without delay. All flexor tendons were exposed. The soldier was wounded on 6 September 1944. Eight days later, the wound was completely covered by an abdominal pedicle graft. The last photograph shows the arm 6 weeks following injury. The value of an early pedicle graft in an injury such as this cannot be exaggerated.

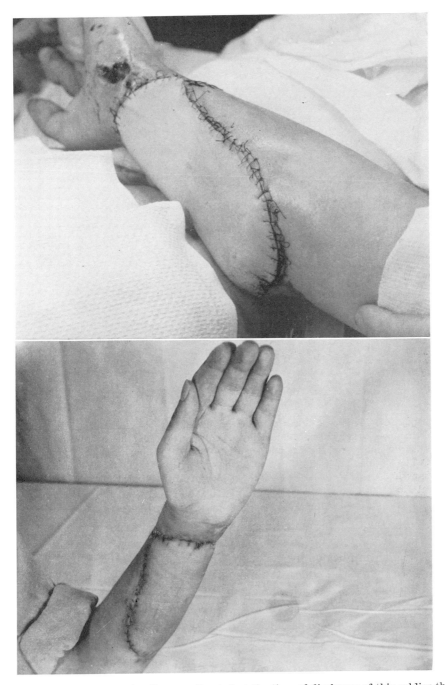

FIGURE 206.—Continued.   It was estimated at the time of discharge of this soldier that he would get about 85 percent return of function of the hand. Without the pedicle graft, there would have been complete loss of function. (Case of Capt. William W. L. Glenn, MC, and Lt. Col. Eugene M. Bricker, MC, 22d General Hospital.)

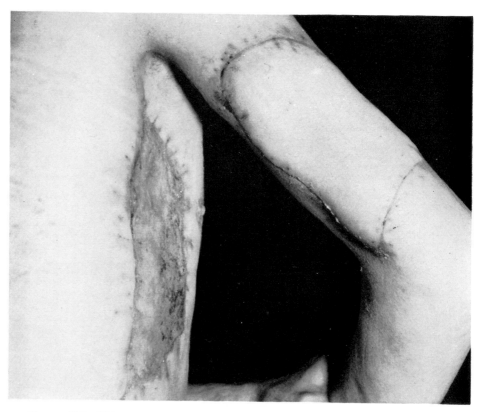

FIGURE 207.—This case illustrates the end result of replacement of a large soft-tissue loss of the upper arm by use of an undelayed pedicle graft from the chest wall. In planning all undelayed flat grafts, the size and position of the base is obviously of very great importance. The size of the base in this case demonstrates the extreme which sometimes may be necessary if a graft is to be successful. (Case of Maj. Clifford LaV. Kiehn, MC, 117th General Hospital.)

One factor that accounted for the use of the lower leg so frequently as a means of accomplishing crossed leg pedicle grafts was that many of these wounds were complicated by associated fractures (fig. 209). It was a frequent occurrence that a pedicle graft might be urgently needed, but its application was almost impossible because of an accompanying fracture. A great deal of ingenuity was exercised in solving these problems. In some cases, it was justifiable to consider applications of the graft as being more important than primary consideration of the fracture. Properly applied plaster splints could sometimes be made to hold the fracture in position during application of the graft. The use of Anderson splints was resurrected to help solve these problems, and they were found to be of distinct value in some cases for maintenance of position during the period of preparation of the wound and application of the graft (fig. 210). The splint was left in place only until the graft was completed, a matter of 3 or 4 weeks, after which it was removed and the generally accepted methods of treating fractures were instituted from this point on.

Very few delayed flap grafts were done. Obviously, if delay was necessary, the job might just as well be done in the Zone of Interior. However, there were a few instances in which the procedure could be simplified and the certainty of a satisfactory outcome increased by delaying the pedicle graft. This would often be done while the wound was being prepared to receive the graft.

Tubed pedicle grafts were found to have very little application in solving the needs of early grafting in a theater of operations. Even when the time element was of no importance, tubing of the graft was considered to be a superfluous procedure.

Pedicle grafting was not used for facial reconstruction in the communications zone. It was felt that this was a procedure better done in the plastic surgery centers in the Zone of Interior.

Summary.—The opportunity of using pedicle grafts in the treatment of complicated war wounds on such a scale as was done in the European theater was a unique experience. There is no doubt that it served a great purpose in the preservation of function in many extremities.

Treatment of Hand Injuries

Plastic surgeons had long been interested in the problems presented by the injured hand. Long before the invasion of Normandy, burned hands and the severe wounds of hands received accidentally in combat training were recognized as acute problems. After the Normandy invasion, it was discovered early that hands were going to form an unexpectedly high percentage of casualties and that the principles involved in treating hand injuries were not generally recognized. The plastic surgeons were then interested primarily in replacing the soft-tissue loss in the avulsed type of injury (figs. 211 and 212). This had been practiced as an early procedure previously at the 298th General Hospital in England. This problem having been recognized, cases were searched for throughout the hospital centers in England and those requiring pedicle grafts were transferred to the hospitals designated for plastic surgery. This accumulation of the severely injured hands in the plastic surgery hospitals led to the logical conclusion that the best method for handling all hand injuries was to place them in special services under interested, qualified personnel.

On 4 September 1944, a memorandum on the subject of development of hand centers (app. II, p. 999) was submitted to the Chief Consultant in Surgery and referred to hand centers in both the communications zone and the Zone of

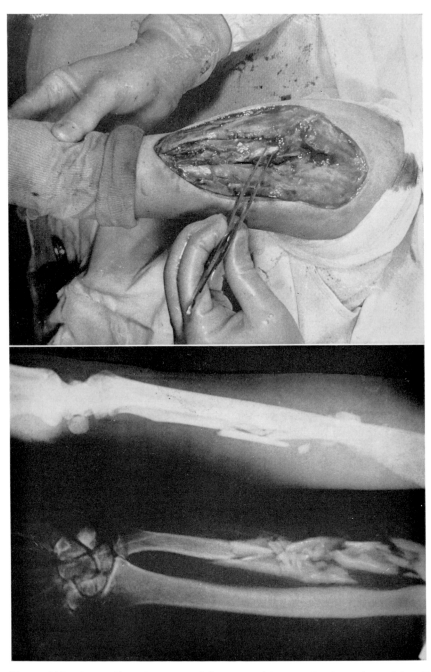

FIGURE 208.—A complicated compound fracture with extensive loss of overlying tissue is converted into a simple fracture by the use of an undelayed pedicle graft. It was found that these grafts could be applied to wounds that far from fulfilled our original concept of how a wound should appear before a graft could be applied.

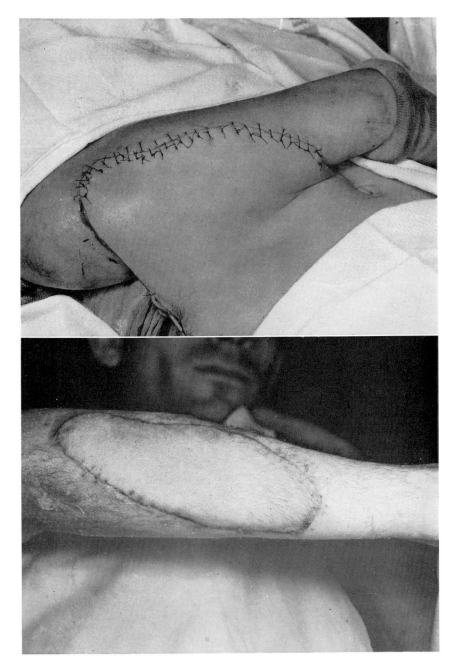

FIGURE 208.—Continued. A vascular type of graft cannot be compared with a free graft that depends on the wound for its own sustenance. A well-planned pedicle graft is a viable vascular dressing that can be considered as carrying sustenance to a wound. (Case of Maj. Clifford LaV. Kiehn, MC, 117th General Hospital.)

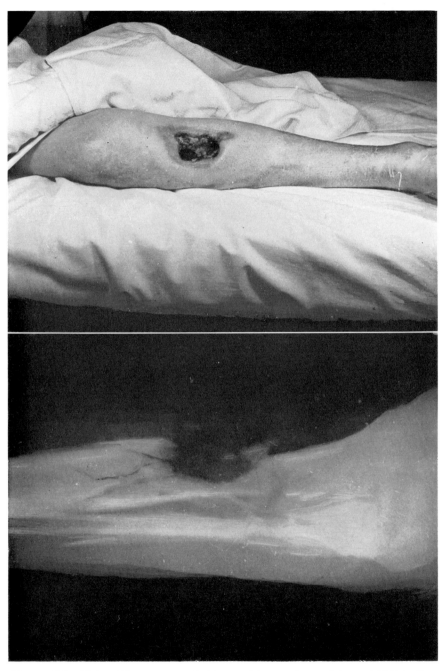

FIGURE 209.—This soldier was wounded by machinegun fire on 5 August 1944 in France. He was evacuated to a hospital center in England where a split graft was attempted on 8 October. It was not until 21 October that the patient was transferred to a plastic surgery center and the pedicle graft applied.

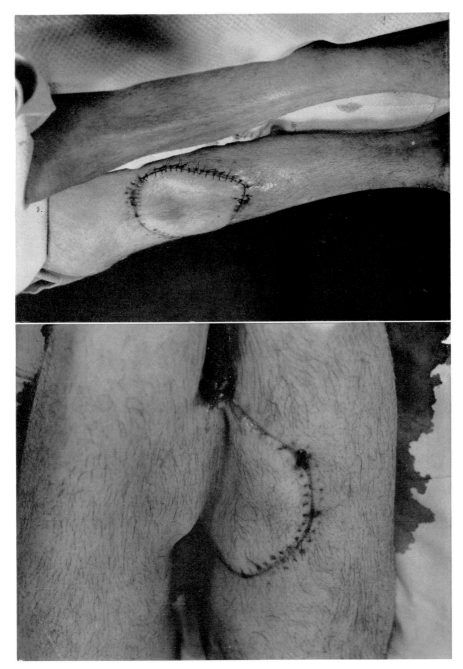

FIGURE 209.—Continued. Ideally, the pedicle graft could have been applied from 7 to 14 days after injury. (Case of Lt. Col. Malvin F. White, MC, 129th General Hospital.)

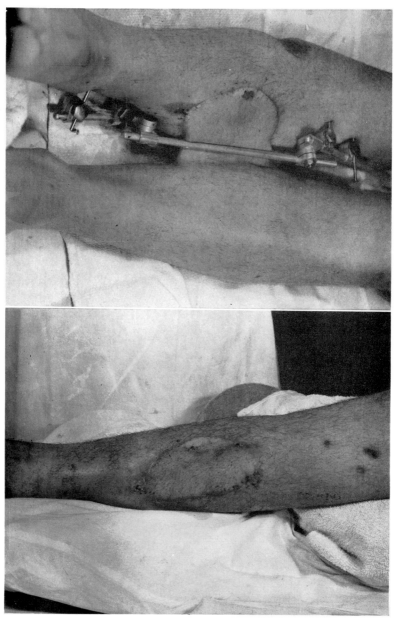

FIGURE 210.—This case illustrates the technique of immediate undelayed cross leg pedicle graft covering a compound defect of the tibia. The Anderson splint was occasionally used in these complicated cases. The splint was dispensed with as soon as a graft was applied. Large, undelayed flap grafts such as that illustrated were possible. The fact that the leg grafts were done with such a low incidence of failures was undoubtedly due, in large part, to the youth of the patients. (Case of Lt. Col. Malvin F. White, MC, 129th General Hospital.)

Interior. Following this, hand centers were developed both in England and on the Continent. It was the aim to have each center under the supervision of both a qualified orthopedic surgeon and a plastic surgeon. With the cooperation of Col. Mather Cleveland, MC,[1] Senior Consultant in Orthopedic Surgery, most of the hand centers were located in the hospitals designated for plastic surgery. Although this was a very definite step forward, it by no means solved the problem of adequate care for hand injuries.

With the start that was made, it is believed that, had the war progressed, the organization would have resulted in a standard of care for hand injuries never before equaled. Unfortunately, this state of affairs was far from being reached by the end of the war. The difficulty resided in the fact that the plastic and orthopedic surgeons themselves had much to learn, and the respective consultants were slow in recognizing the need for fundamental changes in overall policies. The surgeons in the hand centers believed at an early stage that they had reached an impasse because they were not receiving the casualties early enough after the injury. This led to the idea that possibly more definitive surgery should be done at the evacuation hospital level. The standard of care at the evacuation hospital level previously had not been high. Although it may be understandable that the surgeons at the evacuation hospitals were more concerned with injuries of a more serious nature, it hardly justifies the delegation of injured hands to surgeons of the least experience, as was frequently done. In March 1945, a directive was issued stating that hand injuries should be closed after they were debrided in the evacuation hospitals. The results of this policy could never be determined with certainty because the war ended soon after it was put into effect. It is, indeed, doubtful that much would have been accomplished by this change in policy.

Hand wounds with such loss of soft tissue that important underlying structures were exposed fell into the category of those amenable to pedicle grafting. The procedure of pedicle grafting of such wounds had certain shortcomings and limitations, the most notable of which was the unavoidable limitation of motion and poor position often necessary during application of the pedicle graft. With proper care, these objectionable features could, to a large extent, be avoided. It was possible to have good position and active motion maintained during the time the graft was being applied in most, but not all, cases. It took fine judgment to weigh the disadvantages afforded by these objectionable features against the need for pedicle graft and to decide whether the procedure should or should not be done. This author's views at the time on the treatment of hand injuries were set forth in a memorandum, dated 5 March 1945, to Colonel Cleveland, Senior Consultant in Orthopedic Surgery, ETOUSA, (app. I, p. 1001).

---

[1] Cleveland, Mather: Chapter IV, Hand Injuries in the European Theater of Operations. *In* Medical Department, United States Army. Surgery in World War II. Hand Surgery. Washington: U.S. Government Printing Office, 1955.

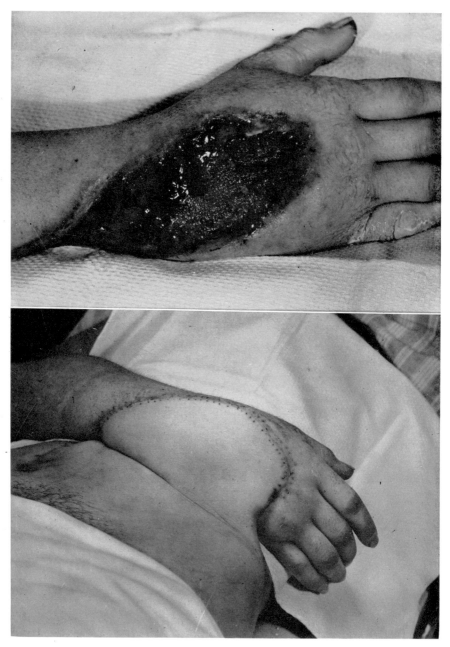

FIGURE 211.—The illustration of a large, soft-tissue loss from the dorsum of the hand, associated with underlying bone injury. Such a wound might conceivably be covered by a split graft. However, the possibilities of return of function and subsequent reconstructive surgery are greatly increased if a pedicle graft is used.

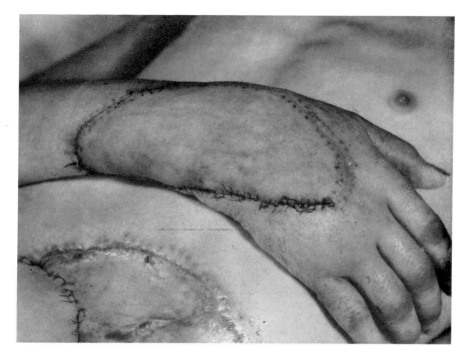

FIGURE 211.—Continued.

Summary.—When one considers all the thought and planning devoted to the preparation for treatment of maxillofacial injuries, burns, and massive soft-tissue injuries, it is surprising that more definitive plans for the treatment of injured hands were not formulated earlier in the course of the war. It was never anticipated that severe hand injuries would form such an important segment of the casualty list. It is perfectly obvious that an anatomical structure as delicate and complicated as the hand requires the most detailed and skilled care if function is to be maintained. Although the late phase of care of injured hands has been developed to a very fine degree, there is no doubt that the very early care could be of equal importance in the preservation of function. Until very late in the war, our overall efficiency in the early care of hand injuries might be compared to that of a plumber trying to service a Swiss watch. This should not obscure the fact that there were two or three surgeons in the European theater who were extremely expert at hand care and who were, to a large extent, responsible for stimulating more interest in this type of injury.

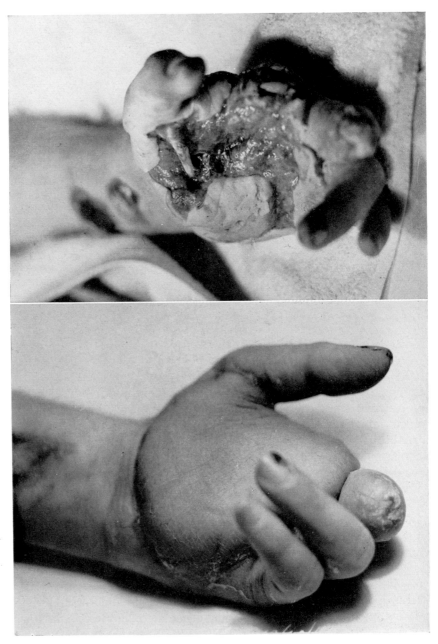

FIGURE 212.—The provision of surface covering through and beneath which subsequent
reconstructive surgery would be possible was of primary importance in the rehabilitation
of the injured hand. However, it had to be applied with a proper perspective and with
consideration of total hand function. In the case illustrated here, the urgent demand
for palm covering in relation to subsequent function is perfectly obvious. (Case of Lt.
Col. B. Eugene Boyer, MC, 53d General Hospital.)

CHAPTER IX

Urology

John N. Robinson, M.D.

Maj. Gen. Paul R. Hawley, MC, Brig. Gen. Elliott C. Cutler, MC, and Col. James C. Kimbrough, MC, organized in ETOUSA (European Theater of Operations, U.S. Army) the finest surgical consultant system the U.S. Army has ever known. The system was initiated with the arrival of U.S. troops in Great Britain and was gradually curtailed after V–E Day. On 5 October 1943, Maj. (later Lt. Col.) John N. Robinson, MC (fig. 213), was appointed Senior Consultant in Urology, ETOUSA, in addition to being chief of urology at the 2d General Hospital.[1] The small volume of troops and the small number of urological cases at this time made this part-time arrangement possible. Soon, however, the volume of work increased so much that it became necessary for the author to devote full time to this job. Thus, he became the only consultant in urology to be appointed at a theater headquarters level during World War II. The general duties of senior consultants in the European theater have been enumerated elsewhere. Briefly, they may be characterized as being "the eyes and ears of the Chief Surgeon."

JUSTIFICATION FOR A SENIOR CONSULTANT IN UROLOGY

How was a urological consultant justified when there were general surgeons available who might possibly cover this field?

First, it is necessary to recall that the development of Specialty Boards and certification had grown between the wars and that urology had become a specialty recognized by the leading societies and medical schools. In ETOUSA, as well as in the U.S. Army as a whole, the many civilian doctors who had volunteered for service were not qualified to do urology when compared with a certified urologist. Hence, with one or two urologists in each hospital and over 200 hospitals in operation, it was natural that there should be a urological consultant. Only one urologist had been certified by the board in the peacetime U.S. Army immediately prior to the period of limited emergency declared in 1939.

Second, in an oversea theater, it was not always possible to use civilian consultants as in the Zone of Interior, and the Army would have been open to criticism if the best specialty care had not been available.

---

[1] Office Order No. 40, Office of the Chief Surgeon, Headquarters, European Theater of Operations, U.S. Army, 5 Oct. 1943.

Third, the general surgical consultants were so busy that they did not have time to attend to the details of urology, did not know the personnel, and, in some instances, were not familiar with certain new developments.

Fourth, the positive reasons for this appointment, from the writer's point of view, were that the urologist in a general hospital had no one to consult, no one with whom to discuss new developments, and no one with whom to air problems. Also, the consultant's visits were often a means of solving problems of a personal nature, especially in making some of the junior officers feel that they were needed and that someone above the hospital level was interested in their welfare. In other words, it helped the morale of these officers. There

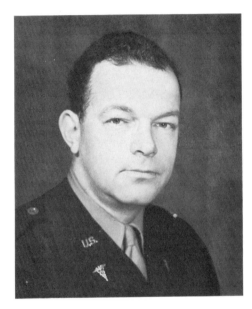

FIGURE 213.—Maj. John N. Robinson, MC.

were also times when the consultant helped in ascertaining the capabilities of a hospital urologist as an aid to the chief of surgery and the commanding officer. The commanding officers of hospitals were always most helpful and cooperative.

Fifth, as the number of hospitals and urologists increased, a need for meetings developed for the purpose of discussing urological problems and new developments and formulating plans for the future. This author organized and held approximately nine of these meetings in Great Britain and on the Continent. Many of these meetings were held at the time of large Allied medical meetings so that urologists in the theater were able to attend both. From 15 to 45 urologists attended these sessions. Much of value came from these meetings; and, needless to say, they would not have been held had it not been for the fact that there was available someone with the ability to initiate and direct them.

Sixth, it is almost impossible to secure accurate and valid statistics after any war is finished. Regrettably, this collection of statistics did not start soon enough in the European theater; but, eventually, worthwhile information, based on reports received from the evacuation, station, and general hospitals in the theater, was compiled. One of the most important reasons for having special consultants was to direct the gathering of medical information. Also, a specialty such as urology needed representation in order not to be left out in planning for the future.

Finally, the writer was of the opinion that, had Colonel Kimbrough, Chief of Professional Services in the Office of the Chief Surgeon, not been a dedicated urologist, there might not have been a Senior Consultant in Urology in the European theater, in spite of all other cogent reasons for appointing such a consultant.

ACTIVITIES OF THE SENIOR CONSULTANT IN UROLOGY

Colonel Kimbrough was the acting urological consultant from 1942, when U.S. Army hospitals first arrived in the United Kingdom, until the appointment of the Senior Consultant in Urology in October 1943. In these early days, supply and administrative considerations were of the first order, with the result that, at the beginning, there was not much urology practiced other than some treatment of gonorrhea and a few operations. Often, the urologist learned to become one of the best foraging officers in the units (fig. 214). At times the British food and equipment were trying, but everyone soon became acclimatized. The first responsibility was to get back to duty every soldier, in preparation for the invasion. After the Senior Consultant in Urology was appointed, monthly visits to each hospital were made; but this soon became impossible due to the increasing number of hospitals.

In this period before the invasion, everyone was busy with the planning and improvisation necessary to take care of expected casualties (fig. 215). Most of this work was routine, but the use of penicillin in the treatment of gonorrhea was of great interest. Its first use took place at the 2d General Hospital, which was located near Oxford, where Dr. Howard E. Florey was developing penicillin for clinical use. At first, small doses of 10,000 units every hour or 2 for 10 doses were given, and then larger doses, until finally a large single dose was accepted as the standard method of treatment. The first war casualties from air raids over the Continent were also received in this period. Data gathered from the operational research unit of the Office of the Chief Surgeon, ETOUSA, showed that, of 147 airmen killed in action, 9.5 percent had injuries to the genitourinary tract in addition to their fatal injuries.[2]

Another important service performed by the urological consultant was the writing and editing in collaboration with Colonel Kimbrough and Maj. Howard I. Suby, MC, of the urological section of the "Manual of Therapy, European Theater of Operations," a guide to the handling of all severe genitourinary injuries.[3]

---

[2] (1) Kimbrough, J. C.: War Wounds of the Urogenital Tract. J. Urol. 55 : 179–189, February 1946. (2) Medical Department, United States Army. Surgery in World War II. General Surgery. Volume I. [In preparation.]

[3] Manual of Therapy, European Theater of Operations, Surgical Emergencies, Section B, VIII. Wounds of the Genito-Urinary System.

During the early days of the invasion, before hospitals could be established on the Continent, Colonel Robinson's duties consisted of visiting hospitals set up along the south shore of England to assure that urology was well taken care of and, as did all surgical consultants, to carry out orders of the Chief Surgeon concerning general surgical matters.   As the hospitals began to function on the Continent, hospital centers began working fully, and, in some of

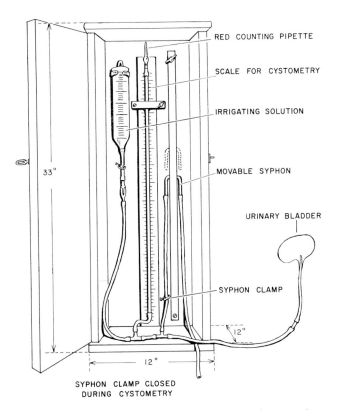

RED COUNTING PIPETTE

SCALE FOR CYSTOMETRY

IRRIGATING SOLUTION

MOVABLE SYPHON

URINARY BLADDER

33"

SYPHON CLAMP

12"

12"

SYPHON CLAMP CLOSED
DURING CYSTOMETRY

FIGURE 214.—A drawing of a portable tidal drainage-cystom-
eter set designed and built in the European theater.

these, special treatment facilities were set up to take care of special problems.   With the exception of neurogenic bladders associated with paraplegics, there was no need for genitourinary special treatment facilities because there were a sufficient number of well-trained urologists.   Thus, all problems could be taken care of in any of the general hospitals (fig. 216).   There was a urologist for all but one general hospital.   All but a few station hospitals had a urologist, and those that did not had consultation available at a short distance. The evacuation hospitals had at least one capable urologist per field army available for consultation.

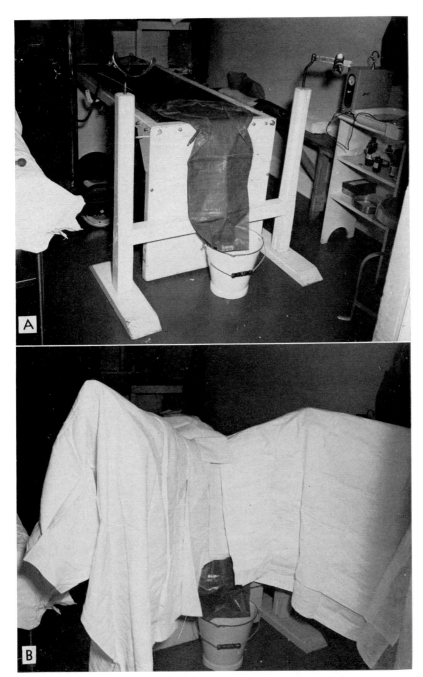

FIGURE 215.—Improvisation at the 38th Station Hospital, Winchester, England, to permit the performance of complete cystoscopy with retrograde pyelography. The 38th Station Hospital was established to act as a transit (evacuation) hospital during the continental invasion. A. Improvised stirrups for ordinary Bucky X-ray table. B. A patient in position, fully draped.

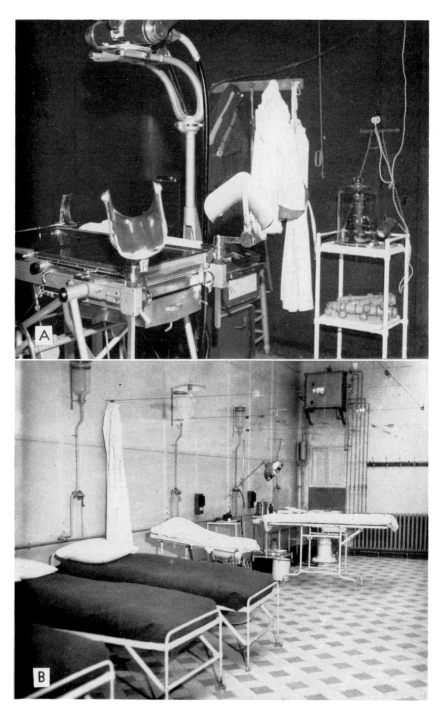

FIGURE 216.—The genitourinary clinic at the 45th General Hospital. A. Cystopyelographic facilities. B. A ward.

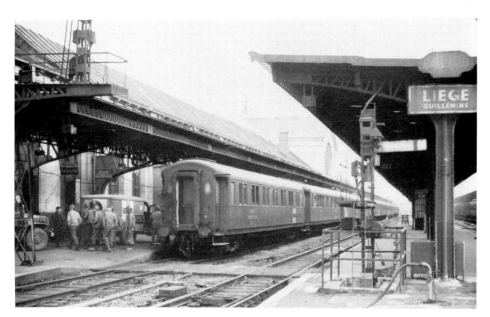

FIGURE 217.—A hospital train being loaded at Liége, Belgium.

During full-scale operations on the European Continent, consultation, inspection, and personnel placing were the primary functions of the writer, as Senior Consultant in Urology. Clinical meetings were held when possible at places where most officers could attend. In between these duties, one of this consultant's interesting assignments was to report on the efficiency of an ambulance train plying between Liége, Belgium, and Paris (fig. 217). Interestingly enough, this ambulance train was commanded by a urologist who liked his work. Getting the soldiers back to duty as soon as possible was still the most important responsibility, and, in this connection, the writer helped to set up urological rehabilitation facilities at the chief rehabilitation center in England. The result was a saving of time in returning a soldier to duty.[4] Much time was devoted to checking on all cases that did not do well and endeavoring to find out how to correct bad results.

During the closing days of the war in Europe, the author gathered some of the theater's top urologists in Paris for the purpose of assembling data and writing about wounds of the genitourinary tract, using as sources their personal experiences and material collected from the hospitals.[5] A final remark about urologic personnel is that more than 200 urologists were working in urology on V–E Day. Twenty-five urologists were not. Many of the latter had been averse to remaining in urology because, by doing so, they would have lost any chances for promotion.

---

[4] (1) Urological rehabilitation was organized by Capt. Marius Russo, MC, at the rehabilitation center at the 307th Station Hospital, Stoneleigh Park, Warwickshire, under command of Col. Frank E. Stinchfield, MC. (2) See footnote 2(2), p. 575.

[5] See footnote 2(2), p. 575.

CHAPTER X

Anesthesia

Ralph M. Tovell, M.D.

When this writer (fig. 218) was requested, in November 1954, to prepare for publication a personal account of his experiences as Senior Consultant in Anesthesia to the Chief Surgeon, ETOUSA (European Theater of Operations, U.S. Army), he was hesitant about acceding to the request, for he realized that it would be difficult to recapture the spirit and anxieties of the national effort during World War II. In addition, failures of memory were likely to occur when one attempted to recall events after the lapse of almost 10 years since the European campaigns had been successfully terminated. He was aware of the fact that he had a copy of a factual account of anesthesiology in the European theater that had been prepared at the end of the war as a part of the medical history of the theater in World War II. Little did he realize the difficulties that would be encountered once he undertook to refer to source material in the preparation of this chapter. When this was attempted, there immediately arose a conflict between the recorded data worthy of publication and the events that would be interesting to those who might read this volume. It is in the shadow of this background that the writer attempts to capture the reader's interest.

CALL TO ACTIVE DUTY

When the United States entered World War II on 7 December 1941, it was expected that the writer would be declared essential and that military service would fall to the lot of members of his staff at Hartford Hospital, Hartford, Conn., who were younger. It was, therefore, with some surprise that he received a call from Col. (later Brig. Gen.) Fred W. Rankin, MC, Chief Consultant in Surgery, Office of The Surgeon General, on 3 July 1942. Colonel Rankin's conversation was very much to the point. Colonel Rankin stated that there was a job he wanted this writer to do and that he would like him to come to Washington to discuss the program. In 1942, Independence Day fell on Saturday. The writer intimated that because of the holiday Colonel Rankin might not want to see him until Monday. Colonel Rankin's reply was specific. He stated that the Office of The Surgeon General was in full operation on Saturday and, as civilians might well realize, there was a war on. The writer reported to Colonel Rankin at 0900 hours on Saturday and was briefed regarding his prospective duties and responsibilities as a consultant in anesthesia in the European theater. The interview ended with the instruction that he return to Hartford and coordinate the program with the medical director and the staff of Hartford Hospital. On Monday, 6 July, the writer called and informed Colonel Rankin that he would be ready to report when orders were issued.

It had been anticipated that the writer would receive a majority. However, when he discussed this matter with Dr. Wilmar M. Allen, director of Hartford Hospital, Dr. Allen expressed the opinion that the rank offered was not commensurate with the responsibilities to be undertaken. It was, therefore, with some satisfaction that the writer subsequently received orders specifying that he would report for duty in the grade of lieutenant colonel. On 20 August he was sworn in as an officer of the Army of the United States, and on 26 August

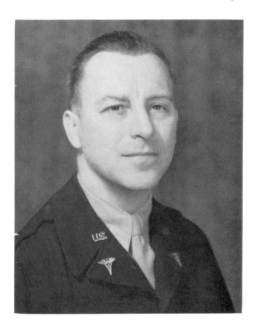

FIGURE 218.—Col. Ralph M. Tovell, MC.

Lt. Col. (later Col.) Ralph M. Tovell, MC, reported for duty in Washington. He was assigned to Walter Reed General Hospital, Washington, D.C., for the usual course of indoctrination which was hyphenated in order to permit him to spend considerable time in the Office of The Surgeon General.

ORIENTATION IN THE UNITED KINGDOM

The author proceeded from New York City to London by flying boat via Halifax, Nova Scotia, and Foynes in southern Ireland. His orders stipulated that the trip be made in civilian clothes. The trip was uneventful until the aircraft landed in the harbor at Foynes. There, the crew found that the tide was running in one direction and the wind was quartering from another. They taxied the flying boat over the choppy water for approximately 45 minutes, during which many of the passengers became seasick even though they had avoided airsickness during the trans-Atlantic trip. At Shannon the passengers were taken to the airport by bus, where they, as a combined force of civilians, Red Cross workers, and Army officers, were required to stand inspection by customs and immigration officers. For this procedure, the author was fortunate enough to stand in line behind a Regular Army colonel. Because three planes had landed within a few minutes of one another, the congestion of passengers awaiting planes for England was considerable. As the travelers were slowly making their way forward to the inspection points, it was announced over the loudspeaker system that all military personnel were to come to the head of the line. This was a rather startling announcement to Army officers supposedly in disguise and particularly so to a lieutenant colonel who had been in the Army less than a month. After a quick whispered conference with the Regular Army colonel preceding him, the two decided that this was no trick leading to internment in a neutral country. The two colonels promptly moved to the head of the line where the necessary formalities were accomplished with dispatch. This incident made a vivid impression on the author, and he was forced to alter his concept of neutrality, particularly of the southern Irish variety. In subsequent conversation with military friends, he learned that there were 150,000 southern Irish in the British Army. He was asked: "Under those circumstances, what kind of neutrality could you expect?"

Soon, the passengers were winging their way to Bristol, England, in a British plane that was entirely blacked out. The trip from Bristol to London was made by train. The author arrived in London at approximately 2300 hours on 25 September 1942 and suddenly was thrust into the utter darkness of the London blackout. It is difficult to describe this consultant's discomfiture. He found himself in a strange land without adequate knowledge of the Army procedure to be followed in finding a billet. However, organization was good, and transportation was at hand for conveyance to the billeting office. It was surprising how well and how easily U.S. Army drivers were able to wend their way through busy streets of a great metropolis pulsating with life in the darkness.

On the morning of the next day, 26 September 1942, the author reported at ETOUSA headquarters, 20 Grosvenor Square. He was informed that he was to be reassigned immediately to Headquarters, SOS (Services of Supply), at Cheltenham, England, a city approximately 90 miles west of London and some 30 miles beyond Oxford. He proceeded to Cheltenham by train and once again went through the prescribed procedure of getting bedded down, this time at the Plough Hotel, a hostelry about 200 years old that, in days long gone by, had been used as a terminal for stagecoaches plying their routes in the Cotswolds district. More recently, the hotel had been occupied by permanent residents including elderly widows and spinsters and a smattering of British Army officers, retired from the Indian Service. This hotel, along with many others in the town, had been requisitioned by British authorities for U.S. Army personnel. In spite of the dislocation of the permanent residents, the reception of a growing horde of Americans arriving to staff a continually growing headquarters was remarkably amiable.

The next morning, the author reported for work, physically ready for it but mentally in very much of a quandary regarding the future. He met his new superior, Col. James C. Kimbrough, MC, who had been assigned the unenviable job, for a Regular Army officer, of riding herd on a group of senior consultants representing the several specialties in medicine and surgery— individuals whom he could not help but look upon as civilians in disguise and who were reputed to be prima donnas in their civilian practice at home. Colonel Kimbrough met the challenge of his assignment with fortitude and with a diplomacy that might be unexpected of a Regular Army officer who had been born in the mountains of Tennessee. His advice and his encouragement were forthright. When all other attempts failed to orient civilians who could not have been other than stupid in their practices at home, he was able to quote volubly from the Bible to illustrate his point. The personnel of the Professional Services Division, Office of the Chief Surgeon, Headquarters, ETOUSA, were indeed fortunate to have as their chief "sheepherder" a urologist, professionally competent and renowned, who spoke in professional medical terms rather than in military jargon. In addition, he was capable of orienting them in military thinking. He guided them through the maze of military procedure, the utilization of which was so necessary in order to accomplish their mission in a growing Army that was preoccupied with tables of organization and equipment. They of the Professional Services Division are ever grateful for his leadership.

This consultant also met Col. (later Brig. Gen.) Elliott C. Cutler, MC, Chief Consultant in Surgery, and Lt. Col. (later Col.) William S. Middleton, MC, Chief Consultant in Medicine, Professional Services Division, Office of the Chief Surgeon, ETOUSA. Maj. (later Col.) James Barrett Brown, MC, Senior Consultant in Plastic Surgery, and Lt. Col. (later Col.) Loyal Davis, MC, Senior Consultant in Neurosurgery in the division, had been resident in the theater for several weeks prior to the author's arrival. They were all very helpful in orienting him in problems they had faced and in problems they knew he would face in the near future. Their help and advice were greatly appreciated because this author, as the first Senior Consultant in Anesthesia appointed in the U.S. Army, had no precedents to follow. Fortunately, great latitude subsequently was allowed him in organizing a program.

EARLY ACTIVITIES AND RECOMMENDATIONS

During this period of groping for information upon which to build, this consultant decided that the best part of discretion was to meet his counterparts in the British Army, the Royal Navy, and the Royal Air Force and in the Canadian Army. He learned that Air Commodore R. R. (later Sir Robert) Macintosh, the Nuffield Professor of Anaesthetics at Oxford University, was senior adviser to the Royal Air Force and that Dr. I. W. Magill of London represented the EMS (Emergency Medical Service) and the Royal Navy. Col. (later Brigadier) Ashley S. Daly, RAMC, was his counterpart in the British

Army. Dr. John Gillies, professor of anesthetics at the University of Edinburgh, was the senior representative of anesthesia in Scotland. Col. Beverly Leech, commanding officer of the 5th Canadian General Hospital and an old friend, was senior anesthetist with the Canadian Army. This consultant immediately made plans for conferences with Colonel Leech and Commodore Macintosh, whom he had known previously.

Through Air Commodore Macintosh, arrangements were made for this author to meet Colonel Daly, adviser in anesthetics to the British Army, whom he had not previously known except by reputation. But Colonel Tovell first visited several of the U.S. Army hospitals and, subsequently, through the cooperation of his counterparts in the British Services, visited British and Canadian hospitals. On 28 October 1942, he submitted Col. J. C. Kimbrough, MC, Director of Professional Services, a report covering impressions gained during one month of duty in ETOUSA, with summary and recommendations. Inspection of several British hospitals, both military and EMS hospitals, had revealed that they were equipped to carry on all phases of anesthesia such as would be conducted in British civilian hospitals, with the exception that, in military hospitals, provision was not made for the use of cyclopropane and carbon dioxide absorption (fig. 219). Endotracheal anesthesia was fully accepted as an essential method. Equipment consisting of laryngoscopes, endotracheal tubes, and connecters were provided for all operating room units. Anesthetic equipment was found to be standardized, and disposable deteriorating rubber parts were found to be interchangeable. Anesthetics were administered by medical officers only, and personnel were of a high order and included many anesthesiologists of either national or international reputation.

Inspection of Canadian hospitals revealed that their anesthetic equipment equaled that seen in civilian hospitals in either the United States or Canada. Anesthetic machines were of American origin, the models were standardized, and they provided for use of carbon dioxide absorption and cyclopropane. Personnel in anesthesia were found to be well trained and adequately able to make an intelligent choice of agent and method to be used under varying circumstances.

Inspection of American military hospitals revealed that equipment for inhalation anesthesia was of British origin and was British owned (fig. 220). Admittedly, the 2d General Hospital, Headington, Oxford, did have one McKesson and one Foregger machine, but they were British owned. Equipment for endotracheal anesthesia was lacking in many hospitals and incomplete in others. Assigned anesthesiologists in units based in the theater were found to be insufficiently trained, and they were, in addition, inexperienced. With the civilian type of practice encountered at the time, they were relatively satisfactory, but, in the opinion of the Senior Consultant, they were inadequately equipped to cope with battle casualties in great numbers. Problems, as reported, were substantially as follows:

1. Medical officers assigned as anesthesiologists in hospitals need further training.

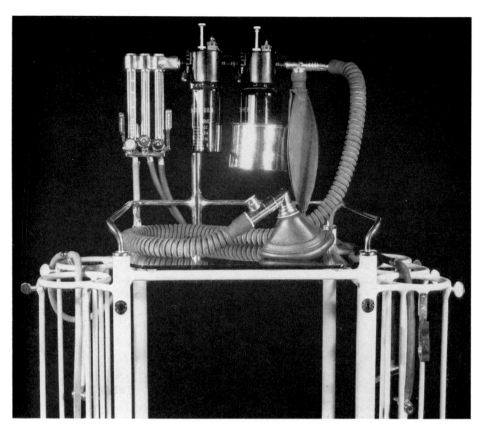

FIGURE 219.—British anesthetic apparatus, seen in British military hospitals in October 1942 and supplied to U.S. Military hospital units arriving in England at that time.

2. Medical officers in hospitals and not assigned to anesthesia need training and experience in order to serve as alternate anesthesiologists to cover demands which would be placed on units upon the arrival of battle casualties.

3. There is need for training corpsmen of satisfactory personality and aptitude in the fundamentals of administering ether by the open-drop method under supervision of an assigned anesthesiologist.

4. Many hospitals functioning in the theater are urgently in need of equipment and supplies.

5. Hospitals moving out of this area for service in an active theater of operations need their equipment checked. Essential items not included in tables of equipment should be added. The need for checking is magnified when it is realized that expendable parts for equipment produced by the several suppliers in the United States are not interchangeable. Equipment is useless if accessories and equipment are not manufactured by the same company.

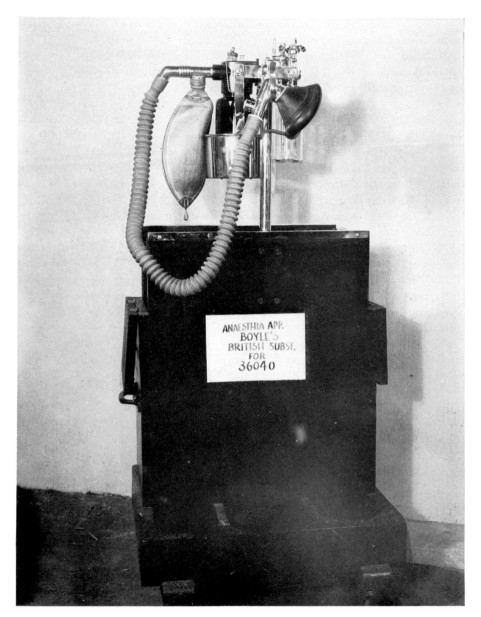

FIGURE 220.—Portable British anesthetic equipment supplied to U.S. Army hospital units in September 1942.

6. Because so much of the equipment in use in the American hospitals is of British origin, there is need for descriptive literature to be made freely available to anesthesiologists with each unit if they are to requisition supplies intelligently.

This summary of problems was followed by a series of recommendations listed substantially as follows:

1. That facilities for training be established at the 30th General Hospital, Mansfield, and at the 2d General Hospital, Oxford, to provide courses in anesthesia for medical officers of the U.S. Army.

2. That two anesthesiologists of teaching caliber in the grade of captain or preferably major be requisitioned from the Zone of Interior to take charge of anesthesia in the above-mentioned locations.

3. That, until such time as one or both of these facilities are functioning, the offer of Air Commodore Macintosh of Oxford to welcome observation of practice of anesthesiology at the Radcliffe Infirmary be accepted and that two medical officers be assigned for periods of one month.

4. That anesthesiologists be advised to train medical officers of their own units in anesthesiology.

5. That anesthesiologists be advised to train suitable corpsmen in the fundamentals of the administration of ether.

6. That endotracheal tubes be approved in principle as essential and that appropriate equipment for endotracheal anesthesia be provided as standard to operating room units in general, evacuation, and surgical hospitals.

7. That the facilities for CO_2 absorption be provided in equipment supplied to general and station hospitals.

8. That equipment contemplated for shipment with hospital units leaving this theater be checked by a competent anesthesiologist.

9. That each hospital unit stationed in this theater be supplied with the following British texts: "Essentials of General Anaesthesia" by R.R. Macintosh and Freda Pratt; and "Recent Advances in Anaesthesia and Analgesia; Including Oxygen Therapy" by C. Langton Hewer.

10. That authorities in Washington be requested to prepare supply lists for anesthetic chests suitable for general, station, evacuation, surgical, and mobile operating units. Anesthetic equipment and supplies issued in units would eliminate the hazards of lack of standardization of equipment.

11. That training medical officers in anesthesia in the Zone of Interior, along the lines planned in civilian hospitals and in replacement pool centers, be facilitated to the fullest extent immediately.

It was further pointed out that these recommendations concerning the practice of anesthesiology would in no way elevate this practice above the standards already established in British and Canadian hospitals in the theater.

On 2 December 1942, a report, entitled "Anesthesia," was prepared for submission to The Surgeon General. Much of the data that had been recorded in the preceding report of 28 October was provided in the report to The Surgeon General. The following points were made:

1. Tables of supply were inadequate to cover the requirements of modern anesthesiology.

2. Machines built by the several manufacturers in the United States were not standardized, and expendable parts were not interchangeable.

3. Descriptions in the tables of supply were inadequate to eliminate the possibility of obtaining a machine built by one manufacturer and accessories built by another. This chance of nonconformity was enhanced by the practice of shipping a gas machine in one crate and equipment of a deteriorating nature (rubber parts) in another (fig. 221).

4. American machines were not equipped to use American and British gas tanks interchangeably.

5. American equipment supplied to hospital units staging in the theater (for North Africa) was not checked by either the anesthesiologists involved or the Senior Consultant in Anesthesia for possible deficiencies due to losses.

The following impressions were stated. The problems involved in supplying British equipment adequate for U.S. Army hospitals in the United Kingdom could be solved in cooperation with medical supply officers in this theater. Anesthesiologists could and would be trained in the fundamentals of the specialty. Anesthesiologists, however, who arrived in the theater inadequately trained and who remained only for a short staging period could not be trained to meet the demands that would be placed upon them in a field of active military operations; that is, the North African theater where operations had opened on 8 November 1942.

The report to The Surgeon General ended with a series of recommendations that seemed important at the time. For instance, it was recommended that a competent consultant in anesthesiology be obtained to function in the Office of The Surgeon General in cooperation with the Personnel and Supply Divisions. It was further recommended that tables of supply be amplified to meet modern requirements; that standardization of suitable equipment for each type of unit be achieved permitting interchangeability of rubber parts, endotracheal equipment, and masks; and that small pieces of equipment not connected with the gas machine (that is, ether masks, airways, tubes, needles, syringes, laryngoscopes, connecters, and drugs—particularly drugs usually supplied in ampules) be listed and supplied as a unit in order to simplify problems in supply. It was requested that the work of the Committee on Standardization, initiated through the efforts of the American Anesthetists Society, ETOUSA, be supported and that, with the cooperation of the Army and Navy, its functions be pushed to their logical conclusion. It was pointed out that this committee included representatives of manufacturers of gas machines and rubber accessories, manufacturers of oxygen and anesthetic gases, and the National Bureau of Standards, U.S. Department of Commerce. Representatives from the Army and Navy, to this consultant's knowledge, had been assigned for each meeting that he had attended before entering on active duty. It was further recommended that this effort be directed toward uniformity of threadings, tapers, openings, and valves and coordinated with projects in the Air Forces for standardization of methods of supply, storage, and administration of oxygen to aircrews. The urgency of augmenting the training programs pertaining to physicians in anesthesia in the Zone of Interior was emphasized, and in addition, it was recommended that the program be

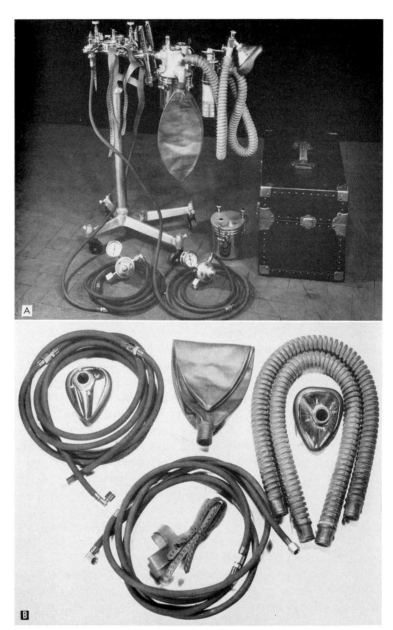

FIGURE 221.—"Marriage" of anesthetic machines and expendable rubber parts shipped separately. A. Portable American military anesthetic machines, assembled after expendable rubber parts shipped in a separate container had been "married." B. Expendable rubber parts which were shipped in a separate container. Because expendable parts produced by American manufacturers were not interchangeable, problems of "marriage" (as usual) were very real.

expanded. This request was a reflection of the fact that hospitals had arrived in the European theater without adequately trained medical anesthesiologists before embarkation for foreign service. The report ended with a request that opportunity be afforded a consultant in anesthesia to observe operation of hospital units in a theater of active military operations in order to evaluate and to report needs in training of personnel, agents and methods to be employed, and equipment to be supplied for future campaigns.

The 2 December report to The Surgeon General was supported by data provided by Capt. Harry K. Shiffler, MC, of the 48th Surgical Hospital, Tébessa, Algeria, then engaged in the North African operations. On 24 November 1942, he reported that his unit had taken over an ill-equipped local hospital and had started work immediately. The operating room was moderately sized, and there were two tables on which the patient and litter were placed. Two patients, therefore, were always being operated on at the same time. It was necessary for him to put the heads of the tables together in a V-shape so that he could give anesthesia to two patients at the same time. For 3 days, only two anesthetists were available, and each took 12-hour shifts. For the first 2 days, only chloroform and ethyl chloride were available. (There were a few cans of ether, but they lasted only a short time.) Since there was a limited supply of chloroform, he had to save it for the longer operations and use the ethyl chloride for the minor procedures. He wrote as follows:

Naturally, as you can readily understand, Lieutenant Marmer and myself were wishing for our own American supplies to come, as neither of us coming from the States had ever had experience with chloroform. There was only one mask available, so I fashioned another out of a Planter's Peanuts can—it worked quite well. Everything was done by the open-drop method, of necessity. * * * As soon as our own supplies arrived, including Pentothal Sodium and ether, we at least had a wider choice. * * * In my opinion, Pentothal Sodium is the most valuable single anesthetic agent for the anesthetist in the field during combat conditions. Unfortunately, we had no 20 cc. syringes; and we had to do all our work with 10-cc. syringes. * * * The laryngoscopes you were kind enough to send me were used to great advantage. I feel that every hospital set up to do surgery should have, as part of its basic equipment, laryngoscopes and endotracheal tubes. * * * It should be stressed that any unit going into action should have plasma immediately available. There is no doubt in my mind that it was lifesaving to many of our boys.

These reports have been cited in detail because they set the stage for future activity to be undertaken in preparation for the eventual invasion of continental Europe. They outlined fundamental problems to be overcome in relation to organization for training of personnel, procurement of standardized equipment, alteration of tables of equipment to meet the needs of the several types of units, and the need for a competent observer to visit an active theater of operations to evaluate the usefulness and possible deficiencies of relatively recently and newly designed American equipment. Some of these problems entailed the establishment of long-term programs, particularly in reference to training of anesthesiologists in the Zone of Interior and in the United Kingdom, and in standardization of equipment involving new designs to permit employment of agents supplied from either American or British sources.

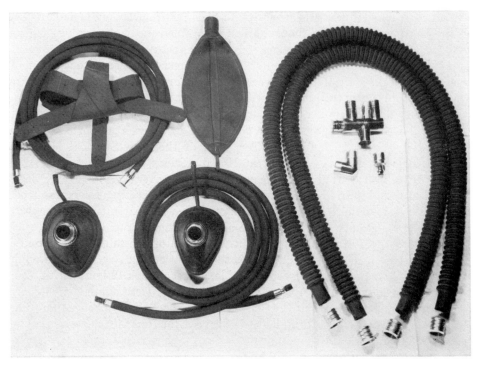

FIGURE 222.—Adaptable substitute expendable anesthetic equipment obtained from British sources.

The one immediate pressing problem was to rectify the situation created by the shipment of gas machines in one crate and equipment of deteriorating quality in another. This situation was due to practice established in the United States on the principle that deteriorating rubber parts packed over a long period of time with nonexpendable equipment would deteriorate and be useless upon receipt in a theater of operations. This principle was well founded, but failure to "marry" deteriorating equipment with nonexpendable equipment at ports of embarkation created a serious situation whereby nonexpendable equipment received in a theater of operations was rendered useless so long as the corresponding expendable parts failed to arrive. This situation was particularly serious for hospital units unpacking their equipment for the first time upon their arrival in North Africa. The situation was less emergent, however, for those units arriving in the United Kingdom because there was an established industry to provide adaptable substitute expendable equipment (fig. 222). The supplies of expendable British equipment, however, were meager, and adaption and procurement were difficult. Another phase of the problem in Great Britain was the adaption of American machines to make it feasible to utilize anesthetic gases supplied in British cylinders. The British Oxygen Co. was very helpful in designing adapters permitting utilization of British deteriorating equipment and in designing adapters (fig. 223) per-

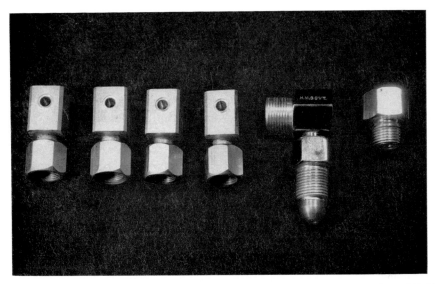

FIGURE 223.—Adapters obtained from British sources to permit utilization of British cylinders on American anesthetic machines. The first four, left, were yoke adapters (US No. 9–NO2101; British No. A3043) required for each anesthetic machine. The bullnose adapter, second from right, made it possible to link a large British oxygen cylinder to an American anesthetic machine. The nitrous oxide adapter, right, served a parallel purpose.

mitting employment of British cylinders on American gas machines. Due, however, to the necessity for time-consuming negotiations through the Ministry of Supply, authorization for procurement of these items was slow. Production, due to shortage of materials and manpower, was also time-consuming. Ultimately, the principle of obtaining expendable supplies through British sources raised the problem of identification of these materials by American anesthesiologists.

The first few months in Britain had been revealing. Making the rounds of hospitals scattered throughout southern England, by car, proved to be a frustrating experience. Roads were blocked with pitifully weak log barriers, and directional signs were completely absent. The citizens were well trained in their refusal to give out any information. It was common experience to inquire of an old "gaffer," who probably had never been more than 20 miles from home, the direction of a town that one knew was within a 3-mile radius. He characteristically replied that he "never heard of the place." If he was particularly well versed in civil defense, he would refuse to tell you the direction to the nearest police station, which was usually your last resort for gaining information. A blanket of fog, which so frequently covers Britain during the autumn months, added to the difficulty of transportation. The English girls who were assigned as drivers from the motor pool were expert and very helpful.

Gradually, a bird's-eye view of problems was gained in relation to anesthesia equipment, supplies, and personnel that would face ETOUSA during the ensuing 2 years. It was indeed fortunate that a U.S. Army destined to invade northern France was based in a country that was highly industrialized. Deficiencies in equipment that were a reflection of the unpreparedness for war at home, and the all too successful submarine campaign against American convoys, could to a certain extent be alleviated by requisitioning substitute items from British sources. Problems in personnel were more difficult to solve, but it was noted that anesthesiologists in the theater were gradually receiving equipment satisfactory to meet fully the needs of military practice. Relatively inexperienced anesthesiologists had improved the character of their work, particularly following temporary duty for the purpose of observing and receiving instruction at British and American hospitals. The anesthesiologists who had arrived with the 3d Auxiliary Surgical Group constituted a pool from which anesthesiologists could be drawn to replace less-experienced medical officers during their periods of absence for training. During this same period, several well-trained and experienced anesthesiologists arrived from the Zone of Interior assigned to units which were to remain in the European theater. This made it possible to plan on using these men as instructors in U.S. Army hospitals and led to the hope that the practice of assigning anesthesiologists to British units for training might be augmented by training anesthetists in U.S. hospitals. It was in this atmosphere that the year of preliminary planning, 1942, ended.

CONSULTANT DUTIES

The Senior Consultant in Anesthesia by this time realized the significance of his duties: To observe, to report, and to recommend to the Chief Surgeon, ETOUSA. The Division of Professional Services, of which he was a part, was without command function but was expected to formulate policies, obtain their authorization, and check on adherence to policies thus established in general, evacuation, station, and field hospitals and later in base sections and hospital centers. His problems were common to those of his associates, each consultant having a set of problems with which he had to deal that were peculiar to his specialty. The work of the Senior Consultant in Anesthesia included visits to hospitals, observation of work being done with criticism and suggestions regarding organization and practice, preparation of reports with recommendations, preparation of material covering policies for issue as directives by the Chief Surgeon, establishment of satisfactory report forms, collection and evaluation of statistical data, and establishment and maintenance of liaison with his counterparts among the Allies.

It was the responsibility of each senior consultant to evaluate the skill of members of his specialty in all types of units in relation to the part which each unit was expected to play. This role necessitated the interviewing of personnel of incoming hospitals. A file system was established containing a summarized medical biography of each officer in the specialty. Notes were added recording observations made subsequently regarding the skill of officers at work. This information was used as a guide in establishing each officer's rating, and it was on the basis of this information that recommendations were made to the Personnel Division, Office of the Chief Surgeon, Headquarters, ETOUSA, when it was necessary to reassign officers to fill vacancies. In the case of anesthesiology, it was also necessary to tabulate the training, experience, and skill of anesthesia nurses attached to each unit.

EXTENSION OF ACTIVITIES IN 1943

Supplies and Equipment for Anesthesia

It was with some dismay that the work of the ensuing months was contemplated, with the realization that the tempo of it would be intensified remarkably as the buildup of the U.S. Army for invasion progressed. During the month of January 1943, a survey of needs for anesthetic and oxygen therapy equipment was completed. A report, entitled "A Consolidated Report Regarding Equipment for Anesthesia and Oxygen Therapy in the ETO," was submitted on 31 January 1943. The salient points in the report concerned the requirements for gas machines and provision of adapters to permit use of supplies of gases from British sources. It was pointed out that British machines in American hospitals permitted attachment of cylinders containing pure carbon dioxide, a practice which in itself was hazardous but which, under circumstances of military effort, was complicated by the fact that British cylinders containing carbon dioxide were painted green in accordance with the British Code of Identification. To an American physician, this color indicated safety and the presence of oxygen. It was, therefore, recommended that supplies of carbon dioxide for anesthetic purposes be withdrawn. Subsequently, arrangements were made with Mr. H. A. Chapman of the British Oxygen Co. that only mixtures of carbon dioxide in 7-percent concentration with oxygen in 93-percent concentration would be made available to American hospitals.

On 27 February 1943, a letter, entitled "Carbon Dioxide For Inhalation," was issued by the Office of the Chief Surgeon over the signature of Col. Oramel H. Stanley, MC, Deputy Chief Surgeon, to base section surgeons and commanding officers of all U.S. Army hospitals. This command letter provided for the recall of all cylinders containing pure carbon dioxide in exchange for cylinders containing a mixture of carbon dioxide and oxygen. Attachment to anesthetic machines of cylinders containing only carbon dioxide was to be discontinued as soon as the mixture was available, and it was specified that carbon dioxide in 7-percent concentration and oxygen could be used for stimulation of respiration when that was required. Hospitals possessing freezing microtomes could still obtain pure carbon dioxide, but under no circumstances was it to be stored with gases for inhalation.

It was necessary on 15 February 1943 to issue Circular Letter No. 27, Office of the Chief Surgeon, Headquarters, ETOUSA, stating that standard U.S. and British color schemes differed and that, in order to identify gases in cylinders, the labels always must be read. Color markings on cylinders were to be considered only to corroborate labels. This was followed with a description of British and American cylinders, including their characteristics, by which they might be differentiated. Information of general interest regarding cylinders and their gaseous contents was given broad distribution.

This problem of identification of gases and cylinders was recognized by authorities outside the Medical Corps. On 20 February 1943, Circular No. 18 was issued by Headquarters, ETOUSA, under the title "Industrial and Breathing Gases and Cylinders." Means and methods of procurement of oxygen as well as acetylene, hydrogen, and nitrogen for industrial purposes was stated. Confusion was subsequently occasioned in medical units by this directive because the color code for oxygen according to British specifications was stated as black. The directive failed to indicate that nitrous oxide cylinders were also black but possessed a different type of valve. The directive also stated: "Where facilities for painting according to British standard specifications are not available, the Requisitioning Officer may request the British Oxygen Company to paint the cylinders. Correct shades and types of paint are available at Headquarters, SOS, ETOUSA, APO–871." This statement failed in the matter of thoroughly assigning responsibility for painting according to the British standard specifications, and at the same time introduced the hazard of error where painting was undertaken by organizations other than the supplier. Another requirement of the directive was that, until all U.S. Army cylinders were repainted to conform to British standard specifications, it was essential that a label clearly indicating the type of gas be securely pasted on the cylinder. To paste labels securely on cylinders stored in the open was impossible, and it was implied that identification of gases and cylinders by means of colored paint would subsequently be adequate. This policy introduced hazards where the American color code definitely conflicted with the British. This directive had originally been issued without the knowledge or concurrence of the Office of the Chief Surgeon. It was unfortunate that distribution included units of the Medical Department.

At the time of the preparation of the "Consolidated Report Regarding Equipment for Anesthesia and Oxygen Therapy in E.T.O.," which was submitted by this consultant to the Director of Professional Services on 31 January 1943, the hazards of a gas attack were very much in the minds of all (fig. 224). The report, therefore, included the recommendation that each hospital be provided with efficient quick-coupling oxygen sets of British origin to provide a minimum coverage of 3 percent of bed capacity in each hospital, additional equipment to be retained in supply depots to cover 2 percent of the bed capacity. This level was set after consultation with Col. William D. Fleming, MC, Chief Gas Casualty Officer, Gas Casualty Division, and Colonel Middleton, chief medical consultant to the European theater. Installation of quick-linkage pipelines was advocated to save shipping and utilize to the best advantage the limited supply of cylinders in time of real need. It was noted that procurement of BLB (Boothby, Lovelace, Bulbulian) masks and regulators had been sat-

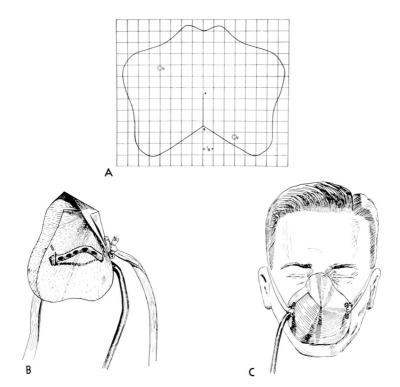

FIGURE 224.—Primitive preparation in 1942 against gas attack. A. A pattern for a face mask to be cut from oiled paper. B. A pattern of a face mask shaped for the administration of oxygen. C. Use of a face mask for the administration of oxygen.

isfactory, but, as a safeguard against gas attack, it was recommended that 3,000 masks and regulators manufactured by the Oxygen Equipment Manufacturing Co. of New York be procured from British sources where they were known to be surplus. Subsequently, 50 units of the oxygen quick-coupling sets (sufficient to supply 500 patients) were received ready for distribution. Fortunately, gas attacks never materialized and the equipment was not used.

The use of oxygen tents was pointed out to be impractical in the European theater because ice was not freely available in quantity and because the administration of oxygen in adequate concentration was incompatible with good nursing care, in the presence of multiple wounds requiring frequent treatment or observation. The logic of discontinuing the import of oxygen tents requiring the utilization of ice was manifest in a country where even chilled beer could not be obtained. Procurement of oxygen tents from the Zone of Interior was discontinued.

During the early months of 1943, anesthetic machines continued to arrive in the European theater with deteriorating rubber equipment. This created a problem of major magnitude. After much difficulty, substitute equipment was obtained from British sources. Some delay was occasioned by lack of standardization between Heidbrink Co. and McKesson Equipment Co. machines on the one hand, and between the machines produced by the Boyle Co. and the Medical and Industrial Equipment Co., both of London, on the other. This lack of standardization necessitated accumulation of four pools of equipment for maintenance purposes and was responsible for no little confusion. Attempts to rectify this situation were without avail for many months, but progress was made through a subsequently established committee, known as the Service Consultants Committee on Anesthetics, which included representatives from the U.S. Army and the several sections of the British Forces as well as the Ministry of Health and the Department of Health for Scotland. In addition, the Canadian Army had direct representation.

Adaption (fig. 223, p. 593) of American equipment to British cylinders likewise constituted a problem. The original estimate of the number of adapters required was predicated on the basis that the major supply of anesthetic machines and apparatus for oxygen therapy would be procured from British sources and would therefore not need adaptation to British cylinders. This calculation was based upon the fact that the outcome of the submarine campaign seemed grim; but, with subsequent marked Allied successes in dealing with submarines, delivery of equipment from the Zone of Interior increased beyond original hopes and the procurement of adapters lagged behind needs thus created. The establishment of Depot M–400 at Reading, England, on 1 February 1943, for maintenance and repair of anesthetic and X-ray equipment, proved to be a real boon. Lt. Col. (later Col.) Kenneth D. A. Allen, MC, Senior Consultant in Radiology, was largely responsible for establishment of this facility. The original need was to staff this depot with personnel skilled in servicing anesthetic and oxygen therapy equipment. Attempts to obtain skilled personnel from the Zone of Interior were without avail. As a result, technicians servicing such equipment were trained in England with the cooperation of the British Oxygen Co. Anesthetic and oxygen therapy equipment distributed to issuing depots throughout the theater was screened through Depot M–400 for completeness. American apparatus so screened had the proper adapters added in order to make possible utilization of either British or American cylinders.

Training

Medical officers trained in anesthesia continued to be in short supply. Training seemed to be the only answer. Problems arising from the supply of unlike pieces of equipment from various manufacturers in America and in Britain made training even more imperative. It was stressed that each hospital should have a trained physician anesthesiologist and an alternate physician to cover for him, and in addition, depending on the size and type of the hospital, should have a sufficient number of assistants to cover periods of peakload. Training by apprenticeship to skilled anesthetists was continued and accelerated through the year. In case of need, arrangements were made for trainees to go on temporary duty for a period of 30 days to hospitals possessing anesthesiologists of teaching caliber where they had sufficient clinical material for purposes of demonstration.

Early in the year, lack of clinical material in U.S. Army hospitals necessitated making an arrangement with British military hospitals and the EMS for augmenting the training and experience of U.S. Army officers. In this effort, Brigadier Daly, Air Commodore Macintosh, and Dr. F. Murchie of the Ministry of Health cooperated wholeheartedly. In all, 99 officers received one or more months of training outside their own unit, and others received instruction and gained experience within their own unit. As the year 1943 drew to a close, it was less frequently necessary to allocate trainees to British hospitals because U.S. Army hospitals contained more clinical material and anesthesiologists of teaching caliber. The program of arranging temporary duty for U.S. Army personnel at British hospitals led to its administrative difficulties, sometimes with respect to rations, other times with respect to the jealousy of hospital commanders in reference to their prerogatives. Apparently, the Senior Consultant in Anesthesia had been less than efficient in laying on the program through the highest international channels. Instead, the arrangements had been made at the operational level. Occasionally, the commanding officer of a British hospital wanted to know why his unit had been invaded by one or two American officers who had arrived without the proper fanfare of announcement. To the Senior Consultant in Anesthesia, it seemed that, if the British had patients and were short of personnel and if the U.S. Army had physicians without patients, temporary duty for American officers to British hospitals was the logical procedure to remedy the situation and at the same time provide for training.

Throughout the year, the Senior Consultant in Anesthesia or his alternate, Maj. (later Lt. Col.) Fenimore E. Davis, MC, presented a 2-hour lecture before each class attending the ETOUSA Medical Field Service School at Shrivenham. The presentation included a discussion and slide demonstration of intravenous anesthesia, drugs for regional anesthesia, and untoward reactions likely to be encountered in accomplishing blocks frequently employed in military practice. Evidences of oxygen want and remedial measures were outlined and stressed. In addition, lectures along similar lines were presented before staff meetings at individual hospitals, on invitation.

Special Reports

In order to improve clinical anesthesia and to provide means for the accumulation of statistical data, two forms for reporting the course of each anesthetic administered were devised and circulated. The smaller form, known as the ETOUSA MD Form No. 55–0–1, was for general use and was designed to fit the EMT (Emergency Medical Tag) envelope. One side of the form provided space for recording the preoperative examination of the patient, and the opposite side was for recording progress of the anesthetic procedure. A larger form, identified as Form 15 E.T.O.—P.S., was similarly designed and was for use in general hospitals using the larger-sized forms throughout their complete reporting system.

A monthly report covering activities of the anesthesia and operating room section was required from each hospital in the European theater by a command letter issued by the Office of the Chief Surgeon on 24 February 1943. Through the cooperation of anesthesiologists in the theater, statistical information was submitted to the Office of the Chief Surgeon for analysis. These data were collected to establish experience factors in reference to agents and methods used and thus provide the Supply Division, Office of the Chief Surgeon, data from which to estimate requirements for future supply. The data also indicated the direction in which emphasis should be placed in the training of anesthetists.

Visit to North Africa

Revision of TM (War Department Technical Manual) 8–210, Guides to Therapy for Medical Officers, issued on 20 March 1942, was under consideration by the Professional Services Division throughout 1943. It became evident that, in order to intelligently prepare such an manual, a tour of observation in a theater of operations actually involved in combat was necessary. Therefore, on 11 September 1943, a request for orders to visit NATOUSA (North African Theater of Operations, U.S. Army) was submitted and eventually approved. The purpose of this trip was to collect data for completion of the portion of the manual on anesthesia and data relating to maintenance of a proper balance in the program for training anesthesiologists and oxygen therapists. Orders were issued on 12 October 1943 by Headquarters, SOS, ETOUSA, and the trip was accomplished between 20 October and 20 November 1943.

A tour of duty in NATOUSA, for observational purposes in an active theater, proved to be interesting and instructive. This author observed hospitals in the vicinity of Algiers, Algeria, and Bizerte and Tunis, Tunisia, in North Africa; Palermo and Catania in Sicily; and Naples and Caserta in Italy. He also went as far forward as divisional clearing stations in Italy. Following his observations in the field, a report was submitted to the Chief Surgeon, ETOUSA, entitled "Impressions Gained During a Trip to NATOUSA and Fifth Army."

The author observed that there was a distinct shortage of trained and experienced anesthesiologists to take care of peakloads of casualties. Some hospitals were without the services of a trained anesthetist. The greatest need for thoroughly qualified anesthesiologists existed in units situated in forward areas, where the severest injuries were seen and treated. It was in the forward areas that anesthetists attached to auxiliary surgical groups were rendering the most and best service.

There was a great need for portable gas machines in each hospital platoon of field hospitals, where intermittent positive pressure was essential for adequate care of nontransportables. A real need for the same types of equipment existed in evacuation hospitals of either the 750- or 400-bed type. An inequality of distribution of portable gas machines and anesthesia sets existed. In this regard, the situation was similar to that which existed in England, but, unlike the European theater, the North African theater could not procure machines from British sources to cover the deficiencies. Distribution of soda lime for the machines was inadequate in quantity. When the need was extreme, Shell Natron was used as a substitute, thus diverting this specialized material into unintended channels. This practice was not without its hazard to both patients and anesthesiologists. Where continued, the use of Shell Natron produced deterioration of already scarce anesthetic equipment. Because of these difficulties, this consultant reported that there was a real need for developing light, sturdy, and freely portable equipment to provide intermittent positive pressure for resuscitation with either air or oxygen, if available. He further stated that this apparatus should be able to clean inflowing air, if and when gas warfare was employed. He believed too, that such equipment should incorporate facility for the administration of ether vapor when desired.

Portable suction apparatus also was scarce, while there was a real need for it in field and evacuation hospitals. Equipment designed in the United States and provided in tables of equipment was satisfactory when electricity was available. Situations were encountered, however, in which portable apparatus, operated manually or by foot action, would have been of value. Such apparatus, aside from supplying the need in far-forward areas, could augment rather than displace existing portable equipment that was electrically operated. In his report, the author suggested that the reversal of the valve system in foot-operated tire pumps, currently in civilian use in England, would be easily possible, and that, with the addition of a vacuum bottle, suitable tubing, and an aspirating tip, the apparatus would be satisfactory.

This consultant soon learned, upon his return, that in the Army one should never make a recommendation unless he is prepared to follow through with it. With the help of Major Davis, who was trained first as an engineer and subsequently as a physician, a sturdy and freely portable piece of equipment was designed (fig. 225) and produced at Depot M–400 to provide intermittent positive pressure for resuscitation with air or with oxygen, if available. This apparatus also provided a facility for the addition of ether vapor when desired. Through the cooperation of Down Bros. of London, medical equipment manufacturers, foot-operated tire pumps, designed to service heavy trucks in civilian use, were altered by reversal of their valve systems, and thus a foot-operated vacuum pump was produced and supplied to augment suction pumps electrically operated in U.S. Army hospitals.

In NATOUSA, anesthesia practice was noted to be circumscribed by the lack of fully experienced anesthesiologists. This led to inexpert choice of agent and method for patients in critical condition. The same shortage tended toward the use of agents and methods beyond the boundaries of their known wisest employment. On the one hand, surgeons advocated and undertook the

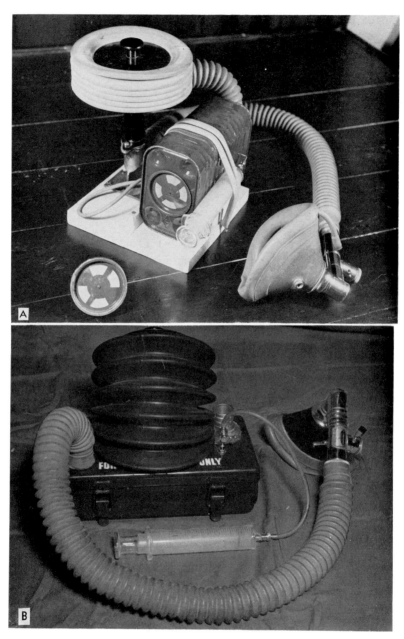

FIGURE 225.—An ETOUSA resuscitator and ether vaporizer, developed at Depot M–400, Reading, England, by Maj. Fenimore E. Davis, MC, and Colonel Tovell. A. An experimental prototype, utilizing a gas mask canister. B. The final type incorporating a first aid kit container in place of the standard gas mask canister. The bellows bag was that originally designed for the Oxford vaporizer. A gas mask canister could be attached to the air inlet, right rear, in the event of a gas attack during operation. Liquid ether was delivered to the vaporizing chamber by syringe.

administration of spinal anesthetics in instances in which, with the services of an expert anesthesiologist, the same surgeons would have elected inhalation anesthesia. On the other hand, there was a tendency to employ Pentothal sodium (thiopental sodium) in contravention of known contraindications because of its ease of employment in periods of peakload. Lack of skilled anesthesiologists, adequately equipped to undertake administration of inhalation anesthetics employing carbon dioxide absorption and intermittent positive pressure administered through an endotracheal tube, accentuated this tendency. The need for conservation of time also dictated the choice of anesthesia. In some instances, erroneous judgment was responsible for subsequent difficulties that would not have occurred had the patients been in as good condition as was first believed. Absorption of morphine administered subcutaneously to patients suffering from exposure and exhibiting peripheral vascular constriction resulted in delayed absorption, and the pain frequently was not relieved. A second dose under these circumstances might be given with similar results; but, when the patient was treated for shock by warming or administration of fluids, or when given an anesthetic, absorption was rapidly hastened and morphine poisoning was exhibited.

An awareness of the hazards inherent in the use of Pentothal sodium in the presence of shock, particularly following hemorrhage, was appreciated. It was recognized that Pentothal sodium was hazardous in the presence of bleeding lesions within the mouth or in the presence of dyspnea from any cause. The use of Pentothal sodium for surgical procedures within the thorax or abdomen was contraindicated. Ether was recognized as the agent of choice for production of muscular relaxation for the recently wounded. Anesthesiologists in the North African theater were of the opinion that availability of cyclopropane was highly desirable, particularly for patients in critical condition. In relation to problems of supply, the value of cyclopropane seemed obvious because the space required to transport cyclopropane in quantity equivalently useful to nitrous oxide would be small in comparison.

The greatest need for portable gas machines existed in field hospital platoons functioning independently and set up adjacent to division clearing stations for the treatment of nontransportables. This circumstance, the author reported, would necessitate supplying field hospitals in the European theater with nitrous oxide, oxygen, and soda lime. He further recommended that provision be made to supply each auxiliary surgical group with 10 portable gas machines, 10 portable suctions, and the necessary gases for them. He suggested that these machines be distributed to those teams assigned to hospital units operating under peakload, and that first priority be given to thoracic, general surgical, and plastic surgical teams. Supplies of these items in hospitals were inadequate to cover the needs of the teams.

Practice in hospitals in North Africa and Italy working under battle conditions demonstrated the sagacity of planning to supply citrated blood from a blood bank established in a rear area. Such procurement made thorough control possible in reference to syphilis, malaria, and jaundice and, at the same time, relieved units in forward areas of the responsibility for setting up local blood banks. This consultant observed that, without the availability of sufficient blood, adequate care of the wounded would be impossible. Upon the author's return to England, this matter was thoroughly discussed within the Professional Services Division, Office of the Chief Surgeon, and plans were laid to establish a centralized blood bank with Maj. (later Lt. Col.) Robert C. Hardin, MC, in charge of the operation. Major Hardin's organization ultimately provided blood for the initial stages of the invasion of northern France. Procurement of blood from troops in England, and later on the Continent, was continued even after an adequate line of supply was established with the Zone of Interior. During the campaigns in northern Europe, Major Hardin's organization continued to distribute blood throughout the theater. If a patient died, his death was attributed either to his having been given too much or too little blood or too faulty administration of the anesthetic. Seldom would surgeons admit deaths were due to wounding, and never, it seemed, would they admit that the surgical procedure was contributory. Major Hardin and the author stood shoulder to shoulder on the same chopping block.

The trip to North Africa was a geographic revelation. The handicaps under which an army in the field worked made a real impression. The disadvantage of a native population that on occasion was less than friendly was observed. The native Arab was seen in his own habitat, with a discerning eye. It was adequately demonstrated that Africa is a cold continent with a hot sun. The trip back to England was more than interesting and a little frightening. When this consultant arrived in Marrakech, Morocco, via plane from Algiers on the return trip, he both expected and desired to be forced to remain there for 2 or 3 days until air transportation became available for the trip to northern Scotland. After a very arduous trip across North Africa to Bizerte, Tunisia, and then on through Sicily to Italy, he would have welcomed time to bask in the sun. Much to his chagrin, upon inquiring about transportation to Scotland, the author was told that there would be a C–54 plane on which he could leave within 1½ hours. He decided to accept the accommodation rather than wait 3 or 4 days or more for another vacancy that might be further delayed by high priorities given to ferry pilots returning to the United States to bring back still another plane.

The trip was uneventful during the first 13 hours. Subsequently, the passengers were told that the aircraft was bucking a headwind and getting low on gasoline. The pilot was forced to break radio silence and asked for permission to approach Scotland over the Irish Sea, rather than fly to the west of Ireland on a course that was usually followed to avoid German fighter bombers based in Brittany. His luck did not hold well. The plane was met over the Irish Sea by a JU–88 which attacked from the rear. It was a physiologically stimulating experience to descend to approximately 500 feet above sea level in the fashion of a falling leaf, not knowing whether the plane was in control or out of it. After the plane landed at Prestwick, Scotland, having been escorted in by two

P–40's, it was discovered that one wing had been pierced by a 20-millimeter shell. The shell had lodged between two wing tanks but had failed to explode. Fortunately, no one aboard was injured. It was theorized that perhaps a Czech had sabotaged the German war effort. This consultant realized that, although he was a noncombatant, he was not a neutral. Not many months were to pass before his status as a noncombatant would be brought into focus again. While he was accompanying a full complement of wounded in a C–47 from France to England, a "trigger-happy" American shore battery, located on the south coast of England, fired at the plane. The flight engineer quickly shot off a couple of identifying flares which were recognized by the gunners below. The firing ceased, and no damage was done. The pilot was exasperated. He said that he had approached the coast in the stipulated manner and was therefore totally at a loss to account for the action of the guncrews.

PREINVASION ACTIVITIES

Many hoped that 1943 would be the year of action. This proved to be impossible; and, instead, the invasion of northern France was delayed until June 1944. The buildup for invasion started with the arrival of units of the First U.S. Army in the theater. It was immediately obvious that an accentuated program for training anesthesiologists was necessary. Three courses were held in 1944 at the 120th Station Hospital, Tortworth Court, the first from 17 to 22 January inclusive, the second from 21 to 26 February (fig. 226), and the third from 20 to 25 March inclusive. A fourth course was held at the 10th Station Hospital, Manchester, Lancashire, for Third U.S. Army personnel during the period 1 to 4 May inclusive. The average attendance was approximately 70, and at least half of the trainees were medical officers. The program was intensive; but, in retrospect, it seems to have been pitifully inadequate. Nevertheless, the writer is still confident that much was accomplished in the way of orientation. The many officers who participated as lecturers deserved commendation for their effort.

D-DAY AND ITS AFTERMATH

It is a well-known historical fact that D-day occurred on 6 June 1944. On 23 June, the author reported to the Chief Surgeon his impressions gained since D-day. It was with real satisfaction that this consultant was able to state that in all echelons anesthetic equipment had been adequate with only a few shortages of one or another article in isolated instances (fig. 227). Likewise, oxygen-therapy equipment had been adequate to meet the immediate need on the Continent. Once again, however, the problem of supply had raised its ugly head. Adapters for use on British cylinders were found to be lacking in some units equipped with complete hospital assemblies shipped directly from the Zone of Interior. Fortunately, adapters were available to cover these deficiencies. American cylinders were still being used in many fixed facilities in the United Kingdom. As a result, Col. Silas B. Hays, MC,

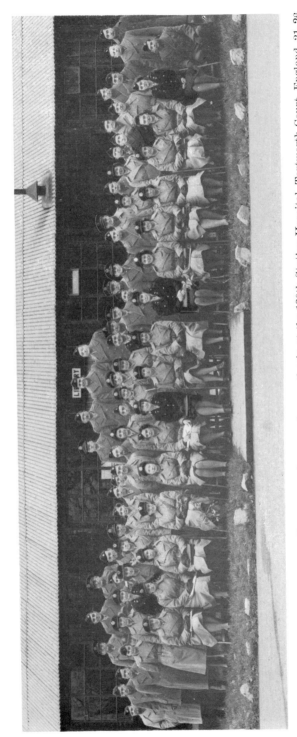

FIGURE 226.—Student officers attending a second course in anesthesia at the 120th Station Hospital, Tortworth Court, England, 21–26 February 1944.

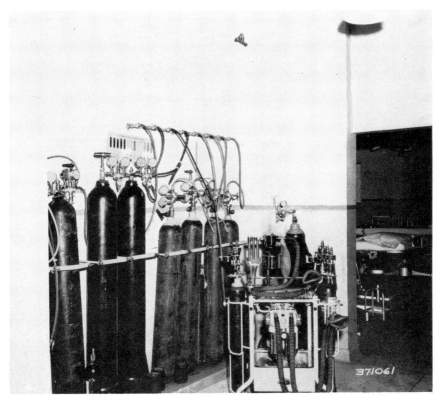

FIGURE 227.—Central oxygen and nitrous oxide manifolds which supplied the four operating theaters at the 298th General Hospital (University of Michigan unit) at Frenchay Park, near Bristol, England. An anesthetic machine of British origin is in the right foreground.

chief of the Supply Division, Office of the Chief Surgeon, recalled both empty and filled cylinders from U.S. hospitals in the United Kingdom for transportation to the Continent. The 130,000 beds distributed in over 100 hospitals in the United Kingdom were supplied with gases contained in British cylinders. The most evident need for equipment during the first fortnight of the invasion was for suction apparatus. Tables of equipment were not adequate to cover needs. American equipment could not be used in Britain in wards wired with 230 volts without utilization of transformers, and transformers were not freely available. The need for foot-operated suction, first recognized in North Africa, was once again evident.

Pentothal sodium was the agent most frequently used in all echelons and with general satisfaction and safety. In certain isolated instances, anesthetists had been influenced to use this drug under unwarranted circumstances, such as the incision and drainage of a phlegmon of the neck. Spinal anesthesia was used in general hospitals providing definitive treatment but was seldom used for the treatment of those recently wounded. This consultant received the impression that, although fluids had been freely administered, undertreatment rather than overtreatment existed. In one area at least, supplied from British sources, blood in relation to plasma was being used in the ratio of 10 units to 1. At the time, this was considered a nonjustifiable depletion of supplies of blood, but, as the campaign progressed, the need was more and more easily justified.

VISIT TO NORMANDY

During the first week of July, this consultant visited hospitals in Normandy, and a report of observations was prepared. He noted that some evacuation and field hospitals were in the process of packing in preparation for moving forward while other hospitals still remaining in operation were working beyond the limits of their capacity. One 400-bed evacuation hospital had 520 patients on its second day of operation, with a preoperative backlog of 250 to 300. This was due to a special circumstance: Its normal line of evacuation was over Utah Beach and the airstrip intended for evacuation of the wounded was needed for fighter squadrons. It was recognized that evacuation by hospital carrier might take as long as it would take to work down the backlog of preoperative patients. A problem in sorting, therefore, existed in regard to selection of patients to be transported by surface carrier to Great Britain and patients to remain with the unit for surgical treatment.

A platoon of the 13th Field Hospital was visited and found to be not too busy. It was supported by two teams from the 3d Auxiliary Surgical Group. Equipment was adequate to meet needs with the exception that Shell Natron canisters were lacking for closed-circuit oxygen therapy apparatus. These teams had had no deaths on the operating table. A neighboring unit, the 16th Field Hospital, Normandy, France, was attached to and working with the 67th Evacuation Hospital, while awaiting the arrival of equipment. This unit had been in active operation in Egypt. The 47th Field Hospital, Normandy, France, was likewise awaiting the arrival of its equipment, which its personnel knew lacked gas machines and equipment for oxygen therapy. This unit, originally belonging to the Third U.S. Army, had arrived last and had been assigned to the First U.S. Army. This circumstance accounted for failure to obtain those supplementary items authorized for First U.S. Army units in the European theater. A lack of coordination between the efforts of attached auxiliary surgical group teams and the personnel of a platoon of a field hospital was in evidence. Two units never do well under one roof unless the commanding officer of the facility has full coordinating control. This matter was reported for policy decision in relation to field hospitals.

Pentothal sodium was being used in approximately 75 percent of the operations. Oxygen was frequently given for support. For the longer procedures, nitrous oxide and oxygen was given, and ether was employed to produce relaxation. The muscle relaxants of the curare series were not available at the time.

It was also quite the usual practice for hospitals to prepare atropine-morphine and Pentothal sodium in bulk. This practice resulted in the conservation of valuable time, facilitated preliminary medication in the operating room, and eliminated haphazard premedication in wards. In order to time properly the administration of preliminary medication with the beginning of an operation, it was necessary to give atropine and morphine intravenously in the operating rooms. Because Pentothal sodium was being prepared in bulk, the prevailing practice of procuring Pentothal sodium in small 1-gram ampules seemed extravagant in terms of supplies and also in the time required to make the preparation. This consultant suggested that Pentothal sodium might well be obtained in 10-gram ampules and that distilled water for its dilution could better be supplied in bottles containing 500 or 1,000 cc. In one instance, faulty filling of a cylinder constituted a problem. An officer of the 3d Auxiliary Surgical Group reported that a cylinder, marked "Oxygen" and painted black with white neck like its British standard, contained—in actual fact—carbon dioxide. When the gas was employed, it produced cyanosis following a period of hyperpnea. This was recognized, the contents of the cylinder were emptied, and the cylinder was returned for refill. No patients suffered. This circumstance was another facet of the overall problem of identification of gases in cylinders.

Some deaths had occurred in which anesthesia was considered to be contributory. In these instances, inhalation anesthesia was as frequently blamed as when Pentothal sodium was employed. Vomiting with aspiration during the induction of anesthesia was recognized as a major hazard. It was noted that the critical interval in which anesthetists should be interested was the time between eating and wounding, rather than wounding and operation, because digestion was inhibited immediately after wounding. This author advised that accidents due to aspiration could, in some instances, be prevented by initiating vomiting prior to induction of anesthesia. Attempts to wash a stomach with a Levin tube in place had given only partial protection.

Plasma and blood were being used in the ratio of 1 to 1. In order to conserve blood, which was limited in supply, this consultant expressed the hope that the ratio of plasma might be raised to 2 units for 1 of blood. Along this line, he also noted that, during hot weather or when patients were perspiring or vomiting, there was a very real need to replace chlorides by the administration of normal saline. A common complaint was that the needles in plasma sets were too small in caliber to permit the administration of blood. The air vent in the blood bottle was too short to reach above the surface of the fluid. Filters became clogged with fibrin. Pressure was necessary to maintain flow of fluid. The valves of blood pressure bulbs, used to create pressure, became clogged. It was recommended that the Office of The Surgeon General be informed of difficulties due to small-caliber needles and be requested to include larger, size-16 needles in plasma sets.

Arrangements for the treatment of shock seemed to entail some confusion. There was a general tendency toward failure to isolate patients requiring major effort in the treatment of shock. As a result, officers were confronted with patients in widely dispersed parts of preoperative tents and failed to treat shock adequately. This consultant advised that it was desirable to segregate patients needing major effort in the treatment of shock in order that the medical officer in charge might be able to keep them under his direct supervision at all times. He further advised that an officer with mature experience be assigned to these duties. Surgeons found it impossible to maintain continuity of observation between operations. It was with these matters in mind that a senior consultant ended his first tour of duty to the Normandy beachhead on 8 July.

MOVE TO THE CONTINENT

On 28 August 1944, movement of the Professional Services Division, Office of the Chief Surgeon, to the Continent began. Travel was accomplished by train to the marshaling area near Southampton, thence by boat to Utah Beach, and lastly to Headquarters, Communications Zone, at Valognes, France, by truck. The group was delayed for 3 days en route at the marshaling area because the ship on which it was scheduled for transport to France had no accommodations for females. The party included two, the chief nurse and Capt. (later Maj.) Marion C. Loizeaux, MC. The party was subsequently assigned to a Victory Ship, carrying some 1,500 troops, packed like sardines in a can. The passage across the English Channel occupied 24 hours because of the circuitous route that the ship was forced to take in order to avoid minefields. Off Utah Beach, the travelers were transferred to a tender. This transfer necessitated climbing down a rope net to the deck of the tender which was in constant motion. For a landbound Army man, this was a new experience. Fortunately, the operation entailed no injuries to any of the group. From the tender, the members walked ashore over the hardstand, getting no more than their feet wet. The evidence of sunken ships and the litter of destruction on the beach were still present, reminding all of the contrast between the ease of their landing and the difficulties in the original invasion by shock troops.

As they proceeded inland, it was obvious that the Army had accomplished a great deal in clearing away the bits and pieces of gliders forced to land in fields that were too small because all the larger fields had been well planted with "Rommel's asparagus," posts approximately 8 feet long imbedded upright in the ground at regular intervals. The purpose was to prevent the very landing that occurred in spite of this enemy action. It was amazing how thoroughly an Army in combat was able to clean up its new backyard in the less than 6 weeks that had elapsed between this consultant's first trip to the beachhead in early July and the permanent transfer of the Office of the Chief Surgeon in August. Not only had the superficial evidence of destruction occasioned by the invasion been removed, but the fields had been cleared of mines as well. This total area had been cleared to provide space for incoming troops and the buildup of a major supply base.

The headquarters remained in Valognes only a few days. At this time, the advance of the Allied armies was extremely rapid. Orders were received to move to Paris. This city continued to be the location of European theater headquarters throughout the remainder of the fighting in northern Europe. The first entry into Paris was memorable. Although the city had been secured a few days prior to the arrival of the headquarters group, the elation of the populace was very much in evidence. The author was intrigued to learn that he had been assigned a billet in the Hotel California. Subsequently, after a tour of hospitals in the then existing forward area that required approximately one week for its accomplishment, he returned to the Hotel California to find that it was completely occupied by the Women's Army Corps. His gear had been moved out. He was temporarily dismayed with the idea that he would never see it again. The personnel of the billeting office, however, were completely efficient. They informed him of his new assignment, and there were equipment and personal belongings, completely intact with not one item of importance, collected during 2 years' sojourn in England, missing.

ACTIVITIES DURING THE FINAL CAMPAIGNS

Thereafter, the work of the Senior Consultant in Anesthesia was divided between the Continent and installations in the United Kingdom Base. With the establishment of hospital centers in the United Kingdom Base, a consultant in anesthesia was nominated for each of the seven centers. The author expected that, during the remainder of 1944, and until the termination of the campaigns in northwestern Europe, his work in the main would be confined to facilities (60,000 beds) on the Continent with the hospital center consultants functioning in the United Kingdom. The medical officers to whom this responsibility was delegated were as follows:

Center	Officer	Hospital assignment
I	Capt. Gilbert Clapperton, MC	67th General Hospital, Musgrove Park, Taunton, Somerset
II	Capt. Lawrence F. Schuhmacher, Jr., MC	140th General Hospital, near Ringwood, Hampshire
III	Capt. Arthur LeeRoy, MC	154th General Hospital, near Wroughton, Wiltshire
IV	Capt. Charles Burstein, MC	160th General Hospital, Stowell Park, Gloucestershire
V	Capt. Milton H. Adelman, MC	155th General Hospital, near Hanley, Worcestershire
VI	Capt. Jasper M. Hedges, MC	137th General Hospital, Otley Deer Park, near Ellesmere, Shropshire
VII	Capt. Phillip E. Schultz, MC	7th General Hospital, North Mimms, Hertfordshire

As rounds of hospitals and auxiliary surgical groups were made, it was apparent that accessory equipment beyond their authorized allowances would facilitate their operations. The primary need was for a manually controlled apparatus for resuscitation which would supply intermittent positive pressure without the necessity of having cylinders containing oxygen. The second need was for a suction apparatus that was foot operated rather than electrically driven. At the same time, it was realized that the allowance of gas machines to evacuation hospitals and field hospitals was inadequate to meet their needs. During the last quarter of 1944, it was agreed that the authorized allowance of these items should be increased so that each 400-bed evacuation hospital would have four gas machines and each 400-bed field hospital would have six. In November, this author was notified by the Supply Division, Office of the Chief Surgeon, that 1,000 units of foot-operated suctions had been received, 500 from Down Bros., London, and 500 from the Zone of Interior. These units were distributed, one unit to each general and station hospital, two units to each evacuation hospital, and three units to each 400-bed field hospital. The latter made available one unit to each of the three hospital platoons in the field hospitals. Distribution at this stage of the campaign was difficult on an automatic basis, and not until all units learned of the availability of these units for suction were requisitions placed for them.

Following practices established in the immediate preinvasion period, hospital commanders and their chiefs of surgical service were urged, throughout the year, to assign medical officers and nurses for training in anesthesia and oxygen therapy within their units where trained anesthesiologists of teaching caliber were available. Admittedly, there was some reluctance to follow this advice with enthusiasm, but in many instances it was undertaken with ultimate benefit accruing after the units were assigned their combat support missions. In September 1944, the lack of anesthetists in forward areas, particularly in evacuation hospitals, was creating a bottleneck in the treatment of the wounded. Anesthetists to meet attrition were not available. It was therefore proposed to the Surgeon, United Kingdom Base, that 25 general and station hospitals possessing qualified anesthesiologists of teaching caliber be ordered to undertake the training of one medical officer and one nurse in anesthesia. Col. (later Brig. Gen.) Charles B. Spruit, MC, Surgeon, United Kingdom Base, endorsed this program. Letters were written to the 25 selected hospitals advising each commanding officer immediately to assign a medical officer and nurse from his unit to full-time training in anesthesia with the understanding that when training was completed one or both individuals would be subject to reassignment to units in greater need of their services. In November 1944, 10 general hospitals arrived in the United Kingdom from the Zone of Interior without coverage in anesthesia. Officers made available through the training program were assigned to these new units or to units already in operation requiring only minimal skills in anesthesia. In the latter instance, the more skilled anesthesiologist of the operating unit was reassigned to the new general hospitals. The rate of attrition among anesthetists throughout the theater was increasing due to illness, fatigue, and nonbattle injury. The pool of anesthetists in training was being rapidly depleted. It was therefore recommended to the Surgeon, United Kingdom Base, that in each instance in which a trained anesthetist was moved his replacement was to be similarly trained and oriented in anesthesia. Thus, the training program was perpetuated.

Because fatigue became evident among anesthesiologists of auxiliary surgical groups and those assigned to evacuation hospitals, the policy was established in October 1944 that medical officers over 40 years of age be permanently reassigned from forward units to fixed facilities in the communications zone. A second phase of the program rotated younger anesthesiologists in forward areas to fixed facilities in the communications zone for a period of 60 days and sent anesthesiologists forward from fixed hospitals for a similar period of temporary duty in forward area hospitals. As a result of this exchange program, the experience of anesthesiologists involved was broadened, and each had an opportunity to observe at first hand the problems of the other.

Throughout the year until closure of the school, a lecture, illustrated by slides on anesthesia and oxygen therapy, was delivered before each class for medical officers at the ETOUSA Medical Field Service School, Shrivenham. The practice, which had been initiated in 1943, of holding conferences for anesthesiologists immediately after each monthly meeting of the Section on Anesthetics of the Royal Society of Medicine in London was continued throughout 1944. Interesting clinical topics were presented by selected members, after which open discussion of problems was encouraged. By this means, use of agents and methods tended to become standardized for the benefit of the sick and wounded. Copies of three films, prepared by Dr. I. W. Magill and Dr. G. S. W. Organe of London under the sponsorship of Imperial Chemical Industries, Ltd., were made available as training aids through the Army Pictorial Service. These films dealt with ether anesthesia, endotracheal anesthesia, and intravenous anesthesia. Throughout the year, they were shown to many groups. Attempt was made through the Office of The Surgeon General to obtain copies of training films produced in the Zone of Interior, but information was subsequently received that shipment of these training aids overseas was not possible.

As the war progressed in Europe, lines of communication lengthened tremendously and the battlefront became far flung, extending from The Netherlands through Belgium and Luxembourg and eventually to southern France. The problems of observation, supervision, and control of anesthetic practice grew tremendously as the battleline was extended. Even changes in climatic conditions from the heat of summer to the cold winter of 1944–45 created new problems. The character of wounds and injuries changed. The incidence of exposure was magnified. Frostbite and trenchfoot became prevalent. It was necessary to caution that doses of morphine given as preoperative medication for seriously wounded patients should be small. It was further emphasized that morphine must be administered with caution to the walking wounded, to patients to be evacuated by air, or in the presence of jaundice, craniocerebral injuries, pneumothorax, hematothorax, or pleural effusion. With the arrival of cold weather, the hazards of morphine poisoning were accentuated due to slower absorption in the presence of shock. The syndrome became evident when patients were warmed and were given fluids to alleviate shock.

It was necessary to issue an administrative memorandum that the administration of spinal anesthetics would in all instances be undertaken by medical officers only, although care of the patient during the operative procedure might be delegated as the situation warranted. The use of spinal anesthesia was discouraged except for definitive late treatment of wounds involving the buttocks and lower extremities.

Material covering the subject of intravenous administration of procaine hydrochloride had been prepared and distributed to the Senior Consultants in Maxillofacial Surgery, Neurosurgery, Orthopedics, and Dermatology with the request that the method be cautiously tried in suitable instances. It was known that it was feasible to inject a dilute solution of procaine hydrochloride intravenously in order to obtain relief from pruritus associated with jaundice. It was considered that patients with severe burns might be similarly helped without the production of respiratory depression. Sedation in the presence of involvement of the tracheobronchial tree due to inhalation of smoke and noxious vapor was recognized as a difficult problem. The incidence of burns proved to be much lower in the European theater than had been contemplated. Opportunity was afforded to give limited trial to the use of procaine hydrochloride administered intravenously. Reasonably satisfactory sedation was obtained in many instances. This experience led to the administration of procaine hydrochloride for sedation in the presence of conditions other than burns. In patients with fractures recently confined within a cast that included both the trunk and either a leg or arm, the administration of procaine hydrochloride intravenously alleviated restlessness due to the marked restriction of movement. It was subsequently noted that reduction of swelling and edema occurred in surprisingly rapid fashion. Orthopedists found it necessary to change casts at shorter intervals in order to compensate for the rapid reduction in size of a leg.

As the incidence of trenchfoot increased, utilization of sympathetic block became more frequent. During the first 5 months after D-day, sympathetic block was reported employed in 1,300 instances for an overall incidence of 0.94 percent. Its employment in the presence of vascular injuries associated with marked edema was helpful. It was subsequently shown that utilization of sympathetic block in the presence of cold exposure of extremities or trenchfoot was essentially noncontributory to improvement. Statistical data regarding the incidence of utilization of other anesthetic agents and methods have been reported elsewhere.[1]

    [1] (1) Tovell, Ralph M.: Problems in Supply of Anesthetic Gases in the European Theater of Operations, U.S. Army. Anesthesiology 8 : 303–311, May 1947. (2) Tovell, Ralph M.: Problems of Training in and Practice of Anesthesiology in the European Theater of Operations. Anesthesiology 8 : 62–74, January 1947. (3) Tovell, Ralph M., and Barbour, Charles M.: Comparative Uses of Pentothal Sodium in Civilian and Military Practice. Lancet 67 : 437–443, December 1947.

The problem of promoting anesthesiologists became more acute throughout the year, and no solution was found. A new table of organization and equipment No. 8–550 for 1,000-bed general hospitals had been promulgated by the War Department on 3 July 1944 stipulating that anesthesiologists be in the rank of captain. In August 1944, this consultant commented to the Chief Surgeon, ETOUSA, that there was a distinct correlation between the existing shortage of anesthesiologists and the lack of opportunity for advancement in rank. Medical officers had no incentive to qualify as anesthesiologists because of the existing limitations. He also pointed out that modern anesthesia demanded adequate training and experience if the lives of the sick and wounded were to be adequately protected. He stressed the fact that anesthesiologists were responsible for the safeguarding of equipment in operating rooms, the training and control of personnel, and the supervision of central supply and oxygen therapy as well as the administration of anesthetics. The author therefore recommended that in order to provide an incentive for medical officers to qualify as anesthesiologists and in order that qualified anesthesiologists of long standing in the theater might receive the recognition they deserved, an urgent request for a change of the new table of organization to provide for a majority for at least one anesthesiologist in each 1,000-bed hospital be submitted to The Surgeon General.

The problem of promotions was not limited to general hospitals. The situation in auxiliary surgical groups became acute, particularly in those groups that had been overseas for 2 years or longer and had served in Africa, Sicily, Italy, and France. In the 3d Auxiliary Surgical Group, there were 21 anesthesiologists with 2 years of service who had no opportunity under existing tables of organization to improve their rank, no matter how long the war lasted. The situation was depressing to their morale in view of the fact that they had seen junior surgeons of less training and experience become chiefs of surgical teams and gain the rank of major. These anesthesiologists had been caring for nontransportables in field hospitals, their skills were recognized and appreciated by their associates, but this appreciation was not reflected in the tables of organization. It was evident that a general overhaul of tables of organization was warranted.

Miscellaneous activities continued to occupy a great deal of the time of the Senior Consultant in Anesthesia. He attended meetings of the Medical Research Council in London, particularly those dealing with blood, blood substitutes, and shock. Several meetings of the Service Consultants Committee on Anesthetics held at 1 Wimpole Street, London, afforded an opportunity for the interchange of information among consultants to the Ministry of Health, Scotland; the British Army, the Royal Navy, and the Royal Air Force; EMS hospitals; and the Canadian Army. Liaison through these meetings was particularly valuable. Meetings of the Inter-Allied Conference on War Medicine were also attended. The Senior Consultant in Anesthesia also attended two meetings of British and American consultants, one held in Paris and the other in Brussels.

From time to time throughout 1944, material was prepared for submission to the Office of The Surgeon General regarding the adequacy of equipment and supplies for anesthesia and oxygen therapy. This material was forwarded in ETMD (Essential Technical Medical Data) reports that proved to be an important medium for the submission of information to the Office of The Surgeon General. On 29 January 1945, a memorandum was submitted to Colonel Cutler regarding the preparation of sterile solutions of procaine hydrochloride from bulk supplies of the drug. It was pointed out that two deaths had occurred, one following the subcutaneous infiltration of procaine hydrochloride (presumed) for the investigation of a severed peroneal nerve and the other during the administration of a sympathetic block. These deaths had occurred at different hospitals. At the hospital where the death occurred following subcutaneous injection in the popliteal region, another patient exhibited convulsions of a severe nature but recovered under appropriate therapy. It was pointed out that the prevailing practice of supplying procaine hydrochloride in bulk led to difficulties in preparation and identification of solutions of proper concentration and sterility, particularly in field and evacuation hospitals. Sterilization was carried out either by boiling in a water bath or by autoclaving. Frequently, excessive heat tended to minimize the anesthetic effectiveness of the resulting solution. As a result, there was a tendency to use a stronger solution than was justifiable for infiltration. Under these circumstances, toxic doses were rapidly approached. It was recommended that serious consideration be given to a change in policy in supplying procaine hydrochloride. It was believed that many of the sources of hazard would be eliminated if the drug were supplied in ampules containing 1.0 gm. in 5 cc. of solution. Such ampules could be sterilized by immersion in any approved colored antiseptic solution. The proper dilution could be achieved using either sterile water or sterile normal saline in quantities of 95 cc. to produce a solution of 1.0 percent or 195 cc. to produce a solution of 0.5 percent concentration. This was the type of material that was submitted in the ETMD reports.

The ETMD reports moved on a "two-way street." Difficulties encountered in the use of piperocaine hydrochloride (Metycaine Hydrochloride) for spinal anesthesia were reported. In the ETOUSA Manual of Therapy, issued 5 May 1944, a table of dosage for tetracaine hydrochloride (Pontocaine Hydrochloride) and procaine hydrochloride combined, procaine crystals dissolved in spinal fluid, and Metycaine Hydrochloride in spinal fluid was outlined. The dose of Metycaine Hydrochloride was limited to a maximum of 140 mg. Difficulties in the use of Metycaine Hydrochloride were experienced, and, as a result, the use of Metycaine Hydrochloride was discouraged and supplies were allowed to dwindle. The Office of The Surgeon General was acquainted with these problems because parallel difficulties had been experienced in the Zone of Interior. On 16 June 1945, a memorandum from the Supply Division to the Professional Services Division drew attention to Section VI of War Department Circular No. 134, dated 4 May 1945, which stated that Metycaine Hydrochloride would no longer be employed in Army hospitals in any form. Major Davis, acting for this author, replied to this memorandum on 18 June 1945 and advised withdrawal of Metycaine Hydrochloride from issue in the European theater.

Material submitted for the ETOUSA Essential Technical Medical Data Report for the month of April 1945 included a statistical summary of anesthetics administered during the period 1 June–31 December 1944. Comment regarding this summary was as follows:

Although field blocks including local infiltrations were employed less frequently during November and December 1944 than they had been in the previous five months, the incidence of employment of specific regional blocks increased in all types of hospitals, the greatest increase being in evidence in evacuation hospitals; and significantly in evidence in Field Hospitals. The overall average of employment of specific regional blocks increased from 1.43 percent to 2.57 percent. This, too, is considered to be a development in a desirable direction because with proper organization of the section on anesthesia, the time lag between operations can be decreased. Patients maintain full control of their own airway, dehydration through vomiting is not increased as it may be after inhalation anesthesia, nursing care is kept at a minimum and patients are immediately evacuable, if that is necessary.

Incidence of employment of sympathetic block increased in all types of hospitals with the exception of field hospitals. This was in the main due to the increased incidence of "trench foot." Present opinion regarding the efficiency of sympathetic block for the treatment of trench foot is extremely guarded. It is felt that in no instance did the accomplishment of a sympathetic block tend to increase the patient's debility insofar as his injury was concerned. In the vast majority of instances, however, it could not be thoroughly established that accomplishment of sympathetic block improved the patient's rate of recovery. One death occurred during the accomplishment of stellate ganglion block undertaken for relief of peripheral vascular inadequacy of the upper extremity. This death was probably due to inadvertent injection of procaine within the dural sheath where prolongation of the sheath existed and protruded through the foramen.

* * * * * * *

Pentothal supplemented by other anesthetic agents was the method that was employed more frequently in November and December than in the previous 5 months in all types of hospitals except field hospitals. Statistical data in relation to field hospitals has not been broken down on the basis of their working status, but it is known that throughout November and December a greater number of them were working as Communications Zone units doing station hospital work. In many instances, these units so employed lacked the benefit of skilled anesthetists where auxiliary surgical teams were not attached.

* * * * * * *

It is obvious from these statistical data that the best qualified anesthetists should be assigned to auxiliary surgical groups and evacuation hospitals. * * *

Changes in T/O&E 8–580, 31 January 1945, for 750-bed Evacuation Hospitals are also considered to reflect experience encountered in this theater. However, inclusion of only one nurse anesthetist is inadequate to meet the needs for 24-hour operation of 10–12 operating tables. Six nurse anesthetists for such a union represents the minimum number required and then it would be necessary to orient three or four other nurses into the intracacies of anesthesia or else depend upon augmentation by personnel from auxiliary surgical teams. Experience has been that seldom is it necessary for 750-bed evacuation hospitals to be thus augmented. In the 2d Evacuation Hospital, 10 nurses have been oriented in the administration of anesthetics.

* * * * * * *

Comment in a similar direction was made with regard to 400-bed evacuation hospitals. It was stated that four nurse anesthetists were required as a minimum to staff such a unit during active operations in spite of the fact that a 400-bed evacuation hospital was frequently augmented by auxiliary surgical teams.

Subsequently, statistical data covering the period from 1 January through 31 May 1945 were submitted in the semiannual historical report prepared by Major Davis in this consultant's absence on a trip to the Zone of Interior, undertaken on 28 May 1945.

This sketchy account of activities during 32 months in Europe would be completely inadequate without comment upon a trip to the concentration camps in Weimar and Nordhausen, Germany, within a day or so of their capture by units of the U.S. Army. Information had reached Headquarters, ETOUSA, in Paris, regarding the deplorable condition of the unfortunates incarcerated there. A small group of consultants, including this author, flew to Weimar to investigate the situation. Upon arrival, the group first visited the pathologic museum, featuring tattooed skin taken from victims. The group learned that approximately 51,000 individuals had died within the electrified wire enclosure after 1 January 1945—many of them from starvation, others by hanging, and still others in the furnaces that had been erected immediately above the gas chamber. A pile of human ashes, 6 feet high, was seen. The condition of the inmates of the several barracks defied description. Starvation, superimposed upon tuberculosis, was universal. These humans wore masks that were immobile and expressionless; they appeared not to care whether they lived or died. Their diet of 600 calories per day was immediately increased, but any undue increase produced a dehydrating, fulminating diarrhea. Deaths continued to occur all too frequently following liberation. In order to take care of the children, it was necessary for the U.S. Army to divert a 400-bed evacuation hospital for this purpose alone.

The situation at Nordhausen was bad, but not as bad as at Weimar. In the Nordhausen internment camp, the internees had been forced to work in the underground factories producing V-1 and V-2 missiles. For this reason, the caloric intake of the workers had been maintained at a higher level; nevertheless, the death rate had been high. Arrival of new and more healthy individuals had been scheduled to meet the attrition. This was cheaper than feeding the working force adequately. It was brought home to the group of consultants, once again, that the capacity of man's inhumanity to man was infinite.

VICTORY IN EUROPE

When V–E Day arrived, this author was in London. The joy exhibited by the British was real in a restrained way. Seeing the lights go on, even though they were turned on, of necessity, in haphazard fashion, was a memorable experience. The next day the author flew to Paris, and because of some confusion in the announcement of V–E Day the French people were one day late in their celebration. Therefore, he had the opportunity to participate again in this gala event. He spent the evening observing the festivities. At 2300, he was walking down the Champs Élysées when he noticed that a group consisting of a man, a woman (apparently his wife), a 14-year-old boy, and a woman who appeared to be the boy's grandmother were observing him specifically and with keen interest. This author, in turn, observed that after a hurried conversation among the four the younger woman was summoning courage to speak to him, a complete stranger. This she did, in English.

She, Madame Cloup, stated that her family had noticed by his insignia that the author was a medical officer. Her husband was a surgeon, practicing urology. They would be honored, she continued, if the author would accompany them to their home for an "after-the-theater" dinner to celebrate the victory. Colonel Tovell was touched and pleased to be thus singled out for participation in their victory party. He accepted rather hesitantly because he knew of the short rations that existed among the French population in Paris. He explained that he had just recently completed dinner but that he would be very happy to accompany them and join in their celebration. Madame Cloup surmised his thoughts and explained that her friend (the older woman in the group) had just arrived from Normandy, where food was more plentiful, and that she had brought a roast of beef which they wished to share with him. The author accompanied them to their flat on the Left Bank of the Seine where he was entertained royally. A friendship was established that has been maintained by sporadic communication throughout the years.

AFTER V–E DAY

Victory in Europe brought with it, its problems. The war was not over; Japan still remained to be defeated. Problems of selection and redeployment had to be met. It was realized, ridiculous though it may seem, that, during the period of redeployment of medical officers to other theaters, a new training program in anesthesia and oxygen therapy should be set up. On 19 May 1945, this consultant submitted a memorandum to the Training Division, Office of the Chief Surgeon, outlining the proposed program. It was necessary geographically to divide the program into two sections, one for the Continent and another for the United Kingdom.

On the Continent, certain hospitals, designated as teaching units for anesthesia, were to have one medical officer trainee and one nurse trainee. Active training was for a period of not less than 3 months, the military situation permitting. Trainees were subject to reassignment in the hospital center in which they were trained on the recommendation of the hospital center's consultant in anesthesia. Names of trainees in excess of local requirements, who were declared ready for reassignment by the hospital center's consultant, were to be available for reassignment on recommendation by the base section consultant in surgery or the Senior Consultant in Anesthesia, Office of the Chief Surgeon,

ETOUSA. It was the intent to continue this system at the specified hospitals as long as clinical material was available and teaching anesthesiologists remained assigned. It was further planned that monthly conferences would be held at each hospital center at the discretion of the center consultant in anesthesia. Presentation of papers, exchange of ideas, and discussion of problems were thus to be made possible. In addition, the center consultant was to be authorized to make rounds of each hospital in his area in order to check on the organization, practice, and training within the section on anesthesia and operating rooms of each unit. Furthermore, each hospital center was to receive four medical officer trainees and two nurse trainees on temporary duty from communications zone and field army units for a period of 1 month's training in anesthesia and oxygen therapy. As a part of the training program, it was proposed that during operating periods trainees observe or work as apprentices under the supervision of the chief anesthesiologist of the particular facility. In order to support the senior assigned anesthesiologist in this training program, it was further proposed that one medical officer of recognized teaching ability be ordered from field army units to each hospital on a temporary duty status. In this manner, a pool of demonstrators and lecturers could be established.

For the United Kingdom Base Section, a similar program was suggested and initiated. The ETOUSA Society of Anesthetists was reactivated and held monthly meetings in London at the Royal Society of Medicine headquarters. Major Burstein of the 160th General Hospital was chairman. Since there was a shortage of anesthetists in the United Kingdom Base Section, and, since those available had been closely tied to their work over a period of months, they needed relief. On the other hand, anesthetists assigned to field army units needed to gain general hospital experience in the administration of anesthetics and the organization of the section on anesthesia and operating room. It was, therefore, recommended that anesthetists from auxiliary surgical groups and evacuation hospitals be given a tour of temporary duty for 60 days in United Kingdom Base hospitals. The program in the United Kingdom was expandable beyond that possible on the Continent. The offer of anesthesiologists in British universities to participate in the retraining program of the U.S. Army was accepted with gratitude. It was therefore recommended that authorities of the University of Edinburgh be contacted through Dr. John Gillies, Royal Infirmary, Edinburgh, to establish courses for anesthesiologists in C and D categories on the basis of 30 days' temporary duty for classes not to exceed 20 medical officers. It was postulated that similar arrangements could be made at Glasgow through Dr. Andrew Tindal. Similar facilities, it was suggested, could be made available through Professor Macintosh, head of the Department of Anaesthetics, Oxford University.

Imperial Chemical Industries, Ltd., had undertaken to produce training films in anesthesia and resuscitation. Three films, entitled (1) "Open Drop Ether," (2) "Endotracheal Anaesthesia," and (3) "Intravenous Anaesthesia," had been available to the U.S. Army in 1943. Arrangements had been made with Army Pictorial Service to copy these films and to reduce them from 35 mm. to 16 mm. for distribution to hospitals. In the interval, Imperial Chemical Industries, Ltd., had produced five other films. Four of these were reviewed by the Senior Consultant in Anesthesia and were considered appropriate for the U.S. Army training program. As a result, it was recommended that the Army Pictorial Service make three copies of each of these new films for distribution to hospitals on rotation. On 18 May 1945, the day before the proposals for the training program were submitted, this consultant had previewed a film produced in the United States, entitled "The Physiology of Anoxia, the Basis for Inhalation Therapy." It was recommended that three copies of this film be obtained from Washington at the earliest possible moment, one copy to be allocated to the United Kingdom Base, one copy to be made available for purposes of training in the Paris hospitals, and the other copy to be made generally available through the film library.

In furtherance of the plans submitted, courses in anesthesia were arranged at Radcliffe Infirmary, Oxford, and at the University of Edinburgh. Various hospital centers on the Continent also conducted anesthesia courses. The Faculty of Medicine, University of Paris, cooperated in this work furnishing cadavers and a dissecting room where the technique of regional anesthesia could be demonstrated. Maj. Paul W. Searles, MC, 5th General Hospital, was in charge of this effort.

Duties associated with termination of the campaign, collection of statistical data, establishment of the new training program for anesthetists, and selection of personnel for reassignment to another theater of operations occupied Colonel Tovell immediately after V–E Day. On his return to the Zone of Interior late in May he held conferences with interested chiefs of service in the Office of The Surgeon General, after which he attended a meeting of the American Board of Anesthesiology in New York City and assisted in the conduct of the oral examinations. On 17 July 1945, he received orders relieving him of duty as Senior Consultant in Anesthesia in the European theater. On this same day Maj. Lloyd H. Mousel, MC, was appointed Consultant in Anesthesia to The Surgeon General, but Colonel Tovell continued to serve in an advisory capacity until 15 October 1945, when he was relieved from active duty. Late in December of the same year he was invited to join the Veterans' Administration, of which Maj. Gen. Paul R. Hawley had just become Chief Medical Director, as Chief Consultant in Anesthesiology. The passage of Public Law 293, on 3 January 1946, which established the Department of Medicine and Surgery, Veterans' Administration, made it possible to formalize the invitation.

The story of anesthesiology in the European Theater of Operations has been told fully and frankly, with the hope that if another war comes, the documentation of lessons learned during one major war will contribute to the effective use of this specialty in another.

Part II

THE PACIFIC AND ASIA

CHAPTER XI

Pacific Ocean Areas

John B. Flick, M.D., Forrester Raine, M.D., and Robert Crawford Robertson, M.D.

Prior to August 1944, the Pacific theater of war was divided into three parts: SWPA (the Southwest Pacific Area), SPA (the South Pacific Area), and CPA (the Central Pacific Area). Each of these areas had its U.S. Army component. In SWPA, there were USAFFE (the U.S. Army Forces in the Far East) and USASOS (the U.S. Army Services of Supply). In CPA, the Army component was known as USAFICPA (the U.S. Army Forces in the Central Pacific Area) and in the SPA, as USAFISPA (the U.S. Army Forces in the South Pacific Area). Overall command of the areas encompassed by CPA and SPA was placed upon Adm. Chester L. Nimitz, U.S. Navy, whose headquarters was known as CinCPOA (Commander in Chief, Pacific Ocean Areas). This command corresponded to that of General Headquarters, SWPA, with its commander in chief, General of the Army Douglas MacArthur, U.S. Army.

SURGICAL CONSULTANTS

Col. Wm. Barclay Parsons, MC, was Consultant in Surgery, Office of the Chief Surgeon, USASOS, SWPA, and Col. Ashley W. Oughterson, MC, Consultant in Surgery, Surgery Section, USAFISPA. Both were on a full-time basis. Col. Forrester Raine, MC, was surgical consultant in USAFICPA, in addition to his duties as Chief, Surgical Service, 147th General Hospital, on the outskirts of Honolulu. Also in the Central Pacific Area, functioning as consultants in addition to other duties, were Col. Robert Crawford Robertson, MC, Consultant in Orthopedics, and Lt. Col. Leslie M. Garrett, MC, Consultant in Roentgenology. Colonel Robertson was Chief, Orthopedic Section, 219th General Hospital, Oahu, T.H., and Colonel Garrett, Chief, Roentgenological Service, 218th General Hospital, Fort Shafter, Oahu.

USAFPOA (the U.S. Army Forces, Pacific Ocean Areas) was set up as an administrative overall command in approximately August 1944 to compare with that of CinCPOA. At that time, USAFISPA and USAFICPA were reduced to the level of base commands under the jurisdiction of the USAFPOA. At the same time, the area then known as the "forward area"—the Marianas group of islands and, subsequently, Ulithi, Angaur, and Iwo Jima—became the Western Pacific Base Command. During the Ryukyu Islands campaign, Okinawa, Ie-jima, and adjacent smaller islands were under the jurisdiction of the USAFPOA. Later, in June 1945, the USAFPOA became USAFMIDPAC (the U.S. Army Forces, Middle Pacific), a subordinate command under the overall Army command, AFPAC (Army Forces, Pacific).

When the USAFISPA became a base command, Colonel Oughterson was placed on temporary duty at the Surgeon's Office, Headquarters, USAFPOA, as full-time Consultant in Surgery. Colonel Oughterson served in this capacity from August 1944 to December 1944, when he went to the Philippines. In February 1945, Colonel Oughterson returned from the Philippines, was assigned to the Western Pacific Base Command, and became Consultant in Surgery there. He remained until June 1945, when he was ordered to the Medical Section, General Headquarters, AFPAC, as Director of Research and Consultant in Surgery.

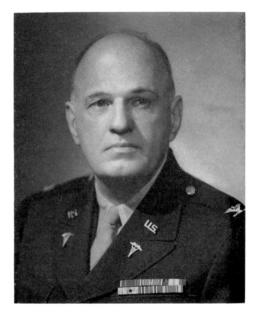

FIGURE 228.—Col. John B. Flick, MC.

The Tenth U.S. Army, whose headquarters and some of whose medical units had been staged on the island of Oahu, T.H., subsequently was sent to Okinawa. This army had the following consultants in the field of surgery: Col. George G. Finney, MC, Consultant in General Surgery, Lt. Col. (later Col.) Harold A. Sofield, MC, Consultant in Orthopedic Surgery, and, after arrival in Okinawa, Lt. Col. (later Col.) Douglas B. Kendrick, Jr., MC, Consultant on Whole Blood and Shock.

Col. John B. Flick, MC (fig. 228), became Consultant in Surgery, USAFPOA, on 1 April 1945. At this time, the surgical consultants were Colonel Oughterson for Western Pacific Base Command, Lt. Col. (later Col.) Willis J. Potts, MC, for South Pacific Base Command, both on a full-time duty basis, and Colonel Raine for Central Pacific Base Command, on a part-time duty basis.

Colonel Robertson became full-time Consultant in Orthopedics, USAF-POA, on 31 May 1945.

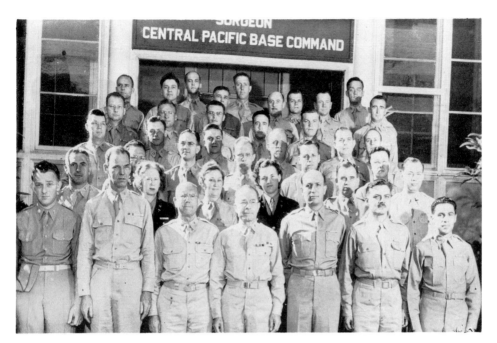

FIGURE 229.—Col. Paul H. Streit, MC, Surgeon, Central Pacific Base Command (front row, center), and his staff, 1944.

In May 1945, Lt. Col. (later Col.) Edward J. Ottenheimer, MC, replaced Colonel Oughterson as Consultant in Surgery, Western Pacific Base Command, in addition to his duties as Chief, Surgical Service, 148th General Hospital, Saipan. It was obvious, however, that it was impossible for Colonel Ottenheimer to function satisfactorily in either position in this dual capacity. In mid-July 1945, Colonel Ottenheimer was appointed Consultant in Surgery, Office of the Surgeon, Western Pacific Base Command, on a full-time basis despite the fact that he could ill be spared from the 148th General Hospital. Upon the cessation of hostilities, Colonel Ottenheimer was called to Headquarters, USAFPOA, to supervise the writing of the medical history of USAFPOA and USAFMIDPAC.

Prior to 1 April 1945, the surgical consultants to the Surgeon, USAFPOA, were on temporary duty from general hospitals with the exception of Colonel Oughterson, who was on temporary duty from Headquarters, South Pacific Base Command. It was not until 29 May 1945 that the allotment for officers in the Surgeon's Office, USAFPOA, was increased from 17 to 47, which enabled the assignment of the requisite number of professional consultants. The professional consultants in the Surgeon's Office, Western Pacific Base Command and Central Pacific Base Command, were on temporary duty from general hospitals. This policy made little difference in the Central Pacific Base Command (fig. 229) which was so located that the professional consultants in the Surgeon's Office, USAFPOA, were available for advice, and the pressure

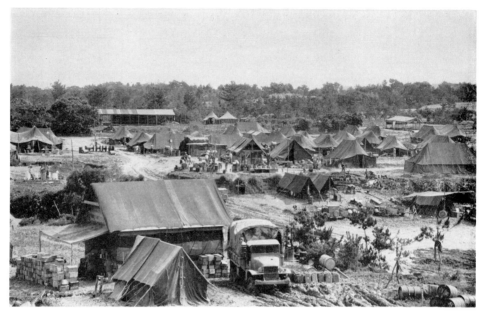

FIGURE 230.—The 76th Field Hospital, Okinawa, Ryukyu Islands, June 1945.

of work was not so great as in the more forward areas. In the Western Pacific Base Command, however, the need for a full-time consultant in surgery was great and urgent during the fighting for Iwo Jima and Okinawa (fig. 230). The great distances to be covered in the Pacific and the need for close observation of the hospitals doing a large volume of surgical work made it imperative that a surgical consultant be appointed on a full-time basis there. Constant watchfulness of practices in caring for casualties and in their evacuation to areas further back was necessary. The surgical consultant at Headquarters, USAFPOA, acted in an advisory capacity and in liaison to the Surgeon, USAFPOA. It fell to the lot of the base command surgical consultant to follow recommendations made, and to see that policy was carried out.

The policy of using Medical Corps officers from general hospitals for part-time or full-time service on temporary duty at various headquarters deprived the hospitals involved of the services of an officer, usually one of outstanding professional ability. Since there was a shortage of specialists throughout USAFPOA, these officers on temporary duty could not be replaced in the hospitals to which they were assigned from a professional standpoint; neither could they be replaced numerically, because of the rigidity of the tables of organization. Furthermore, this practice interfered with promotions.

DUTIES OF THE CONSULTANT

It was evident from the start that the duties of the consultant encompassed more than strictly professional work. The quality of surgery depended upon many factors, but the most important were the proficiency and distribution of personnel. Also of importance were the indoctrination of medical officers in the methods and policies of military surgery, the checking of equipment, and the clinical supervision of work in the hospitals. In addition, the consultants acted as technical advisers to the theater surgeon. Not the least of the consultants' duties was to listen with a sympathetic ear to the problems of their fellow medical officers serving in the Armed Forces.

Liaison between the Army, Navy, and Army Air Forces left much to be desired. This was evidenced in many ways, but particularly in the evacuation of casualties. On one occasion, orders for the surgical consultant to visit the Marianas Islands forbade him to visit Advance Headquarters, CinCPAC (Commander-in-Chief, Pacific), during the period of temporary duty. This occurred at a time when several joint problems had become acute. Despite orders to the contrary, conditions made possible a visit to CinCPAC advance headquarters, and in justice it must be said that the surgical consultant was received and the joint problems were discussed.

Unless the consultant gained the confidence and received the wholehearted cooperation and support of the theater surgeon, his duties were futile.

PERSONNEL

Shortage of Medical Corps Officers

Almost throughout the war, the strength of professionally qualified Medical Corps officers in POA was inadequate to the needs for the high type of professional work which was the goal of all concerned. It was only by extending efforts almost to the breaking point of the individual during certain periods that the goal was attained. The tables of organization of numbered general hospitals were inadequate for the type and volume of work demanded for the care of casualties in the operations in POA. For example, it was necessary in the forward areas for all hospitals to maintain a perimeter guard against enemy infiltration of the hospital site with the organically assigned personnel at hand. This was true in the Marianas until V–J Day. On those islands where Army personnel were admitted to Navy hospitals, the burden of preparing the payrolls, providing the clothing, recopying the admission and disposition forms, profiling, and so forth, of these patients fell to the lot of the nearby Army hospitals on whose rolls they were administratively carried. On 27 July 1945, the 204th General Hospital, Oahu, was responsible, from the administrative standpoint, for 934 Army patients in Navy hospitals on Guam. At the same time, there were 1,908 patients occupying beds in the 204th General Hospital. The burden was too great for the tired staff of the 204th General Hospital. The matter was presented to the Chief of Staff, Western Pacific Base Command, and it was suggested that a team be organized with qualified personnel taken from each hospital in the Marianas and attached to Headquarters, Army Garrison Forces, Guam, to relieve the 204th General Hospital of this administrative burden. This was done. Had similar personnel for guard, finance, refrigeration maintenance, and the like, been furnished, as planned, the problems would have been solved.

The number of Medical Corps officers authorized for numbered general hospitals was particularly inadequate for the workloads imposed during active operations against the enemy. Ultimately, this was corrected in part by augmenting these hospitals with special teams, but this did not take place until the Ryukyu Islands campaign was almost completed. Eleven special teams arrived in the Marianas Islands and three in Oahu during the month of June 1945. In the meantime, the staffs of busy hospitals were reinforced with medical officers from the staffs of hospitals less busy. Medical Corps officers from Army Air Forces medical treatment facilities, from Navy hospitals, and from ships in harbor were pressed into service. Teams were organized on the spot, sometimes composed of Army, Navy, and Army Air Forces medical officers. Their services were invaluable. In hospitals predominantly surgical, the internists became members of shock teams and surgical ward officers.

The actual number of Medical Corps officers in POA was close to the authorized allotment, but there was a shortage of specialists. This was no doubt due chiefly to a shortage at the source of supply on the mainland, but, in part, the shortage was due to factors that crept in during the early days of the Pacific campaigns and that later were difficult to correct. The theory that a Medical Corps officer should be able to serve in any capacity had no small part to do with the shortage. This theory was definitely disproved to all as the war progressed, but, in the meantime, position vacancies were filled with officers not professionally qualified for the positions to which they were assigned and were given job classifications instead of professional proficiency classifications. Such practices created a problem which was difficult to solve. The rigidity of tables of organizations, the problems of rank and precedence, and a confusing chain of command added to personal troubles. There were no pools of Medical Corps officers from which to draw. There was a shortage of specialists on the basis of authorized strength in every category. There was no rapid method of requisitioning and securing personnel urgently needed.

A study of the rosters of all professional units in the USAFPOA made in June 1945 showed shortages of specialists on the basis of authorized tables of organization as follows:

Military Occupational Specialty	Shortage
3105 Gastroenterologist	7
3107 Cardiologist	12
3113 Allergist	12
3303 Medical Laboratory Officer	17
3306 Radiologist	16
3151 Thoracic Surgeon	2
3131 Neurosurgeon	12
3152 Plastic Surgeon	3
3153 Orthopedic Surgeon	13
3106 Ophthalmologist & Otorhinolaryngologist	28
3125 Ophthalmologist	2
3115 Anesthetist	28

There appeared to be an overage of officers classified "3150, Medical Officer, General Surgery," but this was only apparent and not real. The explanation was obvious when this group was studied. It included all Medical Corps officers who had had, or claimed to have had, any training in surgery whatsoever. Many of these were not qualified to fill vacancies to which they had been assigned.

The study of the personnel situation that was made in June 1945 by no means represented a true picture of shortages on the basis of actual needs. A further consideration was the length of time many of the Medical Corps officers had served in the tropics or semitropics with consequent impairment of their efficiency. The needs were evident, but there was no way of meeting them at that time.

Requisitioning Medical Corps Officers

Requisitions for Medical Corps officers were made by theater units through channels. These were screened by Headquarters, Replacement Training Command, USAFPOA, and at regular intervals were sent by that headquarters to the War Department. Medical officers with a classification "3100, Medical Officer, General Duty," were being used to fill specialist vacancies, and additional officers with the "3100" classification were being requisitioned by units. Seldom were specialists in any other category requisitioned by units. The theater surgeon could only advise; he could not screen requisitions. Therefore, he could not correct deficiencies in the flow of personnel from the mainland.

It was not until the summer of 1945 that the professional consultants were able to screen requisitions for Medical Corps officers and advise the Medical Section, Headquarters, Replacement Training Command, concerning them. At that time, 30 officers with the classification "3100" had been requisitioned by theater units. It was known that there existed an overage of officers classified "3100" and a shortage of officers classified as specialists. Thereupon, it was agreed to requisition 30 specialists and, when they arrived, to assign them to hospitals where specialist shortages existed in exchange for officers who were classified "3100."

Classifying Medical Corps Officers

The classification coding of all Medical Corps officers in USAFPOA was begun toward the end of 1944 and was continued through the winter of 1945. Classification and coding were done principally by evaluation on the basis of questionnaires. Later, officers were reevaluated after personal contact and observation of their work. It was not uncommon to find that several classifications had been entered on the qualification record of an officer in accordance with the position that the officer held at the time of recording. Finally, revaluation on the basis of personal observation by the consultants led to many changes in classification and to the transfer of officers and brought to light the fact that the shortage of specialists was even greater than that which appeared in the initial study of the situation.

In compliance with a letter directive, dated 1 July 1945, from Brig. Gen. B. M. Fitch, by command of General Douglas MacArthur, to commanding generals in AFPAC, concerning Classification of Medical Corps Officers, a new classification survey was made. This consisted of the completion of a new WD AGO Form 178–2 and AFPAC MD Form No. 1 on each medical officer. The base command consultants and the USAFMIDPAC consultants recommended a classification by indorsement on each form. Final classification was determined by General Headquarters, AFPAC.

Surveys in Relation to Rotation

As early as the first week in July 1945, a survey of Medical Corps officers in the Middle Pacific from the standpoint of their service rating scores was completed. This was done in order to envision losses and prepare for reorganization when the announcement of a given "critical score" would permit many medical officers to rotate home. In August the survey was repeated, with consideration of three additional factors: age, length of service overseas, and length of total service—all of which had a bearing in determining "adjusted" service rating scores for rotation.

Personnel of Medical Units in Transit

The professional consultants of Central Pacific Base Command and USAFPOA (later USAFMidPac) inspected all medical units passing through Oahu from the standpoint of professional proficiency of the staff and adequacy of equipment. If necessary, replacements were made with Medical Corps officers taken from hospitals or other medical organizations within the Central Pacific Base Command or other base commands. This arrangement was far from satisfactory since it weakened base command units. But replacements could not be secured from the mainland without great delay, and it was imperative to send units forward with at least the minimum of specialists and as good a staff as could be assembled without wrecking the staffs of the fixed installations in the communications zone. After V–E Day, certain units originally destined for the European theater were sent to the Pacific. Frequently these were short of specialists, and it was impossible to supply them from personnel already in the Pacific.

Morale

Suitable assignment was perhaps the most important single factor in maintaining good morale. A medical officer would tolerate hardships if occupied by work in which he was interested and for which he had aptitude and training. Medical conferences, journal clubs, and attendance at medical meetings all bolstered morale, as did the establishment of library facilities (fig. 231) and the circulation of medical journals. Joint medical meetings

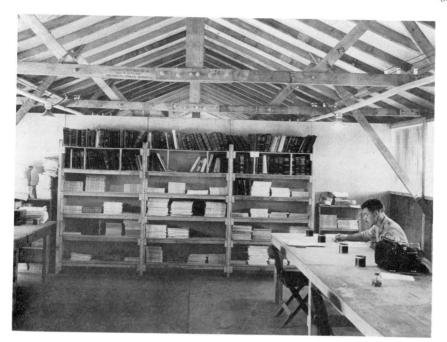

FIGURE 231.—Medical Library, 39th General Hospital, Saipan, 1945.

of Army and Navy medical officers were held on most islands. The programs usually were well thought out and excellent. Consultants participated whenever possible. The oversea installations were adequately supplied with medical textbooks and journals. However, facilities for a library and conference room were not always created.

Living conditions and recreational facilities varied greatly in each hospital and on each island (fig. 232). Housing, recreational facilities, and clubs were of prime importance on small islands in uncomfortable climates. It was evident that these things influenced the morale of personnel. Military necessity—the construction of essential military projects—was the reason given for not obtaining these facilities where they did not exist.

On Guam at the 204th General Hospital, the quarters in which the officers lived were crowded; because of shortage of personnel, there was no charge of quarters on duty; there were few recreational facilities; and there was no club. The comparison with Navy facilities on the same island made these deficiencies stand out sharply in contrast.

In some instances, notably on Saipan, medical officers were housed in relatively primitive quarters and hospital construction had not been completed. These factors played an adverse role from the morale standpoint of medical personnel.

In personal notes taken by the surgical consultant, he recorded that long periods overseas without any definite knowledge as to their prospects of being replaced was influencing the morale of medical officers.

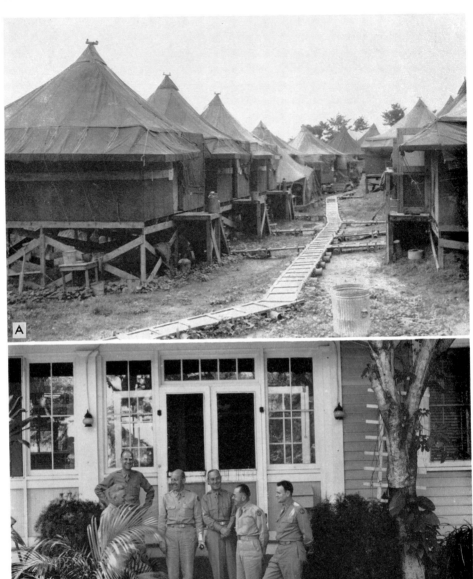

FIGURE 232.—Living conditions and recreational facilities. A. Officers' quarters on Okinawa, August 1945. B. The Officers Club, Fort Shafter, Hawaii. Brig. Gen. John M. Willis, Surgeon, USAFPOA, extreme left (behind palm fronds), and Col. Paul H. Streit, Surgeon, Central Pacific Base Command (second from right), 1944.

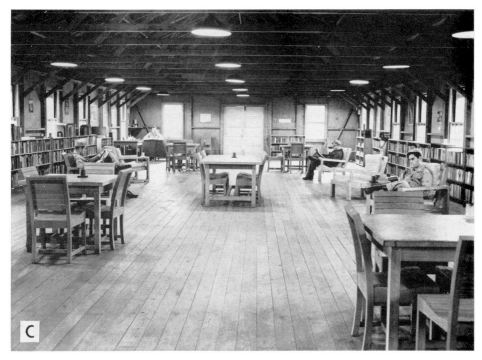

FIGURE 232.—Continued. C. The library of the 129th Station Hospital, Hawaii, 1944.

Promotions and Rank

It was sometimes necessary to transfer officers who merited promotion because of their training and experience and for whom there were no position vacancies on the staffs of the hospitals to which they were assigned. This was particularly true of personnel in affiliated units. The assignment to hospitals of medical officers who had attained relatively high rank in line organizations but who had not had training or experience to equip them to head services or sections in hospitals remained a problem throughout the war. No satisfactory solution as to their use was found, and they continued to block the promotions of those more professionally proficient.

EDUCATION AND TRAINING

Indoctrination of Units in Staging

The medical units on the Hawaiian Islands, assigned or ultimately to be assigned to the Tenth U.S. Army, were given instructions by the consultants of USAFPOA as well as by the consultants of the Tenth U.S. Army. This was accomplished by informal talks and demonstrations on surgery in the combat zone (fig. 233). In addition, teams were organized from general hospi-

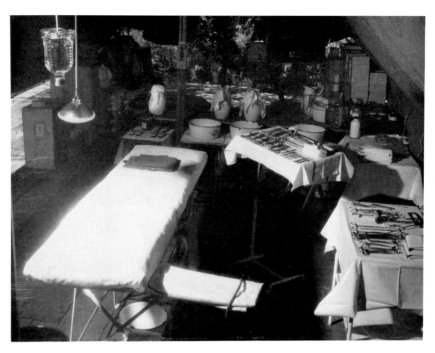

FIGURE 233.—An exhibit, for instruction purposes, of an operating room set up in the field, Hawaii.

tals staging at Oahu and went forward to augment the staffs of field hospitals designated for the assault phase of the Okinawa operation. At this time, no teams were available from the Zone of Interior.

School of Anesthesia

There was a shortage of medical officer anesthesiologists throughout USAFPOA. The shortage in this specialty was as great as, if not greater than, in any other. It was felt by this surgical consultant that every hospital at which surgery was being performed should have assigned a medical officer trained in anesthesia and put in charge of the operating room and anesthesia section. Toward this end, the first school of anesthesia was established at the 148th General Hospital on Saipan in June 1945. Instruction was carried out under the direction of the consultant in anesthesiology from the Surgeon's Office, USAFPOA. Students for the course were obtained from the 23d Replacement Depot, 8th Convalescent Hospital, and from surgical specialty teams whose officers assigned to anesthesia had had little or no formal training in this specialty.

It was felt by the surgical consultant that too little emphasis had been placed on the importance of anesthesia for the management of battle casualties

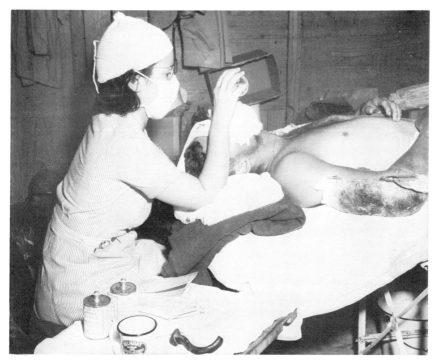

FIGURE 234.—A nurse administering ether anesthesia by the open-drop method, prior to the amputation of a gangrenous arm at the 69th Field Hospital, Okinawa, May 1945.

in USAFPOA, especially in the forward areas. In most hospitals, nurses with some training in anesthesia were in charge of the anesthesia section (fig. 234). These, however, had had little or no training in endotracheal anesthesia, and did not have the necessary knowledge of physiology and pharmacology to direct difficult anesthesias such as in thoracic surgery and neurosurgery.

Because of the shortage of anesthesiologists, nurse anesthetists were obliged to administer spinal and intravenous anesthetics.

CENTERS FOR SPECIALIZED TREATMENT

On Oahu, the 147th General Hospital was designated as a center for thoracic surgery and the 218th General Hospital, for neurosurgery. The former had a thoracic surgeon and the latter a neurosurgeon on the staff. During the Okinawa operation attempts initially were made to admit all fractures of the femur to the 147th General Hospital. This plan was abandoned because the burden became too great for the staff of a single general hospital to handle.

In June 1945, preparation was made for fabrication of artificial eyes at the 218th General Hospital. The necessary personnel had already been trained

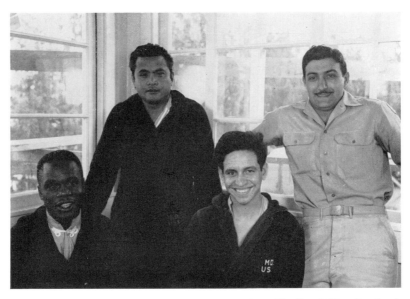

FIGURE 235.—Patients at the 218th General Hospital, Fort Shafter, T.H., after having been fitted with plastic eyes, August 1945.

on the mainland. On 3 July, a directive was published concerning the artificial eye program directing that patients throughout USAFMIDPAC be transferred to the Central Pacific Base Command (218th General Hospital) for custom-made final prosthesis (fig. 235). Certain other hospitals in USAFMIDPAC were designated for ophthalmic surgery and were supplied with conformers for use following eye enucleations. These were the 148th General Hospital, Saipan; 204th General Hospital, Guam; 232d General Hospital, Iwo Jima, Volcano Islands; 233d General Hospital, Okinawa; and the 374th General Hospital, Tinian. The shortage of ophthalmic surgeons made it necessary to limit the number of hospitals designated for this type of work.

During the Okinawa operation, triage was accomplished at the ports of debarkation on Saipan Island, Marianas Islands, and, as far as possible, patients requiring specialized surgery were sent to those hospitals designated for the purpose (fig. 236). The scarcity of specialists in certain categories made this imperative. Thus, during the early part of the Okinawa operation, the 148th General Hospital received all patients arriving in Saipan with thoracic wounds (fig. 237) and wounds involving the brain and spinal cord. The cases of peripheral nerve injuries were too numerous to assign to a single hospital which had only one neurosurgeon on the staff. Later, when the 39th General Hospital, Saipan (fig. 238), was functioning, it was designated as the island neurosurgical center and a center for burns, and the 148th General Hospital remained the center for thoracic surgery. The 369th Station Hos-

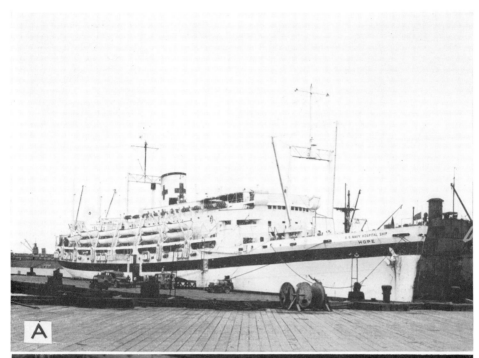

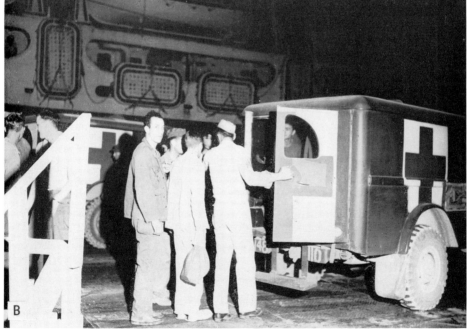

FIGURE 236.—Debarkation activities at Tanapag Harbor, Saipan, in the spring of 1945.
A. The U.S.S. *Hope* being unloaded. B. Patients boarding an ambulance of the 148th
General Hospital, Saipan Island, Marianas Islands.

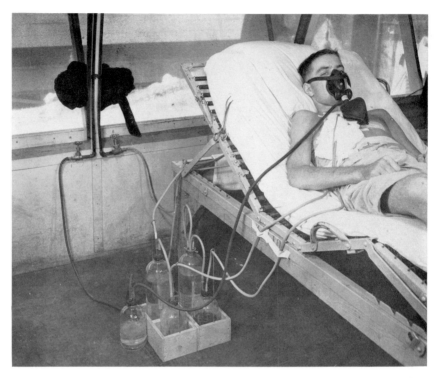

FIGURE 237.—Postoperative care of a patient after thoracic surgery, 148th General Hospital.

pital, Saipan, was utilized for battle casualties having soft-tissue wounds and for minor orthopedic conditions.

At Guam, the 204th General Hospital was designated a center for thoracic surgery. On this island, neurosurgical patients were sent to one of the Fleet hospitals until the arrival of a neurosurgical team on 15 June 1945, when they were cared for at the 204th General Hospital.

On Tinian, Army casualties were admitted to the Navy Base Hospital and to the 374th Station Hospital, there being no Army general hospital on this island until the middle of May when the 374th Station Hospital was designated a 1,000-bed general hospital. It was never possible, however, adequately to staff the 374th General Hospital from the professional standpoint for the care of battle casualties. Thoracic surgery patients arriving on Tinian were cared for at the Navy hospital, where a thoracic surgeon was on the staff. Patients with lesions of the brain and spinal cord, if transportable, were transferred to Saipan. This arrangement was not satisfactory, but all available beds were needed and had to be used. Fortunately, the number of casualties debarked at Tinian was not great.

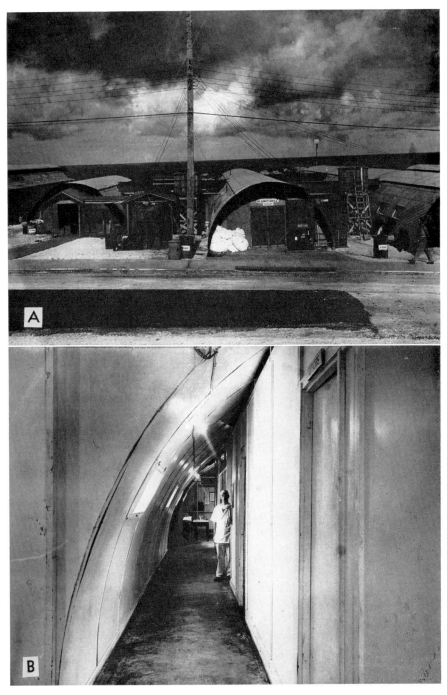

FIGURE 238.—The 39th General Hospital, Saipan, 1945. A. The exterior, showing quonset construction. B. A corridor leading to operating rooms.

DIRECTIVES CONCERNING PROFESSIONAL PRACTICE

Official medical publications (other than books or journals) and directives were universally scarce in USAFPOA. This was noted by The Surgeon General on his visit of inspection early in 1945. The matter was taken up in Washington, and improvement was effected. However, as late as August 1945, War Department Technical Bulletin (TB MED) 147, concerning management of battle casualties, which had been issued in March 1945, had not been distributed to Medical Corps officers in Guam and Tinian. Saipan had received an allotment of this publication and distributed it to that island only. None were left over for the other islands in the Western Pacific Base Command.

Apparently, medical publications were being sent promptly to USAFPOA and Southwest Pacific Area, but there were deficiencies in distribution. In the case of the Southwest Pacific Area, for a number of months, initial distribution involved mailing of publications to a number of points in the widely dispersed area. Redistribution was, in turn, accomplished to subsidiary facilities and units. At certain bases, such as Hollandia, Adjutant General publication depots were established, but the lack of manpower continued to interfere with getting the publications out. This was true all along the lines of communications from depots to bases and to field army units.

In the case of USAFPOA prior to 1 March 1945, initial distribution of publications was by mail from the Zone of Interior to a single Adjutant General depot on Oahu. This depot, however, merely distributed these publications to the major technical services, with each service handling the distribution of publications and forms pertaining to them. This decentralization was put into effect at the request of the theater Adjutant General because of lack of space, personnel, and experience by the Adjutant General depot in this area. After 1 March 1945, initial distribution was by mail from the Zone of Interior to a number of bases, facilities, and units, as in SWPA. It was planned to establish a central Adjutant General depot on Oahu to take over the initial distribution within a specified area of all War Department publications and forms, and the filling of requisitions from all activities and units in the USAFPOA which had been handled on a decentralized basis. To the best knowledge of the authors, this was not accomplished during the war. During the Okinawa operation, very few medical officers on Okinawa or in the Marianas had seen the aforementioned TB MED 147. A number of important directives, however, including "Surgery in the Combat Zone," were written, reproduced, and widely distributed by the Surgeon, USAFPOA.

The distribution of advance copies of directives to the various headquarters was satisfactory and kept the consultants informed concerning the professional policies of The Surgeon General. Even though directives reached hospitals, there was no assurance that they would reach the individual members of the staff or would be read by them. Thus, it became the responsibility of the consultants to see that policy was carried out.

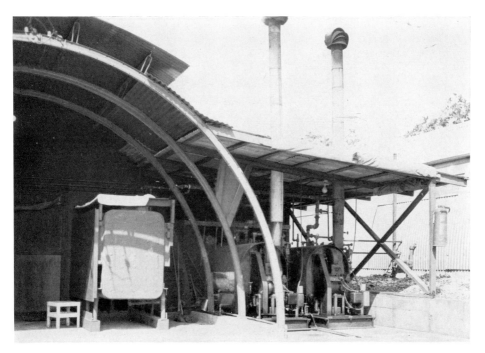

FIGURE 239.—An exterior view of a sterilizer and steam boilers at the 148th General Hospital, Saipan, 1945.

VISITS TO HOSPITALS

The consultants made ward rounds much as a chief of service would make in a civilian hospital. Patients were examined, dressings removed, records perused, and cases discussed. Not infrequently, rounds, begun on the wards, ended in the library or laboratory. Rounds not only served to evaluate a medical officer's professional ability but to test his knowledge of policy. Every physician entering the Army needed indoctrination in Army policy concerning military surgery. Not infrequently, he would resist directives until the rationale of policy was made clear to him. He continued to be an individualist and wished to be convinced that certain procedures, which in his civilian experience were satisfactory, were not necessarily so in Army practice.

Inspection of the operating rooms, of operating-room technique, of sterilizing equipment (fig. 239), of instruments, and of operating-room records were included in the visit. The X-ray departments were inspected, not only in reference to equipment and quality of work but also with respect to protection of personnel from undue exposure to X-rays (fig. 240). In several hospitals, where lead sheet was not available, the substitution of sand-filled partitions was a practical improvisation which on test was found to be effective. Equipment for surgery, including sterilizing apparatus, for the most part was good. This also applied to anesthesia equipment. There was an ample supply of portable

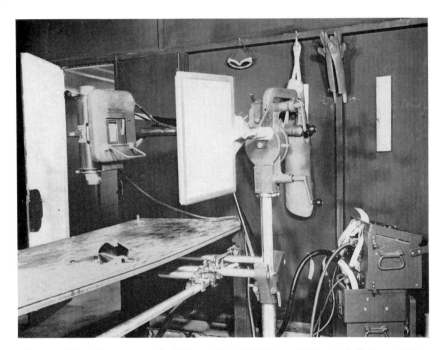

FIGURE 240.—Fluoroscopy facilities at the 148th General Hospital, Saipan, 1945.

operating-room lights. Ceiling lights for operating rooms had to be improvised and installed by hospital personnel in the majority of the facilities in the forward areas. Fluorescent tubes, usually eight in number, mounted in suitable ceiling fixtures was the most common type of ceiling light in use. Lamps removed from portable field surgical lights also were used as ceiling lights.

Air conditioning of operating rooms was an important consideration in the hospitals of the Marianas Islands. There, the heat was so intense in the operating rooms, usually quonset huts, that those working in them were dehydrated and exhausted in a few hours—so much so that it was necessary to put the operating-room personnel on a salt regimen. Air conditioning was not installed until toward the end of the Okinawa operation in the Army hospitals at Saipan. It had not yet been installed in the operating rooms of the hospitals on Guam and Tinian when the war ended. Air conditioning in the operating rooms of the 148th General Hospital (fig. 241) at Saipan brought the temperature down to 84° F.—cool in comparison to outside temperatures. It appeared that but few of the engineers who were available understood the installation or maintenance of air-conditioning units. Those installed on the outside of surgical buildings, exposed to the sun, stopped functioning frequently and had to be adjusted. When fresh air was brought in from the outside the heat of the air threw too great a burden on the machines. It was necessary to recirculate the air in the building. A service team composed of members well trained in air conditioning was needed.

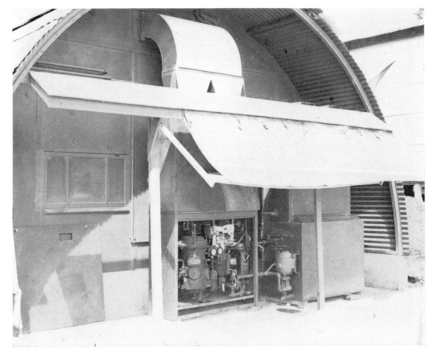

FIGURE 241.—Exterior installation of air-conditioning equipment at the 148th General Hospital, Saipan, 1945. Note the makeshift canopy to protect the equipment from strong sunlight.

THE OKINAWA OPERATION

The lack of evacuation hospitals and a shortage of well-qualified surgical specialists at Okinawa gave rise to serious difficulties in properly caring for casualties during the Okinawa operation. It was the consensus that each division should have been supported with field and evacuation hospitals and that "blown up" field hospitals did not functionally take the place of evacuation hospitals. The surgical teams did excellent work, but were too few in number. All hospital staffs were well indoctrinated in the use of blood (fig. 242). Shock was well managed by teams organized from among available internists and they did valuable work. Tents which were equipped to deal with shock and to prepare patients for operation were set up in close proximity to the surgical operating tents. Equipment included oxygen apparatus, materials for blood determinations by the copper sulphate specific-gravity method, and the Levin type of stomach tube as well as the usual materials for the emergency care of the wounded. A Levin tube was introduced in all patients with suspected penetrating wounds of the abdominal cavity. Priority for operation was established for casualties urgently in need of it by those in attendance in the "shock tent."

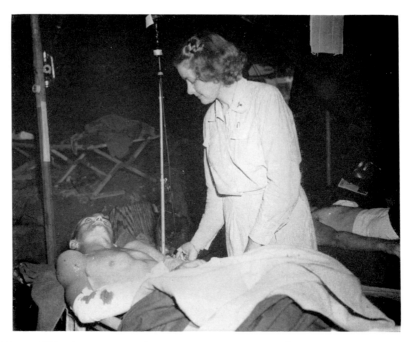

FIGURE 242.—A nurse, one of the first group to land on Okinawa, checking the administration of whole blood to a casualty at a hospital in close support of the fighting, April 1945.

Several patients with vascular wounds were seen whose amputations should have been performed earlier than they had been. The fault may have been due to failure to observe patients closely enough following ligation of vessels, to depending too much upon the efficacy of sympathectomy or parasympathetic nerve block, or to an effort to save a few additional inches of an extremity. One such patient was seen who went into profound shock on the sixth or seventh day, from which he died without amputation. He had had a ligation of the common femoral artery followed by lumbar sympathectomy, and the seriousness of his condition was not recognized until he was moribund.

There was considerable discussion concerning the desirability of attempting repair of arterial injuries and the need for arterial suture material, Blakemore vitallium tubes, and heparin in the hospitals of the forward areas. It was believed by the surgical consultants, however, that more harm than good might come of it unless such work was limited to certain hospitals staffed with surgeons trained in vascular surgery and the work could be done on an investigative basis. Had the war continued, the establishment of centers for vascular surgery, staffed by qualified surgeons, would no doubt have been recommended.

The field hospitals did not have a sufficient number of trained anesthetists. They had an inadequate supply of anesthesia machines, suction apparatus, and oxygen therapy equipment. There was no shortage of oxygen in large cylinders, but there was a shortage of reducing valves, flowmeters, and high-

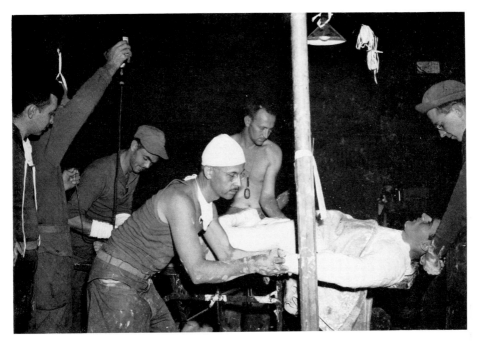

FIGURE 243.—Treatment at the 69th Field Hospital, Okinawa, in May 1945.

pressure tubing. It was the impression of the Consultant in Surgery, USAFPOA, that oxygen therapy should have been used more extensively in the management of shock. There were not enough reducing valves to use oxygen for many patients at the same time. The shortage was partially overcome by borrowing reducing valves from ships.

Shortages in medical equipment were due in part to limitations imposed on the amount of shipping because of military necessity.

The specialized professional teams assigned for the Okinawa operation included two general surgical, one neurosurgical, and two orthopedic teams. All of these teams were not up to authorized strength. None of them had with them the equipment authorized for specialized teams.

A critique of the Okinawa operation stated with respect to field hospitals (fig. 243):

Experience with field hospitals revealed in certain instances notable deficiencies in selection of personnel and in the training of the unit. Insufficient attention had been paid to the professional qualifications of officers designated for responsible positions on the medical and surgical services. Organization and direction of the laboratory service was inadequate and the technical quality of the work poor. Training of the personnel in the operation of the unit as a hospital had been neglected. This was particularly true of the organization and instruction of shock teams. Many of these deficiencies have been corrected by transfer and exchange of officers and by professional instruction on the ground.[1]

---

[1] The Report of Surgical, Medical, and Orthopedic Consultants for Operational Report of Okinawa Campaign, 30 June 1945.

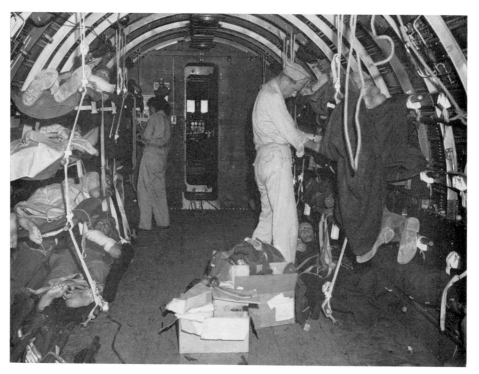

FIGURE 244.—Patients being prepared for air evacuation by converted C–54, Okinawa, July 1945.

The activity of the consultants of the Tenth U.S. Army did much to correct deficiencies. Despite criticisms herein contained, the quality of the medical service in the Okinawa operation in general was good.

During the Iwo Jima operation, casualties were evacuated principally by ship to Saipan, overflowing the hospitals there and leaving beds vacant on Guam and Tinian. During the Okinawa operation, air evacuation began on D+8 and finally surpassed evacuation by ship (fig. 244). Planes debarked at Guam and almost none at Saipan or Tinian. At this time, the hospitals on Guam were overwhelmed. All attempts to control evacuation of casualties in the Marianas Islands in accordance with the beds available on each island failed. This had a very definite influence on the care of the wounded and, through fatigue, on the morale of personnel.

In a few instances consultants traveled as observers on ships evacuating wounded from Okinawa to the Marianas Islands. In this way, valuable information was gained concerning treatment given casualties in the forward areas and their condition upon evacuation.

The routing of ships appeared to have been done without due consideration for facilities or vacant beds in the hospitals on Saipan, Guam, or Tinian. Sufficient notification of the time of arrival of patients at a port was not given.

In some instances, between five hundred and a thousand patients arrived without previous notification, which led to confusion. Failure in properly "tagging" patients led to improper triage.

During the Okinawa operation, the 148th General Hospital cared for the majority of the serious casualties brought to the island of Saipan. The 39th General Hospital was not ready to receive patients until the campaign was well underway. The 148th General Hospital was used exclusively as a surgical hospital and was so organized with the formation of shock, plaster, and traction teams. Surgical teams were formed with officers assigned to the staff of the 148th General Hospital, with Marine Corps and Air Force medical officers from local installations, and with Navy medical officers from ships in the harbor. Nine surgical operating teams worked around the clock in shifts.

As the Okinawa operation progressed and hospital beds in the Marianas became filled, the policy of retaining patients with fractures of the femur temporarily was abandoned. Patients with compound fractures of the femur were treated by debridement of the wounds if this had not been done, by secondary debridement if this was indicated, by skeletal traction, and, in suitable cases, by secondary closure of the wounds 7 to 10 days after primary or secondary debridement. Because of the need for beds, these patients, during the height of the campaign, were evacuated to the rear before the fractures were "frozen." Casts were applied, and Kirschner wires were removed before the patients were evacuated.

In the Marianas, circular casts were not split owing to the prevalent climatic conditions and their instability when this was done. On the other hand, patients were not evacuated after the application of casts until the danger of interference with circulation was past.

The impression gained in the Marianas and at Oahu was that surgical patients who had arrived during the Okinawa operation had been better treated and were in better condition than patients arriving during the Iwo Jima operation.

In the Marianas, of necessity, battle casualties were sent to station hospitals as well as to general hospitals. An effort was made to admit only the less seriously wounded to station hospitals, but, on occasion, the seriousness of wounds was not recognized. This was particularly true of wounds of the buttock that had penetrated the rectum and of vascular wounds. The latter were not recognized until progressive extravasation of blood produced noticeable swelling in the region of the wound. The station hospitals were visited frequently by consultants who advised on treatment and transfer of seriously wounded patients to general hospitals. It was evident that the professional qualifications of staff members of station hospitals did not meet the necessary requirements for the care of the seriously wounded. Directives dealing with hospitalization of battle casualties were published by Western Pacific Base Command, and by the Surgeon's Office, USAFPOA, but could not be followed always since at times the urgent need for beds demanded that those vacant in station hospitals be utilized for battle casualties.

During the height of the Okinawa operation, it became necessary to relieve medical officers in the hospitals on Saipan of nonprofessional duties. This was accomplished by directive from the Office of the Surgeon, Headquarters, Island Command, Saipan. Medical officers, badly needed for surgical work in the operating rooms, were being given such duties as the censoring of mail. It was directed that officer patients convalescing in hospitals be used for this purpose; also, that property accountability and other nonprofessional duties be assigned to nonprofessional personnel.

During July and the early part of August, hospitals in the Marianas Islands were visited by the Consultant in Surgery, USAFMIDPAC, and the Consultant in Surgery, Western Pacific Base Command. All medical officers were revaluated from the standpoint of the positions to which they had been assigned, and replacements, when indicated, were advised. Suggestions were made regarding medical supplies and equipment from the standpoint of the heavy load anticipated in future operations. At this time, the hospital center at Tinian was in the process of construction.

HOSPITAL CENTER AT TINIAN

The hospital center at Tinian comprised five 1,000-bed general hospitals. The facilities for surgery, the establishment of centers for specialized work in individual hospitals, the assignment of personnel, and the need for and requisitioning of specialists were discussed and planned in detail with the commanding officer of the hospital center. It was expected that 70 percent of the beds of the center would be devoted to surgery. The tentative plan for professional service in surgery envisioned a division of work in units as follows:

Unit 1. Neurosurgery, abdominal surgery, orthopedic surgery, and urology.

Unit 2. Amputations, burns, general surgery, orthopedic surgery, and urology.

Unit 3. Thoracic surgery, maxillofacial surgery, ophthalmic surgery, general surgery, orthopedic surgery, and urology.

Unit 4. Internal medicine and medical specialties, general surgery, orthopedic surgery, and urology.

Unit 5. Neuropsychiatry and neuropsychiatric patients requiring surgery.

Each hospital was designated as a center for specialized work, and in addition—with the exception of Unit 5—would have cared for general surgery, orthopedic surgery, and urology. The surgery performed in Unit 5 would have been limited to surgery which arose in neuropsychiatric patients, most of which would have been in connection with self-inflicted wounds. This plan did not necessitate major changes in hospital staffs. An acting director of surgery was selected. This officer was to have been responsible for the overall supervision of the surgical services throughout the hospitals comprising the center and in control of the surgical teams assigned to it.

Twenty-eight surgical operating rooms would have been available in the four hospitals designated for surgical work. On the basis of the Okinawa operation, it was expected that approximately 140 surgical operations would be performed daily when the next military operation was under way. It was estimated that each surgical team on a 12-hour shift would average eight operations per day. On this basis, 17 surgical teams would have been needed. Nine of these teams were to have been requisitioned, and eight were to have been organized from the staffs of the five general hospitals composing the center. Teams were to have made up for the lack of certain specialists on the hospital staffs.

Plans included a request that an Air Transport Command liaison officer be assigned to the center on a full-time basis to facilitate evacuation of patients by air.

It was planned also that the Consultant in Anesthesiology, USAFMID-PAC, would organize the anesthesia section and remain at the center for the early part of the next military operation.

Work on the hospital center was discontinued with the cessation of hostilities.

NOTES AND FORMAL REPORTS

The Consultant in Surgery, USAFPOA, made daily notes concerning visits to hospitals. These were too wide in scope and often too personal to submit as formal reports, but they were the basis for formal reports. Formal reports were sent through medical channels beginning with the commanding officer of the hospital visited and ultimately reaching the Surgeon, USAFPOA. Only those things were reported formally which could not be dealt with locally, or which were informative in a general way and upon which it was felt that the base command surgeon might wish to comment by indorsement. At the end of a visit to forward areas, the personal notes of the consultant were read by and discussed with the Surgeon, USAFPOA, often with other members of the headquarters staff in conference. Thus pertinent matters observed by the consultant came to the attention of the operations, personnel, and supply officers in the Surgeon's office. These matters were dealt with at once. Not infrequently, on visits to forward areas, notes were sent directly to the Surgeon by courier. In the last month of the war, formal reports were not made. Detailed notes, however, were kept and submitted to the Surgeon upon return of the consultant from the Marianas Islands.

JOHN B. FLICK, M.D.

CENTRAL PACIFIC AREA

Examination of the situation in the Central Pacific Area in the fall of 1942 revealed that the principal problem was a dearth of trained professional personnel. There was only one other diplomate of the American Board of Surgery in the area and, in addition, over the next 3 years, only three other

Fellows of the American College of Surgeons in general surgery were in the area. With this personnel, five general hospitals and nine station hospitals had to be manned.

Since additional trained surgeons could not be expected to arrive in the area, the first important task was an appraisal of all the existing surgical talent followed by the training of these men in order to provide adequate surgical care of patients. All medical officers in the area who had had as much as one year's residency training in surgery were interviewed. The medical officers of divisions training in the area were interviewed and, where it seemed desirable for the good of the service, exchanges were made to augment somewhat the percentage of at least partially trained surgeons. When it was felt advisable, officers were placed on temporary duty at the 147th General Hospital for a 4- to 8-week period of observation so that their surgical skills could be more accurately determined and, in addition, so that they themselves could have a "brush-up" period in surgery. During 1943 some 10 or 12 such temporary assignments were made, and during 1944 more than 30 officers were rotated through the surgical service of the 147th General Hospital with a view to enhancing their previous surgical training (fig. 245). Since some of the station hospitals were more than 1,000 miles from their nearest neighbor, it is obvious that consultations on individual problems were impossible and that the fate of the patient rested with those who were immediately available.

Besides the deficiencies in trained surgical personnel, there were very few corpsmen who had been trained for operating-room duty. Since some of the smaller station hospitals were going to forward areas where no nurses would be available, it was felt that the training of corpsmen in surgical techniques was most important. Accordingly, a training school was set up at the 147th General Hospital for corpsmen in operating-room techniques. These men were put through an intensive two months' course, and it was very gratifying, as well as surprising, to see what excellent scrub nurses they made at the end of that period. Actual figures were not available at the time of this writing, but there must have been at least 50 enlisted men so trained during the course of the war.

The war in the Central Pacific Area was under the command of the Navy and at no time was there an appreciable number of fixed Army hospitals assigned to the care of frontline casualties. This meant that virtually all the casualties received in the general hospitals in the Hawaiian Islands arrived there from 2 to 4 weeks after they were wounded. This naturally posed an entirely different problem from that encountered in the North African and European theaters. It was fortunate that, during early operations on the coral islands, there had been no appreciable fertilization of the ground and gas bacillus infections were virtually unknown. Furthermore, it was found that initial debridement could be carried out 3 weeks after wounding with surprisingly good results. The ideal time for secondary closure of those wounds which had been debrided was, of course, lost during the period of transportation. But again, it was found that secondary closure could be satisfactorily accomplished at the end of 3 weeks' time instead of at the end of from 6 to 10 days.

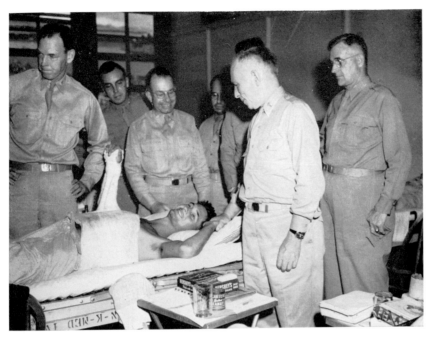

FIGURE 245.—Maj. Gen. Norman T. Kirk, The Surgeon General, making ward rounds in the 147th General Hospital, accompanied by Gen. John M. Willis (right), Colonel Streit (center, behind patient), and Col. Forrester Raine, MC (left).

The percentage of complicated chest wounds was, the writer fears, considerably higher in the Central Pacific Area because aspirations of hemothorax and even pneumothorax were, as a rule, delayed for 3 or 4 weeks. This necessarily increased the number of decortications that had to be done to achieve satisfactory respiratory function. These decortications were started in the Central Pacific Area at about the same time as in the North African theater and yielded excellent results.

The type of wounds received in the Central Pacific Area differed materially from those in other theaters. In at least the first 2 years of the war, attacks were all against small coral atolls and the little artillery the enemy had was knocked out by Naval bombardment (fig. 246). Wounds, therefore, resulted predominantly from small-caliber bullets, small-caliber mortars, or hand grenades. Japanese hand grenades were much lighter and splintered into much finer particles than did the U.S. Army grenades, so that on the whole wounds did not show the great destruction of tissue which typically occurred with high explosives. This may well account for part of the reasonable results attained in spite of delayed debridement.

The technical bulletins emanating from the Office of The Surgeon General were of the greatest assistance. They permitted personnel in the Central Pacific to profit by the experience earned from the management of a tremendous

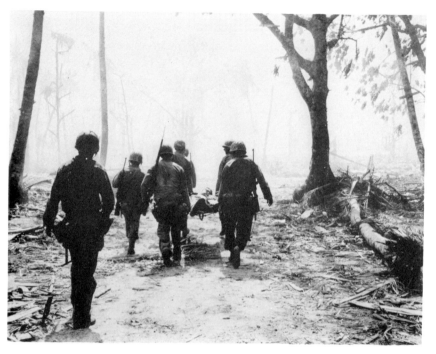

FIGURE 246.—Litter bearers of the 7th Infantry Division, bringing in a wounded soldier, Kwajalein, February 1944. Note the great destruction of vegetation.

number of casualties without having to go through an appreciable period of trial and error themselves.

The largest number of casualties handled over a short period of time by the Central Pacific Area general hospitals occurred following the Saipan, Guam, and Tinian battles. These casualties were evacuated from the islands by hospital ship and landed at Kwajalein for care and transshipment to the hospitals on Oahu. These casualties numbered 2,900 during June and July of 1944. The small station hospital at Kwajalein was enlarged to a 1,400-bed hospital with virtually no addition of medical personnel and did an excellent job of screening, emergency treatment, and transfer. Among these casualties were approximately 60 with severe chest wounds who, it was believed, could not be evacuated safely by air at the altitudes usually flown. With the marvelous cooperation of the Air Transport Command, two planeloads of these patients were flown to Oahu at under 4,000 feet. Since this was below the usual cloud level, this air evacuation was carried out without utilization of refined navigational aids. But, happily it can be said that planes and patients arrived in good shape, none the worse for their trip.

So far as the author is aware, no new developments or outstanding contributions to surgical knowledge emanated from the Central Pacific Area. It was demonstrated many times, however, that, in spite of an inadequate number of fully trained personnel, satisfactory end results could be achieved in the management of casualties who were received long past the ideal time for treatment. It was believed that this accomplishment resulted from foresight in anticipating the future and in attempts at training the many who arrived with inadequate training before entering the service.

FORRESTER RAINE, M.D.

CONSULTATION IN ORTHOPEDIC SURGERY

The uncertainty of the United States' participation in World War II ended at Pearl Harbor on 7 December 1941. As an Infantry veteran of World War I, and a long-time Medical Reserve Officer of the Arms and Service Assignment Group, this author, Lt. Col. (later Col.) Robert Crawford Robertson, MC, received a telegram that day requesting his early active duty. On 26 December, a representative of The Surgeon General telephoned the author inquiring if he would like assignment to Hawaii as orthopedic consultant. Orders to Letterman General Hospital, San Francisco, which then contained many Hawaiian casualties, soon followed. The kind and considerate help of Lt. Col. (later Col.) Oral B. Bolibaugh, MC, Chief, Orthopedic Section, Letterman General Hospital, was invaluable in initiating the author into the professional and administrative problems of a large military hospital. Colonel Bolibaugh soon left to assume command of an evacuation hospital and later rendered outstanding service in the Mediterranean and European theaters.

On Friday, 13 March 1942, aboard the U.S.S. *Republic*, this consultant entered Pearl Harbor, a "graveyard of once proud ships" where intense repair activities were everywhere evident. At Fort Shafter, Oahu, T.H., he reported to Col. (later Brig. Gen.) Edgar King, MC, Surgeon, Hawaiian Department, whose farsighted planning, combined with the outstanding cooperation of the civilian doctors in Hawaii, had resulted in superior medical service during and following the surprise attack of 7 December. Colonel King was an officer with long service in the Regular Army. One of his basic convictions was: "He is a medical officer, he can do anything."

Hawaiian Department, 1942

The major Army hospitals on the island of Oahu were Tripler General Hospital (later the 218th General Hospital), where Maj. (later Col.) August W. Spittler, MC, was Chief of Surgical Service; and Schofield Station Hospital (later North Sector General Hospital, and eventually 219th General Hospital), where Maj. (later Col.) Leonard D. Heaton, MC, was Chief of Surgery. Major Spittler and Major Heaton were superior officers of the Regular Army who had rendered outstanding service during and following the raid. Their kind cooperation and help in the problems of medical supply, planning, personnel and patient evaluation, and the professional management of battle and garrison casualties were of the greatest aid in making the transition from an orthopedist in private practice to a staff orthopedist in an oversea theater.

The Hawaiian Department at the time expected another attack by the Japanese and was serving as an oversea defense area. Numbered general and station hospitals arrived and established on the islands of Oahu, Kauai, Maui, and Hawaii. Tables of organization did not meet local needs, and provisional hospitals were established on these islands as well as on Molokai and Lanai. Throughout the early years of the war, many provisional units found it difficult to receive authorization for obtaining necessary personnel. As a result, many medical officers were placed on temporary duty at various installations to meet needs as they arose.

The year 1942 was spent chiefly in organizing to meet anticipated needs. A shortage of specialized personnel immediately became apparent. This remained the major problem throughout the war. The shortage of orthopedic surgeons authorized by tables of organization in June 1945 totaled 13 (26 percent). The assignment of Maj. (later Lt. Col.) John R. Vasko, MC, to Tripler General Hospital, Honolulu, and the arrival of 1st Lt. Robert W. Ray, MC, with the 147th General Hospital early in 1942 established a firm foundation for orthopedic care in the Department. Both of these officers demonstrated outstanding professional ability and retained their assignments as chiefs of the orthopedic sections in these hospitals throughout the war. Staffing, equipping, and planning within the various hospitals of the islands was further complicated by the various provisional hospitals considered necessary because of the terrain and anticipated attack. Plans had to include provision for the care and evacuation of wounded on each island and by ship among the islands in case of attack.

In the summer of 1942, reports were received that there was an unusual incidence of delayed union and nonunion in fractures treated in the military hospitals. Reports of all fracture cases showing delayed union or nonunion were obtained from the various hospital commanders and a personal check was made of all of these cases. No evidence was found to substantiate these reports.

Among this consultant's early duties were the evaluation and assignment of personnel, the formulation of professional procedures in accordance with the evacuation policy of 120 days, the providing of surgical support for a regimental combat team in amphibious operations, the inspection of the proficiency of all numbered hospitals and all tactical medical units in first aid procedures, the establishment of facilities for orthopedic alterations on shoes by a quartermaster shoe repair shop on each of the islands, the changing of automatic medical supply items, the establishment of emergency and expansion facilities within military and civilian hospitals and ships in all of the islands in anticipation of attack, and the marking of tourniquet cases in the field. Employees of Hawaiian contractors who were performing construction work for Army expansion plans received Army medical care to include preemployment physical examinations by teams composed of Army medical officers and subsequent medical care given in Army medical facilities.

In June 1942, the Hawaiian Department received a few Army air and ground casualties from the Battle of Midway. The Navy casualties, who were far more numerous, were seen through the courtesy of the commanding officers of the various Navy hospitals. The shortage of specialized personnel experienced by the Army was not then, and never became, apparent in the Navy hospitals in the Pacific Ocean Areas. During the late 1930's, the splendid Navy medical service had commissioned into its Reserve Corps in advanced grades many doctors from the staffs of medical schools and teaching hospitals. The outstanding men so obtained formed a magnificent pool at the outbreak of the war. In the author's opinion, the Army would do well to consider similar methods in future Reserve planning.

Circular letters issued by the Office of The Surgeon General were extremely helpful during 1942, as were subsequent Essential Technical Medical Data reports and War Department technical bulletins in standardizing new professional methods and in the management of garrison and battle casualties.

The organization stage was fairly complete by fall of 1942. On 5 November 1942, this consultant was assigned as chief of a separate orthopedic service at North Sector General Hospital, Oahu, T.H., in addition to his duties as orthopedic consultant, Hawaiian Department. General King's instructions were: "You will keep me informed of the orthopedic situation from front to rear at all times."

Replacements from the mainland arrived in large numbers. Many were in the 40-year-plus group and presented various problems, chiefly those centering about unaccustomed physical activity. The majority were recruits of only 1 or 2 months' service, and outpatient services at the hospitals became extremely heavy. One muscular Texan who was inducted into the Army one month after injuring his leg was seen as an outpatient one month later in one of the Department's hospitals. X-rays showed a complete oblique fracture of the proximal end of the tibia and neck of the fibula, with slight displacement of fragments and with very good callous formation. Upon his being questioned, he revealed that he had received no medical care and had performed full duty, including hikes. He stated: "They think I'm yellow, Doc, but I just can't take those long hikes very well." The "low backs" presented a major problem which continued throughout the war. Department policies were established as follows:

1. In the absence of objective physical and X-ray findings, treatment will be given on an outpatient basis.

2. Hospital cases will be disposed of on an individual basis, and as many as possible will be returned to limited service within the Department if they are unable to perform full duty.

3. No case will be returned to the mainland in the absence of definite pathology.

These policies continued in effect throughout the war, and proved very effective.

By the end of 1942, many senior regular medical officers had been rotated to the mainland for reassignment, chiefly in command positions. Several infantry divisions had arrived, the 25th Infantry Division had departed for the South Pacific Area, the Department's numbered hospitals were well established, and they were set up for emergency and expansion needs, including the treatment of gas casualties. The cooperation of the commanding officers, chiefs of surgery, and the orthopedic section chiefs in the various hospitals was excellent. Their problem cases were freely presented, and "hideouts" were very infrequent. The Battles of the Coral Sea, Midway, and the Solomon Islands had disclosed that the Japanese were brave men, but not invincible. The Hawaiian Department's primary problem continued to be the procurement of specialized personnel.

Central Pacific Area, 1943

The new year, 1943, was ushered in by the following instructions from General King: "You keep a check on all the hospitals in this Department and transfer any case to the general hospitals as indicated without consulting me." General King believed that additional orthopedic surgeons should be developed within the Department instead of their being requested from the mainland. Search was made of personnel records and repeated many times throughout the war for officers suitable for such development. When available, they were transferred to a general hospital for training.

Largely because of the relatively low hospital workload and the absence of combat casualties, there developed a marked tendency on the part of several hospitals to attempt professional procedures beyond their professional capacity. This was corrected by directives listing the type of cases to be referred to general hospitals for definitive treatment.

The braceshop at North Sector General Hospital was developed and served the Department. Cases requiring braces were referred to that hospital for fitting and application of the brace.

Analysis of the outpatient clinics disclosed a very large number of foot cases. Because of this a spot check of eight companies or the equivalent was made by an orthopedic team. Findings indicated such poor foot care that a Department directive was issued emphasizing the duties of unit commanders in preventing and correcting this problem.

First aid fracture procedures, including splinting, were checked at the various hospitals on admission of each patient. Instructions were issued requiring a report to the Department Surgeon of all cases evidencing unsatisfactory care. Only an occasional unsplinted case appeared thereafter. Standard and improvised splinting and first aid management of fractures was checked in each tactical unit. These inspections were personally conducted, and many amusing incidents were encountered. One incident occurred in a battalion medical detachment of an antiaircraft artillery regiment. Improvised methods for treating a simulated compound fracture of the femur were requested of two soldiers. When their job was completed, a small gauze bandage had been wrapped about the mid-thigh. A large wooden stake had been driven into the ground in the region of each axilla, and each foot had been tied to a similar stake for "traction" and for "still more traction."

Internal derangements of the knee, including many unusual cases of osteochondritis dissecans, were seen in quite large numbers in all of the general hospitals. Functional results permitting return to full duty were disappointing following surgery. Fifty individual cases were personally followed up after surgery and formed the basis for a command directive published 6 July 1944 restricting arthrotomy of the knee to carefully selected cases.

Recurrent dislocation of the shoulder joint was also a difficult and fairly frequent problem. Surgery was considered only if the dislocation was seen by a medical officer. Initially the Nicola type of operation was favored, but followup disclosed recurrences in an estimated 40 percent following return to duty. Bankart's operation was first employed in 1943. The results of both types of operation were so generally disappointing that surgery thereafter was restricted to carefully selected patients who were returned to limited service.

Fractures of the carpal scaphoid were very numerous. Fresh cases responded well to conservative cast treatment and were returned to duty. Ununited fractures which were symptomatic and did not respond to conservative or to operative procedures (an entirely satisfactory surgical procedure was not developed) were placed on limited service.

Following several requests for authority to visit the outlying islands of the Department, Colonel Robertson went in June 1943 as representative of the Department Surgeon with a general and special staff group from the headquarters staff of Maj. Gen. Robert C. Richardson, Jr., Commanding General, Hawaiian Department. The group visited Canton, Christmas, Palmyra, and Fanning Islands. Small defense units held each of these islands. Medical personnel were adequate. Each island presented individual problems, but, in all, the medical plans both for garrison and for providing medical support in the event of an enemy assault were considered sound. This trip was most informative and stimulating, as it introduced new thoughts regarding the problems of medical reinforcement in case of enemy attack, and the management and evacuation of casualties on an isolated island target.

On 14 August 1943, the Hawaiian Department became USAFICPA. During the same month, Brig. Gen. Hugh J. Morgan, Director, Medical Consultants Division, Office of The Surgeon General, visited USAFICPA and presented his observations in other theaters. He stated that penicillin was a promising drug and would be made available. And, in October, small amounts of penicillin did become available through the courtesy of good friends in the U.S. Navy. It was in January 1944 that the command obtained its first supply of penicillin through Army sources.

Because of troop concentrations on the island of Oahu, including the 7th Infantry Division which had arrived following its capture of Attu, the orthopedic outpatient clinics became very large, each clinic frequently handling in excess of 100 cases daily. This number of outpatients combined with the limited orthopedic staffs seriously interfered with hospital care. At an informal meeting with the surgeons of the 6th, 7th, and 40th Infantry Divisions, it was agreed that the problem could best be solved by the following measures: (1) Giving minor orthopedic care in the clearing company of each division, and referring only more serious cases to a hospital; (2) restricting to 50 the number of hospital outpatient clinic cases on each of the 3 outpatient clinic days each week; and (3) formation of a reclassification board within the area for disposition of division cases rather than boarding them through the hospitals. These measures proved effective.

On 7 November 1943, the Hawaii Chapter of the American College of Surgeons gave a most delightful scientific and social program for Fellows in the Armed Services. In the same month, General King directed that each combat division be furnished an officer trained in the management of fractures. He accepted the suggestion that each division provide one medical officer for training in fracture management during its stay in the islands and that this officer accompany the division on its departure. This plan was adopted, and subsequent personal observation of the professional skill displayed by many of these men during combat was gratifying.

Formally organized orthopedic training programs were established in December 1943 to take place in designated general hospitals on the island of Oahu for officers and enlisted personnel. The courses were made available to selected medical personnel of divisions and other tactical units. This policy paid off handsomely in subsequent combat operations as well as in the fixed hospitals. Largely because of the success of this program, a similar training program was later established for all Army medical officers by order of the Commanding General, USAFPOA, dated 20 October 1944.

During the latter part of 1943, the 204th General Hospital was without an orthopedist because of the shortage of trained personnel, and orthopedic cases were directed to other hospitals. It was again recommended that the Surgeon, USAFICPA, requisition three orthopedists with professional qualifications for section chiefs to be assigned to the area's large fixed hospitals, where the orthopedic census averaged about 25 percent of the total hospital census. The surgeon of each incoming unit was contacted for an officer with surgical background suitable for further orthopedic development, but rarely did such a man become available.

A few battle casualties were received from the Gilbert Islands operations. Analysis of 127 cases admitted to hospitals on Oahu showed wounds of the extremities, spine, and pelvis in 90, or 70.8 percent, of the cases. Practically all were wounds inflicted by small arms. The standard of treatment in the forward area was good. No case of cast constriction, major amputation, or gas gangrene was seen. Sulfonamides were given en route. Limited air evacuation was used in this operation. Initial impressions were favorable. The author requested authority to participate in the coming invasion of the Marshall Islands but was refused.

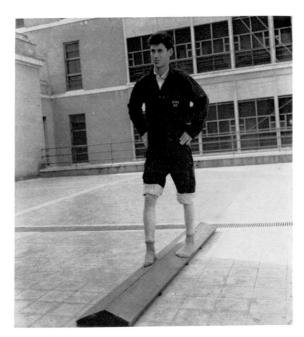

FIGURE 247.—The courtyard of the 147th General Hospital. A patient exercising on a walking board.

By January 1944, the orthopedic training program in the general hospitals was organized on a 13 weeks' basis, and several officers were attached to Tripler, North Sector, and the 147th General Hospitals (fig. 247).

The Marianas and Leyte, 1944

The first group of casualties from the Marshall Islands arrived on 12 February 1944. At North Sector General Hospital, 173 were received, of which 43 were orthopedic cases, chiefly patients with wounds inflicted by small arms. Many had received initial definitive treatment aboard ship. By Navy standing operating procedure, the medical officers of each ship decided prior to combat the principles and methods of treatment which would be followed during the action. This procedure was quite in contrast to the professional methods as prescribed by The Surgeon General of the Army and, in combined operations, resulted in confusion between the medical services. Colonel Raine, area surgical consultant, Col. Charles T. Young, MC, Consultant in Medicine, Office of the Surgeon, USAFICPA, and the author checked the 646 wounded in the various hospitals, and made the following observations:

1. Selected cases were given plasma or blood shortly after wounding.

2. Sulfonamide therapy was well administered en route.

3. Clinical records and X-rays did not accompany the patients to the rear area hospitals, but arrived several days later.

4. Wound debridement was unsatisfactory in 13 percent.

5. Closed wounds were found in 13 percent. Of these, 60 percent were infected.

6. Wounds treated by open methods rarely showed infection.

7. Amputation stumps were not treated by traction. Fifty percent were closed by flaps and were infected.

8. There was no gas gangrene or tetanus.

9. Splinting was good.

In the joint report, the three officers recommended that the area surgeon further emphasize directives that had been published on methods of treatment and that agreement be obtained with the Navy on methods of wound management. This consultant was convinced that consultants should accompany each invasion and attempt to supervise the management of patients on the target. Lt. Col. (later Col.) Laurence A. Potter, MC, Surgeon, 7th Infantry Division, and an outstanding field medical officer, with experience in Attu and the Marshall Islands, concurred, and so recommended to General King.

A prominent visiting civilian consultant to the Navy was impressed by the Stader splint, which was used quite extensively in that service. After checking this method of treatment with several Navy orthopedists and seeing their cases, this consultant recommended to General King that the Army obtain the item for evaluation in each of the command's fixed general hospitals. The Surgeon General disapproved this requisition. Time proved him correct in so doing because of the numerous late complications which followed.

In the spring of 1944, Maj. John J. Cawley, Jr., MC, a "graduate" of the USAFICPA orthopedic training program, was assigned to the 204th General Hospital, which was for a time without an orthopedic section. He reorganized the section, continued as chief throughout the remainder of the war, and rendered superior service.

In the hospitals, it was possible accurately to forecast combat operations by the increased number of self-inflicted gunshot wounds of the extremities. When self-inflicted wounds became numerous, it was positive evidence that an operation was pending. Unfortunately, nearly all of these cases were reported by investigating boards as "Line-of-duty, yes."

On 15 May 1944, the author submitted a letter to General King requesting temporary duty on a combat mission "for the purpose of supervising and assisting in the care of orthopedic casualties." Four days later, he was unofficially advised that his request had been favorably considered.

The shortage of orthopedic personnel continued to be acute. General King advised this consultant that orthopedists were not available from the mainland. Again the qualification card of each medical officer in USAFICPA was reviewed in a search for prospects. Training programs in the general hospitals were functioning well, but practically all of the officers in training were on temporary duty for only a few weeks and then moved on with their divisions. Nevertheless, two excellent men for development and permanent retention in orthopedic assignments were obtained. They were Capt. (later Maj.) Arthur M. Faris, MC, a diplomate of the American Board of Obstetrics and Gynecology, from a military police battalion; and Capt. (later Maj.) Lawrence L. Hick, MC, from the 7th Medical Battalion.

Brig. Gen. Earl Maxwell, formerly Surgeon, USAFISPA, and Colonel Sofield, formerly Orthopedic Consultant, USASOS, SPA, reported to Headquarters, USAFICPA, as the South Pacific Area was closing. Colonel Sofield reported that USAFISPA had four general hospitals, three large station hospitals, and a total of nine orthopedic board diplomates. This relatively large number of certified orthopedists was present because USAFISPA had affiliated units. In USAFICPA, there were no affiliated units, and, as a result, there were only two orthopedic board diplomates.

The Marianas operations

On 4 July 1944, the first battle casualties from Saipan arrived—six evacuated by air. By 14 July, the orthopedic census at North Sector General Hospital totaled 336, of whom 78 were battle casualties. On 15 July, General King directed this consultant to go to Kwajalein to supervise the management of the cases arriving there from the Marianas operations. On the author's arrival on Kwajalein, he met Lt. Col. Byron A. Nichol, MC, Island Surgeon; Brig. Gen. Clesen H. Tenney, Island Commander; and Capt. Robert F. Sledge, MC, USN, Atoll Surgeon. The island hospital—Provisional Station Hospital No. 2, commanded by Maj. (later Lt. Col.) Maximilian C. Kern, MC—was reinforced by personnel of the 51st and 52d Portable Surgical Hospitals, just arrived from the South Pacific and without recent clinical experience. The instructions were to evacuate the first 50 cases received each day to Guadalcanal station hospitals because the Oahu hospitals were filling up.

There were 1,314 Army hospital beds on Kwajalein, obtained by using the newly erected Army Air Forces barracks for emergency and expansion facilities. All hospital enlisted personnel were made available for professional work when one officer and enlisted personnel were detailed from tactical units to operate the hospital messes, run water details, and so on. The Navy operated all atoll hospitals except Kwajalein. Penicillin and volunteer blood donors were available. Colonel Nichol and the author agreed that white (14-day) cases be retained on Kwajalein, blue (15- to 60-day) cases be evacuated to Guadalcanal, and red (60-plus day) cases be evacuated to Oahu, insofar as practical. On 30 July, Kwajalein received 291 battle casualties from the hospital ship, U.S.S. *Solace*. Casualties remaining on board were taken to the Navy hospital on Burton Island. On the same day, 50 casualties came in by air. Cases arriving at the Army hospital were almost entirely Marines, who for the most part had been well treated, although many of the spica casts were broken and very few amputation stumps were in traction. A few instances of inadequate debridement, primarily closed wounds, tightly packed wounds, unnecessary excision of skin, unsplit casts, anklet traction still in place, and several cases of anerobic cellulitis were encountered. Four aircraft were available for further evacuation out of Kwajalein each day—two for Oahu and two for Guadalcanal. These were C–54's, and each had two flight nurses and was equipped to carry a total of 32 litter cases. The vast majority of patients were evacuated from Kwajalein by air. On 3 August, General Tenney advised that the Kwajalein hospital beds would be limited to 450 upon arrival of additional units who would require the Army Air Forces barracks for housing. Atoll beds after arrival of these units were to be: Kwajalein 450, Roi 450, Burton 450, and Carlson 150. Reserve Army medical supplies were stored on Carlos Island, where it was possible to establish 300 additional beds, if necessary, but transportation to that island was by boat only. On the same day, 50 casualties arrived from Tinian, many requiring blood transfusions.

On 6 August, this consultant sent a memorandum to Col. Eliot G. Colby, MC, Surgeon, Army Garrison Force, Island Command, Saipan, reporting the condition of cases received on Kwajalein. After one week, with practically no battle casualties, a radio was sent to General King requesting temporary duty in the Marianas. The author, meanwhile, visited Makin, one of the Gilbert Islands, where Maj. Robert D. McKee, MC, was Island Surgeon and commanding officer of the 1st Station Hospital, which served the island and evacuated to Kwajalein. Personnel and supplies were adequate. On return to Kwajalein, the author learned that hospital ships were expected on 20 August. On 16 August, reports were received that the wounded were being well evacuated from Kwajalein. On 19 August, this consultant received radio orders from General King to proceed to the Marianas.

Colonel Colby was Island Surgeon, Saipan, where island spraying with DDT was first done. The 369th Station Hospital was operating, and the 148th General Hospital was just getting established. The evacuation policy was 30 days. This consultant immediately saw patients, checked supplies, reviewed surgical principles and methods, and discussed the effects of the 30-day evacuation policy with the staffs of these two units and with Colonel Colby. On 24 August, the author proceeded to Guam where Capt. John B. O'Neil, MC, USN, was surgeon of the V Amphibious Corps (fig. 248). The 77th Infantry Division with the 36th Field Hospital, operating a forward and a rear section, and the 289th Station Hospital, which was just establishing facilities, formed the Army contingents of this corps (fig. 249). Neither of these hospitals had an officer trained in fracture management. Combat operations were practically at a standstill because of mud. DUKW's (amphibious trucks, 2½-ton cargo) were useful in the evacuation of wounded (fig. 250). Dengue fever was epidemic. Evacuation within the division was temporarily impossible because of the mud. The author reviewed cases and professional management at the 36th Field Hospital. It was impossible to visit the tactical units. Captain O'Neil, in discussions, emphasized the need for qualified medical personnel in the combat zone and for a directive covering professional management in combat operations. On return to Saipan, minor recommendations regarding personnel and supplies were made to Colonel Colby.

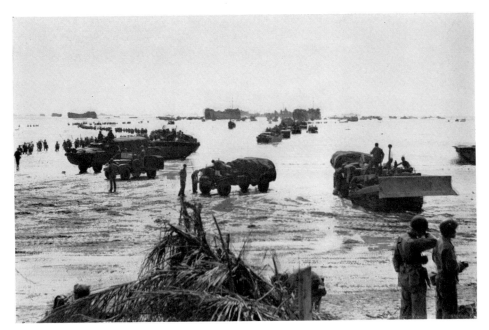

FIGURE 248.—The landing on Guam, 23 July 1944.

Return to Hawaii

On reporting to General King, this consultant's major recommendations were that:

1. Additional specialized medical officers be obtained to staff properly the large hospitals.

2. All training courses for Medical Department personnel emphasize principles and methods to be employed in the combat zone.

3. Refresher courses in the large fixed hospitals be of at least 6 weeks' duration.

4. Consultants discuss anticipated problems of the combat zone with medical officers of tactical units shortly before their departure on combat missions.

5. Mobile surgical teams be made available for use in combat, forward, or rear area hospitals as required.

6. Officers of the Army Nurse Corps be made available to mobile hospitals soon after their establishment.

7. Air evacuation from the combat zone be supervised by an air evacuation officer.

8. The use of blood transfusions be increased in the combat zone.

9. An attempt be made to obtain skin traction methods in the management of amputation stumps of Army personnel treated aboard ships.

10. Further use be made of consultants in the combat zone.

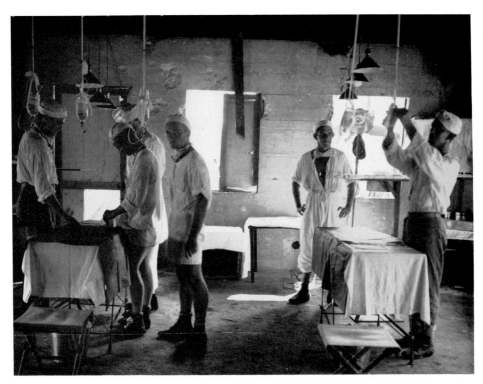

FIGURE 249.—An operating room, established in a building that had been recaptured from the Japanese, Guam, July 1944.

General King then stated that the author was full-time orthopedic consultant for USAFPOA, the command's new designation, and relieved him of duty at North Sector General Hospital. General King ordered the author on temporary duty to the XXIV Corps as an observer for a coming operation and said that a request for leave on the mainland would be in order upon the author's return to Hawaii. Major Faris, another "graduate" of the orthopedic training program, was designated this consultant's replacement as Chief, Orthopedic Section, North Sector General Hospital. Colonel Oughterson (formerly surgical consultant in the South Pacific Area) was the new Consultant in Surgery, USAFPOA.

On 21 August, Brig. Gen. Raymond W. Bliss, Office of The Surgeon General, and Brig. Gen. Fred W. Rankin, Chief Consultant in Surgery to The Surgeon General, visited Headquarters, USAFPOA. They had no specific recommendations for the command's orthopedic problems.

On 2 September 1944, this consultant discussed the pending operation with Colonel Potter, Surgeon, XXIV Corps, and Lt. Col. (later Col.) Robert J. Kamish, MC, Surgeon, 7th Infantry Division. The author was to be a working observer, acting initially as orthopedic consultant to the 7th Division and later as the Corps orthopedic consultant. On the following day, he made

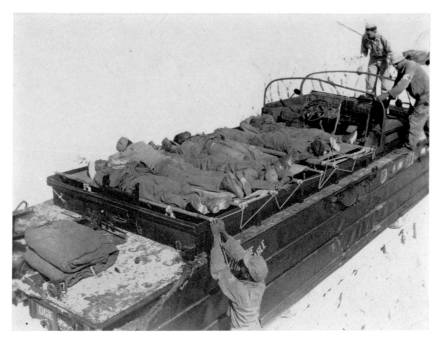

FIGURE 250.—Casualties being loaded on DUKW's for evacuation.

final rounds at North Sector General Hospital with Major Faris and found that several of the knee cases that were closed with cotton had extruded sutures. The author also met with the staffs of all the available mobile surgical hospitals that would be attached for the operation and discussed orthopedic principles and case management.

On 12 September 1944, this consultant reported aboard the U.S.S. *J. Franklin Bell* in Pearl Harbor. On 14 September, a meeting was held with the senior medical officers of all participating ships and the key medical officers of the 7th Division. These officers, including the author, planned, discussed, and agreed upon the medical policies and the principles and methods of treatment and evacuation to be followed in the operation. Particularly emphasized in professional care were early adequate initial surgery, open treatment of wounds without tight packing, traction on amputation stumps, cast fixation of fractures and severe soft tissue injuries, and the use of penicillin.

The force departed Pearl Harbor on 15 September. On the following day, the target was officially announced to be the island of Yap, Caroline Islands, and all were briefed on the operation. Three hours later, it was announced that the target had been changed. The task force arrived at Eniwetok, and 4 days later the new target was announced to be Leyte, Philippine Islands, and D-day, 20 October 1944. Now, the XXIV Corps would become part of the Sixth U.S. Army under Lt. Gen. (later Gen.) Walter Krueger.

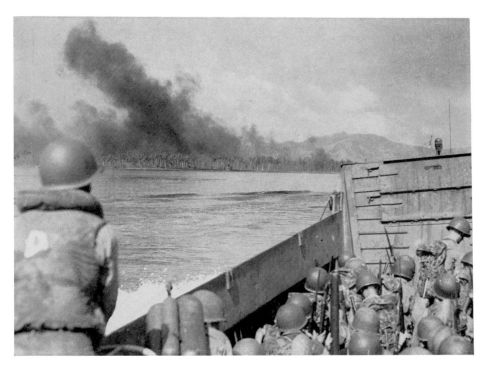

FIGURE 251.—The shoreline of Leyte Island at the invasion point, as seen from an incoming LCVP, 20 October 1944.   The smoke is from the naval bombardment.

On 3 October, the force arrived on Manus, Admiralty Islands, where the new medical plans were discussed with Colonel Potter and Colonel Kamish.   By his personal request, the author was to go ashore on D-day with a collecting company.   The force left Manus on 14 October.

Leyte, Philippine Islands

On 20 October, the Pacific was calm as a millpond.   The force entered Leyte Gulf about dawn.   The Japanese sent out an occasional welcoming committee of a Zero or a torpedo bomber flying low.   All that this consultant saw were shot down.   By plan, the XXIV Corps assault wave which included one platoon of Company C, 7th Medical Battalion, was to go in at about J+4 or J+5 (hours) on call.   Personnel were loaded into LCVP's (landing craft, vehicle and personnel), which circled briefly, then formed up on the line of departure abreast the bombarding ships.   At J+25 (minutes), the LCVP in which the author was riding was on Beach Yellow 2 at Dulag (fig. 251). When the assault force newspapers appeared a few days later, the official version was: "Our troops in their desire to close with the enemy, at times overran their line of departure."

The collecting company established in the remains of the church (which faced the square) and evacuated to the medical shore party, which in turn evacuated by LCVP to ship (fig. 252). At about 1500, the collecting station was joined by Captain Minden and his surgical team from the Clearing Company, 7th Medical Battalion. The team established itself inside the church and began definitive treatment for nontransportable military casualties and severely wounded civilians (fig. 253). Shore-to-ship evacuation stopped before dusk, and, as the collecting company and surgical team were the only medical units behind the 184th Infantry, the group worked throughout the night. The Japanese attacked the 184th Infantry shortly before dawn with infantry and tanks, as the regiment was warned they would. Both the U.S. Army and the U.S. Navy turned their full firepower onto the attacking Japanese, which made a deafening but magnificent display of coordinated fireworks in the dark. On the following day, the clearing company arrived and established its station, and the collecting company moved forward. Two surgical teams from the 76th Station Hospital, Leyte, soon joined the collecting company, which then established a station with a military section for emergency surgery and a civilian section for definitive care.

While with the 7th Infantry Division or with the XXIV Corps, this consultant observed professional methods or assisted in patient care in a battalion aid station of the 184th Infantry, all companies of the 7th Medical Battalion, 69th Field Hospital, Leyte, 76th Station Hospital, Leyte (fig. 254), 165th Station Hospital, Leyte, and the 394th Clearing Company of the 71st Medical Battalion (Separate). Several of the mobile hospitals were not unit loaded, and their supplies were widely scattered on the various Corps beaches, causing much delay in getting them established. All medical units established their own perimeter of defense. Personnel of the 51st and 52d Portable Surgical Hospitals were used as surgical teams to reinforce clearing companies and field hospitals. Blood was obtained from patient and volunteer donors. Because of nearby airfields, ammunition dumps, and artillery positions, several of the medical units received enemy fire of various types, which caused numerous casualties among their personnel. On 24 October, this consultant was slightly wounded in the left thigh by a shell fragment, and a walking cast was applied from ankle to groin.

Upon leaving the XXIV Corps, the author reported to Headquarters, Sixth U.S. Army. The surgeon, Col. (later Brig. Gen.) William A. Hagins, MC, was a delightful gentleman with the wisdom of having participated in the establishment of 14 previous beachheads. He felt that clearing companies reinforced with surgical teams and evacuation hospitals provided the best medical support for divisions in amphibious operations. Within the X Corps, the 1st Field Hospital, Leyte, the 2d Field Hospital, Leyte, and the 3d Field Hospital, New Guinea, were establishing hospitalization facilities, while their surgeons were active with surgical teams reinforcing clearing stations and evacuation hospitals. The 36th and 58th Evacuation Hospitals were established

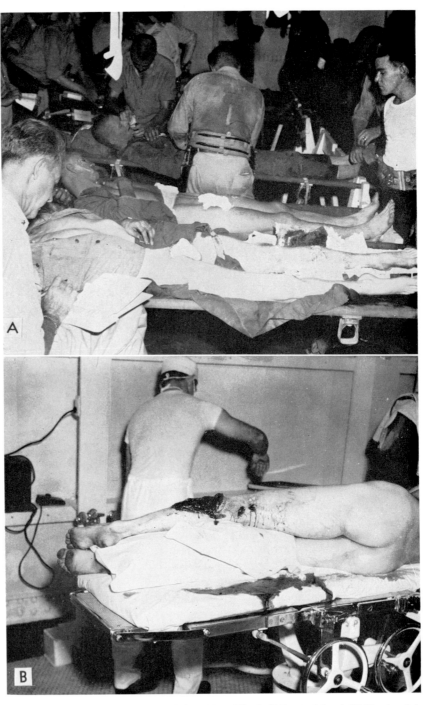

FIGURE 252.—Casualties aboard the U.S.S. *J. Franklin Bell*, Leyte Island, Philippine Islands, 20 October 1944.   A. The officers' wardroom.   B. The operating room.

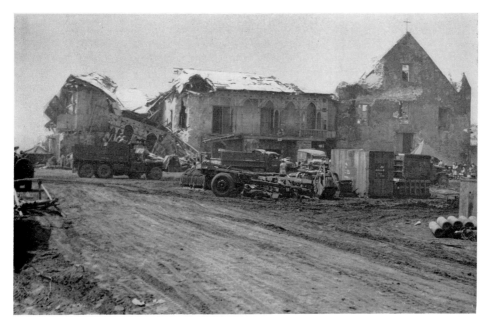

FIGURE 253.—A church used by the 7th Medical Battalion as a collecting and clearing station with an attached surgical team, Leyte Island, 24 October 1944.

near Tacloban, Leyte. This consultant was greatly impressed with the evacuation hospitals. Both received patients on D-day, were fully established by D+3, were staffed with well-qualified specialists, and received whole blood daily by air. A few selected female nurses were with these two hospitals and were of great value, particularly in postoperative care and in raising the morale of the patient.

From Leyte, this consultant proceeded to Peleliu Island, Palau Islands, where combat operations were in progress. The 17th Field Hospital, Peleliu Island, in addition to serving the Marine assault force, was operating as a link in air evacuation between Leyte and Biak.

Major conclusions formed during these operations were:

1. Because of attacks on ships, blackout conditions, vagaries in the weather, and other unforeseen circumstances, medical plans for operations in the future should include provision for complete definitive surgery to be furnished ashore.

2. Four surgical teams should be attached to each division clearing company.

3. Each combat division should be supported by one evacuation hospital, semimobile.

4. Station hospitals, when employed as evacuation hospitals in combat, must be supplemented by surgical teams.

5. Personnel of portable surgical hospitals were best employed as surgical teams and for providing postoperative care.

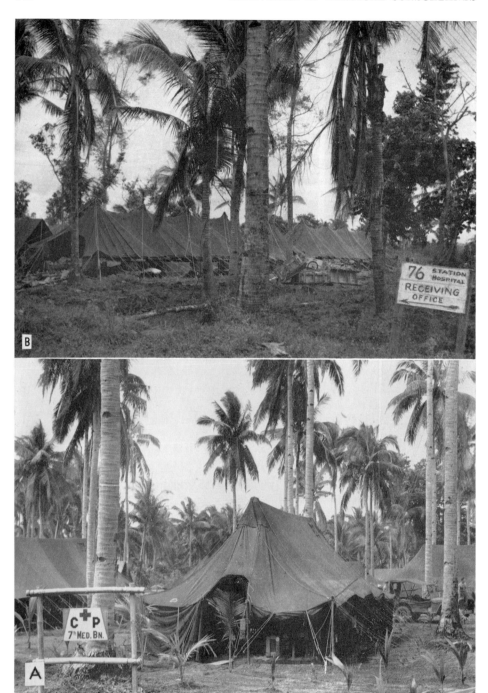

FIGURE 254.—Some 7th Infantry Division and XXIV Corps medical installations on Leyte visited by Colonel Robertson. A. Command Post, 7th Medical Battalion. B. Tents of the 76th Station Hospital, Leyte.

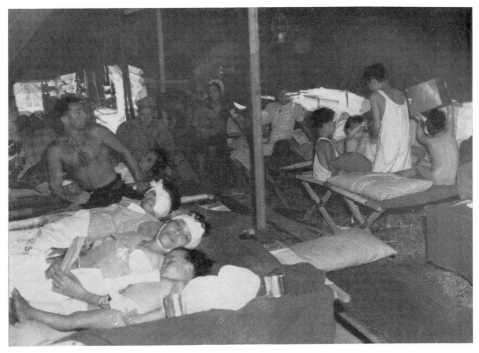

FIGURE 255.—Surgical ward of the 165th Station Hospital, Leyte Island, showing numbers of civilian patients, November 1944.

6. Well-trained surgical teams were of great value at all levels within the combat zone.

7. Medical personnel assigned to units entering combat should receive training in small arms to include the carbine.

8. Unit loading and unit control of supplies on the beaches was essential.

9. Civil affairs units should be established early to assume full medical care of civilians, thus freeing the medical service of tactical units of this additional burden (fig. 255).

10. Army Nurse Corps officers should be brought to the target on call of the surgeon of the combat forces.

11. Medical and dental officers of company grade and selected officers of field grade should be rotated between mobile and fixed medical units on a 12 months' basis.

12. Use of the Thomas' arm splint should be discontinued in the combat zone.

13. New tents should be obtained that can be properly blacked out and yet permit work to continue within.

14. Morphine should be administered only by Medical Department personnel.

15. Refresher courses given in large fixed hospitals resulted in improved surgical care on the target.

16. Refresher courses given in rear area hospitals for medical officers of tactical units should further emphasize procedures and techniques to be employed in the combat zone.

17. Training courses in the large rear area hospitals for selected enlisted men should further emphasize training in the handling of trauma.

18. Consultants should be attached to each combat force.

In addition to these recommendations, the author brought back a renewed love and admiration for the combat soldier, regardless of his color, flag, or religion.

Hawaii again

On return to Headquarters, USAFPOA, in November, this consultant found that General King had been rotated to the mainland and Brig. Gen. John M. Willis had replaced him. Lt. Col. William B. McLaughlin, MC, a diplomate of the American Board of Orthopaedic Surgery, from the South Pacific, was the new chief of the orthopedic section at North Sector General Hospital and doing superior work. Patients in all Oahu hospitals were receiving excellent care. Battle casualties found in a station hospital were transferred to a general hospital.

General Willis recognized that the prevailing shortage of orthopedic personnel was acute and approved requisitioning the necessary personnel from the mainland. He also approved this consultant's writing directly to Col. Leonard T. Peterson, MC, Chief, Orthopedic Branch, Office of The Surgeon General, and to Lt. Col. John J. Loutzenheiser, MC, Consultant, Orthopedics and Reconditioning, Ninth Service Command. Personal letters were written to each of them asking about the condition of patients on arrival on the mainland. Mobile orthopedic teams were requested by General Willis. Personnel for the four that were to be formed were selected by the author. He continued to give talks on orthopedic management in the combat zone before numerous tactical, mobile, and fixed hospital units.

Back to the United States

Finally, this consultant submitted his request for temporary duty and leave to the Zone of Interior. The request was approved. On 18 December 1944 he left Oahu, and on the following day at Letterman General Hospital, San Francisco, Calif., he checked the condition of patients evacuated from the Pacific with the Commanding General, Brig. Gen. Charles C. Hillman, and his chief of surgery, Col. Russel H. Patterson, MC. Both reported that patients arrived in good condition. Their chief criticism was the manner in which hands were splinted.

The author arrived at his home on 23 December, in time for Christmas and a happy reunion with his family. He gained 14 pounds during the first 2 weeks at home.

By invitation of Colonel Peterson, this consultant visited Battey General Hospital, Rome, Ga., and made rounds with him and Maj. (later Lt. Col.) James J. Callahan, MC, Consultant in Orthopedic Surgery, Fourth Service Command. The principles and methods of treatment seen were essentially those that had been followed in the Pacific. Hoping to find additional orthopedic personnel for USAFPOA, the author requested 10 days' temporary duty in the Office of The Surgeon General. The request was approved, and he proceeded to Washington where much time was spent at Walter Reed General Hospital. Several of the Pacific wounded and other old friends were seen. With Colonel Peterson, he reviewed the qualification cards of all orthopedic surgeons available for assignment and found no prospects for USAFPOA.

Okinawa, Victory, and Demobilization, 1945

In San Francisco, it developed that air transportation would mean a delay of at least 2 weeks. As this consultant had been alerted for the next operation, he returned to Pearl Harbor aboard the U.S.S. *Okanagoan* (APA 220) on her maiden voyage.

On Oahu, he found that General Willis was in the forward areas with Maj. Gen. Norman T. Kirk, The Surgeon General of the Army. The author saw all orthopedic cases in the general hospitals on Oahu, and received his anticipated orders for temporary duty as observer with the Tenth U.S. Army for Operation ICEBERG (Okinawa). In the Tenth U.S. Army, Col. Frederic B. Westervelt, MC, was Surgeon; Colonel Finney, surgical consultant; Col. Walter B. Martin, MC, medical consultant; and Colonel Sofield, MC, orthopedic consultant. Colonel Oughterson was to be surgical consultant and Col. Benjamin M. Baker, MC, medical consultant of the forward base area with headquarters on Saipan. General Maxwell was to accompany the invasion forces and become Surgeon, Army Garrison Force, following the operation. Lt. Col. (later Col.) Moses R. Kaufman, MC, theater psychiatric consultant, and the author were to go with the task force in addition to being assigned as Tenth U.S. Army consultants. There were no evacuation hospitals. Each division was to have one field hospital, with two portable surgical hospitals and four surgical teams attached, to act as an evacuation hospital. A directive, "Surgery in the Combat Zone," was to be issued to all medical units of the Tenth U.S. Army. When General Kirk and General Willis returned from the forward areas, the utilization of consultants in the various zones of the theater was discussed with them (fig. 256).

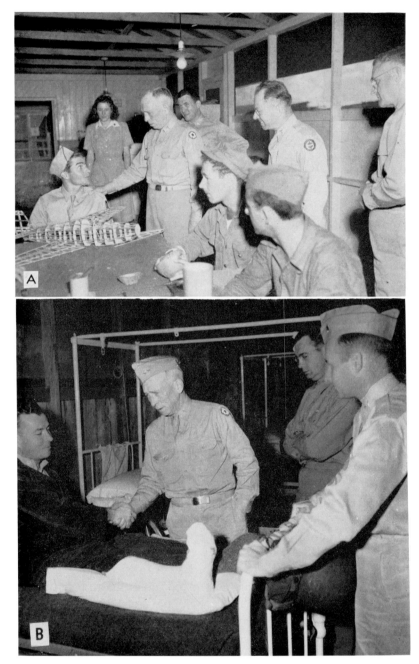

FIGURE 256.—Maj. Gen. Norman T. Kirk, touring the Middle Pacific. A. An occupational therapy shop of the 129th Station Hospital convalescent center. General Kirk (with hand on patient), Colonel Streit (second from right, standing), and General Willis (extreme right). B. An orthopedic ward of the 22d Station Hospital, Oahu, T.H.

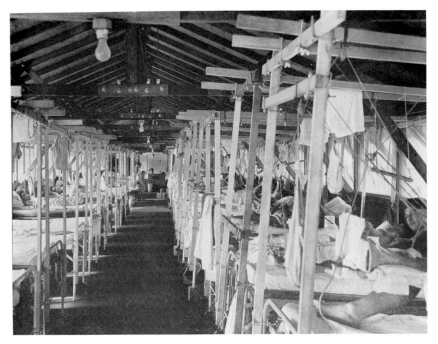

FIGURE 257.—An orthopedic ward at the 39th General Hospital, Saipan.

The Okinawa operation

On 5 March 1945, this consultant boarded the U.S.S. *Montauk*, assistant command ship, and arrived at Saipan on 13 March. At the 39th and 148th General Hospitals and the 369th Station Hospital, he reviewed cases and medical plans for Operation ICEBERG. Orthopedic cases were to be treated only at the 39th and 148th General Hospitals, where it was hoped that all fractures of the long bones could be held until "frozen" (fig. 257). At Tinian, where Captain Mueller, USN, was Island Surgeon, the author discussed with the combined Army and Navy medical officers the medical plans for care of battle casualties.

This consultant left Saipan in a convoy with the 2d Marine Division. The target day was officially "Love Day," 1 April 1945 (Easter Sunday), and H-hour was 0800. On "Love Day," the sea was calm, and the day, clear. The amphibious assault feint of the 2d Marine Division was beautifully executed. Then the convoy continued to the landing beaches on the west side of the island. The power of American industry as evidenced by the many new types of ships engaged was amazing (fig. 258). The assault waves met little resistance. The author remained aboard ship, where occasional air attacks were received. On 4 April, he visited the hospital ships, U.S.S. *Comfort* (Army) and U.S.S. *Solace* (Navy) and reviewed professional methods. He also visited Landing

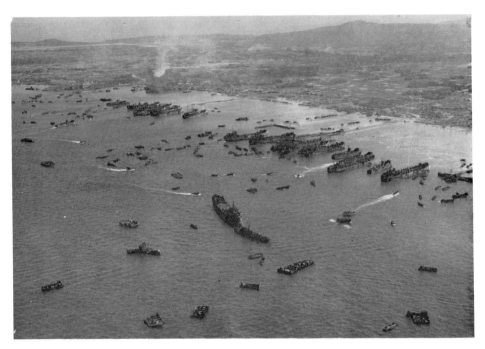

FIGURE 258.—The ships that carried men and supplies to Okinawa, 4 April 1945.

Ship, Tank, Hospital Ship 929, which was serving as the force blood bank until the blood bank could be established ashore and as the control ship for medical supplies and casualties.

On 5 April, this consultant went ashore where he saw Colonel Potter, Surgeon, XXIV Corps; Lt. Col. Byron B. Cochrane, MC, Surgeon, 7th Infantry Division; Maj. Homer P. Struble, MC (who had excised the author's shell-fragment wound on Leyte) and many other old friends (fig. 259). The 31st and 69th Field Hospitals were not fully operational because of supply difficulties. The author was instructed to serve as consultant with the XXIV Corps. Colonel Sofield was to serve in a similar capacity with the III Amphibious Corps and with the Tenth U.S. Army. The XXIV Corps, moving south on Okinawa, had established contact north of Naha. On 6 April, the author again went ashore. As he left the beach to return to his ship, the first organized Japanese kamikaze (suicide) attack on the ships began and continued for about 5 hours. The LCVP, during the return to the ship, was a perfect ringside seat. The kamikaze corps was not a suitable assignment for a coward.

On 8 April, the author reported to Headquarters, XXIV Corps, and served with the Corps through 6 May. He assisted in the organization of shock wards; supervised and participated in the postoperative care of patients and in their general management; held informal discussions on professional methods with the various tactical and hospital units; corrected on the spot errors observed; and prepared indicated directives for the Corps surgeon.

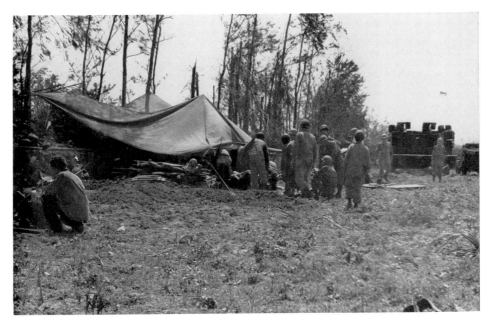

FIGURE 259.—An aid station on the beach at Okinawa, L-day, 1 April 1945.

Many of the wounds were caused by multiple shell fragments, and they were very severe and destructive. On 16 April, he submitted a report on the medical situation to General Willis.

This consultant served with and visited the following units: All battalion aid stations of the 105th and 106th Infantry, 27th Infantry Division; the aid station of the 3d Battalion, 165th Infantry, 27th Infantry Division; regimental aid stations of the 17th, 32d, and 184th Infantry, 7th Infantry Division; Companies A, B, C, and D (52d and 66th Portable Surgical Hospitals attached) of the 7th Medical Battalion; Companies A, B, C, and D (96th and 98th Portable Surgical Hospitals attached) of the 102d Medical Battalion (fig. 260); Companies A, B, C, and D (51st and 67th Portable Surgical Hospitals attached) of the 321st Medical Battalion; the 31st and 68th Field Hospitals; the 394th Clearing Company of the 71st Medical Battalion (Separate), which was operating two holding platoons for evacuation from shore to ship; and the Evacuation Center, Tenth U.S. Army.

The experienced units for the most part established themselves rapidly, functioned efficiently, and evacuated promptly. The Clearing Company (Company D), 7th Medical Battalion, was outstanding, largely as a result of the experience acquired in several previous campaigns and the wise training of its personnel. It was the only division clearing company in the XXIV Corps that had early X-ray facilities, and it possessed the only barber, hot shower, and laundry seen during the author's stay on Okinawa. With this company, Captain Minden continued his superior surgery and was a constant inspiration

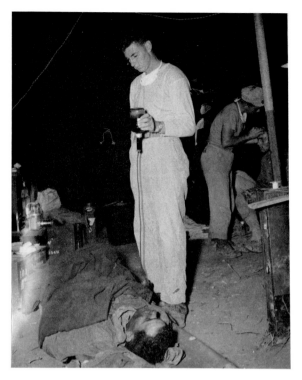

FIGURE 260.—Whole blood being administered to a
casualty at a clearing station of the 102d Medical
Battalion, Okinawa, 21 April 1945.

to all who witnessed his work. The field hospitals were slow in establishing
adequate shock facilities and postoperative care for the large numbers of seriously wounded which they received, largely because of inexperience. Shore-
to-ship evacuation was often long delayed because of darkness, air attacks on
the ships, or weather conditions. The mobile orthopedic teams rendered professional care of superior quality. Medical supply difficulties were markedly
reduced over previous operations. The medical control ship greatly simplified
the evacuation of casualties from the shore to the proper ship and the movement
of medical supplies from ships to the proper beach. The copper sulfate method
of hematocrit determination was used in all clearing companies. Whole blood
and oxygen were used in the 7th Infantry Division at the collecting station
level and proved to be of great value.

It was felt that informal meetings with the medical officers of all units and
on-the-spot correction of errors were particularly valuable functions for consultants during combat. Meetings within the divisions were normally held at
the clearing company and were attended by practically all officers of the division medical battalion and the regimental medical detachments. The consultant received many invaluable viewpoints and suggestions during these meetings

and will always be grateful for the opportunity he had to learn from these indispensable men. The chief difficulties encountered stemmed largely from the fact that there was an insufficient number of trained personnel on the target. In correcting this deficiency, the attachment to army hospitals of excellent specialized teams obtained from the Navy hospitals that did not operate as units was of the greatest value.

On 8 May, this consultant was released from temporary duty with the XXIV Corps and Tenth U.S. Army and reported aboard the U.S.S. *Relief*. After seeing cases and discussion with the surgical staff, he sent a memorandum to the Surgeon, Tenth U.S. Army, concerning the condition of patients as received and seen aboard ship. Surgical principles aboard ship did not vary appreciably from those followed in Army facilities on land, except that traction was rarely applied to amputation stumps. At Guam, all patients were unloaded and taken to the hospitals of their respective services.

The author then visited all fixed army hospitals on Saipan, Tinian, and Guam during the period 15–27 May, and each orthopedic case was seen and discussed. Because of a shortage of hospital beds and personnel, it appeared these hospitals could not long continue to hold patients with fractures of the long bones in traction until "frozen." The author made the trip from the Marianas Islands to Oahu by evacuation aircraft. Excellent patient selection and care was observed.

Experience in this campaign resulted in the following major recommendations:

1. Medical officers with high professional qualifications should be assigned as far forward as possible, normally at clearing company level.

2. Refresher training in fixed hospitals should be given on every possible occasion to officers assigned to mobile medical units.

3. In the training of mobile hospitals preceding combat, additional emphasis should be placed on living in the field under combat conditions, rapid establishment of facilities for the reception of large numbers of patients, the treatment of shock, postoperative care, rapid evacuation, and the provision of professional care on a 24-hour basis.

4. Company grade and selected field grade Medical Department officers should be rotated between fixed and mobile units, preferably after 12 months' service.

5. Air evacuation is particularly desirable for major fracture and amputation cases.

6. Halftracks serve well as ambulances in exposed areas because of their protection against near misses and small arms fire. The chief limitation is their capacity of only one litter case.

7. Female nurses should be brought to the target as soon as the danger of their being captured by the enemy has passed.

8. Theater consultants should continue to accompany each invasion force.

Following his return to Oahu on 28 May 1945, this consultant visited the various hospitals where he checked and found the care being given patients to be excellent. Great improvement in patient care was apparent in all echelons during the Okinawa operation. This improvement was the result of the increased number of trained personnel on the target, the availability of whole blood, improved methods in the management of wounds and shock, and the increased use of air evacuation. Because of the shortage of hospital beds in the theater, it was not possible to hold the numerous casualties with fractures of the long bones until the fragments were frozen in traction, as had been planned. These casualties had to be evacuated in casts by air to the mainland.

General Willis was very critical of this consultant's long absence in the combat zone. Even after he explained the situation on the target and pointed out that it was on the target, rather than in the rear areas, that mortality and morbidity were reduced, he remained in obvious disfavor until a letter of commendation arrived from Colonel Westervelt, Surgeon, Tenth U.S. Army. General Willis added a nice indorsement, brought it to the author in person, and then asked if he would like to go on the next operation. This consultant was restored to favor.

Preparations for invasion of Japan

Major activities now centered about medical plans for the invasion of Japan. The author met with all medical officers of the 98th Infantry Division; with the staffs of the 317th General Hospital, the 97th and 98th Station Hospitals, and many of the island's fixed hospitals. Using prepared talks and informal discussions, he stressed the space and other requirements for the treatment of shock and hemorrhage, the importance of making hematocrit determinations, the required standards of resuscitation prior to and following surgery, the necessity for adequate initial surgery and the splinting of fractures and soft-tissue wounds, the need for adequate postoperative care, and the value of air evacuation. Field conditions in combat were also emphasized before the mobile hospitals. Motion pictures of surgery during the Okinawa operation were shown and discussed at a meeting of the Air Transport Command surgeons at Hickam Field and before the staffs of several other tactical and fixed units. This consultant made several visits to the 8th Station Hospital, which operated the reconditioning center on Oahu (fig. 261).

On 1 July 1945, USAFPOA was redesignated USAFMIDPAC, and placed under General Headquarters, AFPAC, with General MacArthur in overall command. During July, Colonel Potter arrived from Okinawa en route to the mainland for temporary duty and leave. He concurred in Colonel Robertson's formal report on Operation ICEBERG and brought news of mutual friends, some of whom had been killed in action, and many of whom had been wounded.

On 25 July, this consultant observed a dry run by the recently arrived 86th Evacuation Hospital, which was attached to the 98th Infantry Division. An informal discussion was then held with the staff regarding combat zone surgery.

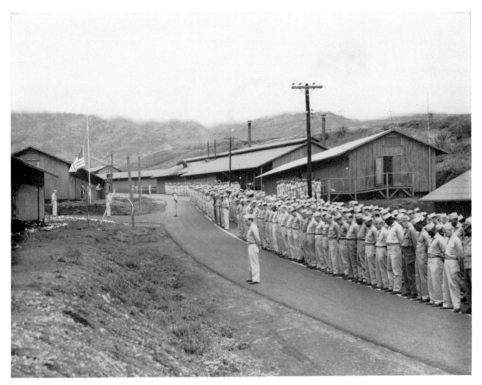

FIGURE 261.—The 8th Station Hospital, Hawaii. Formation, to mourn the death of the Commander in Chief, President Franklin D. Roosevelt.

Thereafter, the author had frequent informal discussions jointly with the Surgeon, 98th Division, and the Commanding Officer, 86th Evacuation Hospital, regarding their particular problems in the approaching operation. The orthopedic surgery detachments were busy on temporary duty at the 218th and 219th General Hospitals. A hospital center was being organized in the Marianas.

In addition to plans for the invasion of Japan and consultations in the various hospitals of the Central Pacific Base Command, this author was occupied with various other staff duties. There were reports to General Maxwell listing the orthopedic qualifications of the officers of the general and station hospitals assigned to him on Okinawa. He made personnel studies of the orthopedic surgeons, Central Pacific Base Command, which showed that there were present only 37 of the 50 authorized by tables of organization. He served as a member of a reclassification board on the military occupational specialty classification (professional and administrative) of all Central Pacific Base Command medical officers. In addition, he was a firing member of the Surgeon's Office pistol team, which finished 10th in the field of 15 entries from the general and special staff sections in the headquarters pistol tournament.

Victory and demobilization

The atomic bomb on Hiroshima caused much excitement. On 14 August came the big news that the war was over! During the next few weeks, this consultant received several letters from medical officers with long and outstanding combat experience stating that they were being retained in division medical units doing no professional work while newly arrived officers with only 9 months' internship were being assigned to hospitals. General Willis, while sympathetic, felt that men with combat experience should be retained in tactical units as there might yet be need for them in this capacity.

On 1 September, the author presented a paper entitled "Management of Orthopedic Battle Casualties in the Pacific" with slides showing the care of wounded from battalion aid stations to rear area general hospitals. This presentation was before the Hawaii Chapter, American College of Surgeons. The slides were made from motion pictures taken for the official medical history, most of which were taken by Capt. Ted Bloodhart, SnC, and were very complete.

Plans were rapidly developed to reduce medical installations and personnel. Colonel Ottenheimer was assigned to the office to edit the theater medical history. On 17 September, the 40-hour week became effective. Aside from working on the orthopedic section of the history, duties were very pleasant with much golf and swimming. Colonel Potter, en route back from the mainland, visited before returning to the XXIV Corps, destination Korea. Col. Elbert DeCoursey, MC, Consultant in Pathology, AFMIDPAC, and Col. Verne R. Mason, MC, Medical Consultant, AFMIDPAC, left for Japan to join Colonel Oughterson in the study of the medical effects of the atomic bombs. The author's orders for release from active duty appeared on 17 September. He completed the orthopedic portion of the medical history and turned it over to Colonel Ottenheimer.

On 24 September 1945, the author boarded the U.S.S. *Azalea City* destined for San Francisco. On 1 October, the returnees changed from khaki to olive drab uniform. All hands were on deck, silent and thankful as the coast neared. The underside of Golden Gate Bridge was lovely. Inside the harbor, a "Welcome Home" ship with flags flying and bands playing circled the U.S.S. *Azalea City* several times, an unexpected and joyous welcome. Never before had "The States" appeared so beautiful.

Summary

The Pacific Ocean Areas, commanded by Adm. Chester W. Nimitz, U.S.N., consisted of numerous widely separated small islands. The duties of USAFPOA, commanded by General Richardson, were those of a defense force operating a training and staging area and maintaining a base for, and conducting, amphibious operations. Cooperation among medical officers of tactical and fixed medical units, line officers, and medical officers of the Navy was excellent. As a consultant assigned to Headquarters, USAFPOA, the author received authority to move and act within the theater in keeping with his assigned duties.

The major problem throughout the war was the procurement of adequately trained personnel. The deficiency in trained personnel was met in part by training courses for selected individuals who subsequently served in tactical units and in the mobile and fixed hospitals. The shortage, particularly noticeable in the early invasions, was corrected in part by the assignment of qualified individuals and orthopedic teams to task forces. In attempting to correct the overall theater shortage, the Surgeon, USAFPOA, was most cooperative in approving recommended transfers and assignments for the more optimum distribution of available surgical talent.

Another difficulty arose from the fact that combat operations in the POA were joint operations involving both the Army and the Navy. The Surgeon General of the Army directed principles and methods of treatment which would result in high standards of professional care and uniformity of methods throughout the Army. In the Navy, principles and methods of treatment were established at the local level. The differences in professional management between the two services did not occasion friction at unit levels during combat or garrison duty, but the differences were quite apparent to the other service when large numbers of casualties were handled by one service. Such differences can only be corrected centrally, either in Washington or at the theater level by issue of similar directives to all services. Casualties were as a rule evacuated to fixed hospitals, operated by their respective services, rather than to the hospitals, regardless of the service, best suited for the management of their particular pathology. When separate hospitals are maintained in the same area by the several services, the formation of interservice hospital groups and the assignment of casualties, irrespective of service, to hospitals staffed for their various specialized needs should result in improved case management and in economy of medical personnel.

The third major difficulty was in establishing facilities during combat with sufficient trained personnel and beds to provide complete 24-hour care on the target. The need for 24-hour service was indicated in many instances because of the unavoidable delay in evacuating from shore to ship, and was most marked in the early phases of an invasion. During combat, the need for trained personnel was greatest on the target. When combat ceased, the need was greatest in the forward and rear area fixed hospitals. These varying needs were best met by the use of mobile specialized teams transported by air.

Medical officers who were assigned to tactical units lost much of their specialized professional skill during their long periods of inactivity, while officers assigned to rear area fixed hospitals often possessed skills which were in greatest demand in the combat zone. The first mentioned deficiency was met in part by the establishment of refresher courses in rear area hospitals to which officers assigned to tactical units were attached for varying periods of time prior to their entry into combat. The second deficiency was overcome by the limited transfer of personnel from fixed to mobile hospitals. The initial definitive surgery received by a severely wounded man was usually the most important single factor in determining his survival or eventual disability. This treatment should be given as soon as possible after wounding. For these reasons all physically able company grade medical officers and selected field grade officers should be rotated between tactical and fixed installations after a period of one year. Mobile hospital commanders should be carefully briefed on and envision situations which their units are likely to encounter in combat, and, during training, these units should prepare for such conditions. Areas particularly to be stressed were: Unit loading and care of supplies in the combat zone; rapid establishment of facilities for the treatment of large numbers of wounded; establishment of adequate shock, X-ray, surgical, and postoperative facilities; and rapid definitive treatment and evacuation. There was no substitute for combat experience. The best alternative was wise briefing by experienced officers with combat experience.

Pertinent technical and professional information should be disseminated to all units and individuals and carefully studied prior to combat. This goal was never fully attained, largely because invasions conducted in the Pacific Ocean Areas were combined operations, participating units often mounting from widely scattered areas of departure. This difficulty was in part corrected by the activities of consultants on the target.

Members of the Army Nurse Corps proved invaluable in mobile hospitals, from both a professional and a morale viewpoint. They should be brought to the target on call of the surgeon of the task force.

Air evacuation was extremely valuable because of the great distances covered by lines of evacuation in the Pacific Ocean Areas. Orthopedic cases were particularly suitable for evacuation by air. When personnel or hospital facilities are limited in an oversea theater, major fractures and amputees should be evacuated by air to the United States soon after initial definitive treatment.

Consultants, as special staff officers, must be free to move about and act both in advisory and professional capacities throughout the entire command.

ROBERT CRAWFORD ROBERTSON, M.D.

CHAPTER XII

Southwest Pacific Area[1]

Wm. Barclay Parsons, M.D., I. Ridgeway Trimble, M.D., and George O. Eaton, M.D.

JULY 1942 THROUGH AUGUST 1944

This portion dealing with the activities of Col. Wm. Barclay Parsons, MC (fig. 262), as the surgical consultant in USASOS (the U.S. Army Services of Supply), SWPA (the Southwest Pacific Area), covers a period preliminary to the engagement of large bodies of troops in combat; namely, from July 1942 through August 1944, when the writer returned to the Zone of Interior. At the beginning of this period, U.S. Army combat elements in Australia consisted of two National Guard divisions, a few assorted antiaircraft and warning batteries, engineer regiments, and a small number of Army Air Forces pursuit and bombing squadrons. At the end of the period, the air forces had grown markedly, the Sixth U.S. Army had been organized, and the Eighth U.S. Army was being activated. In the beginning, an invasion of Australia by the enemy was assumed to be a real possibility, which fortunately did not eventuate. Gradually, the Allies established a foothold in New Guinea, and when the Japanese attacks on Milne Bay and over the Owen-Stanley Mountains toward Port Moresby had been repulsed late in 1942, the ground and air forces began the long tough road that led eventually to the Philippines.

General Characteristics of Operations in Southwest Pacific Area

It seems pertinent to review some of this history because the conduct of combat conditions in the Southwest Pacific Area was strikingly different from that in other theaters. The bases in Australia were far apart, as were those in New Guinea (map 2). For a long time, the number of troops engaged was comparatively small, and tropical disease of different types was for a time an important military problem.

The first combat with the enemy was the Buna, New Guinea, operations, lasting from October 1942 to early January 1943. This was fought over almost unbelievably difficult terrain consisting of jungle swamps enjoying, if

---

[1] See Activities of Surgical Consultants, Vol. I, chapters XVII and XIX for information relating to the Sixth and Eighth U.S. Armies, both of which served in the Southwest Pacific Area during World War II. See also chapter XIII, From Auckland to Tokyo, of this volume for the activities of Col. Ashley W. Oughterson, MC, who served as a surgical consultant in the Southwest Pacific Area temporarily during the initial stages of the invasion of the Philippines and was later assigned as surgical consultant at Headquarters, U.S. Army Forces, Pacific.—J. B. C., Jr.

that is the word, an annual rainfall of about 12 feet, where, before Atabrine was available, malaria caused five casualties for each man wounded in action. For most of the Buna operations, only two regimental combat teams were engaged. Their components, at times, fought as companies and sometimes as squads. Transportation was at a premium. There were two grass airstrips on the north side of the Owen-Stanley Range that would accept a C–47 type of aircraft with difficulty. Flying was possible between Port Moresby and the north coast at Dobodura (fig. 263) only during the morning hours because of the daily blanketing of the mountains by clouds and the coastal area by rain each day

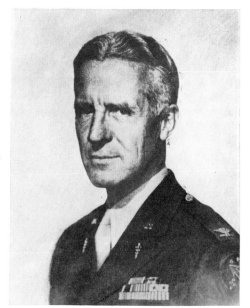

FIGURE 262.—Col. Wm. Barclay Parsons, MC.

by noon or earlier. There were few roads or tracks, and usually the wounded had to be brought back from the front on native-type litters, carried by four natives, after emergency treatment at a 25-bed portable surgical hospital (fig. 264). This litter carry frequently took as long as 8 hours through swamp and jungle to the nearest 50-bed station (fig. 265). The casualties had to be taken thence by air to either a 750-bed evacuation or a 100-bed station hospital at Port Moresby to await transportation to Townsville, Australia, by air or freighter. From Townsville, they were taken by air or exceedingly slow train on a narrow gage railroad to one of the general hospitals in Brisbane, Gatton, Sydney, or Melbourne. Fortunately, battle casualties were few because of the limited scope of combat activity, and the surgical caseload did not rise to really large proportions until the invasion of the Philippine Islands. As a matter of fact, considerable hospitalization facilities were planned and construction had

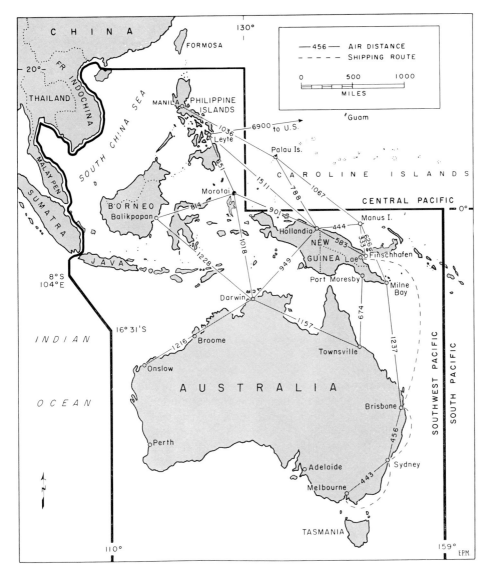

MAP 2.—The Southwest Pacific Area.

started in eastern New Guinea, but these were abandoned before completion because of the rapidity with which the strategic situation changed.

The experience at Milne Bay was an excellent example of preparation for a need that could have been of major proportions but never materialized. After the Buna area was secure, a base was established at the small harbor of Oro Bay (fig. 266) and a major base was begun at Milne Bay with its commodious deepwater harbor (fig. 267). Early in 1943, clearing of land, mosquito

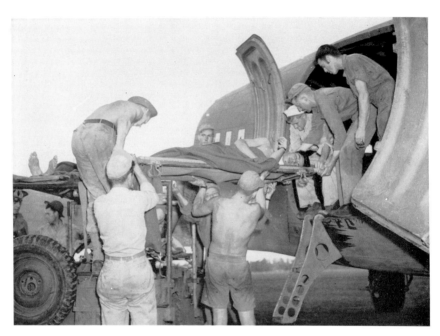

FIGURE 263.—Wounded, being transferred from litter jeep to C–47 aircraft at Dobodura, New Guinea, for evacuation to Port Moresby, March 1943.

control, and pier and airfield construction were started. Two general and some 200- and 500-bed station hospitals were included in the plans. Before either general hospital was completed, however, the war had moved 1,500 miles away. The Allies then held Finschhafen, where construction was going on apace, and Milne Bay was abandoned, as it did not lie in a convenient line of supply or evacuation. These facts are mentioned to indicate the general mise en scène composed as it was of great distances, a rapidly advancing combat area, and, fortunately, comparatively few battle casualties.

Interpersonal Relations

The Medical Department has often sensed an apparent reluctance on the part of line officers to encourage certain measures that the Medical Department strongly feels would contribute to the greater fighting efficiency of the troops. This seemed to hold true in the Southwest Pacific Area until a medical crisis arose that threatened the successful prosecution of the war. In December 1942 before the virtue of Atabrine had been established and the drug made available, the incidence of malaria in the small force stationed at Milne Bay was at the unbelievable rate of over 1,000 per 1,000 per annum. This occurrence, plus the fact that in the Buna operations there were over 8,000 casualties from malaria, made imperative some prompt action to institute medical measures against this new and threatening enemy. General Headquarters, SWPA, appointed a joint American and Australian medical commission to deal with this problem. Their mission was successfully accomplished. The important point from an administrative standpoint was the fact that the carrying out of proper Atabrine administration was made a command responsibility. It is certain that this circumstance improved beyond measure the relationship between the line and the Medical Department.

On the other hand, the relationship between the consultants (including the author) and the medical officers of the Regular Army was slower to improve. At the time of this writing, and presumably for the future, the role of the consultant is well established, well understood, and appreciated. For some time, it was clear that the Surgeon, USASOS, SWPA, had no inkling of the role of the consultant and in fact resented his presence, although, in fairness to him, it was doubtful that he had ever received proper briefing. For some weeks, there was reluctance on his part to allow this consultant to travel for the purpose of visiting various hospitals in a professional capacity. He insisted, instead, upon strict Army-type inspections. Gradually, by emphasis and persuasion, these inspection tours were officially changed to "instructional visits" and were so specified in travel orders. This change resulted in an abrupt change in the reception accorded the surgical consultant by area and base commanders and by the hospital commanders who, with few exceptions, were Regular Army officers during the first year. All these men had quite naturally resented another adjectival inspection but were glad to welcome someone whose sole, or at least major, interest was the care of patients.

As mentioned earlier, the situation in the Southwest Pacific Area during the first 2 years consisted of three elements: Great distances, limited combat activity, and a resultant relative excess of hospitals. The total number of hospitals was not great, but the available space was useful until malaria was controlled. Later, hospital facilities were in excess of the surgical load until the invasion of the Philippines. One of the problems that this fact produced for the surgical consultant was the maintenance of morale among many highly trained general and orthopedic surgeons in the various hospitals who complained, with considerable justice, that they had joined the Army to use their skills and experience for the benefit of the wounded soldier but were idle, or nearly so, month after month. Many of the hospitals were at great distances from headquarters and other installations were in what seemed to the personnel to be both God- and Headquarters-forsaken spots. The execrable climate, the lack of recreational outlets, inactivity, and a feeling of uselessness were major factors in the deterioration of morale. A visit of several days by the consultant as often as possible to one of these "neglected" areas seemed to be refreshing and stimulating to the local staff, even though no matters of much surgical importance might have been involved. A similar need for close liaison between the Office of The Surgeon General and the theaters of operations is discussed later.

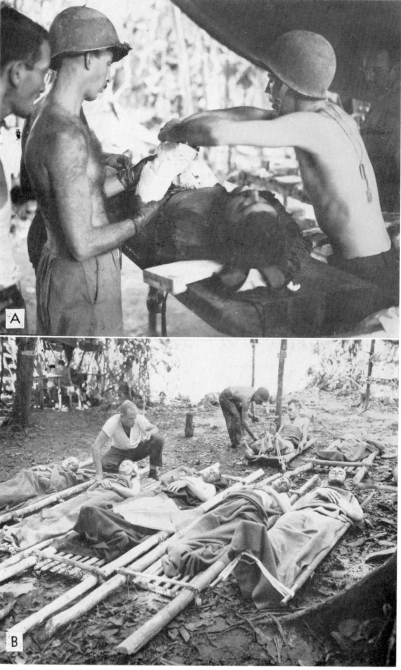

FIGURE 264.—Portable surgical hospitals on New Guinea. A. Maj. George A. Marks, MC, treating an American soldier at the 5th Portable Surgical Hospital in the Buna Mission area, December 1942. B. The 4th Portable Surgical Hospital, 800 yds. south of the Buna Mission, December 1942.

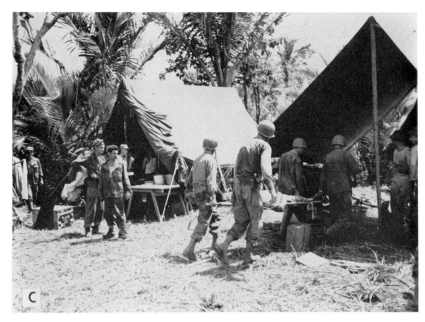

FIGURE 264.—Continued. C. The 12th Portable Surgical Hospital, about 4 miles below Sentani Airstrip, New Guinea, April 1944.

Hospital Units

To understand the local geography in reference to the distances involved, it may be helpful to superimpose mentally the map of Australia and New Guinea on one of North America. If one places Melbourne at New Orleans, one would find Sydney in North Carolina, Brisbane in Delaware, Townsville in Maine, Port Darwin near Winnipeg, and New Guinea over Nova Scotia. From below Sydney northwards the railroad network was narrow gage, often only single track, on which trains ran at a leisurely pace. From Brisbane to Charleville, where there was a small station hospital near a magnificent airfield constructed in anticipation of a Japanese invasion of Australia, the distance was about 400 miles. The train required 22 hours to travel this distance as it sped along at not quite 20 miles per hour. Later, as air transport became available, travel by rail became unnecessary and the transportation of patients became more rapid and more comfortable.

With this brief geographical review it may be useful to note the location of the hospitals before, as well as after, the development of large bases in New Guinea. During the first year, there were four affiliated general hospitals in Australia—the 4th from Western Reserve at Melbourne, the 118th from Johns Hopkins at Sydney, the 142d from the University of Maryland at Brisbane, and the 105th Harvard unit at Gatton, some 40 miles west of Brisbane (fig. 268).

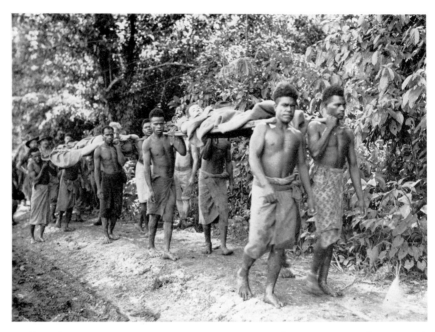

FIGURE 265.—Australian soldiers wounded in action near Sattelberg, New Guinea, arriving at a casualty clearing station after 24-hour litter carry by native bearers.

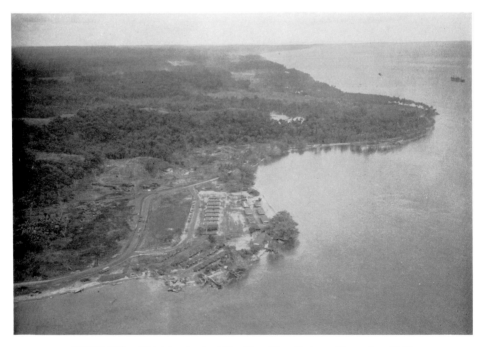

FIGURE 266.—The base area at Oro Bay, New Guinea, December 1943.

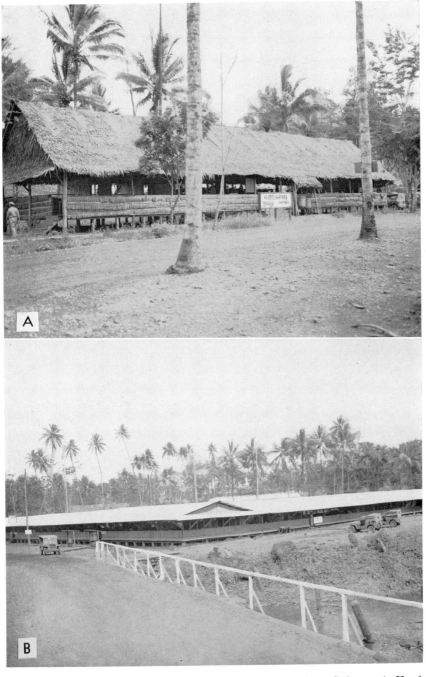

FIGURE 267.—The development of a major base at Milne Bay, New Guinea. A. Headquarters, Base A, 30 January 1944. B. Base A operations building, 5 October 1944.

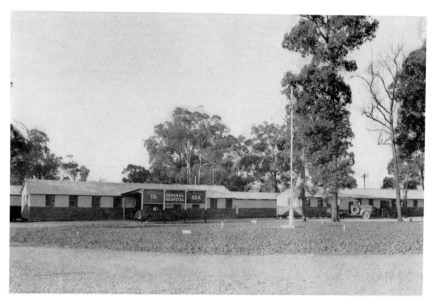

FIGURE 268.—The 118th General Hospital, Sydney, Australia, 8 July 1943.

Four other general hospitals, three affiliated, were assigned to the theater later on. The New York Hospital unit (the 9th General Hospital) arrived in mid-1943 and after a wait at Brisbane set up on Goodenough Island in the Trobriand Islands, near Milne Bay. In 1944, the University of Wisconsin's 44th General Hospital was assigned to a point near Townsville where it functioned in a mild way before moving onward, and the Presbyterian Hospital unit (13th General Hospital) was established at Finschhafen. One nonaffiliated general hospital and the 47th General Hospital from the College of Medical Evangelists were stationed temporarily at Milne Bay (fig. 269), but they arrived just as the Milne Bay base section began to close down, and later were moved forward.

The Southwest Pacific Area was fortunate in having two 750-bed evacuation hospitals. The 10th Evacuation Hospital was moved to Port Moresby before the Buna operations and proved an important holding place for casualties from the Buna area on their way to Australia (fig. 270). The 1st Evacuation Hospital functioned at Rockhampton in the Townsville area near a divisional training area before going to Oro Bay early in 1943.

Station hospitals were scattered about near cities such as Brisbane, Townsville, and Cairns, and near landing fields such as Cooktown, Charleville, and Port Darwin. In New Guinea, they were at Moresby, Dobodura, Milne Bay, Oro Bay, Lae, and Finschhafen. When New Britain was invaded and the attack up the coast was started, station hospitals were at Cape Gloucester and Arawe on New Britain. The first leapfrogging north of Finschhafen brought units to Saidor and then to Hollandia before the attack at Leyte (fig. 271).

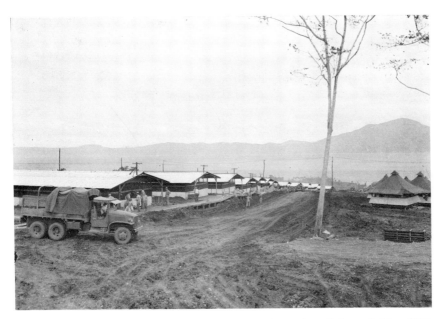

FIGURE 269.—The 47th General Hospital, Milne Bay, New Guinea, 9 May 1944.

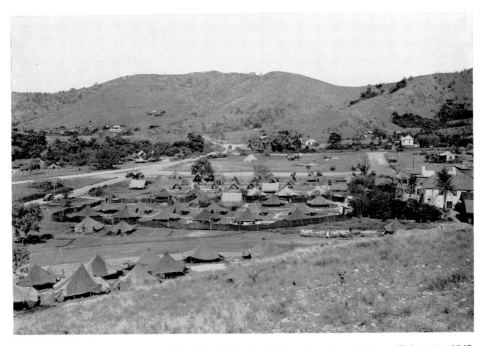

FIGURE 270.—The 10th Evacuation Hospital, Port Moresby, New Guinea, February 1943.

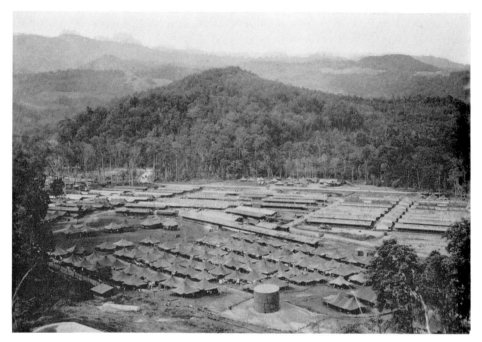

FIGURE 271.—The 27th General Hospital, Hollandia, New Guinea, 1944.

Expansion of Consultant Staff

Until the spring of 1943, although the distances were great, it was possible for the surgical consultant, with the aid of Maj. (later Lt. Col.) George O. Eaton, MC, the orthopedic consultant, to visit all hospitals in the theater frequently enough and with sufficient time at each place to become well acquainted with the personnel and to influence the care of wounded by personal consultation at rounds, by staff conferences, and, from time to time, by communication from the Office of the Surgeon, USASOS, SWPA. An enlarged staff of consultants was purposely not established in the early period for two reasons. In the first place, the clinical load and the number of hospitals was not too heavy for the surgical and orthopedic consultants to cover adequately because, after a few months, it was possible to move the injured by air whenever desirable to all areas under the control of USASOS, SWPA. In the second place, it was considered wise to keep in units those men who later on might be needed to head surgical or orthopedic services, or to act as assistant consultants. Late in 1943, the bases in New Guinea began to increase in size with the activation of the Sixth U.S. Army, great increases in air force strength, and the arrival of new hospital units. It then became necessary to appoint two assistant consultants. Lt. Col. (later Col.) I. Ridgeway Trimble, MC (fig. 272), and Maj. (later Lt.

Col.) George A. Marks, MC, were selected for these positions. They were placed on temporary duty from their affiliated units to different areas in New Guinea with 2 or 3 bases under each man. This arrangement furnished detailed consultative activity to the various rapidly growing base sections and also afforded the senior consultant opportunity to cover the entire area and, when necessary, to function within individual units.

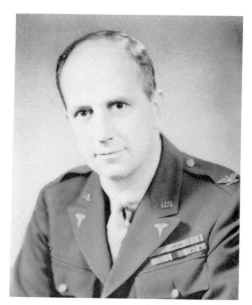

FIGURE 272.—Col. I. Ridgeway Trimble, MC.

Teaching Functions of a Surgical Consultant

The two major functions of a surgical consultant in a theater of operations were, first, to insure the employment of accepted surgical principles and proper surgical techniques in the care of the wounded, and, second, to place available personnel in key positions in the most advantageous manner. Two methods of instruction were used; namely, direct contact and written directives. The directives were distributed to all units to correct errors that had occurred, or in anticipation of their occurrence. In the early period, it was comparatively simple to travel throughout the area, even though each trip covered three or four thousand miles, to visit all hospitals and to discuss in staff meetings problems of surgical therapy as the particular point in the chain of evacuation occupied by each unit affected such treatment. After about 12 months, new units began to arrive so frequently from the Zone of Interior and at such widely spaced points that assistant consultants were needed to assay their professional quality and to brief them promptly. This briefing immediately on arrival was most constructive. It impressed on the personnel the fact that there was a consultant interested in them and their professional performance, and it was educational in that these newly arrived medical officers had but little knowledge of war surgery in general. In particular, they had no appreciation of the influence transportation bore upon the repair process in a wound. Until the time arrived when the wounded soldier could be held for a considerable period at a relatively advanced unit where definitive treatment could be given, the emphasis in instruction had to be placed on the simplest basic principles of wound treatment, such as treatment of shock, thorough debridement without undue removal of bone fragments, approximation of divided nerves, loose packing, and effective immobilization for transportation.

An example of how such instruction bore fruit follows. The surgical consultant met a small evacuation hospital at Milne Bay on its arrival from the Zone of Interior and just before it embarked for the attack on Manus in the Admiralty Islands. This unit was composed of fairly well trained surgeons but could not boast the presence of a single board diplomate on its staff, and none of them had ever heard a shot fired in anger. A directive had been published covering the basic principles to be followed in the care of wounds in a combat area such as that which faced this unit. At a personal conference with the staff, the surgical consultant had an excellent opportunity to discuss the subject in detail, to indicate what was required of the incoming surgeons, and to review the operations that should not be undertaken and the reasons for the policy. Perhaps as a result of this briefing, the casualties returned by that unit were handled in a superior manner. Shortly afterwards, the surgical consultant was invited by the Sixth U.S. Army to visit units of that army. This was the first time that any consultant from USASOS, SWPA, had been invited to the army area, and, shortly thereafter, Maj. (later Lt. Col.) Frank Glenn, MC, was appointed as the Sixth U.S. Army surgical consultant.

Utilization of Surgical Manpower

Portable surgical hospitals.—There were eventually several affiliated general hospitals in the Southwest Pacific Area. There has been considerable discussion as to the wisdom of forming such units, particularly in reference to the concentration of a large number of highly trained personnel in one unit. In the experience of the Southwest Pacific Area during this period, these units were of the greatest service. Not only was the care of the wounded in the affiliated units of superior caliber, but these units also furnished a pool of talent available for drafting into key positions. During the Buna fighting, where the movement and placement of even the smaller regularly constituted hospitals was impracticable, portable surgical hospitals were developed (fig. 273). They were formed from the personnel of the affiliated units. These small surgical hospitals did a magnificent job, and later others were formed for some of the larger station hospitals. Still later, when the consultant could influence the shifting of personnel, other individuals were drafted to fill certain key positions. A striking example of how effective such a drafting could be and how useful it was to have a pool available was indicated by the experience with a station hospital at Port Moresby which had a distinctly inferior rating. The hospital commander was replaced by a medical officer of the Harvard unit, and the chief of surgery, by a surgeon from the New York Hospital unit. These two individuals in positions of responsibility transformed this station hospital in a few months from perhaps the worst into one of the best in the theater.

Surgical teams.—Another important use of available personnel was accomplished after the arrival of Brig. Gen. (later Maj. Gen.) Guy B. Denit as Chief Surgeon, USASOS, SWPA. He brought with him a refreshing change of attitude, as any recommendations made to him by the consultant received immediate study, and those approved were put into effect. For example, as it was certain that no auxiliary surgical group was to be sent to the Southwest Pacific Area, this consultant had tried for a year to get approval of a plan to organize surgical teams in the larger hospitals for reinforcement of whatever small hospitals might be committed in the area of combat. General Denit's predecessors had refused to sanction this plan. They had been unable to comprehend its usefulness and had been afraid of losing control of the personnel. General Denit, however, at once foresaw the probability of the need for more manpower in the forward hospitals and knew that orders could be worded to prevent the stealing of personnel. One or more teams, each consisting of medical officers, nurses and enlisted men, were thereupon organized in all general, the two 750-bed evacuation, and certain larger station hospitals. These teams, with their own instruments, were to be on call for orders placing them on temporary duty wherever, and for as long as, the need for them existed, and until the parent organization might require their services. This arrangement had the virtue of flexibility in that many hospitals in the rear could readily spare one or more such teams for service in a forward unit during the early stages of an operation, while a later exchange could be effected as needed or desired. Exactly this same plan had been used most advantageously by the American and British Medical Departments in World War I and was being used successfully by the Australians in the Southwest Pacific Area.

Which units might be committed to the combat area could not be foreseen at this time. There was only one field hospital in the theater, but the Southwest Pacific Area had one medical regiment, the various components of which had acquired experience in a station hospital at Port Moresby (which hospital they had built themselves) and had also operated small station and portable hospitals in New Guinea and New Britain. It was expected that some of these units, as well as some smaller evacuation hospitals, might be the hosts, as it were, of these teams. The second section of this chapter contains a discussion by this consultant's successor of how they functioned.

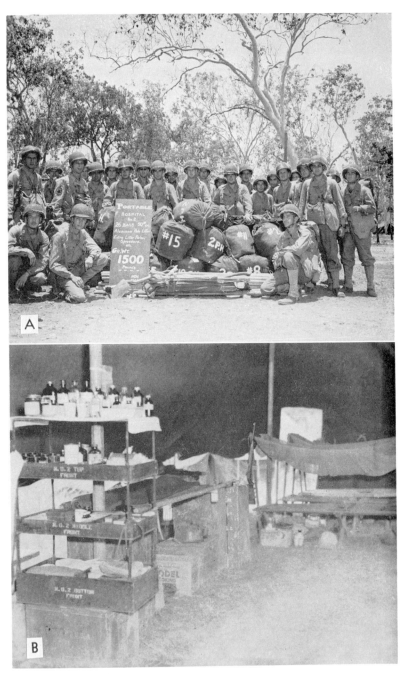

FIGURE 273.—Development of portable surgical hospitals. A. Test results with the 2d Portable Surgical Hospital proved the impracticability of equipment for hand carrying by individuals. The weight limit of impedimenta per individual was reduced from 60 to 40 pounds. B. The equipment setup for medical casualties.

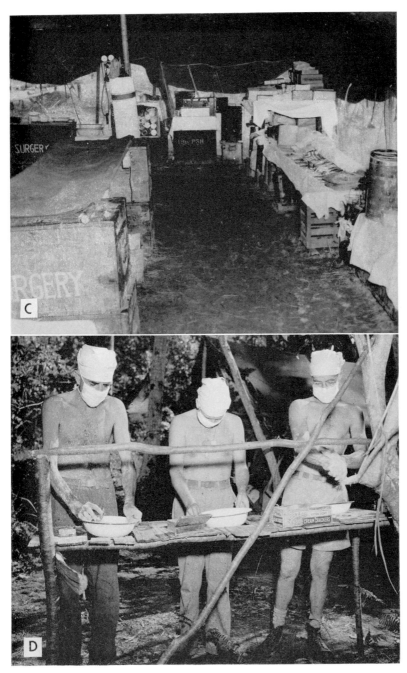

FIGURE 273.—Continued. C. The equipment setup for surgical casualties. D. The scrub setup of the 24th Portable Surgical Hospital at Morobe, New Guinea, 24 April 1943.

Equipment

In general, the equipment was satisfactory, but the smaller hospitals, particularly the portable surgical hospital, lacked an orthopedic table. The surgical consultant, therefore, designed and had constructed locally two types of aluminum tables. One was similar to the original Hawley table; the other was a light, collapsible model, packed in a box approximately 5 feet long by 18 inches in cross section.

Plasma and Whole Blood

Dry plasma was always in good supply, but early in 1943 whole blood became available from the first-class blood bank established in Sydney by the Royal Australian Army Medical Corps and the Australian Red Cross. The blood supplied was pooled O type, processed in accordance with the highest standards, packed in ice in a double-walled sheet metal box, and shipped by air. Because the casualties were limited in the early period, the supply of blood was adequate. The thermos bottle effect of the double-walled box served to keep the ice frozen until arrival at New Guinea, and the time taken in transit was reasonable until the combat area had moved far away. Before the attack on Hollandia (where casualties were minimal) an arrangement with the Seventh Fleet made blood available from the bank established on a converted LST (landing ship, tank). Well before the attack on the Philippines, plans had been made for the air shipment of blood from the Zone of Interior.[2]

Liaison With the Office of The Surgeon General

There was a distinct feeling at the time, which is confirmed in retrospect, that the liaison between the consultant in a theater and the Chief Consultant in Surgery to The Surgeon General could and should have been closer. This liaison could have been by frequent letters and by less frequent personal visits by the Chief Consultant in Surgery himself or by one of his assistants. There was, unfortunately, an impenetrable barrier between the various theaters through which information should have passed freely—information of a professional rather than a military nature—as to the problems faced and the measures devised to deal with them. It is certain that the experience gained in any one of the theaters would have been of benefit elsewhere. This communication, of course, should have been in both directions, and, if authorized by The Surgeon General, it could not have been objected to by the theater surgeon. At least one visit of reasonable length per year by the Chief Consultant in Surgery or his representative would have been most welcome, and, it is believed, constructive. Such visits would have given the opportunity to exchange much information not suitable for transmission by correspondence.

The Chief Consultant in Medicine to The Surgeon General did make one lengthy visit, passing several days at various hospitals and including several areas in New Guinea. This visit was valued most highly by the medical

---

[2] Medical Department, United States Army. Blood Program in World War II. [In press.]

services of these hospitals, and it is believed that the experience was educational for the Chief Consultant in Medicine. Unfortunately, the Chief Consultant in Surgery was able to pay only one fleeting visit, so that he never became thoroughly aware of the local situation in general or particular, and there was no opportunity for quiet, leisurely discussion by which many lesser and certain major matters could have been clarified.

Military Rank of Consultants

One cannot be sure as to the importance of military rank for consultants, but it seemed reasonably certain that a more flexible table of organization for the staff of a theater surgeon would have been advantageous, that the surgeon in the theater should have had the rank of major general, and his chief consultants, the rank of brigadier general. In this respect, it was interesting to observe the ranks held by the senior medical officers in the Australian Army. Their surgeon general was a major general, even though there were but nine Australian divisions, and three of his consultants held the rank of brigadier. Also of interest was the fact that in the Australian Army there was no line drawn between the medical service and the combat forces such as that which existed in the U.S. Army between the SOS and field armies. This homogeneous arrangement led to smooth coordination, and one could not help but wonder as to a possible loss of effectiveness in the American organization under the existing system. Also, it was believed that the higher rank held by the Australian consultants was a large factor in their greater freedom and power.

Summary

In summary, one cannot be certain as to many of the problems that may appear in a future conflict, should one arise. Many unforeseeable conditions will of course have to be faced, although the peculiarities of the different areas of almost the entire globe as they may affect combat troops are now well-known and can therefore be taken into consideration in the plans for such a conflict. There are three points that the writer would, however, like to emphasize. First, a flexible table of organization for the professional services in the headquarters of any theater, liberal both as to numbers and as to ranks, would insure worthwhile freedom and prestige to the theater surgeon and his consultants. Second, it seems desirable to urge freer communication between the Office of The Surgeon General and the theater consultants and to emphasize the importance of personal contact at least once a year between the chief surgical consultant in the Office of The Surgeon General, or one of his associates, and the surgical consultant in a theater of operations. Finally, and of most importance, the consultant system at the end of World War II was well established and must not be allowed to lapse, as it was allowed to lapse between World Wars I and II. If the consultant system is continued with strength and enthusiasm, there will be in any future conflict immediate effectiveness of professional influence, hand in hand with the purely military development of the Medical Department.

WM. BARCLAY PARSONS, M.D.

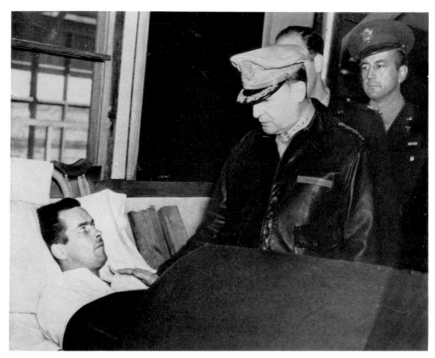

FIGURE 274.—Lt. Col. I. Ridgeway Trimble, MC, accompanies Gen. Douglas MacArthur
on a visit to a hospital in Australia.

AUGUST 1944 THROUGH JANUARY 1946

In August 1944, Lt. Col. (later Col.) I. Ridgeway Trimble, MC, succeeded
Col. Wm. Barclay Parsons, MC, as Consultant in Surgery, Office of the Chief
Surgeon, USASOS, SWPA (fig. 274). This consultant continued to serve as
surgical consultant to the Surgeon, AFWESPAC (the U.S. Army Forces,
Western Pacific) after USASOS, SWPA, was absorbed into this organization
in June 1945. In October 1945, he assumed the same position at General
Headquarters, AFPAC (Army Forces Pacific), continuing in it until 27 January 1946, when he and the Consultant in Neuropsychiatry left Japan, the
last of the wartime consultants to return to the Zone of Interior.

The Consultant System

In December 1943, when it had become apparent that a single surgical
consultant could not cover the widely dispersed medical activities in the Southwest Pacific (map 2, p. 689), the author had been placed on temporary duty in
the area surgeon's office, as assistant surgical consultant to Colonel Parsons.
In this capacity, he visited the hospitals at Port Moresby and Milne Bay
(Bases D and A) in New Guinea (maps 3 and 4).[3]

---

[3] Colonel Trimble's experiences before his assumption of his duties as assistant consultant and,
later, as Consultant in Surgery to the Surgeon, USASOS, SWPA, may be cited as typical of the
experiences of many medical officers. Since 1940, he had held a commission as lieutenant colonel,

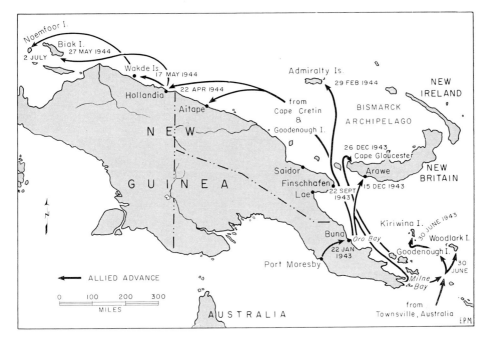

MAP 3.—The Allied advance from Townsville, Australia.

Medical Corps Reserve, in the 18th General Hospital, the affiliated unit of the Johns Hopkins Medical School where Colonel Trimble was assistant professor of surgery. When the 18th General Hospital was divided into two units in April 1942, he became chief of the surgical service in the second unit, the 118th General Hospital. This hospital left Baltimore on 20 April 1942 and, after 10 days at Camp Edwards, Mass., was sent to the Port of Embarkation, San Francisco.

Up to that time, the Hopkins unit had been merely a paper organization, with no military training other than occasional meetings and lectures. It had had no active duty and no sustained, practical, realistic military indoctrination. When it left Baltimore, it had no enlisted cadre, and its personnel consisted of only medical officers and nurses. When the unit sailed from San Francisco, it had its full complement of personnel, but they were without training, and training could not be provided en route. The crowded conditions on shipboard (three other affiliated general hospitals, a dozen station hospitals, and all their equipment were also among the organizations transported on the U.S. Army Transport *West Point*), and the necessity for almost continuous messing and for frequent boat drills, as well as the prohibition against lights, made any instructional work of a major nature during the voyage entirely impossible.

The 118th General Hospital landed in Melbourne, Australia, on 4 June 1942. Ten days later it was moved to Sydney, where it was set up at the Royal Prince Alfred Hospital, one of the teaching hospitals of the University of Sydney. For about a year, this unit was the only U.S. Army hospital in New South Wales to care for Army, Navy, and Air Force patients. The work was chiefly of the station hospital type, though some combat-wounded casualties were received, among them a few Filipinos who had been brought out of the Philippines on the S.S. *Mactan*, the only hospital ship to leave the islands before their surrender. These patients had been cared for in Australian Army hospitals before the 118th General Hospital began to function.

The next battle casualties received came from Buna-Gona on New Guinea. When a permanent installation for the 118th General Hospital was set up, as part of a hospital center constructed at Herne Bay, Australia, 25 miles south of Sydney, with Lend Lease funds, the surgery was derived chiefly from troops staging in the Sydney Base Area and was still chiefly of the station hospital type. The only battle casualties received were brought in by Australian hospital ships and were chiefly patients who required late orthopedic care.

Colonel Trimble's first real contact with battle casualties was therefore in December 1943, when he went on temporary duty for 4 months as assistant surgical consultant in the Office of the Surgeon, USASOS, SWPA. His experience duplicated that of many other medical officers who, when the need arose, were able to transfer their fine training and broad experience in civilian surgery to the military situations they encountered.—J. B. C., Jr.

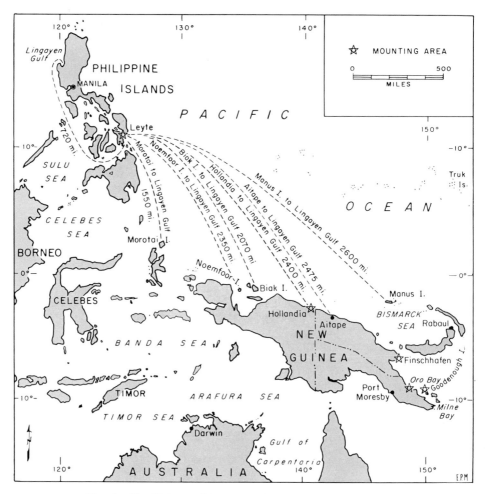

MAP 4.—The distances from mounting areas to Lingayen Gulf.

Although the original plans for the consultant system worked satisfactorily enough with this expedient and others, it would have been better if the table of organization for Headquarters, USASOS, SWPA, had been so set up that the consultant section could have been enlarged as needs increased. Originally, there had apparently been no real appreciation of the services which could be rendered by consultants. The situation changed when General Denit became Chief Surgeon in January 1944 and as his position and authority were widened in the successive reorganizations which occurred in the Pacific in 1945 (fig. 275). General Denit, who had served in the North African theater before his appointment to the Pacific, was thoroughly cognizant of the accomplishments of the consultant system in that theater and of the improvement in the care of battle casualties that had been effected through the system.

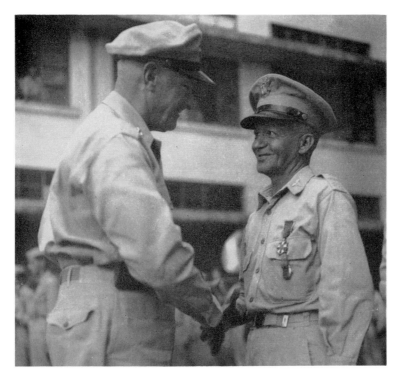

FIGURE 275.—Maj. Gen. Guy B. Denit receiving the Legion of Merit from Maj. Gen. James L. Frink, Commanding General, USASOS, Manila, Philippine Islands, 1 May 1945.

However, it was not until after the organization of AFPAC, in June 1945, that a satisfactory table of organization for consultants in surgery was set up in the Pacific (chart 6). Even this plan, though in a sense it went from poverty to riches, was still a compromise because it provided for no consultants in the various specialties at the top level of AFPAC. The compromise could not be avoided. General Headquarters insisted upon such a small staff at this level that there were spaces for only three consultants, one in medicine, one in surgery, and one for special research projects. Initially, upon organization of General Headquarters, AFPAC, the late Col. Ashley W. Oughterson, MC, was assigned to fill the positions for both the consultant in surgery and special research projects. It was planned, therefore, to resort again to the expedient of temporary duty and to bring various surgical specialists assigned to AFWESPAC from that headquarters to General Headquarters, AFPAC, as they were needed for special periods.

Before it became necessary to put this plan into effect, the Japanese surrendered—on 14 August 1945 (fig. 276). A surgical and an orthopedic surgical consultant remained on duty at Headquarters, AFWESPAC. Colonel Oughterson had a particular knowledge of, and interest in, wound ballistics. Almost as soon as he arrived at General Headquarters, AFPAC, the first atomic bomb

CHART 6.—*The table of organization for consultants in surgery, U.S. Army Forces, Pacific*

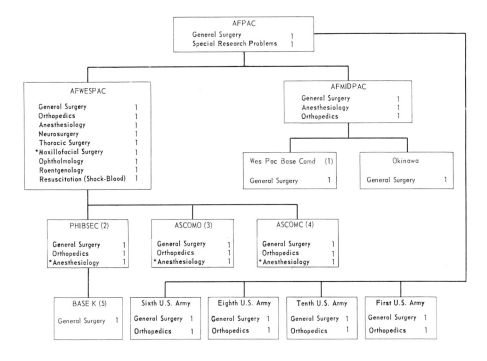

*May be assigned to hospital.

1. Western Pacific Base Command, Saipan. 2. Philippine Base Section, Manila. 3. Army Service Command O, logistical support command for the Sixth U.S. Army. 4. Army Service Command C, Logistical support command for the Eighth U.S. Army. 5. Base K, Tacloban, Leyte, Philippine Islands.

was dropped, and he immediately assumed the responsibility for special studies of the casualties at Hiroshima and Nagasaki.

A consultant in anesthesia was never appointed in the Southwest Pacific Area. Maj. (later Lt. Col.) Forrest E. Leffingwell, MC, was appointed in May 1945 to survey anesthesia practices in hospitals in the Philippine Islands and to act as part-time consultant at Headquarters, AFWESPAC. While he performed these duties, until November 1945, Major Leffingwell also continued his duties in anesthesia in the 80th General Hospital in Manila.

Functions of the Consultant

When the author was appointed Assistant Consultant in Surgery, Office of the Chief Surgeon, USASOS, SWPA, his duties were to visit the hospitals in the bases in New Guinea (fig. 277), evaluate the surgical personnel in them, evaluate the professional care that casualties were receiving, and make recommendations to the Chief Surgeon based on these observations.

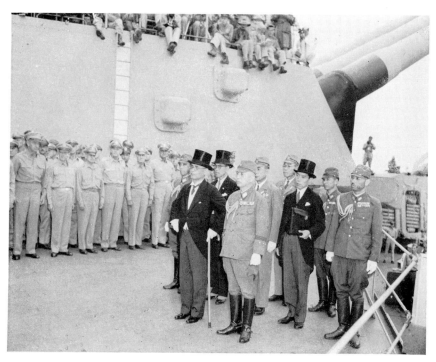

FIGURE 276.—Japanese emissaries arriving aboard U.S.S. *Missouri* in Tokyo Bay to sign surrender terms, 31 August 1945.

When he assumed his duties as Consultant in Surgery, Office of the Chief Surgeon, USASOS, SWPA, in August 1944, in succession to Colonel Parsons, his functions were considerably broadened. The chief function of the surgical consultant in this office was to advise the Chief Surgeon on ways and means of giving the most expert professional care to wounded soldiers. The most efficient way of accomplishing this result was the correct evaluation and placement of surgical personnel (pp. 714–719).

Other duties of the Consultant in Surgery included maintenance of close liaison with all offices of the Medical Section, Headquarters, USASOS, SWPA, especially those responsible for medical planning, evacuation, hospitalization, supply, and personnel; instruction of newly arrived personnel in the principles of the surgical care of battle casualties; correction of surgical errors by indoctrination and demonstration; dissemination of information secured from other theaters and the Zone of Interior; compilation of data for ETMD (Essential Technical Medical Data) reports; planning for medical support of future operations; and constantly striving to formulate plans to prevent the occurrence of casualties and to improve the care of the wounded. Because of the vast distances and the difficulties of communication in the Southwest Pacific (map 2, p. 689), the Consultant in Surgery, when he left the Office of the Surgeon, SWPA, had to be prepared to function independently for long periods of time.

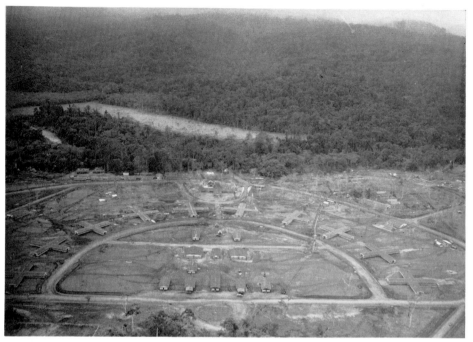

FIGURE 277.—The 10th Evacuation Hospital, Oro Bay, New Guinea, December 1943.

Because of his interest in the condition of the battle casualties whom he had observed at Hollandia after they had been evacuated from Leyte early in that campaign, this consultant received permission from Headquarters, USA-SOS, SWPA, to go to Leyte on the hospital ship *Comfort*, to make first-hand observations there. The ship arrived on 14 November, "Bloody Sunday," the day of the first Japanese suicide (kamikaze) raids, and he operated all night with the Navy surgeons on the LST 464, assisting in the care of the casualties.

After a 10-day stay on Leyte, this consultant flew back to Headquarters, USASOS, SWPA, in Hollandia, to organize the surgical teams which had been offered to Brig. Gen. William A. Hagins, Surgeon, Sixth U.S. Army, and had been accepted by him for the remainder of the operation on Leyte and for the invasion of Luzon (p. 726).

After he had landed on Leyte, the author learned that army hospitals coming ashore were having considerable difficulty in setting up because, almost as fast as they selected appropriate sites, these sites were taken over by line or other troops (fig. 278). He was able to have this situation altered by the sort of fortunate personal contact that accomplished so much in this and other theaters of operations. Instructions were promptly issued from General Mac-Arthur's headquarters, which were then at Tacloban, Leyte, that medical units were to have first priority on sites that they selected. To follow this up, this consultant wrote to General Denit, and had the letter hand-carried to him, suggesting that it would be well to send medical officers of high enough rank to Leyte at once, to prevent a repetition of this particular difficulty.

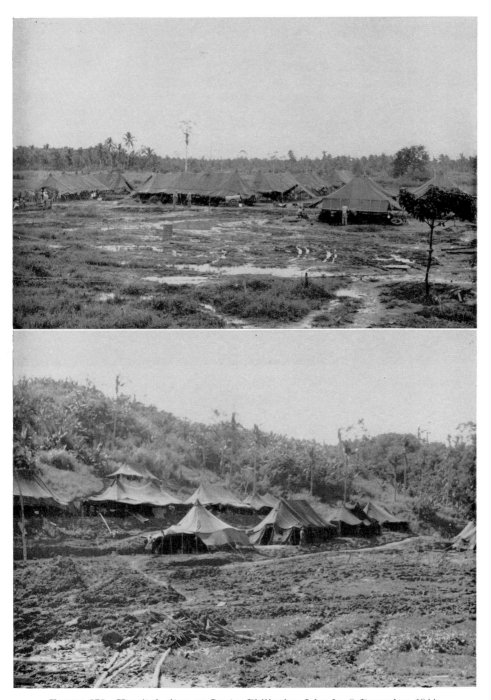

FIGURE 278—Hospital sites on Leyte, Philippine Islands, 8 December 1944.

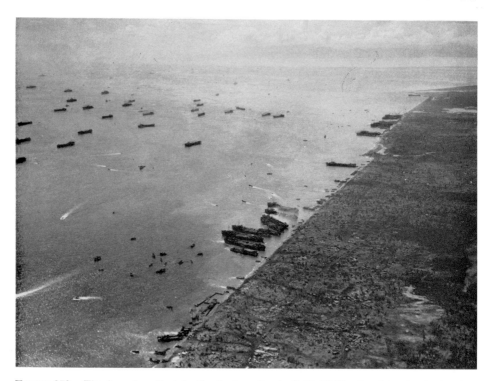

FIGURE 279.—The invasion fleet in the harbor, Leyte Gulf, Philippine Islands, 22 October 1944.

The author also, indirectly, achieved another change that was not a real medical responsibility by pointing out to Col. Roger O. Egeberg, MC, aide to Gen. Douglas MacArthur, an unnecessary tragedy which had occurred in the harbor at Leyte (fig. 279). A troopship, loaded with Air Force personnel, had lain at anchor for 13 days and then had incurred very heavy casualties from a Japanese suicide raid. The troops had not been landed before the raid because of lack of protection ashore from the heavy tropical rains. An order was at once issued from General MacArthur's headquarters that thereafter troops were to be landed as soon as their ships reached Leyte Gulf, whether or not they had to stay out in the rain when they went ashore.

Evaluation and Assignment of Personnel

Evaluation of personnel

The second surgical consultant in the Southwest Pacific Area, like the first, had no more important duty than the evaluation and assignment of surgical personnel. His task was more difficult, however, for, after the first hospitals with outstanding surgical talent reached the theater in 1942, there were no further increments of such caliber, and few, if any, replacements on any superior level of ability. Except for consultants, no other fully trained ("A–

3150" or "B–3150") surgeons arrived in the Southwest Pacific Area during the 3 years of active fighting there. Since no trained surgeons were made available as casual replacements to the end of the war, it was necessary to reinforce weaker units by taking more experienced personnel from other more richly supplied units.

Shortages of trained personnel could be partly explained by a certain amount of wastage in newly arrived units. It was not possible to remedy this situation throughout the war. Better planning for equipment, transportation, and other details would have shortened staging periods and permitted surgical personnel to be put to work at once. This would have improved the morale of the medical officers, who, quite naturally, resented long periods of enforced inaction.

The chief reason for shortages of personnel, however, was that in World War II, as in previous wars, too little attention was paid to the essential qualifications of medical personnel. Tables of organization were adequate, but the ability of the officers assigned to the various spaces was often not correctly evaluated. As a rule, the assignment was on the basis of rank, without sufficient consideration of the adequacy of professional abilities.

Emphasis on rank was not, of course, a fault confined to the Medical Department of the Army. When surgical help was offered to the Navy for the LST's which were to participate in the invasion of Leyte, it was refused as not needed, on the ground that the ships were adequately staffed, some of them by officers with the rank of lieutenant commander. It is true that all LST's had medical officers on them, but many of these officers were not surgeons, let alone experienced surgeons, and the casualties had to get along with such care as these officers could provide them during the week's trip from Leyte to Hollandia. The classification of medical officers into specialty groups came too late in the war to be helpful in the Southwest Pacific, and experienced personnel were in short supply until the fighting ended.

This consultant, like his predecessor, followed the plan of studying all newly arrived hospitals in regard to qualifications of personnel and recommending such changes in assignment as seemed necessary. As may be expected, the best surgeons were not always those with the best training on paper.

Selection of personnel for portable surgical hospitals (fig. 280) was a major responsibility of the surgical consultant, a responsibility which increased in difficulty as the supply of experienced surgeons dwindled.

As of the middle of July 1945, a month before the surrender of Japan, the 141 hospitals in AFWESPAC (including the Sixth and Eighth U.S. Armies), with 67,000 beds, needed 314 surgical officers to bring them up to authorized table of organization strength (table 3). The 32 surgeons then in the theater with a rating of "B–3150," or higher (table 4), included the surgical consultants in the Office of the Surgeon, AFPAC, and the commanding officers of several hospitals. There were only 14 orthopedic surgeons, 3 plastic surgeons, and 2 neurosurgeons with the rating of "B" or higher. The single surgeon in the

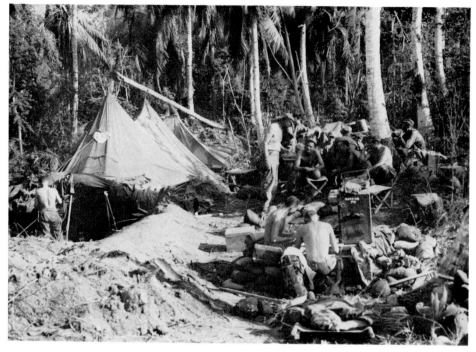

FIGURE 280.—The 8th Portable Surgical Hospital at Yellow Beach, Zamboanga, Philippine Islands, on J+1 days, 11 March 1945.

area with any training in thoracic surgery had a rating of only "D–3150." Because of these shortages, work beyond their abilities often had to be done by medical officers without specialty ratings.

Transfer and assignment of personnel

It was the policy of the Chief Surgeon that all changes of assignment of surgical personnel within the Southwest Pacific Area should be either initiated by the Consultant in Surgery in his office or referred to the consultant for his approval. These instructions were usually carried out, though often after considerable and usually unavoidable delays. When they were violated, they almost always involved company grade officers, and the consequences of their disregard were seldom serious.

The Chief Surgeon's policy was entirely logical, since one of the functions of a surgical consultant was to evaluate the individual abilities of surgical officers, and changes in assignments should not have been made without his knowledge and consent. After his visits to various hospitals, this consultant always reported to the Chief Surgeon his evaluation of each unit as a whole, his recommendations for strengthening it if it was weak, or, if there was an excess of surgical talent in it, for funneling some of it off to strengthen less efficient and less well staffed units.

TABLE 3.—*Shortages of surgical officers in AFWESPAC (including Sixth and Eighth U.S. Armies), 17 July 1945*

Type of hospital	Number of hospitals	Number of beds	Number of surgical officers short of authorized strength
General	29	37, 500	103
Station	36	11, 950	62
Evacuation	14	6, 650	65
Convalescent	1	3, 000	4
Field	17	6, 800	42
Portable surgical	44	1, 100	38
Total	141	67, 000	314

Type of hospital	Number of surgical officers needed by specification serial number [1]											
	3150	3153	3106	3125	3126	3111	3131	3152	3151	3306	3115	Total
General	2	12	16	9	10	7	21	4	4	15	3	103
Station	6	10	22	1	____	9	____	____	____	5	9	62
Evacuation	2	6	6	____	____	6	8	12	13	____	[2] 12	65
Convalescent	2	____	2	____	____	____	____	____	____	____	____	4
Field	11	____	9	____	____	____	____	____	____	8	14	42
Portable surgical	31	____	____	____	____	____	____	____	____	____	7	38
Total	54	28	55	10	10	22	29	16	17	28	[2] 45	314

[1] 3150—general surgeon; 3152—orthopedic surgeon; 3106—ophthalmologist and otorhinolaryngologist; 3125—ophthalmologist; 3126—otorhinolaryngologist; 3111—urologist; 3131—neurosurgeon; 3152—plastic surgeon; 3151—thoracic surgeon; 3306—radiologist; 3115—anesthesiologist.

[2] Corrected figure. The original document showed 14 in this block, which would have made the obviously erroneous shortage of anesthesiologists 47, the shortage of surgical officers in evacuation hospitals 67, and the grand total of shortages 316.

TABLE 4.—*Medical Corps surgical officers in AFWESPAC (including Sixth and Eighth U.S. Armies), as of 15 July 1945, by specialty and rating (qualification)*

Officer's rating	Number of officers by specification serial number [1]										
	3150	3153	3106	3125	3126	3111	3131	3152	3151	3115	Total
B	32	14	8	11	6	10	2	3	0	4	90
C	180	31	15	15	26	23	10	1	0	13	314
D	105	33	9	2	6	8	3	2	1	27	196
None	70	0	2	1	1	3	2	0	0	6	85
Total	387	78	34	29	39	44	17	6	1	50	685

[1] 3150—general surgeon; 3153—orthopedic surgeon; 3106—ophthalmologist and otorhinolaryngologist; 3125—ophthalmologist; 3126—otorhinolaryngologist; 3111—urologist; 3131—neurosurgeon; 3152—plastic surgeon; 3151—thoracic surgeon; 3115—anesthesiologist.

Recommendations for the transfer of surgical personnel sometimes were based on incompetence but more often were based on the lack of experience of the particular officer in a position in which surgical experience was not only desirable but essential. No matter how urgent the transfer might seem, however, its accomplishment was always tedious and was sometimes unsuccessful. The chief causes of delay were distances between units and headquarters and delays at headquarters. Even though written communications were dispatched by airmail, this method in wartime was often slower than ordinary mail in peacetime. For instance, when the author was acting as assistant surgical consultant in the winter of 1943–44, he might recommend, from a base hundreds of miles from headquarters, that a certain officer be transferred. The recommendation would be made to the Chief Surgeon through Colonel Parsons, Consultant in Surgery in the Chief Surgeon's Office; communication took weeks, and, if Colonel Parsons was out of his office, more weeks might elapse before the recommendation could be made and acted upon.

There were also other delays. Before an officer could be transferred, it was the policy to secure concurrence of (1) the base section commander, which in practice meant his surgeon, and (2) the commander of the hospital to which the medical officer to be moved was assigned. The consultant had no authority to order the transfer of personnel. He could only make recommendations, and the hospital commander could think of many justifiable reasons why a transfer should not be made, particularly when it was proposed that a good officer be moved out of the unit.

This excess of military courtesy, which was a wartime development, really amounted to obstruction. Before the war, The Surgeon General exercised a centralized control over all Medical Department personnel and dictated their assignments. The concurrence of post commanders was not necessarily secured in advance. During the war, army commanders had this authority within their armies, and, if the changes recommended were not accepted, there was usually a sound reason, chiefly the shortage of replacements.

Proposal for temporary duty of medical personnel

At the end of December 1944, this consultant proposed to the Chief Surgeon, USASOS, SWPA, a plan to augment the strength of the medical units in the Sixth U.S. Army on Leyte, in which casualties were then being received in such numbers as to require augmentation of the table of organization strength. The plan was that hospitals that found themselves in this situation should apply for additional personnel by requisition, specifying the military occupational skill desired, and that these requisitions would be filled by personnel, on a temporary duty status, from hospitals in the rear that were less active or were building or staging. Hospitals under control of USASOS, SWPA, would make their requisitions to the Chief Surgeon through the base, intermediate section, or base section surgeons. Hospitals under the control of field armies would effect the temporary exchange of personnel within the army command at the discretion and direction of the army surgeon. When the emergency had passed, personnel on temporary duty would be returned promptly to the parent organization.

The plan was approved informally by the Surgeon, Sixth U.S. Army, but was disapproved by the Chief Surgeon, USASOS, SWPA, who feared that officers on temporary duty would be retained too long in an army area when they might be needed in their own units or might be permanently lost to their own units and thus pass out of USASOS, SWPA, control.

When this plan was proposed, it was estimated that 40 percent of the hospitals in the area would be inactive for one or another of the reasons mentioned. This estimate was much too high, but the proportion was still considerable, because of the character of military operations in this area. Had the plan been approved, it would probably have added six or eight trained general surgeons and the same number of trained orthopedic surgeons to the hospitals in the Sixth U.S. Army area. The number would have been no larger because so many surgeons had already been withdrawn from general and station hospitals to serve on surgical teams, and, for this and other reasons, these hospitals had already been stripped to the bare bone in professional personnel. Even this small number of competent surgeons could, however, have been assisted by less experienced surgeons, and the plan would have helped to overcome the acute shortages of trained personnel that frequently existed in army areas.

Training Policies and Problems

Long before World War II, the whole subject of the proper treatment of battle-incurred wounds had been well discussed in the official history of the U.S. Army Medical Department in World War I. Not many World War II surgeons were familiar with these volumes (although General Denit carried the surgical volumes ashore with him when he landed in North Africa). The information contained in these volumes, with the proper modifications for the advances in the management of shock, anesthesia, antimicrobial therapy, and similar subjects, could well have formed the basis of the directives concerning medical care promulgated in World War II. Few surgeons in the Southwest Pacific Area knew that this history existed.

Practical training

Didactic instruction was of great value in the indoctrination of newly arrived units, but actual experience was necessary to convince most surgeons of the fundamental differences between civilian and military practice. The misunderstandings were universal. It was remarkable to note the sameness of the errors committed by surgeons inexperienced in military medicine, even though they were experienced and competent in civilian practice.

Primary suture of wounds, inadequate debridement—particularly of innocent-appearing perforating wounds of large muscles, tight packing of wounds, and undue reliance on bacteriostatic agents were among the cardinal errors.   It was hard to make surgeons without combat experience realize that transportation of the combat casualty from one facility to another was inevitable and that his care must be geared to that fact.   A procedure which would have been reasonable and appropriate in civilian practice, when the patient could remain in bed until his wounds were healed, was therefore not safe in military practice in forward hospitals from which the soldier must be transported to the rear.   Transportation under the happiest circumstances induced fatigue and further shock.   The jolting caused shifting of fascial planes, with resulting hemorrhage or the collection of fluid in dead spaces, which was an invitation to infection.   All of these possibilities were enhanced by the methods of evacuation necessary in the Pacific (fig. 281).

Personal visits to hospitals by consultants were found to provide the most effective form of teaching, and a large part of the consultants' time was necessarily spent away from the Chief Surgeon's Office.   In a theater in which hospital units were in isolated bases, these visits were especially appreciated by the hospital staffs.   For one thing, they indicated the official interest of the Chief Surgeon in the problems of all the hospitals and their staffs.   For another, they provided opportunities for discussion of professional problems. The liaison thus established between the consultants and the base surgeons proved most useful.   The base surgeons came to rely upon the opinion of the consultants concerning the care and disposition of patients, as well as the placement of personnel.

New units arriving in the theater were met at the staging areas by the consultant.   Meetings were held with the surgical staffs, and the surgical policies of the theater were discussed.   Whenever possible, surgical officers were placed on temporary duty with active hospitals, so that they could obtain instruction in special problems and could see for themselves how battle casualties must be managed.

Hospital units designated to accompany a task force were always visited whenever possible by the surgical consultant before departure.

The training courses in various specialties provided by the Medical Department in the Zone of Interior were excellent.   However, judgment and skill cannot be learned in a matter of weeks, and most of the officers who had taken these courses were still inexperienced and required careful supervision. It was repeatedly observed that the selection of officers for these courses was not as wise as it might have been.   It would have been better, for instance, to train experienced general surgeons for neurosurgical duties rather than, as happened in a number of instances, give the courses to officers who had had little surgical experience or none at all.   It was later found that the consultants in neurosurgery in the Office of The Surgeon General had also arrived at this same conclusion.

Except in anesthesia, no attempts were made at training in the surgical specialties in the Southwest Pacific Area.   This single attempt was limited to the training courses in anesthesia given at the 118th General Hospital, at the request of the Chief Surgeon. The 4-month period of instruction covered the physiology and pharmacology of anesthesia, care of anesthetic equipment, and special techniques. There were 22 hours of lecture. The practical part of the course consisted of the administration of anesthetics, under supervision, to between 100 and 120 cases for each graduate. The courses were discontinued in July 1944, because of shortages of surgical cases in the hospital. When the selection of students for this assignment was judicious—as it sometimes was not—the graduates proved both capable and useful.

It was recognized early in the fighting in the Southwest Pacific Area that some means must be devised by which tours of active hospital duty could be provided for inexperienced medical officers serving in units in which no real clinical experience or training was possible. The basis of planning was that officers who were assigned as battalion surgeons or to remote dispensaries or who were engaged in duties that were chiefly administrative should be transferred temporarily to hospitals in which they might receive the necessary training, while officers in those hospitals would serve as their exchanges. The refresher courses in the designated hospitals were to include anesthesia, ophthalmology and otolaryngology, general surgery, orthopedic surgery, roentgenology, and general medicine and allied specialties.

These plans were discussed vigorously at intervals, but they were not implemented until Manila was taken and Luzon was secured, chiefly because of the long distances, shortages of transportation, and difficulties in radio and postal communications in the Pacific. Early in August 1945, 50 medical officers from the Sixth and Eighth U.S. Armies were finally placed on detached service in general hospitals on Luzon for the purposes just described.[4] They had scarcely begun their work when both armies were alerted for occupation duty in Japan and they had to be recalled.

Dissemination of information

It would have been extremely profitable if exchange of information concerning policies, techniques, and professional experiences had been permitted directly between the medical section of a field army headquarters and that of USASOS, SWPA, as well as between the Southwest Pacific Area and other theaters. As it was, all of this information was transmitted by way of the Office of The Surgeon General. It was slow in reaching the Pacific and even slower in seeping down to the surgeons who needed it most. Much of this information was also not as detailed as it might have been.

Bases in New Guinea, including Port Moresby, Milne Bay, Oro Bay, Lae, Finschhafen, Hollandia, and Biak, all had their own medical societies, as did the bases at Tacloban on Leyte and in Manila (fig. 282). Medical meetings were difficult to hold because of the conditions prevalent in the area, but, in retrospect, they could have been more widely utilized than they were. Ward rounds and seminars should also have been more widely employed.

---

[4] Circular Letter No. 31, Office of the Chief Surgeon, Headquarters, U.S. Army Forces, Pacific, 28 July 1945, subject: Training Program For Medical Officers.

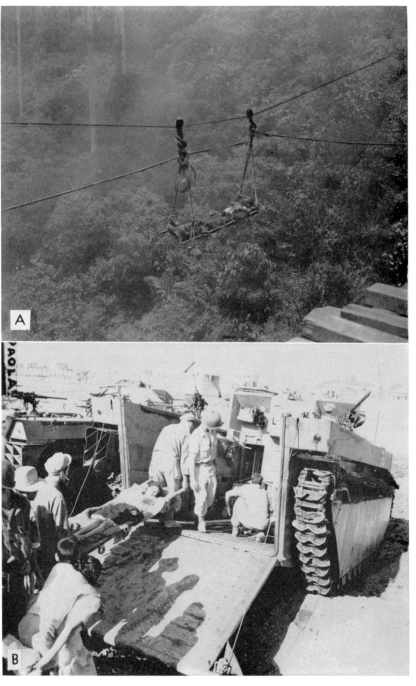

FIGURE 281.—Methods of evacuation in the Southwest Pacific Area, 1945. A. Litter carry over deep ravine by cables. B. Amphibious tanks (Buffaloes).

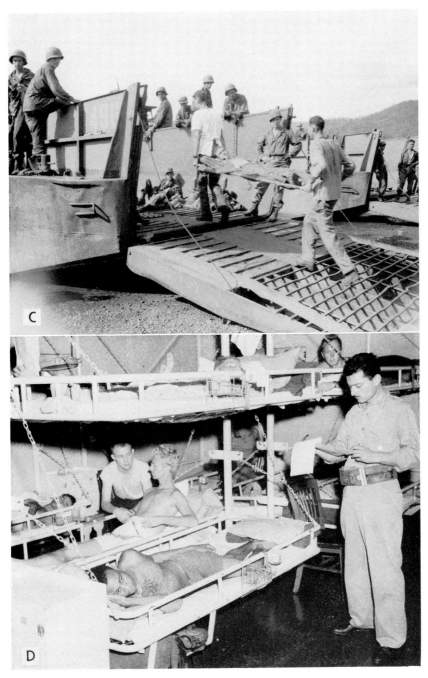

FIGURE 281.—Continued.   C. Landing craft.   D. A hospital ship.

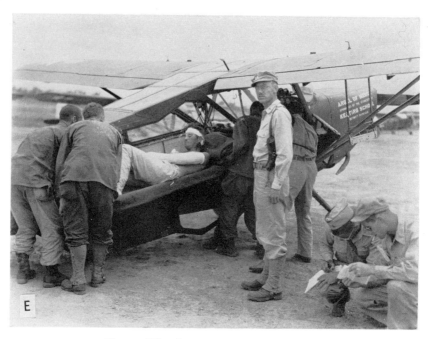

FIGURE 281.—Continued. E. Light aircraft.

The professional training of inexperienced medical officers in the Southwest Pacific would have been greatly simplified if texts and journals had been provided in much larger quantities.

Directives.—In the Southwest Pacific Area, as in other theaters, the varied training of medical officers and their range of surgical experience, ranging from a great deal to none at all, required that specific instructions be issued for methods of treatment of wounded casualties. Medical information was issued in the form of technical memorandums, prepared in the Chief Surgeon's Office, USASOS, and published over his signature.

Before these official memorandums began to be issued, standing operating procedures were issued on various levels—by hospital commanders, division surgeons, corps surgeons, and base surgeons. They were chiefly based on information secured from hospitals that had treated large numbers of casualties. Localized standardization of sorts was thus developed, and objectionable and questionable practices were generally prevented, but there was no true uniformity of management of casualties until the official directives just mentioned began to be issued. These memorandums were based not only on the previous experience in the theater but also on the experience of other theaters as relayed to the Southwest Pacific Area in the form of ETMD reports.

The distribution of these reports in the Southwest Pacific Area was not good. This consultant did not know of their existence until August 1944, and

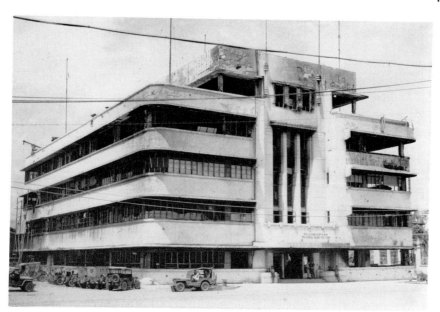

FIGURE 282.—Headquarters, Philippine Base Section, Manila, Philippine Islands, 25 May 1945.

his own lack of knowledge reflected the general lack of knowledge of other medical officers concerning them. Once the ETMD reports were called to the attention of medical officers, they cooperated in producing material for them, and much valuable data were thus secured. It was the policy, as far as possible, to use the names of contributors, in fairness to them and also because of the stimulus thus provided to further production.

When the Consultant in Surgery finally learned of the existence of the ETMD reports, he suggested that whole articles, or abstracts of articles, of special value which appeared in them be reprinted in pamphlet form each month, either by the Office of The Surgeon General or in the area, and be distributed to officers performing surgery. The plan, which was suggested on a worldwide basis, proved impractical in the Southwest Pacific Area because of the rapid movement of Headquarters, USASOS, SWPA, to Hollandia in September 1944, to Leyte in January 1945, and to Manila in the following April.[5]

---

[5] There is an unfortunate lack of detailed data on various types of combat-incurred injuries from hospitals in the Southwest Pacific Area. This experience suggests that a standard form should have been provided for all of the theaters for the reporting of monthly battle casualties from each medical treatment facility. Such a form could have contained the information in more detail than was required in the official forms in use, without, at the same time, being so detailed as to impose an additional burden on medical officers already overwhelmed with work. There was no machine records unit in the Office of the Chief Surgeon, SWPA, at any time, and, even if it had been available, reports received from individual hospitals varied so widely that they could not have been fitted into a theater pattern.

Surgical Teams

As pointed out elsewhere (p. 756), the concept of surgical teams was not accepted in the Southwest Pacific Area until April 1944, shortly after General Denit had become Chief Surgeon, USAFFE (U.S. Army Forces in the Far East), and SOS, SWPA. The teams which were then formed on paper were offered to the Surgeon, Sixth U.S. Army, by General Denit in the summer of 1944, for the invasion of Leyte. The offer was declined, and no surgical teams were used to supplement the medical units scheduled to support the landings of 20 October. Shortly afterward, this decision was reversed, and four teams were placed on temporary duty with the Sixth U.S. Army, with the understanding that they would return to their original stations when the need for them had ceased. The value of the team concept was so evident that other teams were requested for support of the field and evacuation hospitals which landed in Lingayen Gulf in January 1945. In all, 23 teams were used in this invasion, and others landed elsewhere, with units of the Eighth U.S. Army. It was part of the author's duties as surgical consultant to provide the personnel for these teams.

The objections originally raised to the use of surgical teams when they were first proposed by Colonel Parsons in 1942 had been chiefly by medical personnel with limited clinical experience. The objections did not prove valid. Testimony from forward units was that the presence of these teams, far from being resented by organic personnel of field and evacuation hospitals, was welcomed. The second objection raised to the team system, that personnel constituting them would be lost permanently to the parent organization, also did not materialize; it was obviated by correctly written orders.

Although surgical teams filled an appreciable portion of the surgical breach in the last months of active fighting in the Southwest Pacific Area, auxiliary surgical groups would have been more satisfactory for a number of reasons. They were better organized. Their personnel had generally had better training and more experience, and were therefore of more even ability. Finally, the morale factor could not be ignored. The great weakness of surgical teams as they were constituted in the Southwest Pacific Area was that their makeup depended entirely upon the decisions of the commanding officers of the hospitals from which they were derived. Some of these commanding officers simply used the opportunities thus afforded to get rid of undesirable personnel. Many of the officers who served on the teams were well trained and highly competent, but commanding officers, quite naturally, did not willingly release their best surgeons. Therefore, the teams, like the staffs of portable surgical hospitals, though competent on the whole, represented a very uneven array of talent.

Specialized Hospitals

In both Australia and New Guinea, from 1943 on, a considerable amount of specialization was practiced in hospitals. Several bases were large enough to justify the establishment of hospital centers, one or more of the hospitals being devoted to particular specialties.

When the idea of specialized hospitals in Hollandia was first proposed by this consultant, the chief of the Professional Services Division, Office of the Chief Surgeon, USASOS, did not regard the idea as practical because of the long distances between hospitals and the extremely poor roads. The idea was revived in Leyte but again was not regarded as practical in view of the bad weather, the poor roads, and the difficult terrain. In retrospect, it seems to have been an error not to have pressed the idea more vigorously at an earlier date in the Southwest Pacific Area, in view of the excellent results obtained by this method in the Mediterranean and European theaters.

The author's suggestion that casualties be moved from Leyte and Mindanao to Manila for specialized treatment was also not accepted because the officer in charge of the evacuation section in the Office of the Chief Surgeon, USASOS, SWPA, considered that evacuation from that city to the Zone of Interior would present undue transportation difficulties. Actually, these difficulties did not occur, and failure to accept the plan was unfortunate. Because of the delay in their utilization, hospitals in Manila played no part at all in the care of combat casualties, being utilized only for staging and for the care of station hospital type patients. The hospitals in Leyte, meantime, were seriously overcrowded, and their staffs were greatly overworked.

A limited form of specialization became effective in February 1945, when casualties with chest injuries were directed, as far as possible, from Luzon to the 118th General Hospital on Leyte, while surgeons from other units were brought over, as admissions required, to this hospital on temporary duty.

It should be emphasized that the idea of specialized hospitals to handle special types of wounds, including fresh wounds, like a number of other ideas which did not win acceptance, was proposed by the theater Consultant in Surgery on the basis of his own observations and his clinical experience. The idea was rejected in an office in which planning was largely by tables and charts, and usually by officers whose clinical experience was limited and who lacked firsthand knowledge of the surgical situation in forward areas.

Equipment

The theaters of operations in the Pacific were generally regarded as the stepchildren of the war, and in a sense they were, though the vast distances and the difficulties of communication between them and the mainland always had to be taken into account. In spite of the obstacles which had to be overcome, equipment was, on the whole, very satisfactory. Smaller hospitals frequently complained of the lack of certain items, but the explanation usually was that these items were not on their tables of equipment and were not needed for the mission of hospitals on this level.

Nonstandardized items could usually be procured when a real need for them could be shown, though there was often a considerable delay before they were received.

Clinical Research and Investigation

No outstanding surgical research was accomplished in any of the Pacific areas, in contrast to the outstanding investigations in such medical fields as malaria, dengue fever, scrub (bush) typhus, and schistosomiasis.

Original plans for the Southwest Pacific Area did not include formal research studies. The need for an organization for the correlation and encouragement of both clinical and laboratory research was, however, promptly evident, and in 1943 Col. Maurice C. Pincoffs, MC, Consultant in Medicine, USASOS, SWPA, requested, through the Chief Surgeon, that a medical general laboratory be provided for this purpose. In March 1944, word was received from the Office of The Surgeon General that such a unit would be sent to the area. Because there were a number of medical officers in the theater with interest and training in investigative work, as evidenced by their previous accomplishments, it had been requested that the laboratory arrive with certain table of organization vacancies, to be filled by these officers. This request was complied with. Inability to secure necessary priorities and other factors delayed the arrival of the unit, and it was not until August 1944 that the 19th Medical General Laboratory debarked from the United States, designated to arrive in the Southwest Pacific in September.

From the surgical standpoint, it had always been considered highly desirable that the laboratory unit coming to the area should be operated in combination with hospital facilities. After considerable discussion among the consultants involved, it was decided to use for this purpose the 250-bed 12th Station Hospital, which was duly transferred from Australia to Hollandia.

With the assistance of USASOS engineers, plans were drawn up to house the laboratory and the hospital under one roof. Plans were also made for changes and additions required to make the portable hospital buildings, suitable for use in Australia, satisfactory for scientific investigative purposes in tropical New Guinea. A high priority was secured for the large amounts of material and extra equipment required for these new purposes. The necessary items were secured through the Office of the Chief Quartermaster, SWPA, then located in Sydney, Australia, and were placed aboard a liberty ship destined for Hollandia. During this period, steps were taken to locate personnel within the area who could contribute to the project.

In spite of these careful plans, nothing came of them. Not long after the arrival in Hollandia of the 12th Station Hospital, the 19th Medical General Laboratory, and the material and equipment just described, the tactical program for the invasion of the Philippines was so stepped up that the investigative project had to be curtailed. The 19th Medical General Laboratory was, however, established as planned at Hollandia (fig. 283).

Development of Body Armor for Infantrymen

Almost as soon as the author entered service, he became interested in the possibility of protecting particularly vulnerable areas of the body by the development of some sort of body armor for the chest and abdomen of infantrymen,

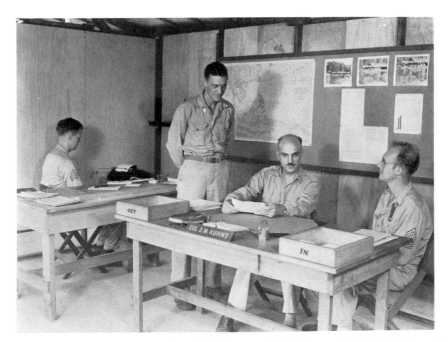

FIGURE 283.—Col. Dwight M Kuhns, MC, Commanding Officer, 19th Medical General Laboratory, Hollandia, New Guinea, March 1945.

just as helmets had been developed for the protection of the head. In September 1942, while still in Australia, he learned that the Japanese were testing an armored vest on their troops in New Guinea (fig. 284). Eventually, after a great deal of effort in various quarters, he was able to procure a specimen vest through the kindness of the commander of an Australian destroyer. In the meantime, Col. (later Brig. Gen.) Percy J. Carroll, MC, then Surgeon, USAFFE, had been informed of this consultant's project and had expressed great interest in it.

The Japanese vest was an ingenious article. It was made of metal plates, set in canvas, was buttoned on in three overlapping sections, and weighed a little over 5 pounds. Tests showed that this vest, which was designed to protect only the anterior chest, could resist missiles shot from machineguns and pistols at velocities of 800 f.p.s. Metal construction was obviously essential. Tests with vests of plastic material available at that time showed that they were easily pierced and fragmented by the .45-caliber automatic pistol and the Thompson submachinegun.

From the Japanese model, the author constructed a protective vest made of six large overlapping metal plates that had been molded on a man 5 feet 7 inches tall and weighing 150 pounds (fig. 285). The vest covered more of the region of the collar bones, upper breast bone, flanks, and lower abdomen than the Japanese vest.

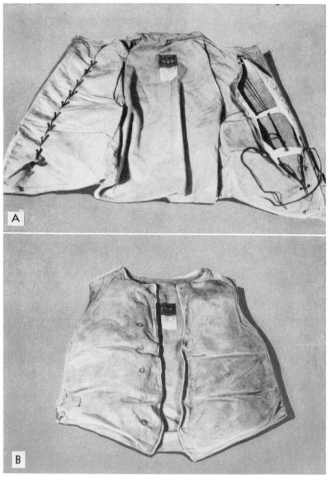

FIGURE 284.—A captured Japanese armored vest. A. The vest open.
B. The vest closed.

On 25 March 1943, the author sent to Brig. Gen. Clyde C. Alexander, USASOS, SWPA, a summary of his studies on protective body armor. In this communication, he recommended that a vest "constructed along the lines of the captured Japanese vest" be produced for U.S. Army infantrymen. In June, upon request, he sent his set of Japanese body armor to the Chief Ordnance Officer, USASOS, SWPA. In December, also upon request, he submitted the vest which he had designed to the Chief Ordnance Officer, USASOS, SWPA, to be sent to the Chief of Ordnance, War Department, Washington.

In February 1944, upon request of Maj. Gen. (later Gen.) Nathan F. Twining, Commanding General, Fifteenth U.S. Air Force, the vest was submitted through channels to the Surgeon, Fifteenth U.S. Air Force. General Twining had become interested in it while he was a patient in the 118th General Hospital.

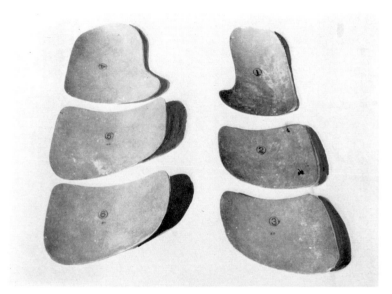

FIGURE 285.—Metal plates designed by Colonel Trimble for a protective vest.

In April, a complete set of blueprints of this vest was made in the Office of the Surgeon, Fifteenth U.S. Air Force. Also in April, at the direction of the Chief Surgeon, USASOS, SWPA, a complete report on the body armor which he had devised was submitted by this consultant to the Office of Scientific Research and Development, Washington, with an indorsement by General Denit.

On 4 August 1945, in a memorandum to General Denit, Chief Surgeon, AFWESPAC, the author summarized conferences he had had in Washington with various officers in the Office of the Chief of Ordnance, Army Service Forces, and with Brig. Gen. Edward S. Greenbaum, USA, Executive Officer, Office of the Under Secretary of War. He learned during these conferences that 8,000 vests, 4,000 in a light and 4,000 in a heavier weight, were then on their way to AFPAC by ship and that an additional 100,000 of the heavier variety would become available about 1 September. A recommendation that 400,000 more be produced without further delay had not yet been acted upon.

The surrender of the Japanese on 14 August 1945 made unnecessary the use of the protective vests sent to the Pacific. It is not likely that these vests would have proved satisfactory. They were constructed as a sort of overhead apron, with a front and back, and were very awkward to put on and take off. More important, the basic idea of protective overlapping plates had been discarded entirely.[6]

---

[6] The story of the development of body armor in the Pacific, with illustrations, and its subsequent development and use in the Korean War, is told in greater detail in: Medical Department, United States Army. Wound Ballistics. Washington: U.S. Government Printing Office, 1962. It is unfortunate that the wearing of protective armor was not pushed as vigorously in World War II as it was in the Korean War. The use of protective armor would undoubtedly have saved many lives.—J. B. C., Jr.

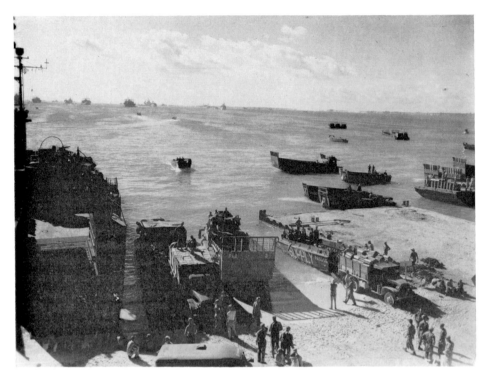

FIGURE 286.—Red Beach, Los Negros Island, Admiralty Group, 7 October 1944.

Amphibious Landings

When the author assumed his duties as surgical consultant, succeeding Colonel Parsons, in the Office of the Chief Surgeon, USASOS, SWPA, the next military move was to be the occupation of Morotai (Operation INTERLUDE), to be followed a month later by the first Philippine operation, then planned for the island of Mindanao (Operation KING I).

Planning for Morotai operation

The experiences gained in the medical support of amphibious landings in previous operations were immediately investigated by this consultant (fig. 286). His review included not only the reports of the landings in various portions of the Southwest Pacific Area but also the reports from the European theater in which Maj. Gen. Paul R. Hawley, Chief Surgeon, had summarized the medical experiences of the D-day landings in France.

In his report, General Hawley repeatedly emphasized the outstanding part played by LST's in the provision of medical service for the invading troops. These ships were used as both aid stations and hospital ships; each of them carried an experienced surgeon, 2 young Naval medical officers, and about 20 hospital corpsmen. Hundreds of casualties from the beaches received their first medical care on them. Casualties with abdominal wounds were operated upon on them, with excellent results. Ships' personnel assisted in the care and feeding of the wounded during their off-watch periods. Returning LST's transported about 90 percent of the total casualties evacuated during the early days of the operation, sometimes carrying as many as 150 to 300 on a single trip.

On 6 September and 8 September 1944, in memorandums addressed to the Chief Surgeon, USASOS, SWPA, through the Chief of Professional Services, this consultant commented on the plans for the Morotai operation in the light of the D-day experience in Europe, and made the following recommendations:

1. Medical collecting and clearing company personnel should land with the assault waves during combined operations. This recommendation was based on General Hawley's criticism that during the landings in Normandy, only the 1st Division sent its medical troops in early; the clearing company that landed with it cared for the division casualties and for casualties of combat teams on either side of it for the first 24 hours.

2. Experienced surgeons should accompany the clearing company personnel. They could be selected from the list of surgical teams, each consisting of two surgeons and six enlisted men, submitted by the Chief Surgeon, USASOS, to the Sixth U.S. Army and the Seventh U.S. Fleet.

3. LST's to serve as hospital ships, especially staffed and equipped and clearly marked to indicate their mission, should go in to the beaches as soon as the task force commander deemed it suitable. These ships should not be used for cargo purposes; they should be ready to take on patients immediately and not have to wait until their cargoes were unloaded on the beaches.

4. An experienced surgeon and two assistant surgeons should be on each LST to be used for hospital purposes. Present plans of the Seventh U.S. Fleet called for an experienced surgeon on every fifth LST and a junior medical officer, with two Navy corpsmen, on each of the other LST's. The beachmaster was to direct casualties who in his opinion needed major surgery to the LST's carrying experienced surgeons. The author considered this plan practical only if the LST's not staffed with experienced surgeons were to be used only to transport casualties from the beaches to hospital ships lying a mile or two offshore for definitive surgery. If casualties were to be kept aboard LST's for any length of time, it was essential that they be staffed by experienced surgeons. The details of the plans were not clear in this respect.

5. Portable surgical hospitals with the best trained surgical staffs (the 1st, 3d, 5th, 16th, and 23d) should go ashore about the sixth wave. Evacuation hospitals would go ashore later, the time of their landing depending upon the security of the position.

6. Army surgical teams could be used to supplement Navy medical personnel aboard the LST's. The professional training of the Navy medical officers was not clearly known, but reports suggested that they had had relatively little surgical experience.

7. Evacuation by air of casualties given definitive care in portable surgical hospitals and evacuation hospitals should begin as early as possible. In Normandy, although no air evacuation had been anticipated before D+7 and it was not expected to be significant before D+14, air evacuation began on D+3.

8. An ophthalmologist should be available promptly, as previous experiences had shown that there would be numerous eye injuries.

9. Regularly scheduled conferences should be held by representatives designated by the Chief Surgeon, USASOS, SWPA, and the Senior Medical Officer, Seventh U.S. Fleet.

Planning for invasion of Leyte

The Morotai operation, because of General MacArthur's strategy in outflanking the Japanese, was accomplished on 15 September 1944 without casualties. Operation KING I, the landings planned for the southern Philippines, was therefore canceled, and Operation KING II, the invasion of Leyte, was advanced to 20 October 1944.

The plan was that, during the assault phase of these landings, all casualties requiring immediate hospitalization would be evacuated by assault Naval craft, APA's (attack transports) and Geneva-protected hospital ships. To accommodate the casualties, certain changes were made in the structure of the LST's and the APA's. LST's, each staffed with a surgical team of three officers, were to care for 75 litter and 75 ambulatory wounded each. LST's without surgical teams were to transport 15 litter and 15 ambulatory wounded each. APA's with four medical officers were to transport 150 litter and 250 ambulatory wounded each. Naval medical personnel were to provide definitive surgical care to casualties en route from the target area to the New Guinea bases.

This consultant, with the approval of General Denit, visited the Senior Medical Officer, Seventh U.S. Fleet, several weeks before A-day, to review with him the plans for care of the wounded and the professional qualifications of the Army and Navy medical officers scheduled to provide definitive care. As already mentioned, the records indicated that most of them had little or no surgical training. The Senior Medical Officer had no detailed record of the professional qualifications of the Navy personnel assigned to this duty, but he stated that he was certain that they were competent. He added that some of them were lieutenant commanders. The offer made by the author, on behalf of General Denit, to supply experienced Army surgeons for duty on the LST's and APA's was declined.

The elaborate system planned for the Morotai operation by the Navy had been further expanded for this operation. The wounded would be transferred to the LST's with due regard for the nature of their wounds and the specialized personnel aboard the ships, whose presence would be indicated by different kinds of flags. The beachmaster was to decide where the individual casualty belonged and was to start him on his way to the appropriate ship.

The difficulties in this plan seemed obvious, and the author pointed them out. They included the extent of the beaches; the confusion of battle, which would make identification of particular LST's difficult if not impossible; the frequent multiplicity of wounds, which would make it difficult for a lay person to decide which of the injuries was the most important; and the possibility of hostile air attacks. It was thought that all of these conditions would so complicate this specialized plan of triage as to make it impractical, as indeed it proved to be.

On 5 October 1944, in another memorandum to the Chief Surgeon, USASOS, SWPA, the surgical consultant stated that the Navy planned to use LST's for hospital purposes only after the cargo was removed. He recommended, as in an earlier memorandum, that these ships should be in the landing force, ready to receive casualties immediately and not after the removal of their cargo, since a very large number of casualties might well occur during the assault on the beaches. He also recommended again that every LST, instead of every fifth ship, carry an experienced surgeon pointing out the efficiency of this plan in the Normandy landings. He recommended that several portable surgical hospitals, staffed with experienced surgeons, be placed on the LST's which would act as hospitals during the invasion. He further recommended that the portable hospitals serve as hospitals throughout the landing operation.

Report on Leyte invasion

ETMD reports from the Southwest Pacific Area for December 1944 described the early surgical care during the Leyte invasion as follows:

In the first phase of the landings, casualties injured on landing craft, after being given primary care, were transferred to LST's and attack transports staffed with surgical teams (fig. 287). Those injured on shore were treated by battalion and regimental aid stations; they were given plasma as necessary, and the usual first aid measures were carried out (fig. 288).

As the task force units moved inland, medical collecting and clearing companies began to function. Casualties received primary treatment almost immediately after wounding, and then, with little delay, were put aboard LST's, where blood was available and definitive surgery was undertaken. Although seven LST's were offshore on D-day with surgical teams aboard, only two were primarily hospital ships. The others could not take over the care of patients until their cargoes were landed. Attack transport ships could be unloaded faster than LST's, and they were therefore the first ships to leave Leyte with casualties.

The 7th Division Clearing Company was ashore by H+6 and performed approximately 150 definitive operations within the next 48 hours. From D-day until D+4, however, most definitive surgery was done on Navy craft

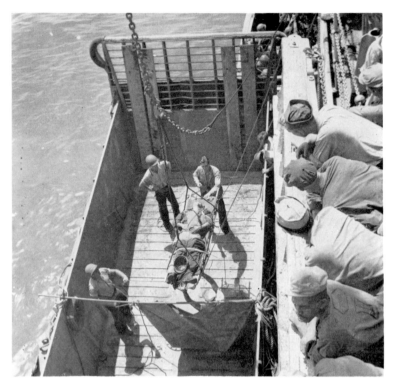

FIGURE 287.—An American casualty being loaded aboard ship in Leyte
Harbor, 20 October 1944.

offshore. When the wounded were near the beach, the timelag between wounding and first aid was a matter of minutes. The wounded were then carried almost immediately to LST's for definitive surgery, which sometimes was done
within 1 or 2 hours after wounding.

In the second phase of the invasion, the distance ashore along which the
LST's were distributed was greatly increased, and the perimeter extended as
much as 15 miles in depth. Mobile aid stations and clearing stations were kept
well up near the line, and, at first, the wounded received both first aid and
definitive care promptly. As the distance to the beaches increased, 12 hours
sometimes elapsed before definitive treatment on an LST followed primary
care (fig. 289). Torrential rains, in addition to distance, played their part
in the increased timelag.

The ships that had taken part in the original operation soon became
crowded, and some were sent back to the bases well loaded. Not enough then
remained to take care of casualties from the shore as well as the considerable
number wounded in the harbor in the Japanese suicide raids. Later, it was
possible to evacuate casualties to APH's (transports for wounded) and hospital ships.

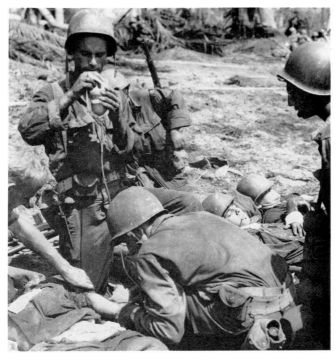

FIGURE 288.—First aid measures being carried out at an aid station on the beach at Leyte, 20 October 1944.

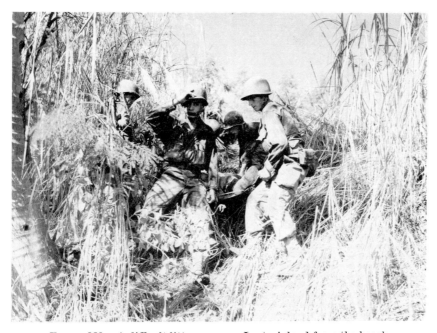

FIGURE 289.—A difficult litter carry on Leyte, inland from the beach.

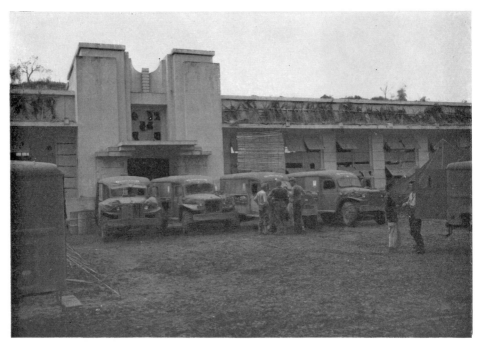

FIGURE 290.—The 58th Evacuation Hospital at Tacloban, Leyte, Philippine Islands, 26 October 1944.

In the third phase of the landings, field and evacuation hospitals were set up; the 58th Evacuation Hospital (fig. 290) was in full operation in a school in Tacloban on D+4 and had begun to function 48 hours earlier. Some hospitals were delayed in opening because the tactical situation did not permit unloading of their equipment.

After D+6, most definitive surgery was done in hospitals on shore (fig. 291). In order to keep beds clear for casualties, the hospitals continued to evacuate patients from rear areas to the LST's, where they remained until hospital ships arrived; if a hospital ship was in the harbor, patients were taken directly to it. Air evacuation to New Guinea and Saipan began on D+6 and was in regular operation after D+16 and D+21, respectively.

The landings at Leyte presented a problem not encountered in any previous amphibious landings in the Southwest Pacific; for 38 days, large numbers of casualties continued to occur in the harbor, from bombing and strafing by enemy planes. Both first aid and definitive care for these casualties were supplied by LST's, APA's, and APH's. In the remaining landings on the Philippines, the care of casualties during the assault phase was relatively simple because all enemy airfields within operating radius had been effectively destroyed by U.S. Navy and Army Air Force planes before the landings.

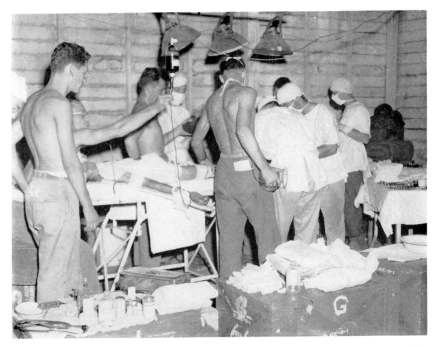

FIGURE 291.—Definitive surgery in a portable surgical hospital, Leyte, Philippine Islands.

LST 464, which had been converted for hospital purposes, and LST 1025, which had a surgical team aboard but had not been converted, carried heavy surgical loads from D-day on (fig. 292). These two ships, the Sixth U.S. Army surgeon stated, "saved their lives" before sufficient hospitalization was set up ashore to care for the casualties of the invasion.

This consultant, after his experience at Leyte (p. 712), concluded that the LST, properly altered, admirably fulfilled the needs created by the new tactical situation that had developed there. The great advantage was that, when it was thus altered, it was primarily a hospital ship—not a cargo ship, used secondarily for hospital purposes. It could therefore remain on station in the harbor and be available for use at all times. A large hospital ship in the harbor would have served the same purposes, but the risk of its being hit, with a resulting heavy loss of life, made such an arrangement unwise.

Planning for invasion of Japan

Preliminary medical planning for the projected OLYMPIC and CORONET invasions of the Japanese islands were begun by General Denit's directions in May 1945. The first of these landings, on Kyushu, was scheduled for 1 November.

On 8 May 1945, the author addressed a memorandum to General Denit, a summary of which follows.

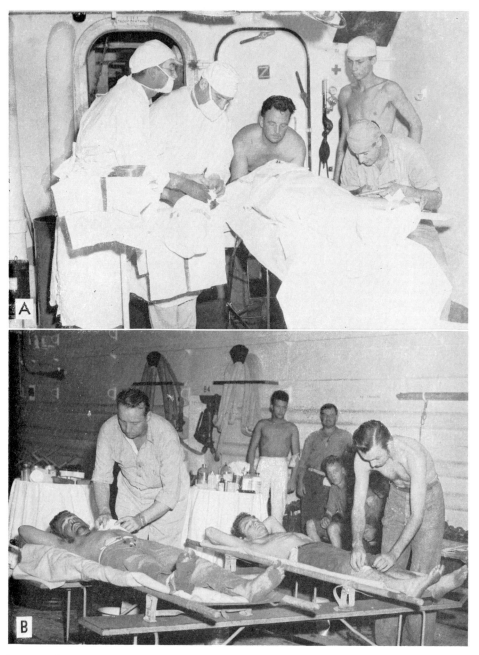

FIGURE 292.—An LST handling a surgical load during the Leyte invasion. A. An operating room set up in troop quarters on the middle deck. B. A treatment station on tank deck.

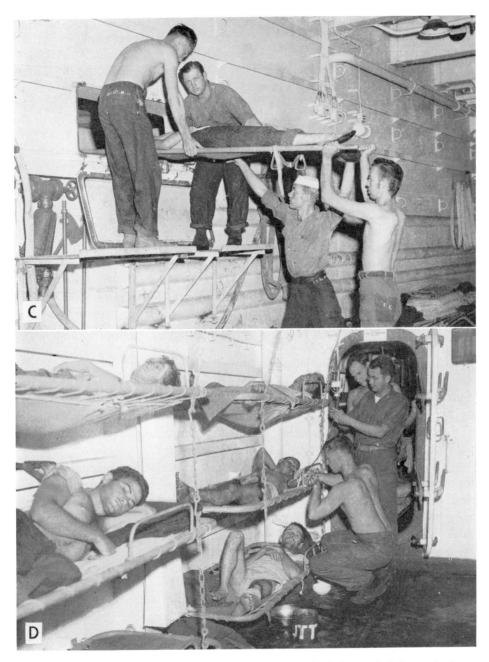

FIGURE 292.—Continued.   C. Casualty scuttle from tank deck to surgical teams in troop
    quarters.   D. Litter arrangement in troop quarters.

An amphibious landing anywhere within range of undestroyed Japanese air bases would be attended by daily attacks of enemy planes upon allied troop and supply ships. Resulting casualties would be heavy. LST's and APA's with surgical teams aboard would take care of casualties on D-day through D+2, but then after having discharged their cargoes, they would pull out, and their surgical teams would no longer be available. Large hospital ships of the Geneva type would run too much risk by remaining in the harbor. The establishment of hospitals on shore would not solve the whole problem, for distances would be great, landing on beaches often difficult, communications poor, and transportation scarce for some time.

This situation was first encountered on Leyte (p. 738). Immediately after that operation, recommendations were made by the Office of the Chief Surgeon, USASOS, SWPA, at this consultant's suggestion, to The Surgeon General by letter and to the senior medical officers of the Seventh U.S. Fleet and 7th Amphibious Force, by interview, that multiple small ships, of the station hospital type, based on the LST 464 model, be maintained in the harbor at all times in all similar future operations. Lessons from the invasion of Leyte and from the Okinawa operation, then in progress, indicated that renewed and stronger representations should be made for greatly increased numbers of this type of hospital ship to care for Army and Navy casualties in all future combined operations.

On 10 May 1945, this consultant sent to General Denit a statement from the Basic Concept of Operation OLYMPIC and pointed out that it was not clear in it whether the 15 LST's planned as a minimum were to be equipped as hospital ships, like LST 464, and would be staffed to render definitive care. The statement that they would "administer emergency treatment and sort patients for further evacuation" implied the contrary.

The author recommended that these points be clarified. In his opinion, repeatedly expressed, the value of these ships rested entirely upon (1) their availability in the harbor day and night, and (2) the provision on them of adequate equipment and competent staffs to provide definitive major surgical care. On 14 May, the Medical Section, General Headquarters, concurred in the proposed use of the LST's; those ships whose primary function was to provide definitive surgical care would be differentiated from those with minimal equipment and surgical teams.

On 28 June 1945, in response to a request from the G-4 Section, General Headquarters, AFPAC, to General Denit, this consultant and Lt. Col. (later Col.) Harold A. Sofield, MC, orthopedic consultant in the Office of the Surgeon, AFWESPAC, submitted recommendations for General Denit's approval and transmission to the G-4 Section, General Headquarters, AFPAC. A summary of these recommendations follows.

1. The use of the LST as an auxiliary hospital ship is of the greatest importance in the care of casualties sustained in an assault landing; in the care

of casualties sustained on shore for the first 2 or 3 days, while hospitals are being established; in the care of casualties sustained on ships during the ensuing days or weeks as the result of enemy air attacks; in evacuation parallel to the beach when roads are obstructed; in triage of the wounded; and in the maintenance of a supply point for whole blood and medical supplies.

2. The proposed role of the LST in the forthcoming operation should be clarified. At this time, it is not known whether the LST's to be used will be of the hospital type, such as LST 464, or only secondarily for hospital use, such as LST 929. It is also not known whether the LST will act as a hospital ship primarily; will carry troops and cargo and, after unloading, accept patients for definitive major surgery while transporting them to a rear base; or will act as a sorting station and evacuation point and be used for definitive surgery as an emergency measure only. If the plan is to use the Geneva type of hospital ship employed at Leyte, which retired from the combat area as soon as casualties were received, a number of LST's of the 464 type should be provided, to function as station hospitals in the harbor and provide specialized care for harbor and beach casualties. If attack transports are to be employed as hospital ships and remain with the assault shipping, they would provide definitive care for these casualties, and the LST's could be of the 929 type, functioning as sorting and evacuation points and doing only emergency definitive surgery.

Previous experience has shown that two LST's per assault division are necessary to provide minimum coverage. If the APA's are to retire from the assault shipping, LST's of the 464 type should be provided in the ratio of two ships to one of the 929 type. If the APA's are to remain in the area, this ratio could be reversed. The number of LST's specified would be in addition to those equipped and staffed to transport wounded from the target area back to a base area.

3. A careful study should be made of the professional qualifications of surgeons designated to do definitive surgery. Army personnel should be freely offered to the Navy when additional experienced surgeons are needed. The experience of the Normandy landings showed that one experienced surgeon and two assistants should be on each ship on which definitive surgery is to be performed. The surgical personnel of all Army APA's should be carefully reinterviewed and strengthened by the Surgeon, Port of Embarkation, San Francisco. If, in the opinion of the surgical consultants, these staffs are not adequate, surgeons from AFWESPAC should be placed on board on recommendation of the Chief Surgeon.

On the recommendation of this consultant, Col. Douglas B. Kendrick, Jr., MC, who had inaugurated the blood program in the Office of The Surgeon General and who was then serving as consultant in blood and transfusion with the Tenth U.S. Army on Okinawa, was placed on temporary duty in General Denit's office, to make plans for the supply of blood for the invasion of Japan. Colonel Kendrick was also to organize auxiliary blood banks in Manila and on Okinawa to supplement the supply from the United States via Guam in case difficulties of transportation reduced the supply. Lt. Col. Mark M. Bracken, MC, Chief of the Laboratory Service, 27th General Hospital, was placed on temporary duty to work with Colonel Kendrick on the implementation of these plans.

Colonel Bracken was also directed to form medical teams, each consisting of two medical officers and four enlisted men, from the general hospitals in the theater, to serve as shock teams in field, portable surgical, and evacuation hospitals, and clearing companies. This was an entirely new idea in the Southwest Pacific Area, suggested by the surgical consultant to increase the usefulness of the surgical teams by removing some burdens from them, so that they could pursue exclusively their work of operating on the wounded.

The planning for the invasion required a knowledge of troop strengths, military objectives, the nature and amount of medical support, the airfields to be designated for evacuation, the naval plans, and other vital data. General Denit's office was given free access to all information, and the medical planning was based on full military knowledge.

The surrender of Japan in August 1945 made it unnecessary to continue the planning for Operation OLYMPIC. Planning for Operation CORONET had not yet begun. To show, however, the immense size of the projected medical support, as well as the variegated duties and opportunities of a consultant to help in the whole theater planning, the following memorandum for General Denit, prepared by this consultant in Washington on 4 August 1945, is quoted:

My dear General:

1. In my notebook marked "Surgery", which I have left with Colonel Baker, is the latest information on such items as Blood Plan, Briefing of Hospitals, Body Armor, Hospital Personnel Equipment, Task Force Study, and Trench Foot.

a. In the Whole Blood Plan, Major McGraw of The Surgeon General's Office made certain suggestions, as are attached [not reproduced]. A letter from Colonel Robinson to you states that the Navy will cooperate in every way with Kendrick's plan.

b. I have talked with Colonel Studler of the Ordnance Dept. about Body Armor. A Major Shaw from his office, and a Captain of Infantry, are already in Manila with samples of armor. With Colonel Voorhees I interviewed General Greenbaum in the Office of the Secretary of War. After the conference General Greenbaum prepared a radio for General Somervell's signature addressed to General Styer of AFWESPAC, stressing the favorable opinion of the War Department about the armor and asking for early information as to the Theater's needs for it. The latest information on the subject is contained in my file.

c. Information on the Hospital Equipment problem which you asked me to take up is contained in this file also in a letter to you from General Bliss on the subject.

d. Personnel. Satisfactory arrangements have been reached about surgical consultant personnel, and Colonel Carter is having their orders cut. The 5th Surgical Auxiliary Group should be in the Theater at the present time. Hospitals arriving in the next few months are:

Hospital		*Expected Date of Arrival*
Evacuation	5 (Five)	August
Field	10 (Ten)	August
Station (250 Bed)	3 (Three)	August
Auxiliary Surgical Group	1 (One)	August
Evacuation	6 (Six)	September
Convalescent	1 (One)	September
Clearing Companies	16 (Sixteen)	September
Collecting	5 (Five)	September
Ambulance	16 (Sixteen)	September
General (1,000 Bed)	41 (Forty-one)	September
Station (750 Bed)	5 (Five)	September
Station (500 Bed)	16 (Sixteen)	September
Evacuation	9 (Nine)	October
General	10 (Ten)	October
Medical Professional Group	1 (One)	October
Station (500)	4 (Four)	October
Evacuation	5 (Five)	November
Station (500 Bed)	1 (One)	November
General (1,000 Bed)	41 (Forty-one)	"Later"

The importance of sending personnel in advance of T/O hospitals to which they are attached was emphasized to Dr. Ginsberg. He was likewise advised of the urgent need to send replacements for medical officers in the Pacific with three or more years' service overseas. Three hundred and fifty (350) medical officers from the European Theater have been discharged from the service, although they do not have so high a number of service points as do officers still left in the Pacific Theater. In spite of Congressional pressure, it would be fairer to keep men from the European Theater in the Army on duty in the Z.I. to release men from the Z.I. to go to the Pacific as replacements.

e. Task Force Study. One of the points which I asked Colonel Robinson and Colonel Kendrick to try to settle in our absence from Manila was the consent of the Navy to use Army surgical teams on ships carrying battle casualties not staffed with experienced surgeons. In a recent communication to you from Colonel Robinson it is stated that the Navy has agreed to this arrangement. The date of arrival of Geneva Convention hospital ships at the target has not yet definitely been established.

f. Trench Foot. Colonel Gordon and Major Shaw from The Surgeon General's Office are already in Manila. Colonel [Gordon] was Chief of Preventive Medicine in ETO.

Postsurrender Responsibilities

The Japanese surrender

Almost immediately after the first U.S. troops landed in Japan and assumed their occupation duties, General MacArthur issued an order directing them to carry no firearms. Events proved the wisdom of this directive. The surrender of Japanese troops was so complete and so final that neither mass nor isolated acts of violence occurred after it. As a result, there were no more battle casualties, and occupancy of surgical wards consisted of patients injured in traffic accidents and street fights. Burns from gasoline-driven equipment were also frequent.

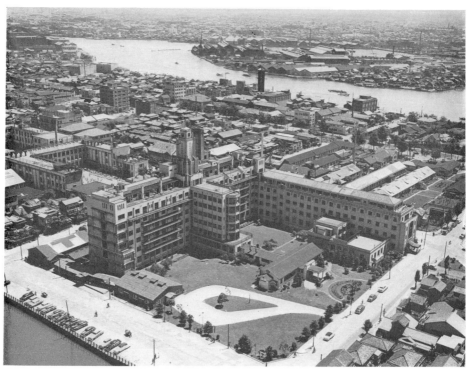

FIGURE 293.—The 49th General Hospital (formerly St. Luke's Hospital), Tokyo, Japan.

This consultant's chief problem after the surrender was to spread available surgical personnel, with adequate training and experience, over the larger Japanese islands of Honshu, Kyushu, and Hokkaido, as well as Formosa and Korea. This became his responsibility when he was transferred, late in October 1945, from the Office of the Surgeon, Headquarters, AFWESPAC, to the Office of the Surgeon, Headquarters, AFPAC. Early in December, he proceeded from Manila to Advance Echelon, AFPAC, in Tokyo, from which point he visited all the U.S. Army hospitals in Japan from the most northern at Sapporo on Hokkaido to the most southern at Sasebo on Kyushu (fig. 293).

At this time, the pressure for discharge of troops and other military personnel had begun to be applied in the Zone of Interior, and the process which General Eisenhower was later to describe as "demobilization by demoralization" had already begun. Specialists were in exceedingly short supply, and great care had to be exercised to utilize them wisely. The rapid transportation of patients to centers in which specialists were available or the movement of specialists to isolated areas to meet major emergencies was not practical because of poor roads, indifferent rail service, and closure of all air service during the winter. This made it necessary to staff more hospitals than would otherwise have been required with surgeons who were capable of giving definitive care in the event of major emergencies. It was a wasteful use of personnel but was the only possible plan under the circumstances.

One of the principal emergencies after the occupation of Japan was motor traffic accidents, which were frequent and serious on the narrow, poorly lighted roads traversed by a population untrained in the alertness and rapid reflexes required by modern motor cars. In November 1945, admissions from this cause were at an all-time high. At one time, traffic accidents accounted for 38 percent of all surgical admissions at the 165th Station Hospital, with compound fractures heading the list. It was not unusual to receive 5 or 10 patients at a time over the weekend, as the result of a single accident. On one occasion, 38 Japanese prisoners of war were received en masse when the vehicle in which they were being moved was overturned.[7]

Obligation in the Philippines

An unfortunate result of the rapid withdrawal of U.S. Army troops from the Philippines at the end of the fighting in the Pacific was the hardship it worked on the Philippine Army, including the Scouts. Medical care of these troops was very poor at this time, as was the medical care of guerrillas and civilians, because of the almost total destruction of medical services during the Japanese occupation. Those who were aware of how many American lives had been saved by Filipino troops and civilians, often at great cost to themselves, were much disturbed by the situation.

After observing these conditions, this consultant made certain recommendations to the Surgeon, AFPAC, 7 December 1945, as follows: (1) Provision of additional technicians to supplement the single technician then working in the braceshop set up in the 313th General Hospital in Manila; (2) provision of additional technicians to instruct Philippine Army personnel in the operation of the braceshop sent to the Philippine Army from the Zone of

---

[7] Colonel Trimble, as a result of these experiences, considered the whole question of traffic accidents so serious that, on his return to the Zone of Interior in the spring of 1946, he addressed a memorandum on the subject to The Surgeon General, through the Director, Surgical Consultants Division, Office of The Surgeon General. In it, he pointed out that at the time of writing traffic accidents were responsible for the great majority of deaths within the Army, for the largest proportion of seriously ill patients in hospitals, and for an incalculable amount of morbidity and permanent deformity. These accidents, he continued, were largely preventable, and, while accident prevention was a function of the Provost Marshal's Office, he believed that the Medical Department should assume a share of the responsibility, if only because of its responsibility for the management and end results of these injuries.

Colonel Trimble recommended that a special committee be appointed, under the jurisdiction of the Preventive Medicine Division, Office of The Surgeon General, to study the problem along epidemiologic lines and to formulate definite and vigorous directives based upon the findings of this study. The memorandum concluded with the statement that, since commercial transportation companies were able to hold their drivers to strict accountability in the matter of accidents, it was unrealistic to assume that the Army, with its far tighter control and discipline of personnel, could not achieve even better results. A similar program had been effective in the Southwest Pacific Area when it was set up in the fall of 1944.

No action was taken on these recommendations, on the ground that in the Zone of Interior safety committees were already in existence at each post and station and that a medical officer with advisory responsibility was usually assigned to them.—J. B. C., Jr.

Interior; (3) transportation of the 20-odd Scouts then in need of prosthetic appliances to amputation centers in the Zone of Interior, for necessary plastic procedures and fitting of prostheses; and (4) provision of a supply of prostheses, with a fully trained technician to take the measurements for them, to provide for personnel in the Philippines in need of surgical care after amputation.

It was not considered possible to implement these recommendations at this time, but later, in April 1946, a complete unit was sent by The Surgeon General to establish an amputation center for Filipino personnel.

Japanese Prisoners of War

Until the invasion of the Philippines, U.S. Army medical officers had no extended contacts with Japanese prisoners of war. This was partly because prisoners were not taken in large numbers and partly because they were chiefly the responsibility, from the medical standpoint, of the Australian Army Medical Department. As the number of prisoners increased, large camps to handle them were established on Leyte, Luzon, and the smaller islands of the Visayan group. American medical officers were then detailed to these camps.

Management of a typical camp

Since all prisoner-of-war camps were managed on the same general plan, the experience of the 174th Station Hospital may be cited as typical. This hospital took over hospital facilities at New Bilibid Prison from the 21st Evacuation Hospital on 2 June 1945. The report from which most of the following data are summarized was prepared at the request of this consultant by Maj. Joseph T. Kauer, MC, chief of the surgical service.[8] Other data have been obtained from the report of the official inspection of the station hospital at the prison on 2 and 3 November 1945 by a committee of medical officers of which the author was a member.[9]

The experience at this camp may be accepted as typical of the experiences of all similar camps.

During the peak of activities after V–J Day, additional facilities had to be provided at Luzon Prison Camp No. 1 at Canlubang, 5 miles away from New Bilibid, and the personnel of the 174th Station Hospital had to be augmented by personnel from the 136th General Hospital (fig. 294). When the facilities were enlarged, the policy was set up of treating all surgical patients and all of the more seriously ill medical patients at New Bilibid. Other medical patients and convalescent patients were assigned to Canlubang. Medical, surgical, and neuropsychiatric patients were segregated.

---

[8] Essential Technical Medical Data, U.S. Army Forces, Pacific, for October 1945, appendix E, subject: Medical Experiences in Luzon P.O.W. Camp No. 1.

[9] Col. I. R. Trimble, MC, Surgical Consultant, for Army Forces, Pacific, through Surgeon, Base X, and Chief Surgeon, Army Forces, Western Pacific, 7 Nov. 1945, subject: Surgical Care Afforded Japanese Patients at the 174th Station Hospital, New Bilibid Prison, and at POW Camp No. 1 (Canlubang).

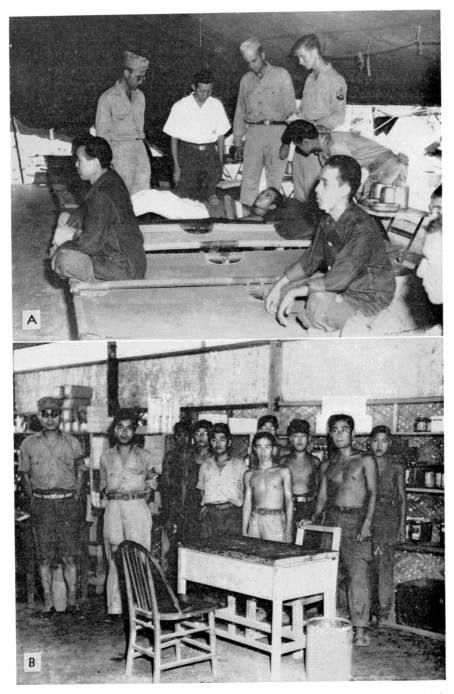

FIGURE 294.—Prison Camp No. 1 at Canlubang, Luzon.   A. Colonel Trimble (second from right, standing), inspecting the condition of a patient.   B. Medical supply.

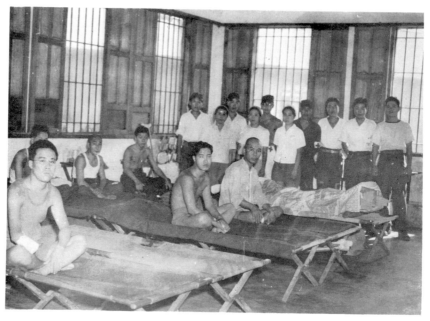

FIGURE 295.—Japanese prisoner patients and ward attendants in New Bilibid Prison, Luzon.

New Bilibid Prison, located 21 miles south of Manila was a Commonwealth of the Philippines institution, built in 1936. The long building in which professional activities were housed and which had formerly been used as a hospital contained 4 wards of 75 beds each; 3 general operating rooms; an operating room for orthopedic surgery; a supply room for sterile supplies; the X-ray department; the dental clinic; and the laboratory and pharmacy (fig. 295). Sewage facilities were modern and the water supply was adequate. This was generally true throughout the camp, even in the tented areas; improvisations were only occasionally necessary.

Between 2 June and 31 October 1945, 10,684 prisoners of war were admitted to the hospital at New Bilibid. The peak census was 5,672 in October. These patients were predominantly Japanese, with a small proportion of Formosans and Koreans. During this same period, 56,000 prisoners of war and internees were confined in 11 compounds at Canlubang. At the peak, the daily average sick call was 12,500, chiefly for skin diseases, malaria, and beriberi.

Surgical equipment and instruments were those standard for a U.S. Army station hospital. Medications were drawn from the standard Army supplies provided in medical depots. Routine laboratory examinations were performed at the prison. Specimens for special or complicated tests were sent to the 19th Medical General Laboratory in Manila. All inmates of both camps received rations equivalent to those given hospitalized American soldiers. Multivitamin powder was included in all diets, and additional vitamin therapy was prescribed as indicated (fig. 296).

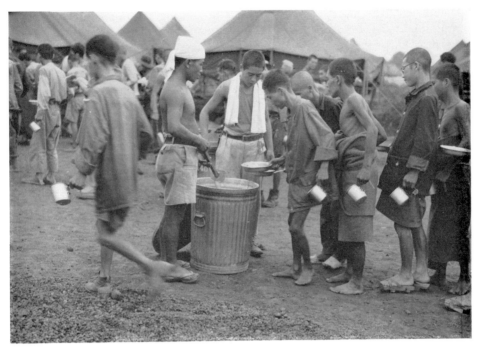

FIGURE 296.—The serving of a meal at Prison Camp No. 1, Canlubang, Luzon.

Professional personnel

At a typical peak time during the operation of New Bilibid and Canlubang camps, the professional surgical personnel at New Bilibid consisted of a chief of service with a rating of "B–3150," a surgical ward officer, a radiologist, an anesthetist, and two Dental Corps officers. The hospital census rapidly outstripped the ability of U.S. Army personnel to care for it. At one time, only two medical officers were caring for 1,900 patients, many of whom were critically ill.

To meet the shortages in personnel, Japanese medical officers, nurses, and corpsmen were pressed into service as rapidly as possible. Before V–J Day, there were only eight Japanese physicians at the prison; they had been taken prisoners when their hospital ship, which was functioning as a troop transport, had been captured in the East Indies. During the peak period, 117 Japanese medical and dental officers were utilized in both camps. Of the 58 officers assigned to New Bilibid, 28 ranked as surgeons, although only 8, including a well-trained otolaryngologist, an ophthalmologist, a gynecologist, and 2 dentists, had had any appreciable training according to American standards.

Physicians.—Japanese techniques differed widely from those employed in the United States, and the Japanese approach to all medical problems also differed widely. The physicians paid much less attention to history taking than American physicians. They were inclined to group all illnesses into broad general categories according to the presenting symptoms. Physical examinations were cursory, and, until the Japanese medical officers were taught otherwise, they examined dirty surgical cases only at a distance, regarding any other course as beneath their professional dignity. Their approach to all surgical problems was stereotyped, and they were influenced by their past general experience far more than by an independent consideration of the physiological and pathological features of the special case under consideration.

Japanese physicians needed a great deal of education in operating room techniques, beginning with the preservation of sterility. They were familiar with techniques of local and spinal analgesia, but only two or three had ever seen intravenous anesthesia administered, and none of them had had any personal experience with it. They were also unfamiliar with modern anesthetic machines. They were ignorant of the indwelling nasal catheter, continuous intestinal decompression, and closed drainage in empyema.

Penicillin meant nothing to them either as a name or as a therapeutic agent. They used sulfonamides according to standard practices but did not hesitate to place sulfathiazole powder into direct contact with nerve tissue. The use of whole blood and plasma in malnutrition and the use of plasma for burns and hypoproteinemia were outside of their experience. They relied on physiologic salt solution for intravenous therapy and treated shock by the intravenous administration of camphor. Burns were treated by the tannic acid method.

All of these practices were obviously based on German medical practices in vogue 40 years earlier. When they were discussed with them, the Japanese officers repeatedly made the point that these practices were far more suited to their economic status than the modern and elaborate system brought back by the occasional physicians who had received their training in the United States. Their interest in these modern practices was, however, intense. They fully realized that Germany was no longer the fountainhead of medical knowledge and that the pace of professional attainment in the immediate future would be set by the United States.

Nurses.—Nurses were in such short supply at New Bilibid that even when they were augmented by Japanese nurses, they could be assigned only to wards in which surgical patients and the most seriously ill medical patients were cared for. The work of these Japanese nurses was generally satisfactory. The seven nurses who had been trained at St. Luke's Hospital in Tokyo and who were used in the operating rooms compared favorably, in training and ability, with U.S.-trained nurses.

Clinical considerations

The prisoners of war received at New Bilibid Prison fell into two general groups, those received before the Japanese surrender and those received later. Many of the patients admitted to the hospital wards before V–J Day came from U.S. Army hospitals, and their good condition was in marked contrast to the status of the prisoners taken directly to the prison camps, most of whom were in poor nutritional condition by U.S. standards. Of the 2,395 surgical patients, about 50 percent had sustained gunshot wounds of various types without fractures; 14 percent had gunshot wounds with fractures associated with osteomyelitis.

After V–J Day, combat wounds became increasingly less frequent, and the chief patient load consisted of civilians, including women and children, some 300 or 400 of whom came out of the Luzon hills each day. All of them were placed on suppressive Atabrine (quinacrine hydrochloride) treatment for malaria as soon as they were admitted. Many of them were suffering from irreversible nutritional and deficiency diseases. Their condition suggested that of inmates of German concentration camps, and numbers of them died within a few hours of admission.

Surgical conditions.—None of the patients with combat-incurred wounds had received adequate care by U.S. Army standards. No wounds had been debrided, and all degrees of suppuration and gangrene were observed. Fractures, if they were splinted at all, were immobilized only crudely, with bamboo splints. Very few combat-incurred wounds could be managed by early secondary closure, regardless of the time at which they were seen, because of the patients' general status. Malnutrition and deficiency diseases presented a most unfavorable background for the management of all surgical conditions. The treatment of these diseases, in fact, had to take precedence over all but the most dire surgical emergencies.

Anemia and hypoproteinemia, even after intensive therapy, retarded the response to ideal surgical management. Whole blood was used liberally in these cases, donors being obtained from healthy prisoners of war on work details. Women and children with severe hypoproteinemia were treated by plasma transfusions. There were no serious reactions to these methods.

A few late closures of combat-incurred soft-tissue wounds were done with good results, but most wounds of this kind were handled better by skin grafting than by excision and closure. Results of skin grafting were, surprisingly, about as good as among U.S. Army casualties.

A number of cases of tetanus developed, as was to be expected under the conditions. Two patients died from this cause a few hours after they had been admitted, and there were two other later deaths in the remaining thirteen cases. Therapy was by standard measures.

There were also four cases of gas gangrene, one of which was fatal. One of the remaining patients required amputation of the leg, but the other two responded to wide incision, in one instance of the lower leg and in the other of the upper arm. All of these patients received antitoxin.

As a matter of necessity, most surgery after V–J Day was done by Japanese medical officers, U.S. Army surgeons limiting themselves to the most serious procedures, such as intestinal surgery. During the June–October period of the operation of the camp, there were 110 major and 706 minor operations, and 245 casts were applied. The lack of surgical experience and judgment of Japanese medical officers was reflected in the 33 appendectomies done by them in October for supposed acute disease. Only 11 of these patients really had acute appendicitis, and the elementary notion of aseptic technique possessed by the Japanese surgeons was evident in the 12 percent incidence of infected wounds.

Beriberi abscess.—An entirely new clinical entity (new, at least, to U.S. Army medical officers) was observed in many of these patients, so-called beriberi abscess. The infection, which occurred on the lower extremity, usually in the anterior tibial area or on the dorsum of the foot, began as an extremely soft, fluctuant swelling. Neither rubor nor calor was present, and tenderness was not significant. When the swelling was incised, subcutaneous pus was released; only in longstanding cases was the fascia involved. The pus was thick, yellow, and of the typical *Staphylococcus* type, but the etiology was not established, for the circumstances were not favorable for bacteriologic studies and none were made. The abscess cavity was lined with necrotic subcutaneous tissue, and in no instance could a definite wall be demonstrated.

As a rule, these abscesses appeared in extremities that were or had been the site of serious nutritional edema; in two instances, the edema was so intense that necrosis of the skin occurred. Their etiology was never clarified. It was concluded that edema, although it was probably not an essential predisposing factor, apparently favored the growth of organisms which had entered the skin by way of the abrasions and scabietic lesions so prominent among these patients.

Evaluation of medical care

Upon orders of the Chief Surgeon, AFPAC, the prison camps at New Bilibid and Canlubang were visited on 2 and 3 November 1945, by a committee of medical officers consisting of Col. Albert R. Dresibach, MC, chairman; Lt. Col. Clarke H. Barnacle, MC, recorder; and the author.[10] The objective of the inspection was to determine whether the medical care and general treatment of sick and wounded Japanese prisoners of war and internees at these installations accorded with the provisions of the Geneva Convention. The committee report was entirely favorable; both medical care and general treatment, including the diet provided, fully conformed with these provisions. Not a fly was seen in either camp.

The findings of this committee were in agreement with those of Brig. Gen. Hugh J. Morgan, and Col. Francis R. Dieuaide, MC, who had visited the camps previously as representatives of The Surgeon General, U.S. Army.

These formal reports confirmed the information obtained on informal attempts to gain some idea of the attitude of the patients in the camps toward U.S. Army personnel and of their reaction to the treatment which they were receiving. Interpreters were directed to make inquiries along these lines at times when U.S. medical officers were not on the wards and were also instructed to report on conversations among the patients.

---

[10] See footnote 9, p. 748.

Without exception, the patients were very grateful. Some said that discipline in the U.S. Army must be very strict, since they had never seen a commissioned or a noncommissioned officer strike a patient. Many expressed amazement that American medical officers themselves examined and dressed their wounds; in the Japanese Army, this was the duty of the corpsmen. They also expressed amazement that American medical officers answered night calls.

These and other instances of what Western physicians conceive of as only normal medical care were to these prisoners signs of kindness and consideration which were evidently unique in their experience. Their army training had led them to expect only brutality and neglect from their own nationals, and propaganda had led them to expect the same kind of treatment from their U.S. and other Western conquerors.

Lessons of the Pacific Fighting

Certain conclusions set down by the surgical consultant in the Southwest Pacific Area after his return to civilian life may be summarized as follows:

1. It is strange that such an obvious principle as that of early and expert definitive surgical care was not automatically adopted at the beginning of World War II, when experts in the various surgical specialties joined the Army in such great numbers. It was slow to be adopted in the Southwest Pacific Area, chiefly because the value of the consultant system was slow to be realized. Consultants were assigned to headquarters in the smallest possible numbers. There were no consultants to the armies operating in the Southwest Pacific until after the landings in Leyte, in October 1944. The surgical consultant in the Southwest Pacific Area was permitted to participate in the attack on Leyte but was refused permission to accompany the transports in the attack on Luzon. More intimate contacts between theater and Army consultants and surgeons would have enhanced the efficiency of medical care of casualties.

2. At the beginning of the war, there were only a handful of expertly trained clinical surgeons in the Regular U.S. Army. To the end of the war, there was still a scattered lack of appreciation of the difference between a medical officer *designated* to do surgery and a medical officer *trained* to do surgery. In the Pacific, at least, there was only slow realization of the extreme importance of the wisdom of sending experienced surgeons of mature judgment into forward areas and assigning younger, less experienced surgeons to base hospitals, where they could work under supervision.

3. The chief duty of the surgical consultant in the Southwest Pacific Area was the assignment of good surgeons to serve as chiefs of surgery in the portable hospitals supporting the various landings. This was an extremely difficult task because of the paucity of well-trained surgeons in the Pacific; practically all of them were sent to the Mediterranean and European theaters, or were in the Zone of Interior.

4. The vast distances in the Pacific greatly complicated medical care of casualties. Sometimes 2,600 miles separated the target area and the point from

which an operation was mounted. In hops to small, isolated islands, there was no such thing as a chain of evacuation. Definitive surgical care had to be given on the spot. Specialized hospitals were accepted as a practical possibility only after the Philippine invasions.

5. Distances in the Pacific also made communication extremely difficult. Brig. Gen. Elliott C. Cutler, MC, Chief Consultant in Surgery, Office of the Chief Surgeon, European Theater of Operations, U.S. Army, stated that he could sit at his desk at headquarters in London and within a few minutes reach by telephone the commanding officer of any hospital in England or on the Continent. In the Pacific, even radio communication was not possible, and most business had to be conducted by mail. Attempts to transfer medical officers might take a month or more. A visit by plane to hospitals in the various bases might take a minimum of 2 weeks, partly because of waiting for priorities and the vagaries of the weather; the visit itself was likely to consume the smallest part of the time period.

6. Evacuation of casualties in the Pacific fighting was always a problem. Portable surgical hospitals were sometimes miles ahead of the artillery pieces going into the jungle. The hospitals would follow the infantry and set up a few hundred yards from the enemy. Evacuation was necessarily a complicated process. It was first by litter, sometimes borne by natives but more often by Army litter bearers because the natives did not like to go forward. Then native litter bearers would take over later. Sometimes, evacuation was by ox-drawn cart or by amphibious vehicle.

Air evacuation, which was an outstanding success and solved many of the problems of transportation in the Pacific, came late in the war.

7. Surgical teams were proposed very early in the Pacific fighting by Colonel Parsons, first Consultant in Surgery in the area, but the plan was not accepted until April 1944. Auxiliary surgical groups never served in the Pacific; all of them were sent to the Mediterranean or European theaters. Portable surgical hospitals helped to solve the problems of forward care of casualties but did not prove an entirely acceptable solution. Specialized hospitals, as already mentioned, were not permitted until the Philippines were invaded and never really fulfilled their possibilities.

8. The difficulties of surgical care of casualties in the climate, terrain, and vast distances of the Pacific areas were probably never fully realized in the Office of The Surgeon General because there were no really intimate contacts between that office and the Pacific. The single visit, during the course of the hardest fighting, was by the Consultant in Surgery in that office and was very brief. The only other visit, by The Surgeon General, was also brief and did not occur until after the Philippines had been almost secured.

9. The difficulties under which medical care was accomplished in the Pacific are unlikely to occur again. For one thing, the value of the consultant system is now fully appreciated in the Medical Department of the Army and is firmly established in it. For another, the Medical Department has set up

residencies in its largest hospitals in the various specialties and is thus assured of a supply of fully trained medical officers in the event of another emergency.

10. Far and away the most valuable surgical lesson learned by the U.S. Army Medical Corps during World War II was not the use of penicillin, or of large quantities of whole blood, or of evacuation by air of the wounded—great as these advances were. The most valuable lesson was the realization of the validity of the concept, well known to all trained surgeons, and also learned and then forgotten by the Medical Corps after World War I, that the mortality and morbidity of combat casualties can be reduced to a minimum only when mature, highly trained surgeons are available in forward areas of combat.

The consultant's own experiences, both triumphs and disappointments, and the similar experiences of others, bear out this concept. Any acceptable plans for surgical support of future operations must follow the same principle. If any plans contain even the possibility of delay on the availability of immediate, definitive surgical care by surgical experts, they should be discarded forthwith.

I. Ridgeway Trimble, M.D.

ORTHOPEDIC SURGERY

Maj. (later Lt. Col.) George O. Eaton, MC, reported for active duty on 20 April 1942 as chief of the orthopedic section of the 118th General Hospital (fig. 297). Less than one month after activation, the unit proceeded to the west coast and embarked for oversea duty. After approximately one year of hospital duty at Sydney, Australia, Major Eaton received orders placing him on duty in the Office of the Surgeon, USASOS, SWPA, as the Consultant in Orthopedic Surgery. Headquarters at that time was at Sydney, Australia, but was almost immediately moved to Brisbane, Australia, approximately 500 miles closer to the combat zone in New Guinea with still some 1,700 miles intervening.

Functions and Activities

The orthopedic consultant served first under the direction of Col. Wm. Barclay Parsons, MC, Consultant in Surgery, USASOS, SWPA, and later under Colonel Parsons' successor, Col. I. Ridgeway Trimble, MC. He was charged with the responsibility of care of wounds of the extremities and spine, in addition to nonbattle injuries, which were at least 10 times as frequent. The nonbattle injuries closely resembled civilian practice as regards clinical management, except that transportation and evacuation policies had to be integrated with treatment of fractures and soft-tissue injuries.

At the beginning of the war in the Pacific, the reason for having consultants was little understood by those in command positions. When reporting into a base in the forward area, courtesy, convention, and orders required his reporting to the commanding officer as well as the base surgeon. It was the exception rather than the rule that the mission of the consultant met with the enthusiastic approval of those key officers. The fact that the consultant's

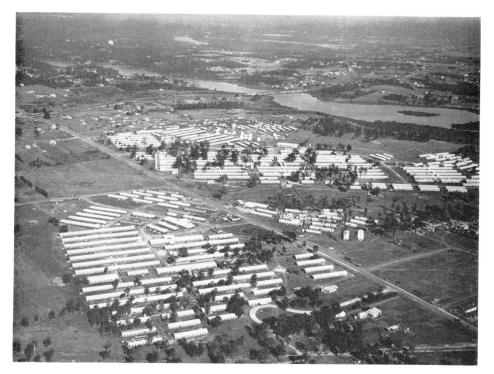

FIGURE 297.—Base 7, Sydney, Australia, and the 118th General Hospital, 1943.

report with its estimate of caliber of local efficiency was reported to the theater surgeon, but not back to the base, protected the consultant but at the same time tended to make him rate as a necessary nuisance, somewhat analogous to an uninvited guest. In forward areas, the consultant had to use various forms of hitchhiking and was usually dependent on the hospitality of the unit being visited. A visit from a consultant was often rated by the recipient as an inspection, and indeed at times the consultants were under orders to include an estimate of the quality and operation of utilities, mess, and other activities only remotely related to the surgical care of patients.

The fact that there was no provision in the tables of organization for consultants further added to the difficulties under which they worked. If a medical officer was assigned to a headquarters for duty as a consultant, his chance of promotion was essentially nil. Administrative officers, rather than consultants, were given priority for any promotional opportunities. Consultants of low field-grade or company-grade rank had less influence with a full colonel commanding a hospital or serving as a base surgeon.

There were several affiliated general hospital units in the Southwest Pacific Area that were replete with very high-grade medical talent from a medical school. One such unit was left so far behind the center of activities that it had almost no patients. When the orthopedic consultant tried to persuade the commanding officer to permit the reassignment of two of his three good orthopedic surgeons to units that had none, his answer was that his unit represented their alma mater and was not to be molested no matter how urgent the need was elsewhere.

The Southwest Pacific Area included all Australia plus New Guinea and the nearby islands. A consultant's travel was almost entirely by air. The usual procedure was to request approval to make a consultant trip when such a move was indicated, and orders were generally promptly approved and issued. Such a trip would include visiting all army hospitals in a given area, so long as they were operated under command of USASOS, SWPA. If the unit were under command of the Sixth U.S. Army or the Eighth U.S. Army, the USASOS consultants were out of bounds unless especially invited by the army command. A visit to a general hospital would consist of a 1-, 2-, or 3-day visit, seeing all cases, approving or criticizing management of cases, giving teaching ward rounds, spreading information as to newer development in the management of specific problems, and, sometimes, explaining the rationale of directives and technical memorandums. In smaller units such as station, evacuation, and field hospitals, the orthopedic consultant's obvious duty sometimes was to teach a medical officer who was not especially or adequately trained in orthopedics how to manage the usual orthopedic problems. It should be mentioned in passing that the station hospitals, field hospitals, and evacuation hospitals performed essentially identical missions in the Southwest Pacific Area. The smaller units seemed to value the visit of a consultant and made him feel very much needed. The opportunity for teaching by working several days with an incompletely trained medical officer presented itself very frequently and was utilized to the great advantage of the patient (fig. 298).

Management of Patients With Low Back Complaints

The Southwest Pacific Area was a wide geographical area, and this fact led to the development of many minor changes in the treatment of the wounded and injured because of geographical factors and evacuation policies. It was necessary to develop a working rule for the management of patients with low back complaints. The incidence of such complaints seemed to increase whenever service became less attractive and sometimes when it became more hazardous. Some of the younger medical officers who were incompletely trained did not feel free to take on the responsibility of sending a patient back to duty if he was complaining of disabling, low back pain.

It became necessary to define by a technical memorandum the recognition of spondylolisthesis by X-ray examination and how to avoid making a diagnosis of spondylolisthesis when none was present. Spondyloschisis was also frequently discovered in the study of a patient. In the case of spondylolisthesis, the recommendation was made that such patients be evacuated to the Zone of Interior for disposition, with the application of a supporting plaster jacket and with the lumbar spine in mild flexion for transportation if pain was severe

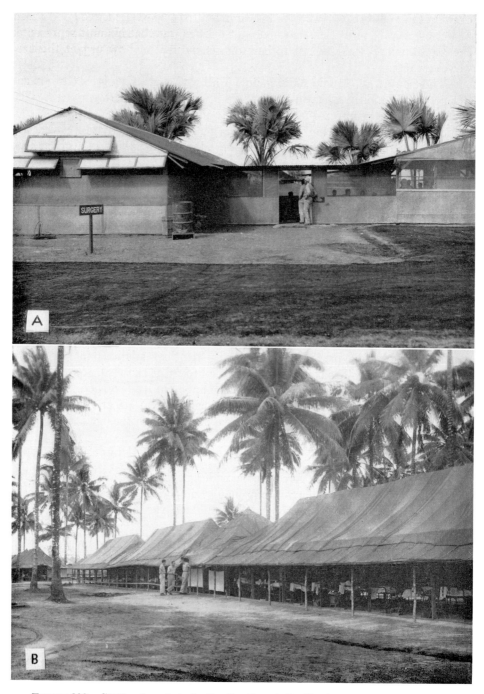

FIGURE 298.—Station hospitals in the Southwest Pacific Area. A. The operating pavilion of the 13th Station Hospital, Mindoro, Philippine Islands, February 1945. B. The 155th Station Hospital, Morotai, 2 June 1945.

or displacement very marked. A patient with preslipped spondylolisthesis, or spondyloschisis, if the condition was accompanied by moderate or severe complaints, was also recommended to be returned to the Zone of Interior.

Congenital anomalies of the spine (such as spina bifida occulta, sacralization of lumbar vertebrae unilateral or bilateral, lumbarization of sacral vertebrae, six lumbar vertebrae, ununited accessory ossification centers in the transverse or posterior spinous processes) were found with approximately the same frequency in patients with or without low back complaints. The discovery of such anomalies was not sufficient reason to hospitalize or change the duty status of the complainer, and it was necessary to spread the word that the discovery of such anomalies was not to be given weight when deciding on the disposition of a patient. It was recommended that the degree and reality of the disability in the function of the back, as determined by positive physical findings, should in such cases be the basis for decision in regard to return to duty, reassignment, or evacuation to the Zone of Interior. The rule was gradually developed that the medical officer would use the diagnostic facilities at his command for the investigation of a low back complaint and, if insufficient positive objective findings developed, the officer was to send that soldier back to duty rather than to send him to a rear and larger hospital for more exhaustive investigation of his complaint.

Evacuation Policy

In the early part of the war, the evacuation policy was determined by the relative frequency of opportunity to send patients back to the Zone of Interior by water. Air evacuation had not yet been developed. Consequently, the policy was that a patient who could not probably be returned to duty in 90 days should be tagged for evacuation to the Zone of Interior. It frequently happened that the patient would remain in a rear base hospital for 30 to 60 days awaiting transportation by ship to the Zone of Interior. As transportation facilities improved and as air evacuation became more prevalent, the evacuation policy was gradually reduced to 60 days, then to 30 days, and even less.

Transportation of Fractures

The following rules were laid down in the treatment of fractures admitted to any unit forward of the hospital that would give definitive treatment prior to evacuation to the Zone of Interior. Three essentials were named: (1) The treatment of shock, (2) care of the soft part wounds, and (3) immobilization for transportation. It was estimated that about 68 percent of battle wounds were of the extremities. About one-half of these were fractures, so that some 34 percent of battle wounds were compound fractures. Attention to length and alinement, although desirable, was not stressed if it jeopardized any of the three main essentials, prolonged the operative time, or involved manipulations which predisposed to infection. The main difference between military and civil practice was the necessity for transporting the soldier. Transporting involved jolting which caused shock, shifting of the tissue planes, bleeding, the accumulation of fluid in dead spaces, and infection. A lapse of 2 or 3 weeks after infliction of the wound was not too long a delay before the successful restoration of length and alinement could be obtained in the ordinary compound fracture encountered in combat. This statement is not to be taken to mean that the bone wound was unimportant. The first stage of bone repair depended on vascularized tissue from the surrounding soft parts. The later stages involved actual bone repair from the bone ends which therefore had to be in contact. After transportation to a hospital where the patient could be kept for the required period, the bone wound assumed importance equal to that of the soft parts. Since all major fractures required prolonged hospitalization, they were to be evacuated to the rear as soon as their condition permitted.

The Thomas' splint was useful for the transportation of cases of femoral fracture from the battalion aid station to the first hospital for definitive treatment. It was not recommended and was not used for further transportation to rear echelon hospitals as it did not provide the essential complete immobilization. Any of the methods of applying traction through the Thomas' splint during extended transportation were unsatisfactory. The Tobruk splint, which was developed in the famous defense of Tobruk in the Middle East, was publicized for a while as an excellent method of management of compound fractures of the femur but proved to be entirely unsatisfactory. Properly applied, a one-and-a-half spica cast was the method of choice for the transportation of femoral fractures, and other long bone fractures were transported in a solid plaster cast which was split the entire length of the limb. In applying the cast the optimum position of the fragments was obtained if easily accomplished, but it was again emphasized that, for transportation, immobilization was relatively of far greater importance than the position of the fragments.

To avoid the needless and often harmful frequent changing of casts, a note was made on the field medical record as to any anticipated or feared complications, or if, on the other hand, evacuation without changing the cast could be expected with confidence. Plating and operative fixation of fractures in any of the forward units was discouraged because of the likelihood of infection and the danger of damage in transportation. The journey to the base hospital was begun by the patient with a compound fracture after shock therapy had been completed, the wound had been debrided, and the fracture immobilized. In the early days of the New Guinea campaign, the distance was about 1,500 air miles, and evacuation might be by ship or plane with numerous stops and ambulance rides en route. Stops would be made at military hospitals, and a tendency developed to change the cast at each stop in order to observe and report the condition of the wound. For this reason, the rule was made that a patient would not be subjected to change of cast if his temperature was normal, the injured limb comfortable, and the circulation in the toes or fingers normal. This rule proved to be satisfactory and practical.

All patients with compound fractures had a normal expectancy of not returning to duty within 4 months and were therefore destined to complete their convalescence in the United States. Treatment in skeletal traction of compound femoral fractures in forward units, such as field and evacuation hospitals, had to be discouraged and eliminated. There was too much risk of attack by air, in which case it would not have been possible to put the patient into a protective slit trench. Thus, the only place in the oversea theater that a compound fracture of the femur could be safely treated in skeletal traction was at the rear base hospitals, out of reach of possible enemy air attack. In the later days when air evacuation became available, the patient was returned to the Zone of Interior in his plaster spica cast by air evacuation and put up in traction after arrival and assignment to a hospital in the United States.

The experience in the Southwest Pacific Area with the immediate open reduction of simple shaft fractures was not good, and the routine use of open reduction and fixation as an elective method of treatment was discouraged and frowned upon. In the forward areas, in field hospitals operating under tents, in the jungles, or around air strips, contamination and infection played too big a role to justify the hazard of open reduction as contrasted with the relative safety of closed reduction.

The transportation of compound fractures of the humerus in traction by means of hanging casts proved to be so unsatisfactory that the Air Transport Command announced that such patients would not be accepted for evacuation. The lack of immobilization led to swelling, bleeding, and pain and markedly increased the problems connected with the evacuation of such patients. The only exception to the rule of not transporting patients in traction was in the case of guillotine amputations. The maintenance of continuous, even traction of the skin during evacuation of amputees was considered to be of the highest importance to the end result of such cases. The use of elastic traction proved to be more effective in maintaining a continuous, even traction during evacuation. Accordingly, an elastic cord for traction was provided through medical supply sources, and this item became available on requisition for use in the transportation of amputees. The cord was constructed of multiple rubber fibers and was supplied in a length of from 8 to 12 inches, which was sufficient length for a single case.

Classification and Selection of Patients for Evacuation

In order to expedite the evacuation of major clinical problems to rear area general hospitals for further study and treatment, station, field, and evacuation hospitals were advised to classify selected cases for evacuation to a general hospital. The evacuation of such cases was ordered not to be interrupted at subsequent station hospitals en route except when the patient's condition was such as to require immediate interruption in the transportation journey. The fact that the general hospital type of treatment was indicated was shown by placing "GH" in red on the roster immediately preceding the name and number of the patient and on the face of the field medical jacket just above the patient's name. In general, major orthopedic conditions, including fractures

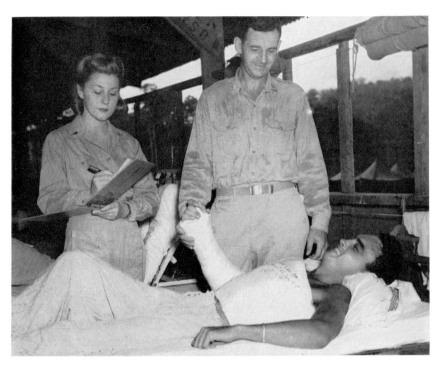

FIGURE 299.—An orthopedic casualty in the 54th General Hospital, Hollandia, New Guinea, after evacuation from Leyte, January 1945.

requiring more than 60 days of hospitalization, were classed as "GH" cases (fig. 299). In cases of chronic low back complaints, chronic joint complaints, and chronic foot complaints, if no positive objective findings appeared after study (including X-ray, laboratory, and psychiatric investigation), and when complaints were disproportionate to the organic findings, it was recommended that the patient be returned to duty with reassurance. Only in the case of repeated admissions were such patients to be evacuated to a general hospital for further study, treatment, and disposition.

Summary and Recommendations

In the Southwest Pacific Area during World War II, any question of contact of the consultants with the Office of The Surgeon General was strictly informal and unofficial and, understandably, was frowned upon. The Office of The Surgeon General could perform a very useful function in a more or less global type of war by acting in the capacity of transmitter of information gained by experience in other theaters. Each theater will have its own peculiar problems, and it is difficult to see how the Office of The Surgeon General could appreciate or could advise in such problems unless it had firsthand experience with such specialized matters. Statistics of World War II will show a marked improvement over those of World War I in the rate of survival and the escape from permanent crippling disabilities of individuals suffering wounds of the extremities. This improvement will be primarily the result not of advances in chemotherapy but rather of advances in shock therapy and in wound management. Further improvement will be possible.

The command and administrative branch of the Medical Corps must take a more active interest in the clinical welfare of the patient. The visit of The Surgeon General to the Pacific areas in the early months of 1945 was a most powerful and pleasant stimulus to the average professional medical officer. Here was the highest ranking medical officer in the Army of the United States on a tour of inspection, making clinical bedside rounds, and giving helpful instruction and criticism to the ward officer. The consultant system, begun in World War I and enlarged in World War II, is the key to improving the quality of medical service rendered to patients. Particularly in the more forward areas, the average young surgeon is loaded with more responsibility than he has been trained to assume. He is notably conscientious and anxious that his patients should receive the best possible treatment. He is unable to follow the patient's progress after evacuation. Circulars and memorandums have a way of not reaching him. Only by the visits of consultants can he learn of his errors and of new methods and procedures.

Military surgery has made great strides, but even more progress will be made if more emphasis is placed upon the quality of professional accomplishment. Command and administrative officers in the Medical Corps should look upon the consultant as a teacher rather than an inspector and should not use the consultant to check on activities other than those directly related to the welfare of the patient. Provision should be made in the tables of organization for appropriate rank for consultants. Officers commanding medical units should be expected to place a high degree of importance on the quality of the medical care the patient in his unit receives instead of being nearly entirely concerned with the impeccable management of utilities and visits of Inspectors General.

GEORGE O. EATON, M.D.

CHAPTER XIII

From Auckland to Tokyo

Ashley W. Oughterson, M.D.

INTRODUCTORY NOTE

The material in this chapter is derived from the official wartime diary of the late Ashley W. Oughterson, M.D., and is presented in substantially the form in which the then Colonel Oughterson prepared it. The original plan was for Dr. Oughterson to write this chapter, from his diary and other official papers. With his untimely death, that plan became impossible, and, since no one else possessed the information, the best solution seemed to be to use the material he had recorded during the war.

Dr. Oughterson, Clinical Professor of Surgery at the Yale University Medical School, entered active duty in the Medical Corps of the U.S. Army in January 1942 as a lieutenant colonel (fig. 300). His first assignment took him to the Army Medical School, Walter Reed Army Medical Center, Washington, D.C. From April to June 1942, he was at Lovell General Hospital, Fort Devens, Mass., as chief of the surgical service. He was next assigned to the 39th General Hospital, a medical unit sponsored by and affiliated with the Yale University Medical School. The unit was staged at Camp Edwards, Mass., and was subsequently shipped to New Zealand, where it established facilities at Auckland in November 1942. Colonel Oughterson served as chief of the surgical service of the 39th General Hospital until March 1943, and then as hospital commander until July of the same year.

It was after this experience that Colonel Oughterson received his first assignment as a surgical consultant. As the tempo of fighting in the Pacific accelerated, he was moved from one key assignment to another, wherever the services of a medical officer of his capabilities were urgently needed. As a result, Colonel Oughterson eventually served as a surgical consultant in every major command in the Pacific theater of war. His account may overlap portions of others in this section on the activities of surgical consultants in the Pacific areas, but his outlook and perspective differed somewhat from those whose interests were perhaps more parochial. Related accounts are also presented in chapters XVII and XIX of "Activities of Surgical Consultants, Volume I" of this historical series. These chapters, by Dr. Frank Glenn and Dr. Frank J. McGowan, respectively, pertain to consultation in surgery in the Sixth and Eighth U.S. Armies, which served in the Southwest Pacific Area.

The diary material has been compiled and edited by Maj. James K. Arima, MSC, and Pfc. Jacques Kornberg of The Historical Unit, U.S. Army Medical Service, but editing has been kept to a minimum.

Since this account was prepared, for the most part, from handwritten notebooks maintained by Dr. Oughterson during his war service, as Editor-in-Chief of the historical series, I considered it advisable to have the manuscript reviewed by the former chief surgeons of the commands in which Dr. Oughterson served. They were Brig. Gen. Earl Maxwell, MC, USAF (Ret.); Maj. Gen. John M. Willis, MC, USA (Ret.); and Maj. Gen. Guy B. Denit, MC, USA (Ret.). These reviewers were asked to verify the general authenticity of

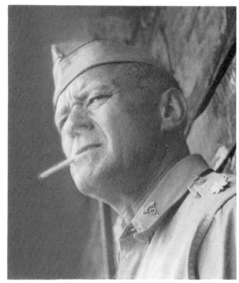

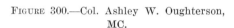

Figure 300.—Col. Ashley W. Oughterson, MC.

Colonel Oughterson's statements, and, especially, to add any comments wherever their broader knowledge of the events discussed might place the data in better perspective for the reader. They were also asked to review the manuscript in the light of subsequent events, just as Dr. Oughterson might have done had he lived to do so himself.

The general comments of these reviewers follow in this introductory note. Their comments on specific passages are included as footnotes in the appropriate places. The reviewer making the comment is identified by his initials.

With respect to the entire manuscript, General Maxwell commented:

I have made very few corrections or comments since it [the diary] was so typically the thoughts of such a great organizer. To change the wording or to delete some of his caustic remarks I think would detract from the entire theme of the manuscript.

I will assure you that the entire diary is exactly the thinking of a mature mind on a very difficult subject. Dr. Oughterson, or "Scotty" as we all called him, believed in saying exactly what he thought and I believe if he could have edited this manuscript he would still think and write the same context.

General Willis wrote:

I do not mean to be disparaging toward Colonel Oughterson's service, because I think he did a magnificent job. I do not, however, believe that he realized that the tactical use of medical units had been a subject of study by experienced officers ever since the end of World War I, nor do I believe he realized that these tactical units were "personneled" by officers of little military experience, and necessarily there were many square pegs in round holes and vice versa. These could only be "fitted" by removal from one place to another, involving transportation which was at a premium.

* * * I firmly do not believe in placing the highly experienced surgeon in the Battalion Aid Station or even an Advanced Surgical Hospital. I think they could be of greater use to a greater number further back.

In explanation of the latter point, General Willis noted: "[Dr. Oughterson] entered active duty * * * with a wide experience in peace-time general surgery. Unfortunately, there were too few such qualified surgeons and even fewer who were available to the Military Service." Had the type of surgeons Dr. Oughterson desired been provided, as he advised, in sufficient numbers "to man the Clearing Stations, the Portable Surgical Hospitals, the Field Hospitals, and the Battalion Aid Stations, the evacuees at the general hospitals, both advanced and at home bases, would have suffered, and many of those still training would never have arrived at the front to relieve the tired and wounded already engaged in combat."

General Willis also noted that certain conditions in the western Pacific in late 1944 and early 1945, upon which Dr. Oughterson had commented adversely, existed as a result of policies and practices in effect before his (General Willis') arrival on the scene, and "everything by that time had been formulated and was going." Moreover, General Willis informed me in a telephone conversation on the Oughterson diary in February 1959: "* * * I arrived in Hawaii around the middle of November in '44 and left there on the 31st of January or the 1st of February with Kirk, Simmons, and Welch and that group down there and went over to the South Pacific. Of course I didn't have anything to do with the South Pacific—but it [the tour] did include Saipan and those places, so I went with them to see that, and, being with them, I had to go all the way around."

Another point is evident from General Willis' remarks, that, when Colonel Oughterson was himself in the Marianas, he might not have been fully aware of the planning that was going on in Hawaii and also might not have appreciated the time required to put theater plans into effect so that results would be noticeable at the working level where he was. He might, General Willis thought, have taken into more consideration the fact that many of the problems that faced the medical service in the Pacific existed, and continued to exist, as a consequence of circumstances outside the control of the Medical Department.

Finally, General Willis wrote: (1) "The early sections of Col. Oughterson's report deal with observations, comments and criticisms without giving the credit to the younger and perhaps less talented medical officers who were working in the most unfavorable conditions, but nevertheless were giving everything they had"; (2) "The routine ½ gr. of morphine, the too-tight plaster bandage, the poorly kept records and the failure to transmit them with the patients were the results of 'hurried-up training' at the home training centers, but such was necessary because of the pressing need of replacements;" and (3) the slow evacuation sometimes evident in the Pacific was "the result of the lack of sufficient transportation and the distances involved."

General Denit's comments were as follows:

Thank you for letting me see Colonel Oughterson's manuscript. I am glad it is to be published. I think it is very interesting. I wish I had been able to keep notes as he did.

My general comment is that I am not inclined to take exception to anything he has to say. After all he gives the picture as he sees it.

Let me say here about any medical history of the Pacific Areas, the organization of the Pacific was so complicated that in order to understand how the medical services functioned, one would have to study the overall administrative volumes of the history of each headquarters of the Pacific Areas. To do this would require many months of study. Therefore, to write a correct history and to find out who did what in the various medical headquarters would be impossible unless one had had experience in all areas of the Pacific. Now take General MacArthur's headquarters. He did most of his fighting with so-called task forces. The CG of the task force, most often General Krueger, but not always by any means, would determine his needs to carry out his missions. This of course included medical units. I *sometimes* got a chance to review and comment but no amount of pleading could change things if the CG, task forces, ruled otherwise. Of course I never thought enough medical means were provided. Often I was right.

Then when the means in way of organizations were provided, the task force commander would not force his engineers to build minimum facilities for the hospital. Hence my remark [p. 852] that the Army wouldn't obey orders. Many times, in fact at all times the engineers were way behind schedule in helping the medical service *build its* own hospitals. But such is war in the jungles. No one who hasn't experienced it can believe the difficulties encountered.

For instance * * * the Signal Officer * * * was next to General MacArthur and had his ear. In every area he got the high ground for radio; I took what was left. Not only that, but he said our X-ray and diathermy machines caused interference with his sending and receiving communications, so we had to be a certain distance from his installations. Hence the *frog ponds* for hospital areas. In truth, though, all areas at certain seasons in the tropics are mud holes.

I wish it were possible for me to tell of how the complex organization made it impossible for the Chief Surgeon of the American Forces in the SWPA [Southwest Pacific Area] and USAFFE [U.S. Army Forces in the Far East] to force upon the various commands his ideas. Even when his recommendations to GHQ were accepted they were not carried out by the task force commanders. Possibly in a number of instances tactical considerations governed.

I will say this. The medical service knew what it wanted, its planning was good, and, considering all factors, the medical service of the Southwest Pacific Area was superb. General MacArthur said so repeatedly.

    *   *   *   *   *   *   *

I had a great admiration for Colonel Oughterson and gave him the job of "thinking" and advising me on how surgery and care of the wounded could be improved. I didn't want him to have any administrative authority. I wanted him to (1) see, (2) think and (3) advise. Often when one tries to correct he loses his value as an adviser.

    *   *   *   *   *   *   *

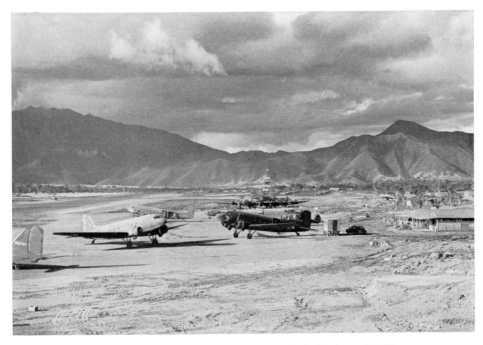

FIGURE 301.—Tontouta Airfield, New Caledonia, August 1943.

The use of Colonel Oughterson's diary was necessary, as already noted, because of the information contained in it and not available elsewhere. In the light of the comments of the chief surgeons under whom he served, its publication in essentially the form in which it was written by him during his wartime service seems even more justified.

Col. JOHN BOYD COATES, Jr., MC, USA
Editor in Chief

Auckland, Friday, 6 August 1943

Orders today from COMGENSOPAC [Commanding General, South Pacific], permanent transfer to USAFISPA [U.S. Army Forces in the South Pacific Area].[1]

Nouméa, Wednesday, 11 August

Took off in a B-24 at 0730. Down at Tontouta Airfield, 1400 (fig. 301).

Quartered at Nouméa [Headquarters for USAFISPA was at Nouméa, New Caledonia] in the Grant Hotel Central which I am told was formerly a house of ill repute (fig. 302).

---

[1] U.S. Army Forces in the South Pacific Area was established in July 1942 with responsibility for the administration, supply, and training of the U.S. Army ground and air troops stationed in the South Pacific Area.

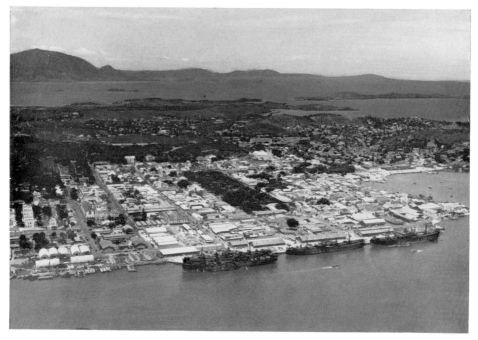

FIGURE 302.—Nouméa, New Caledonia.   An aerial view of the central part of the city.

Saturday, 14 August

Looked over the medical supply situation with Colonel Stuart [Col. Samuel E. Stuart, MC, Deputy Surgeon, USAFISPA].   Met Maj. Gen. Robert G. Breene, chief of SOS [Services of Supply].   "We are fighting the Japs, not each other."

Monday, 16 August

Visited the 31st Station Hospital. Poor site—hot—construction fair. Records fair.   No monthly records are kept on surgery.   Excellent equipment. They are having trouble with skintight plaster casts.   A vaginal insufflator is needed.

Espíritu Santo, Tuesday, 17 August

Arose at 0200.   Drove to Tontouta Airbase.   Arrived at Espíritu Santo Island [New Hebrides].   Visited the 25th Evacuation Hospital, Chicago group—excellent.   Casualties are arriving here with dirty wounds.   Lt. Col. (later Col.) Willis J. Potts, MC, the chief of surgery, wants a proctoscope, Berman locator, smaller catgut, plaster knives, shears, Roger Anderson pins, light bulbs, lead letters for X-ray, jars for sutures.   He has too many silver clips.

Wednesday, 18 August

Made rounds at the 25th Evacuation Hospital.   Saw about 35 patients. Maj. (later Col.) Harold A. Sofield, MC, is in charge of orthopedics.   They do elective operations on patients remaining on the island—knees, removal of large chondroma. Very few infections have occurred.

Visited the 122d Station Hospital.

Guadalcanal, Thursday, 19 August

Off at 0800 in General Owens' [Brig. Gen. Ray L. Owens, Deputy Commander, Thirteenth Air Force] plane. Arrived at Guadalcanal at 1130. Lunch at Thirteenth Air Force with Maj. Gen. (later Lt. Gen.) Nathan F. Twining [Commanding General, Thirteenth Air Force]. Then to Service Command Headquarters, Col. Russel J. Caton, MC, Surgeon. Watched LST [landing ship, tank] unload 200 patients on the beach. Most of these were wounded on Monday. Today is Thursday; thus 72 hours have elapsed. Most of the wounds were dressed in a short time except for the 20 caught on Baanga Island (?) for 4 days without medical care. Need better facilities on the LST.

Visited the 21st Medical Supply, "Hicks' Guadalcanal Pharmacy." Captain Hicks is a livewire from Shreveport, La. Visited the 20th Station Hospital. The buildings are thatch tents with grass and canvas, which last about 3 months here. This is actually a 500-bed hospital with facilities for 840 beds. The operating room is of the quonset type. They are doing little elective surgery, but have done a few open reductions in the past. This island already has miles of good road. The drainage system is improving.

Went to the 52d Field Hospital, which has done most of its major work under Major Baker—well trained. Saw a patient who had suffered a compound fracture of the tibia yesterday at 1100, on an island off New Georgia. He was brought here by boat and SCAT [Service Command Air Transport] in 24 hours. A good debridement had been done, dry gauze left in place.

New Georgia, Saturday, 21 August

Up at 0330 and drove to Henderson Field. Took off at 0530 in a transport plane. Landed at Segi, a small airstrip built in 10 days on the lower end of New Georgia.[2] The Russells are beautiful, and at 0630 the view from Segi is the most beautiful that I have seen in the South Pacific. We were joined by another transport and took off for Munda with four fighter escorts. The airfield is in good condition except for the litter of Japanese planes and materials (fig. 303). Drove over some of the worst roads I have ever seen to headquarters of the XIV Army Corps. Met Maj. Gen. Oscar W. Griswold [Commanding General, XIV Corps]. Talked most of the morning with Col. Franklin T. Hallam, MC, surgeon to the XIV Corps—a fine person doing a grand job. He needs more help to do it.

Drove to Laiana Beach in the afternoon, through a devastated area, and was amazed at the size and number of Japanese foxholes at about every 30 feet or less. Shellholes were almost continuous. Materiel and firepower played

---

[2] The capture of New Georgia Island with its important Munda Airfield was accomplished by Maj. Gen. Oscar W. Griswold's XIV Corps. The first landing in force was made 30 June on nearby Rendova Island. Elements of the 37th and 43d Divisions then landed on New Georgia enveloping the western end of the island. After our forces were reinforced by troops of the 25th Division, Munda was captured on 5 August.

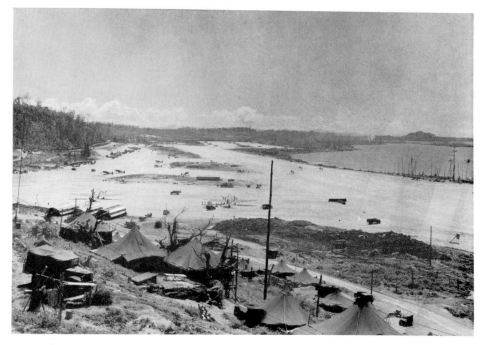

FIGURE 303.—Munda Airfield, New Georgia.

an impressive role in getting the Japanese out with so few casualties on our side.   There was an estimated 4,000 to 5,000 Japanese [there were 9,000 Japanese troops defending New Georgia] on this island, but it took the better part of three divisions to get them out.   Many Japanese skeletons were lying about in their clothes.

Visited the clearing station, 37th Division—100 patients—well run (fig. 304).   These clearing stations require either a full complement of personnel or outside help, in order to set up.   In island warfare they sometimes assume the function of surgical or field hospitals.   The 37th has about 100-plus cases of diarrhea per day, returns more than 40 per day—more than most clearing stations.   Must look into the sedation that is being employed here.   Ten thousand units antitoxin being given as prophylactic for gas gangrene.   Chest wounds are well handled.   There are no nets in use here.

The clearing station is surrounded by barbed wire on which tin cans have been placed.   Some Japanese have raided the hospital.   War here appears to be more vicious than in most places.

Patients are evacuated to the beach through 3 to 5 miles of circuitous roads (fig. 305).   An LCT [landing craft, tank] takes them to the 17th Field Hospital on Kokorana Island.   From there they are transported by LST or by SCAT to Guadalcanal.   The trail for jeeps and ambulances is very rough.   Some with severe fractures die as a result of the ride.   Very impressed by

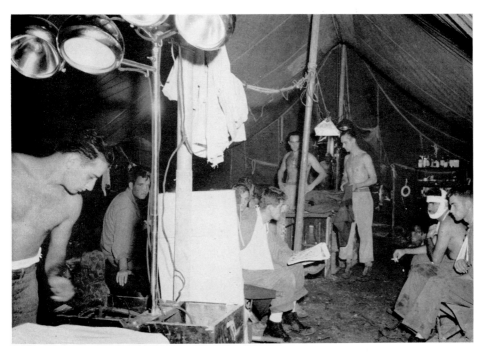

FIGURE 304.—A clearing station, 37th Division, August 1943.

"carryall" which will go through mud that the jeep cannot maneuver. The boats should have regular schedules for stopping along shore to transport the wounded. As it is now, the wounded must take their chances on the supply boat reaching them in time.

Colonel Hallam—"War neurosis starts with the poor officer who cracks up—for then the men go."

Staying here at headquarters at the eastern end of Munda strip on a hill overlooking Rendova Island. Most of nature's creatures here are harmless, except for man. Many flies get in your mouth, but mosquitoes are very rare. There are red ants in the area, but they don't bother us much. Some masks have been found that were used by the Japanese for terrorizing purposes. This climate is hot and wet; everything molds, including the feet. No wonder fungus infection is a problem.

Here is one place where folks don't want to wear medals or anything else to distinguish themselves. Everybody from the general on down wants to be as inconspicuous as possible. The wounded do not complain and are quiet. I suppose there is relief in the knowledge that they are out of it now. My impression is that this is a good Army, with wonderful equipment, which moves forward slowly, and ponderously, but inexorably. It is amazing how the jungle is transformed into "civilization," at least superficially.

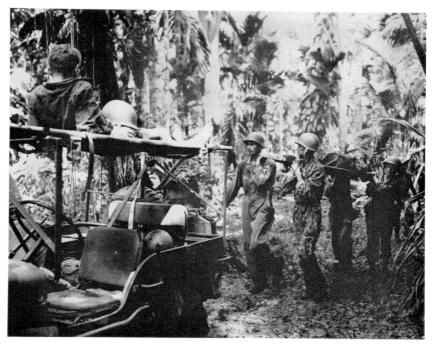

FIGURE 305.—Evacuation to beach by litter bearers and by jeep, New Georgia, 1943.

Sunday, 22 August

Drove to Headquarters, 25th Division—Lt. Col. Raymond H. Bunshaw, MC, Regular Army, is division surgeon. The roads are almost impassable. The clearing station is with headquarters in a hollow 1½ miles from Munda Field. The food here is only fair. There are flies everywhere. Operating tents are screened with mosquito netting. Bunshaw says that ear dermatitis is caused by swimming in streams.

Owing to the fact that the clearing station is split up, one platoon being on Vella Lavella Island, the other on Guadalcanal, they are short of equipment. Bunshaw lost three surgeons to Guadalcanal and is short of both surgeons and men. Most of the doctors are young and inexperienced. Colonel Bunshaw says that he needs two surgeons for each platoon. He thinks that rotation of 3 to 4 months is not enough.

Captain Silverstone, in charge here, says that they use a lot of oxygen, but have no apparatus. Should clearing stations have a rebreathing outfit and so save the O_2? Suction apparatus is also badly needed. A folding Mayo table is urgently needed. Water is a problem here as it must be transported to this spot, and the roads are in bad condition. Water is now being brought in by 5-gallon cans. Why not have a canvas storage tank to tide them over when roads and weather are bad? They need a gasoline washing machine too,

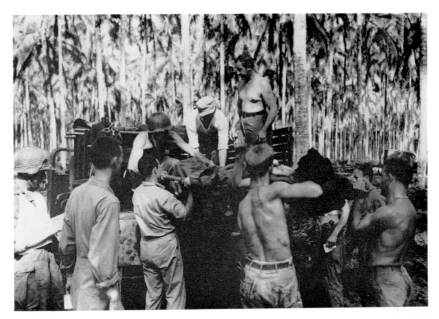

FIGURE 306.—A 2½-ton truck evacuates casualties to the beach, New Georgia, 1943.

and a refrigerator for serums. Many eyeglasses are broken and because of this the men must be evacuated or placed on limited duty.

The mud is knee deep; the woods are thick, hot, and steaming, but not real jungle. Because of the greasiness of this mud, hobnails are needed for the stretcher bearers. The wounded are evacuated here from as much as 5 miles away—some through swamps—and 2 days are sometimes required for a litter to get through. The ½-ton ambulance does not have enough power to get through these roads; the ¾-ton is okay (fig. 306).

War neurosis is less in this division than in others. This is because of better leadership; 40 percent of the officers are Regular Army. Both Colonel Bunshaw and Colonel Hallam believe that weak leadership is the chief cause of war neurosis.

Kokorana Island, Monday, 23 August

The road to the front is closed to all but engineer and signal troops, so I decided to go with the patients who were being evacuated to the 17th Field Hospital at Kokorana Island, which is off Rendova Island and about 14 miles from Munda (fig. 307).[3] We left the 25th Division clearing station at 0830 and arrived at the 17th at 1230. The boat trip was pleasant for a well man, but there were no facilities for the patients. I climbed from the LC [landing

---

[3] The 17th Field Hospital arrived on Russell Island on 31 March 1943 and received patients the first day. On 16 July and 25 July 1943, the 1st and 3d platoons, respectively, left to take part in the New Georgia operations, while the 2d platoon continued to operate a 100-bed hospital on Russell Island.

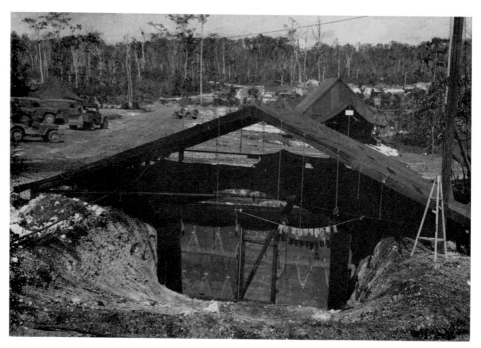

FIGURE 307.—A screened underground operating room at the 17th Field Hospital, after its
move to New Georgia, 27 October 1943.

craft] to an LCT and then to shore, only to find that we were at the 118th
Medical Battalion. So we embarked again to find the 17th Field. This
moving about is tough on very sick patients.

The 17th has a beautiful location in the middle of a coconut grove. The
climate here is cooler and dryer than New Georgia. This hospital has been
bombed and strafed. Six or eight tents were knocked down by 500-pound
bombs, and eight corpsmen were killed. They have done an impressive job.
Two operating rooms have been built underground, but again there is no screening. The mess tent is screened, but, as in all these places, the tables are not.
Why not have a little more screening in order to protect the food? The flies
swarm on the food, though somehow diarrhea has not become a problem here.
However, the 37th Division clearing station has had a lot of diarrhea. Major
Willis [Maj. James G. Willis, MC], the surgeon, is cognizant of the fact that
too many dressings are taken down, but this appears to be necessary since
there is no way to tell if they have been properly done at the forward area.
Many wounds are dressed 4 to 6 times before definitive treatment is given.
Undoubtedly, many wounds are infected in this manner. There is little reason for screening a division clearing station and not screening the succeeding
stations where dressings are done. I have not seen a mask here, and yet sore
throats are frequent among the medical personnel. Instruments are kept in
sterilizing solutions, usually alcohol.

Evacuation has been a problem in this area. The LST's carry supplies which they land at another island, and they do not like to remain around here too long. They do not always take the time to run over to the 17th. The movement of patients from island to island, or along the shore, is not under unit or Army control. This lack of organization results in many delays. Can this movement be correlated with the Navy? The suggestion that more surgery be done on the LST appears unsound only because not enough good surgeons could be obtained for this purpose. Why not?

Tuesday, 24 August

Remained at the 17th Field today. Talked long with Colonel Bell, the commanding officer. The morale of this outfit is low; the old problem of rotation and promotion.

Many ear conditions here, canal furuncles and fungus. It is thought to be due to the moisture in the air and not due to swimming. Many of these ears appear to be filled with scaly exudate. It occurs in both the healthy and the malnourished. Another problem is refractions. There are many broken spectacles and new cases requiring refraction, but no sets. Tonsils all bled, so they gave up operating on them. They want tuning forks to test hearing. There is a need for sulfamicro drugs for wound dressings. They must also have more ready-made splints, sealing dressings against flies and ants, and soap solution. The orthopedist says that cases arrive in good condition except during a push. A few cases have arrived in a state of shock. He has seen a few skintight plasters. He believes that a portable Hawley table would be of great help in the field hospital.

Visited the 25th Division casualty setup adjacent to the 17th Field, in charge of Major Klopfer. The clinic is excellent. This unit really functions as a convalescent camp, since many patients enter from the 17th Field without a diagnosis. Those with war neuroses may be kept here for one month to see if they can make use of them.

Major Klopfer believes that one month is too long a period to keep men in the line. The men may have only three hot meals during the whole time. They get little sleep and they must fight all day. As he said, "it takes a superman." He finds that a considerable number of the war neurosis cases are due to exhaustion. He thinks the situation would be helped by shorter periods at the front. The men should also be able to look forward to something in the way of relief after the job is done. Malingering is not high here.

Conversation with Capt. Benjamin A. Ruskin, MC, a psychiatrist. He divides neuropsychiatric cases into two categories: Group I, those who have had trauma; and II, those who are afraid of trauma. The functions of these psychiatrists seem to be: (1) Sorting out the patients who can be saved, (2) educating officers and enlisted personnel, and (3) therapy. They do not appear to have enough diversional activity; more books, movies, and games are needed.

Rest camps should be set up only where these activities can be provided.   The morale of the 25th Division is poor because of the length of time away from home plus the long campaigns.   Efficiency is dropping rapidly.

New Georgia, Wednesday, 25 August

Left Kokorana Island at 1030 on a mail barge from Munda Beach.   We were accompanied by boats of all varieties: personnel barges, LC's, LCT's, et cetera.   All kinds and combinations of uniforms were to be seen.   Some men were stark naked; others wore only a hat or shoes.   One sergeant had all sorts of insignia on his hat.   Asked why, he said that they all came in handy, depending on where he was.   A boatload of men went by looking more like a band of pirates than soldiers.   One man in a mottled jungle suit appeared in our boat.   Someone asked him a question.   He promptly lay down, saying "I don't know or give a damn,"—and went to sleep.   We arrived at XIV Corps headquarters, 1400, to find that Colonel Hallam has been down with dysentery for the last 3 days.

Although it had been on the same site for 1 month, the 17th Field Hospital on Kokorana had screened only the mess building, and that just partially.   It would have taken very little more to have screened the entire mess.   If not with screen, mosquito bars would have done for 1 month.   The latrines were open and poorly constructed.   Operating and dressing rooms were not screened.   No effort has been made to improve conditions, although it is true that they have been expecting to move.   Since only a minimum of lighting is available, everyone goes to bed at 1830.   The 25th Division operating room is screened with a mosquito bar, although they are working under more difficult conditions.

Thursday, 26 August

Slept soundly in spite of an alarm and the sounds of 105 mm. guns shooting over our heads.   However, this morning my head feels as though it had been pounded.   Went over to the 37th Division clearing station (fig. 308) and also visited the 43d Division.   Men of the 37th say that they are handicapped because the clearing company does not function as a unit.   They are more short of enlisted men than officers, although the new T/O [table of organization] cuts their enlisted strength even more.   Whenever they have had to move, they have had trouble in getting help to set up and have not been able to get bulldozers.   Help is most needed in the initial stages, for screening, etc.   *Anopheles* are getting worse in the Laiana Beach area, and there is not enough mosquito bar for screening.   There has also been some trouble and confusion in connection with priority of location for the clearing station, and some unnecessary moves were made.   Headquarters seems to decide on one location and then change its mind.   Lt. Col. Hobart L. Mikesell, MC, is division surgeon [acting].   He thinks that the triangular division splits up medical personnel too much for island warfare.   Could doctors be obtained by substituting MAC [Medical Administrative Corps] officers to do the routine administrative tasks in the collecting company, since these units function chiefly during battle?

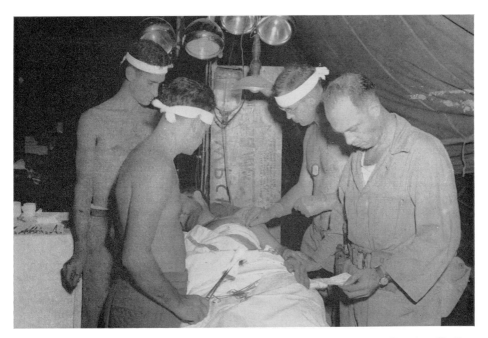

FIGURE 308.—A surgical team completing a thoracic operation at the Clearing Station, 37th Infantry Division.

The men of the 37th Division came on New Georgia with inadequate equipment, for some things had to be left behind. Many left their bags behind, hence they do not have enough socks, shoes, etc. They need a refrigerator for serum and cold drinks, and a washing machine. The sterilizers are too small. How to blackout! Allowed four basic instrument sets, they found out that they only had two. There are no batteries for lights, but they are short of bulbs anyway. Splints and litters tend to run out. Wire ladder splints are needed. No screening anywhere, neither in latrines, mess or operating room—and flies are swarming. I wonder if they do enough debridement?

Guadalcanal, Friday, 27 August

Batteries in headquarters camp began a barrage at 0430, and I was sleeping in the corps surgeon's tent on a small hill directly in front of the guns. Japanese planes came over and bombed us at 0530. They did not hit the field, so I took off at 0800.

We made an unexpected stop at Russell Island, so I got out to visit another platoon of the 17th Field, which is in command of Major Addison, who is also the island surgeon.[4] They need an intensifying screen for the X-ray, as the X-ray generator fluctuates too much. The incidence of malaria on Russell is more than was anticipated. Dental work is behind, and some patients

_____
[4] See footnote 3, p. 777.

are evacuated because of the lack of dental facilities. A dentist reported here today. There is not much surgery to be done here. They have done only one major surgical operation this month and a moderate amount of minor surgery. Malaria and dentistry are the big problems. The splitting up of these field hospitals takes away a certain amount of equipment and cuts the personnel, particularly corpsmen. As a result, these hospitals leave much to be desired.

In this rapidly moving front of island warfare, a field hospital cannot stay put very long. As a result, they do not put much effort into keeping up to the highest possible standards and tend to get into slovenly habits. The 1st and 3d Platoons of this hospital were located on Kokorana instead of at the forward area on New Georgia, thus adding 4 to 5 hours' delay to the care of casualties. The hospital has remained there for nearly a month, though this location is not particularly invulnerable. It has been bombed and had 8 or 9 deaths—more fatalities than even the dressing station on Georgia. With better forward clearing stations and LST's with an adequate operating room, the field hospital here would act primarily as a holding and evacuation station.

I caught the 1530 plane for Guadalcanal and met Capt. Richard A. Kern, MC, USNR, and Cdr. Theodore E. Reynolds, MC, USNR, medical and surgical consultants for the Navy. There was an enormous amount of destroyed Japanese shipping between Florida Island and Guadalcanal. The loss of materiel and personnel must have been very great. This was the show that definitely stopped the southward advance of Nippon. The Canal is one great dust cloud and fairly cool in contrast to the steamy heat and mud in New Georgia. I put up at the Service Command in a new screened and floored tent. The eternal cry is "screening."

Saturday, 28 August

I spent the day going about with Captain Kern and Commander Reynolds. Visited several Seabee installations and they are splendid. Their ingenuity is astounding. Washing machines were improvised out of gasoline drums. The Seabees and the LST ships are the greatest innovation I have seen in this war.

Filariasis has now been found here. Some native villages still remain as close as one-quarter of a mile from the camps. This may be a problem (fig. 309). The Navy experienced a severe amount of dysentery on landing here. Again, screening is the answer. More dental equipment and dental officers are needed here too. This seems to be true in all echelons.

I visited the Mobile 8 [U.S. Naval Mobile Hospital No. 8]. Capt. William H. H. Turville, MC, USN, is commanding officer. He is an intelligent, able disciplinarian, who has built the best naval hospital I have seen in the South Pacific. The total area covered is 79 acres. The hospital is of prefabricated construction. It took 2 months to build, and has 400 patients at the moment; it is expanding, however, to a 1,500-bed hospital.

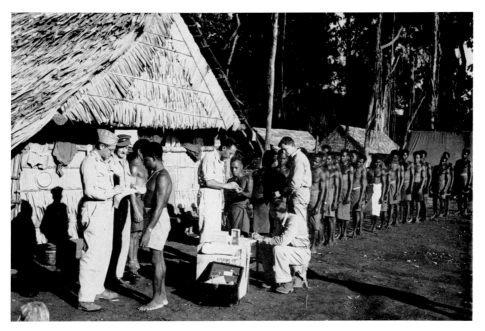

FIGURE 309.—Blood specimens being taken to determine the index of malaria in a native labor camp near a military base, Guadalcanal, August 1944.

Sunday, 29 August

On this rainy day I am plagued by a head cold and diarrhea. I visited the 24th Field Hospital. Lt. Col. L. B. Hanson, MC, is the commanding officer. He is one of the finest commanding officers I have seen in any hospital. His unit has not yet seen action. They are a hand-picked group of men with varied talents. In ingenuity they compare favorably with the Seabees. A field hospital is supposed to have 150 tons of equipment. Hanson now has about 300-plus, including cement, lumber, screening, two refrigerators, one large reefer (freezer), numerous engines, an ice cream unit, etc. This looks like the Army's number one field hospital. The generators furnished to the field hospitals are inadequate for the load. Not enough mess equipment or carpenter tools are being supplied.

Twenty-plus cases of gangrene occurred during the month of July at the 20th Station Hospital and the 52d Field Hospital. A tremendous amount of debridement was done at the 52d Field Hospital. Why so much here—more should be done forward?

Monday, 30 August

Spent the day at the 52d Field Hospital. The location is not too good. The site is hot, on low ground, and on the dusty side of the road. It has an advantage in being between two airstrips, affording the use of a Japanese powerplant and water supply. The hospital is now in command of Major

Baker, who is well trained and has good judgment. The orthopedist is also good. Tents are built off the ground. The operating room is well screened with good fly locks. This hospital has an adequate amount of screening, which is well distributed, except that the mess kitchen and mess tables are located in separate tents, while they should be combined. The patient is sprayed before he enters the hospital. He is marked "today" for dressings. A large sterilizer was obtained, since the pressure cooker was too small. The sterilizer is heated on a field range. They refill bottles and make their own sterile water with an autoclave. They have averaged about 325 patients per day and use about 3,000 gallons of water per day, kept in tanks which last from 2 to 3 months. The 14 Japanese treated here have been good patients. The only cases of tetanus seen have occurred among them. Many patients are waiting for new spectacles.

It seems that the splinting done in the forward echelon is frequently inadequate to immobilize and does not extend over the adjacent joints; for example, the ankle. Applying one layer of sheet wadding and then plaster, would be a better method. The area should be shaved and washed with green soap and water. Debridement is frequently inadequate, dirty clothing and dead tissue are not removed, and hemorrhage is not adequately controlled.

In the beginning of the New Georgia campaign many of the wounded never went through a clearing station, and treatment was delayed for from 48 to 96 hours. The 17th Field was established about 4 weeks after the landing on Rendova, and patients were then evacuated in much better condition. Before this there were, for example, casualties with the femoral artery and vein severed that were not ligated upon evacuation.

LESSONS OF THE NEW GEORGIA CAMPAIGN

There is, in general, too much dependence on sulfonamides and not enough on debridement. There is a tendency to dump sulfonamides into wounds that are not deeper than 1 inch. The same is true for larger wounds in the application of debridement. One doctor here found that spores and grams and rods are common in these wounds and sometimes exist in almost pure culture. The only complications caused by sulfonamides were seen in five or six cases of suppression of urine with blood, and all of these cases recovered. Some through-and-through wounds have come in with a sponge in either end (plug), held in by a catgut suture.

Fifty percent of the tags attached to the patients are useless, and rarely do they contain clinical information. The chief question that is to be answered is what was done when, and when the wound needs a dressing. The people here would like to know what eventually happens to the gas gangrene cases and if any new ones develop later on.

I have now collected data on 20 cases of gas gangrene from the 52d Field and 20th Station Hospitals. There appear to be at least two underlying reasons for the occurrence of gas gangrene:

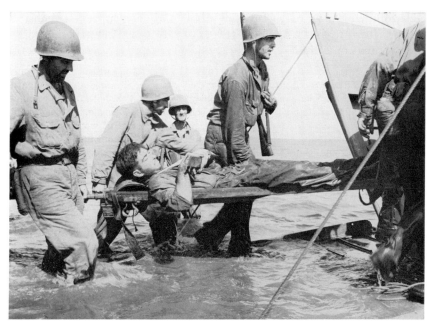

FIGURE 310.—A casualty of jungle fighting being loaded aboard a Higgins boat for evacuation by sea, New Georgia, July 1943.

1. The reasons of organization and administration, which contribute to delay in the treatment of the sick and wounded. Hence, the failure to provide adequate medical care in the forward areas during the New Georgia campaign. Some of this was probably unavoidable and was caused by such incidences as the bombing attack on the beachhead shortly after the invasion. With the difficulty of communication in island warfare, there are plausible reasons why all patients do not go through a clearing station. However, this lack of medical facilities resulted in long delays in the treatment of casualties. Although sulfanilamide was applied rather routinely in the early stages, this did not prevent gas gangrene. However, gas gangrene occurred only in very severe wounds.

2. Professional care was at times inadequate due to: (a) Failure to appreciate the importance of thorough debridement—in many instances it was superficial only, (b) failure to control hemorrhage, (c) inadequate cleansing with razor, soap and water, (d) doctors in clearing stations said that patients were in too great a state of shock to permit more thorough debridement; also, the number of casualties that passed through the clearing stations were at times greater than could be cared for adequately, and (e) patients transported on LST's to Guadalcanal received inadequate care. The trip lasted from 20 to 24 hours. Only one doctor was assigned to each boat, and there were no adequate facilities for operating or dressing wounds (fig. 310).

The following is an extract on the problem of gas gangrene from the sanitary report for July 1943, Headquarters, XIV Corps, Forward Echelon, New Georgia Occupation Force:

Hospitals in rear areas began to report, early in July, the occurrence of gas gangrene among battle casualties arriving from the New Georgia area. Immediate investigation as to the probable causes of gas gangrene infections was undertaken, both by the rear echelon of the Corps at Guadalcanal and by the forward echelon at New Georgia. It was found that the main causes were lack of early debridement, primary closure of wounds, tight packing to prevent hemorrhage, and a lapse frequently as long as 72–96 hours from time of injury before definitive treatment could be instituted at Guadalcanal.

Immediate steps were taken to minimize the incidence of gas gangrene among battle casualties. The division in combat at that time was notified of the occurrence and probable causes of the gangrene. Large quantities of gas gangrene antitoxin were sent to New Georgia with instructions to administer prophylactic doses wherever indicated. Medical facilities aboard LST's, which carry patients to the rear areas, were increased by the Navy.

It should be remembered that, while the occurrence of gas gangrene among battle casualties is unfortunate, division medical service was the only source of medical treatment of battle casualties in the New Georgia area during the first 28 days of July. Facilities for definitive surgery were lacking north of the Guadalcanal-Russell Islands area. The 24–36 hour trip by LST from the combat area to Guadalcanal, during which time the wounds were not redressed, except in emergency, provided an excellent incubation period.

The establishment, toward the middle of July, of the policy that all casualties should be cleared through the division clearing station before evacuation to the rear on the LST's, did much to prevent long journeys to the rear by casualties who had received only aid station care. The arrival during the latter part of July of 21 medical officer replacements and elements of the 17th Field Hospital did much to provide adequate early surgical care, and the occurrence of gas gangrene was reduced to a minimum.

FRANKLIN T. HALLAM
Colonel, Medical Corps

It should be noted that the above use of antitoxin is of questionable value. It should in no way minimize the surgical care (debridement). The increase of medical facilities on LST's (September 1) consisted of two doctors instead of one. Their facilities were still inadequate.

Tuesday, 31 August

A boy was riding on the fender of a truck when a bullet from a machinegun, one of ours, hit him in the back. He was instantly paralyzed. This happened at 1700. He arrived by plane at the 52d Field Hospital at noon next day. A boy, the tail gunner in a B–24 on a bombing mission on Bougainville, parachuted from his burning plane, and was strafed by the Japs. He was shot through the belly and the right side, and had a large exit wound just to the right of his spine. There were six perforations of the intestine and the missile had passed medial to the right kidney. He was operated on at the 20th Station Hospital within 2½ hours and is doing well this afternoon. A boy, belly gunner on a bomber, was shot through the upper third of the left leg. Both veins and arteries gone, and a compound comminuted fracture—amputation was necessary. He was operated on within 3 hours and is doing well. Air transport of the sick can accomplish wonders, but it should not supplant proper

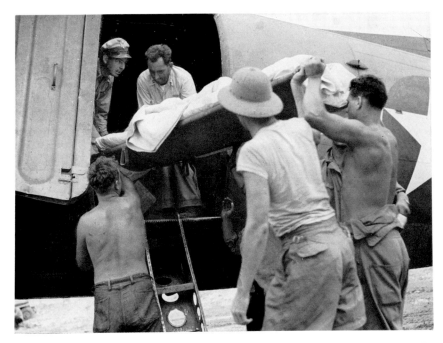

FIGURE 311.—Evacuation by C–47 transport plane from Munda Airfield, New Georgia, August 1943.

surgical care in the proper place, which is still forward (fig. 311). A detonated dud hurt no one but a cook 200 yards away in the messhall. The fragments took out both eyes and the bridge of the nose, passing very cleanly sideways. He is in good condition and wants to know about his eyesight.

Spent the day at the 20th Station Hospital. Col. Harvey Laton is commanding officer. They landed on Guadalcanal January 16th, and took patients on the 24th. They have been flooded out once. The area is low and hot and unsuitable for a station hospital.

Colonel Rosenzweig, a gynecologist, is chief of surgery. Captain Kluger, orthopedist, is young and very good. He states: "All wounds with gas gangrene gave evidence of hasty treatment and inadequate debridement." They are short 1 officer and 40 men. The ophthamologist emphasizes the need for spectacles. More than 100 men are waiting in the convalescent camp for spectacles. Major Lechen, an otolaryngologist, wants to know about doing tonsils. Infected ears have been cultured and a variety of fungi found. The incidence of optic neuritis and choroiditis is out of proportion. There have been many cases of concussion deafness, and a set of tuning forks is needed to differentiate the degrees of deafness. The lab needs facilities for anaerobic cultures. Pyrogallic acid is in demand. The dentist is short of articulation sets.

It is desirable to have a well-qualified surgeon in the forward echelon for each of the following jobs: Neurosurgery and thoracic, orthopedic, and general surgery. The latter is the most important. Too much assembly line treatment occurs in forward hospitals. The extension arm splints were found to be no good.

This hospital appears to be doing a good job. Their records are fair; eye, ear, nose and throat care is okay; the X-ray service is good; the lab is fair; the food is fair; the library is good. Staff meetings were held formerly but are irregular now.

Wednesday, 1 September 1943

Visited the convalescent hospital under Major Kellefer, an orthopedist. They have not begun to keep systematic records yet. I talked to him about this. He thinks that 80 percent of the war neuropsychiatric histories are poor; that sorting is done on snap judgement. The chief problem in choosing psychiatrists is separating the sheep from the goats. He raised the question of reclassifying doctors at home.

The 43d Division attacked Rendova on 1 July. The beach was bombed and strafed by the enemy on 2 July. There were more than 350 casualties. No clearing station had been set up, and the casualties were loaded directly onto an LST. For some reason the LST could not get off, and all the patients were transferred to another LST during the night. The 43d never had a clearing station on New Georgia Island.

Major Barker, medical inspector of the 37th Division, is down with dysentery at the 20th Station Hospital. Barker thinks that some of the dysentery contracted was due to the use of halazone tablets. How many tablets to a canteen would be safe? Look up the division sanitary reports.

The 37th Division medical service was operating with a shortage of 8 officers and 100 enlisted men. The eight officer replacements had no field training but were put out into the field nevertheless, and one of them cracked up within 24 hours. One officer and six enlisted men were killed.

Lt. Col. James H. Melvin, MC, Surgeon at the Service Command here, and Major Barker both agree that a force medical supply unit should accompany the infantry in island warfare. Many of the units lost part of their supplies during the landing, and there was no source of replacements short of Guadalcanal. Captain Hicks, 21st Medical Supply, agrees that it would also simplify his problem. He found it impossible to get supplies to the various isolated units whose supplies would get lost on some island, since frequently he did not know where they were. Recommend that the force medical supply unit function as in quartermaster exchange of property on LST's. The problem here is chiefly one of making litters and blankets available for the wounded. Since the men must frequently sleep in foxholes, it is to be expected that cots or litters may be used for casualties, and allowance should be made for this in the exchange of supplies. This new plan, by giving a division the things it needs when they are needed, would avoid burdening the divisions unduly.

All agreed that since clearing stations frequently function as field hospitals, they should also be provided with washing machines. The 24th Field Hospital has three. There is no time to build these things during a "push," when they are most needed. Improvisations of all sorts can be done in a quiet time, but by then the need has largely disappeared and the damage has been done.

Thursday, 2 September

Spent the day reading, arranging transportation, writing, and treating my feet for the "rot."

Espíritu Santo, Friday, 3 September

I rose at 0300, although we did not leave the airfield until 0630. Arrived at Espíritu Santo [New Hebrides], 1030. Called Colonel Morgan Berry, MC, and stayed with him. Met Lt. Col. Benjamin M. Baker, MC, medical consultant for this command, who was on his way north to the Canal. He has worked chiefly on the problem of malaria. I attended a session of the Espíritu Santo Medical Society, which meets every other Friday. The hospital staff put on a good program. Reports were given on: Subphrenic abscess, malaria and dengue, internal derangement of the knee joint, anesthesia—very good.

Capt. Richard A. Rose, MC, 321st Service Group, wants a transfer for duty as an anesthesiologist. I talked to Captain Miller, who was on an LST that was bombed and sank off Vella Lavella Island. He agrees that they need an operating room aboard, preferably on the side forward where the carpenter shop is. This side is relatively quiet and easier to lightproof. Better arrangements should also be made for keeping food dry.

The loading of patients must be planned out before the boat comes in, so that those who are seriously wounded will be put in the proper place and receive earlier attention. Miller suggested that two men be used for this purpose, one of whom would remain at the landing point. He says that two doctors aboard the LST would not be enough, and that four to six corpsmen were needed, two of whom should be of top caliber. These measures would apply only at the time of a "push."

I talked with Colonel Potts and Major Sofield regarding a policy on leaves. Six months or more of continuous duty in the islands seriously affects morale. Moreover, some men have been here longer than others due to lack of replacements. It is also important to keep up the morale of the men who treat the sick.

Saturday, 4 September

I spent the morning on the wards with Colonel Potts and Major Sofield. I saw a compound fracture of the lower third of the humerus with a hanging cast, and unfinished at that. There was a knee case that had to be reoperated. What was supposed to be a cyst turned out to be a ruptured muscle. Evidently more information must be entered on the EMT [Emergency Medical Tag]. Baker left today. We will meet again in Suva [Fiji] on the 18th. I am scheduled to fly to Nandi [Fiji] on the 15th.

I saw another disturbing case. This soldier had been wounded in the arm late one afternoon during the New Georgia fighting. The wound was dressed almost immediately. He was evacuated the next morning at 1000 and reached the 17th Field Hospital at 1500. Only the 25th Division clearing

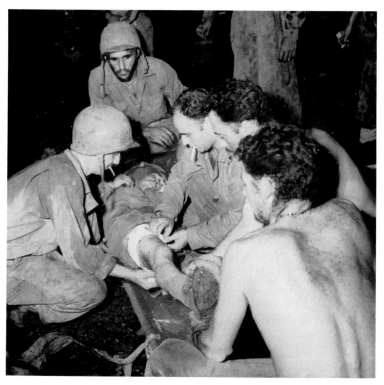

FIGURE 312.—An aid station on Rendova Island, Solomon Islands, 12 July 1943.

station had moved forward on New Georgia. If just one platoon of the 17th had been near the beach, he could have been debrided. Debridement with anesthesia wasn't done at the 17th, although he was there for 4 days. He was then sent to Mobile 8 on Guadalcanal, where a Roger Anderson splint was applied. From there he was sent to the 25th Evacuation Hospital [Espíritu Santo]. He continues to have fever and a great deal of pus from his wound.

Folding fracture tables are needed for field hospitals.

MANAGEMENT OF CASUALTIES IN THE NEW GEORGIA CAMPAIGN

1. First aid treatment was usually promptly received by the injured (fig. 312). The delays that did occur were usually unavoidable. A shortage of litters and of hobnailed shoes for the litter bearers was partially responsible for the delay.

2. Clearing Stations.

a. They get little or no help to set up at a time when casualties are coming in heavy, and do not have enough time with the help available to give adequate care to patients in a "push."

b. Supportive treatment appears to be good.

c. Debridement is inadequate in many cases because the men are pressed for time. Furthermore, some of them do not even understand the principle of debridement. Not enough soap and water are used. More instruments and a larger sterilizer—or preferably two sterilizers—are needed. More good surgery is needed in the clearing station and nothing should be spared to make this possible. In island warfare the field hospital may be so far from the clearing station that many serious cases must receive definitive treatment here. Better sorting of cases at the clearing station and a more efficient system of transportation to the field hospital is needed.

d. Records on the EMT are poorly kept. Enlisted men should be trained to put down what was done, and when the next dressing is due.

e. Fracture treatment is poor and is characterized by inadequate debridement, inadequate immobilization, and inadequate use of plaster.

f. Sanitation methods must be improved. The screening of messes should include the space set aside for eating. Flies are present in abundance. The operating tents must be screened.

3. Field hospitals should be placed as far forward as possible. The inadequacies mentioned above with regard to treatment in the clearing station apply to the field hospital too. The field hospital should go in with a full complement of supplies. Dividing up of supplies has proved a serious drawback in many instances. They should have help immediately on landing, in order to set up one good-sized bomb shelter. The clearing station or the field hospital should be located on or near the beach, in order to have the best possible liaison with the LST's.

4. Hospitals that are to be used in the line of evacuation should have more clearly defined locations. If station hospitals are to be used in evacuation, their personnel should be picked accordingly, with at least one first-class surgeon. The less well trained men should be used in hospitals that are off the direct line of evacuation. The 25th Evacuation Hospital is too far back now to perform the functions of an evacuation hospital.

Sunday, 5 September

I spent the day with Harper [Lt. Col. Paul Harper, MC, Malaria Control Unit] and Sapero [Cdr. James J. Sapero, MC, USN, CINPAC] who are doing a fine job. Commander Sapero was teaching in the Navy school in Washington before the war and has had some experience in malaria work. He was ordered out here during the thick of the crisis, when 16 percent of the men who had landed here [Efate Island, New Hebrides] were in the hospital as a result of malaria, the noneffective rate growing steadily. They had a so-called commission on Efate Island when he arrived, which did not even know to look for breeding places of *Anopheles* but set out to destroy all mosquitoes. Malaria control is just now getting under way, 1 year from the time of our arrival here. Only one educational directive has been published, and a command directive is just now being written. Sapero should be encouraged and his work recognized.

Monday, 6 September

Visited the 25th Evacuation Hospital—Col. Morgan Berry is commanding officer. They have two good orthopedists. Maj. Harold A. Sofield is chief orthopedist. He could be used as a consultant in the teaching program, being put on detached service at first. The orthopedic and surgical service in the 25th Evacuation is well covered, so that this is not entirely unfair to Colonel Berry. At the 25th Evacuation Hospital, 35 percent of the casualties are fractures, of which 93 percent are compound, 15 percent femur. Next to general surgery, the biggest surgical problem is orthopedics. However, Lt. Col. Willis J. Potts, the chief of surgery, is well qualified. He is a competent surgeon and a good administrator with a pleasing personality. The 25th Evacuation Hospital is a well-run hospital doing professional work of a high quality.

UTILIZATION OF MEDICAL FACILITIES IN A THEATER OF OPERATIONS

In general, the surgical care of the wounded does not appear to be badly done, and the Medical Department is doing a good job under difficult circumstances. However, there is room for improvement.

1. The problems are: To provide the best possible early treatment for the wounded at the front during the "golden hours"; to insure the same high quality of treatment all along the line of evacuation.

The above can be accomplished by:

a. Planning good locations for facilities to be set up promptly when needed, and a well-organized system of transport.

b. Adequate trained personnel: Since we are short of trained personnel, this problem resolves itself into one of distribution of the best-trained personnel in key positions. The distribution of personnel along the line of evacuation must be such as to make them available to the greatest number of patients. This means that the line of evacuation must be planned out carefully, since the number of trained specialists is limited. Transportation under conditions of battle does not always allow for the proper sorting of casualties. The first wave of patients that arrived on Guadalcanal were transferred to hospitals on the basis of the seriousness of the case in relation to the condition of the roads and distance of the trip. This whole problem might have been eliminated by the proper location of facilities. Furthermore, not enough consideration was given to the personnel available at these hospitals. Thus, if only one orthopedist or neurosurgeon is available at a certain hospital, the patients that fall under these specialties should be sent there. This sorting should be a function of the island or service command surgeon, and should not be done solely on the basis of the number of beds available. However, if there is only one hospital on an island, this procedure is not necessary. Economy of supplies and personnel is one of the advantages of centralizing hospital facilities.

2. Medical officers, especially those in the forward echelons, should receive some instruction in the care of wounds and the treatment and trans-

portation of fracture cases. These are the two major problems in the care of battle casualties, and it is here that instruction is most urgently needed. In order that this instruction may reach personnel in as short a time as possible, the instructor should visit the forward echelons. It would be particularly desirable that they first visit troops and installations that are about to go into action.

3. Since there are extreme fluctuations in the casualty load in island warfare, a more flexible medical service should be provided. This can best be done by using surgical teams, operating under the direction of the corps surgeon. Such teams could be drawn from hospital installations in the rear echelons, provided that these are kept up to strength.

4. The policy of promoting officers in order to fill the T/O (table of organization) of an installation—even when the best available men are chosen— has often resulted in placing officers in positions which they were not qualified to fill. The promotion of any medical officer to the grade of lieutenant colonel or colonel, should receive very careful consideration from both the professional and the administrative standpoint. The essential problem is to find posts that they are qualified to fill. When they are not qualified for such posts, either professionally or administratively, the question of promotion should be precluded.

It has rained buckets all day and night.

I visited the 122d Station Hospital, which is making excellent progress. Major Camp has built a well-designed surgery, though it is much larger than is necessary for a 500-bed hospital. They expect to open the surgery in 2 weeks. The personnel of this hospital is young and enthusiastic, but not well qualified.

Capt. Gilbert N. Haffly, MC, of the 25th Evacuation Hospital, an excellent EENT [eye, ear, nose and throat] man, is training a general practitioner to do EENT work in this hospital. Captain Haffly says that nose and throat maladies constitute 65 to 70 percent of his work. Not a single paracentesis has been done here so far. He does not think anyone with a chronic ear condition, or with a history of recent ear trouble, should be taken in the Army. Exposure to a tropical environment results in an acute exacerbation of chronic trouble. Otitis externa is a big problem. Haffly intends to report further on this. He recommends the application of 1 percent thymol in 50 percent alcohol, or thymol iodide powder. He does not think that this inflammation is contracted by swimming in the local waters.

It was raining by the bucketfull all day, and all flights were grounded. My plans to travel to Efate must await the favorable decision of the gods. I spent the afternoon talking with the Navy consultants, Captain Kern of Philadelphia, the medical consultant, and Commander Reynolds of San Francisco, the surgical consultant, and with Cdr. Emile Holman, MC, USNR, and Lt. Cdr. James C. T. Rogers, MC, USNR. They have just returned from Tulagi and Florida Islands [the Solomons].

Surgical and medical care for the Marine Raiders appears to be a very difficult problem, since they carry so little medical equipment. They do not even carry a stretcher—nothing but fighting equipment and a little food. Losses in the 4th Marine Raider Battalion, which made initial assaults on New Georgia, were: 33 killed, 134 wounded, 170 medical casualties, or 48 percent casualties, of which almost half were surgical cases. In the action at Bairoko Harbour [New Georgia Island], there were approximately 600-plus casualties. Four hundred were evacuated by PBY ["Catalina"] flying boats, one hundred by APD [transport (high speed)] fast destroyer transport, and one hundred by LST. The second wave of Raiders carried some dressing station, but these did not usually get set up until some 2 or 3 days later. Hence there is very little substantial treatment until the wounded are evacuated to Guadalcanal.

While at the Mobile 8 Naval Hospital, I heard it stated that, since practically all head wounds, most chest wounds, and the majority of the belly wounds turn out to be fatal, these casualties should be considered lost and no attempt be made to save them. Someone added that perhaps this was the right thing to do and that only the minor cases should be treated. The point here, I suppose, is to utilize personnel and equipment as efficiently as possible. I objected, for I believe that every effort should be made to save lives, if this can at all be done without materially jeopardizing the outcome of the war. We must consider that morale would go to pot in a hurry if the soldier thought that in certain instances no attempt would be made to save him. It is true that many men have been wounded and a few killed while trying to save a wounded man. I know of one instance when three were killed by Japanese snipers while trying to help one wounded man. The Japanese use our casualties as bait for a kill.

Captain Kern thinks that the men should be instructed to crawl for cover when wounded. The white dressing of a wounded man makes a beautiful target. The Japanese have foreseen this and use a green triangular dressing as a covering. Some of our men smear mud over their dressings so that they are not conspicuous. Another practice to correct is that of giving all of our wounded one-half grain of morphine. Because of this, many walking cases are converted into litter cases. Kern is much concerned over the absence of camp sanitation. Piles of tin cans, partly filled with food, act as fly breeders.

The Navy badly needs 6-inch prepared plaster. That is the first thing I have heard of that the Army has, and that the Navy doesn't have. The Navy has given us just about everything else, and perhaps we can help them out in this case. The Navy has been well supplied with washing machines, refrigerators, tables, quonset huts, and what-have-you. Their equipment for tropical warfare, as one New Zealand officer, Colonel Twhigg [Col. John M. Twhigg, New Zealand Army Medical Corps] remarked, includes, "everything that opens and shuts." However, Reynolds and Kern observed that the greater mobility of Army equipment is an important asset and that the Navy is not prepared to move fast. However, most of the comforts of tropical warfare are furnished by the Navy.

Kern and Reynolds are both in favor of surgical teams, particularly as the Navy has a surplus of doctors in their rear echelons. They told me about some Marine divisions, which among their medical staff did not number a single qualified surgeon. On the whole, their care of the wounded and their organization of evacuation lines is in a worse state than the Army's. We are still making many of the mistakes of the last war and are not getting all of the square pegs into square holes. These Navy people are beginning to recognize, I think, the importance of having adequate medical facilities on the LST's. However, "the skipper would never give up his carpenter shop." We will see what happens.

Efate, Wednesday, 8 September

I left Espíritu Santo Island this morning at 1000, had lunch at the Efate Island airstrip, then drove to headquarters of the island command at Vila. Headquarters is situated on a fine hill overlooking a beautiful harbor. Colonel Carroll is the island surgeon—a pleasant fellow. The 48th Station Hospital is under the command of Lt. Col. (later Col.) Lester F. Wilson, MC. It is the only large Army medical installation on the island. Parts of two platoons are set up on the far side of the island to act as a field clearing station for emergencies.

U.S. Naval Base Hospital No. 2 is the largest hospital on the island and has a beautiful location on a hilltop. It is well equipped and well run, although I am a bit skeptical of some of their talent. They now have some 700 to 800 patients, half of which are Army personnel. Most of the patients from the 20th Station Hospital, and the 52d Field Hospital, both at Guadalcanal, have been evacuated here. There has been some trouble with records and some friction with the 48th Station Hospital. The Navy does not send their records along with the patients. I don't see any reason why hospitals should keep the records of their patients. Certainly all of his records, and not only the EMT, should accompany the patient. There are a great many orthopedic cases here.

The 48th Station Hospital is being enlarged to a 500-bed hospital and has about 300 beds at present. Colonel Wilson is a general traumatic surgeon and does some surgery. The hospital has a beautiful site on the hillside overlooking the harbor view. Most of the buildings are quonsets, with a boardwalk running between them. The messes are excellent, clean, and well screened. Good planning is everywhere in evidence. A very good medical supply unit, the 24th, is part of the hospital. The staff was drawn mostly from the 12th General Hospital, which is the Northwestern [University] group. They are young but energetic. The chief of the medical service is good. The chief of surgery, Major Douglas, is young but well grounded. Unfortunately, they have no orthopedist. Captain Lindberg, laboratory head, is excellent. Morale is good.

They are having trouble with their water supply—inadequate filter. The proctoscope bulbs are all out, owing to line fluctuation. Can a Castle light battery be used instead? They have a good GU man, but no cystoscope for him to use. It has been on order for 6 months. Is there one at Nouméa? They are out of 2½ percent sodium citrate ampules. Their needles and sutures are too large. Check on maintenance at Nouméa; this is a general complaint. Opium powder is needed for the pharmacy, and more class IV supplies for the laboratory: beakers, flasks, glassware. They also want washing machines and gaskets for sterilizers.

Colonel Carroll says that the dental problem is considerable here. Seven to ten percent of new arrivals from the States have deficient teeth, but the hospital is short of dental equipment. They have seen three cases of yaws among Army personnel here.

Captain Lindberg has found that low glucose tolerance occurs in cases with jaundice and small livers. He needs brown sulphaline. He has a new, quick, thick-smear Giemsa stain—takes 10 minutes.

I saw a femur fractured up to the trochanter that had been kept here 12 weeks. The fellow also had a compound fracture of the wrist and hand. He should have been evacuated, since they have no orthopedist here. But apparently the boats do not come in often. Why can't air evacuation be used for these cases?

I left Efate at 1400 and arrived at Nouméa, 1615 hours, with Charles G. Mixter. He says that only 50 percent of their planes are used for the evacuation of patients. Personnel is available, but the planes are being used for other than ambulance transport purposes. There is too much of this lack of good management. I have observed plenty of patients who would benefit by air evacuation. This source of assistance has been neglected, however, simply because people don't get together on these problems.

Nouméa, Thursday & Friday, 9 & 10 September

I spent these two days getting organized here at headquarters, writing reports, letters, etc. Two eye magnets are available for shipment. I took up the question of screening with Major Moore of the Engineers. How much should a hospital or medical installation take with them to the forward areas?

Saturday, 11 September

Worked on reports today. I received a splendid report from Major Barker, the 37th Division Medical Inspector. His findings sounded as though I had written them up myself. It is amazing how closely our observations have coincided.

Wednesday, 15 September

I was supposed to be in Fiji today and have my orders to proceed there. But it seems as though fate orders otherwise. Went for a 5- or 6-mile walk with Paul Harper Sunday evening and felt fine. I had on a new pair of shoes. Awoke that midnight with a very severe shaking chill. It was so severe that I could not get out of bed for some time. By morning the chill had subsided, although I knew I was not quite all there when they took me to the hospital. I thought surely it was malaria, but to my amazement it turned out be a lymphangitis. It is now subsiding. I suppose it will be a week before I get going again.

Friday, 17 September

Sulfadiazine is certainly amazing. I now learn that I came in here quite balmy with a temperature of 104—my WBC [white blood count] was 19,000 on Monday. I now feel fine but Captain Dietrich won't let me up. He has done a good job of keeping tabs on my blood count, urine, etc. My blood level was 5.5, but WBC fell to 3,000, so he stopped the drug. I have a little residual redness, soreness, and swelling of the right leg. But I don't think there is any thrombosis, although the captain thinks differently.

Brig. Gen. Fred W. Rankin [Director, Surgical Consultants Division, Office of The Surgeon General] just walked into my room. He is along with a troop of Senators, and they wouldn't leave him alone long enough to let him chat with me. The Senators, as usual, were all interested in people from their own State. He has been to Australia. Colonel Pincoffs [Col. Maurice C. Pincoffs, MC] is Chief of the Professional Service [Headquarters, USAFFE] and, he says, a trouble shooter for Col. (later Brig. Gen.) Percy J. Carroll, MC [Chief Surgeon, USAFFE]. Fred doesn't think he is as much use there as he would be in the job of consultant. Fred says he wants to stop the practice, among soldiers, of self medication with sulfonamides, but is a little afraid of public opinion. I wish he had stayed longer, for I could have told him a lot of things. However, it is nothing that he could do much about. I presume it is our job to try to straighten things out.

Tuesday, 21 September

Discharged from 27th Station Hospital today (fig. 313).

Listened to a talk by Maj. Gen. Brehon B. Somervell, Commanding General, Army Service Forces. He says that in 3 months we will have as much shipping available as we did at the beginning of the war, but that it will be next spring before our facilities for passenger shipping reach that stage.

Wednesday, 22 September

Spent the day writing directives on medical specialty boards, and on debridement and the care of wounds. Had a conference with Captain Kern and Commander Reynolds of the Navy.

Fiji Islands, Thursday, Friday, and Saturday, 23, 24, 25 September

Arose at 0300 hours—turned my ankle in the dark. Arrived at Tontouta Airfield 0500, from which we flew to Plaine de Gaiacs, New Caledonia. Had fresh eggs for breakfast. Took off at 0945. Arrived at Fiji at 1430. Nandi [on the western side of Viti Levu Island, the largest island in the Fijis] is in a valley surrounded by high mountains. The grass is green and the island appears fertile. Talked with a captain who had been at the 39th General Hospital as a patient. He was stationed at Bora-Bora, Society Islands, with the 8th Station Hospital, 280 beds. There are only about 1,500 men stationed

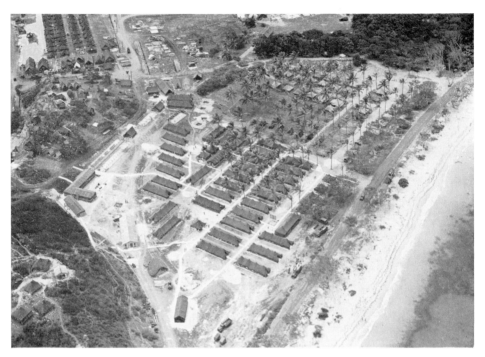

FIGURE 313.—An aerial view of the 27th Station Hospital, New Caledonia, February 1943.

there now, and about 35 to 50 in the hospital, which has 10 officers. Three officers would be plenty now. Colonel Sherwood plans on sending those patients who have been here over 1 year back to the States, because of the prevalence of filariasis. Certainly no replacements are needed here or possibly some could be taken out.

Monday, 27 September

Flew from Nandi to Suva [on the eastern side of Viti Levu Island] in a New Zealand de Haviland. We went above and through the clouds, over mountains, and then down through a hole into Suva. I prefer to take my chances over the ocean. Checked into the Grand Pacific Hotel. Met Ben Baker and Colonel Dovell, island surgeon.

Tuesday, 28 September

Spent the day at the 18th General Hospital—a grand crowd. The hospital is on the grounds of Victoria College, the Fijis' institution of higher learning—a fine location.

They need masks, bladders for the anesthesia machine, intratracheal anesthesia sets. They have five National field sterilizers we can have, and an extra 230 kv. electric sterilizer. They also have horizontal autoclaves, utensil sterilizers, and hot water sterilizers—all of them run on steam. The supply unit is well equipped.

They have done a fair amount of work but less than the 39th General Hospital and not enough to keep the men busy or happy. Much of their work is ordinarily done in a station hospital. These hospitals are chiefly taking in malaria patients from the Americal Division. They have more surgeons than they need for the work they have been doing. It seems that through ignorance of the functions of the different types of hospitals, the 142d General Hospital was originally set up in the field. Eventually, it was brought over to Suva. Now, however, there are two general hospitals at Suva. Colonel Dovell thinks that the 7th Evacuation Hospital, part of which is on Tongatabu, South Tonga, is of no use at Nandi and that it should come over to the Suva area to function as a convalescent hospital. While it is true that there should be a convalescent hospital at Suva, the personnel of the evacuation hospital should not be used for this purpose.

Wednesday, 29 September

Spent the day at the 142d. Lt. Col. Murray M. Copeland, MC, is commanding officer. Lt. Col. Harry C. Hull, MC, is the chief of surgery (fig. 314). Their physical plant, an old New Zealand hospital, is better than that of the 18th General Hospital. Very little surgery is being done. There are 160 patients, with space here for 450. They still work on a 60-day evacuation policy.

They have no intratracheal closed-tube anesthesia set, no Roger Anderson splints, or tincture of Belladonna; are short of sodium morrhuate, phenobarbital, resorcinol, sodium citrate ampules $2\frac{1}{2}$ percent, aluminum sulfate, traction bows, and wood applicators. Gigli's saw and Steinmann pins are of poor quality. They have an extra water bath setup and three National field sterilizers. Their biologicals are getting out of date.

Thursday, 30 September

Back at the 142d General Hospital. An excellent orthopedist here. They are about to lose two men from their surgical staff of nine. The mess is excellent. As at the 18th General, all of these men are anxious to go to the front with a surgical team. Colonel Dovell thinks that it is a great mistake to send good men to the front where they may be lost. However, he can be convinced.

Friday, 1 October 1943

Left Suva in the morning with Col. George G. Finney, MC, and Col. Murray Copeland and drove to Nandi via the Queen's Road. Had a pleasant luncheon on the beach with Colonel Dovell and Miss Donohue [Lt. Regina M. Donohue, ANC], Chief Nurse at the 142d. Arrived in the evening at the 7th Evacuation Hospital, which is situated in a delightful valley near a mountain range, about 10 miles from the Nandi Airport and 18 miles from the dock. Lt. Col. Robert B. Lobban, MC, is commanding officer. Lt. Col. McKelvie is chief of medicine, and Maj. Robert S. Ackerly, MC, is chief of surgery. They came from the States last spring, first to Tongatabu and then to Fiji. They never functioned as an evacuation hospital and have done very little surgery. They acted as a station hospital in demalarializing the American Division.

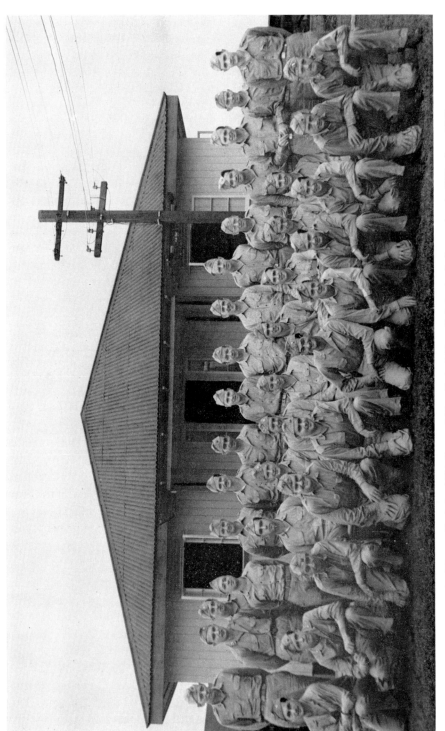

FIGURE 314.—The staff of the 142d General Hospital at New Caledonia, before going to Fiji, June 1943.

A good staff, but no talent to spare. Most of their surgeons are young, with few specialists and no orthopedist. This hospital was first built by the New Zealanders and is now partly under wood and canvas. Had dinner—good food with sauterne.

Saturday, 2 October

Made the rounds at the 7th Evacuation Hospital. They need portable lamps, microscopes (now have one field microscope), antigen for Kahn test, homatropine, and pyrogallic acid. They have a portable orthopedic table, which could be used with a Hawley table. Scissors are of poor quality. Two utensil sterilizers, the 240 and large field sterilizer, have been acquired. No special anesthetist is assigned here. They would like Lt. Fred Dye, who is with the Americal Division.

Visited Lt. Col. James F. Collins, MC, Division Surgeon of the Americal Division. Appears to me to be a fine person doing a good job, and he has plenty of ideas which he promises to put down on paper. He is now short 15 men, and 6 of his doctors are sick. He believes that the old system of three clearing companies is better than the present one clearing company setup.

I put George Finney on a plane and spent the night at the 71st Station Hospital, which is now under construction on a good location. They will be ready to take patients in 2 weeks and could even do so now. Lt. Col. Anthony Ruppersberg, Jr., MC, an obstetrician, is commanding officer. He is energetic and is doing a fine job. The hospital will have 250 beds and eventually expand to 500. They need an EENT man. Check with the possibility of getting Bodein from Americal. Are they getting the journals here? Major Heyer, chief of the medical service, wants an EKG machine. Carbon dioxide tanks with proper connections for frozen sections are needed in all general hospitals.

Sunday, 3 October

Drove from Nandi via the King's Highway to Suva (180 miles), thus circling the island.

SUMMARY OF THE FIJI TOUR

1. Hospitals.

a. The 18th General Hospital is about to expand to a 1,000-bed T/O. They have excellent talent. Should this hospital be enlarged, however, it would take considerable building.

b. The 142d General Hospital is also about to expand to a 1,000-bed T/O. They also have excellent talent. This hospital is on a good site, which can easily absorb some additional construction.

c. The 7th Evacuation Hospital should be divided up in order to provide a convalescent hospital, and could be best placed in Suva in the camp partly occupied by the Quartermaster. The remaining units of this hospital could be utilized to supplement the 142d General Hospital, or to form a smaller evacuation unit.

2. At present there are approximately 2,500 beds on Fiji and too much concentration of medical and surgical talent. One general hospital, the 142d,

with a capacity of from 1,000 to 1,500 beds, one convalescent hospital with 2,000 beds, and one station hospital on the north side of the island would be ample. This would leave from 3,500 to 4,000 beds on Fiji and free the talent of the 18th General Hospital for assignment nearer the zone of combat.

3. At least two well-equipped surgical teams can be provided from Fiji. Colonel Dovell tends, as usual, to push off the less-qualified and less-experienced men for duty at the front. We should first give it a try with the best men.

Nouméa, Monday, 4 October

I was up at 0400, took off at 0600 in a GI clipper ship, landed at Espíritu Santo 1100 hours, then to Efate, and arrived at Nouméa 1500 hours.

Sunday, 10 October

Hal Thomas [Lt. Col. Henry M. Thomas, Jr., MC] arrived yesterday on his way to the Southwest Pacific as medical consultant. I'm still working on directives and hope to finish up in a few days. Ed Ottenheimer [Lt. Col. (later Col.) Edward J. Ottenheimer, MC, Chief, Surgical Service, 39th General Hospital] says he will send us Claiborn [Lt. Col. Louie N. Claiborn, MC] and Post for the surgical teams.

Tuesday, 12 October

Completed the gas gangrene directive. Experimented with insufflators for sulfanilamide; perhaps I can stop its too liberal use in wounds. Met Colonel Ward, who is going to Fiji. Col. (later Brig. Gen.) Earl Maxwell [Surgeon, USAFISPA] is off on a trip to New Georgia and will try to straighten out the morale of the 17th Field Hospital. He will see Maj. Gen. Robert S. Beightler of the 37th Division and lay plans for our next move.

Wednesday, 13 October

Dinner last night at Mobile 8 with Jack Carmody [Lt. (later Cdr.) John T. B. Carmody, MC, USNR] and Frank Hauter. Mobile 8 has a new clubhouse with a large fireplace and a bar. Drinks are the best ever. Ten to fifteen cents is what they charge. Chatted with Captain Dearing after dinner concerning plans for Bougainville, our next major military objective.[5] He is a very pleasant fellow. General Rankin met him at the hospital.

Sunday, 17 October

Spent yesterday at the 8th General Hospital (fig. 315) with Colonel Miller. They have no urologist and con use a major or a captain. He might be exchanged for an anesthesiologist whom they could train here. They also have no neurosurgeon.

The problem in Army medicine is, as in civilian medicine, one of getting the right man in the right place at the right time. Here, under the conditions of

---

[5] Bougainville was to provide the Allied forces with important airfields from which Rabaul and the remaining Japanese installations in the Solomons could be neutralized. New Zealand troops occupied two islands in the Treasury group of the northern Solomons late in October. The 3d Marine Division of the I Marine Amphibious Corps landed on 1 November at Empress Augusta Bay in western Bougainville. On 11 November, elements of the 37th Division entered the line. On 15 December, command of the beachhead passed to the American XIV Corps, which had been reinforced by the Americal Division.

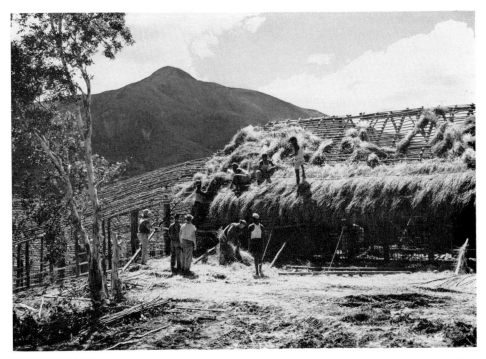

FIGURE 315.—Construction of a native-style barracks for the 8th General Hospital, New Caledonia, September 1943.

island warfare, we are trying to make each island a unit in itself, with all branches of medicine adequately covered. But there are just not enough qualified men to go around. This is particularly true for the forward hospitals. Field hospitals have had to perform the work of evacuation hospitals in these areas. I've seen three divisions here without one competent surgeon. Hence it is no wonder that the early treatment of wounds is not good. It would take a lot of shifting to change the situation, and they are a little loath to move people for fear of not getting their cooperation.

One of the great difficulties of getting adequate personnel in the right places is due to the fact that too many high-ranking officers have been promoted without the proper professional qualifications. Every commanding officer wants to promote the officers in his own organization. Even some old Army men look more to their own organization than to the good of the service. Moreover, I am very, very doubtful of the wisdom of having affiliated units. This results in too great a concentration of talent. The area surgeon does not feel free to move these men about.[6] Hence there is no way of strengthening the weak spots in the command.

---

[6] Colonel Oughterson has answered his own criticism: "There are just not enough qualified men to go around". They are all "agglutinated" in the affiliated units, and it is difficult to pry them out. See also p. 823.—J. M. W.

Tuesday, 19 October

Lt. Col. Paul Kisner, MC, and I left Nouméa in a staff car at 0730 to drive to Plaine de Gaiacs, a distance of 160 miles. The road beyond Bouloupari was very rough. We arrived at Bourail, Headquarters, New Zealand Forces, South Pacific, at 1200 and had lunch with Colonel Twhigg. I acquired a new pair of New Zealand army boots, and then on to Plaine de Gaiacs at 1600. We looked over the hospital there and had a good supper.

The 331st Station Hospital now has 50 beds and 50 more that are almost ready for occupancy. Maj. Hugo A. Aach, MC, is commanding officer and has one lieutenant who assists him. He is doing a good job developing the hospital. Laboratory facilities are meager. He has had quite a number of accidents from the ATC (Air Transport Command) base. Eight patients with burns have been treated, one of whom died. The grounds are very dirty, and under these conditions burns treated with paraffin can easily become infected, as these did. They soon after adopted the practice of bandaging these burns. His equipment is good and he has no needs except for more medical personnel.

After supper we drove back to Bourail where we stopped at the New Zealand Hospital. Up at 0500 and arrived back at Nouméa, noontime. During this 2-day trip, I wore the seat out of a new pair of cotton trousers. There is no argument about trauma aggravating pilonidal cysts.

Friday, 22 October

Visited the 31st Station Hospital today. Lt. Col. Corren P. Youmans, MC, is commanding officer. This is the breakdown of the University of Minnesota hospital group after a change in T/O. There are five young and energetic surgeons here. They should have a chief of surgery sent in if they are going to expand to a 500-bed hospital. Not that the young men are bad, but they are immature.

Six hundred patients have been transported here by air since 15 September. These are seen at Tontouta Airfield by the 31st Station Hospital men. The sick cases are kept at the 31st Station Hospital and the others are sent on to the 8th General Hospital. Many patients who have recently been operated on have been shipped down here. These surgeons are objecting to what has been done at other hospitals. A directive is needed regarding records and X-ray procedures. They think that too many cases with simple ailments are being evacuated. Besides, patients with psychosis are being sent down with an organic diagnosis, which throws them off the trail here and obviously makes treatment more difficult. This is a rather dirty hospital, hot, and on low, mosquito-ridden grounds.

Espíritu Santo, Monday, 25 October

I left this morning with Ben Baker on a Navy flying boat. Left at 1200. Sandwiches and coffee served en route. Stopped at Efate—Havannah Harbour is full with battlewagons. Arrived at Espíritu Santo, 1730 hours. Stayed at the 25th Evacuation Hospital.

Tuesday, 26 October

Saw Lt. Col. Arthur G. King, MC [Surgeon, Service Command]. He is not doing a bad job—efficient. Sofield's orders arrived (assigning him to SPA [the South Pacific Area] as orthopedic consultant). The 10th Medical Supply Depot under Capt. E. Lucas is doing better and is nearly all undercover. Found three anesthesia chests and two field sterilizers. Visited the 122d Station Hospital. Major Camp seems the head here and he has done a good job planning. The hospital now has 500 patients, although capacity is rated at 1,000.

Guadalcanal, Wednesday, 27 October

Arose at 0400 and after a good breakfast of ham and eggs we took off for Guadalcanal in a B–24 Liberator.

Arrived at Guadalcanal 0930 and reported to the 37th Division headquarters. Met Col. Edward J. Grass, MC, a pleasant division surgeon from Washington, D.C., who was very cooperative. He plans on using surgical teams in the collecting stations. This should work out well, since there is a collecting company with each combat team. For a second echelon hospital, we shall use the clearing station. Will the combat operation be such as to make this practicable? Distance is the determining factor. Major Bliun, Commanding Officer, Company D, 112th Medical Battalion, is a fine fellow. There is the utmost spirit of cooperation, and I think that the venture will succeed.

The supply problem has not been cleared up. Plaster of paris in cans has been issued in quantity for the combat teams, but only 24 dozen bandages are on hand. We will change that. Prophylactic kits are still being issued, with no females within 1,000 miles of here. Other uses have been found for them, such as covers for pistol barrels, watches, and pocket drug kits. Started Atabrine therapy today. Two ships were sunk offshore carrying power generators for the 37th Division. Mono was taken by the Marines today.[7]

Thursday, 28 October

Went over the supply question with Lieutenant Rhodes, medical supply officer of the 37th Division. The maintenance lists are not adapted to this area. There is a surplus of some items; for example, mops, prophylactic kits, tons of cotton, and not enough of other items. What good are mops with no floors to mop? We talked about the plan for surgical teams. Since they still do not grasp the principle of time relationship in the treatment of casualties, it will take a lot of conversation to convert them. There will be trouble getting lighting facilities, since there are no generators.

Visited Capt. George Ellis [Capt. James W. Ellis, MC, USN], Surgeon, 1st Marine Amphibious Corps, at the old Imperial Japanese Headquarters—a lovely site on the beach. Emile Holman [Cdr. Emile F. Holman, MC, USNR, Surgical Consultant, 1st Marine Amphibious Corps] was there as a consultant surgeon to the Marine Corps. They plan to evacuate serious casualties from Bougainville to Vella Lavella Island by destroyer, which again means from 3

---

[7] See footnote 5, p. 802.

to 4 hours by boat, and a total delay of approximately 8 or 12 hours. It will be interesting to compare Army methods with those of the Navy in this operation. Only the two anesthetists, Lieberman and Rose, have arrived so far.

Friday, 29 October

Plans today for the movement of three combat teams. The plan is to use surgical teams in the collecting stations. The two surgeons, one anesthetist and two corpsmen of the surgical team, with its extra equipment, will be attached to the four officers and men of the collecting company.

We have no generators for the collecting company, so I have spent the day in pursuit of three light generators and so far have found none. Major Smith, a pleasant fellow from the Engineers, offered one 5-kilowatt generator weighing 1,800 pounds—a fine piece of equipment, but a white elephant to move. Eleven generators were lost in the two boats the Japanese sunk off the shore the other day. Why do they still put all their eggs in one basket? The Navy doesn't have any either, so they say. The Seabees are making three plaster supports for shoulder spicas, using heavy steel since it is the only thing available. Weight could be saved by using an alloy.

Acquired a carbine today. This is a fine outfit: Colonel Grass, surgeon; Maj. John Bliun, commanding officer of the clearing company; and Vic Kolb, an excellent officer. They put on a fine review this afternoon.

Saturday, 30 October

Went to see the the the 117th Engineers about digging in for operating rooms, and so forth. Surgeons for the teams arrived today. They are Shackelford, Watson, Manwell, Post, and Troland. Three anesthetists, Schulman, Rose, and Lieberman, and a bacteriologist, Michael, also arrived (fig. 316).[8]

Monday, 1 November 1943

Navy started shelling Bougainville yesterday. Had conference with General Beightler [Maj. Gen. Robert S. Beightler, Commanding General, 37th Division] and staff this morning.

Friday, 5 November

A busy few days, mostly spent in gathering supplies. Eighty-eight hundred pounds of supplies were supposed to arrive on the *Currey* and did not. Headquarters, USAFISPA, informed us by radio that they were put on the boat. After I had given them a reply, we received a radio saying that the supplies had been found and were to be shipped by air. Yesterday 34 of 48 boxes arrived. Today they were sorted and put aboard ship. Almost all personnel were on board today. Don't know where I am supposed to be, but I will board the *President Adams* tomorrow.

The cooperative spirit and morale of this division, and of the officers and men of the forward area, appear wonderful. The soldiers are not worried about the outcome of the war, but they are full of doubts and fears for the

---

[8] So far as they could be identified, these officers were: Capt. William G. Watson, MC, Maj. Edward J. Manwell, MC, Capt. Charles E. Troland, MC, Capt. Harold C. Schulman, Capt. Max Michael.

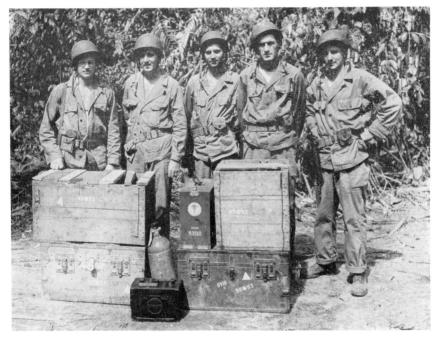

FIGURE 316.—Surgical team with equipment (left to right: Capt. William G. Watson, MC, Capt. Charles E. Troland, MC, surgeons; Capt. Harold C. Schulman, anesthetist; Sgt. William F. Marsden, Sgt. Murray M. Lemish, technicians), Bougainville, 13 December 1943.

future. The bold confidence of a century ago, or even of the last war, is not to be seen. They are not sure why they are fighting. They want to go home, since they feel they have done their bit. Nevertheless, they carry on.

Saturday, 6 November

1445 hours. Since I could get no information as to what ship I was supposed to go on, I stayed ashore last night. We had an air raid at 0100. Went to the beach this morning and found Captain Ellis, Senior Medical Officer of the 1st Marine Amphibious Corps, and General Craig [Brig. Gen. Charles F. Craig, Assistant Division Commander, 37th Division] sitting on their jungle packs. So I finally climbed on and went out with them to the *Adams*, where I was put in a large stateroom next to General Gage of the Marines and General Craig of the 37th Division. The room is equipped with a fine shower bath and a fan. Had a fine lunch of iced tea, spaghetti, meat sauce, and apricots. The table was set with napkins and a white tablecloth. I have to pinch myself to realize we are off to invade Bougainville. There are about 20 ships in sight, and the destroyers and cruisers are gathering around, so it won't be long before we are off.

We intend to use the surgical teams with the collecting stations, though this may be too far forward. Ideally the surgical teams should be behind the collecting stations, but General Beightler is afraid of isolating the teams and leaving them open for infiltration. The Engineers have promised to dig us in with bulldozers, if the road comes up with us.

The weight and transportation of equipment is a big problem in island warfare. Each team has a 250-pound chest full of instruments, et cetera. In addition, I have provided sterilizers, autoclaves, anesthesia machines, suction, generators, orthopedic tables, etc. The equipment should be as light as possible for this type of warfare. For example, the horizontal field sterilizer weighs 350 pounds crated. Equipment could be permanently attached to a light truck without great loss, since the truck engine could be used to run the generator. So far I have seen no operating installation where a truck could not get to. However, one disadvantage to a truck would be the difficulty of digging in and the fact that it might be damaged as a result of bombing. This campaign should enable us to discover the best method of handling our equipment.

It is obvious that the clearing company T/O is not adapted for this type of warfare in which combat teams operate independently. The clearing company has one set of equipment and two clearing platoons to be divided into three small hospitals, which is impossible. I would suggest that, given this situation, each combat team should operate as a self-sufficient unit with one collecting station and two small hospitals for each team. Two hospitals are needed in order to "leapfrog." If need be, the collecting stations could be combined with the two hospitals, one of which would operate as a surgical hospital, and the second would care for routine cases not requiring skilled surgery. Thus, if there is a danger of infiltration, they can be combined: hospital number one with number two, or number one with the collecting station. A field hospital can be used to back up the division, both as a rehabilitation camp and to hold patients for evacuation. We will watch this operation to see how the arrangement functions.

The *President Adams*, Sunday, 7 November

We left Guadalcanal last night at 0100, just as the moon went down. I had a good sleep in spite of the fact that it was hotter than Hades, even with the fan working. This morning we had a wonderful breakfast of ice-cold grapefruit, ham, eggs, toast, and coffee. I can't tell how large the convoy is, for the ships extend further than I can see. We are sailing up through The Slot. New Georgia is on our left and Choiseul Island will soon be on the right. The news says that the Japanese are sending down large convoys from the Truk Islands naval base. A lovely day, with a gentle roll to the sea and lots of flying fish. Apparently we have plane protection from the adjacent islands.

Bougainville, Monday, 8 November

Bougainville, 1400 hours. An uneventful night, but hotter than Hades; cloudy and raining, so there was no bombing. A lovely clear morning—could not see land yet. It appears that we came straight in. The cargo ships are in line, with destroyers on either side. The island has a beautiful skyline with rugged mountains and two volcanoes that are said to be active. One of them is directly behind the landing point [Empress Augusta Bay]. Our guns are firing west at the Japanese lines, where they landed several barges last night. As far as we know they have no artillery. We were ordered to land at 0850, and in less than an hour there was nobody left on board but the crew and some supplies.

The terrain near the beach is lava sand, with some swamp behind. However, it is fairly dry now. Tremendous confusion on shore, but after about two hours we found the clearing station and the collecting station. We will stay put here for the night until a plan of the campaign is given us. At 1100 hours, the Japanese came over. I guessed that there were about 25 to 30 planes, later found out there were 70. The ships had 15 minutes' warning and pulled out to sea. The sky seemed full of ack-ack and planes. I hear that one of our ships was hit but stories fly so thick and fast that you can't tell what is really happening. Hal Sofield just came up and told me to put in my diary: "The *Adams* was hit in the stern a half hour after we debarked." The boys already have the barbed wire up around the clearing station. I have dug a foxhole and put my jungle hammock in it, since we must all stay underground at night.

Tuesday, 9 November

There has been very little infiltration of Japanese. Only a few casualties. The 37th is to take the left half of the perimeter. The Marines have a clearing station in this sector, and so far are doing the surgery under poor conditions. They don't have screening and the debridement is very crude. There is a division hospital (3d Marine Division, I Marine Amphibious Corps), with a Dr. Bruce [Lt. Cdr. Gordon M. Bruce, MC, USNR], an ophthalmologist from New York, in command.

Wednesday, 10 November

Some trouble today on the right flank, about 90 Marine casualties. The beach along the left flank is being evacuated by amphibious tanks. I saw returning tanks, loaded with our dead. We are not yet set up for operating, although fortunately it would make little difference if we were. The planning of this clearing station has been noticeable by its absence, partly due to lack of information, and partly because we are waiting to take over after the Marine division hospital moves out. Finally found Captain Ellis of the Marines in his headquarters about 100 yards behind us in this extraordinarily dense jungle.

Thursday, 11 November

0800 hours. Armistice day and a good joke on the well-known human race. On the present model, all days will eventually be armistice days. Six hours of bombing and strafing last night, from 2000 to 0200, with many humorous situations and much shouting and conversation in one syllable words. Some fellows stayed in the foxhole, but with a little practice, I found I could beat the best of them in the race back. The only trouble was that the first in was at the bottom of the heap. The landing craft carrying the Marines

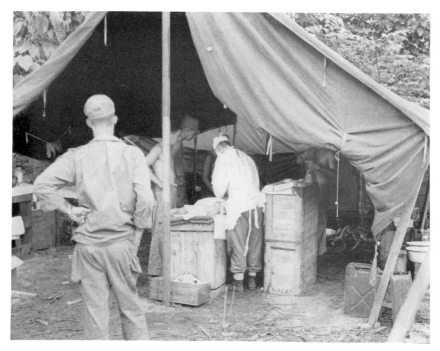

FIGURE 317.—A surgical team at work 5 days after the landing, Bougainville,
13 November 1943.

for the main attack on the island took more than 60 casualties. A destroyer
and numerous barges are said to have been sunk.

Friday, 12 November

Bombing last night was limited to an attack on the LST's. There is a
question as to whether surgical teams will work under the present arrangement. This is a good outfit with a fine cooperative group of men (fig. 317), but
after 5 days here we still have no adequate surgical setup and nothing screened,
not even a latrine. The surgical team, not being a separate unit, can
do nothing. It would be better for the surgical team to go in as a unit with
its own command responsibility. Without good surgical care, this outfit would
have been sunk if there had been a large number of casualties. Captain Ellis
has changed the evacuation policy again. This time evacuation is to be to
Vella Lavella Island by boat and PBY ["Catalina" flying boat] but again this
is too late for definitive surgery. It must be done on this island to be effective.
Admiral Halsey [Vice Adm. William F. Halsey, Commander, South Pacific
Area, and Commander, South Pacific Forces] was here this morning.

Saturday, 13 November

0800 hours. The convoy with the 129th Infantry Regiment is coming in.
Yesterday we moved to the edge of the [Koromokina] River. The woods here
are infested with every kind of bug as well as mosquitoes. I awoke this morn-

ing with six of them inside my net. Air raids last night at 8, midnight, and 2, 3, 4 and 5 in the morning.

Sniper fire getting closer this morning. The NCO's at the far end of one tent started shooting at what they said were Japanese. The Japanese had infiltrated through this area at the beginning of the week, and shot at the corpsmen in the Marine hospital. I was not too confident and so got out my carbine. The orders are to shoot anything outside the area that moves. Hence, the boys are likely to try out their guns. Some of the Japanese snipers are brought down by this method, and, of course, if one of our boys moves about out there after dark, he can only blame himself for the consequences. The Japanese infiltrates in the night and usually climbs a tree to await his opportunity at daylight. One of them waited until the middle of the day when there were plenty of people about the hospital, and then opened up with a machinegun. Fortunately no one was killed, but several were wounded. This is of course suicide for the Japanese, for he never gets away after that. The 129th Infantry came in, but could not land all its men owing to the high surf. Ben [Baker] and Kaufman [Lt. Col. Moses R. Kaufman, MC, Consultant in Neuropsychiatry, USAFISPA] arrived.

There is dissension between the surgical team and the clearing company. The surgeons were restless because of the slow progress and lack of organization. Surgical patients were coming in, and the surgeons were not being asked to see them. The clearing station personnel, who are not surgeons, were attempting to do the work in the same old fashion. I have asked Hal Sofield if he can get the teams organized and build an operating room. We have been here 6 days with nothing much to do, and still no adequate operating room. There is no provision for blood transfusion, no hemoglobinometer or microscope. These were to be brought up later. I am not yet sure how this experiment of ours will work out. This is a loyal outfit, and for anyone to show them up is of course disastrous. Even though they admit they are not first-class surgeons, nevertheless, the demonstration of this in front of their own company is too much for them to take. I am inclined to think that surgical teams must function as separate units under a separate command. They cannot be held responsible for good surgery without good surgical equipment, and it appears that the teams do not have enough authority to get things done. The unit should have the responsibility under the division surgeon for all surgery in the forward area. Clearing stations, which are without first-class surgeons, cannot be expected to turn out high caliber work.

Sunday, 14 November

We are experimenting with putting one surgeon and one anesthetist from each team with the collecting station and using three of our surgeons with the three doctors in the clearing station, all this in the interest of harmony. I am putting up General Breene's sign, "We are fighting the Japs and not each other." Hal has been working on the surgery. He has it above ground in a tent. General Beightler came over and immediately perceived that being situated next to the antiaircraft guns was not the right place for us. We will move in 10 days, but having a surgery is worthwhile even for so short a time.

The Japanese are trying to come over here through two mountain passes.

Monday, 15 November

We opened the surgery today although it is not yet screened. The plain facts are that the medical men of this outfit do not believe in the bacterial theory of disease, or, if they do, they do not appreciate its significance. It is almost hopeless to expect that directives or conversations will quickly change the prevailing concept of surgery. I have yet to see a surgeon who did good surgery at home do bad surgery in the Army. It is my opinion that the sloppy surgery I have observed in the Army is merely a reflection of sloppy surgery in civilian practice.

The *Talbot*, Guadalcanal, Wednesday, Thursday, 17, 18 November

Sofield and I were at the beach at 0730 in order to go to Vella Lavella with patients. A Japanese attack came at 0800. I don't know how many planes there were, for the air was full of both theirs and ours. It was fascinating to watch the 90-mm. shells following the planes. The marksmanship was very poor, for the crews were not leading the aircraft sufficiently. They were too excited and shot at anything in sight.

We finally put off for the *Talbot*, an APD (transport, high speed), and had the 40 patients aboard by 1030. For some reason, we circled around until 1400. Then we started out for Vella Lavella, at 22 knots.

When we approached Vella Lavella, our orders were changed and we went on to Guadalcanal, arriving at 1000. Hence, the trip by fast destroyer transport took about 24 hours. There was only one doctor on the ship, and operating facilities were meager. Patients were carried up and down steep companionways—no way to treat an acute belly. The captain said this was a usual performance and that the schedules of the APD's were not correlated with the needs of the wounded. Two patients have died in transit. Both were in shock when put aboard. We went to the 37th Division rear echelon headquarters, where Colonel Moore gave us some beer and clean clothes, and then to the 20th Station Hospital.

Friday, 19 November

The 20th Station Hospital has poor morale and is doing poor surgery. The least that should be done is to give them a strong commanding officer and a good surgeon.

Saturday, 20 November

The 25th Division needs more doctors. They now have 35 and should have 49. They could then send out two anesthetists to train others. The 21st Evacuation Hospital is being set up, as is also the 137th Station Hospital. The 9th Station Hospital has not yet opened its surgery. Sofield and I talked to all the doctors on Guadalcanal today, including Army surgeons at the 20th Station, 137th Station, and 21st Evacuation Hospitals.

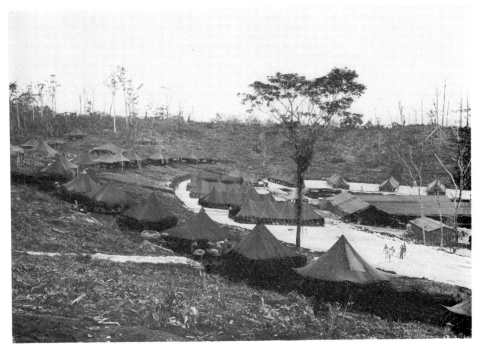

FIGURE 318.—"Probably the best constructed, laid out, and equipped field hospital in the Army"—the 24th Field Hospital, New Georgia, 27 October 1943.

Sunday, 21 November

Spent the day packing, washing, and trading. Colonel Hallam came over to visit me. The XIV Corps is moving to Guadalcanal and then to Bougainville.

New Georgia, Monday, 22 November

Off at 0500. Stayed at XIV Corps headquarters. The transformation of Munda since my last visit 2 months ago is amazing. The airfield is enormous and there are good roads, quarters, et cetera. Saw Colonel Melvin, who drove us around and arranged a meeting of the island surgeons at the 24th Field Hospital for 1800.

The 17th Field Hospital now has a much better setup and they have profited by experience and example. The morale is better. The 24th Field Hospital, which is on the edge of the airstrip, has a most elaborate layout (fig. 318). Built in a sort of amphitheater cleared of all trees, the buildings form a horse-shoe. The buildings extend out, like a series of terraces, giving the hospital the appearance of a stadium, especially when seen from the air. This is probably the best constructed, laid out, and equipped field hospital in the U.S. Army. In fact it is so well and thoroughly set up that it can no longer be called a field hospital.

The new T/O does not allow enough corpsmen for evacuation of casualties by litter carry, which is so important in tropical warfare. This has often resulted in late treatment with loss of life or limb and prolonged convalescence. It should illustrate the impossibility of laying down a standard T/O for a world-wide war fought under varying conditions. The surgical teams should carry more than two medical technicians—possibly six. Men sent into the area fresh from the States should not be sent directly to divisions in combat. One-third or one-half of them will usually show up poorly.

There is a general request from doctors for some sort of postgraduate training, since many of them have done nothing but administrative work since the war started.

A urologist and a neurosurgeon are needed at the 8th General Hospital [New Caledonia]. They need three-way stop cocks for anesthesia. Order book, "Fundamentals of Anesthesia," for distribution here. Emergency Medical Tags and indelible pencils are needed. Records of the patients come down late. Division will not send the service records of their men to hospitals because they are afraid of permanently losing their hospitalized personnel.

The 109th Station Hospital [New Caledonia] has 24 officers, and it should have 33. They want Lieberman and need a Medical Administrative Corps officer, an EENT man, and some more enlisted men. An optometrist is needed for both the 17th and 24th Field Hospitals. The 43d Division is short eight medical officers, two dentists, and a large number of enlisted men.

The evacuation from Bougainville was planned by Captain Ellis of the Marine I Amphibious Corps. While at Guadalcanal, we were told that everything was settled and that casualties could be evacuated by APD in 3 to 4 hours to Vella Lavella Island. Just before leaving Guadalcanal, Ellis said this was all off; that all work would be done at Cherry Blossom [Bougainville], and the Army could have the installations at Vella. On arriving at Cherry Blossom, we saw that all of the work was not being done there. Some patients were being taken directly to APD's and transported to unknown destinations. I later met someone who had just come from Vella Lavella. He told me that they had not received a single patient there. Moreover, the trip from Bougainville to Vella takes 10 to 12 hours and not 3 to 4 hours. Emile Holman was there, tearing his hair out.

Tuesday, 23 November

The above was written while sitting on the beach at New Georgia. We took off in a Higgins boat. The youngster in charge drove to the wrong side of the marker, ran on a reef, and then finally deposited us on shore. After a 4-hour wait, we got another boat that took us to Ondongo Island. Cordially received by the Marines, we were treated to excellent food, had clean towels, and slept between sheets in one of their quonset huts. Tomorrow there will be a plane to take us back to Bougainville.

Bougainville, Wednesday, 24 November

We took off at noon with General Harris [Brig. Gen. Field Harris, USMC, Commander, Air Command, North Solomons] in a Dumbo (patrol bomber, "Catalina") with a very competent pilot who had been decorated at Midway.

Escorted by 10 fighter planes, we arrived at Bougainville in 1½ hours without incident.

They have made great progress here, and the clearing stations have been moved. The boys had many stories of bombing, strafing, and shelling. Ben [Baker] produced the head of a 90-mm. ack-ack shell, which came through his tent and punctured his rubber mattress.

The Marines reported having had eight cases of gas gangrene. Their evacuation is not completely controlled, and some of the patients have been put on the boat without receiving prior treatment. A considerable number of patients died in transit. Colonel Melvin told me of 12 on one LST. Two died on an APD from Bougainville. *A complete and unified control of evacuation from an island is necessary.*

Thursday, Thanksgiving Day, 25 November

Only one plane dropped its bombs on us last night. The Japanese have some artillery in and are shelling the beach. We had a fine Thanksgiving dinner; very good turkey with stuffing, cauliflower, peas, mashed potatoes, pumpkin pie, luscious biscuits, and coffee. I ate too much as usual.

The construction on the island is developing very rapidly. Planes are now making emergency landings and takeoffs.

Friday, 26 November

Last night we were shelled by Japanese artillery and today everyone is digging deeper. There is still inertia about getting patients underground. They are screening the operating room today (fig. 319). The surgical teams must have the responsibility for building and operating the surgery and furnishing its supplies. Supplies, such as screening, sandbags, et cetera, should not be left under the supervision of any other branch of the service. Experience shows that they are not likely to be on hand when needed. Furthermore, these supplies should go in with the first wave, when casualties are likely to be heavy.

Saturday, 27 November

Last night, the first night on Bougainville without an alert, I had a wonderful, cool, refreshing sleep on my air mattress. Army casualties are still light here. The doctors of the 37th Division have requested that we give nightly lectures on medical topics.

Sunday, 28 November

An uneventful day. Listened to Chaplain Kirker [Lt. Col. Kirker, 37th Division chaplain] talk on "True and False Truth." I remarked that the boys seemed very interested. "That group was christianized by bombs before we got here," said he.

Monday, 29 November

Went out on the right flank to visit a battalion of the 145th Infantry Regiment, who are with the Marines. Went up to within 500 feet of the frontlines, but I could see no Japanese, probably owing to the fact that the land is a dense swamp except along the beach. About 1,000 Marines struck the beach [Koiaris Beach] below here last night. They suffered 40 percent casualties and were lucky to get back with the help of a destroyer. Last night the Japanese shelled

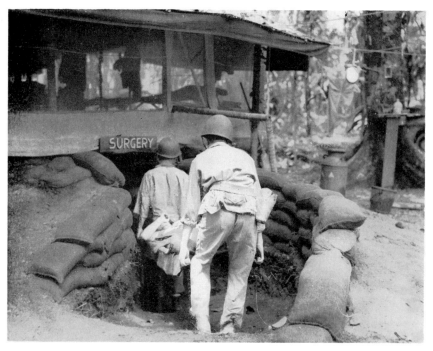

FIGURE 319.—A screened and dug-out operating room, Bougainville, December 1943.

the beach with 8-inch naval guns, location unknown. They hit a gas dump which caused a tremendous fire. Puruata Island [off Empress Augusta Bay, Bougainville] is certainly one of the most bombed and shelled of islands.

Thursday, 2 December 1943

Nothing new, not even the rain. Talked to a group last night on planned health and had a good response. It seems that mobile surgical trucks would be very useful here.

Sunday, 5 December

Everything okay in Cherry Blossom so I decided to return to Cactus [Guadalcanal] for further organization. Had dinner last night with General Beightler, General Craig, and General Krueger [Lt. Gen. (later Gen.) Walter Krueger, Commanding General, Sixth U.S. Army], and they are well pleased with the surgical teams, with our teaching, et cetera (fig. 320). There has been a lot of discussion about how to keep doctors happy while they are in the service, and the consensus is that it is generally impossible.

We have come down to the beach for a Dumbo. No one knows when it will come or where it will go, and the pleasant part of it is that no one seems to care a great deal. The uncertainty and variability of our movements serve to throw the enemy off, but it is amazing how much does get done in this situation.

Fresh supplies of meat, oranges, et cetera, are being unloaded today. The food on the whole has been very good, and there are some excellent cooks and bakers here. Sanitation is not all that it should be, owing to the laxity of the medical officers and their failure to appreciate the importance of good sanitation. There were almost no flies when we first landed; now there are swarms of them. Even after a month very few messes have been screened. However, we have had no dysentery problem.

The mobile surgical units, mounted on trucks, would be a tremendous asset in this kind of warfare. This type of setup would save much labor, while providing facilities in the early stages of combat. I have yet to see a place where a hospital was needed that could not be reached by these trucks.

The foreign body localizer is valuable, but it should be constructed to stand up under damp tropical conditions and function on a battery. A blower is needed to dry plaster casts.

Guadalcanal, Monday, 6 December

Took off from Cherry Blossom in a Catalina yesterday at 1600. We skirted the edge of the island with 10 fighters, then over to the Treasury Islands, and landed at Ondongo at 1730. There were no planes going to Munda, so we started out in a personnel boat. With the aid of a light, great caution, and good luck, we made a landing in pitch dark at 2030. Colonel Hanson came down to take us to the 24th Field Hospital, where we had a good meal and quarters.

This morning we took off by SCAT for Guadalcanal. Colonel Caton is using the 21st Evacuation Hospital for all initial admissions on the island. Patients are distributed from there to the other hospitals. Visited Colonel Taber at the 52d Field Hospital.

Tuesday, 7 December

Two years today since Pearl Harbor. What would people in the States have said if they were told at the time of Pearl Harbor that in 2 years Japan would have achieved most of its imperial aims and have conquered the Philippines, Malaya, and the Dutch East Indies, and that all we would have taken back were two or three islands in the Solomons that few had even heard of before.

Spent the day with Paul Kisner at the 20th Station Hospital. He is already beginning to bring order out of chaos. He wants a chief of surgery, for he cannot raise the level of surgery by himself. He also wants a laboratory man, a trained lab technician, and an eye man.

Visited Mobile 8 and talked about debridement and gas gangrene. They have had about 300 compound fractures with 20-plus cases of gas gangrene, resulting in 2 deaths. The estimate is that 8 to 10 percent of the patients with compound fracture have gas gangrene. Treatment was conservative for the most part. The cases from Bougainville came in with either poor debridement or none at all. I saw some cases, in which the patient had not even been shaved.

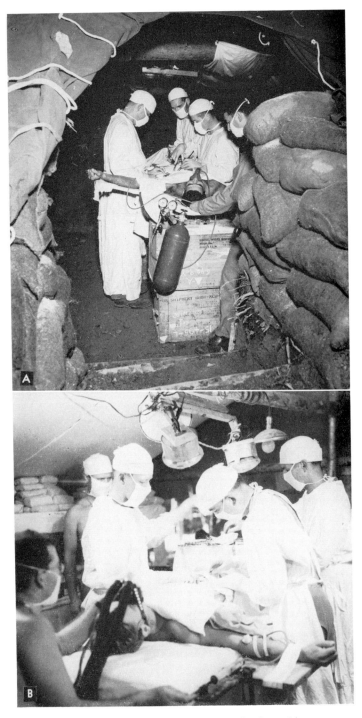

FIGURE 320.—(*See opposite page for legend.*)

Nouméa, Wednesday, 8 December

Off at 0830 for New Caledonia with freight cargo including a 5,000-pound Allison motor. It was raining, and we went up over 10,000 feet to get out of the bad weather—very bumpy ride. I kept wondering what we would do if the motor got loose. However, we landed at 1430 without mishap, and once again sat down for cocktails at the Grand Hotel Central.

Friday, 10 December

Much surprised and pleased to receive a promotion to full colonel today. It looks as though Hal Sofield will be assigned with me as orthopedic consultant.

Tuesday, 14 December

Spent the last 2 days trying to get boat passage to Fiji, but gave up owing to the weather and will try NATS [Naval Air Transport Service].

Wednesday, 15 December

Found out that Ben Baker and Kaufman had returned. Heard that mobile surgical hospitals were on the way. Will they have qualified surgeons? Read Churchill's [Col. Edward D. Churchill, MC, Consultant in Surgery, North African and Mediterranean Theaters of Operation, U.S. Army] report on North Africa. His problems are the same as those met in this theater.

Fiji Islands, Thursday, 16 December

Off at 0800 for Suva, arrived 1330.

Saturday, 18 December

Flew to Nandi where I was met by Colonel Ruppersberg, 71st Station Hospital. While at supper, much to my surprise, in walked Gen. George C. Marshall. He stayed for a few minutes and rushed on. He appears to be vigorous and full of energy. I talked to the hospital staff this evening.

Sunday, 19 December

Went to the 7th Evacuation Hospital in the morning, and gave a talk there at lunch time; then to American Division headquarters from 2 to 4 o'clock for a talk; after that back to the 71st and a talk from 6 to 8 in the evening.

Monday, 20 December

Flew over to Suva this morning and spent the afternoon at the 142d General Hospital. Talked to the 182d Infantry [American Division] in the evening, about to embark for Cherry Blossom. The 142d General Hospital has a fine plant, and I am told that the Fiji Government proposes to take it over after the war. This hospital is doing a good job in pilonidals. They had a large number of corneal ulcers among the survivors of a torpedoed ship (fig. 321). The exact cause of this is unknown and the really bad ulcers cause permanent damage.

FIGURE 320.—"They are well pleased with the surgical teams." Bougainville. A. A surgical team operating in its underground surgery. The floor is about 4 feet below ground level; the sides are built up with sandbags, and it is roofed with heavy logs. (Left to right: Capt. Charles E. Troland, MC, Assistant Surgeon; Sgt. William T. Marsden, Scrub Nurse; Capt. William G. Watson, MC, Chief Surgeon; Capt. Harold C. Schulman, MC, Anesthetist.) B. A surgical team, operating in a clearing station, 17 December 1943. Note the improvised lighting and the use of combined intravenous and endotracheal anesthesia.

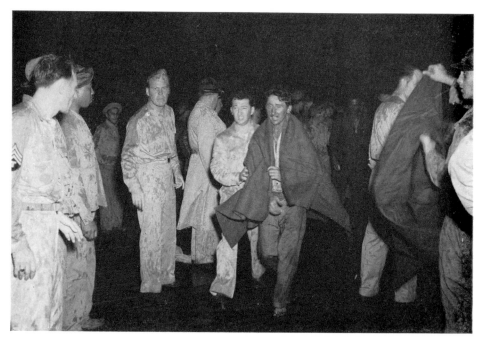

FIGURE 321.—Survivors of the torpedoed U.S. Army Transport *Cape San Juan.* Col. George G. Finney, MC (left center), Commanding Officer, 18th General Hospital, Fiji Islands, supervises transfer of survivors ashore, New Caledonia, 14 December 1943.

The Medical Corps officers of the 182d Infantry wanted to know why they were kept out here away from home for 3 years when so many people were sitting at home. When this campaign is over they are turning in their resignations [sic]. They want postgraduate work after the war, and the AMA has done nothing about it.

The British authorities (minor officials) have shown reluctance to co-operate in sanitation and venereal disease control. Many of the water supplies are contaminated, and there have been outbreaks of dysentery. "I've drunk this water for 20 years, and it is good"—in spite of the bacterial count. It is against the law to examine food handlers here. Prostitution is ignored by the Home Officer, although it exists everywhere.

Tuesday, 21 December

Toured the 142d General Hospital. It is a good institution. They need an otolaryngologist and cannot spare a surgeon.

Nouméa, Monday, 3 January 1944

Since my return to New Caledonia, I have been very busy checking on personnel. We still have a great dearth of qualified surgeons. The men we have are a cross section of American surgeons. We have many specialists, such as gynecologists, whom we must put in charge of station hospitals; and it is unfair to expect too much of them. There is still too much concentration of talent in the affiliated hospitals, which appears to me to hinder the total war effort. Such men may set a high standard in these hospitals, but, as in civilian life, they have too little influence on the total problem. Their influence is even less than it would be were they in civilian life, for these rear area hospitals cannot function as educational centers. The portable surgical hospitals, as judged so far, are not fulfilling their function, because they lack qualified surgical personnel. No amount of good surgery in the rear can make up for poor surgery at the front.

Wednesday, 5 January

I am starting an educational program—have acquired a 35-mm. projector and am now having film strips made. It seems to me that this has great possibilities. I have designed a fly net to be used inside the tent.

Met Captain Hook [Capt. (later Rear Adm.) Frederick R. Hook, MC, USN], Chief Force Surgeon, Navy. He is a fine person with a good knowledge of surgery and a determination to get things done—the best of the lot. Surgery in this neck of the woods will unquestionably improve under his influence.

Guadalcanal, Tuesday, 11 January

Off at 0500, island hopping to Bougainville. Left Tontouta Airbase, my first stop, at 0900. Arrived at Espíritu Santo, 1200. Left at 1300, arrived Guadalcanal, 1700. Stayed with Colonel Caton at the service command. He is dubious of the 137th Station Hospital, and the 9th Station Hospital has not yet proven itself surgically. The 21st Evacuation Hospital is now ready to move forward.

Bougainville, Wednesday, 12 January

Up at 0400 and left Henderson Field at 0530. Landed at Munda where we picked up a fighter escort and left again at 0810. Arrived in Bougainville at 1000 and landed on the new bomber strip. There has been an amazing transformation on this island in 6 weeks. Forty miles of roads have been built.

Thursday, 13 January

Went over the supplies of the portable surgical hospital with Colonel Hallam. Together they weigh 8 tons, so our next problem is to break them down for at least three purposes: (1) To function intact (adjacent to a clearing station or in a stable situation), (2) to function adjacent to a collecting station in a forward area—capable of being easily broken down and relocated, and (3) to function over distances and thus be air transportable. Max Michael will instruct on blood transfusions and falling-drop protein method [for hematocrit determination].

Visited Colonel Collins, division surgeon, at the American Division. They have an excellent operating room setup, neat and screened. They have no definite scheme yet for a convalescent camp. Each division plans on operating its own camp, and there must be a third one for the nondivisional units. This setup has its advantages in that the doctors know the men from their division. But no one has considered the inefficiency of operating three camps when one would do.

The 52d Field Hospital is being set up. Major Davidson, a bright young chap, is Chief of Surgery. He may do all right, or better. The surgical teams left Bougainville this morning.

Saturday, 15 January

I've been giving talks every night. The 37th Division has had an increase of neuropsychiatric patients and raises the question of a correlation between this and the use of Atabrine. The mosquito net tent has proved a success. We will need 15 per division for a start, though the tents will have to be reinforced at the top and at the door. Collecting companies should have a larger sterilizer (14- or 20-inch) and blood pressure apparatus. They need a small autoclave, for these units often occupy isolated positions. Each clearing station needs a horizontal field sterilizer. Many of the gas casualty kits have deteriorated and need replacement. Ambulance headlights should be sent up for the American, and five sets should be supplied to each division. The American needs Mayo stands. They could use an anesthetist. They have Stokes litters, which should be provided for the other divisions.

I visited the frontlines today and could see the Japanese positions. This is beautiful mountain country, and I was amazed at how well our positions have been dug in. Some of the aid stations were right on the rifle line.

Those wounded while out on patrol have a bad time, for a litter carry through the jungle takes 8 or 10 hours. Each battalion should have about 30 more men for litter bearers as it takes 8 men to carry back 1 casualty over this rugged terrain, and the battleline is so thin that infantrymen cannot be spared for this purpose (fig. 322). There are no natives here that could be used as carriers.

Sunday, 16 January

Hal and I spent the Sabbath watching the bombing of "Unknown Hill." As I went up to within 100 feet of the line, we were greeted by strains of "Vienna Waltz." This came from the 145th Infantry and I have never seen a more spic and span outfit. Everything on the frontline is clean and in its proper place, sanitation is perfect, and the food is superior. The climax of the morning was the large bamboo settee constructed by the command post, with its sign, "for visitors only."

Wednesday, 19 January

I have been giving talks each evening. Each night brings the air raids and the need to get up and take cover. Those who are protected in foxholes are almost 100 percent safe. The papers have stated that there is no malaria on Bougainville, yet the 3d Marine Division came down with malaria at an almost 1 to 5 ratio.

The portable surgical hospital needs electric headlights, gowns, caps, and half sheets. Having no generators or sinkers, they are forced to function close to the clearing station.

Guadalcanal, Thursday, 20 January

Left Bougainville this morning without a fighter escort. Since one plane recently disappeared with all on board, everyone must now wear lifebelts. No

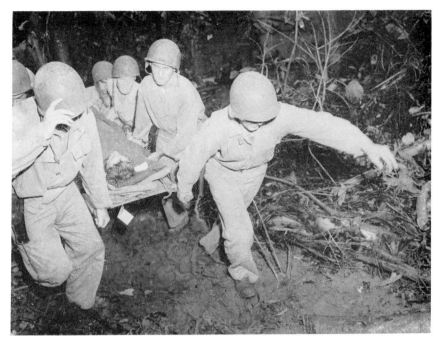

FIGURE 322.—Difficulties of litter carry over the rugged terrain of Bougainville, March 1944.

smoking is permitted on the plane, and the auxiliary gas tanks have been removed. I have been troubled with prickly heat and with generalized skin edema, so I am not displeased to leave this buggy place where the bugs are more abundant and bigger than anywhere else. We went nonstop to Guadalcanal. Went to see Colonel Caton and then to stay with Paul Kisner at the 20th Station Hospital, where Hal [Sofield] was put to bed with boils on his fundament.

Friday, 21 January

Visited 21st Medical Supply. Sent suction apparatus and sterilizer to Americal Division and sterilizer to 52d Field Hospital. Supplies are coming in very slowly, and there is a considerable amount of loss. Apparently people are helping themselves along the line.

Saturday, 22 January

Visited Colonel Bolend, commanding officer of the 21st Evacuation Hospital. He is one of the finest commanding officers I've met. "No man should command a unit from his home town," said he, to which I agreed. Very few people can be really objective in such a situation, particularly if they must go back to the town to live with these same doctors. Difficult situations have arisen where some bad appointments have been made in order to keep the peace. So far, I can see nothing to justify the affiliated unit and a great deal that speaks against it. Besides, talent should not be concentrated to the extent that it is in the affiliated unit, from which it is extremely difficult to transfer personnel. A good distribution of qualified doctors is essential to the welfare of the Armed Forces. Colonel Bolend has his hospital well covered from every angle and can spare three surgeons. We could use such men on our surgical teams.

Sunday, 23 January

Visited the 9th Station Hospital. Colonel Walker says that he and his men have lost their pep—and they have. There are 14 officers here who have been out of the States for 2 years, and they certainly need some new blood. The 20th Station Hospital needs three surgeons—a chief of surgery, an assistant chief, and a genitourinary man.

This afternoon we had a meeting of the portable surgical hospitals. Three of them are good and the other three cannot be used, for they lack qualified personnel. I cannot understand why such unqualified personnel are given rank and sent out here to do a job they cannot do well.

Monday, 24 January

Visited 40th Division headquarters. Major General Brush [Maj. Gen. Rapp Brush] is commanding general. The division surgeon, Colonel Ghormley [Lt. Col. (later Col.) Verne G. Ghormley, MC] is a fine person. He says that they have already weeded out the senile and incompetent. This looks like a good outfit, but Ghormley says that the exact quality of the surgeons is an unknown factor. Much equipment is still lacking: Three number 2 chests so that the clearing company can be split up for the three combat teams, three anesthesia sets, X-ray apparatus, 5-kw. suction generator, Mayo table, instrument table, laundry or washing machines, refrigerator, and reefer.

The National Guard divisions range from good, indifferent, to bad. The medical personnel of those I have seen have, in the initial periods of their operation, always had poor leadership, which resulted in unnecessary loss of life among our men. This tragic situation is due to the two types of men kept on as division surgeons—the senile and the incompetent. It apparently takes about 2 years to get rid of these people. Commanding generals usually do not know enough about medical problems to be able to do anything about this stumbling block. One cannot blame them. One commanding general, who is a good tactician and has splendid morale in his division, does not know the difference between general hospitals and field hospitals. I have never seen a commanding general who did not want to do the best job possible. But, just as they do in civilian life, some unqualified and incompetent doctors sell themselves on the basis of their personality or loyalty. There should be some method of weeding out such division surgeons before going into combat, so as to avoid the unnecessary sacrifice of human life.

Espíritu Santo, Wednesday, 26 January

Plane yesterday to Espíritu Santo. Visited the 122d Station Hospital. They need an EENT man and a young orthopedist. They are also short three doctors, but two could hold them for now. Moreover, the hospital has 21 nurses of 2-years-plus service, of whom 10 are sick at present. There is a question as to whether promotion of nurses should be done on the basis of 50 percent of T/O strength or 50 percent of actual strength. As for technical difficulties, there is a dust problem in their operating room.

Thursday, 27 January

Visited the 31st General Hospital. The hospital is on a beautiful site overlooking the bay and shows promise of development. They are building the surgery and have not as yet taken any surgical patients. The chief of surgery is a proctologist.

Nouméa, Friday, 28 January

Off at 0330 by NATS to Nouméa, where I found a pile of mail and other documents waiting for me.

Sunday, 30 January

Conference with Captain Hook, Captain Kern, Commander Reynolds, and Emile Holman. The Navy is loathe to adopt the idea of consultants, since they have not had the long experience with this type of work that the Army has had. Captain Hook says that they must "go slow." They would be pioneering and would have to proceed by trial and error. The Navy likes the surgical team idea and wants to use it on its next move. We should supply them with material on this subject.

Guadalcanal, Saturday, 11 March 1944

This book has been neglected this past month owing to several factors. For one, I suffered a pigskin heat rash and probably some mental depression. I have been engaged in a long struggle to get some things done. The major projects I've been trying to push through are adequate record and filing systems, on which the general [General Maxwell, Chief Surgeon, USAFISPA] finally agreed to back me. I think that he remained very skeptical though, and I hope that I have not asked for too much. The following information on each patient should be recorded: Name, serial number, diagnosis (according to nomenclature), operation performed, total days in hospital, and disposition. This will enable me for the first time to answer some questions on surgery. The Surgeon General's Office has been asking repeatedly for information which we could not hitherto furnish. A study on wound ballistics has been organized. Ben [Baker], Hal [Sofield] and Max [Michael] got off to New Zealand, and 10 days later, after my work was cleaned up, I joined them.

The 39th General Hospital, with formal flower gardens, is spic and span as an insane asylum. The interior is also shipshape. I wonder what the feeling of the staff will be when they go home to the ordinary dirt of civilian hospitals. It was good to see all my friends again—good for the ego. Col. Don Longfellow, MC [Commanding Officer, 39th General Hospital, U.S. Army Forces, Pacific], did not want to part with Eddie [Colonel Ottenheimer, Chief of Surgery, 39th General Hospital], so we may take Frick on our next move.

I left Auckland via NATS stopping 4 days at Headquarters [Nouméa] to catch up on some last minute things. Then I was off to Guadalcanal, leaving Tontouta at 0830 and arriving at Guadalcanal, 1600. We had a warm front and some very rough weather between Espíritu and Guadalcanal. It was raining hard at Guadalcanal when we arrived, and I went to the 20th Station Hospital with Paul Kisner.

At Guadalcanal, I went over plans and supplies with Colonel Ghormley, Surgeon, 40th Division—a superior fellow. Saturday night festivities were the best in the Pacific and better than the majority of New York clubs. The local talent is amazing and in sharp contrast to the very average talent sent down from the States. Saw Emile Holman, Bruce, Calloway, McMaster and Rogers. They still know little of the plans.[9]

Monday, 13 March

Finney, Sutherland, Hull, Greiner, McQuinton, Troland, and Sofield arrived today. I spent the day chasing supplies. Saw Colonel Lobban and his staff playing poker in the mud, and I extracted three X-ray technicians and two stenographers from the group.

Wednesday, 15 March

Worked on final preparations and went with Colonel Ghormley, Ben [Baker] and Moe [Kaufman] to visit Captain Hughes of the I Marine Amphibious Corps, who told us that the show was off. Apparently, final plans had been completed as of midnight last night. Quite a letdown! Reasons unknown.

Saturday, 18 March

The FOREARM plan being off, our plans are changed, and the extra surgeons are greatly disappointed. Had cocktails and a swim with Admiral Halsey and then saw General Harmon [Lt. Gen. Millard F. Harmon, Commanding General, USAFISPA], who had just returned from Cherry Blossom and is having trouble with his knee. I had a talk with General Harmon and had no trouble in convincing him that a wound ballistics study was desirable, and he wired instructions.

Sunday, 19 March

Everyone is feeling optimistic over the recent change in plans, for it looks as though many lives might have been lost.

Tuesday, 21 March

The wound ballistics team will go to Bougainville by order of General Harmon and at the request of General Griswold of the XIV Corps. Persistence certainly paid off in this case. The team consists of Harry Hull, surgeon; Dan Greiner, pathologist; Frank Sutherland, surgeon; two enlisted men; and one photographer (fig. 323).[10]

---

[9] The plans were for the proposed invasion of Kavieng, New Ireland, Territory of New Guinea, referred to hereafter by its code name, FOREARM. On 12 March, the Joint Chiefs of Staff canceled the Kavieng operation. Preparations had been far advanced, however, and the men and ships that were to invade Kavieng had already assembled at Guadalcanal.

[10] See: Oughterson, Ashley W., Hull, Harry C., Sutherland, Francis A., and Greiner, Daniel J.: Study on Wound Ballistics—Bougainville Campaign. In Medical Department, United States Army. Wound Ballistics. Washington: U.S. Government Printing Office, 1962, pp. 281–436.

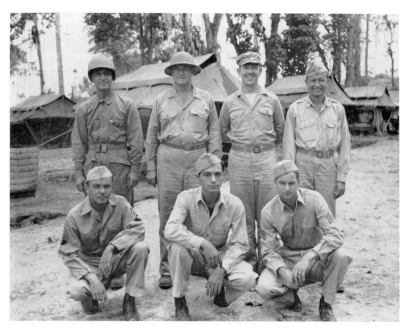

FIGURE 323.—The wound ballistics team at Bougainville. (Rear, left to right, Maj. Francis A. Sutherland, MC, Col. Ashley W. Oughterson, MC, Lt. Col. Harry C. Hull, MC, Maj. Daniel J. Greiner, kneeling, left to right, T/4 Charles J. Berzenyi, T/4 Charles R. Restifo, and Sgt. Reed N. Fitch.)

George Finney, Bill Potts, and Captain McQuinton are staying on to help these hospitals straighten out some of their problems. I found that they were injecting gas gangrene antitoxin into wounds and into the tissue around the wounds, but not introducing enough antitoxin intravenously. Cases were coming down from the front without adequate information on operations or drug therapy. Some had a red blood count of 1.5 million, and some patients have been sent down in poor condition or too soon after an operation. Others, with compound fractures of the humerus, were in hanging casts. Once again it must be concluded that not enough emphasis is being placed on getting the best men into the forward hospitals.

Bougainville, Wednesday, 22 March

Up at 0330 with the ballistics team and off to Bougainville (map 5).[11] We landed at 0830 on the fighter strip, since the other two strips were being shelled. The Torokina fighter strip is also under fire, but is nevertheless functioning. Colonel Hallam met us at the airport—a very efficient, pleasing, and cooperative fellow. He took the team to the 21st Evacuation Hospital for rations and quarters and then showed them his bug and butterfly collection and introduced them to the 37th Division crowd.

---

[11] The fighting had not yet ceased on Bougainville. During March, the Japanese made three unsuccessful attempts to dislodge the American forces from the perimeter that they had occupied.

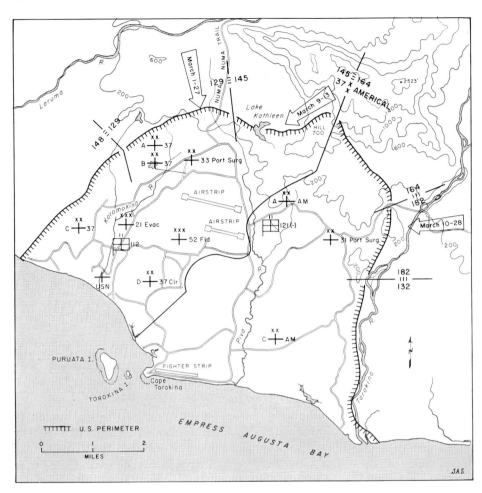

Map 5.—Medical units on Bougainville, March 1944.

Thursday, 23 March

Toured the frontlines of the 37th Division. The collecting station of the 129th Infantry is about 200 yards behind the front, and they have cleared out a beautiful garden here in the jungle with lots of tomatoes, cucumbers, melons, radishes, and some corn.

The Japanese came over the Numa Numa Trail with one-regiment-plus and hit the 129th at a strongly fortified point (fig. 324). Some 400 of them are now being buried by our bulldozers. By climbing over their own dead until our machineguns jammed, they had managed to take some of our forward pillboxes. They would also walk in file straight across a minefield, advancing over the bodies of those who had blown up the mines. However, their losses were too heavy, and except for a few snipers the main body withdrew today. There is no question about their morale and courage. No prisoners are being taken.

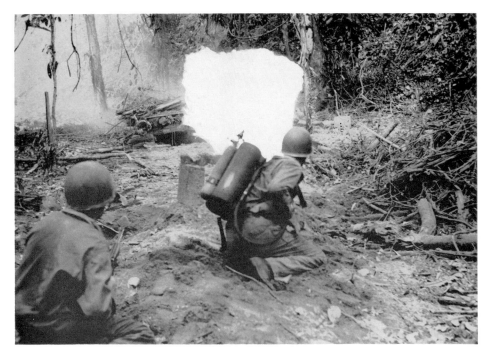

FIGURE 324.—Men of the 129th Infantry Regiment, 37th Division, turning a flamethrower on a pillbox occupied by infiltrating Japanese.

The roads here are good right up to the frontlines, and the wounded are quickly brought back to the evacuation hospital. In the cases of the seriously wounded, the clearing station is bypassed. If the wounded man can be reached, he will find himself in the hospital within from 1 to 4 hours. This is the first time in the South Pacific that an evacuation hospital has been able to function as such.

This particular hospital is in front of the artillery, or rather in the middle, as the 155's and 105's are behind us and the 75's are in front. The 155's go chugging overhead night and day. The chugging noise is made by the wobble of the shell as it passes above. The wobble then diminishes, and the shell moves into a straight path. The sounds coming from this change of motion make it seem as though the shell were falling, although of course it doesn't, and it lands about a mile beyond the hospital.

We also visited Hill 700 where elements of the 145th Infantry are located (fig. 325). This is a very rugged section, and the Engineers have done a really superb job in putting a road right behind the frontline. However, the wounded could not be transported along the road except in armored halftracks because the Japanese have the road covered. It is amazing when one considers that the Japanese tried to attack at this point, for the line runs along a hill which is too steep in spots even to crawl along. They did manage, however, to take the top of the hill, though the ravine below was piled deep with Japanese

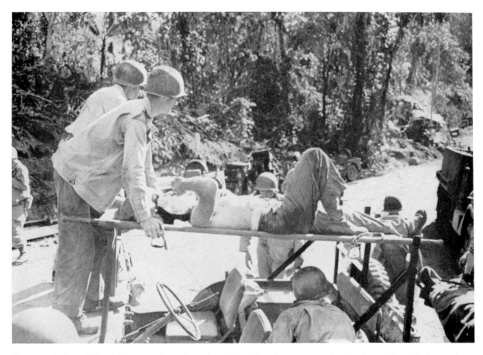

FIGURE 325.—Hill 700, Bougainville, March 1944. A casualty being transferred from jeep to halftrack for evacuation to the rear.

bodies.   Thirteen hundred corpses have been counted and buried so far in the area that our burial parties have dared to cover.   This is an important problem as the unburied attract swarms of huge black flies as big as bumblebees, and the leaves of vegetables are black with them.   The hill was retaken by us at a cost of about 60 dead and 300 to 400 wounded.

We saw General Griswold, Commanding General, XIV Corps, and his chief of staff, General Arnold, who furnished us a vehicle and a driver.   Saw Lieutenant Torrance of the Graves Registration Service, Quartermaster Corps. Our dead, as they are brought to the cemetery, will be detoured a short distance away to the morgue of the 21st Evacuation Hospital where Greiner, the pathologist, with two stenographers and a photographer, will be set up to do his job.

Friday, 24 March

Of all the islands I have visited in the Solomons, Bougainville has the best climate.   The nights are always cool, and a blanket is often necessary.   The air is also dryer because of the sand subsoil that permits good drainage and because of the slight elevation of the land.

The 21st Evacuation Hospital is a clean and well-organized institution. Colonel Allen [Lt. Col. (later Col.) Robert E. Allen, MC], Commanding Officer, was the former executive officer.   Everyone in the XIV Corps is well pleased with them, and they have a good esprit de corps.

We visited Colonel Collins of the Americal who has a splendid clearing station, really more elaborate than is needed. But now that they are getting a number of casualties it has come in very handy for taking in a heavy load. They have underground operating rooms and wards with forced ventilation. This clearing station has been shelled almost daily, and a direct hit was made on the division surgeon's office. Fortunately, he wasn't there at the time. The 52d Field Hospital has also been shelled and took a direct hit on one of its wards. Several patients were wounded although there were no fatalities.

The Japanese hand grenades do not appear to be too effective.[12] It seems that the explosive charge is too small. Five grenades were thrown into one of our foxholes without killing a man, though no one escaped being wounded. Two men are needed to fire our bazooka; the forward man frequently gets powder burns while the man behind may suffer hand injuries. We will examine this problem.

Saturday, 25 March

A small sector of the 129th Infantry was infiltrated the night before last by about 200 Japanese. As a result of this action, 100 of our men were wounded and 30-plus were killed. The ballistics team had more work than they could handle at one time.

The surgical service at the 21st Evacuation Hospital is doing a good job, although the hospital is inadequately designed for the load that it has to carry. For example, the original operating room was made far too small (fig. 326). An operating room in a 750-bed evacuation hospital should provide facilities for eight tables to function at once. It should be centrally located and easily accessible to the laboratory and X-ray. The shock room should be adjacent to the operating room and large enough to hold 30 to 40 patients at one time. When the operating room is placed in front of the artillery, as is the case here, underground wards should be available for at least 200 patients. At the present time this hospital has nearly 100 litter patients aboveground and approximately 120 below ground. Many of these patients are thrown into a state of shock during the process of being transferred underground. Fortunately, shelling and bombing have been light in this particular area. Furthermore, X-ray equipment has been kept together, and one hit could have done away with it all. Part of the X-ray equipment should be located in, or adjacent to, the shock ward, and part in the operating room. This hospital could benefit by instruction on such subjects as sterile technique, the use of plaster, records, et cetera. This will have to be arranged.

Visited the EENT clinic. There are many middle-ear cases, a large number of whom can give no story of how their drum was perforated. One man even had a complete absence of the drum. I believe that a great many men suffer ruptured drums from explosions and do not report this fact. Many of them probably don't recognize any symptoms until their ears become infected.

---

[12] For data on this and other Japanese missiles, see: Beyer, James C., Arima, James K., and Johnson, Doris W.: Enemy Ordnance Materiel. *In* Medical Department, United States Army. Wound Ballistics. Washington: U.S. Government Printing Office, 1962, pp. 1–90.

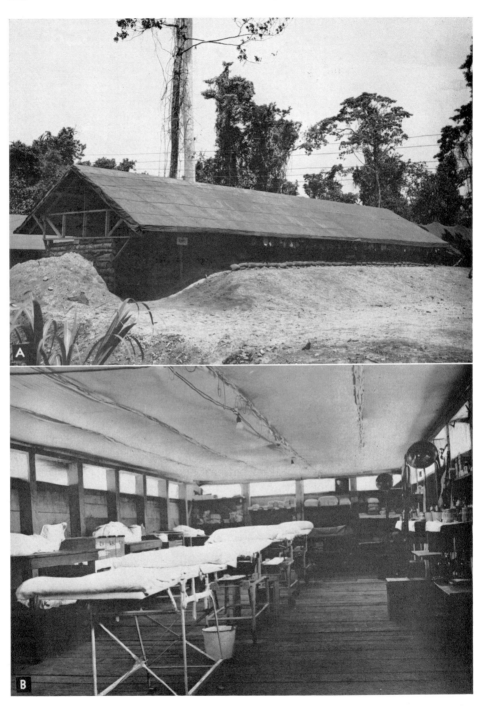

FIGURE 326.—An underground operating room, of the 21st Evacuation Hospital, Bougainville, April 1944.   A. Exterior.   B. Interior.

There are many men in combat who have defective vision and bad hearing, which are particularly dangerous in jungle warfare. I heard about one man who was up for court-martial during the fighting on New Georgia. He had turned his Browning automatic on a patrol returning to our lines, with disastrous results. The fellow could barely distinguish a man at 200 feet, let alone be able to tell the difference between friend and foe.

Saw Maj. Paul Troop of the 145th Infantry this morning. He had a minor wound caused by a "hung bomb" which had caused a tree to burst within the area, killing one and wounding nine.

A Japanese message intercepted yesterday indicated that they would begin an attack. Hence, our heavy artillery barrage last night. Our Cubs have spotted most of their gun positions, and we can only hope that we have knocked them out. Anyway, it appears that we have stopped them for the time being. Yesterday, the Japanese used machineguns to shoot down several of our planes which were flying low over the lines. Americal headquarters is jittery, for the Japanese naval 6-inch guns on Empress Augusta Bay are dropping shells around the general's tent. Everywhere the story of Japanese morale is the same. The Japanese soldier when cornered shouts back that the Japanese Army never surrenders. So far they are right.

Saw Capt. Carnes Weeks [Cdr. Carnes Weeks, MC, USN] who now appears to be Halsey's personal physician. Had luncheon with him and Admiral Halsey several times on Guadalcanal.

The Fiji Scouts are here in force (fig. 327). Their officers are New Zealanders. Both officers and men have won the admiration of all the units here. I just watched a battalion go down the road with a snap that is never seen in our troops. Their casualties are heavy, and the Japanese fear their courage and their ability as natural jungle fighters.

The dead are not coming in so rapidly now, only about 10 to 15 per day, so that Greiner, assisted by Hull and Frick can keep up with the post mortems. Two stenographers are there to take dictation, and they have a photographer there to take the pictures. We have two undertakers who take charge immediately after our work is done. They sew up and wash the body and wrap it in a mattress cover. This project shows earmarks of being a valuable study.

Monday, 3 April 1944

The action is quieting down, although Greiner still averages about six post mortems a day, about half of which are Fijis who were on patrol duty. Opinion differs as to their value as soldiers. They are universally liked, and everyone agrees that they are good on patrol, but apparently they do not stand mortar fire well.

The morale of our troops is high, although we have quite a few neuropsychiatric cases. However, the vast majority of these were neuropsychiatric problems before they entered the Army and cannot serve as an index of the morale of the troops in general. One lieutenant cracked up because he had to lead his men on six assaults of a hill, incurring 50 percent casualties. He felt that he was to blame for the casualties, although he was only obeying orders.

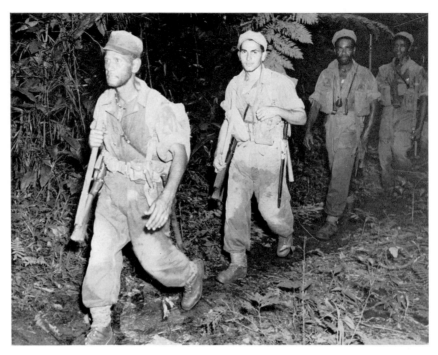

FIGURE 327.—Fiji Scouts returning from patrol into enemy territory, Bougainville, March 1944.

The food here is excellent. Almost every installation now has a garden, and some of these are on a grand scale. Sweet corn, tomatoes, potatoes, onions, radishes, okra, carrots, and the like grow well.

The question of rotation versus leave has now become optional for officers below the grade of lieutenant colonel who have 2 years of oversea service. Most of the doctors prefer rotation to leave. They feel that they have been overseas long enough, 24 to 28 months, and that something has been put over on them by the doctors who have remained at home. The stories of doctors who are "cleaning up" at home does not help morale. This attitude is also in evidence among enlisted men. Obviously, the morale of those serving overseas is in inverse correlation to the income of the people at home. If the income of the civilian population were limited to the corresponding Army income, this factor would be eliminated.

Tuesday, 4 April

Activity is steadily quieting, and nothing is coming in but patrol casualties. Yesterday I completed the initial records of the 37th Division.

Last night, had dinner with Col. Eddie Grass at the 33d Portable Surgical Hospital. Major Tyler, of Denver, is Commanding Officer. This unit wants to stay with the 37th Division. They are set up beside the collecting station and have taken the more seriously wounded who could not stand transportation to the evacuation hospital. They received a direct hit from a 500-pound bomb early in the battle, which wiped out their equipment, including even the pots and pans in the kitchen. All the personnel were in foxholes, and there were no casualties, although the bomb dug a 20- x 6-foot crater. They have been reequipped since then and have only had to contend with mortar fire and sniping. The operating room should obviously have been placed underground. Digging tools and one power saw should be a permanent part of their equipment.

Thursday, 6 April

The cards have been made for all those killed in action and wounded in action on Bougainville since February 15, and some 200 are completed. We found some wooden bullets yesterday. They are said to be used by the Japanese for close-range fighting in order to avoid injuring their own men.

I had dinner last night with General Beightler of the 37th Division. General Griswold, XIV Corps, told me that the 37th was the "banner division" of the South Pacific. General Beightler is one of the world's fine people—simple, modest, and direct. He can also be tough if that is necessary. The general is intent on maintaining high morale and a pride of accomplishment among the men. This is best attained by the careful selection of leaders, fairness, and recognition for a job well done.

NOTES

1. The 9th Station Hospital needs an EENT officer. He will be provided by the 29th General Hospital.

2. Complete field X-ray equipment should be kept in the forward area. In general, more supplies should be kept in the forward area rather than at Nouméa.

3. It should be possible to return an officer from the tropics without a recommendation for either promotion or reclassification. Many of them are inefficient in tropical service and do not fall into either group. Here is a case in which administrative redtape is working against the best interest of the service.

4. More of the following items must be obtained: Scales, blood pressure apparatus, otoscope, sterilizer (Wilmot-Castle), small burners for sterilizer, orthopedic tables; powersaws, axes, and ventilation fans for underground wards and operating rooms; headlights; sclerosing solution for hemorrhoids, eye anesthetic, copper sulfate for phosphorous wounds.

5. Spectacles are still a problem. Do all the men have a second pair?

6. The journals are still not coming through.

7. Replacements should come in early enough for prior training.

8. The Japanese make better use of cover than we do and dig in quicker, using smaller, better constructed foxholes. Every recruit should learn how to dig fast. This is of more value than walking in jungle warfare. The men must also learn to dig deeper and narrower foxholes. They are far too large. Many buttocks wounds are seen in the wards. The soldier must be advised to get his backside down. Careless exposure of the silhouette is too frequent.

We must learn to crawl more often. The Japanese stick closer to the ground. Furthermore, our boys frequently don't wear their helmets on patrol, for they soon find the helmet too tiring.

9. Should patrols (fig. 328) be accompanied by a medical officer? Not unless the medical officer has enough equipment to do more than an aidman's job. Small patrols of less than nine men have an aidman along, and many of them are lost on patrol. One patrol had a battalion aid section of 28 men of whom 10 were wounded in action and 4 seriously. General Hodge [Maj. Gen. (later Lt. Gen.) John R. Hodge, Commanding General, Americal Division] gave orders for a doctor to accompany a reinforced company of 175 men, although no equipment was carried. Citations for medical aidmen are insufficient. However, an infantryman who takes no more risks gets a citation. One battalion commanding officer insisted on bringing back his dead at great risk to the aidmen. Aidmen have been used to carry the dead down from the aid station. Since there are a limited number of aidmen, they should not be used for this task.

10. The 37th Division clearing station performed primary suture of the minor wounds of about 30 men. Almost all healed per primam.

11. More instruction is needed on sucking chest wounds and the proper way of sealing them, which is with a tight adhesive over a pad and gauze, the latter impregnated with petrolatum jelly.

12. Statistics gathered from the 21st Evacuation Hospital:

    41 cases of penetrating chest wounds—12 percent mortality.

    21 cases of sucking chest wounds—18 percent mortality.

    27 cases operated open—29 percent mortality.

Note: Second echelon medical service must have thoracic surgery.

13. We need a movable metal pillbox. It would be of great value in going over a ridge against Japanese positions. A periscope could be attached, so one could look over the ridge. Many Japanese are killed by heavy fire because of their concentration prior to an attack.

14. Captain Dick states that about 5 percent of the men take sulfa tablets by mouth when wounded. It might be better to discontinue this practice entirely, unless they are out on patrol. The full dose, given by a doctor, would more quickly assure an adequate blood level.

15. The Japanese hand grenade is grooved, but does not fragment along its grooves. Having so much powder, it is almost pulverized; hence, its burst is not effective very far. Men sitting in a foxhole in which a grenade has been tossed have been known to put up their feet and come off without serious wounds. However, the blast effect is considerable. Small skin puncture wounds and extensive damage to muscles occur as a result of the blast. A Japanese grenade was seen to go off under a man and lift him 2 feet in the air.

Sunday, 9 April

I was under the impression that the Japanese had finally been driven away, but I was awakened this morning by the shelling of the fighter strip. Last

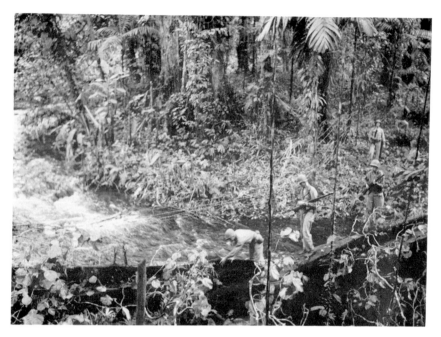

FIGURE 328.—A patrol crossing the Piva River on Bougainville.

night I had a long discussion with the officers. They complain that many hospital staffs are kept inactive over long periods of time. They contend that under such circumstances the men should be sent home, since many planes and ships go back empty. These people refuse to recognize that the difficult problem is to bring men out here. They only see the issue in terms of available transportation back to the States. It was remarked that morale is bad because the Army hasn't been keeping its promise to ship people back on rotation. These men complain that they were not told that the Army's promise would be fulfilled only "if the tactical situation permitted."

Saturday, 15 April

We have been interviewing line soldiers and get much valuable information from privates and noncoms. Many discrepancies having to do with the circumstances in which wounds occur are corrected. It appears that these statements may be taken as about 85 or 90 percent accurate. There is general agreement that every man should know the principles of first aid treatment since regular aidmen cannot get to them at night.

More attention should be given to having better pillboxes, sacrificing camouflage if necessary. The Japanese knew where they were located anyway. Windows on the pillboxes should be screened with chicken wire or, better still, some kind of rubber wire off which the grenades will bounce. The pillbox should slope down at the sides so that the grenades will roll off. Barbed wire should be used more freely. A telephone is needed in every pillbox. These telephones should be attached to the ear in order to leave the hands free.   Our logging trails, which were cut for timber, were used by the Japanese for their main attacks.   Flamethrowers would be useful on the defensive against mass attacks.   A flamethrower with a long hose is more efficient than a tank when the position of the dug-in enemy is known.   Our minefields limit our means of withdrawal, but kill many Japanese.   A bulletproof vest might be useful in this type of warfare.   Inside the pillbox, the noise of firing is intensely annoying, and the helmet makes it even worse.   The 60-mm. mortar shell flare is okay, but the airplane flare is too bright.   The frontlines should be cleared for 300-yard lanes of fire.   The bazooka is very useful against banyan trees.   More men are needed who are trained in the use of bazookas, as many of these guns were available and stood idle.   More Browning automatics are needed, and every pillbox should have one.

Tuesday, 25 April

Went over our results with General Griswold.   He is skeptical about our figures on machinegun casualties, probably because of the gun's highly lethal effect.

Russell Islands, Saturday, 13 May 1944

Off this morning for the Russells.   Went to the 222d Station Hospital. Colonel Currie is commanding officer.   This shows promise of being a fine hospital, and the morale is good.   Visited Colonel Bell at the 17th Field Hospital where the same old problem seems to exist.   Went to the 41st Station Hospital where construction has been stopped.   Colonel McLaughlin [Lt. Col. William B. McLaughlin, MC], Commanding Officer—a fine type.   They need a laboratory officer.   None of these hospitals has a well-trained anesthetist.

Nouméa, Monday, 15 May

I am now back at Nouméa.   Left Bougainville the first week in May for New Georgia Island.   Stopped at Ondongo Island, then by boat to Munda. Stayed at the 144th Station Hospital on New Georgia.   Colonel Haines [Lt. Col. Hilton D. Haines, MC] is hospital commander.

Friday, 14 July 1944

Today is Bastille Day, and tonight the natives are in the square across from Le Grand Hotel Central, beating tom-toms and having a great time shouting and singing—a regular old shakedown (fig. 329).   I felt rather under the weather from around May 15th until early in June, although I kept going. Had no appetite, which caused a loss of weight, and had sporadic diarrhea. Stool examinations did not reveal any ameba.

Hull, Greiner, and Sutherland stayed on to help with the reports.   I have learned how necessary it is to be careful when choosing people for such work, and I would never again attempt it with anyone whom I did not know was definitely interested in the problems.

Admiral Halsey and his staff departed on about June 15th, and General Maxwell, Hal Sofield, and General Harrison left for Washington 5 days later.

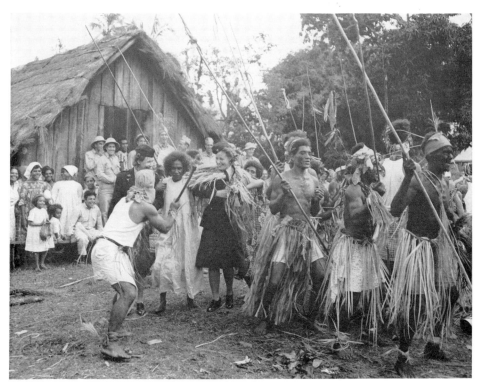

FIGURE 329.—U.S. Army nurses participating in a native dance at Saint-Louis Village, New Caledonia.

Everybody here is full of rumors as to what will happen next, but fortunately I have been so busy that I have not had time to think about it. Around July 1st, Col. Maurice C. Pincoffs, MC, came over from Australia and spent several days gathering data, as New Georgia and Bougainville pass to the SWPA (Southwest Pacific Area).[13] They (i.e., SWPA) either have no regular allotment for consultants, or someone else has filled them, and Col. Wm. Barclay Parsons, MC [Consultant in Surgery, Office of the Chief Surgeon, U.S. Army Services of Supply, SWPA], must be carried as the commanding officer of a hospital. Moreover, being in Services of Supply, they have nothing to do, except by invitation, with combat troops. I realize now what a very fine situation I have had here in comparison. "Pink" [Pincoffs] suggested that the Sixth U.S. Army should have a consultant and asked if I would not consider it. No news has come from Washington so I will sit tight as I have a lot of reports to finish.[14]

---

[13] On 15 June 1944, the islands in the Solomons Group north of the Russells were designated as part of the Southwest Pacific Area.

[14] On 19 June 1944, Colonel Oughterson was awarded the Legion of Merit "for exceptionally meritorious conduct in the performance of outstanding services in the South Pacific Area from 1 December 1942 to 13 June 1944."

Tuesday, 18 July

Heard that we will go under the Central Pacific but do not know as yet what is to be done with the consultants.[15] The ballistics report has been completed except for the typing.

Auckland, Tuesday, 8 August 1944

Today I received orders to go to New Zealand. The plane coming over flew at 10,000 feet, and I was uncomfortably cold in spite of the woolens I wore. Arrived at Auckland at 1600 hours and went out to the 39th General Hospital. Colonel Longfellow is looking well. They have 300 patients, and most of these will soon be gone. The grounds are beautifully landscaped, and the hospital itself is immaculate. It has stood up very well. Gave two talks on wound ballistics.

Nouméa, Saturday, 12 August

Received orders from the Commanding General, South Pacific Base Command, to return. I was having a gastrointestinal series done and had to leave in the middle of the series. Arrived August 15 at Nouméa to find that I have been ordered to Headquarters, USAFPOA (U.S. Army Forces, Pacific Ocean Areas), Hawaii.[16] Eddie Ottenheimer's orders are out, following Colonel Longfellow's okay. He will be invaluable in compiling surgical statistics for the theater. Furthermore, General Maxwell, who has returned, wants to use him as a historian.

Saturday, 19 August

Eddie arrived today, and I have started him on the analysis of surgical records. General Gilbreath [Maj. Gen. Frederick Gilbreath], who is now Commanding General, South Pacific Base Command, has made many reforms, and life for the officers is not generally as pleasant as it was. But there are compensations in better discipline.

Tuesday, 22 August

Drove out to Tontouta and spent the night with Colonel Shope, now commanding officer of the airbase.

Wednesday, Thursday, 23, 24 August, Oahu, T.H.

At 1300 I got on a C–54 coming through from Sydney. These planes are like huge flying boxcars. Arrived at Nandi Airport at 1715 and had supper. Took off at 1815 in a beautiful sunset. Arrived at Canton Island, Phoenix Islands, at 0200. As the plane taxied down to the end of the field on takeoff, it was discovered that the hydraulic system was leaking. This was repaired by about 0600, and we finally took off. We landed at Hickam Field at 1600.

---

[15] The U.S. Army Forces in the Central Pacific Area was the forerunner of the U.S. Army Forces, Pacific Ocean Areas, referred to and discussed later.

[16] USAFISPA was redesignated in July 1944 SPBC (the South Pacific Base Command). USAFPOA was established at the same time as a superior headquarters with jurisdiction over the South Pacific Base Command and what had been USAFICPA (U.S. Army Forces in the Central Pacific Area) which was similarly reduced to a base command, CPBC (the Central Pacific Base Command). Colonel Oughterson was placed on temporary duty as surgical consultant at Headquarters, USAFPOA from the South Pacific Base Command, since there were no position vacancies for consultants of his rank at Headquarters, USAFPOA.

Passed through Army Customs and went out to Fort Shafter, Oahu, T.H. [Headquarters, USAFPOA], where I signed in and looked up Colonel Young [Col. Charles T. Young, MC, medical consultant] who fixed me up for the night in the old Tripler Hospital. Here everyone is dressed up, and there is little evidence of war. Today, Wednesday (having crossed the date line again), I met Brig. Gen. Edgar King (Chief Surgeon, USAFPOA), my new commanding officer. Although he has a fearsome reputation, my first impressions are very good. Colonel Gates [Col. Kermit H. Gates, MC], Deputy Surgeon, is a very busy and pleasant person. Thursday, I visited Lt. Col. (later Col.) Forrester Raine, MC, of Milwaukee, who has been acting surgical consultant for the Central Pacific Base Command. He tells me that there are only four board members in the whole area and that there is a great dearth of good surgeons.

Saturday, 26 August

The general had asked me to write down some of my ideas on the function of a consulting surgeon, which I did and which he approved. He has taken quickly to all my suggestions, and I think that I am going to like working with him. The only aspect of the work that I dislike is that I also have some functions as an inspector. I am afraid that this may strain my pleasant relations with the surgeons. Perhaps this need not happen.

Monday, 28 August

Today I lectured to a medical group and afterward traveled to the northern side of the island to deliver the same lecture to the 71st Medical Battalion. I am beginning to think that my illustrated lecture on debridement must be good, as I could hardly fool all the people all of the time.

Tuesday, 29 August

Spent the day with General Bliss [Brig. Gen. Raymond W. Bliss, Chief of Operations, Office of The Surgeon General, and Assistant to The Surgeon General] and General Rankin [Brig. Gen. Fred W. Rankin, Director, Surgical Consultants Division, Office of The Surgeon General] visiting the North Sector Hospital [219th General Hospital]. Colonel Green [Col. Philip P. Green, MC] is commanding officer, Fisk of Boston is Chief of Surgery, and Robertson [Col. Robert C. Robertson, MC] is Chief of Orthopedics [and Consultant in Orthopedic Surgery, USAFPOA]. Then we were off to the 204th General Hospital of which Col. Tracy L. Bryant, MC, is commanding officer. I had not seen him for the past 25 years. Thence to Doris Duke's and to the Moana Hotel for drinks.

Thursday, 31 August

Off at 0630, visited the jungle course over the Pali [Camp Pali]—a very profitable forenoon (fig. 330). Maj. Bryant Noble, MC, in charge of medicine, is doing a good job. Thence to Koko Head, to visit the field and portable surgical hospitals just out of Saipan. Colonel Pettit—very able. Major Tinker, who is the son of Dr. Tinker of Ithaca, was in command of a portable surgical hospital on Saipan and did a fine job—2 to 5 percent mortality on the

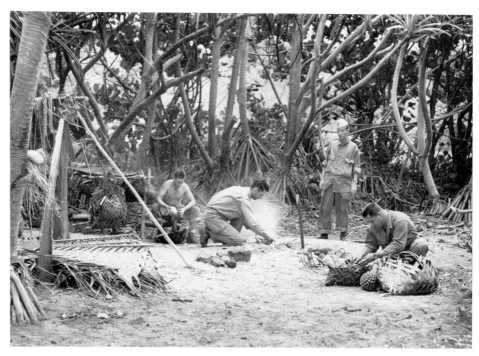

FIGURE 330.—Training in how to live in and on the jungle, at the Jungle Training School, Hawaii.

island. Back to the office and off with General King to a large dinner party for Generals Bliss and Rankin, given by Colonel Streit [Col. Paul H. Streit, MC, Surgeon, CPBC] at the Pacific Club. A good dinner.

Saturday, 2 September 1944

Went out this morning to see General Hodge [Maj. Gen. John R. Hodge, Commanding General, XXIV Corps]—"Old Corkie." The next operation (Leyte Campaign) was explained by Colonel Potter [Col. Laurence A. Potter, MC, Surgeon, XXIV Corps] in a most excellent manner. While there, we received word of an emergency meeting with General King at 1300 hours. Five of us were called; Col. Charles Young, Kester [Col. Wayne O. Kester, VC, Chief Veterinarian, USAFPOA], Lt. Col. Moses Kaufman [now neuropsychiatric consultant for USAFPOA], Diver, and myself. We were brought before a huge table holding 50 items—planning for the next year, involving 50,000 medical personnel. Our conclusions were due immediately, so we had only a half hour to look the situation over. I hope the corrections we made turn out to be right.

Wednesday, 6 September

Still snowed under with work. Checked reports of the Marianas Campaign. The portable surgical hospital, while well adapted to jungle warfare,

appears ill-adapted and wasteful when communications are good. Furthermore, their talent is poor and not as well attuned to needs as is the personnel
of the surgical teams. Generally speaking, the larger installations are more
efficient as regards such things as specialized talent, protection (guards),
laundry, triage, and the treatment of shock. On the other hand, in amphibious operations, size is a limiting factor. The 400-bed evacuation hospital is
about right for these operations, as is also the field hospital if properly staffed.

Talent is wasted by using two smaller hospitals to take the place of one
larger one. Dumbea Valley is a good example of this. Another mistake is
to require station hospitals to do the work of general hospitals, as was the case
on Guadalcanal. The fact is that there were too many station hospitals there,
and, taken individually, they were too small for the job. We now have a 750-
bed station hospital which has been organized by combining three 250-bed
station hospitals. We expect to use it as an evacuation hospital, though the
staff is inadequate. The chief lack is qualified surgeons. I looked over two
portable surgicals and a field hospital and found only two surgeons with ratings
better than "C."

Thursday, 7 September

Talked to the 76th Station Hospital this forenoon. This is a good station
hospital. If this next action is severe, I would expect trouble, for the 165th
Station Hospital is made up of three 250-bed hospitals, and consequently the
personnel is poor. The conversion of several smaller hospitals into a large
hospital is unsound policy. They don't seem to realize that the quality of personnel in a small hospital is, and must be, different than that of a large hospital.
The 69th Field Hospital hasn't any well-qualified surgeon. To expect these
hospitals to function adequately as evacuation hospitals requires more optimism
than I possess. The 51st and 52d Portable Surgical Hospitals are short on
surgical talent. Certainly the portable surgical hospitals are wasteful, and
unless their talent is better than in those I have seen, they only succeed in giving the dangerous illusion that a surgical hospital is available.

The general has been very kind and considerate toward the consultants.
When I told him of the lack of surgical talent, he said: "I didn't know your
standards would be so high."

I looked up some of the anesthetists today, and they are scattered in all
sorts of positions. One of the best, with 6 years' experience, is an executive
officer.

Friday, 8 September

To Koko Head where I talked at the 69th Field Hospital, which is not
too strong in personnel. Spent the afternoon with Robertson who insists that
he wants to do hospital work as well as act as a consultant. Thinks catgut is
better than silk or cotton.

A three-star general here burned his fingers when a matchbox caught on
fire. I went down to see him in response to a call and a two-star general who was
there asked why such high-powered talent was needed for such a little thing.

I said: "I thought perhaps things had gotten so hot that there was danger of a general conflagration." This seemed to please the general to the extent of relieving his pain.

Saturday, 9 September

Visited the new hospital ship *Mercy*, which had Army personnel aboard (fig. 331). Seven hundred patients and only two operating rooms, inadequate for a combat mission. There were only eight medical officers aboard, five of whom are would-be surgeons. The ship should have had the personnel of at least a 400-bed evacuation hospital.

Spent the evening with the general. He is a fine person to work for. Unfortunately, he has not had enough advisers to whom he could delegate responsibility.

Monday, 11 September

Spent yesterday writing a directive on surgery for the forward echelon. The general, to my amazement, insisted I sign it. "It would come better," he said, "from a doctor."

Some doctors are against the use of plaster in the next operation because of gas gangrene. Correcting one surgical mistake with another it would appear. I am more than ever convinced that, as a whole, the amount of gas gangrene is an index of the quality of surgery at the front, and admittedly it was not of the best on Saipan.

Tuesday, 26 September

I am still laboring to get out: (1) An educational directive (none has been issued); (2) a statistical directive (no method exists for gathering statistics on surgery, and one should be set up for POA); (3) a plan for a wound ballistics study (none has been contemplated); and (4) ETMD (Essential Technical Medical Data) reports to this theater, and a plan for developing our own. Discussed some revisions of this plan for ETMD reports with General Bliss. The classification was too high, and subject matter should be concentrated just as in any other medical paper. A consultant, or some one on his staff, should act as editor.

The great shortage in this area is talent. There is only one surgeon here who can qualify as chief of surgery in a 2,000-bed general hospital, and there is a dearth of specialists.

One of the chief functions of a general hospital should be to act as a teaching center; however there is a shortage of good teachers. Very few lives can be saved in a general hospital (area Naval hospital had 1 death in 6,000). The patients die before they reach a general hospital. The shortage of qualified men here is due to the fact that there are no affiliated units. Those from the South Pacific Base Command are tied up by agreement with the Southwest Pacific Area, and personnel cannot be moved although many are idle in that area. The 39th General Hospital has 100 patients.

The portable surgical hospital is too small to function as a hospital and too large to function as a team. It should be disbanded.

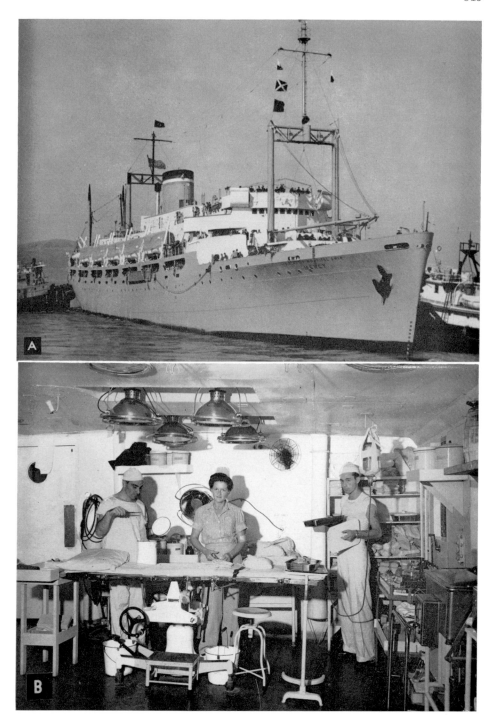

FIGURE 331.—U.S. Army Hospital Ship *Mercy*. A. The *Mercy*. B. Operating room.

Maui Island, T.H., Monday, 2 October 1944

Flew from John Rogers Field to Molokai Island, and thence to Maui Island to visit the 8th Station Hospital. This unit was formerly on Bora-Bora. Lt. Col. Julius Sobin, MC, is Commanding Officer—F.A.C.S., a good surgeon. Chief of surgery is Maj. Charles E. Town, MC. His surgery appears to be good, and he is capable of handling a 500-bed hospital. Capt. Irvin E. Simmons, MC, ENT man, is young but appears capable. Capt. Rosario Provenzano, MC, is in charge of orthopedics—young, but also seems capable. Capt. Leo Tyler, MC, is the anesthetist. This hospital, developed by the 20th Station Hospital from some former school buildings, has barracks-type wards of 750-bed capacity. It has a pleasing location at 1,800 ft., cool, exceptionally well adapted to a station hospital. They now have 600 patients; average census for 1944 was 300. A Marine division is now training here, and they expect an increase in patients. The 250-bed personnel is not enough for present needs, and the Navy has supplied 15 medical and dental officers. The equipment is superior to most general hospitals. In fact, no extra buildings or equipment would be needed to make this into a 500-bed hospital, and their key personnel would be adequate. However, the laboratory does not use the copper-sulfate method. Attended an excellent medical meeting. The staff does not have help enough to offer training courses. They need a dietitian and more enlisted men for the basic jobs.

Hawaii, Wednesday, 4 October

Off to the Large Island [Hawaii] and landed at 1100 hours. Went directly to the 75th Station Hospital, which was organized as a 750-bed and is functioning as a 250-bed hospital. Colonel Underwood of Brooklyn is commanding officer and also functions as district surgeon—a fine fellow doing a good job. Colonel Mayer is Chief of Surgery. He is one of the two or three best-trained surgeons in the CPA (Central Pacific Area). They need a good orthopedist. Pfiffer, general surgeon—young, but has aptitude; Goldman, genitourinary specialist—good; Freidman, ENT—good; Captain Foster (nurse) is the anesthetist. They have one physiotherapist. This service should be developed. One dietitian—good. They need more. The library is good—six textbooks of Christopher and six of Cecil. They do not know the copper-sulfate method at any of these hospitals.

Friday, 6 October

Started off at 0800 to drive around the island through the Kona country. At 1400 we arrived at the 26th Station Hospital on the Parker ranch—35,000 cattle and 10,000 sheep and goats—looks like Wyoming. This hospital has 150 beds and two surgeons. Captain Amstutz is doing an excellent job here. Captain Bigliani, an orthopedist, is assisted by numerous doctors from the Marine division. Cooperation is excellent with the Navy. They need an X-ray man and an ENT man. Anesthesia is done by the nurses—two good ones. Captain Spalletta, laboratory officer, also does cystoscopy. They are doing a lot of work on appendixes and pilonidal sinuses. On the whole they are doing as well as can be expected, and Amstutz is a superior officer.

Saturday, 7 October

Off at 1230 from Hilo and landed at John Rogers Field [Naval Air Station, Honolulu], 1430 hours.

Oahu, Sunday, 8 October

After 6 weeks, I have still not accomplished any of my original projects. There has been a tremendous passing of "buck" slips. It is almost as difficult to get something done here as in a university medical school. The educational directive is under way, stated by G–3 as being long needed. Reproduction of ETMD will be delayed indefinitely, as the photo lab burned down last week. The statistical project is at status quo with more and more excuses developing, such as no help or no room.

There are three ways of determining the quality of medical care: (1) Inspection of hospitals and personnel by consultants and others; (2) statistical record of results (as the cash register is to business, so is the statistical record to surgery); and (3) questions and answers on what the soldier thinks of his medical care. With these three methods correlated, we should be able to determine the quality of medical care and devise means for improving it where needed.

Sunday, 15 October

Still no news from Washington, and General Maxwell is still in New Caledonia.[17] The educational directive is about to be published, so my number one project is done.[18] Must now get out a directive on reparative surgery and another on penicillin. Penicillin has not been used to the extent that it should be. Reports coming in indicate that we are making the same mistakes in medical planning here that were made in the South Pacific one and a half years ago. This also applies to matters other than medical. This theater is fighting its first battles, and, since none of these men have had experience, they must necessarily learn through trial and error.

Sunday, 22 October

Got out the directive on penicillin. We have not been using enough in this theater, and there is confusion as to when to use sulfonamides and penicillin. Arranged program for a territorial medical meeting. Abstracting and getting out ETMD for all hospitals, divisions, corps, and armies—this has not been done before. I'm working on a gas gangrene, anaerobic wound infection report. Have not yet been able to establish a record system.

I would like to go forward, for the flow of Philippine casualties will soon be coming through. The invasion was announced 2 days ago and is going well

---

[17] Brig. Gen. Earl Maxwell had been notified of impending assignment to the U.S. Army Forces, Pacific Ocean Areas; however, when official request had been received in South Pacific Base Command, General Gilbreath had radioed back to the Commanding General, the U.S. Army Forces, Pacific Ocean Areas, that General Maxwell was not available as he had no replacement.—E. M.

[18] The directive published at this time was promulgated by Headquarters, U.S. Army Forces, Pacific Ocean Areas, on 20 October 1944 as Training Memorandum Number 8, subject: Training Program for Medical Officers. Colonel Oughterson later rewrote this directive, adapting the principles in it to Headquarters, U.S. Army Forces in the Pacific, when that command became the superior headquarters in the Pacific.

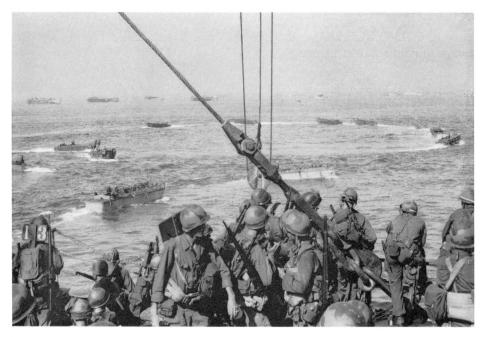

FIGURE 332.—A-day, Leyte Island, Philippine Islands. Landing craft rendezvous for the
assault on Leyte.

(fig. 332).[19] Saw a picture in *Time* of Carnes Weeks with Admiral Halsey. I
envy his seeing the show. Spent a pleasant afternoon at the beach today,
swimming with Colonel DeCoursey [Col. Elbert DeCoursey, MC] and Colonel
Curtis—both fine fellows. This week should bring clarification of the situation here.

Thursday, 23 November

Eddie [Ottenheimer] arrived today with many tales, some new stories.
He certainly was most welcome as I need him to lift my spirits. Things here
have been most discouraging, although I would not have missed the experience,
which is unique in my Army career. I begin to appreciate what is meant by
the word bureaucracy, although I think Marine terms are probably more ex-
pressive. Three months have I labored here and brought forth one directive
on the training of medical officers. All others have been blocked for various
and sundry reasons.

General Willis [Brig. Gen. John M. Willis, Chief Surgeon, USAFPOA]
arrived about 5 days ago. Some personnel have been returned to the States.
One officer, in charge of the personnel of a hospital, never developed anything
worth the name of a department. There was no name file nor classification of

[19] The X Corps from the Southwest Pacific Area and the XXIV Corps from Pacific Ocean Areas
made the landing at Leyte on 20 October 1944 under the operational control of the Sixth U.S. Army.
The customary "D-day" for this operation was formally designated "A-day," and the terms are used
interchangeably by Colonel Oughterson.

personnel. The general filing system in the office was reminiscent of my grand-mother's attic. Things were probably there, but no one could find them. It was not uncommon to find everyone looking very solemn, as though in con-ference, then to discover that they were only looking for a lost document.

The prevailing idea seems to be that the consultant is here primarily to make inspections, write long-winded reports about trivial matters, sit on boards, and see patients. In trying to accomplish something, I have encountered resent-ment and a feeling that I was interfering with things that were none of my business. The consultant takes no part in planning, although the office is making the same mistakes in planning that were made in the South Pacific a year and a half ago. Results: The mortality of wounded on Saipan was twice as high as on Bougainville, and one-third the number of patients returned to duty.[20]

I spent the evening with the general and accomplished much business very pleasantly. My first impression of the general is that he is outstanding in his desire for, and insistence on, a high standard of work. Being new, he of course does not wish to move rapidly against tradition, although he sees the need clearly. This is a fine education on how to win friends and influence people, but not much help yet to the war effort.

Thursday, 30 November

Dinner tonight with George Finney. Says he: "How can we plan when we don't have anything to plan with?"[21] I have now been in this headquarters over 3 months and still have not been asked to take part in future planning; nor after my request, have I been permitted to take part in planning. A field hospital is going in [to the Philippines] with the Marines. They say it will function as an evacuation hospital. The Army says it will not, and I suggest that it should have surgical teams if it is to function. Responsibility is being shifted along. Only God cares for the little fellow! I am wondering when this will crack. It can't go on forever. Once again I must speak to the gen-eral or be derelict in my duty. I would rather be out of the thing than in it and wrong.

Friday, 1 December 1944

Ben Baker arrived today. The role of consultants in the Army needs clarification, and Regular Army personnel must be educated as to the medical problems of a theater. There is only one partially qualified neurosurgeon in this area. The determining factor in the distribution of battle casualties was the number of the doctors available, including those in station hospitals. Anesthesia departments, headed by doctors, have not been established. Essen-

---

[20] Attention is called to Colonel Oughterson's statements on the function of a consulting surgeon (p. 841) and his participation in planning, such as it was (p. 842), written before the undersigned reported for duty. The comments on this instance were made only 5 days after my arrival. Con-sultants working under my command, including Colonel Flick, Colonel Mason, Colonel Loutzenheiser, Colonel Oughterson, and Colonel Ottenheimer, were always consulted on every phase of my duties and at all times were kept aware of any plans involving the medical service.—J. M. W.

[21] I believe Colonel Finney's comment has reference to the lack of "qualified personnel" previously commented on from time to time. Surely that decision had been made prior to my arrival.—J. M. W.

tial Technical Medical Data have not been distributed to hospitals. I suggested that it was by the ETMD more than anything else that the world judged the theater and was met by stubborn incomprehension.

Saipan, Thursday, 7 December

Yesterday, having a chill and after numerous inoculations, I received notice at 2200 to appear at Hickam Field at 0015. We took off at 0130, and, fortunately, being the senior officer on board, I had a bunk. Owing to repeated chills, I stayed aboard until Kwajalein where there was a dismal rain, making this dismal place look worse than usual. I have sympathy for the men whose lot it is to stay in such an unattractive part of the world. Arrived just before dark at Saipan.

Today, with Col. Eliot Colby, MC, Surgeon, Army Garrison Force, Island Command, Saipan, we had a hurried preliminary survey of the island, which is far more attractive than I had anticipated. There was a Japanese air attack this morning, and on getting up I was a bit disconcerted to find no foxholes. Found the colonel in charge of ATC digging a foxhole, asked him why, and he pointed to his teeth marks on the floor. The 148th General Hospital is still in tents although prefabricated buildings are under construction. Headquarters is built in quonset huts, and the labor has been used to improve this and other sites. Colonel Colby says that hospitals have "No. 1" priority, but then "No. 1" becomes subdivided into "a, b, c, et cetera." Visited the supply depot in charge of Captain Phillips. Most supplies are out of doors on the ground, although covered with tarps.

Visited the 369th Station Hospital, where I saw Major Goldsmith who is in charge of a civilian section which will be taken over by the Navy on 1 January. According to Colonel Colby, in the original plan the Navy had designated one medical officer and one corpsman to treat civilian casualties. There were a large number of civilian wounded, even on the beaches. One platoon of the 31st Field Hospital was designated as a civilian hospital. This platoon with 100 beds soon had 880 patients. A second station hospital of 500 beds is under construction adjacent to the 750-bed 369th. This total of 1,250 beds requires a duplicate setup of surgeons, administration, equipment, and so on. This does not seem to be good economy of personnel or equipment, but owing to the difficulty of putting these hospitals together under one T/O they must be set up separately. Certainly T/O changes should be made more easily.

Guam, Saturday, 9 December

Left by plane at 0800 for Guam. Visited the 273d Station Hospital— Colonel Batterton, Commanding Officer. This is a 750-bed station hospital at about 20 miles from the port, but fairly close to the airfields. The hospital is now under construction and should take patients in about 2 weeks.

Tinian, Sunday, 10 December

Visited the 289th Station Hospital, under construction at the edge of the depot field—a splendid location. Quonset hut construction, a 100-bed unit expanded to a 200-bed unit. Maj. Paul S. Read, MC, is commanding officer and also does some surgery. The surgical personnel seems to be about as good as can be expected in a small hospital.

Left Guam at 1900 and arrived at Tinian, passing close to Rota Island which the Japanese still have in their possession. Found Major Shaw, island surgeon—a pediatrician and very energetic.

Saipan, Monday, 11 December

Visited U.S. Naval Base Hospital No. 19 under the command of Captain Mueller, USN. The station hospital at Tinian, the personnel of which have not yet arrived, will be constructed of quonset huts by the Seabees. Shaw had drawn up some very good plans, and this should be a superior station hospital. These two hospitals can provide facilities for 2,000 beds if they get the additional personnel. Flew to Saipan in the afternoon to attend a medical meeting. Pathologist reported findings on autopsies of 60 civilians. About 70 percent were tuberculosis and beriberi, frequently mixed. The next largest group was dysentery and colitis.

Tuesday, 12 December

Drove around the entire island [Saipan] in the afternoon looking at hospital sites. The two general hospitals are toward one end of the island, and the station hospitals are together at the other end. While this is undesirable geographically, it would be unsatisfactory to try to convert the station hospitals into a general hospital. It is understood that all battle casualties will pass through the general hospitals and that the station hospitals will be used primarily for garrison work. The 39th General Hospital is 8 miles from the airstrip, as is also the 148th General; and the 39th is 5 miles from the docks, while the 148th is only 1½ miles from the dock. At present, the 148th General is doing about 40 percent station hospital work. Yesterday, evacuation policy for patients was increased to 60 days for the general hospitals, 30 days for the station hospitals. The 21st Bomber Command has 100 beds to act as a clearing station at the strips, and the ATC has two quonset huts to care for casualties that have arrived or are awaiting evacuation.

Summary of Informal Report to General Willis

There has been a need for sometime for a consultant in this area. The chief problems are: The planning and construction of hospitals; shifting of personnel; and professional questions, especially in relation to the functions of various hospitals.

The 148th General Hospital is now under construction, although they are now functioning in the area under tents. The surgery should be in quonset huts in 2 to 3 weeks. The personnel of the surgical service of this hospital will require strengthening. Further observation at a later date is required for proper evaluation. Approximately 40 percent of the surgery in this hospital involves the garrison forces. Twice the number of beds may be made available for battle casualties by allocating most of the garrison work to station hospitals. This has been discussed with Colonel Colby who has given splendid cooperation.

The 369th Station Hospital, 750 beds, is also under construction and is now functioning in tents in the same area. Lt. Col. Joseph Kuncl, Jr., MC, Chief of Surgical Service, is doing an excellent job, although he is short two Medical Corps officers. The 176th Station Hospital, 500 beds, is also under construction adjacent to this hospital and will be functioning within a few weeks.

I understand the 39th General Hospital is coming here. Neurosurgery and thoracic surgery can be allocated to this hospital, which has qualified specialists. There are also some board members available in this hospital qualified to act as chiefs of service.

I have seen the plans of the 39th General Hospital and there is room for much improvement to insure a better functioning unit. I would strongly recommend that Lt. Col. Edward J. Ottenheimer, MC, be sent here as soon as possible to assist in the planning and construction of this hospital. Colonel Colby concurs and has radioed a request.

With the arrival of the 39th General, the surgical services on this island can be staffed with qualified men, and, with the proper allocation of functions, all specialties could be covered in a superior manner. Guam will be well staffed with qualified specialists, except in neurosurgery.

148th General Hospital.—Of 303 battle casualties received in the 148th General Hospital, Saipan, 149 were evacuated to Oahu and 154 were returned to duty forward. Table 5 shows the number of operations performed during 4 months (August to November, inclusive) in 1944.

TABLE 5.—*Operations, blood transfusions and deaths, by month, at the 148th General Hospital Saipan, Philippine Islands, during the period August–November 1944*

Month	Operations	Blood transfusions	Deaths
August	108	30	6
September	221	10	3
October	248	35	1
November	263	54	1

Leyte, Wednesday, 13 December

Amid wind and rain, arrived at Isley Field, Saipan, 2200 hours. Wet—slept in ATC holding tent for patients. Plane left at 0200. Sat up all night, arrived Tacloban, Leyte, at 1000 hours and circled for an hour before landing. Drove to Tacloban and met General Denit [Brig. Gen. (later Maj. Gen.) Guy B. Denit, Chief Surgeon, USAFFE, and SOS, SWPA, and later Chief Surgeon, AFPAC]. General Denit: "This damn Army won't even obey orders. Supposed to have 12,000 beds by this time and we have only a fraction." I like the general.

Drove to Sixth U.S. Army headquarters and met Col. (later Brig. Gen.) William A. Hagins, MC [Surgeon, Sixth U.S. Army], a Regular Army surgeon (fig. 333). The most outspoken man I have seen in a responsible

position in this war. Says he: "The casualties are not high enough in headquarters." They do not like the PSH (portable surgical hospital) as a tactical
unit, although individual surgeons and units deserve high praise.

Saturday, 16 December

This is a fine country for ducks and it might well be left to them. Instead
we fight over it.

Drove to Dulag. Visited the 165th Station Hospital and skidded around
the mudholes in which it operates. This is a 750-bed station hospital functioning as an evacuation hospital—840 beds available and 899 patients. The hospital is insufficiently staffed to act as an evacuation hospital. Nurses are badly
needed here. Colonel Sneideman, Commanding Officer, appears to be doing

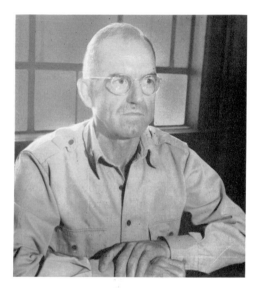

FIGURE 333.—Brig. Gen. William A. Hagins,
Surgeon, Sixth U.S. Army.

a good job under difficult circumstances. Lt. Col. Philip L. Battles, MC, is
doing excellent work on disrupted wounds.

Across the road or pond was the 76th Station Hospital. Colonel Bramble
[Lt. Col. Russell B. Bramble, MC] is Chief of Surgery. This hospital is on
a drier site; it is better laid out, is more compact, and has a splendid underground surgery. Saw many cases coming in from the 36th Field Hospital
across the island, a 2-day trip by road from Baybay. Records were good and
the patients were in good condition. Observed numerous cases described as
trenchfoot, but they do not appear to me to be typical.

The evacuation of patients has not been good. Too many patients have
been evacuated from Leyte. Fifty percent of the Leyte patients sent to Saipan
have been returned to duty in 1 month. However, there were not enough beds
available on Leyte. They were supposed to have 9,000 beds by D+20. Now,
D+60, the only general hospital functioning is the 118th with 600 beds. With
the beds of the station hospitals this adds up to approximately 2,000 beds available. The reasons for this failure seem to stem from rain and the difficult

engineering problems in this area. Hospitals have not gotten help from the Engineers. Also, hospital sites were poorly chosen.[22] Headquarters has one of the best sites along the beach, which I enjoy, but which is not fair to the hospitals and the sick. The evacuation route is hospital to beach, but there is often no LST to pick up the patients. Talked with the skipper of an LST, and he said that the patients were never on the beach when requested. Obviously, an evacuation station should be established on the beach as a holding station to correlate evacuation. Thus, there has been inadequate control of evacuation from the island, and much unnecessary evacuation of patients who could well have recovered here if facilities had been available.

Sunday, 17 December

Went out this morning to visit the *Wasatch*, flagship, and Captain Walker [Capt. Albert T. Walker, MC], USN, surgeon of the Seventh Fleet. Colonel Kendrick [Col. Douglas B. Kendrick, Jr., MC, Special Assistant for Shock and Transfusion, USAFPOA] and I had a long talk with Walker regarding the blood bank. He impressed me with the soundness of his ideas and has a better grasp of the surgical problems of combat amphibious troops than anyone I have seen in the Pacific Ocean Area. Moreover, he has accomplished more than anyone else. We then visited LST 464, which is undoubtedly the finest medical unit afloat. This is an LST that has been converted into a 200-bed hospital ship—clean, good food, laundry, good operating room. Here is the most concentrated and best organized surgical care I have seen in a forward area in the Pacific.

They're doing excellent investigative work on shock and burn patients, whom they have in great numbers. Japanese suicide bombing results in many burns. For burns, they are using plasma and serum albumin in large quantities, all controlled by hematocrit and protein levels—as much as 1,200 units per patient—plus blood. They find serum albumin better than plasma when the condition is severe. They have their own blood bank. The donors are Army personnel who are picked up on the beach. The LST proceeds to pick up patients while the donors are bled, then the donors are disembarked on the way back. Only 1-qt. containers, discarded vacoliter bottles, are used. For pooled group O blood, eight donors are bled into 10-gallon bottles. Nine thousand cc. blood, plus plasma, were given to one patient.[23]

---

[22] I saw these installations when I was with General Kirk and party in February 1945. The locations were miserable but were all that were available at the time. By February, they had either moved or were in the process of moving. I think the medical service did very well, as did the patients with whom I talked.—J. M. W.

[23] Dr. Ernest Eric Muirhead, formerly the director of the blood bank on LST 464, in a telephone conference with Maj. J. K. Arima, 11 December 1958, stated that Captain Walker, surgeon of the 7th Amphibious Force, wanted whole blood and had picked Dr. Muirhead to get it, since Dr. Muirhead had had some experience with whole blood before the war. The Red Cross blood was not then available. So LST 464 was set up in New Guinea and then went to Leyte. According to Dr. Muirhead, they (on LST 464) "had to do with what we had." Two kinds of bottles were used—the 1,000-cc. vacoliter bottles and the 20,000-cc. regular laboratory water bottles. Preservative was made from citrate and dextrose because the ACD solution was not yet available. Any number of donors with group-O blood were bled directly into these bottles, appropriate amounts of citrate and dextrose were added, and the bottles were stored in the ship's walk-in type of refrigerators. The blood was not typed for Rh factor, neither was it titered. In times of stress, transfusions were effected directly from the large bottles, which had been adapted for giving purposes with pressure bulbs.—J. K. A.

Large amounts of citrate may result in carpopedal spasms which are relieved by calcium gluconate. The Navy makes up and distributes sets of copper sulfate for bedside work.

Casualties received earlier were given better treatment than casualties now being received. When the S.S. *Bountiful* took in one load of patients, nearly every compound fracture was infected owing to the poor setup and overloading of shore facilities. The 7th Amphibious Force now has 70 LST's with surgical facilities and 23 surgical teams.[24] Each team is composed of 5 surgeons and 18 corpsmen. These are quickly shifted from one LST to another. This ship [LST 464] also moves about among the fleet, taking cases from ships that have been hit. The LST goes in on the initial landing and remains as a floating emergency hospital. The 60 well-trained corpsmen work most efficiently. The LST unloads its patients to an APA [transport, attack], APH [transport for wounded], or other ship which takes them to hospital ships outside the combat zone. He, Walker, is not informed regarding beds available in the Marianas. See Admiral Laning [Rear Adm. Richard H. Laning, MC, USN, Inspector, Medical Department Activities, Pacific Ocean Areas] about entire theater correlation. Will these LST's and surgical teams later be available for Western Pacific operations?

Captain Walker first described these procedures for the Bureau of Medicine and Surgery in May. They consented to equipping LST's with surgical facilities, but refused to build LST hospital ships on the grounds that conventional hospital ships were being built. They apparently missed the point that hospital ships outfitted in accordance with the Geneva Convention cannot operate in these waters during combat. Three attempts were made to bomb hospital ships, one at night when the ship had to be lit up. Captain Walker asks that I take up the LST hospital ship problem with Admiral Laning. This was the program I tried to institute in the South Pacific a year ago, and which met with Captain Hook's approval but was turned down because of construction difficulties.

Observations on Blood Program

When General Rankin and General Bliss visited USAFPOA, I advocated a blood bank program for all Pacific Ocean areas and suggested that someone who had had experience in the European theater should set it up, Doug Kendrick if possible. Apparently the Navy had also been working on a program, and the first I heard of this was when Blake and Brown came through Hawaii with the blood, on their way West. This had developed into a combined Army-Navy program on the West Coast. The Army was collecting blood in San Francisco and the Navy in Los Angeles. Blood was transported by NATS to Guam under the direction of the Naval District and Capt. Newhouser [Capt. Lloyd R. Newhouser, MC, USN]. The ATC was landing on Saipan, so refrigeration was set up there. But the blood arrived in the Marianas before

---

[24] The 7th Amphibious Force under Rear Adm. Daniel E. Barbey, USN, comprised one of the two attack forces of the Seventh Fleet in the asault on the Philippines.

any real preparation had been made to receive it. Unfortunately, no one in the Pacific Ocean knew about the program, so it got off to a bad start. The Naval surgeons in CINCPAC [Commander in Chief, Pacific Fleet] were peeved but cooperative. When Kendrick and I arrived at Leyte, considerable time and effort was needed to establish cordial relations. Both Army and Navy had had blood banks functioning for some time in the Southwest Pacific, and the LST 464, especially, had performed outstanding service. The people in the Southwest Pacific Area were perturbed that the first they learned of the blood program was from the newspapers. Consequently, their first in-clination was to say that they wanted no part of it. However, in spite of the excellent blood bank already established here, there was a need for still more blood. Many of the hospitals did not know that blood was available. The loss in early shipment of blood to Leyte amounted to approximately 50 percent owing to the fact that arrangements had not been made for proper refrigera-tion or distribution. The chief reason for this loss was lack of ice. There is a need for a directive on the use of blood and an educational program among the medical officers.

There has been a heavy loss of men from the line because of the lack of hospitals. Although the hospitals are here, there are few good sites, and these have been used for other purposes, such as headquarters. Result: Engineering problems are so great that hospital building has been slowed down. Now, D+60, a 15-day evacuation policy is in force. Patients have had to be trans-ported 1,500 miles to the nearest hospital, and since many are returned to duty, time and transportation are lost unnecessarily.

Tuesday, 19 December

Saw Colonel Wills, Base Surgeon, who was very cooperative in helping to arrange the blood program. Visited the S.S. *Mactan*, the last ship on which Colonel Carroll came out of Manila. It now serves as the surgeon's office. Major Steinberg is in charge of planning, another young officer with a large job. The Southwest Pacific Area has 44,000 beds, but about 25 percent of these are inactive due to moving. There are 23 general hospitals. Obviously, gen-eral hospitals are being used for station hospital work, which is one of the reasons that there are not enough specialists to go around.

The overall plan is to support each division with one 400-bed evacuation hospital, one 400-bed field hospital, one separate clearing company, one separate collecting company, one company from the engineer special brigade, and three portable surgical hospitals. Portable surgical hospitals are used because sur-gical teams are not available. The general impression is that the portable surgical hospitals are not adapted to this type of land fighting, but that they are useful as 25-bed station hospitals, for example, to support an isolated airstrip.

Saw Colonel Weston, 44th General Hospital. They were set up near an airstrip. About 600 Japanese paratroopers landed on the strip, and a few nights later reinforcements came in to join them. Our men decided to hold the perimeter, as they had about 200 patients in tents and the road in was im-

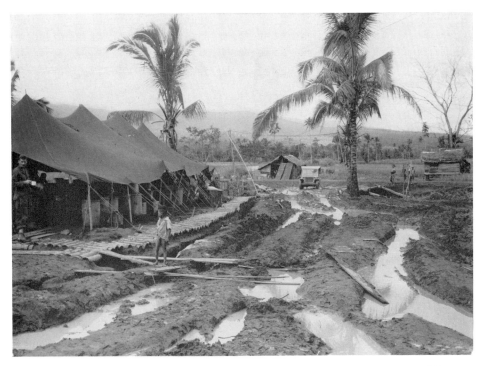

FIGURE 334.—A scene at the 116th Station Hospital, Leyte Island, December 1944.

passable. The Japanese came into a signal company first, and the guards were ordered out to the perimeter. By this time, the Japanese had machineguns set up on three sides of the hospital. There was an all-night fight, and in the morning they found 23 dead Japanese. Two officers of the hospital were wounded. None of the hospital personnel had had training in firearms other than squirrel shooting. The commanding officer suggested, before leaving the States, that they should have such training, and he was told that all the training they would need was in getting into formations, so as to be able to march on and off the trains.

Wednesday, 20 December

Today, I tried to drive to the 44th General Hospital, but the bridges were still out and the roads were impassable. D+60, and no general hospital has been set up as yet to receive surgical patients. Visited the 116th Station Hospital which never took any patients and is now moving (fig. 334).

Saturday, 23 December

Much conversation during the last few days regarding the use of blood and how to get it distributed. Much careful sidestepping to avoid stepping on toes, which have been rendered more sensitive than usual because their owners have missed so many boats. But, slowly the plan is being accepted and cooperation is being achieved. The prima donnas and the weak egos undoubtedly retard military accomplishment. In the Army as in civilian life, if nonmedical men are to assume administrative responsibilities for medical care, they should be educated in medical problems, at least to the extent of being able to identify a competent surgeon.

This morning, I visited the general's (MacArthur's) quarters situated on the beach. Adjacent to these quarters are frame buildings for the staff. The general's house is huge and beautifully furnished.

Sunday, 24 December

Saw Col. Morris Bradner [Col. Morris R. Bradner, MC] of New York. An excellent surgeon who thought he could do more good in this war in an administrative capacity. He was surgeon of the 248th Garrison Force attached to the XXIV Corps. They started for the Palaus from Hawaii, target then changed to Yap, then changed to the Philippines.[25] They were at sea for 54 days and debarked on Leyte D+12. Of this force, apparently only the XXIV Corps was wanted, and now, D+60, the garrison force has not been used and they do not know what their assignment is to be. These hospitals have therefore gone through 4 months of training in Hawaii and have spent 54 days at sea and 2 months on Leyte. Colonel Bradner is discouraged, he has offered his services through the usual channels, but no one seems to want them. Another good surgeon gone to waste in a campaign where surgeons were at a premium.

Monday, 25 December

Visited LST 1018—Lieutenant McDermot, surgeon. They had cut watertight doors between the tank deck and the troop quarters, where they made a dressing room and washing room for patients and an operating room. There was space there for the seriously wounded and 200 patients could be put on the tank deck. Certain equipment was lacking, such as anesthesia machines, water pitchers, and some means of keeping hot soup or coffee. They were staffed with a minimum crew of 2 doctors and 10 corpsmen, which is not enough during an assault. All LST's are to be converted in this manner—they now have 17 converted. In addition, such ships as the LST 464 are needed as floating hospitals.

7th Amphibious Force: 70 LST's, 17 now converted for surgery; No. 464, a hospital LST with complete staff and 60 corpsmen; and 23 surgical teams (5 surgeons, 18 corpsmen each).

Navy doctors say that the initial phase of surgery on land is poorly done. On S.S. Bountiful every CC [compound comminuted] fracture was found to be infected. Captain Walker, 7th Amphibious Force, gets a report—name, rank, and serial number—in all cases of improper handling.

The handling of blood is improving but still needs much supervision. Need a system for dropping blood from "Cubs" by parachute when the roads go out. There is a plan for 96 L–5's ("Cubs") to transport casualties. They can carry one litter and two sitters and operate from an 800-ft. runway.

---

[25] How could anything but confusion result from such a change of plans? Yet the Medical Department had no choice—Yap Island was never invaded!—J. M. W.

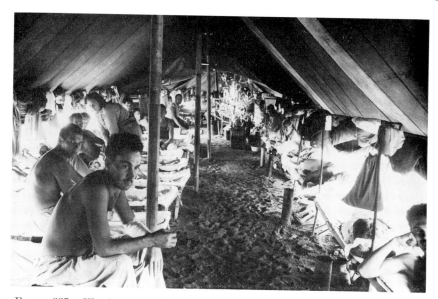

FIGURE 335.—Wards of the 165th Station Hospital, Leyte Island, December 1944.

A better plan for marking hospitals is needed. Some commanding generals are said to be afraid of signs.

Visited Abuyog, the eastern terminal of the road from Baybay. One platoon of a clearing company is here to transfer patients to DUKW's [amphibious trucks 2½-ton] to go to Dulag—about 200 daily. Those who did not stand the trip well (4 hours over bad roads) from Baybay are held here at Abuyog. More serious patients come from Ormoc by boat. Air evacuation from Valencia began on D+60.

Wednesday, 27 December

The 165th Station Hospital (750 beds) was sent in as an evacuation hospital to support the 96th Division. They had two additional surgeons attached. The 76th Station Hospital (500 beds) was to act as an evacuation hospital in support of the 7th Division.[26] Because of the terrain, weather, and tactical situation, these two hospitals were placed adjacent to each other and received patients from both divisions. They were situated about 500 yds. from the beach at Dulag. The site was very poor, so low and muddy that it severely handicapped the functioning of these hospitals.

The 165th Station Hospital usually has about 300 surgical patients, the rest are medical (fig. 335). Since 1 December, they have performed 17 major and 353 minor operations. There were 44 deaths, of which 14 were postoperative (5 abdomen, 9 other) and 30 were nonoperative. The operating room is well set up, but aboveground and without sandbag protection. Wards are of the "T" variety with pyramidal tent junction. Equipment is adequate. This hospital could be improved by a better planned layout. All hospitals that have

[26] The 96th and 7th Infantry Divisions comprised the XXIV Corps and took part in the initial landings at Leyte.

not functioned in the field should receive instruction as to planning from those who have had such experience.

On A+1, 21 October, word was received on shipboard that four surgical teams were needed ashore. They started ashore but were driven off by mortar fire, then went 5 miles down the beach toward Abuyog and landed. They found a few soldiers there who knew nothing of the local situation. They then started up the beach and dug in for the night. Next day they still could not find out who had wanted the surgical teams. They set up at this site on A+4 and immediately received 200 civilian casualties in bad condition. The G-2 [intelligence] was not good, and much of the land and roads that were thought to be usable were actually under water. They had many more casualties than could be handled during the first week, and large numbers were evacuated without being seen. After the first week, by dint of very hard work, they were able to see most of the casualties. However, the job done forward was not entirely satisfactory. Again, this was due to the excessive work that was demanded of the forward installations. Many patients had incomplete debridement. This necessitated the frequent changing of dressings in order to determine the condition of wounds, some of which were labeled "moderate debridement." Since the four surgical teams could not work 24 hours a day, only two surgical teams were operating at a time.

The number of beds available in support of the divisions was inadequate: 750-bed station hospital, 500-bed station hospital, two 400-bed field hospitals—total 2,050 beds. These were situated behind the clearing station to serve three divisions—about 700 beds per division. Result: Large numbers were evacuated from the island who might otherwise have been returned to duty; inadequate surgery and lack of beds prohibited reparative surgery.

There is too much emphasis on planning the rear echelon hospitals. More emphasis is needed on staff planning for hospitalization in forward areas.[27]

Friday, 29 December

Flew over to Valencia, Bohol Island—a former Japanese strip—this morning in a "Piper Cub."

Drove over to Headquarters, 77th Division.[28] The roads were crowded with thousands of natives transporting their household goods on their heads or on the backs of water buffaloes. This migration was coming from the mountains. The GI and the native women were all bathing together in the streams we crossed—danger of schistosomiasis.

Colonel Ivins [Lt. Col. John C. Ivins, MC], surgeon of the 77th Infantry Division, was out. The 95th Portable Surgical Hospital was functioning with the clearing station here. The surgeons of the clearing station were alternating with the surgeons of the portable hospital so that they each did about the same amount of surgery. Reports from the field hospital indicated that the

---

[27] I agree, but task force commanders determined the number of beds in forward areas.—G. B. D.

[28] The 77th Division, which had been engaged in the recapture of Guam, was sent to Leyte in late November 1944 to reinforce the embattled XXIV Corps. On 7 December 1944, it had made a surprise landing near Deposito and had driven through the Ormoc Valley to effect a junction with the 1st Cavalry Division near Valencia, Bohol Island.

surgery of the clearing station was not good and that they were doing other than emergency surgery. Furthermore, the emergency surgery was not well done.

Talked with General Bruce [Maj. Gen. Andrew D. Bruce, Commanding General, 77th Division] who is very medically minded. He says that the foot problem is most important and he wants one pair of socks brought up with the rations each day. He was unhappy with Navy evacuation and stated that 100 wounded men were left on the shore because the boats would not wait. Broken glasses are a major problem. He wants an extra case issued to each man for replacement lenses and frames, especially as he has many men of 35 years or older (average age in the 77th Division, 29 years). Morphine seems to be very beneficial for morale; the surgeon said he had seen no ill effects. General Bruce also wants a bag in the hat for a latrine at night. Evacuation is being done extensively by Cub and this is good for morale. They badly need ambulance Cubs.

Drove to Ormoc, Leyte, to visit the 36th Field Hospital. Lt. Col. Devine [Lt. Col. John L. Devine, Jr., MC] is commanding officer—a superior officer. This hospital is set up in a shelled 16th century cathedral. There is no roof, but the thick walls provided good protection. They will need much equipment and some personnel before their next operation. Generators and X-ray machines are worn out. They need two surgeons capable of heading a team— one general, one orthopedic. They are short 3 officers and 12 enlisted men. Colonel Devine believes that many of the officers and men, having been on five missions, are fatigued. In common with other commanding officers, he emphasizes the need for nurses early in a campaign.

The 36th Field Hospital had 1,884 patients in 17 days, mostly surgical. They averaged 125 per day, 250 patients on the top day. They did definitive surgery mostly—2,600 in a month with three moves. This hospital has kept permanent records for its own use. They are abstracted and typewritten on all field records. The surgical records are superior. They received casualties from the 7th Division, the 77th Division, and the 1st Cavalry Division.

More directives and instruction are needed. Limbs are still being lost due to tight casts. One patient had a cast on over a clove hitch. Result: loss of foot. These hospitals, the 36th and 69th Field had never heard of the copper-sulfate method for protein determination. The 36th Field does not have a qualified anesthetist or anesthesia apparatus.

Saw Colonel Kamish [Lt. Col. (later Col.) Robert J. Kamish, MC] division surgeon of the 7th Division, and talked with General Arnold [Maj. Gen. Archibald V. Arnold, Commanding General, 7th Division]. He is very medically conscious and recommended Kamish for the Legion of Merit. The XXIV Corps under General Hodge has offered full support and recognition to the Medical Corps, and any shortcomings cannot be attributed to lack of support by the commanding generals. Unfortunately, many of the good division surgeons do not and cannot be expected to appreciate surgical principles, since they are not surgeons. Having developed through the field service, they are prone to believe that field surgeons are better qualified to do surgery than is actually the case.

Saturday, 30 December

After seeing Colonel Kamish this morning, I drove to the 69th Field Hospital which has been set up for about a week near the airport at Valencia. The hospital commander is ill and has been evacuated. Maj. Fielding Williams [Maj. Fielding P. Williams, MC] is acting hospital commander. They have no anesthesia machines. This hospital needs at least one surgeon qualified as chief of service. The laboratory has never heard of the copper-sulfate protein method.

Waited at the airstrip and watched a number of patients evacuated by Cub. Compound comminuted fracture of the femur, belly, head wounds, and so on; all evacuated sitting up. They appeared to stand the trip from the clearing station (20 minutes) very well. Ambulance Cubs are needed for economy of operation (three planes needed now where one ambulance plane could suffice) and welfare of patient.

Sunday, 31 December

Spent the night at the 69th Field Hospital and on to the airfield the next day. While at strip, saw General Hodge, Commanding General, XXIV Corps, who stated that he was pleased with the medical service but felt that hospitalization was inadequate. General Richardson [Lt. Gen. Robert C. Richardson, Commanding General, U.S. Army Forces, Pacific Ocean Area] came in, and a guard of honor was present. Came back to Sixth U.S. Army headquarters [the Sixth U.S. Army was comprised of the X and the XXIV Corps] in a "Cub" and spent the afternoon looking over the harbor for Captain Walker.

Monday, 1 January 1945

Japanese started the celebration by bombing last night, and at midnight our boys responded. Felt less safe than in an air raid. Arrangements made for Lingayen operation. I am to go on an LST (H) [landing ship tank (casualty evacuation)] and remain at target.[29]

Aboard LST 1018, Wednesday, 3 January

Boarded the general's crash boat, then on to *Wasatch*, flagship. Left some luggage with Captain Walker who invited me to join him after we reach the target. Left *Wasatch* in search of LST 1018. The coxswain of the boat had received instructions, but got mixed up between true and relative bearings, and we ended up on the opposite side of the bay. We boarded the LST 1018 at supper time after two hours' search.

There is a surgical team aboard of four doctors plus the ship's doctor. This appears to be a capable surgical team that is well organized, but they are

---

[29] The Biennial Report of the Chief of Staff, U.S. Army, for the period from 1 July 1943 to 30 June 1945, to the Secretary of War states: "In the first week of January [1945] a new American assault force gathered east of Leyte, slipped through the Surigao Strait * * * and passed into the Mindanao and Sulu Seas. This American force was treading its way through the heart of the Philippine Archipelago and through waters where the Japanese Navy and air forces had for two years maintained unchallenged supremacy, to invade Luzon by effecting a landing in Lingayen Gulf * * *." D-day was 9 January 1945 and, in this case, was formally designated "S-day."

short of supplies because they were not notified that they were going to function as a hospital ship. Supplies were not available in Leyte, and they could not return to Hollandia or Manus. Furthermore, the other hospital ships have not had the supplies, or they have been reluctant to part with them.

Thursday, 4 January

Clear, set sail at 0600, about 80 ships in sight in the convoy.

1600. Have met a large convoy presumably from Hollandia—numerous battlewagons, cruisers, destroyers, flattops.

1800. Apparently, this convoy is to be about 75 miles long and we have joined up too soon, so we are now going back past innumerable ships to get into position before darkness.

2000. We have now turned around and are heading into Surigao Strait toward a golden glow beneath thick laden clouds.

Friday, 5 January

1400. Sailing through Mindanao Sea—smooth and hot. Bohol fading and Cebu Island can be seen in the distance off starboard.

1830. Negros Island off starboard, like a camel's hump in the clouds—a beautiful golden sunset.

Saturday, 6 January

Negros still off starboard. Smooth sailing through the Sulu Sea.

Sunday, 7 January

Peaceful ships and a clear, bright, hot morning. Japanese attacked at 0600. We are about 8 miles off the lower end of Mindoro Island.

Monday, 8 January

1100. The mountains of Bataan are plainly visible off our starboard. It has been quiet since 0900, and two carriers can be seen between us and Bataan. The convoy plows steadily northward.

Tuesday, 9 January

D-day, reveille 0500.

0600. Up on the bridge; clear starlight with a sliver of an old moon. The dim outline of Mount Santo Tomas on the portside. We are well into the Lingayen Gulf and moving steadily ahead. The dim silhouette of the battlewagons can be made out.

0700. All the battleships opening fire on the portside, followed by the guns on the starboard. We are in the middle. There are two task forces, one off the port (the landing is to be made on WHITE, RED, and BLUE beaches near Mount Santo Tomas) and the other off the starboard bow, preparing for a landing at the town of Lingayen. The shelling starts rather slowly and continues with increasing tempo.

0815. We have moved through the haze nearer the shore, and I can now see the church in Lingayen.

0850. Bombardment continues. Our bombers can now be seen bombing the shore, and great clouds of smoke and dirt shoot into the air in 1-2-3 order. The first wave of small boats loaded from the transports behind us are now passing. They are scheduled to reach the beach at 0930 (fig. 336).

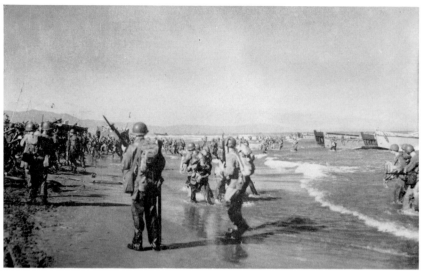

FIGURE 336.—Troops of the 37th Division coming ashore, Lingayen Gulf, 9 January 1945.

0920. The roar is deafening and continuous. The shore has disappeared in a great wall of smoke and fire into which the small boats disappear.

1000. The naval bombardment has nearly ceased, like an intermission when one can relax. From out of the smoke toward the shore comes the sound of distant mortar fire. A great pillar of black smoke appears from the general direction of Clark Field, Luzon.

The smoke is lifting, and once again I can see the shoreline. Everywhere, small boats, like water bugs, are darting hither and yon. The great symphonic overture is over.

Wednesday, 10 January

0500. General quarters; Japanese torpedo boats are among the fleet. Went on deck. Very dark night plus a smokescreen. The Infantry is putting up flares on shore so they can see the Japanese, and we are putting up a smokescreen so the Japanese cannot see us.

0600. Japanese planes overhead, and everybody shooting at things they cannot see.

0645. Another plane raid. This time I saw them diving into the smoke, with tracers going in every direction. Most of the fighting today is in the San Fabian beach section.

Aboard LST 911, Thursday, 11 January

1000. The usual air raid this morning. Went toward shore to visit LST 911 which was unloading on the beach and had a surgical team aboard. A heavy surf—6-foot waves—was running, and I felt and acted like the man on the flying trapeze when boarding this LST.

The 911 had excellent plans worked out for triage, records, and available beds. They have a surgical team of 5 doctors and 11 corpsmen headed by Dr.

Sasnow of San Francisco. They, as well as LST 1018, are short of supplies and equipment for adequate performance in case of heavy casualties. They tried to obtain these from the hospital ships but were unable to do so. Apparently, hospital ships are not fulfilling their function as supply ships. This ship was unable to receive casualties until D+2 as it was not loaded for assault shipping. They have shot down five Japanese planes. As near I can learn, out of some 230 LST's, only one has been hit on this mission, and that by a torpedo. The risk to an LST therefore seems to be slight. Furthermore, they now carry a lot of firepower—ten 20-mm. and seven 40-mm. guns. (Interrupted by another air raid.)

The *Wasatch*, Friday, 12 January

0700. Heavy air raid. This afternoon I went to the *Wasatch* to see Capt. Albert Walker and Lt. Col. Stuart Draper, MC. The latter is a Sixth U.S. Army evacuation liaison officer with the 7th Amphibious Force. I found out that two other LST's are functioning as surgical ships on WHITE beach, where most of the casualties have been received.

Returned to LST 1018, packed my duffle, and returned to the *Wasatch* at Captain Walker's invitation. This is Admiral Kincaid's flagship.

Saturday, 13 January

Visited all the beaches today and went up a river to deliver a Filipino to his family. This chap had 25 years' service in the Navy and had hidden out in Manila for these 3 years. Yesterday he reported to the flagship for duty. He went ashore proudly, dressed in white, to visit his family. On the beaches, the surf was very high, and not one LST was unloading although several were beached. The pontoons were washed up on the shore.

The *Blue Ridge*, Sunday, 14 January

Went with Captain Walker and Commander Klein, who is Walker's assistant, to visit two LST's that are functioning as surgical ships. Water and steam are piped to the tank decks. There are auxiliary lighting facilities and surgical faucets. Steam and water are available in the head for cleaning bedpans. About 50 percent of the cases here have had debridement and casts applied in the clearing station. Some were well done and others poorly. The blood appeared to be in good condition, dated 1 January, "West Coast," and was well refrigerated.

DUKW's bring patients out from the beach and drive them up on the ramp for unloading. However, when weather is rough this may be difficult. The beach setup is splendid. A Navy medical officer and four corpsmen are assigned to the beach. He sets up adjacent to or with a medical company of the special engineer brigade. The engineer medical company designates patients for evacuation and the Naval beach officer is responsible for obtaining the ships and supervising the loading. This plan has been slowly evolved through experience and is the best that I have seen in the Pacific. It could be improved upon with better equipment [in the LST's], such as (1) portable anesthesia machines Heidbrink, (2) intratracheal anesthetic apparatus, and (3) portable orthopedic tables. The personnel of these ships may be overworked, and Army surgical teams functioning on these ships would be of great assistance until shore installations were ready.

This afternoon I heard that the *Blue Ridge*, Admiral Barbey's flagship of the 7th Amphibious Force, was to return to Leyte, so I transferred to her.

SUMMARY OF MEDICAL CARE AND EVACUATION DURING THE LINGAYEN CAMPAIGN

1. The plan.

    a. General objective.

    (1) The distance involved in evacuation made it imperative that definitive surgical care be provided at the target. Emphasis was placed on early and adequate surgical care at the target rather than on speed of evacuation to the rear areas.

    (2) Cooperation of Navy and Army planning was emphasized, and a close liaison was maintained between the commander of the Seventh Fleet and the commander of the Sixth U.S. Army and subordinate units.

    b. Fleet surgical facilities and supplies at combat area.

    (1) Numerous and varied types of vessels carrying combat supplies and personnel to the target were equipped to provide surgical care. Evacuation from the Lingayen Gulf to Leyte was by APH, APA, and LST.

    (2) Near the beaches, main reliance for surgical care was placed on the LST's. Eighteen of these ships had been converted to provide facilities for surgery. Six of these converted LST's were staffed with augmented surgical teams (5 doctors and 18 corpsmen). These ships were under the control of CTF [Commander, Task Force] 77. After unloading, they were to anchor near the flagship for ease of communication. The medical representative of the Commanding General, Sixth U.S. Army, was also aboard this ship. The ships were to remain in the combat area, receiving casualties day and night, and be on call to proceed to beaches or go along the side of damaged ships as needed. One of these LST's was assigned as support for each beach. As they became loaded, and according to the condition of the patient, the casualties were transferred to APA's or APH's for evacuation to Leyte.

    (3) In addition to servicing the ships in the harbor, three PCE(R)'s [patrol crafts, escort (rescue)] were stationed near the flagships. These ships proceeded immediately to any vessel that was hit.

    (4) Whole blood was available from S-day onward on flagships, on any surgical LST, and at reefers on BLUE and ORANGE Beaches.

    (5) Supplies were available, as follows (fig. 337):

Location	Organization	Period of time
WHITE Beach	I Corps Medical Dump	S-day onward
ORANGE Beach	XIV Corps Medical Dump	S-day onward
LST's 564, 118, 704, 202	Medical Exchange Units	S+2 onward
WHITE Beach	21st Medical Supply Platoon	S+4 onward
Dagupan, Luzon	49th Medical Supply Depot	S+4 onward
ORANGE Beach	55th Medical Supply Depot	S+4 onward

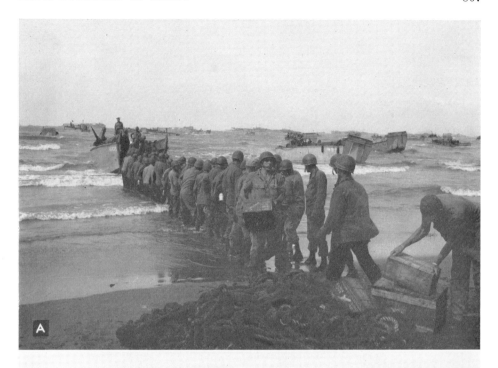

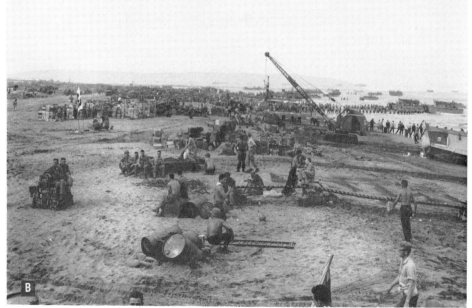

FIGURE 337.—The extent of supply operations, Lingayen Gulf, January 1945.   A. Closeup,
unloading landing craft.   B. Panorama of beach and bay, showing supply dumps.

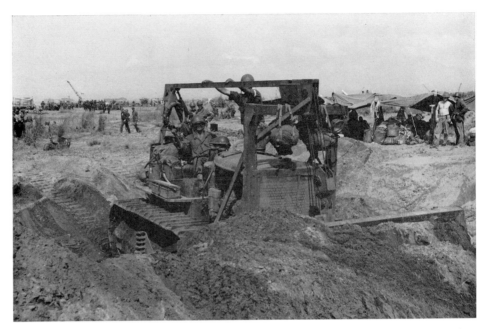

FIGURE 338.—Ground being hollowed out for a bomb shelter and a beach aid station, Lingayen Beach, 11 January 1945.

(6) Beach medical party consisting of one doctor and two corpsmen acted as liaison for Army evacuation from the beach. This officer maintained contact with the beachmaster and the medical company ESB [engineer special brigade] which performed triage for the Army during the early phases of the assault and later acted as a holding hospital on the beach.

 c. Army surgical facilities at combat area.

(1) Each division was to be supported by one field hospital; one evacuation hospital; one clearing company, separate; one collecting company, separate; and one medical company, engineer special brigade.

(2) The medical company of the engineer special brigade was to be the first medical facility ashore. It was established on the beach and remained there, allowing the divisional medical units to proceed inland with the troops (fig. 338). It acted as a holding station on the beach for patients transferred to the LST's and also cared for the casualties that had been wounded on the beach.

 2. The functioning of the plan.

 a. Combat loading of surgical LST's.—In order that these ships may be able to perform their function in providing early surgical care during the initial phases of the assault, it is necessary that they be loaded with combat supplies having an early priority on the beach. One of these ships, transporting bridge pontoons, was not unloaded until S+5. Part of this delay was due to the very heavy surf which prevented the LST's from getting closer than

500 feet from the shore; the remainder of the distance had to be spanned by pontoons.

b. The surf was so heavy that when pontoons could not be maintained only DUKW's were suitable for the transfer of casualties to the LST's.

c. The LST's appeared to be relatively immune from air attack as there were so many more profitable targets. It is likely that LST's are hit only when they become targets of opportunity.

d. The equipment of the surgical LST's could be improved upon by the addition of portable anesthesia apparatus, intratracheal anesthesia sets, and portable orthopedic tables. Those ships acting as surgical stations should also have portable X-ray apparatus. An additional number of pitchers and bowls should be provided to facilitate the distribution of liquids and soup.

3. Observations.

a. The LST converted, equipped, and staffed as a surgical hospital for use during the initial phases of the assault has many advantages:

(1) They provide adequate facilities for early definitive surgery at a time when this cannot be provided on shore.

(2) They provide adequate facilities for handling a large number of casualties (185 casualties) in comparative comfort.

(3) They remove the wounded from the immediate frontline and provide a sense of relative security.

(4) The LST is less likely to be attacked than a larger ship. It carries more firepower than the smaller craft and is less likely to incur serious damage when attacked as a target of opportunity.

(5) When beaching is possible, the transfer of casualties from shore is accomplished with the greatest ease (fig. 339). Transfer of casualties to the deck of APA's or APH's is facilitated from the deck of the LST.

(6) A surgical hospital available to the beach at all times is essential until surgical facilities can be established on shore. This can be provided by the LST with a minimum loss to combat shipping. Inasmuch as several ships are available, they may be dispensed with as the need diminishes.

(7) The presence of such a hospital facility afloat diminishes the need of establishing operating facilities ashore until this can be accomplished adequately and in safety.

(8) There are now 60 LST's converted for surgical use. It is desirable that all LST's be constructed or remodeled so as to be used for patients.

(9) Two types of LST's are needed for surgical care. One functions primarily as a cargo ship, with casualties incidental, and does not remain at the target. A second type, with adequate equipment and a surgical team aboard, remains as a hospital ship at the target.

b. Shore units and control of evacuation.

(1) The beach medical officer and two corpsmen are stationed at each beach and function with the medical company, ESB. The medical company, ESB, performs three functions: Care of beach casualties; triage for casualties

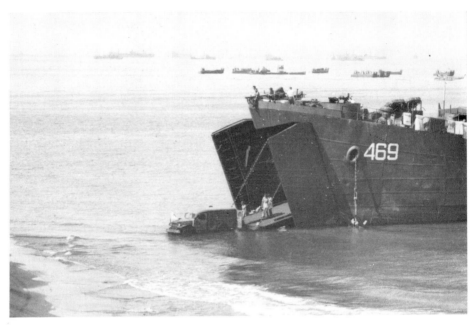

FIGURE 339.—Patients being transferred from an ambulance to a beached LST, Lingayen Gulf, February 1945.

before evacuation; and holding casualties on the beach so that ships do not need to wait for casualties.

(2) The beach medical officer is essentially a traffic officer, for liaison between the Army ashore and the Navy afloat. He is familiar with the surgical ships available and is responsible for seeing that casualties are properly distributed so that ship hospitals do not become overtaxed. For example, when casualties are heavy, minor wounds cannot always be treated ashore and should be sent to any ship that has a doctor aboard, while the serious casualties should be sent to the surgical LST's. When the operation is on a large scale, specialized surgical teams may be spotted on certain LST's.

(3) In heavy surf, as at Lingayen, the DUKW appears the safest means of transporting casualties to ships.

4. Recommendations.

a. Use of medical company, ESB, to act as holding hospital on the beach and for triage.

b. Use of beach medical officer (Navy) to correlate Army-Navy shore-to-ship evacuation.

c. Use of LST's as surgical hospitals. Conversion of all LST's so that they may be used surgically, since the loading and unloading of LST's cannot be controlled according to ship. Certain LST's that have early priority in unloading should be used as evacuation hospitals and remain on the beach until shore facilities are established (one LST to each beach or Army division).

These ships must be adequately equipped for major surgery, including anesthesia.

d. At least one of the surgical teams to be employed (five per division during combat) should function aboard the LST until the shore facility is ready for use.

e. More indoctrination of corps and division surgeons concerning the function of various units, such as clearing stations, surgical teams, field hospitals, and evacuation hospitals.

f. Clearer definition of evacuation policy. Too many men are evacuated who are well before they reach the next echelon.

g. More prompt establishment of convalescent hospitals or units so as not to overutilize the beds of acutely needed surgical hospitals [for those with minor wounds] and so as not to force evacuation of minor wounded from the island.

h. Clearer definition of policy concerning priority for hospital sites and assistance in construction. When hospitals are expected to provide their own construction, they should have the requisite equipment.

Saturday, 13 January

Set sail at 1700 with two APA's and a convoy of destroyers. This should be a fast trip.

Leyte, Wednesday, 17 January

Not one single Japanese attack. Today we passed a slow convoy going south and another one going north. The Sulu Sea seems like an American lake.

Tonight Admiral Barbey invited me up on the bridge for a chat (fig. 340). He is known as "Uncle Dan the amphibious man." The admiral is a large, dark-complexioned man with a friendly, jovial, simple direct manner. He is medically curious and deserves great credit for his cooperation and enthusiasm in developing the medical service for amphibious warfare. He thinks the Japanese conceded the Philippines after the Leyte Campaign, and that Luzon will be only a delaying action while they marshal their forces for the next line of defense.

Sailed into Leyte Gulf and over along the coast of Samar, then straight into our anchorage in front of Tolosa. It began to rain, and I went ashore to what was left of Sixth U.S. Army Headquarters with the Admiral's jeep. The storm increased and reached typhoon proportions during the night.

Thursday, 18 January

Went down to stay in the 118th General Hospital. In the mud and confusion of construction, I had a fine talk with Col. Jim Bordley [Col. James Bordley III, MC] and his colleagues, in the middle of their frog pond.

Peleliu Island, Friday, 19 January

Signed out at Sixth U.S. Army. Boarded plane at Tacloban Field at 1000 hours. Landed Peleliu Island [Palau Islands] at 1400. Went directly to the 17th Field Hospital, now under Navy management. Its chief function is to act as a transfer or holding point at the field. Still raining, but the island is coral and not muddy. Cordially received by Commander Kelley, pediatrician.

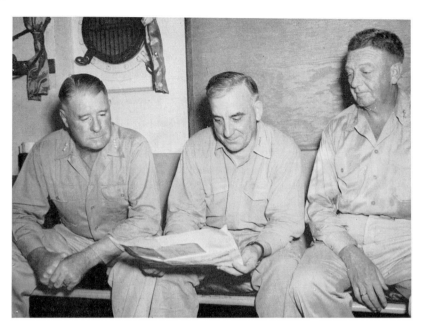

FIGURE 340.—Aboard U.S.S. *Blue Ridge*, 3 January 1945. (Left to right: Maj. Gen. Innis P. Swift, Commanding General, I Corps; Vice Adm. Daniel E. Barbey, Commander, 7th Amphibious Force; and Maj. Gen. Leonard F. Wing, Commanding General, 43d Division.)

After cleaning up I was taken to [U.S. Naval] Base Hospital No. 20 and shown the sights of Bloody Nose Ridge. There I found Emile Holman, somewhat lonely, a bit discouraged, but carrying on. As usual, a fine type of quonset hut construction—1,000 beds. There is no anchorage here, and the only casualties coming in are expected by air.

Guam, Saturday, 20 January

Off at 0945 hours, and arrived at Guam at 1515 hours, after severe rough weather. Amazed at the transformation here since my last visit. After Leyte the air terminal here looks like Grand Central Station, and the paved roads are impressive. Went directly to the 204th General Hospital.

Sunday, 21 January

The 204th General Hospital is set up in tents, with the exception of the operating room, laboratory, X-ray, and nurses' quarters. Their semipermanent installation is being built. They are now operating more than 1,000 beds but at present have only 150 patients, owing to the fact that evacuation to Guam by ATC will not begin until 1 February. This hospital is one of the best set up tent hospitals I have ever seen.

Guam, Friday, 26 January

Have spent the last 4 days recuperating from a cold and visiting the 373d Station Hospital.

Saipan, Monday, 29 January

Arrived at Saipan. Saw Colonel Longfellow and learned of the arrival of the 39th General Hospital. He had sent in an advanced party from Auckland. Ottenheimer had not been sent forward to check on the plans.

Wednesday, 31 January

Construction started on the 39th, and ground cleared. Some of the best level land was not used for the site. No thought to future expansion to 2,000 beds.

Friday, 2 February 1945

Have spent the last 3 days at the 148th General Hospital, which is slowly evolving into a hospital. Construction has been very slow. It still has only a 1,000-bed capacity (total beds available on Saipan, 2,000). Airfields and headquarters have priority.

Saturday, 3 February

Worked on logistics and visited the 369th Station Hospital a well planned and constructed hospital. Colonel Lubitz [Col. Benjamin Lubitz, MC], the commanding officer, was formerly surgeon with the 27th Division.

Monday, 5 February

Visited the 176th Station Hospital, a stone's throw from the 369th. Both have excellent quonset construction. Why two station hospitals should be placed so close together is beyond me. They care for garrison troops scattered over the island. Since these hospitals are not geographically suited for this purpose, they wish to combine them into a general hospital for casualties, thereby correcting one mistake with another. This would entail an unnecessary duplication of skilled personnel as well as equipment.

Tuesday, 6 February

Radio today assigning Baker and me to the 204th General Hospital [Guam]—as this is the only hospital with vacancies for full colonel—and to temporary duty with the Surgeon's Office, Western Pacific Base Command.[30] Also, a teletype for me to return to Headquarters, USAFPOA, by 15 February.

En route to Oahu, Hawaiian Islands, Thursday, 8 February

At 0615, just daylight, we got off and flew all day. At 1800 we landed at Kwajalein, and a nice Navy lieutenant came on board and said that they would give us dinner on the plane and that we could leave in half an hour if it was all right with me. As though I would have nerve enough to tell the Navy what to do! So we left at 1900, and I played poker with four aviators until 0300 of the same day, because we had crossed the dateline. I then went to sleep soundly on my air mattress on the floor until they poked me to tell me that we were starting down. At 0600, with the east in a pink glow, we landed at Johnston Island.

---

[30] The Western Pacific Base Command was activated on 25 April 1945. Included in this command were Army units on Saipan, Guam, Tinian, Iwo Jima, Peleliu, Ulithi, and Angaur Islands. The Western Pacific Base Command was subordinate to Headquarters, U.S. Army Forces, Pacific Ocean Areas.

En route to Saipan, Friday, 23 February

Arrived at Fort Shafter, Oahu, and found Eddie Ottenheimer very industriously acting as consultant, working on history, personnel, etc. Ben Baker was about to leave for Saipan. Many new officers have arrived. The port still has a peacetime atmosphere and everyone is griping about the red tape, et cetera. Most of my time was spent in helping to put together a concise directive for the Tenth U.S. Army on surgical care in the combat zone.[31]

Finally, I got the orders through and escaped with Eddie as though from an asylum. We took off on 22 February at 2300 hours. The nurses who were liberated at Luzon were at the field on their way to the States. The band was there playing "Show Me The Way to Go Home" and other similar tunes, and everyone wore leis.

Saipan, Saturday, 24 February

Spent the day touring the island with General Kirk [Maj. Gen. Norman T. Kirk, The Surgeon General], General Simmons [Brig. Gen. James S. Simmons, Director, Preventive Medicine Division, Office of The Surgeon General], General Willis, and General Jarman [Maj. Gen. Sanderford Jarman, Commanding General of the Army Garrison Forces, USAFICPA and USAFPOA].

Found that only one operating room was functioning at the 148th General Hospital. We spent the remainder of the day trying to get some semblance of organization. We transferred large numbers of the 39th General Hospital staff and a large number of nurses. These changes were quickly accomplished with the support of General Kirk and General Willis.

Note [written, apparently, sometime between 24 February and the next entry, 15 March]: The hospital was soon running on a 24-hour basis with four operating teams working continuously, averaging 60 majors per day. In all, 2,200 [sic] serious casualties were treated, with a mortality of 1.1 percent. Considering the circumstances and the character of the casualties received, this was a splendid record.

Had a meeting with Ben Baker, Colby, General Willis, and General Kirk this evening. Discussed evacuation policy with Willis, with a view to avoiding the loss of shipping and manhours brought about by having to evacuate patients to Oahu, nearly 4,000 miles away.[32]

NOTES ON RECOMMENDATIONS FOR MAJOR GENERAL KIRK

1. The essence of good surgical care in the Army is to get the right man at the right place at the right time, in adequate numbers and with adequate equipment. None of this can be accomplished without planning. Consultants in the Pacific Ocean Areas have not been consulted in planning as of 10 February 1945. The efforts of a consultant who has not taken part in planning are

---

[31] This directive, the subject of which was "Surgery in the Combat Zone," was promulgated by Headquarters, U.S. Army Forces, Pacific Ocean Areas, on 27 February 1945. Colonel Oughterson was later to rewrite this directive at Headquarters, U.S. Army Forces, Pacific, where it was published in that command's *The Journal of Military Medicine in the Pacific*, September 1945, pp. 11–23.

[32] The situation was corrected.—J. M. W.

chiefly limited to trying to lock the stable door after the horse is gone. Under these circumstances, there is a great danger of the consultant assuming a one-sidedly critical attitude, since there is little left for him to do. His mission in planning, to improve the care of the sick and wounded, is blocked at the source.

2. Clinical research, for the benefit of the sick and wounded in this war and in future wars, is a responsibility of the Medical Department of the U.S. Army. It is recognized that the first responsibility is the care of the patient, but there is an equal responsibility for investigative work which will improve the care of the patient. Theater surgeons should be made aware of their responsibility in this field.

3. The essence of good surgical care is to provide good surgeons. The limited number of good surgeons available requires planning in the distribution of skilled talent. Surgeons can be conserved by careful planning of the geographical distribution of hospitals, the size of hospitals, and the type of hospitals. Two or more smaller hospitals should not be used where one larger hospital can do the work. This policy has resulted in a great waste of highly skilled medical talent as well as equipment. Also, the less-skilled surgeon can function satisfactorily in a station hospital, if he is limited to the station hospital type of work.

4. There has been too great a tendency to keep skilled surgical talent in the rear, whereas the most difficult surgical tasks are to be found in the forward area. The wounded soldiers who die, usually do so at the front. Greater mobility of these surgeons through the use of surgical teams is recommended.

5. In the vast stretches of the Pacific Ocean there are a great number of hospitals, large and small. The leapfrogging of these hospitals may involve distances of a few hundred miles or as much as 4,000 miles. Between the time the hospital ceases to function and the time it receives casualties at its new location, several months to a year may elapse. In this manner the 7th Evacuation Hospital was inactive for at least a year. This results in a great loss of highly skilled manpower, as well as a lowering of the morale of the unit. At the same time, the shortage of medical officers, nurses, and technicians in the forward areas has been increased. Air transport should be used to make this idle manpower available.

Saipan, Thursday, 15 March 1945

The major part of the Iwo Jima casualties have now been treated. Plans are now being laid for Operation ICEBERG [the Ryukyus offensive, 25 March 1945]. The shortage of personnel has necessitated that the hospital facilities on this island be organized as a hospital center. Furthermore, the small number of medical casualties has made it necessary to nearly abolish the medical service. Colonel Colby and Colonel Baker have given full cooperation in the face of most trying circumstances. All medical cases are to be transferred to the 176th Station Hospital which, together with the 94th Field Hospital, has five psychiatrists plus other personnel, and functions as a station hospital for medical cases. This frees the 148th and 39th General Hospitals, plus the 369th Station

Hospital, for surgical cases. The 148th General will take any surgical cases except for neurosurgery, while the 39th will take any surgery, but not thoracic cases. The 148th will have a thoracic team, and the 39th will have a neuro-surgical team. The 369th Station Hospital, which is short of qualified surgeons, will handle only soft-tissue wounds.

Thursday, 22 March

The chief of the surgical service, 148th General Hospital, Colonel Cornell, has been transferred to chief of surgery, 176th Station Hospital. He deserves great credit for the cooperative spirit and equanimity that he has shown under these trying circumstances. Colonel Ottenheimer was made chief of the surgical service of this hospital and again demonstrated his rare capacity for surgical organization and judgment. Colonel Bishop became chief of surgery at the 39th, and Major Sutherland was transferred to the 148th General, leaving Major Claiborn at the 39th as assistant chief of surgery. Captain Post and Major DeSopo were placed on temporary duty at the 148th to strengthen the thoracic team. This has necessarily weakened the 39th General, but still leaves it with the strongest professional staff in the Marianas.

A meeting was held with General Kirk, General Willis, Colonel Colby, Colonel Baker, Colonel Oughterson, and Colonel Welsh [Col. Arthur B. Welsh, MC, Deputy Chief, Operation Division, Office of The Surgeon General] regarding the medical problems of the Army in the Western Pacific. The question of the medical support of the Tenth U.S. Army was discussed. It was agreed that this was inadequate, but I am not sure that the shortage and seriousness of the situation was fully realized. The need for hospital beds in the Marianas was discussed, and the great shortage of beds was pointed out. The need for investigation of wound ballistics (requested in a previous letter by The Surgeon General), shock, and related problems was discussed. The meeting adjourned after assurances had been made that everything possible would be done.

I made a visit to Guam and found the situation there comparable to the situation on Saipan. However, no effort at triage has been made here. Control was in the hands of the Navy. Had a long conversation with Captain Anderson [Capt. (later Commodore) Thomas C. Anderson, MC, USN], Admiral Nimitz' surgeon, who was most cooperative. The Army does not have the specialized personnel necessary to provide adequate care for the patients on Guam. Only by making Guam a hospital center can adequate care be provided. General Kirk agreed to the consolidation of small station hospitals as a means of saving personnel, and to the use of surgical teams and the inactivation of portable surgical hospitals.

Friday, 23 March

Received word that 5,000 additional beds may be put on Tinian Island—source of personnel unknown. At least some arithmetical facts are sinking into the planners' minds. Had a conference today with the Commanding Officer, 148th General Hospital, and with Colonel Colby, Colonel Ottenheimer, and Colonel Baker. The problem discussed was how to use the engineers in converting the 148th from an old broken-down farm in appearance and function to a modern hospital. There are inches of mud and dust in the wards and operating rooms. CinCPac has ordered A–1 priority for hospitals, and not without reason.

Thursday, 29 March

The Tenth U.S. Army has been with us. George Finney, Hal Sofield, Doug Kendrick, Ben [Baker], and I, are in the same pyramidal. All that was needed was a little aisle between the bunks. My orders to go along (to Okinawa) have been canceled, much to my chagrin. They sailed on the 27th. The best that can be hoped for is that casualties will be light.

Guam, Sunday, 1 April 1945

I went to Guam with "Red" Milliken. Stayed at the 204th General Hospital. Colonel Bryant is doing a superior job. This is one of the best organized and planned hospitals, and certainly the best Army hospital in the Marianas. It appears that the Navy has given preference of materials and workmen to its own hospitals. The Army hospitals are not as well equipped as the Navy's, which appears to be the Army's own fault. There appears to be little justification for the great difference, since both Army and Navy hospitals must perform the same functions.

Had a very satisfactory chat with Admiral Laning, Navy medical inspector for Pacific Ocean Areas—a practical, forthright, capable officer. His observations on the Iwo campaign bear out mine on the Luzon campaign, and corrective measures are under way. There was much delay at Iwo in getting casualties from the beach to the ships, which the small boats had trouble contacting. Besides, the medical teams aboard the APA's were inadequate, both in number and quality of surgeons, to cope with the situation. The admiral says that the APA should not be used as a hospital ship, and that we must have more hospital ships. However, as Captain Walker so aptly enunciated, the primary consideration must be that of providing definitive surgical care on the spot, and not that of insuring speedy evacuation.

Visited Tom Rivers [Cdr. Thomas M. Rivers, MC, USNR] and his MRU [Naval Medical Research Unit] No. 2 which is under construction and promises to be de luxe. Rivers was burning with indignation as his first request for research was for a chemical analysis on a ton of beer. Requests for help in investigation far exceed his capacity. His interest in problems with the natives is overshadowed by the Navy demand for military medicine.

Carter [Lt. Col. George G. Carter, MC] started as Chief of Medical Service in the 204th. Woodruff [Maj. William W. Woodruff, MC] has many interesting chest cases and many hemothorax cases needing aspiration. Very few of these cases (Marines) were aspirated, due to lack of adequate surgical help at the front.

Saipan, Wednesday, 4 April

There is, today, no hospital on Saipan able to do elective surgery. There are plans to make a hospital center on Tinian, with an additional 5,000 beds. It appears that the medical bed requirement of the Marianas is finally being recognized. However, it should be noted with emphasis that to date no consultant has been used for medical planning by the Surgeon's Office, Pacific Ocean Areas.[33] Many lives have been needlessly sacrificed. The hospital planning could have been greatly improved, and both medical and nonmedical personnel could have been more efficiently utilized.

Friday, 6 April

Lt. Col. Pete Bishop came to see me regarding the morale of the 39th General Hospital. They complain that they are not getting a fair break in construction and personnel, which is a complaint common to all hospitals. It appears that their primary need is for leadership among themselves. Some don't like this and some don't like that, and they fight with the engineers doing the construction. One hopes that with the coming activity most of their problems will vanish.

Manila, Tuesday, 15 May 1945

John Flick [Col. John B. Flick, MC, Consultant in Surgery, USAFPOA] arrived, and for the past month I have had a delightful time traveling over the Western Pacific Base Command. The formation of this command has been in process for some time. The new command of the Pacific, MacArthur and Nimitz, was announced, the WPBC [the Western Pacific Base Command] (p. 873) was announced immediately afterward.

John Flick and I visited all the institutions on Guam and were in agreement as to what should be done, but JF asks continually: "What can be done about it?" There are not enough station hospital beds on Guam, yet it is proposed to change the 373d Station Hospital, which is miles from the port, into a general hospital, and without personnel to staff it. One of the chief sources of wasted personnel in the Pacific Ocean Areas has been the failure to distinguish between the personnel and functions of a general and station hospital.

We journeyed on to Tinian. Colonel Shaw is here, doing a splendid job as island surgeon. He has no inferiority complex and seeks advice wherever he can find it. Result—splendid planning. Had a long conference with General Kimball [Brig. Gen. Allen R. Kimball] who emphasized two important points: Plan for what you want in the future and don't try to do it by hidden figures; and the need for recreational facilities (morale and physical). Don't send out people—we have them to burn—but send the equipment we don't have.

Went to Iwo Jima, referred to as a "solidified burp." It is almost as desolate as the atolls of the South Pacific. Colonel Currey, Island Surgeon, is doing an excellent job.

There are three hospitals on this small island—the 38th Field, the 41st Station, and the 232d General Hospitals. Certainly the two smaller hospitals should be combined.

---

[33] Colonel Flick was surgical consultant at Headquarters, U.S. Army Forces, Pacific Ocean Areas, at this time, and he was consulted in all planning as were the other consultants at the Headquarters. Colonel Oughterson's comment is not a fact.—J. M. W.

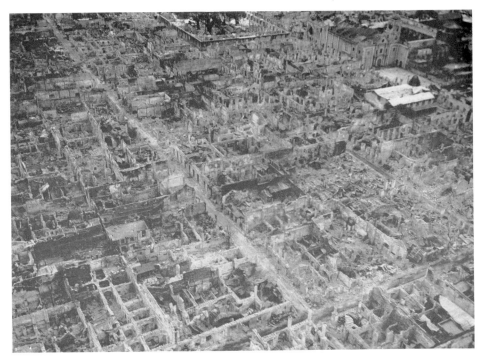

FIGURE 341.—Destruction in the Walled City, Manila, May 1945.

Returned to Saipan and found radio orders giving Ben [Baker] and myself to Headquarters, USAFFE in Manila.[34] Left by NATS on 23 May at 2230, and arrived at Manila the next morning at 0800. The plane circled the city and gave us a good view. While large areas of destruction were visible from the air, it still appeared that most of the city was intact (fig. 341). When we drove through the city we got the reverse impression. Signed in and was quartered in the Avenue Hotel. This hotel is one of the few not totally destroyed.

Tuesday, 29 May

Everything here at present is in a state of flux until the new commands are organized. Met General Denit who is full of enthusiasm about my future job to the point where I am loath to think of going home immediately.

Wednesday, 30 May

Colonel Robinson [Col. Paul I. Robinson, MC] and Major Bouldvan of the USAFFE Board came up to see me about the wound ballistics report. They were very enthusiastic about the study that was done and entered whole-heartedly into plans for a future study. In contrast to the attitude in the Pacific Ocean Area, this was as May flowers to a summer drought, and no

---

[34] The U.S. Army Forces in the Far East, commanded by General MacArthur, was the highest strictly U.S. Army command in the Southwest Pacific Area.

salesmanship was required. Spent the remainder of the day trying to rewrite a directive for surgery in the combat area.

Monday, 4 June

Drove out to Sixth U.S. Army headquarters with Earl Moore [Dr. J. E. Moore, Civilian Consultant in Medicine (Venereal Disease) to The Surgeon General], Lt. Col. Tom Sternberg [Lt. Col. Thomas H. Sternberg, MC], Chief, Venereal Disease Control Division, Office of The Surgeon General, and Major Bouldvan of the USAFFE Board. General Hagins was in his usual good form. After lunch we discussed wound ballistics about which he [General Hagins] is very skeptical, but I left him the Bougainville report and will return in a week for discussion.

Saturday, 9 June

Have been engaged for the last few days in surveying the need for civilian medical care in Manila. This has become necessary from a military standpoint because civilians are occupying many beds in military hospitals. The Philippine civil affairs office originally tried to provide such hospitalization. But their efforts have proven to be inadequate to the need.

Even before the war, hospital beds were inadequate to meet the demand. Approximately 4,000 beds were available. In addition, there was one 1,500-bed hospital for the insane with 3,000 patients. The Japanese set these inmates loose, and most of them are said to have starved, although their exact status is unknown. At present, there are 1,419 provisional hospital beds for the mentally ill, part of which are in the old hospital for the insane, and the remainder in schools. There are 2,457 government beds and 1,163 private beds, many now occupied by nonpaying patients. On 1 July, the private beds will all revert to private-paying patients, leaving approximately 3,800 government beds available.[35]

The Quezon Institute for Tuberculosis—1,500 beds before the war—was always full (fig. 342). The TB death rate was very high. At present the lowest reported TB death rate for Manila has been 80 per week, and the highest was 200.[36] However, it is known that the rate exceeds this number.

The former director of the Quezon Institute, Dr. M. Conizares, is now medical adviser to President Osmena. General Valdez, chief of staff of the Philippine Army, member of the cabinet, and politico, is said to be the best doctor in the Philippines. Some think it would be better if the Army controlled the hospitals and tackled the health problem on the islands. The problem is one of admitting civilians to Army hospitals in those cases in which life-saving procedures must be employed, and of providing facilities for those cases.

---

[35] The Japanese allowed such scant rations that most of the patients in the hospital for the insane were said to have starved. Theer were about 300 left alive when we took over. I am very doubtful as to the figures he gives for the number of civilia nand governmental hospital beds for civilians in Manila, which seems too high. However, I know of no way now of obtaining more accurate estimates for that period. (Letter, Dr. Maurice C. Pincoffs to Col. John Boyd Coates, Jr., MC 8 Feb. 1959.)

[36] The Civil Affairs headquarters at this time estimated the population of Manila at approximately one million. (Letter, Dr. Maurice C. Pincoffs to Col. John Boyd Coates, Jr., MC, 8 Feb. 1959.)

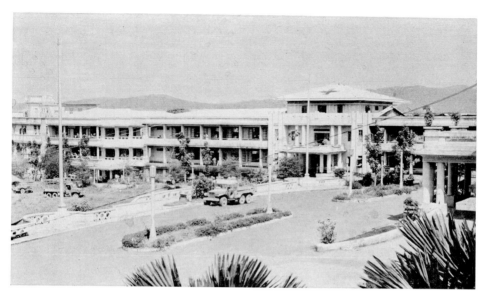

FIGURE 342.—Quezon Institute, Manila.

The facts are:

1. There are approximately 2,000 nonmilitary personnel in U.S. Army hospitals in the Manila area. These fall into two groups:

a. Filipinos (civilians and veterans of the Philippine Army and guerrillas).

b. Other nationals, more than half of whom are medical cases.

2. A survey of patients at the 120th General Hospital (Santo Tomas) (fig. 343) on June 1, revealed the following:

Nationality	Total number of patients	Number who can pay
American	45	[1] 11
Filipino	31	7
Other nationality	56	18
Total	132	20

[1] American veterans.

3. At the 80th General Hospital (Quezon Institute), there were 6 civilians out of 94 non-U.S. Army patients, and the remainder were men who belonged to various components of the Philippine Army and guerrillas and who required long periods of hospitalization. Surgical cases, 40; tuberculosis, 36; psychosis, 15; typhoid, 1; and leprosy, 2.

4. At present, the number of beds provided for the care of civilians in the city of Manila is 5,000 (government 3,837; private 1,163). At the same time, 4,488 of these beds are occupied. This may be considered as full capacity, as it leaves only 10 percent for distribution. Furthermore, no other beds are available for tuberculosis cases or for the insane, who together occupied approximately 5,000 beds in the prewar period.

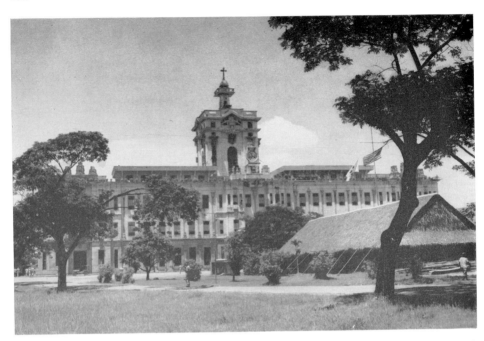

FIGURE 343.—The 120th General Hospital, Santo Tomas University, Manila, June 1945.

5. Other civilian hospitals, such as the Philippine General Hospital (fig. 344), have undergone severe damage. This institution formerly had 1,200 beds and is now functioning with only 236 beds. The government is unable to obtain labor or materials to recondition this hospital. Most of these buildings could be made available with only minor roof repairs, using salvage material. A few of them would require new roofs. This type of reconstruction would provide beds with less labor and material than new construction.

6. We are now authorized to make contracts for the care of Philippine veterans, which includes the Philippine Army and guerrillas. These contracts will be let with the Philippine hospitals to help finance their running expenses. The quality of the care is not high and is uncontrolled. It's sort of like pouring money down a rathole, but there appears to be no other short-term solution.

Monday, 9 July 1945

Had a siege with bad teeth and a hospital sojourn in the 49th General Hospital. I am now assigned as Surgical Consultant, AFPAC, but the general [Denit] has other plans for me.[37] He wants me to function as a surgical adviser responsible to him and without administrative responsibility. He wishes to call me a director of surgical research, which I oppose as a title. Have re-

---

[37] In April 1945, the operational and administrative authority of General of the Army Douglas MacArthur was extended to all U.S. Army Forces in the Far East and mid-Pacific areas. As his operational and administrative headquarters for these forces, General Headquarters, U.S. Army Forces, Pacific, was established. At this time, U.S. Army Forces, Pacific Ocean Areas, was redesignated U.S. Army Forces, Middle Pacific, a subordinate command under Headquarters, Army Forces, Pacific.

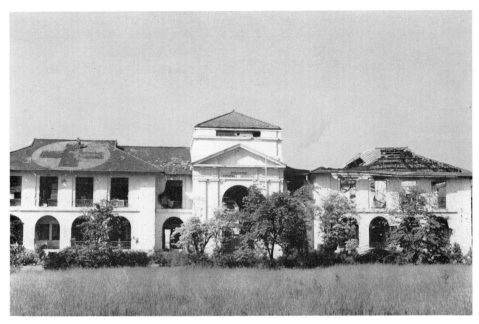

FIGURE 344.—The main entrance of the Philippine General Hospital, Manila, October 1945.

written a directive on surgery in the combat zone as well as a directive on anaerobic wound infections. Have also completed a program for the training of medical officers. The general has asked for a program that will put surgery in his theater on the map, and I have suggested the following:

    1. Publications.
        a. Medical bulletins to be started for dissemination of information.
        b. ETMD to be organized.
        c. History.
All three to be placed under one competent Medical Corps officer.
    2. Training Program for all medical officers to consist of:
        a. Instruction in a hospital.
        b. Instruction in a school of tropical and preventive medicine.
    3. Development of personnel files to show:
        a. Each unit with MOS [military occupational specialty] classifications.
        b. Personnel in each specialty and assignment.
        c. Cross index by name and specialty.

We are now short of personnel, but no one knows how much or of what kind. Consultants should be responsible for checking assignments and recommending reassignment. Moreover, personnel should be interchangeable on a theater basis [assignment controlled by theater headquarters?]. At present, lower echelons may change the assignment of key personnel. Promotion should not be made into a position unless the officer is qualified. This is very difficult to prevent as a commanding officer will usually promote on other bases.

4. *Records.*—A uniform report on individual cases by the chiefs of all the surgical services. Reports should include all deaths and complications, and their causes. A report should be made on each illness or injury on duty, and each death or discharge to the States. The report would be incorporated with machine records based on the standard Army diagnosis.

5. *Planning of operations.*—Consultants should be used in planning. Their advice must be given more weight so that the facilities and personnel commensurate with the mission to be performed will be made available.

6. Consultants should be heeded on plans for anesthesia, ophthalmology, neurosurgery, reconditioning.

7. *Specialization.*—Hospitals should specialize in specific battle casualties and diseases. This will result in better care and a greater opportunity to study diseases.

8. Research investigation of special problems in missile ballistics, body armor, shock, et cetera, should be initiated.

Friday, 13 July

We had a long teletype conference with the Surgeon General's Office for the purpose of finding out why, when we ordered 550 medical officers, they sent us 12. We had a lot of conversation but never found out the reason for the deficit. They said that they would answer by mail.

Monday, 23 July

Have been working the last week trying to get up enthusiasm for a study of body armor and missile ballistics. Splendid cooperation from Colonel Alexander, President, Pacific War Board.

Tuesday, 24 July

Gave some data to Col. Roger Egeberg [Col. Roger O. Egeberg, MC, Aide-de-Camp (Medical) to General MacArthur] in the hope that we may get General MacArthur accustomed to the idea of attaching a missile ballistics team. Working on trenchfoot and wet-cold projects.

Wednesday, 25 July

It appears that, for most people, becoming accustomed to a new idea is like a woman with a new hat. It all depends on what other people think of it.

Friday, 27 July

Today, Japan turned down our surrender terms. Most of the betting here is that the war will end within 3 months.

Visited Sixth U.S. Army headquarters, and spent the night at ASCOM [Army Service Command, SWPA] headquarters. Will try to coordinate the machine records with USAFWESPAC [U.S. Army Forces, Western Pacific, successor on 20 June 1945 to USASOS (the U.S. Army Services of Supply), SWPA] and the training program of USAFWESPAC with ASCOM and the Sixth U.S. Army.

Wednesday, 1 August 1945

Today I flew out to Cabanatuan, Luzon, to visit the 43d Division medical battalion. We flew along the edge of the mountains on the way there and spotted a small group of Japanese who ran off at great speed.

Had lunch with General Wing [Maj. Gen. Leonard F. Wing, Commanding General, 43d Division] of Burlington—a rugged, popular fellow. Listened to the usual complaints about not having enough medical personnel, of always going in short, and then attaching portable surgical hospitals, the personnel of which could not be sent into the field. They had been visited by the army consultant only once.

Monday, 6 August

Feverish activity to get the trenchfoot program underway. General Denit left it in my charge. The Quartermaster had already gotten out a wet-cold directive.[38] Since the quartermaster activity is primarily for the purpose of preventing trenchfoot, I have developed a program that combines information on the preventive medicine aspects and the clothing aspects of the problem in the following way:

1. A letter from the commander in chief to the commanding generals of all higher echelons emphasizing the importance of the problem and telling them what trenchfoot is.

2. A letter from General Denit to all division commanders emphasizing the command responsibility.

3. A medical directive to doctors.

4. The use of information and education facilities.

    a. Directive for training officers, telling them how to do the job.

    b. Booklets for all soldiers.

    c. Movies—shorts combined with entertainment.

    d. Use of radio for short programs combined with entertainment.

    e. *Yank Magazine* and news releases.

Morotai Island, Indonesia, Tuesday, 7 August

A Japanese hospital ship was captured in the Banda Sea and brought into Morotai Island, Indonesia. With Col. Hollis Batchelder of the U.S.S. *Mercy* to assist, I was dispatched to Morotai by special plane, arriving at Morotai at 1600 hours. We reported to Maj. Gen. Harry H. Johnson, Commanding General, 93d Infantry Division. He is National Guard from Houston, Tex., and a forceful pleasant Texan who gave us real southern hospitality, and as good a steak dinner with hot biscuits as I have ever had. Colonel Jackson is his chief of staff.

Wednesday, 8 August

Went with the division surgeon, Colonel Melaville [Lt. Col. Eugene F. Melaville, MC], to see the port director, Commander Harrison, who gave us permission to board the Japanese hospital ship, *Tachi Bana Maru*. This ship had been intercepted in the Banda Sea on 3 August. A destroyer flotilla had gone out for this purpose.

Verne Lippard [Lt. Col. (later Col.) Vernon W. Lippard, MC] just came up to tell me the radio announced that the Japanese have accepted the Potsdam ultimatum.

---

[38] Medical Department, United States Army. Cold Injury, Ground Type. Washington: U.S. Government Printing Office, 1958, appendix H, p. 533.

After boarding the Japanese hospital ship with a walkie-talkie [radio], they [the boarding party] found contraband and summoned an armed boarding party to take charge. There were so many Japanese (1,600) on board that they did not dare go below to search. The exterior of the ship was marked according to the rules of the Geneva Convention. The patients were sleeping on mats spread on top of the cargo, which was mostly contraband and consisted of boxes and bales that were packed with rifles, machineguns, mortars, grenades, and ammunition. Boxes were marked with large red crosses.

There were no seriously ill patients aboard, and all personnel walked off the ship. About a dozen were examined on the dock and sent to the 155th Station Hospital with diagnoses of beri beri, malaria, and fever of unknown origin. There were no wounded, and there was only one surgical patient with an infected leg ulcer. The patients, about 1,500, were said to be the slightly ill. On the whole, they appeared healthy and well nourished.

We visited a compound where 97 officers were interned. They were polite, said they were satisfied with their care, and that no one was sick. A visit to another compound of enlisted men showed several sick men. The chief surgeon of the ship said that he did not know that the boxes and bales contained contraband. No records were available to prove whether these had been bona fide patients before embarkation, and the confusion on shipboard was such that records could not be located. Looting by sailors undoubtedly caused part of the confusion. The ship was in a wretched sanitary condition. The stench was terrific. Clearly, this is a violation of the Geneva Convention.

Manila, Thursday, 9 August

Flew back. Left Morotai at 1000, arrived on Leyte at 1500 hours.

Monday, 13 August

Peace seems near, and speculations are mixed as to whether the Japanese will accept. Certain it is that the majority of people here, as well as at home, are tired of war.

Wednesday, 15 August

News that the Japanese have accepted the ultimatum, which included the proviso that the Emperor may remain. The morning news contains the Emperor's rescript to the people, which, true to form, contains no admission of guilt or moral and spiritual defeat. It only speaks of the military decision against them: "The enemy has used a new and cruel bomb * * * and to continue would mean the total extinction of human civilization." This clearly puts the onus of destroying civilization upon us. "Such being the case, how are we to atone ourselves before the hallowed spirits of our ancestors? By working to save and maintain the structure of the imperial state. Unite your total strength * * * so ye may enhance the glory of the imperial state." We are so tired of war that we accept these words as meaning a pledge of demo-

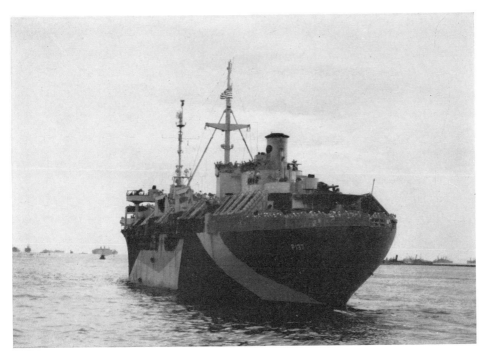

FIGURE 345.—U.S. Army Transport *General Sturgis* departing Manila harbor for Japan, 26 August 1945.

cratic government. Truly, so far we have gained a military decision only, not their ultimate defeat.

Tokyo-bound, Saturday, 25 August

Boarded the U.S. Army Transport *General Sturgis* today at 1500 hrs. General Denit had returned, and I drew the lucky number for this trip. So, with 24 hours to pack and gather up what information I could, I am off for Tokyo (fig. 345).[39]

---

[39] Almost immediately upon his arrival in Tokyo, Colonel Oughterson was named chairman of the AFPAC group that was to participate in the Joint Commission for the Investigation of the Effects of the Atomic Bomb in Japan. The other two groups of this joint commission were the Manhattan Project Group, headed by Brig. Gen. Francis W. Farrell, and a group of Japanese doctors and scientists, headed by Dr. Masao Tsuzuki of Tokyo Imperial University and the Japanese National Red Cross. The formal report of the commission was edited by Colonel Oughterson in Washington and published under the auspices of the National Research Council. (See: Oughterson, Ashley W., and Warren, Shields: Medical Effects of the Atomic Bomb in Japan. New York: McGraw-Hill Book Co., Inc., 1956.)

CHAPTER XIV

India-Burma and China Theaters

A. Stephens Graham, M.D.

On 5 January 1945, Lt. Col. (later Col.) Herrman L. Blumgart, MC, and Lt. Col. (later Col.) A. Stephens Graham, MC (fig. 346), proceeded from Headquarters, Second Service Command, Governors Island, N.Y., to Miami. There they boarded a transport plane and flew by way of Bermuda, the Azores, North Africa, and the Middle East to New Delhi, India, arriving at Headquarters, USFIBT (U.S. Forces, India-Burma Theater), on 28 January 1945.

Late in November 1944, they had been given the opportunity by Maj. Gen. Norman T. Kirk, The Surgeon General, U.S. Army, to become the first professional consultants assigned to the India-Burma Theater. Since there was a pressing need for these consultants, as had been indicated in the Kelser Mission report [1] submitted to The Surgeon General on 18 November 1944, General Kirk desired to send officers with prior experience in this field. At the time, Colonel Blumgart and the author were serving as Consultant in Medicine and Consultant in Surgery, respectively, Second Service Command, where they had pioneered as consultants somewhat more than a year previously. Moreover, the author had served in an oversea combat area—the North African theater—as chief of surgical service of a 2,000-bed general hospital. Therefore, he had had experience in the care and disposition of battle casualties. As one of the organizers of the 45th General Hospital, an affiliated unit of the Medical College of Virginia, Richmond, the author had, early in 1942, served a tour of duty under Col. Norman T. Kirk, MC, then Chief of Surgical Service, Walter Reed General Hospital, Washington, D.C. Under the guidance of Colonel Kirk and Col. Arden Freer, MC, Chief of Medical Service, Walter Reed General Hospital, the chiefs of medical and surgical services of the units affiliated with Harvard, Yale, Maryland, and Johns Hopkins Universities and with the University of Maryland and the Medical College of Virginia had completed the organization of their units and had received indoctrination in the operation of a general hospital.

The author's assignment to USFIBT was contingent upon the action of the disposition board of Fort Jay Regional Hospital, Governors Island,

---

[1] Report, Brig. Gen. Raymond A. Kelser, and Col. Robert H. Kennedy, MC, to The Surgeon General, 18 November 1944, subject: Report of Medical Department Mission to China-Burma-India.

N.Y. This board, fortunately, changed his physical status to general duty from duty limited to the continental United States. In December 1943, the disposition board of Walter Reed General Hospital had established the limited duty status after Colonel Graham had been evacuated to the Zone of Interior from the North African theater in November 1943.

There were other experienced service command consultants who had not had a tour of duty overseas and who were most anxious for this particular assignment in the India-Burma Theater. This was particularly true of Col. R. Arnold Griswold, MC, formerly Consultant in Surgery, Fourth Service

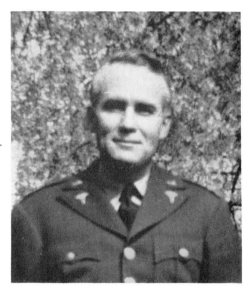

FIGURE 346.—Col. A. Stephens Graham, MC.

Command. At the time, Colonel Griswold was Chief of Surgical Service, Walter Reed General Hospital. Unfortunately for these officers, Headquarters, USFIBT, refused to accept consultants in grades higher than lieutenant colonel. For the first time in their Army careers, Colonel Blumgart and the author were pleased that long-awaited promotions had not materialized. These came later.

Two weeks prior to departure, Colonel Blumgart and the author spent several days in Washington where they were intensively briefed on the medical situation in the India-Burma and China Theaters by officers in the Office of The Surgeon General. The briefing included a careful study of the previously mentioned report of the Medical Department Mission to China-Burma-India. The Mission was composed of Brig. Gen. Raymond A. Kelser, Chief, Army Veterinary Service (fig. 347); Col. Robert H. Kennedy, MC, eminent New York surgeon, who had served as Chief of Surgical Service, Percy Jones

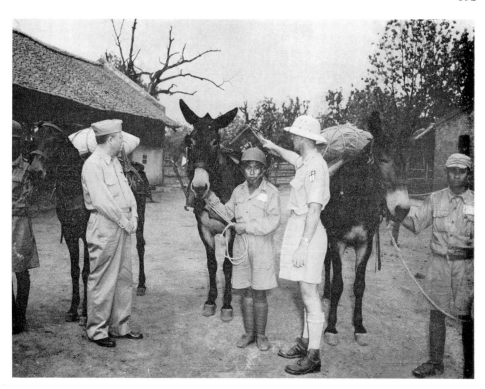

FIGURE 347.—Brig. Gen. Raymond A. Kelser inspecting Ramgarh Training Center, Ramgarh, India, 16 October 1944.

General Hospital, Battle Creek, Mich., and was soon to become the author's successor as Consultant in Surgery, Second Service Command; and Col. Karl R. Lundeberg, MC, Chief, Epidemiology Division, Preventive Medicine Service, Office of The Surgeon General. This highly illuminating report was based on a reasonably comprehensive survey of professional activities in most of the fixed hospitals of the China-Burma-India Theater.[2]   Colonel Kennedy's discussion of deficiencies and irregularities most urgently in need of a consultant's attention materially shortened the period of the author's orientation at Headquarters, USFIBT, in New Delhi and also influenced the sequence of hospitals visited in his initial tour of the theater.

The problems and activities of the surgical officer in the India-Burma and China Theaters can be more readily comprehended in relation to the stated mission of the U.S. Forces in these theaters, the medical service that was developed to support this mission, and the environment in which the personnel operated.

---

[2] War Department orders divided the China-Burma-India Theater into the India-Burma and China Theaters in October 1944.

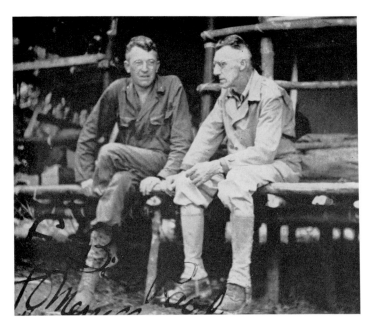

FIGURE 348.—Lt. Gen. Joseph W. Stilwell at his headquarters with
Brig. Gen. Frank D. Merrill.

HISTORICAL BACKGROUND

Mission of U.S. Army Forces in China-Burma-India [3]

Lt. Gen. (later General) Joseph W. Stilwell, USA, arrived in Chungking, China, on 4 March 1942 as head of a military mission charged with improving American assistance to the Chinese. At the suggestions of Generalissimo Chiang Kai-shek, General Stilwell was named chief of staff of the Generalissimo's joint staff, Commanding General of USAFCBI (U.S. Army Forces in China-Burma-India), and Commanding General of the Chinese Army in India (fig. 348). General Stilwell arrived at a most unfortunate period when Chinese, Burmese, and British-Indian Forces were being routed out of almost all of Burma in the fateful Burma Campaign. By the end of May 1942, the Japanese enemy was approaching the eastern border of India and had penetrated well into the Chinese province of Yünnan through the Salween Valley. By their conquest of the heart of Burma, the Japanese were in possession of the southern terminus of the Burma Road and prohibited its use by the Allies.[4]

---

[3] Most of the material for this section was obtained from an official, unpublished historical report in two volumes by Maj. Robert G. Smith, MAC, titled: "History of the Attempt of the United States Army Medical Department to Improve the Efficiency of the Chinese Army Medical Service, 1941–1945."

[4] The Burma Road extended from Rangoon, Burma, to Chungking, China, approximately 1,445 miles. It was made up of a railroad from Rangoon to Lashio, Burma; a new motor road from Lashio to K'un-ming, China, which was constructed in 1937–39; and an old highway from K'un-ming to Chungking.

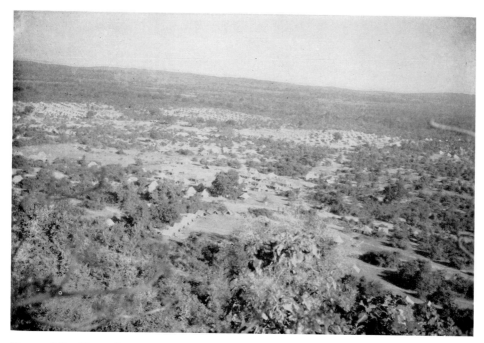

FIGURE 349.—Deogarh training camp of Merrill's Marauders, American combat troops in India-Burma Theater, Hsamshingyang, Burma, 10 December 1943.

In China, there was a desperate scarcity of everything but manpower. It was on the basis of China's dearth of material but abundance of personnel, therefore, that the United States was to attempt to fashion help for the faltering Chinese Army. American efforts were to center upon the dual mission of providing supplies and molding Chinese manpower into an efficient war machine. These missions were to be accomplished by taking remnants of the Chinese Fifth Army, which had fallen back into India, and those of both the Chinese Fifth and Sixth Armies, which had retreated into Yünnan; regroup, equip, and train them; and assign them to a campaign to reconstitute the Burma Road as the vital overland artery between China and her allies.

From a sheer physical standpoint the undertaking—the second Burma campaign—was prodigious.[5] The plan, as it developed, involved three elements: (1) Chinese troops, trained and equipped by Americans but led by Chinese, were to strike westward from Yünnan Province to clear that section of the Burma Road which lay within the border of China; (2) simultaneously, Chinese troops, also trained and equipped by Americans, and a few American troops (fig. 349), both under the command of General Stilwell, were to drive down the valleys of northern Burma and construct a new road, as they pro-

---

[5] This second Burma campaign was later officially designated as the India-Burma Campaign and extended from 2 April 1942 to 28 January 1945. It was followed by the Central Burma Campaign, 29 January 1945 through 15 July 1945.

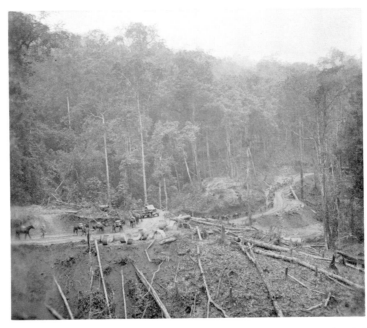

FIGURE 350.—Merrill's Marauders moving up along a newly constructed
section of the Ledo Road.

gressed, from Ledo in Assam, India, to join with the China section of the
Burma Road at Mong Yu, Burma, just within the Burma-China border
(fig. 350); and (3) the British, at the same time, were to operate from the
Chin Hills in northwestern Burma—between Burma and India, push eastward,
and disrupt Japanese lines of communications between north and south Burma.

The fighting for all three elements was of a most difficult nature, being
conducted in mountains, jungles, and valleys. It involved, as one medical
officer assigned to the project described it, a kaleidoscope of mud, shortages,
malaria, overtaxed equipment, rain, disappointment, heat, language difficulties, shifting priorities, jungle fighting, discarded plans, landslides and
homesickness.

A decision to extend their efforts to a large-scale program was reached by
the Americans in the fall of 1944 when it became apparent that the mission
to reopen the Ledo-Burma Road (later Stilwell Road) probably would succeed, but that the Japanese might be waiting at the China end of the road to
greet the first convoy arriving there. As the Japanese pointed the prongs of
their offensive toward Kuei-lin, the approaches to K'un-ming, key supply
terminal for shipment over the Himalayan "Hump" into China, and the approaches to Chungking, provisional Chinese capital, appeared to be open and
exposed to the enemy. The total collapse of the China war effort was not
beyond the realm of possibility.

At this critical point, the War Department suddenly recalled General Stilwell, Commander-in-Chief, USAFCBI, on 19 October 1944 and 5 days later, on 24 October, reconstituted the theater as two separate theaters, China and India-Burma. Maj. Gen. (later Lt. Gen.) Albert C. Wedemeyer was appointed Commanding General, USFCT (U.S. Forces, China Theater), and Lt. Gen. Daniel I. Sultan, formerly Deputy Theater Commander, was named Commanding General, U.S. Forces, India-Burma Theater. China thereby became the operational arm of the American Asiatic effort, and India-Burma became the supply and administrative base for the operation. Only India possessed open ports, Karāchi and Calcutta, for receiving Allied materials. Both theaters continued as integral and subordinate elements of the overall high com-

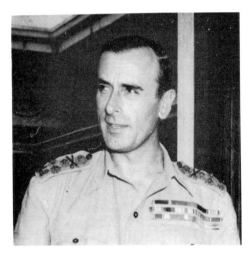

FIGURE 351.—Admiral Lord Louis Montbatten.

mand, the Southeast Asia Command, under the Supreme Allied Commander, Admiral Lord Louis Mountbatten (fig. 351).

In China, American ground troops were only used for advisory, logistic, and training purposes. In Burma, no more than two regiments of American troops with supporting arms and services, exclusive of air forces, were committed to battle. Service troops, including medical units, filled gaps in the Chinese Army, which lacked specialists. The average strength of U.S. Forces in China-Burma-India during 1944 was 168,700. They were spread thinly over the entire area. The various commands and units were engaged in the stupendous task of transporting personnel, supplies, and equipment over long supply lines between the ports of India and the fronts in Burma and China (fig. 352), principally by means of air transport. They had to construct, maintain, and operate the Stilwell Road, gasoline pipelines, and the communications system which connected India, through Burma and across the Himalayas, with K'un-ming, China. Large numbers of troops carried out these service and construction operations under hazardous conditions instead of in

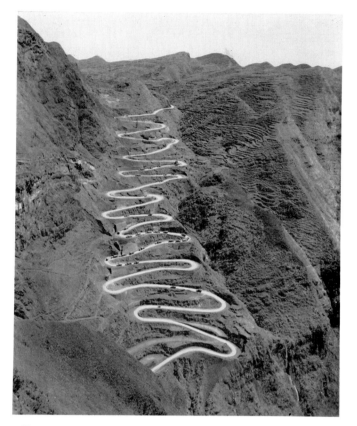

FIGURE 352.—A U.S. convoy, operating between Changi and Kuei-yang, China, ascending the famous 21 curves at An-nan (Ch'ing-lung), China, 26 March 1945.

relatively quiet rear areas, as is normally the case. There were monsoons, almost impenetrable mountain jungles, mosquitoes [6] and myriads of other pests, and active interference by the Japanese troops.

Medical Activities of U.S. Army Forces in China-Burma-India

Theater surgeon's office.—When General Stilwell assumed command he named as his theater surgeon, Col. Robert P. Williams, MC. During the period of the Burma Campaign, Headquarters, USAFCBI, was normally at Chungking, but actually most of the time of the personnel was spent in the field or at Rear Echelon Headquarters, USAFCBI, at Lashio. Later, in the spring of 1942, Rear Echelon Headquarters, USAFCBI, was established at New Delhi, India after General Stilwell's retreat from Burma. In April

---

[6] It has been estimated that in India, the population of which country in 1941 was 388 million, there were between 100 and 200 million cases of malaria and between 1 and 1½ million deaths from this disease each year (Rehn, John W. H.: China-Burma-India. *In* Medical Department, United State Army. Preventive Medicine in World War II. Volume VI. Communicable Diseases: Malaria. Washington: U.S. Government Printing Office, 1963, pp. 347–398).

1944, New Delhi was designated the main headquarters and Forward Echelon Headquarters, USAFCBI, remained at Chungking. Colonel Williams justified his maintenance of the theater surgeon's office at Forward Echelon Headquarters, USAFCBI, in these words:

In all other headquarters the Surgeon's Office is found in the Rear Echelon. That location was tried at the inception of this theater. It did not work, because all major decisions and long-range planning were performed at Forward Echelon. * * * the Chinese Surgeon General, Red Cross, and National Health Administration simply would not do business with an assistant and it placed on the assistant the responsibility of formulation of policy.

Deputy theater surgeon, Col. George E. Armstrong, MC, remained at Rear Echelon Headquarters, USAFCBI, in New Delhi. This arrangement continued until 14 May 1944 when, in accordance with a new theater policy, the theater surgeon and his staff were ordered to reestablish their offices at the main headquarters in New Delhi. When the China Theater was established on 24 October 1944, Colonel Armstrong, who had been moved to Forward Echelon Headquarters, Chungking, was appointed Surgeon, USFCT. In view of the fact that staff officers and responsibilities had been transferred from forward echelon headquarters at Chungking to the main headquarters at New Delhi, the creation of two separate theaters caught the China Theater short of personnel and many other necessities. Colonel Armstrong's staff, inherited from forward echelon headquarters of the China-Burma-India Theater, consisted of two officers and one enlisted man. On 10 December 1944, a rear echelon of Headquarters, USFCT, was established at K'un-ming, and the entire Medical Section, Headquarters, USFCT, moved to that location.

Relations with the Chinese.—By the very nature of its function, the medical service of the U.S. Army Forces in the China-Burma-India Theater was drawn into very close association with both Chinese military and civilian personnel (fig. 353). First of all, the concept of a military medical service had not been firmly established in the Chinese Army. As a matter of fact, for all practical purposes, it was nonexistent. The Americans found it necessary to start at the bottom. An apparent disregard for human suffering and a depreciated concept, which prevailed in the everyday struggle for existence, of the value of human life had been carried over into the Chinese Army. To a Chinese accustomed to seeing Chinese civilians dying along the road with no one paying heed, the sight of Chinese wounded soldiers left to die on the battlefield seemed to cause little outward concern. The soldier was apparently considered expendable, and there was a resultant indifference to the wounded. It followed, therefore, that the medical service of the Chinese Army, whose function it was to conserve life, would be held in little repute.

The Chinese division surgeon was usually a major and a political appointee without adequate medical training. Properly trained and qualified personnel were notoriously scarce. There were few modern medical schools and only one Class-A school in China. Moreover, the available trained personnel were

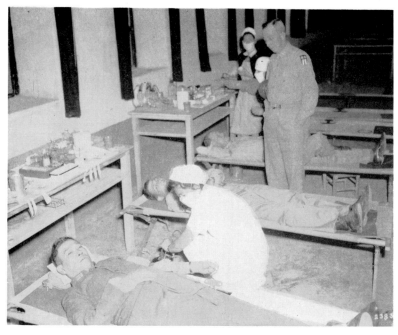

FIGURE 353.—High ranking Chinese and American officers set an example by donating blood at K'un-ming, China.

not being used to the best advantage. Practically all qualified physicians had congregated in the treaty ports at Hong Kong and Shanghai. The hospitals available for military purposes were, in the main, hospitals by courtesy only. The Chinese physicians found no compulsion or inducement to join the military service.

The story of how the U.S. Army helped to form the medical service of the Chinese Forces, as an integral part of the overall plan known as "Operation plan Stepchild," has been recorded in highly revealing and interesting documents.[7] The plan envisioned not only the provision of medical care for the malnourished and the sick-and-wounded Chinese soldier but also the establishment and conduct of technical-training schools in military medical subjects with students who for the most part were lacking in the necessary background or qualifications.

Any officer who might in future wars have to deal with oriental allies will profit from reading Capt. Kenneth M. Scott's "Some Suggestions for Medical Liaison Officers With Chinese Units," on file in The Historical Unit, U.S. Army Medical Service.

---

[7] (1) Smith, Robert G.: History of the Attempt of the United States Army Medical Department to Improve the Efficiency of the Chinese Army Medical Service, 1941–1945, volumes I and II. [Official record.] (2) Medical Department, United States Army. Training in World War II, ch. IV. [In preparation.]

Morbidity.—The U.S. Army medical officer in China-Burma-India was called upon to care for accidentally injured and diseased U.S. Army personnel to a far greater extent than he treated battle casualties. In 1943, when the average strength of U.S. Army personnel in the USAFCBI, was 39,600, there were 49,900 hospital admissions for all causes. Among the total admissions were 4,300 for nonbattle injury and only 200 for battle wounds and injuries. The remaining 45,400 were admitted for disease. During 1944 the average strength rose to 168,700, and during this year there were 173,900 hospital admissions: 157,600 because of disease, 14,500 for nonbattle injuries, and 1,800 battle wounds and injuries.[8] In the same period, however, there were 12,739 Chinese battle casualties admitted to the hospitals of this theater in addition to strictly U.S. Army admissions.

Hospitals.—Battle casualties from the Burma campaigns with a few exceptions received definitive treatment in what was known as the Advance Section, comprised of that territory in upper Assam, India, and northern Burma in the area of the Ledo Road. Hospitals were first established there in March 1943 in the vicinity of Margherita, Assam, India, about 8 miles from the town of Ledo in upper Assam and at the head of the Ledo Road. These were the 20th General Hospital and the 48th and 73d Evacuation Hospitals. By the end of 1943, hospital beds were provided for 3,705 patients by the following eight hospitals: The 20th General Hospital; the 14th (at the 19-mile mark, Ledo Road), 48th, and 73d Evacuation Hospitals, the 25th Field Hospital, Ledo; and the 40th, 42d, and 46th Portable Surgical Hospitals, Ledo, which for a short period functioned as fixed hospitals. This represented somewhat more than half the number of available beds at that time in India and Burma; in China, there were 1,465 additional beds.

The bed capacity of these hospitals in India had by March 1944 increased to 4,310, of which 2,963 were for Chinese soldiers. At the end of March, the 73d Evacuation Hospital moved to Shingbwiyang, Burma, at the 103-mile mark on the Ledo Road, where it was established as a fixed hospital on the sides of jungle hills, 5 miles from a newly constructed airstrip (fig. 354). It functioned as an evacuation and station hospital for American and Chinese troops and also as a general hospital for the Chinese.

During June 1944, the 69th General Hospital and the 28th, 32d, 34th, 35th, 50th, and 53d Portable Surgical Hospitals arrived in Ledo. The general hospital was established at Margherita, several miles from the 20th General Hospital, and the portable surgical hospitals were flown over the Himalayan "Hump" to support the Y-Force operating in the Salween River area.[9]

---

[8] Provisional data based on sample tabulations of individual medical records, Medical Statistics Division, Office of The Surgeon General.

[9] The Y-Force consisted of Chinese Army units operating in Southern China and Along the French Indo-China border; the Infantry and Field Artillery Training Centers at K'un-ming; the Technical Service School at Ch'ü-ching (Kütsing), China; the Medical and Veterinary School at Ta-li, China; traveling instructional groups; and the Burma Road Engineers.

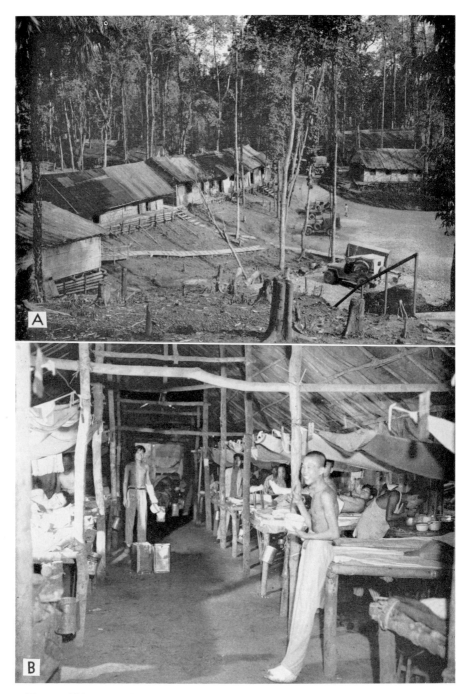

FIGURE 354.—The 73d Evacuation Hospital, Shingbwiyang, Burma, at the 103-mile mark on the Ledo Road. A. The headquarters and registrar's offices. B. A Chinese surgical ward.

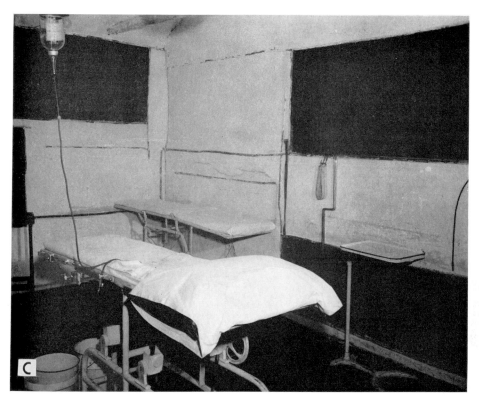

FIGURE 354.—Continued.   C. An operating room.

The entire fighting in Burma was jungle warfare (fig. 355). The usual doctrines of medical evacuation could not be utilized. The use of well-equipped, mobile evacuation hospitals situated relatively close to the fighting line, as was possible in the European theater, was totally out of the question here. The burden of early surgical care of battle casualties fell, in the early days, to the Seagrave Hospital Unit [10] and the 151st Medical Battalion, and later to the portable surgical hospitals. These portable surgical hospitals were small units with 4 officers and 35 enlisted men. Many times these units were divided into two groups to operate in two different areas. Their men often had to march all day on a jungle trail, then set up at night, and immediately start operating upon the wounded. They were inadequately equipped owing to the fact that their entire equipment had to be carried on their backs or by a limited number of horses, except for the supplies dropped by parachute.

---

[10] The Seagrave Hospital Unit was created by Dr. Gordon S. Seagrave, an American missionary to Burma since 1922, from the personnel of the American Baptist Mission hospital at Namhkam, Burma. Consisting initially of Burmese doctors and nurses, it was later augmented as necessary for various missions by the attachment of U.S. Army personnel and units. Dr. Seagrave was at first given an honorary lieutenant colonelcy in the British Indian Army and was later commissioned as a major in the U.S. Army Medical Corps. Still later, he was promoted to lieutenant colonel, Medical Corps.

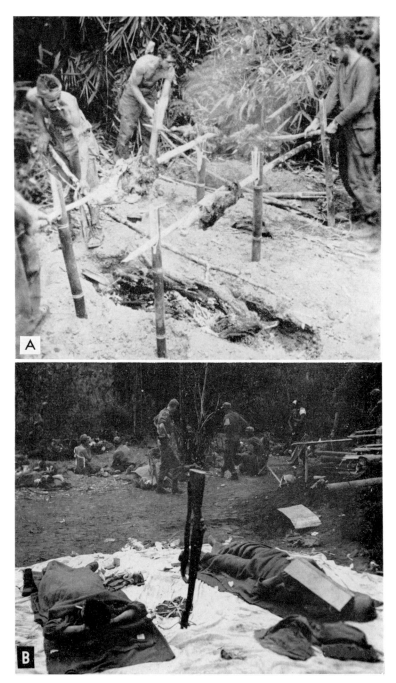

FIGURE 355.—Medical support of a jungle operation in Burma. A. Men of the Medical Detachment, 1st Battalion, Merrill's Marauders, barbecuing deer meat for the wounded, near Hsamshingyang, Burma, April 1944. B. An aid station along the Burma Road, February 1945.

Most of the work in the portable surgical hospitals was done at night since litter bearers usually brought in patients after dark. Except for occasional instances when portable units were relatively fixed, all operating had to be done with the aid of an ordinary flashlight. The fact that battle casualties of the Burma campaign had such excellent medical care and experienced such a low mortality is largely due to the men who worked in the portable surgical hospitals.[11] It was obvious that hospitals working under such conditions could not hold patients. It was equally obvious that few patients would survive transportation over mountain jungle trails and the almost impassable roads from these forward hospitals to the field and evacuation hospitals well to the rear. It was for this reason that the system of air evacuation was perfected.

Air evacuation of the wounded.[12]—At dawn on 15 October 1943, the Chinese Army in India initiated a drive which was to culminate in the reconquest of northern Burma. With the advance eastward into Burma, the Chinese troops were isolated from fixed hospitals in the base by difficulties of evacuation. The road, within any reasonable distance of the area of combat, existed only on engineering blueprints. The Seagrave Hospital Unit and Company D, 151st Medical Battalion, moved in on foot to provide medical service for the Chinese Army in India. With the capture of Shingbwiyang, the first forward airstrip was constructed. It was, however, still frequently necessary to transport patients by litter for several days before this airstrip could be reached. At this point in the campaign, the evacuation period was often as long as from 7 to 14 days from the time of injury to the time of admission at a fixed hospital in the base.

Gradually, as Chinese and American troops (committed in February 1944) advanced through the northern Burma jungle, 20 additional airstrips were constructed to keep pace with the troops. From 6 March to 14 April 1944, the interval between injury at the front and admission to fixed hospitals at the rear averaged 48 hours. Paddy fields were leveled by Chinese combat troops to receive the small liaison planes which were employed to evacuate the wounded, and occasionally sandbars were utilized. The remotest reaches of the densest jungle country in north Burma were penetrated by these planes which landed and took off with wounded soldiers from the most primitive and wholly inadequate strips (fig. 356). Both the planes and the strips were frequently within range of mortar, small arms, and machinegun fire.

The difficulties of evacuation were increased manifold with the onset of the monsoon rains in June. Motor ambulance evacuation came to a standstill. In the valleys, bullock carts with water buffalo "tractors" were employed. Yet, despite flooded airstrips and constant pouring rains, approximately 380 battle casualties reached the Ledo airstrip during June 1944. An additional 900

---

[11] Report, 2d Lt. James H. Stone, MAC, Office of the Surgeon, U.S. Forces, India-Burma Theater, to The Surgeon General, U.S. Army, 30 June 1945, subject: The Portable Surgical Hospitals in Northern Burma.

[12] Official unpublished historical report, Office of the Surgeon, Northern Combat Area Command, U.S. Army Forces, India-Burma Theater, 28 July 1945, subject: A Report Summarizing the Activities of U.S. Army Medical Department Units Assigned to Northern Combat Area Command During the Northern and Central Burma Campaigns.

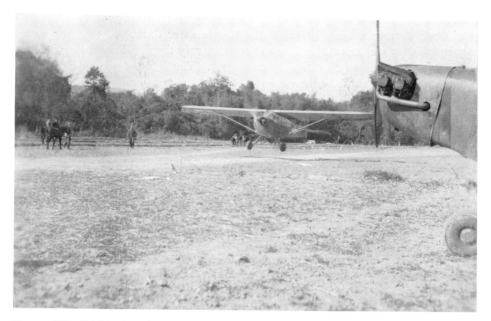

FIGURE 356.—Light aircraft evacuating wounded from a makeshift airstrip near Hsamshingyang, Burma, April 1944.

patients with disease or nonbattle injuries were evacuated from the combat area during this period. In the battle for Myitkyina, 25 percent of casualties arriving at the 20th General Hospital had been injured on the day of arrival (fig. 357).

Quality of surgical care in the India-Burma Campaign.—It was the opinion of surgeons in fixed hospitals to the rear that the quality of surgery undertaken in forward units during the India-Burma Campaign was, on the whole, excellent. When viewed in the light of conditions under which the forward surgery was accomplished, the high percentage of good results represented a remarkable feat of courage, effort, improvisation, and sound, conservative surgical treatment.

In the initial stages of the northern Burma offensive, certain practices no doubt tended to increase both morbidity and mortality rates. But as the experience of surgeons both in the forward and rear areas accumulated, these difficulties were, to a considerable extent, overcome in several ways. On 4 April 1944, the chiefs of the surgical services [13] of the 14th, 48th, and 73d Evacuation Hospitals and the 20th General Hospital were brought together for the purpose of discussing their observations of the care of battle casualties in forward medical units and to formulate recommendations for improvement in the surgical care of casualties by officers in these units. The meeting had been suggested

---

[13] These chiefs of surgical services were: Lt. Col. Willis M. Weedon, MC, 14th Evacuation Hospital; Lt. Col. Kwan Heen Ho, MC, 48th Evacuation Hospital; Lt. Col. Clarence J. Berne, MC, 73d Evacuation Hospital; and Maj. John F. North, MC, 20th General Hospital.

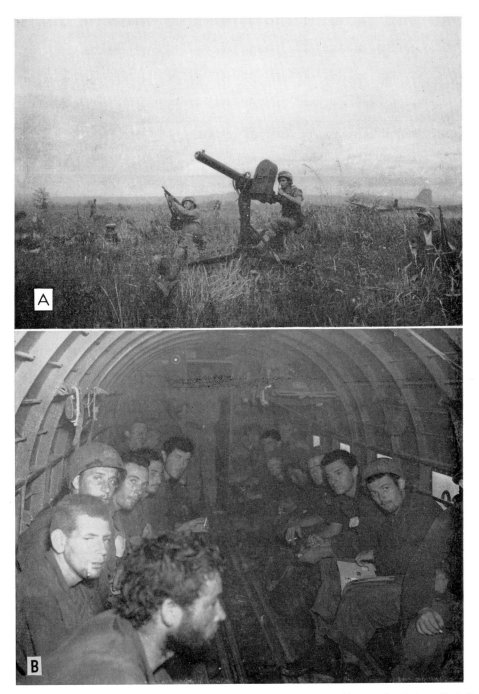

FIGURE 357.—An airstrip at Myitkyina, Burma, May 1944. A. Evacuation being effected while the airstrip is under fire. B. Sick men of Merrill's Marauders, loaded in a C-47 for evacuation.

by Col. Vernon W. Petersen, MC, Surgeon, Northern Combat Area Command, and the officers had been assembled by Col. (later Brig. Gen.) I. S. Ravdin, MC, Commanding Officer, 20th General Hospital. The report and recommendations of this committee formed the basis for a document, "Epitome of Surgical Management," which was distributed by the theater surgeon to forward units.

There is little doubt that the "epitome" on wound management was responsible to some extent for the improvement subsequently noted at base hospitals in the initial treatment of wounds. Officers from these base hospitals observed, however, on visits to forward units that the "epitome" was not too well received. Not only was criticism implied (which was unavoidable), but surgical officers in the forward medical units considered that the proper orientation of SOS (Services of Supply) surgeons in working conditions at the front would have made for more sound, intelligent suggestions based on practical familiarity with the problems of portable surgical hospitals. Similar complaints were made to Colonel Graham when, some months later, he visited these forward units after their transfer to combat areas of China.

These criticisms of the "epitome" were well taken and resulted in an occasional exchange of officers between the rear and forward units. It was recommended that officers assigned to the forward units be relieved from duty at relatively frequent intervals and returned to rear installations for short periods of time. It was believed that, after a month of steady operation under the severe conditions of jungle operations, surgeons of the portable hospitals inevitably grew too fatigued to render the type of service of which they were normally capable. Return to a rear installation would, it was believed, restore the keenness of these officers' capabilities and in the long run result in greater efficiency of the portable surgical hospital. The disadvantage of medical officers working only in one type of unit was that the difficulties encountered by forward units were not appreciated by personnel in the rear, and that, on the other hand, officers at the front were unable to follow up their cases in order to determine the validity of their techniques or to correct errors. The benefits which could be obtained from increased medical liaison were considered to be significant, and efforts were made to achieve it by the exchange of officers as well as by other means.

MEDICAL SERVICES, U.S. FORCES, INDIA-BURMA THEATER

On 28 January 1945, when the consultants arrived in the India-Burma Theater, there were 27 hospitals in active operation: 6 general, 14 station, 4 field, and 3 evacuation hospitals. The total bed capacity of these hospitals was 19,772, and 512 Medical Department officers were assigned the care of 9,819 patients. From a one-man organization in 1942, the medical service had expanded to an organization of 13,780 officers and men.

The theater (map 6) extended west to east from Karāchi, India, to Lashio, Burma, a distance of 2,200 miles.[14] Theater headquarters, at New Delhi, was

---

[14] All distances are expressed in terms of regular Air Transport Command routes between the points mentioned.

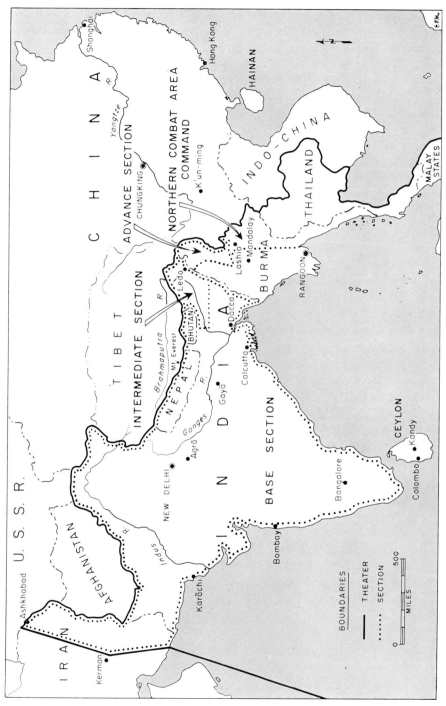

MAP 6.—India-Burma Theater, approximately January 1945.

situated in north-central India, in the Punjab Desert, 650 miles from Karāchi. New Delhi was 1,300 miles from Ledo in the upper portion of the province of Assam, where a number of hospitals were located. The most southerly situated hospital was at Kandy, Ceylon, Headquarters of the Southeast Asia Command (of which the India-Burma Theater was a part), 1,600 miles from New Delhi. The most northerly situated hospital in Burma was at Tagap Ga on the Ledo Road at the 52-mile mark. If the shortest air route between this hospital and New Delhi were taken, one would fly over Bhutan, Tibet (just north of Mount Everest), and the Kingdom of Nepal.

Seventy percent of the hospitals—five general, eight station, the three field, and the three evacuation hospitals—were established in a rectangular area approximately 950 by 450 miles in the extreme eastern portion of India and entirely across northern Burma (map 7). This area was slightly larger than the combined square miles that comprise the 14 eastern coastal States, plus Vermont, Pennsylvania, and West Virginia. It was roughly of the same shape and dimensions. Moreover, it was comparable to the area included in the First, Second, Third, and Fourth Service Commands, as then constituted, or almost twice the size of Texas. The distance from theater headquarters in Delhi to the center of this rectangular area was about 1,200 miles, almost the same air distance from the Office of The Surgeon General in Washington to the center of Texas.

Except for the area of fighting in central and eastern Burma, this vast area encompassing the India-Burma Theater was subdivided into area commands known as the Base, Intermediate, and Advance Sections. The Northern Combat Area Command was comprised of the headquarters and troops conducting operations against the Japanese in the area of construction on the Ledo Road and, later, in central and eastern Burma.

MEDICAL SERVICE, U.S. FORCES, CHINA THEATER

The medical service of the U.S. Army in China had always been badly in need of almost everything: hospital units, qualified personnel (both officer and enlisted), and modern equipment (fig. 358). It was one of the lowest of low-priority theaters. For the most part, the theater had been entirely dependent for logistic support on air transportation over the Himalayan "Hump": Food, clothing, equipment, supplies, high-octane gas for both fighter and transport planes, ammunition, motor vehicles, and so forth. The overland "back door" supply route, the Ledo-Burma Road, and the gasoline pipeline had afforded some relief but conditions were still far from ideal. The first U.S. Army supply convoy entered China over the Ledo-Burma Road on 28 January 1945, the day the consultants arrived in India.

Colonel Armstrong's task of organizing the medical service of the China Theater had been rugged. On 2 November 1944, 5 days after he had been

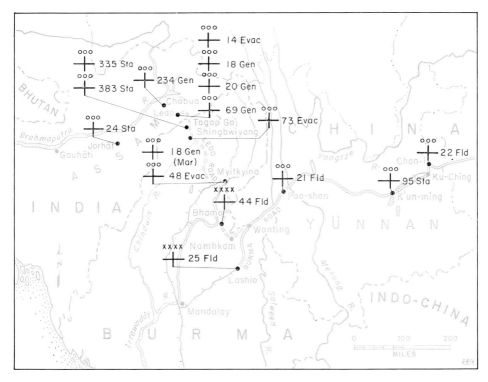

MAP 7.—Services of Supply, U.S. Army, hospitals in India, northern Burma, and China during the first half of 1945.

advised of his appointment as theater surgeon, Colonel Armstrong wrote to Colonel Williams, Surgeon, USFIBT:

Returned to 879 [Chungking] yesterday morning and am now so thoroughly confused that I honestly do not know where to turn. Apparently there are so many big problems to iron out that no one has time to settle any of the little (mine) ones. I am unable to find out whether this office will duplicate all the things done in your office or whether your office will continue to perform many functions for us. Obviously Cavenaugh [Maj. (later Lt. Col.) Robert L. Cavenaugh, MC], Sergeant Copeland, and I cannot go far in running a medical section for a Theater.

A letter from Colonel Williams, which had crossed Colonel Armstrong's in transit had stated the former's views substantially as follows:

As Colonel Williams saw it, very few changes would be required for adequate medical service for both theaters. Practically the only change was that it would not be necessary for Colonel Armstrong to continue reporting to him. However, until circumstances altered things, Colonel Williams intended to send Colonel Armstrong carbons of everything that might interest him. He anticipated that Colonel Armstrong would reciprocate. Of necessity, the two theaters would be so closely booked together that constant interchange would be

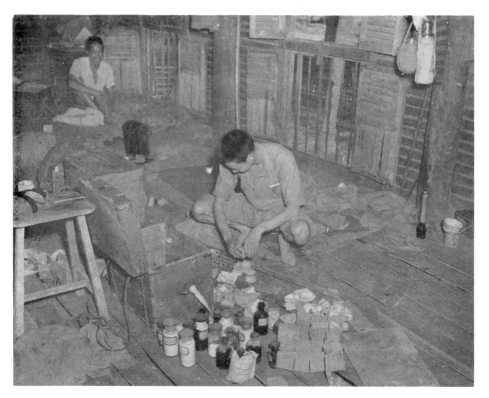

FIGURE 358.—Inadequate medical supplies being sorted at a Chinese medical collecting
station.

required. Colonel Williams intended to make every effort to maintain the
closest cooperation. Anything that he could do he would, just as though they
were still one family.

It was mutually agreed that the Office of the Surgeon, USFIBT, would
render for the China Theater all necessary medical reports and returns, pending the acquisition of additional personnel in the Medical Section, Headquarters, USFCT. By 10 December 1944, when the rear echelon of China
Theater headquarters was established at K'un-ming in Hostel No. 1 and the
entire Medical Section had moved to that location from Chungking, the personnel of the Medical Section, Headquarters, USFCT, had been increased
sufficiently to relieve the India-Burma Theater of all medical functions pertaining directly to China with the following exceptions:

1. *Personnel.*—Because of a lack of port facilities in China, unit and
individual requirements for personnel—both initial and replacements—were
coordinated with those of the India-Burma Theater before their submission
to Washington.

2. *Medical supply.*—For the same reason as cited above, medical supply
requisitions were consolidated with those of the India-Burma Theater.

3. *Hospitalization.*—The India-Burma Theater served as a reservoir for cases from China requiring hospitalization exceeding the established 90-day evacuation policy of the China Theater. Patients en route to the Zone of Interior also had to rely on holding facilities in India-Burma, as no other route was available.

In all other respects, the Office of the Surgeon, USFCT, functioned as that of an independent theater. The theater surgeon's office continued to grow and the staff had increased considerably by the time this consultant arrived in India-Burma. Care had to be taken in accomplishing this not to draw keymen from medical units of the theater, since medical officers and enlisted men were at so high a premium in China that the loss of one man could interfere with the function of an installation. The possibility of replacing him in such a low-priority theater was remote.

The work of the Medical Department, of course, could not wait until all needs had been met. With his limited staff at K'un-ming, and in the early days at Chungking, and with only a skeletal medical organization throughout the new theater, Colonel Armstrong undertook the difficult task of lifting the Chinese medical service from the depths of demoralization and disorganization which attended the threatened collapse of China through the rout of the Chinese Army in southeastern China. At the same time, he had to implement plans for the medical care of U.S. troops who were coming into the theater in increasing numbers.

Inasmuch as the medical service of the USFCT remained throughout the war essentially that of a military mission aimed at improving the efficiency of the medical service of the Chinese Army, it became necessary for the theater surgeon to devote a large part of his time to work with the Chinese medical authorities. These were the Director (Surgeon General) of the Army Medical Administration, and representatives of the National Health Administration, and the National Red Cross Society of China. In addition to these were a considerable number of foreign philanthropic associations with whom the theater surgeon maintained liaison in an effort to coordinate the many diverse aspects of medical service in China bearing on the Allied military effort. In this atmosphere of confusion, division of responsibility and widespread disorganization, it is remarkable that the theater surgeon and his small, but intensely loyal and inspired, staff accomplished as much as they did.

Long before activation of the China Theater, the need for additional hospitalization in China was referred to in communications to the War Department as critical. When, finally, the 70th Field Hospital, designated for China, arrived in the India-Burma Theater in October 1944, it was retained for combat service in Burma until June 1945. In March 1945, two station and three field hospitals were assigned to the China Theater with a total of 1,800 beds. An additional five field hospitals and one general hospital (1,000-bed) were scheduled for transfer to the theater from the India-Burma Theater to make a total of 4,300 fixed beds for the China Theater.

In June 1945, however, when the author departed from the China Theater, there were still only one station and two field hospitals functioning, there were no provisions for establishing a general hospital, and none of the five field hospitals had arrived in China. The most pressing problem was what to do with Chinese casualties, since the War Department would not provide U.S. Army fixed beds for Chinese troops in China, as had been authorized in India-Burma. In China, hospitalization of Chinese troops was considered the responsibility of the Chinese Army Medical Administration. This administration and the Chinese Red Cross established a number of hospitals in the various categories, but practically all of them were woefully lacking in just about everything: Physical faciltes, skilled personnel, supplies, and equipment. The Medical Department, U.S. Army, at the time of this consultant's visit to the China Theater, was committed to care for only casualties near the front who were brought into portable surgical hospitals manned by U.S. Army personnel. The manner in which the portable surgical hospitals functioned is described later in this chapter (pp. 942-945).

FUNCTIONS OF THE SURGICAL CONSULTANT

General Considerations

In addition to the medical and surgical consultants, Maj. John R. S. Mays, MC, Consultant in Neuropsychiatry, Maj. (later Lt. Col.) Richard W. Britt, MC, Reconditioning Officer, and four Medical Administrative Corps officers arrived on 28 January 1945 for assignment to the Office of the Surgeon, Headquarters, USFIBT. Brig. Gen. James E. Baylis, MC, the newly appointed Surgeon, SOS, USFIBT, arrived several days later. General Baylis' last previous assignment had been that of Commanding General, Medical Replacement Training Center, Camp Grant, Ill. Somehow during the period of briefing in Washington and as a result of conversations with officers returned from the theater, some of the newcomers had developed the feeling that their reception at Headquarters, USFIBT, and perhaps even in the field as well, would be somewhat less than cordial. Actually, they were welcomed with genuine warmth, not only at headquarters, but almost everywhere they went in the theater.

There was little doubt that this fine reception was, to a considerable extent, influenced by the character and personality of General Baylis, who was esteemed throughout the Army as an officer of superior ability as an organizer and administrator. He possessed a genius for inspiring subordinates, to whom he delegated great responsibility. He encouraged them to take the initiative in the development of their respective sections in the Office of the Surgeon. He never questioned professional opinions and recommendations of the consultants. The consultants were told to make corrections "on the spot" when they observed irregularities and deficiencies that required prompt action during visits to hospitals. At the same time, they were given to understand that their decisions would be reversed if subsequently it was determined that they had erred. This arrangement in a theater spread out over the entire area of India and Burma, with many installations situated more than a thousand miles from theater headquarters, greatly facilitated and hastened the accomplishment of the consultants' mission. At the same time this implicit confidence in the professional judgment of the consultants had a sobering influence on them in curbing any tendency toward precipitate action of making recommendations without due deliberation.

The functions of the surgical consultant were concisely stated by Brig. Gen. Fred W. Rankin, MC, Chief Consultant in Surgery to The Surgeon General, in the annual report of the Surgery Division for fiscal year 1944, substantially as follows:

The surgical consultants exercise their functions by assisting and advising the service command or theater surgeons on all matters pertaining to surgical practice, including particularly the organization and program of surgical services in medical installations and the quality, distribution, and proper assignments of professional personnel, by providing advice on newer developments in diagnosis and treatment, by stimulating interest in professional problems and aiding in their investigation, and by encouraging educational programs such as conferences, ward rounds, and journal clubs. These consultants are concerned essentially with the maintenance of the highest standards of medical practice. It is their function to evaluate, promote, and improve further the quality of medical care by every possible means, to interpret the professional policies of The Surgeon General and to aid in their implementation.

The formulation of many policies and the making of decisions in regard to the solution of many problems required coordination of the medical, neuropsychiatric, and surgical consultants. Colonel Blumgart and the author were fortunate in that they had, during the preceding year, functioned as a team along with the service command neuropsychiatric consultant in the consideration of many common problems. Major Mays readily fitted into the team, as did the newly appointed chief of personnel in the Office of the Surgeon.

In August 1944, Col. Alexander O. Haff, MC, Surgeon, Services of Supply, USAFCBI, had also been designated deputy theater surgeon and Chief of Professional Services for both the theater headquarters and SOS medical sections. In February 1945, after arrival of the new consultants, these two sections were consolidated and Colonel Haff was evacuated to the United States without replacement. With the position of Chief of Professional Services discontinued, the consultants functioned directly under the theater surgeon rather than through an intermediary chief.

The aforementioned chief of the Personnel Section, Office of the Surgeon, SOS, USFIBT, was Lt. Col. Casey E. Patterson, MC, an officer of high professional attainments. Colonel Patterson cooperated in the consideration of routine professional matters as well as matters pertaining to personnel. In both instances, he screened material before referring it to the consultants.

When the consultants were absent from the office of the theater surgeon, he disposed of all matters except those which definitely required the attention of the consultants. When immediate action was required, he contacted them in the field by telephone, radio, or courier mail. Actually, this organization of the professional services officers with the personnel officer might be described as a committee on professional services and personnel, with the theater surgeon serving as chairman. Its successful operation was insured by the wholehearted cooperation of all members and their ability to discuss problems harmoniously, frankly, and critically. Decisions reached by this group were presented directly to the theater surgeon for consideration. Colonel Blumgart and the author were in a position to compare this simplified organization with the conventional one they had experienced in the Second Service Command, where the chief of professional services undertook activities of a technical and specialized nature with a minimum of consultation with the professional consultants. The simplified system was definitely more satisfactory, at least for the India-Burma Theater. Although no need occurred for the addition of administrative assistants to the professional services organization, such additions could have relieved the specialists of the burden of routine work which would have accumulated in a larger and more active theater.

Soon after the arrival of the consultants in the theater, General Baylis obtained permission of the theater commander to route the consultants' reports through technical medical channels. General Baylis also approved the consultants' recommendation that information copies of these reports be sent to commanding officers of hospitals which had been visited, a practice not hitherto carried out by the SOS or theater surgeons. Almost immediately upon return to theater headquarters from field trips and before formal reports had been compiled, the consultants submitted to the theater surgeon brief, confidential summaries of observations which would require prompt action. If on the tour there were noted deficiencies in physical plants, the need for air conditioning, or other similar nonprofessional matters that required corrective action, a memorandum to the effect was sent to the Chief of Staff, USFIBT.

Considerably less than half of the author's time was spent in the office of the theater surgeon. Here, as a member of the theater surgeon's staff, many activities claimed his time: Preparation of the section on surgery in ETMD (Essential Technical Medical Data) report; review of all publications on surgical subjects reaching the Office of the Surgeon; preparation of material on current surgical problems for the monthly *Field Medical Bulletin, USF-IBT;* preparation of theater circulars, directives, and memorandums on professional surgical subjects; review of clinical records and post mortem findings in all deaths due to surgical causes; review of proceedings of boards of officers; conferences with the other consultants and with the personnel officer; and, finally, compilation of reports on hospitals which had been visited. Moreover, a rather large correspondence was conducted with the Surgeon, China Theater, with commanding officers of hospitals relative to problems of the surgical services, with General Rankin, Chief Consultant in Surgery to The Surgeon General, and with Col. B. Noland Carter, MC, Assistant Chief, Surgical Consultants Division, Office of The Surgeon General. Practically all of these letters, or pertinent portions of them, were brought to the attention of the theater surgeon, or members of his staff, for information, guidance, or specific action.

Editorial Duties

The surgical consultant was responsible for the preparation of the section on surgery in the ETMD report submitted monthly to The Surgeon General. This consultant found that "feeder" reports submitted by hospitals had become routine and lacked material of clinical interest. The theater surgeon, therefore, advised all installations and the headquarters of the various base sections of the type of information desired.

During the visits of the consultants to the various hospitals, further effort was made to stimulate studies of unusual cases. Much valuable material was thereby accumulated and many excellent papers were submitted for publication in medical journals, particularly by officers of the 20th General Hospital (University of Pennsylvania affiliated unit).

The consultants were also responsible for articles or comments in the monthly *Field Medical Bulletin, USFIBT*. The surgical officers of the theater were encouraged to submit reports on their studies, and many of these were published. This bulletin also provided a valuable means of conveying information regarding recent advances in surgery. The policy recently instituted by the former deputy theater surgeon of reprinting in the theater advance copies of important War Department technical bulletins was continued. Distribution of these bulletins to the theater through normal publications channels was extremely slow, and many times essential bulletins never reached the hospitals. Thus, it was most fortunate that the consultants had brought with them the complete medical series of those that had been issued up to the time of their departure from the Zone of Interior. On the other hand, considerable numbers of bulletins consisting of 50 or more pages relating to the water supply of Germany and Czechoslovakia and sanitary data on the Aegean Islands and Finland were received with great promptness.

In some instances, where no suitable official guides or directives were available, appropriate circulars or memorandums were submitted to the theater surgeon and, following his approval, were reproduced and distributed. Restraint was practiced in the number issued. Moreover, the spirit of these publications was that of guidance rather than mandatory direction. Specific directions, however, had to be issued on the transfer of patients to general hospitals and on operations for deranged knee cartilages, chronically dislocated shoulders, and cases of herniated nucleus pulposus. These problems are discussed later.

Review of Clinical Records and Post Mortem Findings

Soon after arrival of the consultants, the theater surgeon approved their request that, in nonbattle casualties, the full clinical records and results of post mortem examinations be submitted to the theater headquarters for review. This practice proved of exceptional value. Theater headquarters was kept informed of some of the most interesting cases. A review of the medical care of the most seriously ill was thereby accomplished, and occasional suggestions were made or deficiencies were noted. Deficiencies were made the subject of correspondence or, more often, a conference with the staff concerned was held on the author's next visit to the installation. It was believed also that this procedure had anticipatory value in that it was generally understood that the clinical record of any seriously ill patient might eventually be scrutinized in the office of the theater surgeon.

SURGICAL PERSONNEL

Personnel Problems

Basic to all other considerations in achieving a high standard of surgical care was the question of personnel. A combination of circumstances prompted the consultants on their arrival in the theater to give personnel matters priority over all other activities. First, Colonel Kennedy, of the Kelser Mission, had personally emphasized to Colonel Graham the need for the consultants to make a prompt survey of personnel. Second, Lt. Col. (later Col.) Durward G. Hall, MC, Director of Military Personnel and Chief of Personnel Services, Office of The Surgeon General, had set a deadline of 1 April 1944 for (1) the execution of the new WD AGO Form 178–2, Supplemental Data for Medical Officers, which had not been accomplished in this theater since its activation, and (2) assignment by the consultants of proper SSN (specification serial numbers) and ratings for all medical officers in the India-Burma and China Theaters. Third was the fact that the personnel officer in the Office of the Surgeon, USF-IBT, was a young first lieutenant in the Medical Administrative Corps. The consultants' initial recommendation to the theater surgeon was the appointment of a highly qualified Medical Corps officer as Chief of Personnel. Colonel Patterson was immediately assigned to this position and proved to be an excellent choice. As has already been remarked, Colonel Patterson and the consultants functioned in a most satisfactory fashion as a committee on personnel and professional services.

Professional Classification of Surgical Officers

The information on the officer's qualification forms and the obsolete Medical Department questionnaire, prepared by the individual officer, was of little value since, in most instances, the information had been entered 2 or more years previously. It was most natural that the classification and proficiency ratings of these officers, based almost entirely on the interpretation of this meager infor-

mation by a nonmedical officer, should result in a number of incorrect classifications and malassignments.

As quickly as the new supplemental data forms were executed and returned
to the Office of the Surgeon, USFIBT, the consultants reviewed them and appended their recommended classifications and proficiency ratings. Since a majority of the officers had been in the theater for 20 months or longer, it was not
surprising that changes were made in almost every instance. In a moderate
number of cases the officers had been incorrectly classified as to their appropriate
specialty, owing to insufficient available data or invalid recommendations of
their commanding officers. A far greater number had been given proficiency
ratings which were either too high or too low. The most significant observation was the fact that many officers had been classified "general duty" who,
through opportunities afforded them by chiefs of surgical services or by their
own diligent application, had acquired proficiency in general surgery or one of
the surgical specialties and because of demonstrated ability deserved a specialty
classification.

Although by 31 March 1945 copies of the newly completed forms, with the
revised classification and proficiency ratings, were ready to be forwarded to
the Office of The Surgeon General, in only 60 percent of instances had the
changes been made on the basis of personal interview and observation of the
officer's professional activities. The theater surgeon, however, informed The
Surgeon General and commanding officers of hospitals that the ratings made
solely on the basis of the newly acquired personnel information were subject
to revision after these officers had been observed by the consultants.

The individual statements of educational training and postgraduate surgical experience were not sure guides to individual surgical proficiency. Certain
surgical officers, for instance, with a wide range of surgical knowledge—some
qualified by an American Specialty Board—lacked conservative, sound, clinical
judgment; others lacked necessary qualities of leadership. Conversely, other
officers with little postgraduate training, who had taken advantage of their
opportunities to acquire proficiency in assignments in the Army as surgical
assistants, were found fully qualified to be chiefs of a surgical service at a 250-
or 500-bed station hospital. The Chief Consultant in Surgery to The Surgeon
General, himself one of the organizers of the American Board of Surgery, repeatedly insisted that absence of certification by the Specialty Boards did not
prohibit inclusion of an officer in the higher proficiency classifications, as "Group
A" and "Group B."

Appraisal of the intrinsic qualifications of the surgical officer could be made
only on the basis of personal observation during actual ward rounds and in
the operating room. This consultant spent at least one and usually many additional hours with each officer on his wards reviewing in detail physical findings,
clinical records, treatment, and administrative dispositions of the patient. Informal discussions of related general subjects formed part of such visits. In
some instances, personality clashes rendered an officer's services ineffective at
a particular installation and could be obviated by assignment elsewhere. Oc-

casionally, the commanding officer of a hospital was encountered who failed to recognize the distinction between efficiency and proficiency classifications. He would question the propriety of the consultant's high proficiency rating in the case of an officer with superior training and demonstrated ability to whom he had given a relatively low efficiency rating. Others were mistaken in the belief that the proficiency rating was influenced by age, rank, length of service, and by the successful completion of advanced Army extension courses conducted for the Officers' Reserve Corps.

Actually, there was a superabundance of officers of field grade in both theaters who, although well versed in the details of Army medical administration, were nevertheless classified as general duty (MOS 3100) medical officers. In civilian life they had begun general medical practice after a 1-year internship. They were too old and possessed too much rank to be assigned as ward officers, yet lacked adequate surgical training and experience to warrant their assignment to positions of responsibility commensurate with their rank. Many, however, had requested such assignments, and a few had become chiefs of surgical services in small station hospitals.

Qualitative and Quantitative Studies

From an initial survey of records in the office of the theater surgeon, this consultant was inclined to believe, as was Colonel Kennedy, that there was an urgent need for many additional medical officers qualified as general surgeons and specialists. Actually, however, as the author was to determine later, there was no lack of capable surgical officers except for a few key specialists, notably experienced orthopedic surgeons. This discrepancy was quite easily explained. First, a large number of officers designated in personnel files as general-duty medical officers had, through earnest effort and careful supervision by highly competent surgeons, become eligible for classification as general surgeons or surgical specialists, "D" or "C." Second, a large excess of surgical talent was concentrated in three affiliated medical units in the Advance Base Section.

These affiliated units were a 2,000-bed general hospital and two 750-bed evacuation hospitals, the latter serving as station hospitals for U.S. Army personnel and as general hospitals for the Chinese. Sixty of the seventy-eight officers assigned to their surgical services were considered capable of undertaking operations without supervision. The census of surgical patients in these three hospitals seldom reached 2,000. This inequitable distribution of surgical personnel was not the fault of the theater surgeon. The trouble stemmed from a policy established in the Office of The Surgeon General around 1939. At that time, written agreements were negotiated with universities in which the university medical schools agreed to organize and staff the professional services of general and evacuation hospitals which were to be activated in the event of war; The Surgeon General, in turn, agreed not to dismember the units except with the consent of the school or the unit itself, or as an urgent military necessity. It is understood that in any future war such a situation as regards personnel in similar affiliated units will not recur.

In sharp contrast to the quantity and quality of surgical officers present in the three foregoing affiliated units in the India-Burma Theater was the situation at three general hospitals in the Second Service Command which the author had inspected during his last month as surgical consultant for the command. These three general hospitals—Tilton, at Fort Dix, Wrightstown, N.J., Rhoads, at Utica, N.Y., and England at Atlantic City, N.J.—had a combined authorized capacity of 6,000 beds. There were 3,889 surgical patients at the time of the survey. Of these, 2,395 were orthopedic cases, mostly battle casualties with multiple compound fractures. All patients were U.S. Army personnel, whereas some 75 percent of patients in the hospitals of the India-Burma Theater were Chinese. Only 37 of the total 62 surgical officers in the Zone of Interior hospitals were classified in categories which would ordinarily permit them to undertake operations without supervision. A quantitative and qualitative comparison of officers assigned to the three hospitals in India-Burma with those assigned to the three hospitals in the Second Service Command showed:

Classification of officers	Number in India-Burma Theater	Number in 2d Service Command
Certified by Specialty Boards	26	16
Qualified for certification	8	4
Classified by consultant, "A" or "B"	32	20
Classified by consultant, "C"	28	17
Classified by consultant, "D"	15	13
Classified "General Duty"	3	12

The disproportionately large surgical staff provided the evacuation hospitals (25 officers each) as compared with the number and quality of officers assigned to other fixed hospitals of comparable size was due to the fact that evacuation hospitals were originally organized to function as mobile field units situated close to and in support of actively engaged combat troops. Employment in this manner would have required a 24-hour operating schedule in which surgical teams would have alternated between surgical activities and periods of relaxation and sleep. The character of the warfare and terrain over which battles were fought in the Burma campaigns precluded the employment of evacuation hospitals in the conventional manner. It was not until near the close of the Central Burma Campaign that a number of these officers were transferred to other hospitals in order to insure balanced, efficient surgical staffs throughout the theater.

By May 1945, through the acquisition of qualified officers, including experienced orthopedic surgeons and other specialists from the United States, and reallocation of officers already in the theater, every surgical service in the hospitals of the India-Burma Theater was satisfactorily staffed. Moreover, the USFIBT was prepared by then to transfer to the USFCT a number of competent surgical officers to offset personnel deficiencies in the China Theater and to replace officers eligible for rotation.

In April and May, a large number of officers became eligible for rotation. Among these were 29 key surgical officers who were due for reassignment in the United States. A brief summary of this consultants' impression of their capabilities was sent to Col. B. Noland Carter, MC, Assistant Chief, Surgical Consultants Division, Office of The Surgeon General. Colonel Carter, in turn, conferred with Colonel Hall, Director of Personnel, in regard to these officers. As a result, by the time these returnees reached redistribution centers, reassignment orders awaited them. The initial success of this process prompted Colonel Carter to request that this information be forwarded in the case of every officer with a classification of "C" or higher.

EDUCATION AND TRAINING

The scarcity of surgical officers—except in affiliated units—sufficiently skilled and personally qualified for positions of responsibility and leadership made it imperative that hospitals be considered as training centers. Key personnel, lost through illness or rotation, could thereby be replaced. An additional incentive for high standards of performance possibly leading to promotion was provided. The accelerated wartime program of civilian medical education frequently resulted in producing young medical officers of considerable innate ability but with meager clinical knowledge or experience. Whenever possible, such officers were assigned to duties under the immediate supervision of mature, seasoned surgeons and, after varying periods of time, were qualified to be chiefs of surgical service in small station hospitals or heads of sections in the surgical services at general hospitals.

The policies governing treatment of various surgical conditions varied greatly from hospital to hospital and indeed from ward to ward. This was due to the fact that the medical officers largely represented a cross section of the American civilian medical profession with widely different types of training experience and personal views and had not received the fundamental directives and guides issued by the Office of The Surgeon General. Few if any TB MED's (War Department technical bulletins, medical) had been received, and but few overall professional policies had been established in the theater. To raise the quality of medical care to the highest possible level, each installation was directed to prepare a list of the TB MED's that had not been received, and adequate distribution was effected. It was further directed that a complete file of such bulletins as well as circulars and other directives issued by the theater surgeon be maintained by the commanding officer and in the offices of the chiefs of medical and surgical services at all fixed hospitals.

The consultants attempted to stimulate professional interest by recommending the establishment at hospitals of a suitable reading and conference room, even when a tent had to be erected for that purpose. Steps were undertaken to supply each installation with its authorized allowance of professional books and periodicals. Through the generosity of the Josiah Macy Jr. Foundation, New York, N.Y., reprints of outstanding articles appearing in current medical periodicals were distributed to the medical officers in the India-Burma Theater.

Medical officers were thereby encouraged to keep abreast of advancing medical knowledge.

Medical officers were urged to review series of cases at their own installations and prepare reports summarizing their experiences. In some instances, these reports were used solely as the basis for a talk at one of the medical conferences, at other times they were found suitable for publication in the *Field Medical Bulletin* or even in current leading periodicals in the United States. A schedule of at least one medical conference a week and one "grand ward round" for the discussion of the most interesting and perplexing cases was established at the various hospitals. The value of such an educational program in providing improved medical care, in heightening the professional interest of the medical officers, and, consequently, in raising the morale was gratifying.

The major portion of the time spent at each hospital by the surgical consultant was utilized in a careful review of medical practice on each of the wards. Each patient was examined, the clinical records were reviewed, and the clinical management was discussed.

PHYSICAL FACILITIES AND EQUIPMENT

Hospital construction.—Hospital construction of every type imaginable was observed: brick, cement (mostly sand and mud), basha, pinewood, teakwood, and tents (fig. 359). A few were excellent, most were highly satisfactory, and with only two or three exceptions, the remainder of the hospital plants were adequate. Some of the units occupied former missionary hospitals. Others moved into administrative buildings of tea plantations and added additional wards of basha construction for patients and erected pyramidal tents for personnel. The basha construction with thatched roof was satisfactory in the climate of India and Burma but it was difficult to maintain in a proper state of repair.

Supply liaison activities.—Evidently there had been a marked improvement in the supply situation following the visit to the theater of the Voorhees Mission in 1944. Although in most installations there was found adequate equipment, in only the 20th General Hospital and a few of the most recently established units was most of the equipment and appliances of the more recent, standard models. Ingenius improvisations were satisfactory substitutes for the standard apparatus in most instances. The relatively few serious deficiencies in equipment which were observed by this consultant appeared in his reports to the theater surgeon with recommendations that the equipment be supplied. Invariably, Maj. Claud D. LaFors, PhC, the medical supply officer in the Office of the Surgeon, USFIBT, a most cooperative individual, handled these requests in a most expeditious manner. Officers in the field were grateful for this service, and unquestionably the professional consultants gained prestige as a result of this and also the manifestations of confidence in the consultants at theater headquarters.

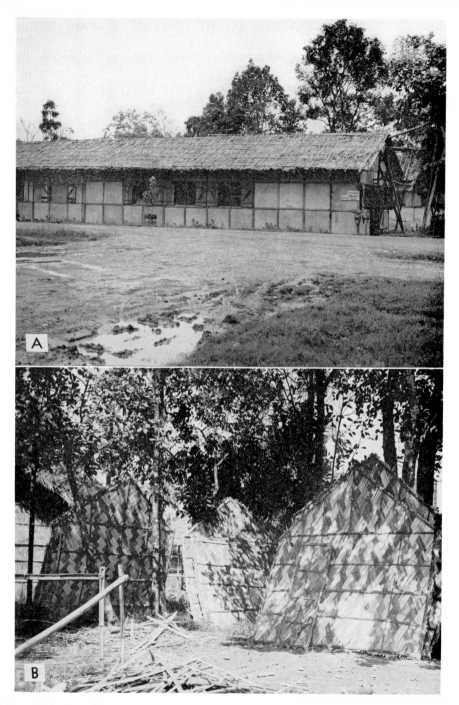

FIGURE 359.—Hospital construction in India.   A. A thatched roof and mud walls.   B. Prefabricated sections for basha construction.

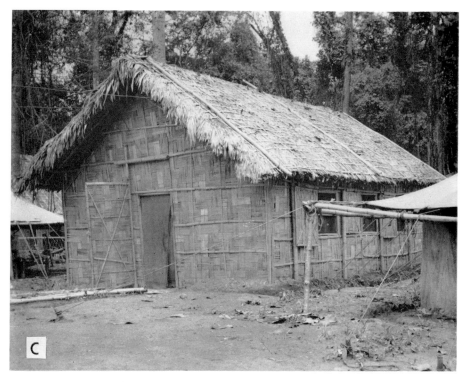

FIGURE 359.—Continued.   C. A basha-constructed ward building.

Cooperative assistance of the same quality was rendered by the Office of The Surgeon General, particularly by Colonel Carter, through whom the author made all his requests for aid.   One of these many requests was for an authoritative statement regarding the stability of penicillin at the high temperatures (110° to 140° F.) to which it was subjected in transit by plane from the United States to India, Burma, and China, when for hours or even days there was a delay at various airports.   Clinical results following the administration of penicillin were not consistent.   This had been observed by Colonel Kennedy on his visit to the theater and subsequently by the consultants.   The question was resolved in 8 days.   The consultant wrote to Colonel Carter, who referred the request to the Laboratories Division, Preventive Medicine Service, Office of The Surgeon General.   The Laboratories Division, in turn, contacted the Food and Drug Administration, Federal Security Administration, and Charles Pfizer and Co. and then sent a report on the matter to Colonel Carter.   When Colonel Carter made it the subject of discussion at the weekly staff meeting, the Supply Service, Office of The Surgeon General, was instructed to issue a directive on the subject and immediately advise the various oversea theater headquarters as to how to proceed in the matter.   This is illustrative of the advantage of liaison between the consultant and the Office of The Surgeon General.   Had the question been processed through normal channels, this matter, which The Surgeon General considered of extreme importance, would not have received such expeditious handling.

Improvised equipment.—This consultant observed, on his initial tour of the theater, remarkable improvisations of equipment. In many instances, the improvisations were almost exact replicas of standard equipment found in hospitals in the Zone of Interior. Particularly striking was the highly satisfactory reproduction of costly, critically scarce apparatus by enlisted personnel at the 69th General Hospital. At the author's request, the hospital forwarded to the theater surgeon detailed blueprints and photographs of these improvisations in order that a manual on their construction and use might be compiled and distributed throughout the India-Burma and China Theaters. Capt. Stanley C. Gillette, MAC, Reconditioning Consultant, Office of the Surgeon, USFIBT,[15] extracted material from this report pertaining to physiotherapy equipment and sent it to all hospitals authorized physiotherapy departments with the recommendation that the apparatus designed to facilitate remedial exercises be reproduced locally and used in conjunction with the reconditioning program. The apparatus to be locally improvised included plans for a Kanavel table, quadriceps exercise table and chest weights, foot inversion board, chinning bar, shoulder wheel, stall bars, shoulder abduction ladder, Sayre head sling, exercise steps, therapeutic bicycle, rowing machine, and whirlpool bath (fig. 360).

On his second tour of the theater, Colonel Graham noted widespread acceptance of this advice to improvise equipment locally. One of the more useful pieces of equipment for the surgical services was an overhead, multibeam operating-room light constructed entirely of salvaged material. In fact most of the improvisations were constructed from salvage, most often from wrecked airplanes and motor vehicles. Perhaps even more practical was the improvised testing equipment used by the ophthalmologists. Equipment unavailable in the theater, and which was accurately reproduced, included Jackson crossed cylinders, illiterate charts, lens centering devices, perimeters, tangent screens, occluders, trial frame wall brackets, and adjustable stools for patients during perimetry and scotometry studies (fig. 361).

Equipment for evacuation hospitals.—The evacuation hospitals perhaps experienced the greatest trouble acquiring adequate equipment. Whereas they gained a large surplus of surgical personnel through functioning as a fixed facility, they were handicapped in that their table of equipment was decidedly inadequate when serving as a station or general hospital. Although some of the deficiencies had been corrected, at the end of the campaigns in Burma they still had not received essential equipment (fig. 362). Requests for this

---

[15] Captain Gillette was one of the four Medical Administrative Corps officers who arrived in the India-Burma Theater with Colonel Graham (p. 912). He was first an assistant to Major Britt and then replaced Major Britt as the theater reconditioning consultant in May 1945, when Major Britt was given command of the 30th Station Hospital.

additional equipment, in accordance with the prevailing theater policy, had to be approved by the War Department. Finally, when the need for equipment in excess of tables of equipment no longer existed, the War Department informed the theater that changes in basic allowances should be accomplished by the theater on the basis of individual needs of the various units since "such a flexibility results in a more efficient medical service and is common practice in other theaters of operation."

SPECIAL PROBLEMS

Transfer of Patients to General Hospitals

The most significant directive pertaining to the surgical service of the theater was issued on 2 April 1945. The directive was entitled "Transfer of Patients to Numbered General Hospitals" and was modeled on WD Circular No. 12, 10 January 1944, which applied to the transfer of patients to named general hospitals in the Zone of Interior. In the course of this consultant's initial tour of hospitals, he had noted that formidable or specialized surgical procedures of an elective nature were being undertaken at field and station hospitals by officers with inadequate formal training or practical experience. There was even less reason for this in the India-Burma Theater than in the Zone of Interior, since, with only two exceptions, these smaller hospitals were situated within several miles of major airfields from which patients could be transported by regularly scheduled evacuation aircraft to general hospitals located not more than 2-hours' flying distance away. Compliance with this directive was uniformly satisfactory, and, in most instances in which the condition of the patient precluded transfer, consultation was requested of a general hospital. In this manner, the quality of professional care afforded patients in the India-Burma Theater was materially enhanced; furthermore, a more equitable and economic distribution of key professional personnel was thus facilitated.

Treatment in Dispensaries

Along these lines there existed one problem for which a completely satisfactory solution was never reached. The same problem was encountered in the Second Service Command, but to a much less degree. Reference is made to the treatment of patients in dispensaries, which in the majority of instances were controlled by the Army Air Forces. Many patients, who should have been transferred to hospitals, were given definitive treatment in these dispensaries. Most dispensaries had established sickbays in which from 10 to 30 beds were maintained. These were, for the most part, operated by general-duty medical officers of recent graduation who had completed an accelerated medical course of 3 years, followed by an internship of 9 months.

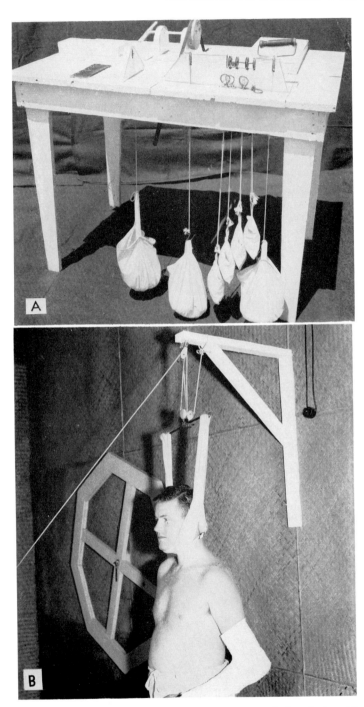

FIGURE 360.—Locally reproduced apparatus designed to aid remedial exercises. A. A modified Kanavel table. B. A Sayre head sling and shoulder wheel.

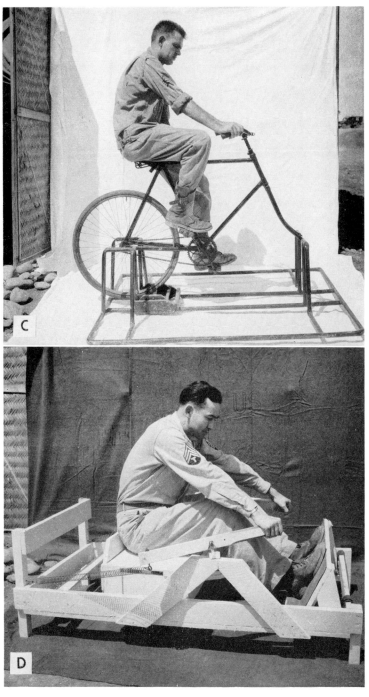

FIGURE 360.—Continued. C. A therapeutic bicycle. D. A rowing machine.

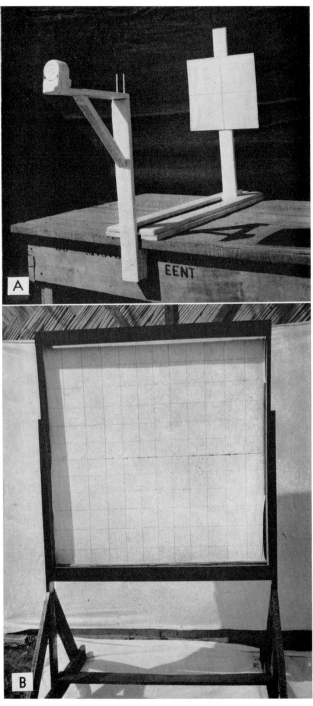

FIGURE 361.—Improvised testing equipment used by ophthalmologists. A. A lens centering device. B. A tangent
screen.

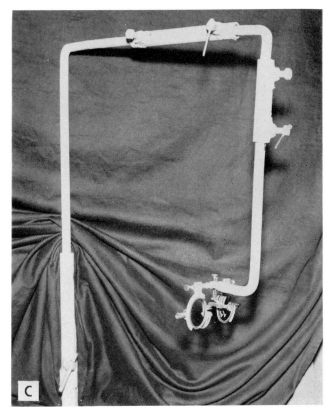

FIGURE 361.—Continued.   C. A trial frame wall bracket.

Scores of patients were observed in hospitals who had been improperly retained in dispensaries, many with peritonitis from a ruptured appendix, others with malalinement of fractured bones which eventually required open reduction, others with severe second- and third-degree burns with infection and contractures, patients with severe local and systemic infections resulting from the late primary closure of lacerations, and patients with many other evidences of poor surgical judgment and treatment of an inferior quality.

This problem was made the subject of a memorandum to the theater surgeon, in which were listed the following recommendations: (1) Inactivate those dispensaries situated within several miles of hospitals or else place these dispensaries under the control of the hospitals which would provide personnel for conducting sick call, (2) prohibit the maintenance of beds in dispensaries except when specifically authorized by the theater surgeon, (3) require dispensaries to render a monthly report listing diagnosis, treatment, and disposition of each patient admitted to a sickbay, and (4) require hospital commanders to report to the office of the theater surgeon all instances of improper treatment in patients admitted from dispensaries.

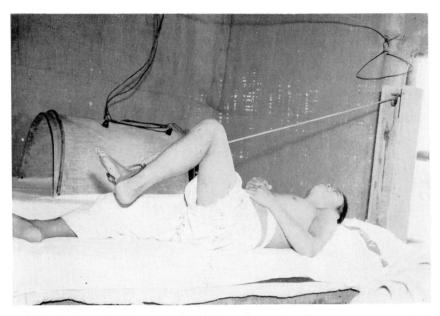

FIGURE 362.—An improvised baker and exercise weight and pulley arrangement at the 14th Evacuation Hospital.

The theater surgeon, in spite of his position, was limited in the actions he could take to correct this situation owing to the relative autonomy of the Army Air Forces in the theater, under whose jurisdiction were most of the dispensaries involved. All elements of the Army Air Forces in the theater, with the exception of the India-China Wing of the Air Transport Command but including the Tenth Air Force, were under the administrative and logistic control of the Army Air Forces, India-Burma Sector, whose headquarters were located at Hastings Mill, Calcutta. Through this headquarters, the Army Air Forces were operationally controlled by the Eastern Air Command of the Southeast Asia Command—a situation which further gave weight to the coequal and separate status of the Army Air Forces in relation to other elements of the Army in the theater. The Army Air Forces in the theater continued to operate their dispensaries on the contention that too many man-days were lost when Air Forces personnel had to be transferred to the fixed hospitals of the theater for the treatment of relatively minor medical and surgical conditions. Some improvement was noted on this consultant's second tour of the India-Burma Theater, but there was much to be desired in the correction of this pernicious situation. As it was earlier stated, no really satisfactory solution of the problem was ever reached.

Treatment of Appendicitis

Another problem which confronted this consultant shortly after his arrival was the relatively high mortality from appendicitis. Practically all of these deaths were in nonoperative cases or in patients who were not operated upon until the appendix had ruptured. It was determined, after a careful study of clinical records and conference with some of the officers involved, that the following factors were influential: (1) The prevalence in Army personnel of diarrheal diseases which mimicked appendicitis, especially amebiasis; (2) retention in dispensary sickbays of patients with appendicitis, many of whom were administered purgatives, until abscess or generalized peritonitis developed (32 such cases were observed during the author's initial tour of hospitals); (3) undue caution of officers who had been criticized by the Surgeon, SOS, USF-IBT, for removal of normal appendixes (hospitals had been instructed that all appendixes removed should be sent to the Central Laboratory for microscopic study). The latter no doubt served as a deterrent to the overzealous young surgeon, but at the same time, it tended to warp the judgment of the conscientious, timid individual who had been officially reprimanded or dreaded such an occurrence.

The combination of abdominal pain, vomiting, and right-lower-quadrant tenderness frequently resulted in the admission of patients with amebiasis to the surgical service. The amebiasis-minded surgeon was not readily deceived, for a history of diarrhea, abdominal tenderness also over other portions of the large bowel, and indurated, tender segments of the large intestines indicated the advisability of stool examination, proctoscopy, and other diagnostic tests. The presence of amebic colitis was, however, no guarantee that the patient did not also have acute appendicitis and require surgical intervention. It was therefore advised that, when any patient showed convincing signs of acute appendicitis, delay in surgery was not to be countenanced. The surgeons were given to understand that, if, after careful study and the use of available consultation, a normal appendix was removed, they would not be criticized or penalized by the theater surgeon. This attitude, it is believed, had a salutary effect on the officers and to some extent was responsible for a diminution in the number of deaths from appendicitis.

Effect of Climate

The consistently high temperatures prevailing in many parts of the India-Burma Theater, the meager recreational facilities, and the isolation of many of the posts had a profound effect on medical personnel. Even in the relatively brief experience of the consultants of somewhat less than a year, it was striking to witness alert, aggressive, enthusiastic medical officers gradually "flatten out" during the second monsoon of their stay. The same influences were apparent in many of the patients.

Heat exhaustion and heatstroke, surprisingly, were not prevalent and constituted a relatively minor problem. During the hot, humid months of the monsoon season, oral afternoon temperatures as high as 100° F. in apparently healthy males and as high as 100.4° F. in females were observed in nonhospitalized personnel engaged in routine activities. Similar elevations among patients were observed in the wards of hospitals in the absence of any other explanation.

The widespread use of sulfonamides, particularly sufadiazine, led to occasional renal complications during the hot season. Every effort was made to impress medical personnel with the necessity of maintaining an adequate urinary output rather than emphasizing fluid intake. Injection of even 3 or 4 liters of fluid a day led, under certain circumstances, to oliguria, hematuria, loin pain, and the like, even when only moderate doses of sulfonamides were administered. Owing to the occasional occurrence of anuria, a circular was distributed which related the advantages of spinal anesthesia in the relief of this state.

COMMENTS ON INDIVIDUAL HOSPITALS

It is difficult, after reading again the author's reports to the theater surgeon on hospitals visited, not to follow a strong inclination to write about each of them. The scope of this undertaking, however, will not permit this, although certain impressions obtained during field trips are reported in later sections of this chapter.

There were several outstanding hospitals in each category, a goodly number of highly satisfactory ones, and only a few definitely mediocre units. Some of the hospitals with the poorest physical facilities were rated by this consultant at the top of the list for performance. That is, esprit de corps was excellent, scarcity of equipment had been remedied by clever improvisations, and the quality of professional care was superior. In others with fine modern physical plants and the latest in equipment, the author found the morale poor and the quality of professional care below standard. The difference very often was owing to the character, qualifications and, or, state of health of the commanding officer and chiefs of services. In seven instances, the consultants and the chief nurse, Lt. Col. Agnes A. Maley, ANC, on their first field trip observed an urgent need for prompt repatriation of hospital commanders. For the most part, they had remained through one too many monsoon seasons and were physically and nervously exhausted. There was also a degree of doubt in some of these cases as to their initial qualifications to command. Replacement of these ill or derelict officers often would alone suffice to improve tremendously both the morale and quality of professional services.

Too frequently, this surgical consultant observed in India, Burma, China, North Africa, and, to a somewhat lesser extent in the Second Service Command, a tendency to assign to administrative posts, including that of hospital commander, officers of field grade rank for whom there was no available clinical assignment commensurate with their rank and military occupational specialty number (usually 3100, general duty). Often they were lacking in both efficiency and proficiency, in aptitude to command, and in administrative ability. Furthermore, it appeared to be somewhat more the rule than the exception in oversea hospitals for a relieved commander to be replaced by the ranking medical officer of the unit, who had acquired his relative position of rank solely by chance and who, consequently, more often than not lacked the qualities necessary to command such a complex organization as a modern army hospital.

FIELD TRIPS, INDIA-BURMA THEATER

Somewhat more than half of this consultant's 9 months in the India-Burma and China Theaters was occupied in field visits to the various installations. Travel was almost entirely by regularly scheduled transport aircraft, although occasionally, as a matter of expediency, bombers or L–5 liaison planes were used. Nearly 200 hours were required to travel approximately 30,000 miles, and probably half as many hours were spent in airports waiting on repairs to planes or, during the monsoons, waiting for what was said to be reasonably satisfactory flying weather.

The isolation arising from the wide dispersion of units and the poor lines of communication made it the more important for the consultants to be regarded as two-way ambassadors between the theater surgeon and the hospitals, interpreting locally the policies of headquarters and acquainting headquarters with the problems confronting officers in the field. For the most part, medical officers had had no opportunity to discuss professional matters with anyone other than their immediate associates and had but little information regarding experience with comparable problems at other hospitals or other theaters. The opportunity to display their own accomplishments was an important morale factor. At many hospitals, the experience and ingenuity of the medical officers provided constructive suggestions which could be transmitted to the officers at other hospitals. Colonel Blumgart said that this function of the surgical consultant as a "circuit rider of good ideas" was probably one of his chief contributions. Through a sincere endeavor to be as helpful as possible, the surgical consultant established confidence among hospital personnel, who accepted suggestions without resentment. In some instances, a surplus of medical talent was present; two or three highly competent surgeons would be found serving in a station hospital. In other instances, however, no surgeon with ability and sound, conservative surgical judgment had been assigned, and it would become necessary to prohibit further surgery in these hospitals until a qualified officer arrived. These instances were, however, relatively few and invariably were immediately rectified by the personnel officer in the office of the theater surgeon in response to a radiogram or telephone call from the consultant.

Advance Base Section No. 3

Soon after his arrival in the theater, this surgical consultant toured hospitals in the Advance Base Section comprised of upper Assam, India, and northern Burma (map 7, p. 908). Most of the battle casualties of the Burma campaigns were hospitalized in this area. Base Section headquarters was at Ledo, where the road of the same name began. The 69th General Hospital was located just outside of Ledo; several miles further along the Ledo Road was the 20th General Hospital (University of Pennsylvania-affiliated unit); at the 19-mile mark of the road was the 14th Evacuation Hospital (New York City Hospital-affiliated unit) ; at the 52-mile mark, at Tagap Ga, Burma, was the 335th Station Hospital; and at the 103-mile mark of the road, at Shing-bwiyang, Burma, was the 73d Evacuation Hospital (Los Angeles County General Hospital-affiliated unit). The Base Section surgeon, Lt. Col. John T. Smiley, MC, a relatively young career army officer, impressed the author as being an exceptionally able administrator.

The 69th General Hospital was an excellent example of what could be accomplished in the organization of a general hospital in a theater of operations when an officer possessing aptitude for command was assigned the task. Evidently, this unit had got off to an inauspicious start late in 1944, at about the time of Colonel Kennedy's visit. Colonel Kennedy was of the opinion that the unit was far from strong and urged the consultants to give it their initial consideration. Subsequent to his visit, Lt. Col. (later Col.) Edward M. DeYoung, MC, a young Regular Army officer, was designated commanding officer, and under his wise and effective direction the hospital became an efficient organization, with the prospects of becoming one of the outstanding general hospitals of the theater.

The 20th General Hospital was unequaled in the Southeast Asia Command. It is difficult to contemplate a discussion of this installation without becoming overwhelmed with superlatives. Suffice it to say that it was outstanding in every respect, and so it should have been, with a hopsital commander of the caliber of General Ravdin—eminent surgeon, educator, and able administrator—and a staff that had remained nearly intact since its arrival in the theater 2½ years earlier, composed of officers practically all of whom possessed superior professional qualification. The physical plant, facilities, and equipment left little to be desired. Particularly impressive were the central supply service, the blood bank, operating rooms, and the unit ward system in which surgical wards were divided into administrative units, each consisting of one or more active and two or more convalescent wards. This hospital, together with the 14th, 48th, and 73d Evacuation Hospitals, performed a noteworthy service in the care of battle casualties during the Burma campaigns (fig. 363).

The 14th and 73d Evacuation Hospitals were also outstanding units, staffed (as has already been related) with an overabundance of highly talented surgeons. Their hospitals were of basha construction and were in a poor state of repair, owing to the monsoons and a predominance of Chinese patients. The 73d Evacuation Hospital was established on the sides of jungle mountains, and all personnel, including the nurses, lived in pyramidal tents. Despite the tremendous handicaps of more-or-less constant rain, mildew, and myriads of insects and pests, these units succeeded in maintaining aseptic conditions while undertaking formidable and highly technical surgical procedures with commendable low mortality and morbidity rates.

The 335th Station Hospital was unique in that the entire personnel of the unit consisted of Negroes. The hospital was situated on the most imposing, and almost the most isolated, site in the theater, with an elevation of about 3,000 feet on a hairpin curve of the Ledo Road and on the side of a hill in northern Burma from which could be viewed a vast expanse of territory including the mountain ranges of Tibet. While visiting the 73d Evacuation Hospital, this consultant was driven in a jeep by Lt. Col. Clarence J. Berne, MC, able chief of the surgical service of that hospital, through 20 miles of almost impenetrable mud to the 355th Station Hospital. Despite its isolation and relative inactivity (its main purpose was to provide medical service for the Negro troops working on the Ledo Road), the morale of this unit was not surpassed by that of any other organization in the theater. Moreover, from the author's observation and those of Colonel Berne, who visited there frequently, it was quite evident that they were rendering superior nursing and medical care.

Base Section No. 2

Base Section No. 2, with headquarters at Calcutta (map 8), contained one general hospital, nine station hospitals, and one field hospital. This base section served the Calcutta district through which port practically all the waterborne supplies for the theater arrived, the 20th Bomber Command, and Air Transport Command installations, a total personnel of about 60,000.

The 142d General Hospital, Calcutta, a unit affiliated with the University of Maryland, Baltimore, Md., took over an already established installation from the 263d General Hospital, which was inactivated in November 1944. There were 2,000 beds established in modern, well-equipped buildings in a 1-mile long area in a rather congested outlying section of Calcutta. Despite the fact that the personnel of this organization were under the impression they were being repatriated on leaving the South Pacific Area after a stay of 29 months, they undertook their new task in a remarkably fine spirit. It was necessary for them to reorganize their staff and expand from a 1,000- to a 2,000-bed hospital. This was accomplished in a highly commendable manner under the direction of the able hospital commander, Col. Murray M. Copeland, MC, himself a distinguished surgeon and formerly chief of the hospital's surgical service. The hospital was outstanding in almost every respect.

It was unfortunate that this unit and the 18th General Hospital, sponsored by The Johns Hopkins University, Baltimore, Md., were redeployed in the India-Burma Theater. Of the 33 Medical Corps officers at the 142d General Hospital, 22 had become eligible for rotation; 48 of this hospital's 83 nurses had become eligible for rotation. All of the personnel of the 18th General Hospital, which had been functioning for more than 30 months in the Fiji Islands, were eligible for rotation to the Zone of Interior. When it was learned that

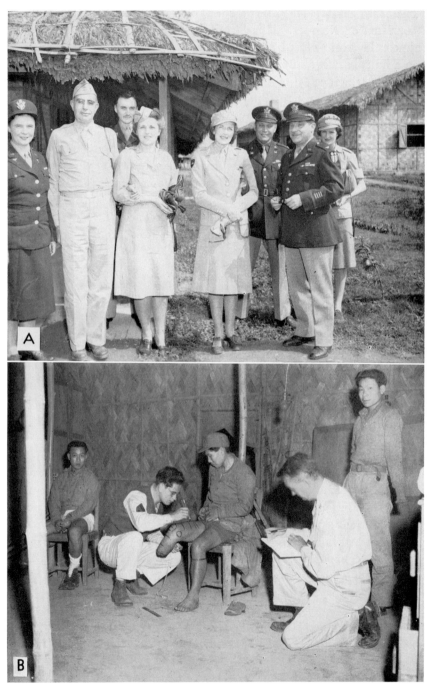

FIGURE 363.—The 20th General Hospital, Ledo.   A. Col. I. S. Ravdin, MC (right front), escorting Lady Mountbatten (center) and other visitors on an inspection of the hospital. B. A Chinese amputee, being measured for prosthesis.

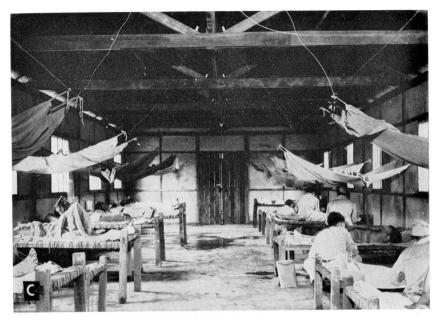

FIGURE 363.—Continued. C. A ward for Japanese prisoners of war.

these hospitals were to be sent to the India-Burma Theater, the theater commander requested the War Department to rotate all the personnel before redeployment was effected. This was not done.

The 18th General Hospital was doubly unfortunate. Its members had served longer in the South Pacific than had the 142d General Hospital. But, unlike the latter unit, which took over a splendid physical plant in the theater's port of debarkation, the 18th General Hospital was required to travel about 800 miles by a train that averaged 15 miles an hour to an abandoned installation on the Ledo Road whose dilapidated structures required almost complete rebuilding (fig. 364). Moreover, the hospital's equipment had not accompanied it from the last station. And, furthermore, the staff had been informed that admissions to their hospital were to be restricted to Chinese soldiers.

Colonel Kennedy of the Kelser Mission, after visiting this unit shortly after its arrival in upper Assam, urged in his report to the theater commander that the entire staff be rotated as rapidly as possible, both for their own good and for the good of the theater. He believed that to retain in the theater two such units would have an adverse effect on the morale of the remainder of the personnel in the theater who were anticipating rotation. Five months later, the author made the same recommendation when the deputy theater commander, Maj. Gen. Frank D. Merrill, solicited his aid in attempting to persuade these people to remain in order to establish a new 1,000-bed general hospital then being built in Myitkyina. The entire unit was rotated in March 1945.

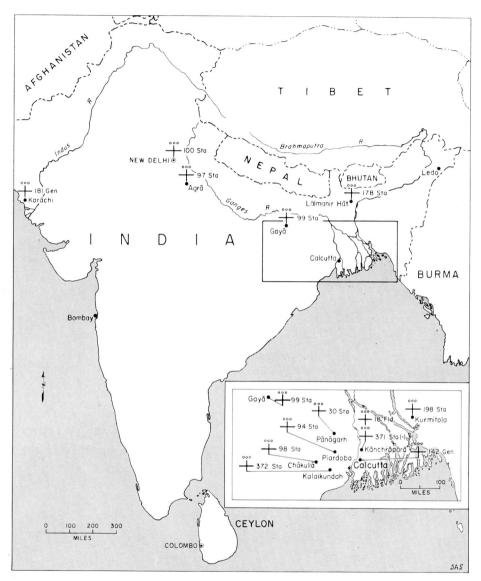

MAP 8.—Selected hospitals of the Services of Supply in India early in 1945, showing concentration in the Calcutta district.

FIELD TRIP, CHINA THEATER

The limited authorization of personnel for the Office of the Surgeon, USF-CT, did not provide positions for consultants. Accordingly, on 5 May 1945, Colonel Armstrong, Surgeon, USFCT, requested of Colonel Baylis, Surgeon, USFIBT, the services of the India-Burma Theater consultants on temporary duty in the China Theater.

Ten days later, on the completion of his first tour of hospitals in the India-Burma Theater, this consultant proceeded by plane over the Himalayan "Hump" to K'un-ming, Rear Echelon Headquarters, China Theater, a distance of about 1,800 miles from Headquarters, USFIBT, in New Delhi. The author's reception in K'un-ming left nothing to be desired. Along with many other visitors to Rear Echelon Headquarters, he was impressed with the spirit of friendliness and cooperation that was more wholehearted than was usually encountered. In great part, it was believed, this spirit was influenced by the character and personality of the Commanding General, Rear Echelon, USFCT, Maj. Gen. Douglas L. Weart, and of the theater surgeon, Colonel Armstrong.[16]

The theater surgeon was optimistic that the consultants would be able, from their observations, to indicate in their reports the most serious deficiencies in personnel and equipment and thus assist in expediting the procurement of much needed relief. At the same time, as was strongly emphasized by Colonel Armstrong, he desired that all irregularities and all evidences of professional incompetence be recorded or brought to his personal attention. He earnestly desired criticism, advice, and help.

Visit to the Combat Area

It had been arranged for this consultant to remain at the Rear Echelon headquarters a few days for orientation, but the day after his arrival the opportunity was afforded him to accompany Col. Benjamin J. Birk, MC, Surgeon of the Chinese Combat Command (Provisional), on a tour of field units in the active combat area.[17] Accordingly, on 17 May 1945, they flew to Chih-chiang, the most forward fighter base after the fall of Kuei-lin, in a Combat Cargo Command plane filled with drums of aviation gasoline. From Chih-chiang they went by jeep over mountains and a makeshift ferry across a river to An-chiang, headquarters of the Eastern Command, Chinese Combat Command.

Although the local military commanders showed little concern over a pincer movement that the Japanese were attempting in this area, they were nevertheless bothered about the considerable number of Japanese disguised as Chinese civilians reported by Chinese military intelligence and the Office of Strategic Services to be in Chih-chiang and An-chiang and the intervening territory. As a consequence, contrary to practices in most other theaters, Colonel Birk and Colonel Graham were issued carbines and pistols and told to display them prominently. All tactical medical units in the combat zone were not only well armed but were also given a special course in the function,

---

[16] Later The Surgeon General, U.S. Army.

[17] The Chinese Combat Command (Provisional) along with the Chinese Training Command (Provisional) comprised the Chinese Training and Combat Command, which was formed as a result of the consolidation in November 1944 of the predecessor Y-Force and Z-Force operations staffs and activities. The new command continued the training and logistic programs in support of Chinese Forces in Central and southern China which had been the missions of the Y-Force and Z-Force.

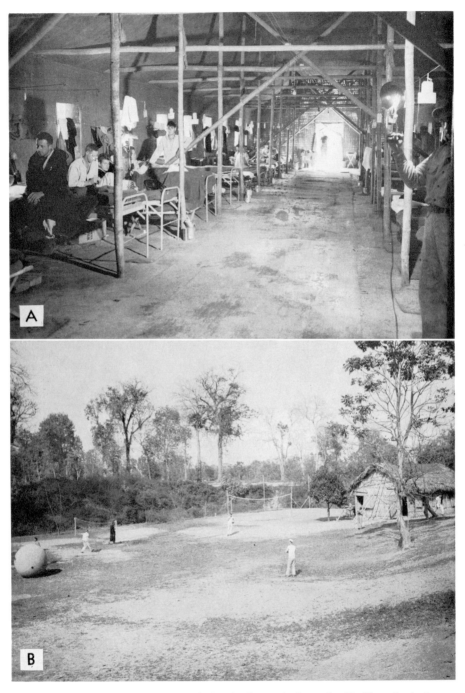

FIGURE 364.—The 18th General Hospital. A. A surgical ward. B. The physical reconditioning area and the occupational therapy building.

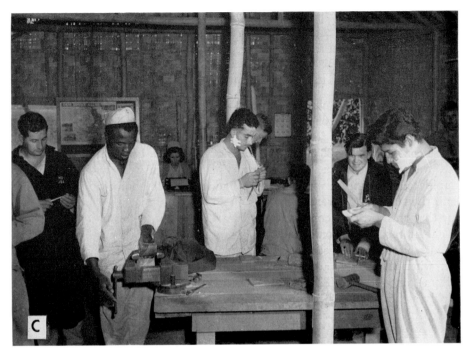

FIGURE 364.—Continued.   C. The interior of an occupational therapy shop.

stripping, assembling, and firing of the various small arms, including the Thompson submachinegun.   Moreover, it was theater policy that the Geneva Cross brassard not be worn, "it having been used as a target by the enemy, often at extreme ranges of automatic fire."

At An-chiang, this consultant reported to Col. Woods King, Commanding Officer, and to Col. Paul G. Hansen, MC, Surgeon, Eastern Command.   During the next 2 days, Colonel Birk, Colonel Hansen, and the author visited all Chinese and U.S. Army hospitals between An-chiang and Tu-chou, along a road to which Chinese casualties were evacuated through narrow mountain files. They saw many Chinese wounded limping along the road with the aid of a stick or rifle, or being supported by, or carried on the backs of, other soldiers.   Still others, unable to walk, were on the ground beside the road.   Their pleas for assistance were ignored by the Chinese soldiers who passed them.   The incongruity of these actions were explained to the author by the Chinese interpreter, who said that the lightly wounded soldier who carried for many miles a more seriously wounded comrade did so because the latter was either related to him or was a member of his squad or platoon.   He might even offer some measure of aid to a member of his company who was in another platoon, but beyond that he would volunteer assistance to no one, regardless of the urgency of the need.

At the most likely points of entry to the road were stationed U.S. Army medical corpsmen to guide or litter-carry casualties to nearby portable surgical hospitals established in tents or Chinese temples or combinations of these two.

The Portable Surgical Hospital

At this time there were only four portable surgical hospitals in the area, and only one section (2 officers and 18 enlisted men) of the 34th Portable Surgical Hospital was then functioning. They had been treating casualties more or less constantly for 36 hours. Scores of wounded, both Chinese and Japanese, were stretched out on the ground surrounding the ancient and quite dilapidated building in which the unit had set up a temporary operating room. Since the two officers were operating on an "assembly line" basis, it was necessary that enlisted men conduct the triage of patients, determining the order in which the casualties would undergo operation. Corpsmen would undress the patients, clean the injured area, accomplish a superficial debridement of wounds, and, when necessary, administer intravenous Pentothal sodium (thiopental sodium) anesthesia. The surgeons progressed along the line of tables as quickly as possible, performing a simple suture of a superficial wound in one, enucleating an eye in another, or amputating a leg or an arm.

The quality of the surgery performed under considerable pressure was, for the most part, highly satisfactory. Working under such trying conditions and in the face of many handicaps, these officers and enlisted men rendered outstanding service (fig. 365). Many lives were saved in instances of the severely wounded and injured, and a considerable number of the lightly wounded were enabled to return to the front after a short period of time.

Certainly this was not the time or place for criticism of surgical judgment or of techniques. From this consultant's observations of officers in action in these small units and from his conversations with them during periods of inactivity, it became clear that most of their surgical training had been acquired, in many instances, in the field by the trial and error method. Even where competent, well-trained surgeons were on duty with the units, they seldom had time to supervise the operating of inexperienced members when there was the great pressure of a large backlog of patients awaiting operation. The author's inclination, soon after arrival in the India-Burma Theater, was to be critical of the assignment to the portable surgical hospitals of so many officers with little or no surgical training and an overabundance of pediatricians, obstetricians, and general practitioners. A study of personnel records of 19 of these units, however, revealed that in well over 80 percent of instances the assignments had been made by the Office of The Surgeon General before they were sent to China-Burma-India. The theater surgeon's error had been to assume that the Office of The Surgeon General had selected qualified personnel for the portable surgical hospitals. Certainly, in any future war only highly skilled young men, preferably under 35 years of age, should be employed in such units.

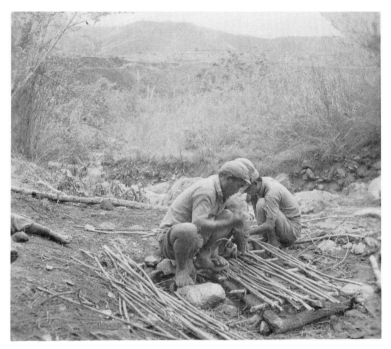

FIGURE 365.—Chinese soldiers constructing an operating table for surgeons of a portable surgical hospital. Japanese positions are on the mountains in the background.

There was much to discourage the personnel of the portable surgical units. For each Chinese soldier they saved, many others died. Some died in transit to their hospital or shortly after arrival because of the long delay in reaching them (many casualties observed by this consultant had been wounded 4 or 5 days previously). Others died after receiving treatment when they failed to survive the trip to fixed installations of the Chinese Army further to the rear. Lt. Col. John H. Sharp, QMC, whose trucks transported these casualties, told the author that on one occasion approximately 200 out of 600 Chinese died in the trucks during their evacuation from U.S. Army hospitals. This was readily understandable since the patients were transported in trucks over rough mountain roads on which there were innumerable hairpin curves. The trucks were driven at high rates of speed by irresponsible Chinese drivers. Moreover, the wounded Chinese soldier, so everyone with whom this consultant conferred agreed, received practically no nourishment throughout the course of his evacuation from the front, except for the short period he remained in the portable surgical hospital. This deplorable situation existed despite the fact that ample supplies of food had been furnished by the U.S. Army to Chinese responsible for feeding patients in transit. Furthermore, it was believed that the total battle casualties and injuries of an entire Chines Army (somewhat larger than the full complement of a U.S. infantry division) could not be properly cared for by the personnel of one half of a standard portable surgical hospital.

A most discouraging observation was the handling of fracture cases, particularly those that had been compounded by shell fragments or bullets. They could not be properly treated in these small units. Those fractures in which union occurred usually presented marked deformity (as observed in Chinese and American field hospitals to the rear) for two reasons: First, there were no X-ray machines available for the portable surgical units; and second, even if alinement was perfect when the plaster cast was applied, the Chinese soldier invariably removed the cast within a few days.

On the basis of the experience of the portable surgical hospital with the Y-Force in the Salween Valley operations,[18] the theater surgeon proposed a revision in the table of organization and equipment for such units to be employed in China. The medical plan had provided for the use of 18 American portable surgical hospital units for the Y-Force. Actually, however, only 10 arrived in time to participate, as 8 were diverted for service in India-Burma. Colonel Armstrong's supporting arguments for the proposed changes were substantially as follows:

The portable surgical hospitals, as originally organized in Table of Organization and Equipment 8–572, were planned for a specific purpose; namely, giving frontline surgical treatment in support of American units in combat. Under this plan, there were always larger hospital units to the rear, which could take care of any medical problems that might arise. In the China Theater, however, the use of the portable surgical hospitals was entirely different. The patients were almost exclusively Chinese soldiers and usually there were no longer American hospitals to the rear which could handle complicated problems. Therefore, it was necessary that portable surgical hospitals also function as field, station, evacuation, and general hospitals (for the Chinese); in other words, they had to be equipped to handle all types of surgical and medical cases and at the same time remain relatively mobile in order to be able to maintain close support of the Chinese units in combat. As mentioned previously, many of these units were split into two sections in order to provide surgical and medical care to the greatest number of Chinese patients, and therefore it was necessary that each section be adequately equipped to operate separately.

Colonel Armstrong indicated changes that should be effected. Four officers, he noted, would be assigned as in the original organization, but, since the units would be split, emphasis should be placed on the assignment of more qualified surgeons. Eleven enlisted men were to be dropped, leaving twenty-two.

At the time of this consultant's visit, there was no indication that the war would end in such a short time, and it was considered an urgent necessity to increase the efficiency of the portable surgical hospitals to the fullest extent,

---

[18] See footnote 9, p. 899.

since the War Department had disapproved the further utilization of fixed beds in U.S. Army hospitals for Chinese casualties. The commanding general of Chinese troops in the Eastern Combat Command expressed to the author his deep concern over the change in policy. His comments paralleled those of the division commander of the 130th Chinese Division, who, according to the American Surgeon for the Y-Force, stated, in effect, that his soldiers were much braver in this campaign than in previous ones because they knew that a portable surgical hospital was close by. The Chinese division commander, it was held, stated also that in previous campaigns the Japanese bullets were not so much of a hazard as the infection resulting from them and that the techniques used by the portable units rendered this danger and fear less important both in actuality and psychologically.

The officers of the portable surgical hospitals that this consultant visited apparently appreciated his visit and the discussions of new concepts in surgical treatment. They expressed the desire, however, to have a surgical consultant assigned to their command who would visit each unit every week or so. The theater surgeon, on the author's recommendation, selected an excellent officer for this post, but before he could start on a tour of duty at the front the war ended. In conferences with the Chinese Surgeon General, Gen. Robert K. S. Lim, a distinguished physician and physiologist who was well known and esteemed in the United States and Great Britain, it was suggested that he arrange for the repatriation of two Chinese surgeons, friends of his and the author's, both highly skilled and possessed of superior surgical judgment, to serve as counterparts of the U.S. Army theater surgical consultant and the contemplated combat area consultant. The suggestion was favorably received, and it is believed that an effort was made to acquire the services of these outstanding countrymen of General Lim, but the plan was never consummated. Practically none of the highly trained Chinese physicians and surgeons, sent to the United States before the war for medical education or for postgraduate training, returned to China during the war.

The Field Hospital

Both the Chinese so-called field hospitals and the U.S. Army field hospitals were visited during this consultant's tour in China.

Chinese field hospitals.—The Chinese field hospitals were primitive. A typical Chinese field hospital was described by the commanding officer of the U.S. 47th Portable Surgical Hospital, I-liang, as follows:

This hospital consisted of several British 'four-man' tents, which are approximately 12 x 15 feet, plus a fairly large adjacent temple, the court sides of which were open. * * * Eight patients were placed in each of the tents, four on each side lying head to head with about a foot of space between each patient. The patient's bed consisted of boards elevated about a foot above the ground on mud bricks. On the boards was placed a thin straw mat. The more fortunate patients had a thin cotton blanket to put over the straw beneath them * * *.

The patients housed in the temple were similarly arranged in the rooms of this building except that in some of the smaller rooms there were large common beds, extending the length of the room, in which several patients were placed.

      *   *   *   *   *   *   *

The food allowance of the patients in the hospital was the same as that allotted for other Chinese soldiers; namely, 25 ounces of rice per man per day. In addition to this, the hospital was allowed 20 Chinese dollars [approximately 25 cents, U.S. currency] per man per day to buy products available on the local market. This was later increased to 120 dollars, but even this didn't buy very much with the marked inflation as illustrated by the fact that an egg cost about 90 dollars and the prices of other products were in proportion.

      *   *   *   *   *   *   *

Nutritional and deficiency diseases comprised a goodly number of the patients in the hospital, and, as can be realized by the above diet which they received, their recovery was not very much enhanced in the hospital.

The nursing care which the sick received was essentially nil. The soldiers assigned to the hospital were technically called nursing soldiers but they had never received any training in these duties. No charts or records were kept on the patients. There was no routine for the giving of medications and other than the bringing of rice into the center of the tent area twice a day for feeding of the patients, no other care was attempted. If the patient had to visit the latrine, which was only a few feet away from the temple and was open, he had to make it under his own power or with the assistance of a fellow patient. The sicker ones being unable to make this journey resorted to the area just outside the tent * * * [or] to the ground in the tent. No water was provided for the patients to wash * * *.

      *   *   *   *   *   *   *

* * * No effort was made to segregate the infectious or contagious diseases. There was no preliminary examination or delousing.

The interest of the Chinese medical officers in the patient was * * * only slightly better than that of the nursing soldiers. They made irregular and indifferent rounds * * * somewhere between ten o'clock in the morning and noon, following which the patients were given drugs which they prescribed. No drug was given without the prescription of the medical officer for each individual dose. As a result of this, regular medication was never given.

There were better Chinese hospitals than this, the author was informed, but in too many instances were many of these conditions reproduced. The Chinese hospitals this consultant visited were about the same as that described. Not once on visits to these places did he see anyone who even claimed to be a doctor, and the nursing soldiers were extremely scarce.

U.S. field hospitals.—On leaving An-chiang, Colonel Birk and the author returned to Chih-chiang, where they visited an Air Force dispensary and two sections of the 21st Field Hospital, only one of which was functioning. The third platoon, situated about 600 miles away, was visited as this consultant returned to the India-Burma Theater. There were among the officers a number of Chinese-American doctors and old China hands, who were former missionaries or sons of missionaries to China. Among these were a number of competent general surgeons, but there was an urgent need for surgical specialists, especially orthopedic surgeons. Moreover, most of the experienced officers were due for rotation, as was the case in the other field hospitals and a number of the portable surgical hospitals.

95th Station Hospital

On his return from the combat area, the author visited the only station hospital in the theater, the 95th Station Hospital, which actually functioned as a general hospital and had been granted the privilege of conducting disposition boards. This hospital was situated on the outskirts of K'un-ming. It was one of the most unimpressive hospitals visited in either theater, from the standpoint of both structure and physical facilities. Most of the station hospitals in the India-Burma Theater were superior to the 95th Station Hospital in almost every respect.

Facilities.—In January 1944, the table of organization had been increased to accommodate 250 patients. On 1 October 1944, the hospital had again been reorganized and designated a 750-bed station hospital. Actually, however, the bed capacity had not exceeded 522 until 10 days prior to this consultant's visit, when it had reached 643. The normal bed capacity had always been lower than the actual census. For instance, on 1 October 1944 there had been 81 patients in excess of normal beds, and on 1 May 1945 there had been an excess of 38 patients. In order to hospitalize these extra patients, it had been necessary to resort to the expedient of installing double-decker beds and cots, which had materially reduced the normal cubic feet of space per patient below the minimum permitted in army hospitals.

Without exception, all of the physical facilities were inadequate as to space and essential equipment. In most instances, they did not meet the normal requirements of a 100-bed station hospital. These included the physical therapy and X-ray departments; the orthopedic, and ear, nose and throat, and eye clinics; the library; wards; and, from the standpoint of essential equipment, the operating rooms as well. Yet, paralleling the increase in patient census, the workload of the clinics and laboratories had steadily increased, although the facilities, which had been inadequate from the first, had not been expanded.

Clinical laboratory.—The clinical laboratory was perhaps greatest in need of expansion. It functioned as a central laboratory for the China Theater, yet the existing facilities were below the minimum requirements for a 200-bed station hospital. Since space for equipment and personnel necessary to accomplish blood chemistry analyses was not available, it had been necessary to send specimens for such determinations to the 234th General Hospital, at Chābua, or the 142d General Hospital, in Calcutta, both in the India-Burma Theater. The pressing need for additional laboratory space, which this consultant, in his report, urged be given priority in the new construction, was emphasized by the high incidence of amebiasis and other diarrheal diseases, typhus, plague, hepatitis, venereal diseases, and other conditions in which diagnosis and guide to therapy were almost entirely dependent on laboratory studies.

X-ray Department.—Although possessing nearly adequate space, the X-ray Department had not been provided adequate protective measures against the radiation hazard for either the X-ray personnel or the patients waiting for examination. Since it was highly problematic when this department would be relocated, Headquarters, SOS, USFCT, was urged to provide as promptly as possible auxiliary protective measures such as lead screens and brick partitions, and, in the new construction, to comply with TB MED 62, 1 July 1944, which prescribed the necessary protective measures. Evidently, this important bulletin had not been received in the theater or SOS headquarters.

A dangerous practice was observed in the X-ray department of this hospital—a practice which had also been noted in a number of station hospitals in the India-Burma Theater. There was a tendency among the less well trained radiologists to employ X-ray therapy to a much greater extent than did the Board-certified, highly competent radiologists in general hospitals. As a matter of fact, in only two hospitals in the Southeast Asia Command, the 20th and 142d General Hospitals, did there exist the two prerequisites to undertaking radiotherapy in a U.S. Army hospital; namely, a radiotherapist certified by the American Board of Radiology and an accurately calibrated X-ray machine (and an apparatus with which calibration could be undertaken at frequent intervals).

Personnel.—The medical officers assigned to the surgical service appeared adequate in number and sufficiently proficient. The acting chief of surgical service was on temporary duty from the 172d General Hospital, which anticipated eventually being established in K'un-ming. It was believed, however, that, in a hospital that possessed the privileges and functions of a general hospital, the chief of the X-ray Department should have had formal radiologic training and extensive experience, if not Board certification. At this hospital, however, the radiologist's sole training had been received in the course of a rotating internship and while conducting a general practice, during which time he had read films with experienced radiologists on an entirely informal basis.

The quality of professional service rendered surgical patients in this hospital, judging from observations made on complete ward rounds, from discussions with members of the surgical service, and from review of many clinical records, was on the whole very satisfactory. There was ample evidence of sound, conservative surgical judgment and competence in surgical undertakings.

Reconditioning.—Physical reconditioning for hospitalized patients had not been instituted at this hospital. At a nearby convalescent facility, however, under the able direction of 2d Lt. Ben Rubin, MAC, who was eminently qualified for the undertaking, a comprehensive reconditioning program for Class-2 and Class-3 patients was being developed and was found to be superior in every respect. It was believed that this program could be of inestimable value in hastening the recovery and return to duty of army personnel. The success of the program was to a considerable extent dependent on the establishment of an effective physical reconditioning program for patients in the hospital. Accordingly, an effort was made to convince the commanding officer and members of the surgical staff of the tremendous importance of their cooperation in this undertaking. In both the China Theater and the India-Burma Theater, this consultant had occasionally met with resistance in attempting to "sell" reconditioning, and it was particularly difficult if the commanding officer did not favor the program. However, units that had finally become aware of the therapeutic value of remedial and conditioning exercises in speeding recovery were enthusiastic converts. Pre-emptory orders from the theater headquarters that such a program be established were not sufficient; it was essential that wholehearted cooperation be obtained from the entire professional staff, the nurses, and the corpsmen of a hospital and that they become thoroughly conversant with TB MED 137, published in January 1945, and the coordination of physical and surgical therapy of orthopedic cases, as described in TB MED 10, published in February 1944.

Failure of Headquarters, SOS, USFCT, to proceed more energetically with new construction that would expand the theater's sole fixed installation capable of undertaking major elective surgery on U.S. Army personnel made the likelihood of a physical plant's being constructed for the 172d General Hospital, committed to the China Theater for June 1945, extremely doubtful. Scarce materials allocated for use in such construction had, apparently, been diverted for other purposes.

Other Hospitals

The 21st and 22d Field Hospitals were also visited. The former, situated at Pao-shan, southern China, was in the foothills of the Himalayan Mountains and was visited on this consultants' return flight to India. The 22d Field Hospital at Chan-i, 100 miles east of K'un-ming, was reached by jeep in the company of Lt. Col. Robert L. Cavenaugh, MC, able executive officer to the theater surgeon and assistant theater surgeon.

In both units there was observed a deficiency in qualified personnel competent to perform major surgical operations. Owing, however, to the excellent character of the officers conducting the surgical services, there had been, in most instances, proper transfer to the 95th Station Hospital of patients requiring the more formidable surgical procedures.

Departure

On the morning of 3 June 1945, this consultant departed from K'un-ming, following a festive evening during which for 5 hours he was honored with a fabulous Chinese dinner of innumerable courses, interspersed with many toasts. The dinner was given by Colonel Armstrong and Gen. Robert K. S. Lim, Chinese Surgeon General, and section chiefs of their respective headquarters.

Return to Headquarters, India-Burma Theater

On completion of his tour of temporary duty in China, the author was discouraged and not at all satisfied that he had materially assisted the Medical Section, China Theater, despite the more than generous expressions of appreciation by the Commanding General and the Surgeon, China Theater, to him personally, and later, in a communication to the Commander and the Surgeon, India-Burma Theater. The U.S. Medical Department in China was woefully lacking in almost everything. There was not a single hospital of modern construction, standard equipment was scarce, and there were too few qualified professional personnel. The whole setup was more in keeping with a mental image of conditions that existed in the frontier days of the Far West or in the South during the Civil War. Mud and filth prevailed everywhere, including K'un-ming.

One was hesitant about criticizing officers who were conscientiously doing their best under most unfavorable circumstances. Although their best was frequently not good enough, it was not their fault that, in many instances, they had been assigned to undertakings for which they did not possess adequate proficiency. On the other hand, the SOS and theater surgeons in the China Theater had no alternative to the employment of personnel sent to them by the India-Burma Theater. And, actually, the latter theater had little superior talent to spare, outside the university-affiliated units that they were disinclined to dismember. It was only natural therefore that, in fulfilling requisitions from China, the Surgeon, USFIBT, did not relinquish his most capable surgeons. In the final analysis, then, it would appear that the shortage of officers in China qualified to perform major operations was due to the War Department's failure in the first instance to assign a sufficient number of officers in this category to the China-Burma-India Theater.

Several weeks after this consultant's return to India, he received a communication from Colonel Armstrong, the substance of which follows:

He was still woefully short of medicos and was trying to persuade the India-Burma Theater's replacement center to facilitate the China Theater's requisitions. Unfortunately, the China Theater at the time had 7 medical officers who had been over there for 30 months, approximately 20 who had "point scores" above 100, and about 8 who were patients in hospitals at the time of writing. Among the medical officers in the China Theater, there were three or four who were over 50 years of age whom Colonel Armstrong was attempting to have sent home under special "WD radio," and the picture was really gloomy.

Two weeks later, the author wrote to Colonel Armstrong as follows:

A great effort has been made by Patterson, Chief of Personnel, Theater Surgeon's Office, and myself to secure for you qualified surgeons classified C– or B–3150, in order to meet your request for eleven so rated, and at the same time assign a sufficient number of officers of same qualification to the 70th and 71st Field Hospitals (prior to transfer to China). In order to accomplish this we have depleted the hospitals of this theater of all but key men and a few qualified limited-duty officers.

A concentrated effort was continued by the consultants and Colonel Patterson, not only to replace promptly officers who were rotated from the China Theater, but to replace them with officers of the highest qualifications available. The war ended too soon to judge the effectiveness of these intercessions, but it was believed that, had the war continued, these efforts would have resulted in a material improvement in the medical personnel picture in the China Theater.

SUMMARY AND CONCLUSIONS

A comprehensive review has been made by this consultant of the activities of the surgical consultant in the Southeast Asia Command, which comprised the India-Burma and China Theaters. Also, the stated mission and activities of U.S. Forces in these theaters has been narrated in order that the problems and activities of surgical officers can be more readily comprehended.

Certain observations and experiences of the consultants would seem to indicate lessons which could be profitably studied by medical officers who might be involved in any future war. Some of the practices of which the consultants were critical were common to all theaters and the Zone of Interior and stemmed from policies formulated in the War Department; others represented policies established in an individual command. Some of the policies which were considered objectionable have been appropriately corrected, others which pose serious problems have not. A brief outline of the more significant lessons learned is here recorded:

1. Improvement in the effectiveness of the consultant system was observed when the position of chief of professional services was discontinued.

2. Similar benefits resulted when the reports of consultants were routed through technical rather than command channels of communications to theater headquarters.

3. Benefits accrued from close relationship between the consultants and the chief of personnel in the medical section at theater headquarters.

4. Supply liaison activities of the consultants between the hospital medical supply agencies were considered decidedly worthwhile by all concerned.

5. Direct communication between the consultants in the theater and the directors of their respective divisions in the Office of The Surgeon General, prohibited in some other commands, proved equally helpful to The Surgeon General and in promoting the success of the consultants' activities.

6. Disadvantages were noted in the theater practice of referring all the way to the War Department, for approval, requests for changes in basic equipment allowances of units functioning in capacities other than originally intended—such as evacuation hospitals employed as station or general hospitals.

7. Failure to send to hospital commanders copies of the consultants' reports with the theater surgeon's indorsement tended to lessen the effectiveness of the consultants' visits.

8. The advantage of making all military units, including the air force, subordinate on medical policies to the theater surgeon was conclusively demonstrated to the consultants of the India-Burma Theater.

9. The unfortunate policy was formulated in the Office of The Surgeon General, prior to the entrance of the United States into the war, that prohibited the transfer of officers out of affiliated hospital units. This policy resulted in the excessive concentration of talented specialized personnel in a few hospitals, while most of the hospitals of the theater woefully lacked competent general surgeons and specialists capable of independent surgery without supervision.

10. Perhaps the most unfortunate practice noted by the consultants in all the theaters in which they served (to a lesser extent in the Zone of Interior) was a tendency to assign to administrative positions, particularly that of hospital commander, officers of field grade rank for whom there was no available clinical assignment commensurate with their rank and military occupational specialty (MOS 3100, general duty). These officers were too often lacking in both efficiency and proficiency, in aptitude to command, and in administrative ability. The solution to this problem, it would seem, is the formulation of a long-range plan during peacetime in which carefully screened reserve officers with aptitude for command are afforded the opportunity to attend special courses supplemented by yearly periods of training directly under highly competent commanders of various types of Army medical installations.

APPENDIX A

OFFICE OF THE CHIEF SURGEON
EUROPEAN THEATER OF OPERATIONS

3 AUGUST 1943

SUBJECT: Surgical Mission to Russia.

TO: Chief Surgeon, European Theater of Operations.

1. Through the British Ambassador to the U.S.S.R., a medical mission was established. The U.S. Army Medical Corps, E.T.O., was asked to participate. A Canadian member was added later. The British Medical Research Council and the British Council assisted in the preparations and organized the transportation.

2. Brig. General Paul R. Hawley appointed Colonel Elliott C. Cutler and Lt. Colonel Loyal Davis as the U.S. members of the mission.

3. Informal instructions to the U.S. members were given by the U.S. Ambassador to the Court of St. James's, Maj. Gen. John C. H. Lee, and Brig. General Hawley. Travel orders were issued by the A.G.O., E.T.O.

4. The purpose of the mission was (1) to learn as much about Soviet military medicine as possible in order that U.S. troops might benefit from the experience, and (2) to cultivate friendly relations with our Soviet allies.

5. The mission * * * arrived at Moscow at 5:45 p.m. July 2, 1943 * * *. It returned by airplane leaving Moscow July 23, and reached the United Kingdom, July 30 * * *.

6. The mission established highly friendly relations with the U.S.S.R. medical authorities, both military and civil. It was warmly welcomed at the Moscow airport by Soviet officials, including two Vice-Commissars of Public Health; was welcomed at a special sitting, by the People's Commissar of Public Health, and shown every courtesy while in Moscow. It was permitted to visit all of the important hospitals in that area. The mission met and had the most friendly relations with Lt. General Smirnov, Chief of the Red Army medical organizaion; [Vice Admiral] Dganaleidge, Chief of the Surgical Division of the Red Navy; [Rear Admiral] Andriev, head of the Red Navy medical service, and Lt. General Burdenko, Chief of the Surgical Division of the Red Army, as well as many other leading medical authorities.

7. *General Medical Responsibility.*

The care of the injured and sick is in two departments in Russia:

A: The responsibility for the care of injured soldiers in the forward areas is that of the Commissariat of Defence and the military medical organization of which Lt. General Smirnov is the Chief Officer, and Lt. General Burdenko the Chief [of surgery]. This included the care of the soldier in combat units, in Army hospitals and through evacuation to the base area.

B: The responsibility for the care of the wounded soldier in the Base Areas, as well as the care of all civilians, is that of the People's Commissariat of Public Health. Some, but not all, base hospitals have army officers as their administrators for purposes of discipline. Each province has an army as well as a civilian representative of the People's Commissar of Public Health in touch with all hospitals within that province. Many of the chief surgeons of the civilian or base hospitals, are officers in the Red Army Medical Service and are in uniform. Officers and men are treated alike in all hospitals and in some hospitals are bedded in common wards, whereas in others there are separate officers' wards.

8. *Organization for Care of Wounded in Red Army.*

A: Wounded are picked up on field by sanitary corps. (Some of these individuals are women who dress wounds and control hemorrhage).

953

B: Battalion Aid Post—A nurse is here who adjusts bandages and gives first aid, administers morphine, sulfanilamide orally and applies splints.

C: Regimental Aid Post—First medical officer is here. Treatment for shock is begun (blood and plasma); better control of hemorrhage; bandages adjusted; novocainization of fractures if very painful; splints applied; tetanus toxoid and morphine given, and gas gangrene serum administered if large and badly lacerated wounds are present. Sulfanilamide placed in larger wounds.

D: Divisional Aid Post (6–8 kms. from front) Consists of a small hospital for emergency surgery only (some abdominal wounds, a few chest wounds and emergency amputations). Carries out the sorting of patients; redressing and adjusting of splints; further treatment of shock (blood and plasma). May add 200-bed mobile hospital at this point or send in additional surgical teams, as military situation demands and justifies.

E: Sorting-Evacuation Hospital (30–50 kms. from front * * * 1,000–4,000 beds) Careful sorting of patients into medical, lightly wounded and serious litter cases. Distributed to special wards in this hospital or to specialized attached mobile field hospitals of 200 beds each for abdominothoracic wounds, extremity injuries, neurological wounds; facio-maxillary wounds; medical diseases or walking wounded. These latter patients may be kept up the line or sent down the line as far as Moscow (200 kms.) but they remain in the Army hospitals and never come under the control of the Public Health Service. (This permits more rapid restoration to active duty.)

F: Evacuation from the above hospitals by train, motor cars or by air. The latter method is reserved for the critically ill patients, special cases (eye), guerrillas (this is a very large undertaking and a major part of the Russian Army), and in special circumstances, depending upon air control and the availability of planes.

G: Air Force and Ground Force personnel cared for in the same hospitals by the same staffs.

H: Organization within Army hospitals is well standardized, set up for a maximum flow of sick and wounded and reveals a high ability for organization. *Example: 200 bed Mobile Field Hospital:*

(a) Admitting Room: This is both for records and sorting. Personnel come in with simple field medical tag pinned on, simple record form filled out and put in envelope; special portion torn off and sent to medical headquarters; colored tag placed on patient (red=surgery, blue=urgent dressing, white=evacuate).

(b) Patient goes to barber if well enough for hair clipping and shaving.

(c) To washroom where clothes are removed and taken away for cleansing and mending. *Patients thoroughly washed.* Separate room for women. (This is one of the major contributions of the Red Army.)

(d) Dressing room—several tables and sterile supplies ready. Patient rebandaged and given fresh clean clothes.

(e) X-ray room.

(f) Operating room for those selected. Up the line only serious cases done. Abdomen, chests and femurs held in hospital for 7–10 days preferably.

(g) A supply of blood (sent from base area refrigerated) is kept in a deep cellar with some ice which is cut in the winter and stored. Blood not used after 3 weeks.

(h) Stretchers are used for cots and two tiers are set upon wooden frames. Ambulatory patients use upper tier. In dressing room and sorting room have an excellent wooden horse which can be broken down by turning a wingnut and can be packed into a very small space.

(i) For each group of frontline hospitals (6–8) there is a laundry controlled by the medical department.

(j) Equipment of forward hospitals: Russian field tent is excellent; 15 feet wide and commonly 30 feet long with excellent windows in walls and often inner cloth lining. Autoclaves, sterilizers, X-ray apparatus, instruments of which a good many are American or British seemed to be sufficient.

Distribution of Beds for Surgery	*Front*	*Rear*
General surgery	91.5	83.0
Neurosurgery	2.9	4.3
Facio-maxillary-plastic	1.6	3.1
Ophthalmology	1.3	2.0
Otolaryngology	0.9	1.3
Neuropsychiatry	0.2	0.1
Amputations	0.9	5.3
Gynecology	0.2	

Distribution of Wounds

Levitt (In charge of hospital for chest, limbs and joints in base
  area) :   *Percent*

Heads	10
Chests	6.7
Abdomen	2.4
Limbs	68–70

Vorshofsky (Chief Surgeon, Western Front) :   *Percent*

Heads	1
Abdomens	2
Chest	4
Arms	40
Legs	35

9. *Principles of Surgical Practice in care of wounded in Red Army.*

A: Excision of wound (debridement) is practiced as far forward as possible, usually
in sorting-evacuation hospitals, but, in instances where great numbers of wounded exist,
this may be done in base hospitals. This is best practiced early, but Russian surgeons
practice excision up to 10–15 days, including compound fractures; relying upon sulfonamides
and immobilization to prevent generalized sepsis.

B: Immobilization of large soft part injuries as well as fractures by wooden splints
(Deitrich) or Thomas type, for evacuation to place of first definitive surgical treatment,
after which plaster of paris is applied. Plaster of paris is put on as early as possible and
is used directly over the wound, "skin tight" and without padding. Not usually applied
before 3 days after injury.

C: Tetanus—Active immunization with tetanus toxoid is practiced. The "booster"
dose is given at the Regimental Aid Post.

D: Gas gangrene—A potent antiserum is used in all serious wounds, usually intravenously. A toxoid is in the experimental stage. Several surgeons told us that the antiserum was not effective.

E: Sulfonamides—sulfanilamide is used both in forward and in base hospitals by
introduction into the wounds, by mouth and intravenously. It is not carried on the person
of the individual soldier. They also have a small supply of sulfapyridine. Observation of
actual patients indicates that they use it more profusely in wounds than we do. A special
form of sulfanilamide in which the preparation is broken down into very small particles by
subjection to ultrasonic wave lengths is used as a cream applied to gauze and placed into
the wound. It is thought to be very efficacious, but it is still in the experimental phase
and is not in mass production.

F: Secondary suture is practiced wherever possible even after 7–12 days. Skin
grafts are used when it seems advisable.

G: Inhalants uncommonly used, usually ether. Novocain commonly used and we
saw many patients incompletely anesthetized writhing in pain. Spinal anesthesia used

chiefly in base hospitals. Hexonal (like Pentothal) used but no gas oxygen machines seen and not told anywhere of its use.

10. *Principles of Practice in Special Fields of Surgery.*

A: Thoracic Surgery—Thoracic wounds treated conservatively. In forward areas sucking chest wounds are closed. Hemothorax treated by tapping; empyema by drainage for three weeks, then 2 or 3 rib fragments are removed and the wounds packed. Only large foreign bodies are removed. Prof. Levitt gave figure of 6.7 percent as proportion of chest wounds. Lt. General Burdenko said that the original mortality of chest wounds (68 percent) had now been reduced to 18 percent. In 1942, only 19 percent of chest wounds were of penetrating type, and of the 12 percent submitted to operation the mortality was 20.5 percent. A simple positive pressure machine was developed by Burdenko (bellows led air via a Wolff bottle (7 cms. of water) to ordinary gas mask).

B: Burns—Use some coagulants (tannic acid and silver nitrate) but prefer open method, in which they dust on a powder containing an anesthetic and an antiseptic (not sulfonamide). Said burns were very infrequent and mostly in air force personnel. Placental extract covering stimulates more rapid covering over with new skin. (??)

C: Fractures—We visited hospitals both in the forward and Base areas where fractures were concentrated. The care given these cases and their results made an excellent impression on us, and since plaster has been the procedure of choice in Russia ever since Pirogoff, in the Crimean War, wrote about its wonderful properties (book published in 1865) we found them masters of this technique. Professor Yudin had cared for over 2,000 fractures in the Finnish war before this war began. Their principles of fracture care are: (1) splint in the field with wooden or wire splints or Thomas' splints. They prefer the Dietrich wooden splint which has an axilla and groin crutch; (2) at sorting-evacuation hospital, or mobile hospital, or base hospital where first definitive treatment is given, all dead and devitalized tissue is widely excised, sulfanilamide is placed in the wound. They often suture the wound open (skin edges to deep fascia) and prefer no gauze packs; (3) "Skintight" plaster is applied without dressing on the wound. They do not transport the cases for a few days. They excise wounds 5–10 days old in the same way and are not afraid of spreading sepsis. Hospitals up the line had good fracture tables and one used a piece of rubber over the dorsum of the foot which was later removed after the cast had set. Casts are not split and never use windows. For best work up the line, a good fracture surgeon with 8 assistants must have three tables going; one for careful preparation, one for the actual operation and one for the application of the cast.

Fracture and Joint Statistics

Time table relation of wounding to surgery (Yudin):   *Percent*

1 to 3 days	1.6
3 to 5 days	24.2
6 to 10 days	36.9
11 to 15 days	21.9
Beyond 15 days	15.4

83 percent

Reasons for changing original plaster cast:

Hemorrhage	2.4
Acute cellulitis	3.1
Sepsis	2.5
Continued fever	7.4
Rising temperature	13.9
Dislocation of fragments	4.7
Soiling of plaster	14.0
Changed at proper time	17.0
Complete recovery in first cast	35.0

	Percent
*Mortality in closed cast*_____	5. 4
Hemorrhage _____	1. 6
General intoxication_____	0. 3
Sepsis _____	2. 9
Tetanus _____	0. 3
Accidental _____	0. 3

Treatment of Joint Injuries

	Percent Mortality
Conservative treatment (drainage)_____	20
Removal of head_____	20
Resection of head and fragments_____	36. 2
Removal of fragments only_____	27

311 Joint cases (Yudin) (Practice excision of knee joint frequently):

Hip joint (75)_____	5
Knee joint (121)_____	6
Shoulder (41)_____	2
Elbow (68)_____	1
Fingers (7)_____	0

Followup study of 500 cases of wounds of joints showed 58 percent incision and drainage and 42 percent resection. Of these 22 percent of the first group were unhealed at 6 months and 28 percent of the resections were unhealed at that time. Arthroplasties were done in 42 percent of the cases incised and drained and in 8 percent of the resections.

D: Supply of Blood and Transfusion Service: The Red Army medical service uses great amounts of citrated whole fresh blood and little plasma. The blood is collected in the larger cities, chiefly Moscow (about 2,000 pints a day and in one hospital bleed 600 people daily). Use excellent technique, physical examination of donors including Wassermann reaction; grouping is done twice; bleed into 250 cc. ampoules with open ends which have rubber tube attachments which are bent over and sealed with paraffin. Blood is refrigerated at 6 degrees C and flown to fronts where it is distributed in refrigerated cars and in frontline hospitals is kept in deep cellars iced at 6–10 degrees C. It is not used after three weeks.

Cadaver blood is still being used at the Sklifossowsky Institute by Professor Yudin. From 1935 to 1943, 2964 cadavers have been bled yielding 5,092 liters of blood. Of this quantity 1,332 liters were discarded (240 for positive Wassermann reaction; 54 for acute bacterial endocarditis; 80 generalized tuberculosis). Bled from jugular vein in Trendelenburg position under aseptic precautions. If yield is small they wash out by injecting Ringer's solution in the arterial side. Sulfanilamide .06 percent is added for preservation. Other medical men do not approve of this method.

At the Central Institute for Blood and Transfusions in Moscow (Director, Professor A. A. Bagdasarov) daily bleeding of donors averages 600 in number. 250 ccs. is taken by gravity method into 2 ampoules (500 ccs. per donor); bleed into citrate solution (using 5 percent sodium citrates). Donors are given a special food ration and some money, but 85 percent of this is given back for airplane construction and other military purposes. Name of donor goes on each ampoule and often is the source of many romances. The donors are largely women. The Central Institute has 79 allied institutions and all plasma and serum is sent to the Central Institute for bacteriological testing before it goes to the army. Transportation to the army and civilian hospitals is by air and motor. The blood is good for 30 days under refrigeration if it is not moved; if transported, 15 to 17 days. Small insulated boxes with ice container hold 4 pints of blood.

Types of fluids used: (a) Whole blood (5 percent citrate and glucose to isotonicity); (b) Salt solution; (c) Special preservative fluid for use with whole blood which renders it useful twice as long as simple citrated blood but it must be added in proportion of 50 percent special fluid (C.I.B.T.) and 50 percent blood. (This C.I.B.T. fluid contains sodium chloride 7.5 grams, potassium chloride 0.4 gms., magnesium chloride 0.1 gms., sodium potassium phosphate 0.208 gms., sodium acid phosphate 0.119 gms., and glucose 10.0 gms. with distilled water to make 1,000 ccs.); (d) Alcohol-sugar solution (Silsovsky's Solution); sodium chloride 7.0 gms., potassium chloride 0.2 gms., magnesium sulphate .04 gms., Vobel's solution 3.3 ccs., glucose 54 gms. distilled water up to 1,000 ccs. (To this is added 80 ccs. of 96 percent alcohol); (e) Dried plasma—add sugar to isotonicity before drying. (Send forward with sterile distilled water, needle and connections. Plasma is kept labelled by groups—if over 750 ccs., it must be used in a compatible group); (f) Federov's solution—80 percent saline and 20 percent serum (not used much); (g) Blood serum—allow this to be made in other institutions but not plasma; (h) Colloid solution from casein—treat casein to detoxify of antigenic and anaphylactic properties, use as 2 or 4 percent solution; (i) Anesthetic and antishock solution—ephedrine, salt solution and codeins (amount not given).

In the army, they use plasma at regimental aid posts and transfusions of whole citrated blood at front hospitals. Believe blood is best treatment for traumatic shock and believe Academician Lena Stern's suboccipital injection of potassium phosphate solution purely experimental.

E: Amputations—practiced as little as possible and rarely in the upper extremities. When done short flap technique and early use of bucket and stick to keep muscles in training. Of amputations done in forward hospitals, 50 percent are reamputed in special centers in base area where prosthetic appliances are specialized in. In such base centers they practice some kineplastic amputations such as forearm with ulna and radius separated for useful stump. They continuously improve prostheses by the utilization of new ideas of the patients who work out individual problems according to the type of future work and the length of the stump. Points of election for amputation are roughly our own. Use button of preserved bone in medullary cavity end of stump.

F: Plastic surgery—Orders are issued in the front areas not to remove bone and skin in jaw and face wounds and not to suture but to leave for experts in base area centers. In facio-maxillary and plastic centers, excellent work is being done, using tubular waltzing grafts well. By the use of early secondary sutures they reduce the plastic work. One specialist, Professor Frumkin, had made 12 new penises out of tubular grafts containing some cartilage from thoracic cage which he waltzed down.

G: Frostbite—The Russian soldier wears woolen wrappings about his feet and thick felt moccasin boots in the winter time. It is in the season of thawing that the large number of frostbite cases occur. Lt. Gen. S. S. Guirgolave, who is accepted as the authority on frostbite in the Red Army, emphasizes the following points:

Damage produced by cold may be divided into the local and general effects. Congelation (formation of ice in the tissues) never follows the local effects even with the descent of the tissue temperature to zero degrees. The pathological processes, and in particular necrosis, are secondary and are a consequence of changes in the viability and metabolism of the tissues and are not an immediate primary effect of refrigeration. The local effects are the result of meteorological and other factors which lower the local and general resistance of the organism, so that the lesions produced are equivalent to those caused by long exposure to intense cold. In the development of the local effects, there is a "prereactive" period during which, by proper treatment, many of the serious lesions can be prevented.

At a body temperature of plus 26 to plus 28 degrees C, the thermoregulatory mechanism of a homeothermic animal ceases to function and it becomes isothermic. An animal, under such conditions, cannot re-establish a normal temperature by normal means and must be actively heated. By a special technique (electro-thermometrie) in which the central nervous system plays a specific and preponderant role, the damaging effects of cold can be reversed. Carbohydrate metabolism, the adrenal glands and the sympathetic nervous system play important roles in this treatment. Intensive and active heating of the frozen parts and of the body must be carried out in line with these pathogenic conceptions in order to treat rationally and prevent the lesions produced by cold. Rapid heating for 20 or 30 minutes causes no damage to the affected parts or to the body. An animal rapidly heated loses less tissue than one slowly heated. Rapid heating has a beneficial effect upon the functions of the cardiovascular and respiratory systems.

Longitudinal incisions should be made in necrotic tissue within 5–6 days and should extend as far as there is no pain or bleeding. In the presence of subcutaneous edematous fluid such an operation (necrotomy) causes a dry gangrene of the part to develop rapidly. If bones are involved amputation of the necrotic portion should be done 6–10 days after injury. These procedures reduce by two to three times the length of time necessary to treat tissue damaged by cold.

H: Neurological Surgery—There are 16 neurological surgeons at the front who have at their disposal 3,200 beds and there are three large hospitals in the rear with clinics which provide 3,700 beds. In other words there are 6,900 beds in the Soviet Union devoted to the care of neurosurgical injuries and diseases. At the front, 2.9% of all surgical beds are for neurosurgical patients, and in the rear hospitals the percentage is 4.3.

Neurosurgical surgeons in the U.S.S.R. have all been trained under the supervision of Lt. Gen. (Academician) Burdenko who dictates and directs all policies and the expression thereof.

The sorting and evacuation of neurosurgical injuries to special hospitals is practiced as far forward as possible in the combat zone and the one neurosurgical group inspected by the mission was on the Vyazma sector in Sorting-Evacuation Hospital No. 290 located about 70 kilometers from the frontline. The maximum distance for evacuation to such a hospital should not exceed 48–72 hours from the receipt of injury. The most seriously wounded are not moved and not operated upon, and it is concluded that they are expected to be mortally wounded cases. Those injured in whom an operation is possible but who are in shock are kept until shock is treated and then evacuated. Hemorrhages and a rise in intracranial pressure are indications for operation on the spot. Neurosurgical definitive care must be located, according to their dictates, at a maximum distance of 2–3 days from the frontline with trained neurosurgeons, neurologist, neuropathologist, ophthalmologist and otolaryngologist in attendance. Evacuation must be rapid, smooth and preferably by air at altitudes not exceeding 5,000 meters. It is agreed that craniocerebral wounds stand evacuation better before than after operation. Postponed operations in well-equipped and staffed hospitals are preferred to immediate operations under poor conditions.

Sulfonamides locally placed in craniocerebral wounds is advocated, but General Burdenko complained that they were not used immediately as systematically at the front as they should be. Sulfonamides are also given to the patients orally and intravenously.

In the first 24 hours after injury 21% were treated in the "First Line"; 20% in the "Second Line"; and 14% in the "Third Line." In the second 24 hours the percentages respectively were 59, 62, and 65 and in the third 24 hours the percentages were respectively 19, 19, and 11. The mortality of craniocerebral wounds in the rear hospitals is 8% and for spinal cord injuries 56%.

Indications for operation in spinal cord injuries are not clear, but they are stated as (a) prophylaxis against infection; (b) symptomatic, and (c) morphological. The clinical conditions for which operation is advised include progressive paralysis, traumatic edema, subarachnoid space block, pain, and meningitis.

The surgical technique employed in the treatment of craniocerebral wounds consists of irrigation of the wound tract with a bulb syringe and suction removal of the blood and injured brain tissue. Treatment of the dural wound is not considered necessary and the lacerated dura is never sutured. Rubber ring pressure dressings are employed to treat cerebral fungi or herniations. Well-encapsulated brain abscesses are removed in toto by electrocoagulation, and drainage is seldom employed. Contrast media for the diagnosis of abscesses and the location of fragments around the abscess are used.

Formalin fixed nerve and spinal cord grafts are used for the repair of large continuity defects in peripheral nerve injuries. The grafts are fixed successively in alcohol, alcoholic ether, alcoholic glycerin, magnesium chloride, and glucose. Twenty-seven patients have been so operated upon, but none of these were presented for demonstration or examination of the results obtained. The microscopic evidence of the experimental studies was not conclusive.

At the Institute of Experimental Medicine, Prof. Propper Graschenko has 150 neurosurgical beds and is conducting problems of clinical research both in the frontline area and at this Institute so that he has continuous control over patients selected for study. He is studying (1) the character of head injuries, their course, and the influence of infection upon the healing of the wounds; (2) the clinical and bacteriological application of sulfonamides to craniocerebral injuries; (3) the diagnosis of early and late traumatic encephalitis and cerebral abscess and (4) the rehabilitation therapy of craniocerebral and peripheral nerve injuries. He has at his disposal an auxiliary microbiological laboratory staff, half of which is at the front and the remainder in the rear zone.

In the short time at his disposal he presented his work upon gas gangrene infections and other anaerobic infections of the brain. Under field conditions, 100 cases of craniocerebral injuries were studied bacteriologically and in 20.3% pathogenic organisms were present; in 24% aerobic organisms were cultured; in 12.4% sporogenic (putrid anaerobes) organisms were present; in 26.8% coccal infections were present; in 16.5% miscellaneous organisms were found. These cultures were made from 48 to 72 hours after receipt of the injury. In 620 cases examined bacteriologically, only 2 were found to be sterile.

After 3 to 4 weeks wounds showed a flora of pathogenic anaerobes in 12%; aerobes in 20%; cocci in 70% and 8 to 10% were infected with putrid anerobes. Of the 20.3% in which pathogenic anaerobes were found, 1.4% died in 6–7 days of severe gas gangrene infections. Subacute anaerobic infection of the brain is found in all large brain fungi, and of 12 such cases, 9 died. Thirty-two cases of chronic anaerobic infection of the brain were studied, and of these 10 died. The course was long 3–4 months, and often encapsulated abscesses formed which often opened on to the surface or into the ventricles with the production of a severe meningitis. In 34 cases of mild anaerobic infection of the brain, there were no deaths.

The types of anaerobic infection of the brain found included *Clostridium perfringens* (*Cl. welchii*), *Cl. sordellii*, *Cl. fallax*, *Cl. oedematiens*, *Cl. oedematiens maligni* and *Streptococcus anaerobius*. A serum is used against gas gangrene infection which is polyvalent and contains *Cl. histolyticum*, *Cl. perfringens*, *Cl. oedematiens* and *Cl. oedematiens maligni*. A prophylactic dose of 10,000 international units is given intramuscularly and therapeutic doses of 3–40,000 units are used intravenously and intramuscularly.

I: New Clinical Methods under Study—

(a) The injection of 70 percent alcohol with 2 percent Novocain solution about fractures in the early days following injury to increase blood supply and to stimulate callus formation. (The mission was not convinced of the usefulness of this procedure.)

(b) The use of placental extract to stimulate healing in chronic wounds or the growth of skin in severe burns.

(c) The use of a cytotoxin made by injecting mesenchymal tissue into a horse and using his antiserum to stimulate the healing of ulcers of the stomach, healing of bone, loosening of scars and stiffness in joints. (The mission was not convinced of the usefulness of this procedure.)

(d) The use of smoke from burning pine wood to stimulate healing (??).

(e) The use of naphthalen (a heavy oil) broken down by ultrasonic method to stimulate healing (??).

(f) Treatment of shock by the suboccipital cistern injection of potassium phosphate solution to stimulate the [vasomotor] centers in medulla. (See article by Lena S. Stern in Lancet Nov. 14, 1942, page 572.)

J: City Accident and Medical Service: Here we saw an excellent demonstration of the Russian ability at organization which surprised us. The Sklifossowsky Institute is the center of this work for Moscow but has 6 or 7 "district" hospitals. All telephone calls come into a central telephone room at this Institute where there are many switch boards and an elaborate system of intercommunication and directing officials. Apparently patients, doctors, police or friends may call in and state facts. Ambulances go out immediately either from the Central Institute or from the nearest hospital to patient after the information is relayed to that hospital. If a doctor is not necessary he does not go on ambulance, but if there has been an accident or if the case is questionable the ambulance contains a doctor, nurse, and driver. As the message leaves the telephone central room in writing, a time clock is started and officials in the room know when the ambulance leaves, for the doctor, nurse, and driver all press separate buttons [which flash lights on in the central telephone room] as they leave. A check list is also kept by director of the time consumed by each operator per case and number of cases per day. Also, the director in a separate room can plug into any line and listen to incoming and outgoing calls. The system, in part, was like that of an Air Raid Warden's set up in some American cities.

K: Gifts to U.S.S.R.—At our original meeting with the People's Commissar for Public Health we spoke of our gifts, letters, etc. Letters cannot be delivered directly to the individual, and conversation with a Russian is safe for him only when some other Russian is present. Two days later Professor Koreisha came to the hotel and took away the penicillin, our letters, and other gifts. General Smirnov, and General Burdenko came to us personally to ask that their thanks be transmitted to General Hawley for his letter. Both stated they would write him in length. General Smirnov toasted a meeting to General Hawley in Berlin as suggested in the latter's letter. No more information regarding the gifts has been forthcoming.

L: Women in Russia: One of the most impressive things is the obvious equality of men and women, and the latter do everything that men do. They are in the Army as soldiers and officers. In the line, we were told there was no woman with a higher rank than colonel. We saw several junior officers with artillery and infantry insignia. In the Medical Service the Inspector General (Brigadier Surgeon Valentina Gorinovskaya) is a woman. Most of the traffic officers all the way from Moscow to Vyazma were women carrying rifles. Trolley cars are run by women. Women help lay car tracks in the city. The nurses not on duty at the 290 Evacuation Sorting Hospital were doing the major share in the construction of the new log houses for future wards.

/s/   Elliott C. Cutler
ELLIOTT C. CUTLER
Colonel, Medical Corps,
Chief Consultant in Surgery

/s/   Loyal Davis
LOYAL DAVIS
Lieutenant Colonel, Medical Corps,
Senior Consultant in Neurological Surgery

APPENDIX B

OFFICE OF THE CHIEF SURGEON
EUROPEAN THEATER OF OPERATIONS

15 May 1944

CIRCULAR LETTER NO. 71

SUBJECT: Principles of Surgical Management in the Care of Battle Casualties.

1. Surgical Echelons.
2. Morphine.
3. Blood Transfusions.
4. "Transportable" and "Non-transportable."
5. Surgical Procedures.
6. Sulfonamide Therapy.
7. Penicillin Therapy.
8. Secondary Closure.
9. General Principles to be followed in the Use of Plaster Casts.
10. Treatment of Anaerobic Infections.
11. Radiology in Forward Area.
12. Identification of Gases in Cylinders.

1. *Surgical Echelons.*

This first paragraph has been extracted, with only minor changes, from a circular letter, Office of the Surgeon, North African Theater of Operations. The policies expressed herein are sound, are based upon experiences in combat and will in general govern the activities of Medical Department personnel in this Theater.

a. The welfare of the patient and the tactical necessity for rapid evacuation demand a clear understanding of the function or mission of each unit of the Army Medical Corps. This is best arrived at by dividing the treatment of a casualty into two stages, primary and definitive. Separate groups of units provide each stage of treatment. In general, the equipment of each group is designed for that purpose only.

b. Stations of the first and second echelons, Aid Stations, Collecting Stations and Clearing Stations, are equipped and staffed for the primary phase of treatment. Arrest of hemorrhage, splinting of the injury, resuscitation measures needed to make the patient transportable, and administration of sulfonamides are the urgent functions of these stations. In addition, the treatment of minor injuries that allow immediate return to duty, is carried out without evacuation. A Clearing Station or functionally similar medical installation, is not designed to provide definitive treatment for battle casualties.

c. It must be remembered that the lightly wounded soldier or a casualty due to accident may regain full combat status within the Theater if proper surgical treatment is carried out, but the Theater may be deprived of his service by faulty surgical judgment. Because a surgical procedure appears simple is not sufficient reason for performing it in a Clearing Station unless the man can be returned to immediate duty without evacuation to the rear.

d. Hospitals of the third echelon, Evacuation Hospitals and Field Hospitals with attached Surgical Teams, are designed to initiate definitive surgical treatment to battle casualties. The more delay there is before reaching this echelon, and the more hands the patient passes through in reaching it, the poorer will be the final results. The evacuation line is *not an assembly line* in which each surgeon does his bit to the patient. It is a *conveyer line*, along the course of which the progress of the patient may be halted to save life or limb, or to render him transportable.

e. Although Field and Evacuation Hospitals with attached Surgical Teams are adequately equipped and staffed to perform rehabilitation operations, they are not designed for this function. Even in quiet times, patients requiring rehabilitation operations will be evacuated to a fourth echelon hospital except when the Commanding Officer decides otherwise, based on knowledge of the tactical situation as well as the surgical aspects of an individual case.

2. *Morphine.*

This note appears because, although morphine is one of humanity's greatest aids in warfare, it is also often misused and frequently given in unnecessarily large and dangerous quantities.

a. *Dosage.* Morphine sulfate gr. ¼ (15 mgm.) is usually adequate; ½ gr. (30 mgm.) may be required and is safe unless repeated. *Always record amount and time of injection.*

b. *Administration.* Subcutaneous or intramuscular injection is employed when a gradual prolonged effect is desired. Massage at the site of injection will hasten absorption. Intravenous injection (gr. ⅛, 8 mgm.) is employed when a rapid effect is desired.

c. *Contra-indications.* The doses of morphine given as preoperative medication for seriously wounded patients should be small (gr. ⅙, 10 mgm. or less). Morphine must be administered with caution to the walking wounded, to patients to be evacuated by air; or in the presence of jaundice, cranio-cerebral injury, pneumothorax, hemothorax or pleural effusions. Morphine will never be used as a sedative for manic or hysterical states.

d. *Poisoning.* Overdosage with morphine is characterized by pinpoint pupils and slow respirations. The outstanding serious effect is anoxia, caused by respiratory depression.

e. *Delayed Morphine Poisoning in Battle Casualties.* Subcutaneous injections of morphine are poorly absorbed in patients who are cold, or who have a low blood pressure and are in shock, under which circumstances pain may not be relieved. As a result, repeated doses given in an attempt to relieve pain may be followed by morphine poisoning when the peripheral circulation is re-established and the unabsorbed deposits of morphine are absorbed rapidly. The intravenous administration of morphine in patients who are cold, or who have low blood pressure and are in shock, will eliminate this problem. Always check for previous administration of morphine and always record the amount and time given.

f. *Treatment of Morphine Poisoning.* Provide a clear airway. Administer oxygen, under intermittent pressure if necessary. A maximal dose of ephedrine, gr. ½ (30 mgm.) administered intravenously, using rise in blood pressure as a guide to dosage, may be employed. Caffein sodium benzoate, gr. 7½ (0.5 gm.) intravenously, may be useful. Empty the stomach prior to development of coma. Stimulate diuresis by means of intravenous glucose. Change position of patient frequently.

3. *Blood Transfusion.*

a. Blood used in the treatment of casualties in shock will ordinarily be administered in the ratio of one part blood to two parts of plasma (one pint of blood to four units of plasma).

b. *Procurement of blood within unit:* Units equipped with the Field Transfusion Kit will follow the instructions contained therein for bleeding lightly wounded and non-combatant personnel and for care of the apparatus.

c. *Procurement of blood from ETO Blood Bank:* Evacuation Hospitals, Field Hospitals, LST's, Holding Units and Transit Hospitals will be supplied with blood from the ETO Blood Bank. All blood from this source is Type O and will not be cross-matched. On the bottle label is an expiration date, beyond which the blood will not be used. The following rules will be strictly followed in the use of Bank blood :—

(1) Blood will be refrigerated constantly between two (2) and four (4) degrees above zero centigrade (+35 to +42 F.) and kept in the dark.

(2) Blood will be removed from the refrigerator and administered cold. It will under no circumstances be pre-heated.

(3) Blood which is allowed to rise above six (6) degrees centigrade will be used within four (4) hours and will not be re-cooled.

(4) All used equipment will be exchanged at time of delivery of blood.

d. *Non-transportable Casualties.*

The *proper sorting* of casualties into transportable and non-transportable classes is of prime importance in evacuation. The following listed types of casualties are usually non-transportable and should be submitted to surgery early. This classification can only serve as a guide, and each individual case deserves separate appraisal.

4. *Non-transportable Casualties.*

a. Wounds of the abdomen.

b. Wounds of the chest which are serious, either because of—

(1) a large sucking wound, or

(2) such massive intra-thoracic hemorrhage that the patient's condition is unsuitable for transportation.

c. Trans-thoracic or abdomino-thoracic wounds. These are often difficult to diagnose and are frequently missed—note that in wounds of the buttock the missile may lodge in the thorax or, similarly, with wounds of the shoulder the missile may lie within the abdominal cavity. If X-rays are available, final lodgement of the missile will make diagnosis easy, but if not, the medical officer must always examine the opposite cavity from wounding to rule this out.

d. Casualties who remain in "shock" after therapy, and whose condition cannot be made suitable for transport. In this group are included multiple fractures, casualties with injury to major vessels, and avascular extremities in which gas infection is likely to occur, and those with concealed hemorrhage.

e. Certain casualties with maxillofacial wounds, where mechanical difficulty in breathing endangers life during transport.

5. *Surgical Procedures.*

a. *Dressings.* Ideally, the primary phase of treatment will be completed in the first unit reached that is equipped to provide it. The dressing is to then be left undisturbed until the patient reaches a third echelon unit for operation. There are certain safeguards and adjustments that must take place en route, but these *do not include inspection of the wound by removal of the dressing unless definite indications for so doing are present.* A compound fracture case may be halted at the Clearing Station for more adequate immobilization or resuscitation, but the wound should not be re-dressed unless necessary to arrest continuing hemorrhage. A wound will not be re-dressed solely for the purpose of re-applying local sulfonamide. Oral administration is sufficient safeguard.

The same principles apply after operation has been completed and the patient is being evacuated to the rear. Uninformed hands do unnecessary dressings. The best safeguard for a patient is an adequate and legible record that accompanies him, which makes it possible for a receiving officer to refer to the record rather than looking at the wound. Infection arising from contamination incurred at the time dressings are changed may make impossible secondary suture of wounds after debridement and arrival at a third echelon unit.

b. *Debridement of wounds.* This is the basis of the proper treatment of all battle casualties. It is definitely more important than chemotherapy, and reliance on the latter must not diminish devotion to the proper surgical treatment of wounds. Use *ample incisions*, practice *minimal removal of skin and bone*, and *maximum removal of all dead or devitalized muscle. Never close primarily wounds debrided under field conditions.* Pack wounds open lightly, *never plug tightly.*

Under favorable circumstances, it is desirable that severed nerves and tendons should be approximated, preferably with metallic or non-absorbable sutures (see Manual of Therapy, European Theater of Operations).

c. *Amputations.* Amputations for trauma will be a circular open (guillotine) amputation at the lowest possible level, followed by the application of skin traction. Skin traction will be applied immediately and must be maintained during all stages of evacuation, including evacuation to the Zone of Interior, and until the stump is completely healed. Skin grafting will not be used as a substitute for skin traction.

6. *Sulfonamide Therapy.*

a. A soldier wounded in action is instructed to take by mouth, as soon as possible, 4 gms. (8 tablets) of sulfadiazine, from his own First Aid packet, except when wounded in the abdomen.

b. The medical officer first dressing the wound should frost it *lightly* with sulfanilamide powder. Not more than 5 gms. (contents of one packet) should be placed in the wounds of any individual, irrespective of the number and size of the wounds.

c. Continue sulfadiazine orally until definitive surgery is instituted. The maintenance dosage is 1 gm. orally every 4 to 6 hours, or 2 gms. parenterally every 8 to 12 hours. Chemotherapy should be given cautiously in the presence of dehydration (for dangers, see Manual of Therapy, European Theater of Operations).

d. Sulfonamide and penicillin therapy will be carried out concurrently.

e. Both penicillin and a sulfonamide should be placed in wounds after definitive surgical treatment (see par. 7h).

f. Sulfonamide therapy will be continued after surgical treatment by oral or parenteral routes, as instructed in the Manual of Therapy, European Theater of Operations.

g. Sulfonamide therapy for *burns* shall consist only of parenteral therapy or local application, *never both.*

7. *Penicillin Therapy.*

a. Penicillin therapy (parenteral) will begin at Clearing Stations, and will be continued at Field and Evacuation Hospitals. Its local use in wounds will begin in Field and Evacuation Hospitals where definitive surgery is carried out.

b. The phrase "Penicillin Treated" will be entered on the EMT or Field Medical Record after the diagnosis in every case so treated. Additional data, including dosage in units, method of administration (parenteral or local) and time and date of administration will be entered on the back of the [EMT] or on Clinical Record form in cases where a Field Medical Record has been initiated.

c. Penicillin is unstable and is best preserved at 4° centigrade. Where refrigerators are not available, keep in *coolest spot possible* and away from sunlight. *Use as soon as possible after removal from hermetically sealed vial,* whether in normal saline or sulfanilamide powder. Vials which are out-dated will not be discarded.

d. Do not use in small superficial wounds of gutter type, or where missile lies close to skin and no fracture.

e. *Parenteral Therapy.*

(1) For *parenteral use* penicillin is dissolved in normal saline. Add 10 cc. *cold* normal saline to 100,000 unit vial of penicillin and inject intramuscularly 2 cc. per casualty. Needles and syringes must not be sterilized by use of antiseptic solutions and must be *cold* because both chemicals and heat inactivate penicillin.

(2) Penetrating and perforating wounds of soft parts: give 20,000 units intramuscularly every 4 hours from Clearing Station through period of definitive surgery and for 48 hours thereafter.

(3) Wounds with *compound fractures:* give 20,000 units intramuscularly every 4 hours from Clearing Station through period of definitive surgery and for 72 hours thereafter.

f. Double above doses, paras. e (2) and (3), where wounds are in region of buttock, perineum, upper thighs and popliteal space.

g. Penicillin therapy may be extended beyond the 48 and 72 hour specified post-operative time, paras. e (1) and (2), if sepsis becomes a major problem.

h. *Local use in wounds* (both soft part wounds and compound fractures) at time of definitive surgery; Dust 20,000 units of penicillin mixed with 3 grams (1 teaspoonful) of sulfanilamide into the wound at the close of the debridement. This is best accomplished by mixing the contents of a 100,000 unit vial with 15 grams (5 teaspoonfuls) of sulfanilamide, and using 1 teaspoonful per wound. All containers must be absolutely *dry and cool* before mixing. Where wounds are multiple, use up to 40,000 units of penicillin in 6 grams of sulfanilamide, distributing proportionately according to severity of wounds. The use of penicillin in wounds is not mandatory but is advisable in all wounds where there is severe destruction of tissue. Should the supply of penicillin be limited, omit local application.

i. Penicillin therapy does not contradict or interfere with sulfonamide therapy.

8. *Secondary Closure.*

a. Although the first principle for the military surgeon to bear in mind is not to close the wound he has freshly debrided, it is essential that he close this wound at the earliest possible moment that is safe. Early closure means limitation of infection and fibrosis, and an earlier restoration to duty. If the primary debridement has been thorough, small wounds may be closed as early as the third day, though the average wound not until the fifth day. Observation of the signs of inflammation, such as discharge, reddening, pain and swelling, will determine whether or not a wound can be closed. It is wiser not to dress the originally debrided wound until the day when secondary closure might be practical, since each dressing invites contamination of the wound. If closure is considered safe, it should be done loosely without undermining the edges or using sharp instruments, and by using retention sutures of silk, or silkworm gut, spaced widely apart and loosely tied. Should mild infection appear, hot, moist dressings may save breaking down of the wound and hasten the healing process. Any signs of severe infection require immediate removal of the sutures.

b. Closure of wounds with fractures should only be undertaken when full penicillin therapy is being practiced and when all the signs of infection are absent.

c. Wounds closed early, before the establishment of granulation tissue or scar tissue, are easier to close than those closed after one or two weeks. In wounds that have been open for a long time, skin grafting is often better than closure by suture. If the original debridement has been practiced with the minimal of skin removal, as suggested above, closure by sutures will be simple.

d. Removal of sutures from such secondary closures should not take place before 10 days unless stitch infection develops. After removal of the sutures it may be wise to maintain approximation of the wound edges with adhesive plaster.

9. *General Principles to be followed in the Use of Plaster Casts.*

a. No circular bandages, dressings, or strips of adhesive shall be used under a plaster cast, as these constrict the extremity and may cause extensive damage if swelling of the part occurs.

b. Adequately padded plasters are probably safer in average hands. Padding should be applied to all bony prominences such as malleoli and heels, knees, particularly over the head of the fibula, wrists and elbows. In addition, sufficient padding should be used over the soft parts to permit some swelling within the cast.

c. *All layers of plaster, sheet wadding or dressings must be cut through down to the skin immediately after the application of a cast following an operation or manipulation. Swelling of the part will occur and, unless all layers of the plaster padding and dressings are cut through, it will be impossible to spread the cast to prevent extensive damage when swelling occurs.*

d. Attention should be paid to the position of the extremity encased in plaster. The foot should be at a right angle to the leg, the knee should be in 10°–15° of flexion, the hip should be in neutral position or slight flexion. The wrist should be supported in neutral position to prevent wrist drop, and the elbow ordinarily is best supported at a right angle. In these positions the patient will transport comfortably, will not take up undue space, and the tendency to develop troublesome fixed deformities will be minimized.

e. A line diagram in indelible pencil should be inscribed on the cast, indicating the approximate location of fracture and position of fragments. The number of the unit, date of injury, date of operation and type of operation should likewise be written on the cast so that if the Field Medical Record is lost, a reasonably satisfactory substitute record will be readily available.

f. Either a platform or a loop or wicket of plaster should be applied to the foot of the cast in order to protect the toes from pressure of blankets, bed clothes, et cetera. Plaster applied to the hand should be trimmed back to the proximal palmar crease to permit full flexion of the fingers and metacarpal phalangeal joints.

10. *Treatment of Anaerobic Infections.*

a. *Gas Gangrene.*

(1) *Types of Wound.* Wounds destroying muscle, either directly or by interruption of the blood supply, are particularly susceptible to anaerobic infections. Such infections are more frequent at the following sites of wounds:—(i) buttock; (ii) upper thigh (compound fracture of femur); (iii) anterior tibial group; (iv) shoulder girdle; (v) short flexors and extensors of forearm.

(2) *Types of Infection.* The following types of infection must be recognized, since they require different therapy:—

    a. Gas gangrene (clostridial).

        (*1*) Diffuse myositis.

        (*2*) Localized myositis.

        (*3*) Cellulitis, "gas abscess."

    b. Gas gangrene (streptococcal), rare.

        (*1*) Myositis.

(3) *Diagnosis.*

a. Clinical. The differential diagnosis among the various types of clostridial gas gangrene and streptococcal myositis must be made to avoid unnecessary radical surgical treatment.

(*1*) *Clostridial myositis, diffuse:* This may develop within 6 hours from the time of wounding, usually within 3 days. The onset is acute with a severe systemic reaction. Locally there is *pain, marked swelling,* frequently *profuse serous exudate, slight gas* formation, *variable odor* of decay and pale or blue-gray appearance of involved muscle. The skin is tense and often white, but may be mottled with a livid appearance if the process is widespread.

(*2*) *Clostridial myositis, localized:* In 5–10 percent of the cases, localization of the process to a single muscle or group of muscles occurs. Symptoms and signs are the same as for the diffuse type.

(*3*) *Clostridial cellulitis:* This process is limited to the immediate area of the wound. The onset is gradual, usually after 3 days, with slight systemic reaction. Locally, there is *abundant gas* formation with a foul odor, slight swelling, and *little local change* of the muscle and overlying skin.

(*4*) *Streptococcal myositis:* The onset is delayed for 3–4 days, and severe systemic reactions do not appear until the late stages of the infection. Locally, there is *marked swelling* with *profuse purulent discharge, slight gas formation,* and *slight odor.* The involved muscle is slightly edematous and the overlying *skin is tense,* often with a coppery tinge. Streptococcal myositis comprises only a few of the cases of gas gangrene.

b. Laboratory. Recognition of infections with anaerobic bacteria is made on clinical findings, which should be checked, where possible, with a smear made from the material in the depth of the wound. A small piece of involved muscle, rubbed on a glass slide and stained by the Gram method, is examined under the microscope. In the presence of clostridial gas gangrene, such smears usually show a predominance of large gram-positive rods. Pus cells are scanty and degenerate. In streptococcal myositis, gram-positive bacilli are absent and in their place large numbers of small-sized streptococci are found among masses of pus cells. Whenever facilities are available, anaerobic wound and blood cultures should be carried out.

The finding of anaerobic bacteria in a wound is not uncommon, and such finding should not influence the surgical treatment, unless there are local clinical signs of anaerobic infection.

(4) *Prophylaxis.* Early, adequate debridement of wounds is the best prophylaxis for anaerobic infections. Debridement where there has been massive destruction of tissues, more particularly in the region of the buttocks, perineum and upper thighs, and where major vessels are injured, must be radical and thorough, using long incisions. If hematoma is present, deep fascial planes must be incised, especially in the popliteal area. Bilateral incisions in the popliteal space just inside the hamstring tendons should be made. The fascia over both heads of the gastrocnemius should be incised—all clots should be evacuated and any continued bleeding controlled by ligature or suture. Gas gangrene antitoxin, sulfonamides and penicillin are not to be considered substitutes for early, adequate debridement. However, where circumstances delay debridement of the wounds mentioned in para. 10. a. (1), for 24 hours or longer, one (1) ampule of gas gangrene antitoxin may be given intramuscularly. Penicillin and sulfonamides are to be used as directed in paras. 6 and 7.

(5) *Therapy.*

a. Surgical. This depends upon the extent of the disease and the type of anaerobic infection. Diffuse clostridial cellulitis is encountered in approximately 80 percent of cases in these categories.

(1) *Clostridial myositis, diffuse:* Amputation as far above visible evidence of involvement as possible *must be carried out immediately,* using the guillotine method, and leaving the wound open.

(2) *Clostridial myositis, localized:* Extirpation of the involved muscle, or group of muscles, should be practiced through long incision.

(3) *Clostridial cellulitis:* Incise the localized process and remove the devitalized tissue. Radical surgery is not indicated.

(4) *Streptococcal myositis:* Extensively incise and drain the involved muscles. Radical extirpation or immediate amputation are not indicated.

b. Serum therapy.

(1) *Clostridial infections:* Three (3) ampules of gas gangrene antitoxin should be given intravenously and repeated hourly for 6 doses (see Manual of Therapy, European Theater of Operations, page 35, para. 27). This may be modified according to the condition of the individual case. Test patient for allergy to horse serum before administration of antitoxin. Adrenalin in a syringe should be at hand.

(2) *Streptococcal infections:* No serotherapy is indicated.

c. Chemotherapy.

(1) *Penicillin:* Give initial dose of 20,000 units, intravenously and 20,000 units intramuscularly, followed by 20,000 units intramuscularly every 2 hours for a period of 3 days. Period of therapy may be modified as seems necessary. Place in the wound 50,000 units mixed in 4 gms. (1 teaspoonful) of sulfanilamide, and repeat at dressings.

(2) *Sulfonamides:* Give 5 gms. of sulfadiazine by mouth initially and 1 gm. every 4 hours.

d. Supportive treatment. Since there is rapid destruction of erythrocytes, frequent whole-blood transfusions will be necessary.

e. All instruments used in anaerobic infections should be sterilized by autoclaving, when available, and the instruments must not be covered with oil, since bacteria surrounded by oil cannot be wetted and therefore are not killed at the usual temperatures.

f. If gas gangrene antitoxin is used, record number of ampules used and name of manufacturer.

b. *Tetanus.*

(1) *Types of Wound.* Any wound, regardless of size or location, is a potential source of tetanus, particularly small puncture wounds.

(2) *Prophylaxis.*

a. Every wounded man will receive 1 cc. of tetanus toxoid, subcutaneously, as soon as possible. This will be recorded on the Emergency Medical Tag, or on the Field Medical Record. If there is no record of the administration of toxoid, or any doubt as to its previous administration, 1 cc. of tetanus toxoid will be given and so recorded.

b. Early, adequate debridement.

c. 1 cc. of tetanus toxoid will be given prior to the manipulation or exploration of an old wound.

d. After appropriate tests for sensitivity, members of Allied Forces (except Canadian), civilians and others will receive 3,000 units of tetanus antitoxin intramuscularly. The Canadian Forces will receive 1 cc. of tetanus toxoid. A syringe containing 1 cc. of 1:1,000 of epinephrine (adrenalin) should always be at hand when tetanus antitoxin is given.

(3) *Signs and Symptoms.* The rarity of this disease must not prevent its recognition. The earlier tetanus is recognized, the more effective treatment will be. The earliest sign is trismus. The patient may complain of pain and stiffness in the neck, back and abdomen. Dysphagia may be present. Localized tetanic contractions are not uncommon.

(4) *Treatment.*

a. *General.* At the appearance of the earliest signs of tetanus, immediate therapy is indicated. All cases must be treated vigorously. The patient should be isolated in a quiet, darkened room.

b. *Control of spasms.* Trismus may be controlled by administration of barbiturates, e.g. Nembutal, which are essentially anti-spasmodic in action. Nembutal, grs. 3 (0.2 gms.) may be given rectally in a well-lubricated capsule that has been perforated several times with a pin. More rapid absorption will be effected if the contents of a capsule are dissolved in water and the solution injected rectally through a catheter of small caliber. The dose may be repeated as required, care being taken to guard against cumulative action and the production of anesthesia. Sodium Amytal, grs. 6 (0.4 gms.) represents an equivalent dose and for treatment over a period of days this drug is to be preferred. Overdosage will be indicated by evidence of hyperpyrexia and incipient atelectasis or pulmonary edema. For spasm involving many muscular groups where anoxia is a feature, administration of Pentothal sodium in 2.5 percent solution intravenously is indicated. The objective is to give just sufficient to control the seizure and to permit effective artificial respiration. From 2 to 4 cc. may be required. Longer acting barbiturates are preferable for prolonged control of spasms, but supplementary administration of Pentothal may be necessary to control acute episodes producing anoxia. For the same purpose, 0.5 gm. of Sodium Amytal, dissolved in 10 cc. of sterile distilled water, may be injected intravenously at the rate of 1 cc. per minute. Avoid use of long acting barbiturates such as Veronal or Luminal because of its cumulative action.

Supportive treatment, administration of saline, glucose and/or plasma, is essential. The prime requisite is to maintain oxygenation, producing muscular relaxation to permit effective respiratory action. All efforts will be defeated if obstruction of the upper respiratory tract is permitted.

Tracheotomy should be performed if laryngeal spasm is causing suffocation.

c. *Antitoxin.*

(1) *Locally.* After appropriate tests for sensitization, 10,000 units of tetanus antitoxin should be used for infiltration about the wound.

(2) *Intramuscularly.* Therapeutic administration of tetanus antitoxin should be early and adequate. After appropriate tests of sensitization, an initial dose of 40,000 units of antitoxin should be given intramuscularly.

(3) *Intravenously.* 20,000 units may be administered intravenously 6 hours after the intramuscular injection. This dosage may be repeated on the second and third

days if conditions require. Extremely large doses of antitoxin are no longer considered helpful.

(*4*) *Intraspinal.* Antitoxin should not be given intrathecally.

d. *Surgical.*

(*1*) *Local debridement.* This is based on the fact that the bacterial anaerobes are the sole source of the toxin. The wound must be widely opened and kept open. Amputation must be considered if other reasoning is suggestive of such a radical procedure. Such debridement should be preceded by the local injection of antitoxin as described in para. *c.* (*1*) above.

11. *Radiology in Forward Area.*

Attention to the following general principles will improve the efficiency of a forward area X-ray service, especially when casualties are received in large numbers.

a. *Housing.* Evacuation hospitals should be arranged to do radiography, fluoroscopy and processing simultaneously. One way to accomplish this is to use a ward tent plus two darkroom tents, one for radiography and one for fluoroscopy, at least the processing tent inside the ward tent. Most hospitals place both within the ward tent. A second inside tent can be improvised from a latrine screen if a second darkroom tent is not available. Improvised duckboards in the darkroom are advantageous. Waiting room for walking cases can be made with empty X-ray chests for seats between the darkroom and fluoroscopic tents, and one low side of the ward tent. Field hospital units have only one X-ray machine, therefore will not require two darkroom tents.

b. *Power.* The utmost skill should be exercised in the care and operation of electric generators. The instructions issued with each generator should be meticulously studied and followed by the radiologist and technicians.

c. *Radiography.*

(1) The field unit X-ray machine on a mobile base can be used beside a table more efficiently if a board or other type of track is improvised to guide the movement of the machine up and down the length of the table.

(2) Positioning should be standardized according to the guide for forward areas furnished each X-ray department by the Office of the Chief Surgeon.

(3) Film drying will be hastened if it can be accomplished outside the darkroom, unless a free current of air can be forced through the darkroom by an improvised light-proof trap. The ventilator alone is inadequate. Item 60120, clips, photographic, will amplify hangers and permit easy stringing of roentgenograms on wires or rope.

(4) Water inlets and drain outlets from the processing units, by improvised hose or pipe "plumbing," will increase the darkroom efficiency.

(5) Roentgenograms should be identified accurately as per existing directives.

d. All patients transferred to other hospitals will be accompanied by their roentgenograms. A filing system should allow easy availability of roentgenograms to those who want to see them and, at the same time, make it possible for them to be accumulated and leave with all patients of a convoy on short notice.

e. There should be a uniform and well-defined policy between the receiving or triage officers and the radiologists as to what type of case will require X-ray examination, and the priority and volume in which they will be sent to the X-ray department. The use of litter bearers to and from the X-ray department should be mutually pre-arranged.

f. Requests for X-rays should be brief and exact throughout the hospital, so that the specific purpose of each request is evident, assuring that the proper technique and positioning can be immediately selected by the radiologist. This will obviate retakes.

g. X-ray examination should only be requested when the findings will affect treatment or, more rarely, the disposal of the patient.

h. *Patients in shock, or threatened shock, should not have X-ray examinations except in rare emergencies.*

i. *Missile Wounds.*

(1) Upper thighs and buttocks—should have additional A.P. or P.A. radiographs of the pelvis and lower abdomen, because complicating involvement is frequently found here.

(2) Thorax—should have additional A.P. and lateral radiographs of the upper abdomen, because of frequency of transdiaphragmatic involvement.

(3) Upper arms, shoulder and neck—should be considered for additional A.P. (or P.A.) radiographs of the thorax to exclude upper lung involvement.

j. *All soft tissue wounds* of the extremities should have an A.P. and lateral X-ray examination of the injured part, including the nearest joint, prior to surgical treatment.

k. *Transportable* cases with wounds of the *face* and *skull* should generally not have X-ray examination until special treatment is available.

l. *Localization of foreign bodies in extremities* is generally best accomplished by A.P. and lateral radiographs. Fluoroscopic orientation by the table device is generally not as practical in extremities as A.P. and lateral radiographs because bandages and wounds prevent marking the skin, and because the surgical approach to the foreign body may not be determined until *after* the X-ray study, and thus skin marking, even when possible, may not be placed on the proper aspect of the extremity. Lateral radiographs of extremities can, and should be made with the patient supine, when turning the patient causes pain.

m. *Fluoroscopy* is seldom as satisfactory as radiography. It is most useful in thoracic cases as an adjunct to radiography, and in localization of foreign bodies in the pelvis where lateral views are impractical and stereoscopy is not available. It is used for other types of cases mainly when facilities for radiography are not adequate to keep abreast of the volume of patients. Fluoroscopy, when not expertly supervised, can be a menace to patients and operators. It should never be attempted until the eyes have been accommodated at least 15 minutes.

12. *Identification of Gases in Cylinders.*

a. Identification of gases in cylinders may be difficult. In order to avoid serious accidents, great caution must be exercised in properly identifying contents of any particular tank.

b. Identification of a gas in a cylinder will be made by the following methods:

(1) By reading the chemical symbol of the gas imprinted in the metal of the valve of British cylinders.

(2) By reading the chemical symbol or name of the gas imprinted in the metal at the shoulder of the cylinder (symbol on British cylinders, full name on American cylinders).

(3) By reading the paper label or tag on British or American cylinders.

(4) By reading the symbol or name of the gas stencilled on or near the shoulder of a British or American cylinder. Arrangements for employing this means of identification have recently been made with the British Oxygen Co. and may not be found on all cylinders for some months to come. Cylinders are also being stencilled in U.S. medical depots.

(5) By interpreting the color or combinations of colors with which British or American cylinders are painted. *Color markings on a cylinder must be considered only to corroborate labels and are never to be used as a single means of identification.* In no instance will the color of valve caps be considered significant.

(6) *To identify gases in cylinders, check for all these means of identification. Unless all means in evidence agree, the gas should not be used.*

For the Chief Surgeon:

/s/ J. H. McNinch
J. H. McNINCH
Colonel, Medical Corps,
Executive Officer.

APPENDIX C

HEADQUARTERS
EUROPEAN THEATER OF OPERATIONS
UNITED STATES ARMY

Office of the Chief Surgeon

8 December 1944

CIRCULAR LETTER NO. 142

GUIDANCE TO DISPOSITION BOARDS

*   *   *   *   *   *   *

2. Attention is invited to Circular Letter No. 124, this office, subject, "Evacuation of Patients to the Zone of Interior," dated 17 October 1944. In the event that there is an insufficient number of 120-day cases to fill lift provided, enough cases will be selected which would fall within a 90-day evacuation policy to make up the deficit.

3. The decision as to disposition should be made as soon after the patient reaches a hospital as possible; i.e., when a diagnosis is made. Hospitals have been lax in this relation and must expedite evacuation. Further guidance, chiefly relating to fractures of long bones, is outlined in Circular Letter No. 131, this office, subject, "Care of Battle Casualties," dated 8 November 1944.

4. The following list of medical and surgical conditions is published for the guidance of Hospital Disposition Boards. It is to be remembered that this list is to be used only as a guide, each case to be decided on its individual merits.

a. Medical Conditions: * * *

b. Surgical conditions. The following list of surgical conditions demand return of personnel to hospitalization in the Zone of Interior.

(1) *Maxillo-facial, plastic and burn cases.*

(a) Severe maxillo-facial injuries associated with loss of tissue, which will require long-term reconstructive plastic surgery.

(b) Extensive loss of oral tissue in an amount that would prevent replacement of missing teeth by a satisfactory denture.

(c) Malignancies about face or mouth which will require extensive surgical treatment.

(d) Deep, extensive burns of the hands and face and extensive burns of other parts of the body.

(e) Wounds of other parts of the body which will require extensive plastic surgical procedures for correction.

(f) Severe compound, comminuted fractures of mandible or maxilla, with or without loss of bony substance.

(g) Patients with deforming but not disabling injuries in whom plastic repair should not be done within the 90-day period.

(2) *Ophthalmic cases.*

(a) Those cases (officers) covered by AR 40–105, par. 9, 14 Oct. 1942.

(b) Those cases covered by MR 1–9, par. 18, 15 Oct. 1942, except "g," also changes 22 Jan. 1943.

(c) Retinitis, pigmentosa, organic night blindness.

(3) *Neurosurgical cases.*

(a) All cranio-cerebral injuries in which there has been gross injury to brain tissue, as in penetrating wound of the head and compound comminuted fracture of the skull, with indriven bone.

(b) All injuries to major motor peripheral nerves. (Disposition of VIIth [sic] Cranial nerve injuries should be decided according to the severity of the disability.)

(c) Tumors of the brain or spinal cord.

(d) Cases of chronic low backache associated with sciatic nerve pain, and accompanied by objective neurological signs. Exceptions may be made in officers occupying key administrative positions and noncommissioned officers with special skills.

(4) *Orthopedic cases.*

(a) All compound fractures of upper and lower extremities involving major joints, or where the infection incident to compounding will not permit solid bony union to occur in four months, or where the healing will cause enough scar tissue formation in the overlying soft tissue to interfere materially with the function of the extremity. This in general will involve compound fractures of humerus, radius and ulna, femur, tibia, and extensive injuries of carpal and tarsal bones, shoulder, elbow, wrist, hip, knee and ankle joints. Possible exceptions may be made in certain selected instances of compounding forces resulting from clean, high velocity missiles where the continuity of the shaft of the bone has not been extensively disturbed.

(b) Simple fractures of femur and tibia, where the continuity of the shaft has been completely broken.

(c) *Extensive* compression fractures of vertebrae with or without dislocation.

(d) Osteoarthritis of joints with disability.

(5) *General surgical cases.*

(a) All cases of proven malignant disease (pre- or post-operative) except those of the integument which seem capable of complete local removal. (Exceptions may be made where surgical excision offers hope of cure and the patient desires to remain in the ETO.)

(b) Perforated gastric and duodenal ulcer.

(c) All complicated cases of cholelithiasis.

(d) Large recurrent postoperative hernias.

(e) Abscess of lung, unless acute and making rapid recovery following operation.

(f) Established vascular disease, such as Raynaud's Syndrome, thromboangiitis obliterans, serious thrombophlebitis with edema and cases with frostbite, immersion foot and trenchfoot in which there is demonstrable severe organic disease.

(6) *Genito-urinary cases.*

(a) All cases of malignant disease except solitary papilloma of urinary bladder.

(b) Kidney.

1. Diseases or injury requiring plastic operation of the kidney pelvis.

2. Bilateral renal disease—calculi—hydronephrosis.

(c) Ureter. Disease or injury requiring secondary or late plastic repair.

(d) Bladder. Neurogenic bladder without definite improvement in 1 month.

(e) Prostate hyperplasia causing symptoms incompatible with duty.

(f) Urethra and external genitalia. Wounds and injuries requiring extensive plastic procedures.

(g) Tuberculosis.

(7) *Otolaryngological cases.*

(a) Hearing loss below a level which makes a patient incompetent for all military duty.

(b) Chronic polypoid sinusitis, *with severe symptoms.*

(c) Allergic rhinitis (severe).

(d) Chronic suppurative otitis media and mastoiditis which requires radical mastoidectomy.

(e) Permanent tracheotomy.

(f) Destructive deformities interfering with mastication, speech and breathing.

(g) Ozena.

By order of the Chief Surgeon:

/s/   H. W. Doan
H. W. DOAN
Colonel, Medical Corps,
Executive Officer

APPENDIX D

HEADQUARTERS
EUROPEAN THEATER OF OPERATIONS
UNITED STATES ARMY

Office of the Chief Surgeon

17 MARCH 1945

CIRCULAR LETTER NO. 23

CARE OF BATTLE CASUALTIES

The following instructions are supplemental to Manual of Therapy, ETO, 5 May 1944; Circular Letter No. 71, 15 May 1944; Circular Letter No. 101, 30 July 1944, and Circular Letter No. 131, 8 November 1944, Office of the Chief Surgeon.

1. *Transfusion Instructions*

a. (1) The following test will be found useful in making differential diagnosis between pyrogenic and hemolytic transfusion reactions. It can be employed with accurate results as early as fifteen (15) minutes after the appearance of symptoms.

(2) *Procedure*

(a) Draw five (5) ccs. of blood from the patient, employing a clean, dry syringe.

(b) Remove the needle from the syringe and eject the blood *gently* into a clean, *dry* test tube.

(c) Centrifuge immediately for five (5) minutes at three thousand (3,000) r.p.m.

(d) Read grossly for presence of free hemoglobin in the serum.

(3) The presence of hemoglobin in the serum is indicative of intravascular hemolysis. The presence of as little as ten (10) milligrams per hundred cubic centimeters will produce a faint pink tinge and can be detected in this manner.

b. *Alkalinization*

Alkalinization is useless in cases in which there is no intra-vascular hemolysis, and will not be carried out in those cases in which the above test is negative.

c. *Deaths from transfusion*

Analysis of reports received shows that one of the major causes of death following transfusion is cardiac overload. The cardiac reserve of patients who have suffered wounds and prolonged shock is definitely lowered. Anuria may also result from prolonged shock. In the attempt to produce diuresis by the administration of intravenous fluids, the cardiac reserve is sometimes exceeded. Ordinarily, three thousand (3,000) cubic centimeters fluid intake daily is sufficient. In the presence of hyperprexia this may be proportionately increased. Blood and plasma received must be taken into account in calculating the total fluid intake.

d. *Sodium*

When sodium salts (citrate) are given to produce alkaline urine, the administration of sodium chloride (physiologic salt) is to be avoided. Dextrose in distilled water may be used to maintain adequate fluid intake. The administration of excess amounts of sodium may produce an alkalosis of a degree resulting in itself in anuria, or the excess sodium may be taken up by the tissues and result in edema.

e. *Care of blood in hospitals*

(1) Blood will be stored in refrigerators at temperatures ranging between two (2) and six (6) degrees above zero centigrade (35.6–42.8 degrees F.).

(2) Blood will not be heated before transfusion.

(3) Blood left unrefrigerated for more than 30 minutes will not be used for transfusion.

2. *Orthopedic Surgery*

a. *Notes for disposition boards*

Under the present evacuation policy to the Zone of Interior, very few simple or compound fractures can be rehabilitated to full duty in this theater. Among the exceptions may be certain fractures incurred by key personnel occupying sedentary positions. A fracture of the clavicle, an undisplaced fracture of the head of the radius or of the lateral malleolus, some fractures of the metacarpal bones, metatarsal bones or phalanges are cited as examples of fractures that may be returned to full duty within the present evacuation policy. There may be a few other instances of minor fractures which will require careful evaluation in order to determine whether there is any possibility of salvaging the officer or soldier involved for further duty in this theater within the time allowed.

Patients requiring elective surgical procedures for internal derangement of the knee joint or recurrent dislocation of the shoulder joint should almost invariably be returned to the Zone of Interior for this surgery. The utmost care should be exercised in arriving at a diagnosis of either of these conditions. A sprain of the knee joint which may be rehabilitated should not be confused with an internal derangement. A recurrent dislocation of the shoulder joint should be thoroughly authenticated before this diagnosis is made.

Osteo-arthritis of a major joint with definite disability as a result should be returned to the Zone of Interior.

b. *Amputations*

Skin traction on amputation stumps must be instituted immediately and maintained adequately and continuously except as stated in par. 5d, of Circular Letter No. 101, this office, subject: "Care of Battle Casualties," dated 30 July 1944. In general hospitals, this traction may be advantageously maintained by a weight suspended over a pulley. This form of traction must also be continuous. The most effective means of maintaining skin traction on the amputation stump during transportation has been described in par. 5e, Circular Letter No. 101, Office of the Chief Surgeon, 30 July 1944. This skin traction should be inspected in each medical unit charged with the care or the evacuation of the patient, and, if found to be inadequate, it should be reapplied immediately.

Closure of amputation stumps by suture or skin graft is not authorized in this theater. Amputees should be evacuated to the Zone of Interior as promptly as possible with skin traction maintained throughout all stages of their journey.

c. *Wounds involving the knee joint*

These wounds have been most satisfactorily treated in the following manner:

(1) A thorough exploration of the joint is performed through adequate medical and/or lateral incisions. A bloodless field should be insured by the use of a tourniquet if there is no associated damage to the femoral or popliteal arteries. The joint is completely irrigated with saline solution which should remove all blood and debris. With adequate retraction, a careful debridement of all damaged tissue, bone, cartilage and synovia is performed with removal of all foreign bodies from the joint cavity. If a meniscus is detached or damaged it should be excised. After further irrigation the synovia and capsule are snugly closed with a single layer of interrupted sutures. If there is loss of capsular substance, the closure may require, in some instances, the utilization of a fascial flap.

(2) After closure of the capsule, 10,000 units of penicillin in 5 cc. of normal saline are injected into the joint cavity. The tourniquet should be released and hemostasis insured by the ligation of all bleeding vessels. The knee joint should be immobilized by means of a plaster of paris spica bandage, knee slightly flexed, with a window over the joint. The joint is aspirated 48 hours after operation, gently washed with saline solution, and another 10,000 units of penicillin instilled into the joint cavity. This procedure may be repeated several times at intervals of 24 to 48 hours if necessary. Parenteral penicillin therapy is carried on throughout this period. The skin wounds may be closed 5 days after primary surgery if there is no evidence of infection.

d. *Compound fractures*

(1) Supracondylar fractures of the femur with sharp spicules of bone which may damage the popliteal vessels should be immobilized with the knee flexed at 20–25 degrees to minimize the danger of this complication. At the time of primary debridement, if there is found to be direct pressure against the popliteal vessels by a sharp spicule of bone, it should be excised. The excised piece of bone should be replaced at the fracture site and not discarded.

(2) *Internal fixation of compound fractures*

A recent report from the Office of the Surgeon General on the condition of battle casualties returning from the ETO has been received February 1945. The concensus of opinion expressed by qualified chiefs of orthopedic sections, chiefs of surgical services and consultants in nineteen named general hospitals in the Zone of Interior was that metallic internal fixation of compound fractures resulted in infection in 25 to 50% of the cases so treated. The metallic fixative agent in all of these infected cases had to be removed. Delayed or non-union has resulted in many of these patients.

In view of the adverse report on the progress of these casualties, internal fixation of compound fractures is prohibited as a routine procedure. It should be resorted to only after a thorough trial of skeletal traction has failed to secure adequate reduction, and after healing of the skin has been accomplished by suture or skin graft. The concurrence of the local orthopedic or surgical consultant will be secured in each instance where internal fixation of a compound fracture is deemed necessary. Combined injuries involving compound fractures and peripheral nerves present special problems. These will be treated at specialized hospitals designated for neurosurgical problems.

3. *Penicillin Therapy*

The following abrogates these parts of Circular Letter No. 71, 15 May 1944, with which it is in conflict.

a. Penicillin therapy will begin at clearing stations.

b. Penicillin therapy will be given to all casualties except those with very minor battle wounds.

c. The use of penicillin locally in all wounds is not required, but its local use in joints and chests is necessary for best results.

d. Data concerning dosage will be recorded on Emergency Medical Tags and Field Medical Record.

e. The distilled water in the plasma set should not be used as the vehicle for injecting penicillin, since it contains citric acid which inactivates penicillin. (Citric acid may inactivate other substances, and the distilled water in plasma sets should not be used except as a vehicle for dried plasma.)

f. The rate of withdrawal of penicillin from supply depots indicates that all wounded are not receiving penicillin as per Circular Letter No. 71. This must be corrected, since there is no more striking advance in the treatment of battle casualties than the relative freedom from infection. In this, penicillin may play a dominant role.

4. *Sulfonamides*

The dusting of a sulfonamide powder into open wounds has proven harmful to early closure of the wound and adds little to the ability of the body to defend itself against bacterial invasion. Such use of sulfonamide powder is condemned hereafter unless there be special indications.

5. *Hernia*

Under the present evacuation policy, all direct and recurrent hernias should be evacuated to the Zone of Interior. Exceptions are for key personnel only.

6. *Chronic Suppurative Otitis Media*

Radical mastoidectomies will be done only on patients in whom there is imminent danger from a spread of infection. This danger is indicated by severe pain around the ear, labyrinthine imbalance, or severe metastatic infection. Other cases of chronic suppurative otitis media and mastoiditis which cannot be treated so that they can return to full or limited duty in this theater within the present evacuation policy will be returned to the Zone of Interior.

7. *Peripheral Nerve Injury*

a. Primary suture of major nerve trunks in war wounds is undesirable and should never be attempted. The contusion of the nerve which invariably accompanies such wounds, precludes accurate trimming of the ends without unnessary sacrifice of tissue. However, when nerve ends can be identified they should be approximated as nearly as possible with a single through and through suture placed not more than 1 cm. from each end. Preferably a fine metallic suture should be used in order that subsequent X-ray examination may visualize the site of the lesion. This fixation-suture is important in that it prevents retraction of the nerve ends.

b. The optimum time for definitive suture is three weeks. Usually at this time it is possible to trim the nerve ends accurately to normal tissue before suture, and the perineurium is sufficiently toughened to permit accurate approximation with fine interrupted sutures.

8. *Gunshot Wounds of the Spine with Neurological Involvement*

Patients with spinal cord injury are the most difficult of all nursing problems. Facilities at the evacuation hospital are not ideal for their care. Therefore, *early* evacuation to fixed hospital installations is always desirable. The following rules for the care of these patients should be adhered to wherever possible:

a. No gunshot wound of the spine should be operated upon in an evacuation hospital when it is possible to transport the patient to a special treatment hospital for neurosurgery within 36 hours from injury. When such evacuation facilities are not available, the neurosurgeon of the evacuation hospital may perform a laminectomy when it is indicated after consultation with the chief of the surgical service and the orthopedic surgeon.

b. Through "holding units" these patients should be sorted for early evacuation to the nearest special treatment hospital.

c. No body cast will be applied in an evacuation hospital solely for the spinal injury. All patients (except those with injury to the cervical cord) will be evacuated in the prone position, care being taken to protect pressure points, especially about the iliac spines. An indwelling catheter will be used until the patient reaches a general hospital.

d. In those cases subjected to operation in evacuation hospitals, movement to a general hospital for nursing care will proceed within 48 hours, condition of the patient and evacuation facilities permitting.

e. These rules do not apply to patients with associated injuries, i.e., chest, abdominal and serious extremity wounds, where the associated lesion may take precedence in treatment over the spinal injury.

f. Cervical cord injuries will be handled according to instruction in the ETO Manual of Therapy, and Circular Letter No. 131, Office of the Chief Surgeon. Traction by either Crutchfield Tongs or Halter is not indicated unless there is fracture-dislocation of the cervical vertebrae. Simple gunshot wounds involving the lamina or the body of the cervical spine do not often require traction.

9. *Abdominal Surgery*

a. *Colostomies*

(1) Wounds of the large bowel should be treated by simple exteriorization of the involved portion, except the rectosigmoid, where the wound in the bowel will be closed and a "loop" colostomy performed above and at the top of the "free" loop. In this instance there must be complete diversion of the fecal stream, and it is advisable to divide the exteriorized bowel transversely and completely at the time of the operation. The distal end may be occluded by a clamp or a suture, as indicated.

(2) The Mikulicz type of procedure has been unsatisfactory in the experience of ETO surgeons and should be abandoned. It has been found to be the cause of post-operative obstruction and much intra-abdominal discomfort. The spur has rarely been sutured over a long enough area, and it is unsatisfactory for complete diversion of the fecal stream. Moreover, Mikulicz developed this operation as an emergency procedure in the early days of abdominal surgery. It is not satisfactory for young people who must live with it for forty years. In the repair of colostomies in base areas, most surgeons have come to complete exteriorization of the lesion and end to end suture in the operative wound. Infection has not resulted from this procedure, and late results are far better than with the Mikulicz type of procedure.

b. Wounds involving the caecum alone or the caecum and ileum require repair of the ileum and caecostomy, i.e., exteriorization of the defect. Ileostomy should be avoided, and double-barrelled opening of ileum and caecum has been proven unwise and undesirable.

c. In concurrent injuries of head and abdomen the abdominal injury takes precedence.

10. *Vascular Surgery*

Every attempt must be made in forward hospitals to repair vascular defects, first by direct suture, secondly by use of improvised tubes or the Blakemore sets. If an extremity can be given some blood for two or three days, even if greatly diminished, collateral circulation will usually develop and save the limb. The repair of the original lesion or an improvised method of getting some blood through the injured vessel need only function therefore for perhaps 48–72 hours.

11. *Notes on Radiology*

a. Unexposed X-ray film can be fogged in many ways. Two important causes are:

(1) By stacking the paste board X-ray boxes flat, either in depots, medical supply departments of hospitals or in X-ray departments. This presses the boxes open and prevents using the bottom film boxes in turn as new ones arrive.

(2) By storing films near a source of heat which is either severe for a short time or above 90 degrees F. for a longer period of time. Cold does not injure X-ray film.

b. All X-ray film will be stored at all times on edge and away from excessive heat.

c. Many kinds of glass can be depicted in the body by regular type of examinations. When glass from mines or other sources is suspected and needs to be located, X-ray examination should be requested. Since radiographs made properly dense with lower kilovoltage will depict still more kinds of glass than high kilovoltage technique, the radiologist

should be notified when glass is suspected.   Fragments from plastic or wooden mines cannot
be depicted by X-ray examination.

12. *The Care of Immobilized Patients* (avoidance of decubiti).

a. Patients who are unconscious or paralyzed, or who are immobilized as the result of
serious injury to the buttock, chest or extremities, need special care.   Such patients cannot
move themselves, and unless moved frequently, serious pressure sores and permanent disabilities will ensue.   Pulmonary congestion resulting from immobility increases the risk of
serious pulmonary complications.

b. Lessening of the disabilities entailed by lack of movement may be accomplished
through instructions to personnel to shift the position of these patients frequently.   Deep
breathing exercises can be conveniently given at the same time that the position is changed.
The attendant nurse or enlisted personnel should move the patient by gently shifting the
position of his pelvis.   Where there is a large buttock wound or heavy cast, more than one
attendant will have to assist in such movement.   The patient can be slightly rolled to one
side, alternating the side on which his weight rests.   Such movement not only relieves the
local pressure which gives rise to decubiti, but shifts the depth of respiration.   It often,
therefore, assists in clearing the respiratory passage through the coughing which may
follow such a change in position.

13. *Maxillofacial Casualties*

a. *Litter Evacuation*

In the litter evacuation of fresh maxillofacial casualties, adequate attention occasionally has not been paid to the proper position for such cases.   Improper position may
result in fatality during evacuation.   Instructions on this matter should be provided all
personnel handling fresh casualties.   Severe cases should be arranged in a prone position
on the litter with the head supported by blankets.   Such position gives the greatest assurance that the airway will be maintained and provides against the danger of aspiration of
blood and oral secretions.

b. *Jaw Fixation for Evacuation*

Par. 1, Circular Letter No. 122, Office of the Chief Surgeon, "Preparation of
Maxillofacial Casualties for Evacuation by Sea or Air," 7 October 1944, is amplified as
follows:

(1) In preparing casualties for evacuation intermaxillary elastic traction should
be reduced to only that amount required to hold the lower teeth in gentle contact with the
uppers when the jaw is at rest.   (Two elastic bands on each side are usually enough to
accomplish this end.)

(2) The traction should be applied in such a manner that it will definitely and
immediately be released by pulling down on a suture passed through the lumen of the
elastic bands.

14. *Thoracic Wounds*

a. *Resuscitation*

(1) Grave thoracic wounds as seen in forward hospitals are commonly associated
with severe pain and shock.   In addition there may be a sucking wound, and a laceration
of the lung or diaphragm.   The cough mechanism may consequently be inadequate in clearing the tracheo-bronchial tree of blood and secretions.

(2) These patients are dyspneic and present signs of anoxia.   Coarse tracheal
rales may be present.   Palpable rales are often felt over the affected lung.   Secretions
should be aspirated immediately, preferably through a bronchoscope or by means of an
intratracheal catheter.   Many of these patients are apathetic or semicomatose and do not
need an anesthetic.   The patients should be moved as little as possible, and aspiration
through a bronchoscope or intratracheal catheter should be done with the patient in a
semisitting position on the stretcher.   Oxygen administration is desirable before and after
aspiration.   When the bronchoscope is used, the flow of oxygen should be directed through
the sidearm of this instrument after the glottis has been passed.

b. *Sucking Wounds*

(1) Debridement of thoracic wounds is aimed at excision of devitalized tissue and removal of foreign bodies, including pieces of splintered rib. This procedure must be done meticulously if the objective of primary closure is to be obtained and if infection of the pleural cavity is to be avoided. The operation should be performed under endotracheal gas-oxygen-ether anesthesia. The wound should not be prepared before the endotracheal tube is in position. Wounds complicated by shattered ribs invariably become sucking during the removal of rib fragments.

(2) The fractured rib ends should be trimmed smoothly and rib fragments bare of periosteum removed. All blood should be aspirated and clots evacuated from the pleural sac. The pleural space should be examined and *all foreign bodies removed* since they usually will cause empyema. Missiles seen in the X-ray film at the level of the 12th rib are frequently in the costophrenic sinus.

(3) It is desirable to remove foreign bodies from the lung and suture lacerations of the latter when the patient's condition permits. Adequate exposure for this purpose can almost always be obtained without additional rib resection by enlarging the wound and making an intercostal extension.

(4) Drainage of the pleural cavity should be established through a stab wound in an intercostal space at the level of the inferior angle of the scapula in the midaxillary line (never through the operative wound). Under field conditions it has been found that the conventional sized catheter becomes occluded quickly. A size 26 or 28 F catheter, or tube, is considered preferable. The tube should be sutured to the skin and connected to a sterile water seal system. It should be removed in forty-eight hours.

(5) The wound should be closed in layers.

(6) Instillation of penicillin, 40,000 units in the pleural sac and aspiration of air from the latter are the final steps in the operation. Air is aspirated preferably from the second interspace anteriorly with the patient lying on his back.

c. *Thoracoabdominal Wounds*

(1) Late complications are common in this group when the right side is involved. These include liver abscess, subdiaphragmatic abscess, empyema, and diaphragmatic hernia. They can best be prevented by proper drainage of the spaces involved.

(2) Wounds of the liver are usually best managed by packing. The packing should be exteriorized through the most accessible point of the body wall below the level of the costophrenic sinus. Foreign bodies in the liver commonly cause abscesses. When accessible, they should be removed.

(3) The diaphragm should be repaired with medium silk.

(4) Intercostal drainage as described in b(4) above should be established.

d. *Hemothorax*

Hemothorax is the most common complication requiring further treatment in rear areas. Frequent aspiration without air replacement is the best prophylaxis against clotting and infection. Following the first operation, 40,000 units of penicillin should be instilled in the pleural space. Patients having a hemothorax should have a final attempt at aspiration before they are evacuated if there is reason to believe residual blood or fluid is present. Aspiration of hemothoraces is often neglected in hospitals passed through in the chain of evacuation. Many aspirations are attempted at too low levels. The most satisfactory point for aspiration is usually at the level of the inferior angle of the scapula at the posterior axillary line. Later, because the lung may become adherent posteriorly, it is commonly necessary to aspirate in the axillary area or anteriorly.

e. *Empyema*

(1) Many patients are reaching general hospitals with empyemas which are already chronic. This is usually due to too prolonged treatment with aspiration and penicillin instillation, to inadequate drainage, or because of retained foreign bodies.

(2) Empyema is best treated by rib resection drainage at the most dependent portion of the cavity. The most advantageous site for drainage is usually the ninth rib at

the posterior axillary line. Mediastinal fixation sufficient to make open drainage safe occurs within ten to fourteen days after wounding.

(3) Postoperatively the patient should sit up at once and be made ambulatory at the earliest possible date.

f. *Intercostal Nerve Block*

The relief of intercostal pain associated with thoracic wounds contributes to a more satisfactory convalescence. The raising of secretions is facilitated, and less morphine is required. This can be accomplished by intercostal injections of 1 percent Novocaine. During the course of operation, readily accessible nerves may be crushed to accomplish this purpose.

g. *Thoracotomy*

(1) Necessity for intrathoracic operative procedures usually occurs in patients having sucking wounds. Such operations can almost always be performed by enlarging the original wound as described in par. b (3) above.

(2) A formal thoracotomy is rarely necessary except in thoraco-abdominal wounds where it is planned to perform both the thoracic and abdominal operation through a single incision.

15. *Closure of Wounds of the External Genitalia*

Experience has shown that wounds of the genitalia, especially the scrotum, tend to break down when they are tightly closed primarily. It is desirable either to leave the wounds open or to suture them loosely.

16. Eye Casualties

a. *Atropine Sulphate*

To prevent the formation of posterior synechia whenever possible, all casualties with evidence of intra-ocular trauma will be treated with one (1) percent sterile atropine sulphate solution or atropine ointment three times per day. Regardless of the evacuation status of the patient, this treatment will be continued until ordered otherwise by an ophthalmologist.

b. *Penicillin and Sulphadiazine in Nonbattle Injuries*

Systemic administration of sulphadiazine and/or penicillin are indicated in penetrating injures to the eyeball or orbital contents exactly as used in other wounds or injuries of the body.

17. *Records*

Field Medical Records must contain all pertinent clinical factors relative to pre-operative and post-operative care. Inadequate records hinder proper care in general hospitals after evacuation of patients from Army areas.

By order of the Chief Surgeon :

/s/ H. W. Doan
H. W. Doan
Colonel, Medical Corps,
Executive Officer.

APPENDIX E

Evacuation by Landing Ship, Tank, From the Normandy Beaches

D. P. Hall, M.D.

Operation OVERLOAD, destined to break the power of Nazi Germany, was directly dependent on landing craft which could transport a grand total of 20,111 vehicles and 176,475 men on an amphibious assault against the shores of Normandy. The LST (landing ship, tank) was said to be the most important instrument of war in the European theater. Sir Winston Churchill once observed: "The destinies of two great empires seemed to be tied up by L.S.T.'s."

On 10 May 1944, U.S. Army hospitals in the United Kingdom received orders from Headquarters, ETOUSA, to send selected enlisted technicians and medical officers capable of performing surgery of trauma to designated channel ports in England for a period of training in the handling of casualties on LST's from the invasion beaches back to English Channel ports.

The LST was the only available craft suitable for the dual role of evacuating large numbers of casualties from the invasion beaches and carrying supplies from the United Kingdom to the Normandy coast. It was wisely decided to equip LST's so that they might carry from 150 to 200 litter and hundreds of ambulatory patients from France back to England. For the actual assault phase of OVERLORD, it was decided to staff a given number of LST's with competent operating surgeons and surgical technicians provided by the Army.

All of the selected army personnel were sent to U.S. Army hospitals on the Channel coast of England to be thoroughly indoctrinated as to their various responsibilities before and during the invasion. The following tasks were specifically stressed for the surgeons: (1) Perform such third-echelon surgical treatment as was practicable, consisting in the main of lifesaving surgery and early debridement of mangled and traumatic injuries; (2) act as surgical consultants to the LST crew. For planning purposes a load of 200 litter casualties was considered to be maximum for an LST. Medical materiel, therefore, was supplied to each LST on this basis. Each LST was provided two standard surgical kits consisting of all surgical instruments that might be used for general traumatic surgery and a medical technician's kit for each technician. In addition, a special surgical outfit which consisted of instruments that might be needed in abdominal or thoracic surgery was issued to each army surgeon. Eight beach bags were provided which contained sufficient battle dressings, morphine, sulfanilamide, and splints to care adequately for the maximum number of wounded. Ten pints of whole blood, biologicals, plaster of paris, dextrose solutions, chemical warfare ointment, and 12 units of plasma were placed on board to be carried on the first trip of an LST to the beachhead. Automatic replenishment of expendable items was to be provided on the return of LST's to the English coast.

During the preparatory phase of organization and training on the Channel coast of England, Lt. Col. (later Col.) Robert M. Zollinger, MC, Senior Consultant in General Surgery for the ETO, visited all training groups and gave wise counsel as to emergencies that might arise and directed the final preparations. Credit for the idea of using rubberized cloth (Batiste) in the place of sterile drapes should go to Colonel Zollinger. This material could be easily cut to any desired dimension and sterilized by boiling for 15 minutes. It proved to be quite an innovation in the more speedy draping and handling of wounds.

On 3 June 1944, all U.S. Army surgical teams were transported to different ports along the English Channel and placed upon waiting LST's. Aboard the LST, each medical officer oriented himself and saw to it that the operating theater, which had been built at the rear of the tank deck, was in order. He also made sure that medical supplies were dispersed at different stations on the LST so that if one source of supply should be destroyed in battle others might be available.

On 4 June, the LST's, with overhead barrage balloons and loaded with combat soldiers, tanks, and vehicles, put out into the English Channel. There was, however, such a heavy gale that, when they made their rendezvous, orders were received to return to port and wait for 24 hours.

On 5 June, the LST's in convoy made for open Channel to become an integral part of the greatest armada in history. There were 9,000 ships and landing craft protected by 702 warships and 25 minesweeper flotillas. Some were destined for Omaha Beach; others, for Utah Beach. Those carrying British and Canadian personnel were routed to Juno, Gold, and Sword beaches.

On 6 June, D-day, almost all LST's were within easy reach of the Normandy coast. Most of them had beached by D+½, and a few were beached later on D+2 day. Disgorging their cargo of combat soldiers, tanks, and vehicles, they were made ready for receiving casualties.

On arrival off Normandy, excitement and tenseness was everywhere very apparent because of going into the battle area under the constant bombardment of the French shore by friendly combat ships with 4-inch to 16-inch naval guns, followed by flashes from the German shore batteries all along the coastline. The first night on the beach was indeed revealing. Some of the LST's had opened antiaircraft fire on German planes against orders for the night. This fire immediately brought about rapid retaliation by the German air raiders, who dropped phosphorous and magnesium bombs along the beach. When the enemy planes ceased their attack at daybreak, many casualties were found on the beach, and the work was cut out for the surgical teams. On Omaha Beach most of the casualties were from the 1st and 29th Infantry Divisions of the U.S. V Corps. Those received and treated at Utah Beach were from the 82d and 101st Airborne Divisions, U.S. VII Corps.

On D+½ and D+2 days, LST's began to receive casualties in larger numbers on the beaches, and routine surgical treatment, such as control of hemorrhage and shock by plasma and whole blood transfusions, was instituted. Fractures were immobilized with splints of plaster of paris. Pain was eliminated by morphine and, when necessary, by ether or Pentothal sodium (thiopental sodium). Infection was combated by the use of sulfanilamide and penicillin; tetanus toxoid and gas antitoxin were given. In any case where there was obstruction of the airway, a tracheotomy was done.

Definitive surgery was done only as a lifesaving measure with careful consideration in favor of conservatism, due thought being given to the possible time interval before definitive treatment could be provided at U.S. Army hospitals on the English coast. Definitive surgery was done in severe chest and abdominal wounds, traumatic injuries of the buttocks, and compound fractures of the extremities with damage to the main blood supply.

Triage became a very important duty of each army surgeon on the beach, as sorting was a necessity in the proper handling and treatment of the casualties. This triage was done so that, upon arrival of casualties from France at the English shore, pertinent information was at hand and available to medical units receiving the evacuated casualties. The wounded were divided into ambulatory and litter cases. The litter cases were further divided into transportable and nontransportable patients. Casualties were classified as transportable when it was considered that they could safely tolerate overland transportation, after debarkation in England, before requiring surgical attention. All those who would require immediate surgical attention and, or, early surgical intervention upon reaching the English shore were classified nontransportable.

An EMT (Army Emergency Medical Tag) was used on all wounded. On the back of this tag, a supplemental record was kept, for use in the event the patient should require definitive surgery. A brief indication of the type of wound, such as head, chest, or abdomen, was placed on the EMT.

Some of the wounded transferred from the Normandy beaches to LST's had received first aid treatment but had lain on the beach for 12 hours in the clothes in which they were wounded. Most wounds were covered by a shell dressing, and few had received any other medication except morphine. Many were dehydrated and anxious because of loss of sleep. Supportive treatment in crossing the Channel to the English hards and quays required much time. Several chest and abdominal wounds necessitated operation. But, by far the greater number were compound fractures requiring immobilization and wounds of soft tissues—including the buttocks—requiring debridement. Because of associated rectal wounds, several colostomies were done on casualties with wounds of the buttocks.

A few German casualties were received. All these prisoners had been poorly treated and dressed, but none had received tetanus antitoxin. Most of their wounds had not been debrided but only packed with petrolatum-impregnated gauze to prevent hemorrhage. Unfortunately, the petrolatum-impregnated gauze became a plug and not a drain. The result was a grossly contaminated wound with an occasional gas gangrene infection. All these wounds were debrided, cleansed, and dressed, and the prisoner patients were given tetanus and gas antitoxin, plus sulfanilamide, en route to England.

Of the wounded received on LST's, the relative regional frequency of their injuries was estimated to be: Extremities, 50 percent; abdominal, 12 percent; thoracic, 9 percent; thoracoabdominal, 1.5 percent; and all other, 27.5 percent.

Many of the LST's caring for casualties made three or four crossings of the English Channel, after which time the Allied invasion forces had gained a good beachhead on the Normandy coast, and airstrips were quickly laid down from which wounded could be evacuated by air to England. Evacuation hospitals and field hospitals were set up at nearly the same time as the airstrips, thus ending the need for LST's as casualty carriers. As a consequence of mission accomplished, all army personnel were ordered back to their respective hospitals.

The army surgeons and technicians who participated in the LST evacuation operations during the Normandy invasion deserve the highest commendation for outstanding courage and devotion to duty under fire. Remember, many had been civilians only a few months before. The writer is sure that the aid, comfort, and lifesaving services given by the relatively few men who made up the surgical staff on the LST's deserve much credit for the reduced mortality and morbidity rate attained among American wounded during the invasion of Normandy.

The Normandy countryside is now green and peaceful. The townfolk of Sainte Mère-Église are free to stroll along Omaha or Utah Beach, but one wonders if they remember the beached LST's, one of the vanguards of their freedom and the refuge of the wounded Yank.

Treatment of Maxillofacial Injuries

(Extract from Manual of Therapy, European Theater of Operations)

A. Primary Surgical Treatment.

    I. General Considerations.

        1. A correlated plan of treatment, if carried out from the time the wound is incurred until definitive treatment is available, will greatly shorten the period of disability of patients with face and jaw injuries, and a larger number will be restored to approximately normal function and appearance than if haphazard methods are followed. Certain things should be done and others should not be done. Hence, attention to these points will save many lives and facilitate later treatment.

        2. The use of local and systemic chemotherapy is indicated as for wounds of other parts of the body. This is particularly important in the treatment of massive wounds involving the floor of the mouth and those associated with compound fractures.

        3. Primary care, points demanding special attention.

            a. Control of hemorrhage.

            b. Provision of adequate respiratory airway.

            c. Temporary approximate reduction and fixation of maxillofacial fractures and adjustment of parts to anatomical position. (Relief of pain, treatment of shock, and other emergency measures as indicated.)

            d. Early evacuation to a hospital for definitive treatment.

    II. Specific Considerations.

        1. Control of hemorrhage.

            a. Control moderate hemorrhage by pressure from gauze compress and bandage.

            b. Hemorrhage not controlled by pack and pressure will require clamps and ligature of the bleeding vessels. In case ligature is not available and clamp is left on, it should be included in the bandage and marked.

            c. In severe hemorrhage, life may be saved by application of digital pressure to a bleeding vessel at a control point in its course, until a clamp and ligature can be applied.

            d. DO NOT increase respiratory difficulty by the application of gauze compress and bandage. Bandages *should not* create backward pressure or traction distally on fractures of the mandible.

        2. Provision of adequate respiratory airway.

            a. Clear mouth and throat of tooth fragments, detached bone fragments, broken or dislodged dentures, and all foreign matter.

            b. Insufficient respiratory airway can be improved by the insertion of a rubber tube through the nose or mouth to the nasopharynx.

            c. Critical cases may require intra-tracheal tube.

            d. Tracheotomy should be done *promptly* if more simple measures fail to provide an adequate airway. In some cases of massive injury about the jaw and pharynx, tracheotomy will be necessary as an emergency life saving measure

            e. In case of collapse of pharynx and floor of the mouth, or loss of control of the tongue, an airway can be maintained by holding the tongue forward. This can be accomplished by passing a suture through the tip for holding it forward. (In extreme emergency cases safety pins have been used to transfix the tip of the tongue.) Fractures of the superior maxillae frequently displace the loose structures downward and backward and definitely interfere with respiration. Bilateral comminuted fractures of the posterior part of the mandible may cause the chin segment to drop downward and backward, likewise causing respiratory interference. In either case, the front of the jaw may be held forward by a simple emergency splint.

      (1) *Material.*

         Wooden tongue depressors, 4
         Adhesive tape.
         Bandage, 2-inch.
         Ligature wire.

      (2) *Construction.*

         Two tongue depressors are placed end to end and are held by two others overlapping them in the middle, all being bound together with adhesive tape.

      (3) *Application.*

         (a) This unit is secured vertically in the frontal region with a circular bandage so that the lower end is projected in front of the mouth. The upper end is attached to the bandage in the occipital region with a piece of tape.

         (b) A wire ligature is attached to the lower teeth or passed around the chin segment of the mandible, and the ends of the wire fastened to the lower end of the tongue depressor piece, either directly or with a rubber band.

         (c) The spring of the tongue depressor piece or elastic traction effectively keeps the anterior segment of the mandible forward. Likewise in cases of backward displacement of the maxillae, forward traction can be obtained by attachment of the upper teeth to the apparatus.

     3. *Temporary approximate reduction and fixation of maxillo-facial fractures and adjustment of displaced parts to anatomical position.*

         a. Institute adequate measures for relief of pain and prevention of shock. Morphine should be administered cautiously to patients with respiratory difficulty and is contra-indicated for patients with associated cranial injuries.

         b. Cleanse wound superficially, removing tooth fragments, detached bone particles and foreign matter.

         c. Displaced parts should be gently adjusted to anatomical position and gauze compress and bandage applied. *Avoid* collapsing bone segments and prevent backward traction on the mandible.

         d. Maxillary fractures and fractures of the adjacent facial bones should be gently supported by stable bandaging. In primary treatment, this stabilization can be improved by the application of gauze compresses and bandages used to control hemorrhage. It is essential to aid at re-establishing the former occlusion of the teeth, therefore all bandages applied should be supportive in this direction. Wire ligatures and suture material, if available, can be applied to the teeth of the same jaw across the line of fracture, to assist in stabilization of parts during evacuation. Multiple loop wiring, with intermaxillary elastic traction for reduction and stabilization of certain fractures, should be accomplished as early as time and facilities permit. Rigid intermaxillary fixation with wire is definitely contra-indicated in primary treatment for any case that might become nauseated or develop respiratory interference during evacuation. Edentulous cases require bandages that gently support the parts and avoid the tendency to collapse the segments. Dentures should be located, if possible, for use with adjustment and splinting of alveolar parts. These should always be transferred with the patient (even if broken).

         e. Stabilization of parts is essential to avoid recurrent hemorrhage, reduce pain and prevent shock.

         f. A stimulating dose of tetanus toxoid is indicated as for wounds of other parts of the body.

     4. *Evacuate patients to a hospital or station where definitive treatment can be provided early.*

         a. Ambulant or semi-ambulant patients with oral or pharyngeal wounds should travel sitting up, if possible.

b. Litter patients should be placed in a comfortable position and prone (face down) so that there is no possibility of interference with respiratory airway or aspiration of fluids.

*   *   *   *   *   *   *

B. Definitive Surgical Treatment.

I. General Considerations.

1. Superficial wounds are classified as those wounds of the face in which there is no evidence of fracture of facial bones, or deep penetration. These wounds, when seen early, may be closed by primary suturing, *provided* they are relatively clean and can be thoroughly cleansed and *carefully* debrided. Severe maxillofacial wounds with loss of tissue, especially those resulting from gunshot, should not be closed by primary suturing. Specialized care should be instituted as early as personnel, time and facilities permit.

2. Anesthesia is seldom required for the initial care of maxillofacial injuries before evacuation to an installation where definitive surgical treatment can be accomplished. When an anesthetic is indicated, first consideration should be given to regional infiltration or nerve block anesthesia for surgical treatment of severe traumatic lesions about the face. General anesthesia may be necessary if trauma involves structures in the nose, mouth or pharynx. Maintenance of an airway and prevention of seepage of blood into the trachea is essential. The use of Pentothal [sodium] is hazardous and is contra-indicated in presence of shock. Inhalation anesthesia is indicated. Introduction of an endotracheal tube, either through the mouth or nose, as conditions dictate, is highly desirable. Maintenance of Trendelenburg position (10°) will protect against seepage into the lung by promoting drainage of blood and secretions into the pharynx where they can easily be removed by suction. Insertion of wet packs into the pharynx is also indicated to establish a closed system. If extensive trauma within the mouth or pharynx is likely to be followed by edema or emphysema, it may be necessary to establish a tracheal stoma prior to surgical treatment of the primary lesion, and to use this avenue of approach for administration of the anesthetic by inhalation and subsequently for aspiration of excess secretions.

II. Specific Considerations.

1. *Reduction and fixation of fractures and adjustment of parts to anatomical position.*

a. Secure consultation and aid of dental surgeon if available.

b. Do not manipulate fractured fragments of maxillae in the presence of fractures of the base of the skull and accompanying injury of the brain until drainage of fluid has ceased and patient's condition approximates normal.

c. Final control of hemorrhage. Use small hemostats and fine ligatures. Ligate locally and not in course of the vessel and maintain maximum blood supply to the parts.

d. The wound should be cleansed thoroughly under the best surgical conditions. Remove all tooth fragments, foreign matter, detached particles of bone and dislodged teeth in line of fracture, since these are elements that invite infection. Do conservative debridement of soft tissues. Excise only tissue that is completely devitalized and tissue which obviously has no chance of survival. Protect nerves, vessels, ducts and glands. The use of small cutting needles and fine sutures placed near approximating skin edges will aid in prevention of suture scars. Skin sutures should be removed early.

e. *Bone particles that still possess periosteal attachment should never be removed, since these small vital attachments may make all the difference between consolidation and new bone formation with restored function, and collapsed fragments with the attendant complications; even comminuted viable bone should be saved.*

f. In cases of massive loss of substance, adjust soft tissue and restore torn flaps to normal position. Suture mucous membrane to skin edges to cover raw surfaces and to preserve skin and mucous membrane. Avoid closures under tension that produce overlapping of fractured ends of bone or collapse of bone fragments. Provide adequate dependent drainage to deep penetrating wounds, and especially those communicating with the mouth. Immediate suture is only advisable in superficial wounds and wounds that can receive proper care within a few hours after injury.

g. Fractures of maxillae and mandible.

(1) Complete roentgenographic studies should be an integral part of definitive treatment.

(2) Aim at re-establishing the former occlusal relationship of the teeth, and ultimate restoration of dental function. Collapse of bone segments should be avoided in cases with loss of structure.

(4) The use of labial arch bars or wiring of the teeth of the same jaw across the line of fracture may be indicated for stabilization during evacuation.

(5) Rigid intermaxillary fixation of the lower teeth to the upper *should not* be used prior to unattended travel. Intermaxillary elastic traction may be used safely for this stabilization since the mouth can be opened in case of nausea and the elastic bands easily removed or tension regulated as indicated.

(6) Immobilization of fractures can be accomplished by the application of intra-maxillary multiple loop wires and intermaxillary *elastics*, for reduction and fixation, when sufficient teeth remain in each jaw. The application of a vertical circular bandage with mild buccal elastic traction may be indicated for auxiliary support of maxillary fractures. (This bandage, made of plastic material, will eliminate the collapsing tendency of ordinary bandage.)

(7) Sectional dental splints of proper design and construction may be used to advantage in the treatment of complicated cases for immobilization when limited function is desirable.

(8) Edentulous fractures require the skillful application of supporting bandages to maintain the parts in proper position, without causing collapse of segments or interference with airway. Dentures are particularly important as they can often be used in connection with supporting bandages or circumferential wiring.

(9) Another method of reduction and retention of edentulous cases, or those with displaced edentulous fragments, is afforded by the application of the extra-oral skeletal pin and bar fracture appliance.

2. Every effort should be made to provide trained personnel for the care of maxillofacial injuries throughout the combat area. Adequate life-saving measures and early treatment are necessary to insure the casualties getting to the hospitals of the next echelon for more definitive treatment. The execution of a well-correlated plan of treatment throughout will not only save life but result in many casualties being returned to duty after a minimum period of hospitalization. End results are of great concern and usually said to be directly proportionate to the nature and character of the early treatment received. Patients with maxillofacial injuries, requiring extended care and reconstructive surgery, should be transferred to the Zone of Interior when the treatment has progressed to such a stage that evacuation can be safely accomplished.

APPENDIX G

Treatment of Burns

(Extract from Manual of Therapy, European Theater of Operations)

A. Primary Surgical Treatment.

I. General Considerations.

1. A high percentage of burns are received accidentally through carelessness and negligence. Efforts should be made to prevent burns by emphasizing the dangers associated with handling gasoline and other inflammable materials, and instituting suitable safety measures.

2. In the early management of a burn casualty, the primary considerations are:—

a. Prevention and control of shock.

b. Prevention of contamination of the burn surface during treatment and evacuation.

II. Specific Considerations.

Initial care.

1. Control of pain by morphine administration. In extensive burns, ½ grain doses of morphine may be necessary. If anoxia is present, large doses of morphine are dangerous, and under such circumstances the dose should not exceed ¼ grain. If the patient is in shock, absorption of subcutaneous or intramuscular morphine may be delayed, in which case repeated doses of morphine should be given with caution. Relief of shock and improvement in peripheral circulation may lead to rapid absorption and over-dosage if morphine has been repeated in such cases. Careful administration of intravenous morphine has the advantage that pain is more promptly and certainly controlled, and the danger of over-dosage from repeated subcutaneous or intramuscular administration is nullified. Doses of ⅙ to ¼ grain, given slowly in 10 cc. of sterile distilled water or saline, and repeated as necessary, is perhaps the safest method of intravenous morphine administration.

2. Early plasma replacement therapy should be instituted. If evacuation cannot be carried out quickly to a place for definite therapy, plasma should be started as part of the first aid measures. If one or two units of plasma can be given *early*, even in the first half-hour, lives may be saved. Quantities of plasma up to twelve units may be required in the first twenty-four hours for extensive burns. If the patient is in shock when plasma is started, the first two or three units should be given rapidly.

3. From the first, efforts should be made to prevent contamination of the burn surface by nose and throat organisms. Those handling the patient should always be masked. If masks are not available, they can be improvised. Aseptic technique, with gloves and instruments if possible, should be used at all times.

4. Casualties with 15% or over of body surface burned should be treated as litter patients immediately.

5. Clothing need not be removed unless too dirty, charred, contaminated or soaked with oil or chemicals.

6. No cleansing or debridement should be attempted in the field. This procedure should only be done in hospitals where complete facilities for definitive treatment are available.

7. Cover the wound with sterile dressings, triangular bandages, or clean sheets. Evacuate to hospital for definitive treatment of the burned area as quickly as possible. Boric acid ointment or Vaseline applied to a grossly contaminated burn complicates the later cleansing of the burn surface. If a local application is considered necessary, 5%

sulfadiazine cream is preferred because of its bacteriostatic effect and its relative ease of removal later if cleansing and debridement are considered necessary.

8. Application of sulfadiazine cream, boric acid ointment or petrolatum to a grossly contaminated burn are *not* to be considered as definitive treatment.

9. Eyes should be gently irrigated with saline or boric solution, and a mild ointment (4% boric acid ointment), or oil instilled. Do not apply sulfadiazine cream to the eyes or lids, since it is extremely irritating to the conjunctiva. The lids should be closed with a pad of dampened gauze over them and a dry one held with adhesive, if possible, as the best dressing for the cornea is the lid. Cocaine or other anesthetics should not be used, as anesthesia of the cornea might lead to damage. If there is evidence of corneal injury, the case requires the attention of an ophthalmologist as early as possible.

10. Severe burns of the hands, or of one hand alone, should be considered as major burns and evacuated to a hospital for definitive treatment.

11. Tetanus toxoid is indicated for all patients with second or third degree burns.

12. Tannic acid, tannic acid jelly, triple dye, gentian-violet, gentian-violet jelly, and other membrane forming applications, should NOT be used.

13. RAPID EVACUATION TO DEFINITIVE TREATMENT SHOULD BE EFFECTED.

B. Definitive Surgical Treatment

I. General Considerations.

1. Each hospital should be prepared at all times with a burn team and a plan for admission, sorting and treatment of multiple burn casualties.

2. In the very early stages the treatment of shock and hemoconcentration takes precedence over local treatment of the burn.

3. Definitive treatment of the burned area is given at the first opportunity presented by the condition of the patient and the presence of adequate hospital facilities. It is aimed at obtaining and maintaining a wound free of contamination and infection.

II. Specific Considerations.

1. *Systemic Treatment*

a. Plasma must be given to maintain blood volume. A simple method of estimating the amount of plasma necessary is that of adding 100 cc. of plasma for every point the hematocrit determination exceeds the normal of 45. Another rough method is that of administering 500 cc. of plasma for each 10% of the body surface burned. The adequacy of plasma administration can be determined by frequent red blood cell, hemoglobin, and hematocrit determinations. An effort should be made to keep the red blood cell count at 5.5 million or below, the hematocrit reading below 50, and the hemoglobin down to 100%. The general condition of the patient, the pulse and blood pressure, are other invaluable guides.

Continued plasma therapy for three or four days may be necessary, and, following this, plasma should be given at intervals to maintain the blood proteins at a normal level.

b. A standard method of estimating body surface burned is by use of the Berkow formula, as follows:

Head	6%
Upper Extremities:	
Both arms and forearms	13%
Both hands	5%
Total	18%
Trunk and Neck:	
Anterior surface	20%
Posterior surface	18%
Total	38%

Lower Extremities:
Both thighs_____ 19%
Both legs_____ 13%
Both feet_____ 6%
Total_____ 38%

c. The need for whole blood transfusion will develop in some cases as early as 2–3 days after the burn is incurred. Plasma is not a substitute for whole blood if secondary anemia is present.

d. A urinary output of 1,000 cc. to 1,500 cc. daily must be established as soon as possible. In the first 24 hours after an extensive burn, it is more important to effect adequate plasma replacement, than to give parenteral crystalloids. During this period it is believed that the salt requirements are met by the salt content of the plasma administered. The daily fluid intake should be maintained at 3,000 cc. to 4,000 cc., and, if parenteral fluids are necessary to reach this level, chief reliance should be placed on 5% glucose in distilled water. Saline should be given sparingly, usually only if there is vomiting or some other cause for salt depletion. As a general rule, not over 1,000 cc. of normal saline should be given over a 24-hour period.

e. During the critical phase (which may last up to 72 hours or longer), the patient must be closely observed for the development of pulmonary edema, shock, morphine overdosage, or the development of cerebral manifestations. Oxygen therapy is often indicated during this period.

f. From the first, the importance of maintaining the nutritional state of the patient should be kept in mind. Every effort should be made to give adequate food and liquids with a high content of carbohydrate, protein and vitamins.

g. A prophylactic dose of polyvalent gas bacillus antitoxin may be given for deep burns at the discretion of the medical officer.

2. *Cleansing and Debridement.*

a. No attempt will be made to clean or debride the burn surface until shock is adequately controlled.

b. The wound will always be treated under standard operating room technique with patient and attendants fully masked.

c. Morphine sedation will be adequate to allow debridement and cleansing of the wound in the majority of cases. Intravenous morphine may be indicated in some instances. If general anesthesia is necessary, first consideration should be given to light intravenous Pentothal sodium. Inhalation anesthesia is contra-indicated if an associated blast injury is present or suspected.

d. In some cases, if the patient is received a short time after the burn is incurred, and if the wound is free of gross contamination, cleansing and debridement may be considered unnecessary.

e. Those burns showing gross contamination should be cleansed with neutral soap and water, and irrigated with saline. Lard, mineral oil or ether, in small amounts, may be used for removal of grease and heavy oil. The cleansing should be done gently with gauze or cotton swabs. Green soap and *brushes* will not be used. The cleansing should include the skin surrounding the burn.

f. Removal of loose shreds of epidermis and large blisters should be done after thorough cleansing. Small blisters may be left undisturbed, or removed, depending on the extent of the procedure necessary and the condition of the patient.

g. Immediate excision and grafting of burns has such limited application that it is not recommended.

h. Debridement should not include excision on loose skin from the *eyelids, ears* or *fingers.* Blisters in these areas may be incised after cleansing.

3. *Dressing.*

a. The burned area should be covered with single strips of fine mesh gauze (44-mesh gauze bandage), impregnated with 5% sulfadiazine cream, boric acid ointment or petrolatum. *Sulfadiazine cream is preferred* because of the early high local concentration of the drug obtained. It does not stand autoclaving and should be prepared at the operating table by spreading thinly on 44-mesh gauze bandage. Sulfanilamide powder may be used with boric acid ointment or petrolatum, but the total dose should not exceed 10 grams. Local sulfonamide therapy is only of value as a prophylactic against virulent infection in the early stages. It is useless after pus has developed from ordinary pyogenic infection of the deeply burned areas. Ordinarily there will be no indication for continuation of local sulfonamide therapy after the first dressing, which, in a favorable case, can be postponed to between seven and fourteen days.

b. The remainder of the dressing will consist of gauze, absorbent cotton, cotton waste, or cellulose. The dressing will be thickly applied over all the burn and will be bandaged on snugly with even pressure throughout. Stockinette or some form of elastic bandage may be used, if available, to maintain pressure. Care should be taken to prevent the pressure dressing from forming an area of constriction. In the case of extremities, the pressure dressing should include the entire extremity distal to the burn.

c. Immobilization of the part by plaster splints placed over the dressing should be effected when possible. Skin-tight plaster casts should not be used. If a complete plaster casing is applied, it should be split to allow for swelling.

d. Burned hands should be carefully dressed with pressure to, and including, the tips of the fingers. The hand should be in the position of function with fingers separated and flexed. Edema is further prevented by elevation, which is best accomplished by overhead suspension attached to plaster arm splints applied over the pressure dressings.

e. Pressure dressings are applied to the face as elsewhere, taking care to protect the eye, pad the ears, and leave an adequate respiratory airway.

f. Genitalia should be covered with 5% sulfadiazine cream and simple dressings. The dressings should be applied in such a manner that they can be changed separately as necessary.

g. Dressings should be changed infrequently in the early stages of a burn, and, if possible, the dressings should be done in the operating room with standard aseptic technique.

h. In some instances it may be necessary to change the dressing at four to five days on a clean and uninfected case, because of external soiling or soaking of the dressing by exudation of plasma. In such cases, it is often satisfactory to change the bulky outer portion of the dressing and not disturb that immediately over the burn surface.

4. *Sulfonamide Therapy*

a. If a sulfonamide is used locally, oral or parenteral administration of the drug should be postponed until adequate kidney function is demonstrated by a daily urinary output of 1,500 cc., and the blood sulfonamide has dropped to a low level. After this period, if evidence of sepsis develops, oral therapy should be instituted and continued as indicated.

b. All cases with moderate to severe burns, that have not had local sulfonamides applied, will be started on oral chemotherapy. Sulfadiazine is the drug of choice for oral administration (sulfanilamide may be substituted). It should be given with caution in the early stage of a burn, and the dose should not exceed 0.5 gram every four hours until the urinary output has reached a normal level. Frequent blood level determination should be done.

5. *Further Care of Burned Surface.*

a. If virulent infection is prevented, healing of superficial burns will take place rapidly.

b. After a period of about two weeks, infection of deeply burned areas by ordinary pyogenic organisms will make frequent dressings necessary in order to maintain cleanliness and promote separation of slough.

c. Wet dressings using saline, boric, Dakin's or azochloramid solution for irrigation should be applied and changed daily.

d. Dressings should be wet before removal.

e. If possible, saline baths should be used for ease of removal of dressings, for cleanliness and to promote active exercises.

f. Unhealed areas should be prepared for grafting, and grafts applied as early as possible. It is often possible to begin grafting within three or four weeks after the burn is incurred.

g. Active motion should be instituted in severe hand burns not later than seven days following the injury. This can be facilitated by removing the dressing and placing the extremity in an arm basin filled with saline.

6. *General Care*.

a. Whole blood transfusions may be necessary as early as three or four days after the burn, and at regular intervals thereafter until the case is healed or grafted.

b. A diet high in calories, *protein*, carbohydrate and vitamins should be maintained.

c. The blood protein level should be observed and kept at a normal level by plasma transfusions as necessary.

d. Careful and sympathetic nursing care is an absolute essential.

APPENDIX H

4 September 1944

MEMORANDUM TO: Colonel Elliott C. Cutler, MC, Senior Consultant in Surgery, European Theater of Operations.

SUBJECT: Recommendation for Care of Hand Injuries in the Zone of Interior.

1. Many severe hand injuries are being seen on the plastic surgery services of the general hospitals in the United Kingdom. An attempt is being made to accumulate these cases from other hospitals into hospitals for plastic surgery, where they can be cared for jointly by plastic and orthopedic or general surgeons. The experience with these cases has given the distinct impression that most surgeons do not realize the possibilities of plastic surgery in obtaining early and adequate closure or covering of the wounds with massive soft tissue and skin loss. Many wounds are left open too long, with the result that prolonged splinting, infection of the open wound, sloughing of exposed bone and tendon, will result in crippling that is out of proportion to the severity of the original injury.

2. Of all cases that deserve special consideration, none are more deserving than hand injuries. It is the responsibility of surgery in this theater to see that the soft tissue loss is replaced early in order to limit progress of the disabling pathological processes that result from an open wound. This procedure should be done *early, before* evacuation to the Zone of Interior. An Article has been submitted to the *Medical Bulletin, European Theater of Operations*, pointing out that hands and other injuries of the extremities that require extensive soft-tissue and skin replacement should be referred to hospitals in which plastic surgery is being done. The number so far subjected to early plastic surgery procedures is only a small percentage of the total that must be in hospitals of the Theater.

3. An increasing number of hand injuries are being sent to the Zone of Interior, following pedicle grafting here. These injuries are of all degrees of severity and many of them will require late reconstructive surgery. The pedicle grafts, in addition to halting the increasing incapacity that results from an open wound, will make it possible for the early institution of physiotherapy and reconstructive operations. The cases will present problems of bone, tendon, and nerve grafting that are completely beyond the scope of the ordinary surgeon. It is very strongly felt that these cases should not be operated upon by any but surgeons who have had some background in this type of work, and in hospitals where the work can be controlled.

4. It is the opinion of this Office that such cases should be accumulated, for their later care, in special hospitals, under the joint care of specialists qualified in this type of work.

/s/ Eugene M. Bricker
Eugene M. Bricker
Lieutenant Colonel, MC
Senior Consultant in Plastic Surgery

999

APPENDIX I

5 MARCH 1945

MEMORANDUM TO: Colonel Mather Cleveland, MC, Senior Consultant in Orthopedic Surgery, European Theater of Operations.

SUBJECT: Treatment of Hand Injuries.

1. The following are the simple principles which I think we should make an effort to see practiced in this Theater in the treatment of hand injuries:

a. Conservative, meticulous, and proper debridement of the primary wound. The wound should not be closed primarily in an evacuation hospital, but displaced skin flaps can be dressed back into place.

b. "Purposeful splinting" always, with maintenance of the palmar arch, and flexion of the metacarpal phalangeal joints.

c. Closure as early as possible, preferably on the third or fourth day. It should be accomplished by secondary closure, split graft, or pedicle graft.

d. Traction only in those cases in which it is urgently indicated, and then for a minimum length of time. The fishhook traction which has been developed at the 22nd General Hospital is probably the best.

e. In some of the severe types of injuries, forget about the restoration of the injured part and concentrate entirely on maintenance of function of what is left. This may mean amputation of an irreparably damaged finger in order to get a healed hand.

f. Active motion should be instituted as early as possible. When the hand is healed, this should be further encouraged by occupational therapy.

g. An effort should be made to avoid the development of a markedly edematous hand with an infected open wound. Proper debridement, proper dressing, proper splinting, and *effective* elevation of the hand will prevent such a development.

h. So long as there is an open wound in the hand, it should be treated aseptically. This means face masks and instruments or gloves, whether the wound is infected or not.

2. The following points are what I consider to be the requirements of a satisfactory hand service:

a. The availability of both an orthopedic and plastic surgeon.

b. The segregation of patients so that they are all together and can receive their exercises simultaneously and benefit by the development of a competitive spirit.

c. Adequate facilities for physiotherapy, with physiotherapists particularly interested in rehabilitation of hands. In a busy center, this may mean additional physiotherapists. There should be special provisions in the physiotherapy department for hand exercising machines, et cetera. If possible, noncommissioned officers who have had hand injuries themselves should be placed in charge of ward exercises.

[s] Eugene M. Bricker
EUGENE M. BRICKER
Lieutenant Colonel, MC
Senior Consultant in Plastic Surgery

INDEX

○